Foundations of Athletic Training

Prevention, Assessment, and Management

SIXTH EDITION

Foundations of Athletic Training

Prevention, Assessment, and Management

SIXTH EDITION

Marcia K. Anderson, PhD, LATC

Professor Emeritus
Department of Movement Arts, Health Promotion, and Leisure Studies
Bridgewater State University
Bridgewater, Massachusetts

With contributions from:

Mary Barnum, EdD, ATC, LAT

Professor
Exercise Science and Sport Studies
Program Director-Athletic Training
Springfield College
Springfield, Massachusetts

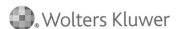. Wolters Kluwer

Philadelphia • Baltimore • New York • London
Buenos Aires • Hong Kong • Sydney • Tokyo

Acquisitions Editor: Michael Nobel
Product Development Editor: John Larkin
Editorial Assistant: Tish Rogers
Marketing Manager: Shauna Kelley
Production Project Manager: David Orzechowski
Photographer: Susan Symonds, Infinity Portrait Design
Design Coordinator: Stephen Druding
Manufacturing Coordinator: Margie Orzech
Prepress Vendor: Absolute Service, Inc.

Sixth edition
Copyright © 2017 Wolters Kluwer.

Library of Congress Cataloging-in-Publication Data

Names: Anderson, Marcia K., author. | Barnum, Mary, editor.
Title: Foundations of athletic training : prevention, assessment, and
   management / Marcia K. Anderson ; with contributions from Mary Barnum.
Description: Sixth edition. | Philadelphia : Wolters Kluwer Health, [2017] |
   Includes bibliographical references and index.
Identifiers: LCCN 2016015373 | ISBN 9781496330871
Subjects: | MESH: Athletic Injuries—therapy | Sports Medicine—methods
Classification: LCC RD97 | NLM QT 261 | DDC 617.1/027—dc23 LC record
available at https://lccn.loc.gov/2016015373

Preface

Four major goals were established for the sixth edition of *Foundations of Athletic Training*. The primary goal was to continue to provide the most current and comprehensive evidence-based content related to the prevention, assessment, and management of injuries and illnesses sustained by physically active individuals. A second goal was to acknowledge the importance and significance of the *Role Delineation Study* (RDS) published by the Board of Certification. The RDS identifies the essential knowledge and skills for the athletic trainer and serves as a blueprint for the development of the certification examination and entry into the profession. As in past editions, each chapter continues to provide critical information that meets or exceeds the specific RDS competencies covered within the chapter. A third goal was to enhance learning potential through the actual presentation of information. In particular, the extensive color art program provides realistic and accurate visualizations of musculoskeletal anatomy, injuries and medical conditions, assessment, and management techniques. The fourth goal also pertained to content presentation. In an effort to continue our tradition of providing special pedagogical features in a visually pleasing format, multicolor borders and formatting have been used to identify critical boxes, application strategies, and tables as a way to highlight key information.

Foundations of Athletic Training has undergone extensive review from leaders in the athletic training field. The review process has been instrumental in enabling us to achieve our goal of developing the most comprehensive text available for athletic training educators and students. The text has been reorganized into seven parts.

Section I, Foundations for the Prevention of Sports Injuries, features new information in Chapter 1 Injury Care and the Athletic Trainer on various new job settings and the integration of emergency medical technicians and paramedics as part of the health care team. Updated information is provided in Chapter 2, Preparticipation Examination and Chapter 3, Protective Equipment. Chapter 4, Protective Taping and Wrapping has added information on the makeup of tape, different types of tape, and the new PowerFlex Taping System.

Section II, Clinical Examination and Diagnosis, includes four new chapters. Chapter 5, Evidence-Based Health Care, discusses evidence-based research as it relates to athletic training clinical practice and is described through a systematic approach to answer clinical questions through the review and application of existing research to improve patient outcomes. Injury assessment has been separated into two distinct new chapters. Chapter 6, Clinical Assessment and Diagnosis, discusses the assessment process for the purposes of developing a complex therapeutic intervention program, detailing the subjective evaluation, objective evaluation, assessment, and plan (SOAP) sequence for an off the field assessment. The new Chapter 7, Acute Injuries: Assessment and Disposition, provides strategies for preventing and preparing for emergency situations and minimizing the extent of injury. Assessment methods for evaluating patients with acute injury are then discussed followed by strategies to remove patients from the injury site following the most current best practices as recommended by the National Athletic Trainers' Association. Finally, the chapter provides a review of the leading causes of sudden death in sports along with the recognition and acute management of these conditions. The new Chapter 8, Assessment of Body Alignment Posture and Gait, describes somatotyping, an overview of posture, information on how to conduct a postural assessment, and how to identify normal and faulty posture and interpret the findings. The second half of this chapter focuses on the principles of gait and gait assessment. Chapter 9, Psychosocial Intervention and Patient Care, has been updated with the most current evidence-based practice in patient care in the psycho-social-emotional domain.

Section III, Therapeutic Interventions, provides updated information on Tissue Healing and Wound Care (Chapter 10), Therapeutic Medications (Chapter 11), Therapeutic Modalities (Chapter 12), and Therapeutic Exercise Program (Chapter 13). As recommended by many reviewers, the joint chapters were rearranged to open with Section IV, Conditions of the Lower Extremity, followed by Section V, Conditions of the Upper Extremity, and finally Section VI, Conditions to the Axial Region. The most current information is provided on concussions, baseline concussion testing protocol, including the SCAT3, VOMS/VORS, and cranial nerve assessments, followed by the graduated return-to-play protocols for patients recovering from a concussion. Within each joint area chapter, assessment has been moved earlier in the chapter to immediately follow the section on prevention of injury. The assessment process continues to follow standard protocol including history, observation, palpation, and physical examination tests (e.g., functional tests, stress tests, special tests, neurological tests, and activity-specific functional tests). Care has been taken to provide sensitivity and specificity scores based on current evidence-based research on many of the stress and special tests. Conditions of the senior athlete and female athlete have been integrated into the regular joint chapters.

Section VII, Systemic Conditions and Special Considerations has been updated with current information on Cardiovascular Disorders (Chapter 24), Neurological Conditions (Chapter 25), Respiratory Tract Conditions (Chapter 26), including the use of a peak-flow meter and asthma management, Gastrointestinal Conditions (Chapter 27), Endocrine Conditions (Chapter 28), and Environmental Conditions (Chapter 29). A new Chapter 30 has been devoted to conditions seen in Athletes with Physical Disabilities. Finally, Common Infectious Diseases (Chapter 31) and Dermatology (Chapter 32) are presented.

PEDAGOGICAL FEATURES

Several pedagogical features continue to enhance the text's usefulness as a teaching tool. These in-text features include:

- **Art and Photography Program.** A color art and photography program supplements the material presented in the text. Using an innovative approach that involves drawings within a human model, the illustrations of musculoskeletal anatomy provide a detailed and realistic depiction of structures.

- **Learning Objectives.** Each chapter opens with a series of learning objectives that identify the key concepts in the chapter.

- **Critical Thinking Scenarios.** Critical thinking scenarios are found at the beginning of most of the major sections in each chapter. These scenarios are intended to encourage the student to critically analyze information and apply decision-making knowledge and skills.

- **Key Terminology.** Important terms are bolded within the text. In addition to the explanation of the term in the chapter, these terms are also defined in the glossary.

- **Critical Information Boxes.** These boxes are interspersed throughout each chapter. They are intended to highlight and summarize important information.

- **Tables.** Several chapters have tables that expand on pertinent information discussed in the text. This format allows a large amount of didactic knowledge to be organized in an easy-to-read summary of information.

- **Application Strategies and Management Algorithms.** In several chapters, field strategies and management algorithms are used to present the clinical application of cognitive knowledge.

- **Application Questions.** At the end of each chapter, a series of injury scenarios and discussion questions are provided to enhance class discussions. There is no right answer because multiple variations of the questions can be discussed by the students. This format allows for a freer expression of knowledge and practical application depending on the work setting, activity, age of the participant, and so forth.

- **Summary.** Each chapter has a summary of key concepts discussed in the text.

- **References.** Updated references are provided. The majority of the references have been published within the last 5 years. The primary exceptions are references to original groundbreaking research.

- **Glossary and Index.** An extensive glossary of terms gathered from the highlighted words in the individual chapters is provided at the end of the book. In addition, a comprehensive index contains cross-references to locate specific information within the text.

ANCILLARY MATERIALS

Online resource centers are available to both athletic training educators and athletic training students on the book's companion Web site at http://thePoint.lww.com/AndersonFound6e.

Instructor's Resource Center

The online resource center is organized by chapters and includes the following:

- **PowerPoint Presentations.** The PowerPoint presentations were developed with an understanding that instructors and students adopt a variety of strategies when using PowerPoint. The slides provide detailed rather than general information, recognizing that it is simpler for an educator to delete rather than add information. In addition, given the tendency of many students to take notes verbatim from a slide, an effort was made to condense the actual wording of statements to streamline the note-taking process. The presentations can be downloaded and customized to meet specific needs.

- **Supporting Lecture Notes.** The lecture notes correspond to the individual slides comprising the PowerPoint presentations. The notes are not intended to serve as an actual lecture. Rather, they are designed to provide the instructor with information that supports the material presented on the slides. As such, the notes include an additional explanation and background information, as well as examples of concepts.

- **Teaching Strategies.** The teaching strategies provide additional experiences and instructional methods to complement the learning process. In particular, the teaching strategies provide an active, problem-solving, and critical thinking approach to learning. For example, Chapters 10 through 19 contain differential diagnosis problems intended to engage the learner in the analysis of clinical signs and symptoms.

- **Reference Materials.** Each chapter contains a variety of materials intended to supplement the information presented in the text. For example, Chapter 1 provides sample forms pertaining to legal considerations. Chapters 14 through 23 include handouts that pertain to the injury assessment process (i.e., history, observation/inspection, palpation, testing). The handouts provide an extensive amount of information in an organized and easy-to-read format.

- **Worksheets.** Using a variety of formats, the exercises in the worksheets require students to demonstrate knowledge and comprehension, as well as to apply, analyze, synthesize, and evaluate information. In addition, some exercises incorporate the use of psychomotor skills. Answer sheets are provided for the worksheets.

- **Image Bank.** A bank of the various illustrations contained in the text is provided.

- **Articles and Web Links.** A list of articles and Web sites that are pertinent to information in various chapters is provided as a supplement for obtaining additional information.

- **Test Bank.** The bank includes more than 1,500 sample test questions composed of multiple choice, matching, true/false, and short answer questions. The program will allow faculty to add/customize their own test questions.

- **WebCT and Blackboard-Ready Cartridges**

Student Resource Center

The online resource center for students will contain two of the same features available through the instructor's resource center—namely, the reference materials and the Web Links. In addition, the student resource center will include the following:

- **Stedman's Audio Glossary.** The glossary available in the text will also be readily accessible online.

- **Articles and Web Links.** A list of articles and Web sites that are pertinent to information in various chapters is provided as a supplement for obtaining additional information.

- **Electronic Flash Cards.** Interactive flash cards can be an effective way to study important terms and concepts. Students will have the option to view cards by term/concept or by definition.

- **Reference Materials.** Each chapter contains a variety of materials intended to supplement the information presented in the text. For example, Chapter 1 provides sample forms pertaining to legal considerations. Chapters 14 through 23 include handouts that pertain to the injury assessment process (i.e., history, observation/inspection, palpation, testing). The handouts provide an extensive amount of information in an organized and easy-to-read format.

- **Quizzes.** Quizzes use a variety of testing formats, including multiple choice and N-wise multiple choice. These formats are similar to those used on the Board of Certification (BOC) examination.

- **Drag-and-Drop Figure Labeling.** The images can be labeled by dragging the correct descriptor to the corresponding element of the figure.

In addition, purchasers of the text can access the searchable Full Text Online by going to the *Foundations of Athletic Training* Web site at http://thePoint.lww.com/AndersonFound6e. See the inside front cover of this text for more details, including the passcode you will need to gain access to the Web site.

Marcia K. Anderson
Bridgewater, Massachusetts

Acknowledgments

The author would like to thank the hardworking and talented staff of Wolters Kluwer. Michael Nobel, John Larkin, and Shauna Kelley who provided enthusiastic support, guidance, and innovative ideas for enhancing this edition of the book. As with any new edition, changes come to the individuals who update and write new chapters. I want to specifically thank Dr. Gail Parr, Professor at Towson University in Baltimore, Maryland for her work over the past decade on this project as a co-author and the individual who developed the online resources for this text and the *Fundamentals in Athletic Training* text. Her contributions were certainly instrumental in the success of this book as a leading athletic training educational text.

I wish to also thank the following individuals who developed new chapters:

Chapter 5, Evidence-Based Health Care, written by Dr. Lisa Juttee, Associate Professor at Xavier University in Cincinnati, Ohio.

Chapter 8, Assessment of Body Alignment Posture and Gait, written by Dr. M. Susan Guyer, Professor of Exercise Science and Sport Studies and ESSS Department Chair & Clinical Education Coordinator of Athletic Training at Springfield College, Springfield, Massachusetts.

Several chapters were also updated by colleagues and friends including:

Chapter 9, Psychosocial Intervention and Patient Care, written by Dr. Victoria Bacon, Clinical Psychologist and Professor of Counselor Education, at Bridgewater State University, Bridgewater, Massachusetts.

Chapter 10, Tissue Healing and Wound Care; Chapter 11, Therapeutic Medications; Chapter 12, Therapeutic Modalities; and Chapter 13, Therapeutic Exercise Program by Pat Cordeiro MS, ATC, CSCS, Assistant Athletic Trainer, Tufts University, Medford, Massachusetts.

Chapter 24, Cardiovascular Disorders; Chapter 25, Neurological Conditions; Chapter 26, Respiratory Tract Conditions; Chapter 27, Gastrointestinal Conditions; Chapter 28, Endocrine Conditions; Chapter 29, Environmental Conditions; Chapter 31, Common Infectious Diseases; and Chapter 32, Dermatology by Dr. Jackie Williams, Program Coordinator, Athletic Training Education, Slippery Rock University, Slippery Rock, Pennsylvania.

In addition to the colleagues working on the chapters, I want to also thank Dr. Dominique Ross, Assistant Professor of Athletic Training & Clinical Education Coordinator at Lasell College, Newton, Massachusetts. Dominique is responsible for updating the Ancillary Materials on thePoint for this project. Her background in clinical education has been instrumental in providing a comprehensive resource center for both instructors and students.

Most especially, I want to thank Dr. Mary Barnum, Professor of Exercise Science and Sport Studies and Program Director of the Athletic Training Program at Springfield College, Springfield, Massachusetts. She has assumed the key leadership role in updating all of the remaining chapters in the text as well as organizing the photography session with Susan Symonds of Infinity Portrait Design from Boston, Massachusetts. Dr. Barnum's knowledge of evidence-based research and clinical skills has surpassed my expectations for the production of this edition. She is a welcomed partner in the project.

A thank you always goes to Dr. Victoria L. Bacon for her kind words and support through another edition of this book, and to Gabby my four-legged union supervisor who waited patiently for her daily walks. I could never do it without them.

MKA

Brief Contents

Contents

SECTION IV Conditions of the Lower Extremity 359

CHAPTER 14 Lower Leg, Ankle, and Foot Conditions 360

SECTION V   Conditions of the Upper Extremity 543

CHAPTER 17 Shoulder Conditions 544

CHAPTER 23 Throat, Thorax, and Visceral Conditions 825

SECTION VII Systemic Conditions and Special Considerations 871

CHAPTER 24 Cardiovascular Disorders 872

User's Guide

CHAPTER OPENING ELEMENTS

Each chapter begins with the following elements, which will help you get off to the right start.

Outcomes

These are the learning objectives that you need to meet after reading the chapter content. (Here's a tip: Read them again after finishing the chapter as a self-test.)

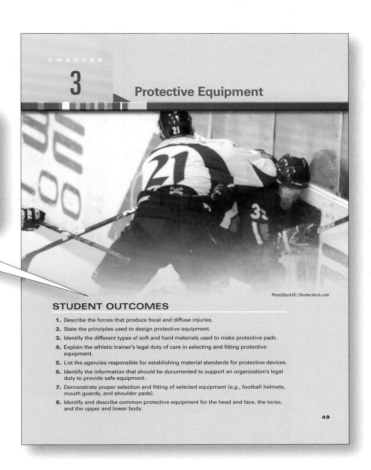

SPECIAL FEATURES

The new and unique aspects of this edition are shown and explained here so that you can make the most out of them.

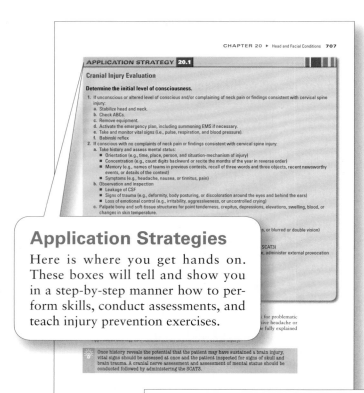

EMS Alerts

Sometimes injuries and medical conditions can become life threatening, so situations in which the athletic trainer should immediately call for an emergency medical services (EMS) response and transport are highlighted and explained.

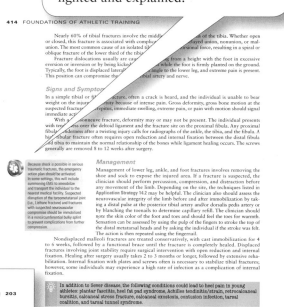

Application Strategies

Here is where you get hands on. These boxes will tell and show you in a step-by-step manner how to perform skills, conduct assessments, and teach injury prevention exercises.

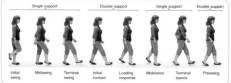

Critical Thinking Questions and Answers

This tried-and-true feature gives you a realistic scenario and then poses a question, which is answered at the end of the section. Use these to practice your critical thinking, problem-solving, and decision-making skills—they'll serve you well in the future.

ADDITIONAL LEARNING AND TEACHING RESOURCES

This textbook features a power companion Web site:
http://thePoint.lww.com/AndersonFound6e

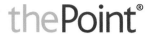

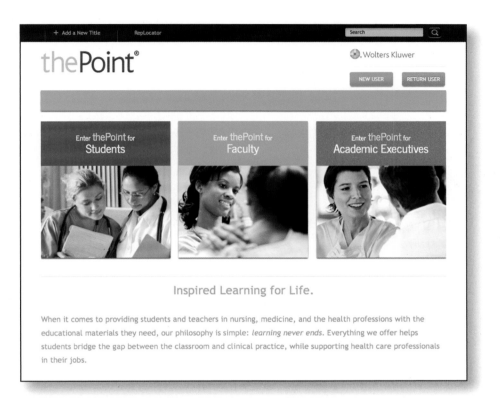

Student Resource Center

- Clinically oriented anatomy images
- Drag-and-drop image labeling
- Audio glossary
- Chapter quizzes
- Electronic flash cards
- Web Links for supplemental information
- Additional reference material, such as boxes, tables, field strategies, and sample forms to support chapters
- **PLUS:** Video clips from *Acland's DVD Atlas of Human Anatomy*

Instructor's Resource Center

- Instructor's manual with testing strategies, lecture notes, worksheets, answers, and handouts
- Test generator
- Image collection
- PowerPoint presentations
- BOC Correlation Chart
- Web Links for supplemental information

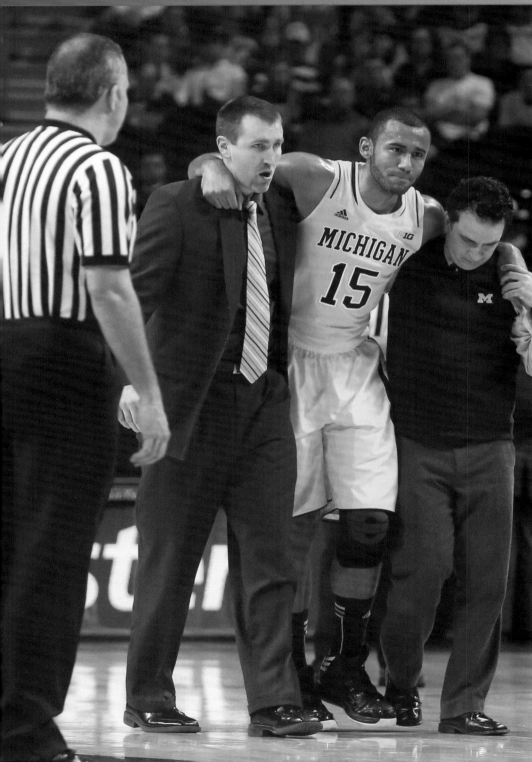

Foundations for the Prevention of Sports Injuries

1 Injury Care and the Athletic Trainer

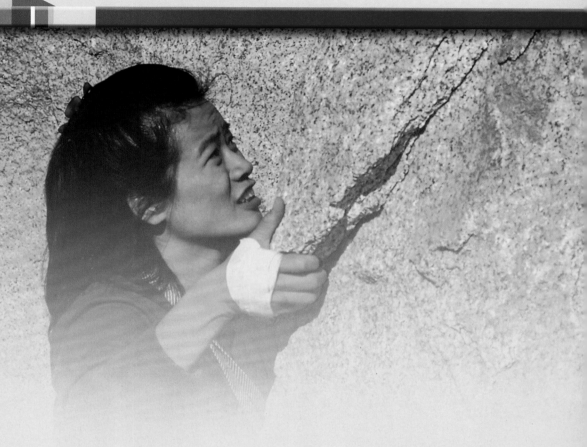

STUDENT OUTCOMES

1. Describe the mission of the National Athletic Trainers' Association (NATA).

2. Describe the mission of the Board of Certification (BOC).

3. Identify the major performance domains of the entry-level athletic trainer as defined in the *Role Delineation Study* published by the BOC.

4. Identify the requirements for earning the ATC (certified athletic trainer) credential awarded by the BOC as well as the requirements for maintaining BOC certification.

5. Explain the basic parameters of ethical conduct and standards of professional practice for athletic trainers.

6. Describe potential work settings for individuals holding the ATC credential.

7. Describe a team approach to the delivery of health care to athletes and physically active individuals.

8. Explain standard of care and the factors that must be proved to show legal breach of that duty of care.

9. Describe measures that can reduce the risk of litigation.

INTRODUCTION

Sport and physical activity, with the inherent risks involved, can lead to injury or illness at any time. Such injuries often are assessed and managed by athletic trainers, who are midlevel health care professionals who, in collaboration with physicians, provide services that encompass the prevention, emergency care, clinical diagnosis, therapeutic intervention, and rehabilitation of injuries and medical conditions of patients who participate in sports, work, and life. This chapter examines the professional practice of athletic trainers, including the function of the National Athletic Trainers' Association (NATA) and the Board of Certification (BOC) as distinct governing bodies for the profession. In addition, information is presented pertaining to a team approach to the delivery of health care for physically active individuals. Finally, legal liability surrounding injury care is presented relative to reducing the risk of possible litigation.

SPORTS MEDICINE

 Should the terms sports medicine and athletic training be used interchangeably?

Sports medicine is a broad and complex branch of health care encompassing several disciplines. Essentially, it is an area of health care and special services that applies medical and scientific knowledge to prevent, recognize, assess, manage, and rehabilitate injuries or illnesses related to sport, exercise, or recreational activity and, in doing so, enhances health fitness and performance of the participant. No single profession can provide the expertise to carry out this enormous responsibility. Rather, professionals from several disciplines play key roles in addressing health care for physically active individuals. These professionals may include certified athletic trainers, team physicians or primary care physicians, orthopedic physicians, physical therapists, emergency medical technicians, radiologists, nutritionists, exercise physiologists, biomechanists, and sport psychologists.

 In many instances, people will refer to "sports medicine" when in fact they should be referring to "athletic training." Athletic trainers are specialists from one of several disciplines within the broader field of sports medicine. As such, the terms sports medicine and athletic training should not be used interchangeably.

ATHLETIC TRAINING

 Why should individuals involved in pursuing a career in athletic training be familiar with the *Role Delineation Study* and the *Athletic Training Education Competencies*?

As medical experts in the prevention, assessment, treatment, and rehabilitation of injuries resulting from physical activity, certified athletic trainers are uniquely qualified to provide health care services to athletes and physically active individuals. While continuing to have a solid presence in the traditional settings of college/university and secondary school athletic programs, athletic trainers have expanded their medical expertise to include clinical settings (e.g., sports medicine and physical therapy centers), offices (e.g., physician extender and hospitals), occupational settings, public safety, performing arts, and the military. It is estimated that more than 50% of athletic trainers work outside the traditional school athletic setting.[1]

National Athletic Trainers' Association

The NATA represents more than 35,000 members in the athletic training profession.[1] Since the first meeting in 1950, the NATA has been responsible for the growth and development of the athletic training profession. In establishing standards for professionalism, education, research, and practice settings, the NATA has played a critical role in the evolution of the skills and qualifications of the athletic trainer. The NATA has used a variety of resources, including public relations, scholarship and research grants, governmental affairs, and annual meetings, to provide an array of services for its members, health care providers, educational institutions, businesses, and the general public.

A watershed landmark for the NATA came in 1990, when the American Medical Association (AMA) officially recognized athletic trainers as allied health care professionals. Another significant indicator of the progress and trends in the athletic training profession became evident in 1999, when the American Hospital Association assigned uniform billing, or revenue, codes for athletic training. This action was followed in the year 2000 by the AMA's designation of current procedural terminology (CPT) codes for athletic training and reevaluation. In 2005, the creation of the NATA Political Action Committee (NATA-PAC) as an incorporated organization signified another pivotal move in the profession. In promoting its mission to serve as a voice for the athletic training profession among federal legislators, the NATA-PAC aims to heighten awareness of the athletic training profession and, in doing so, to increase opportunities for athletic trainers and the individuals they serve.

Board of Certification

The BOC, a separate governing body from the NATA, is responsible for awarding the ATC (certified athletic trainer) credential. The mission of the BOC is "to provide exceptional credentialing programs for health care professionals."[2] In doing so, the BOC safeguards the public by establishing high standards of quality health care professionals through a system of certification, adjudication, standards of practice, and a continuing competency program.

 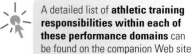 A detailed list of **athletic training responsibilities within each of these performance domains** can be found on the companion Web site at thePoint.

The *Role Delineation Study* (RD) published by the BOC defines the current entry-level knowledge, skills, and abilities required for practice in the profession of athletic training. The RD also serves as a blueprint for the national certification examination. The sixth edition of the RD defines the major performance domains for the entry-level certified athletic trainer as follows[3]:

Injury/illness prevention and wellness protection

Clinical evaluation and diagnosis

Immediate and emergency care

Treatment and rehabilitation

Organizational and professional health and well-being

Injury/Illness Prevention and Wellness Protection

The domain of injury/illness prevention and wellness protection encompasses a broad spectrum of knowledge and skills that address the risks associated with safe performance and function. Such risks range in severity from minor to potentially catastrophic injuries or illnesses. In a similar manner, the strategies used to minimize such risks can vary from relatively simple to complex. General areas in this domain focus on minimizing the risk of injury and illness of individuals and groups through awareness, education, and intervention; interpreting individual and group preparticipation and other relevant screening information (e.g., verbal, observed, written) in accordance with accepted and applicable guidelines; identifying and educating individuals and groups through appropriate communication methods (e.g., verbal, written) about the appropriate use of personal protective equipment (e.g., clothing, shoes, protective gear, and braces) by following accepted procedures and guidelines; maintaining physical activity, clinical treatment, and rehabilitation areas by complying with regulatory standards to minimize the risk of injury and illness; monitoring environmental conditions (e.g., weather, surfaces, client work setting) using appropriate methods and guidelines to facilitate individual and group safety; maintaining or improving physical conditions for the individual or group by designing and implementing programs (e.g., strength, flexibility, cardiovascular fitness); and promoting healthy lifestyle behaviors using appropriate education and communication strategies.[3]

Clinical Evaluation and Diagnosis

The domain of clinical evaluation and diagnosis addresses the responsibilities of the athletic trainer in using standard evaluation techniques and formulating a clinical impression for the determination of a course of action. Evaluation, or assessment, can involve several scenarios, including on-field (or on-site) primary assessment (**Fig. 1.1**), off-field initial assessment, and follow-up assessment. In each situation, the evaluation follows a systematic format that includes obtaining an individual's history through observation, interview, and/or review of relevant records to assess an injury, illness, or health-related condition; utilizing appropriate visual and palpation techniques to determine the type and extent of the injury, illness, or health-related condition; utilizing appropriate tests (e.g., range of motion, special tests, neurological tests) to determine the type and extent of the injury, illness, or health-related condition; formulating a clinical diagnosis by interpreting the signs, symptoms, and predisposing factors of the injury, illness, or health-related condition to determine an appropriate course of action; and educating the individual(s) about the clinical evaluation by communicating information about the condition to encourage compliance with recommended care.[3]

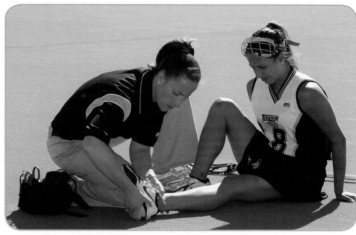

Figure 1.1. Injury assessment. Athletic trainers perform assessments in a variety of settings, including on the field.

Immediate and Emergency Care

The immediate and emergency care domain identifies the role of the athletic trainer subsequent to determining the nature and extent of an injury or illness. Regardless of the setting, the athletic trainer must be prepared to care for and prevent further harm in patients with a variety of conditions. As such, immediate and emergency care could range from coordinating care of individuals through appropriate communication (e.g., verbal, written, demonstrative) of assessment findings to pertinent individuals; applying appropriate immediate and emergency care procedures to prevent the exacerbation of health-related conditions to reduce the risk factors for morbidity and mortality; implementing appropriate referral strategies while stabilizing and/or preventing exacerbation of the condition(s) to facilitate the timely transfer of care for health-related conditions beyond the scope of practice of the athletic trainer; and implementing and directing immediate care strategies (e.g., first aid, emergency action plan) using established communication and administrative practices to provide effective care (**Fig. 1.2**).[3]

Treatment and Rehabilitation

The athletic trainer is responsible for the implementation of treatment and rehabilitation programs appropriate to the diagnosis made during the evaluation and assessment phase (**Fig. 1.3**). The athletic trainer can administer therapeutic and conditioning exercise(s) using appropriate techniques and procedures to aid recovery and restoration of function; administer therapeutic modalities (e.g., electromagnetic, manual, mechanical) using appropriate techniques and procedures based on the individual's phase of recovery to restore function; and apply braces, splints, or other assistive devices according to appropriate practices in order to facilitate injury protection to achieve optimal functioning for the individual.[3]

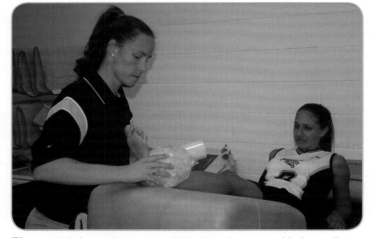

Figure 1.2. Immediate care. Athletic trainers provide immediate care for a variety of conditions, ranging from potentially life threatening to minor musculoskeletal injuries.

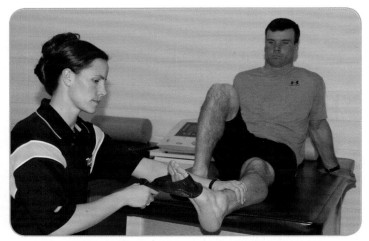

Figure 1.3. Rehabilitation. A major performance domain of the athletic trainer includes the development and implementation of rehabilitation programs.

Organization and Professional Health and Well-being

The domain of organization and professional health and well-being describes the responsibilities of the athletic trainer in developing and executing a series of plans, policies, and procedures to ensure individual and organizational well-being.[3] It is essential that such practices adhere to approved organization and professional guidelines, such as in keeping with the BOC *Standards of Professional Practice* and the NATA *Code of Ethics*. Some aspects of organization and professional health and well-being will be similar regardless of the setting, but when developing policies and procedures, consideration must be given to issues specific to the particular environment. General areas that warrant attention in this domain include applying basic internal business functions (e.g., business planning, financial operations, staffing) to support individual and organizational growth and development; applying basic external business functions (e.g., marketing and public relations) to support organizational sustainability, growth, and development; maintaining records and documentation that comply with organizational, association, and regulatory standards to provide quality of care and to enable internal surveillance for program validation and evidence-based interventions; appropriately planning for coordination of resources (e.g., personnel, equipment, liability, scope of service) in event medical management and emergency action plans; understanding statutory and regulatory provisions and professional standards of the practice of athletic training in order to provide for the safety and welfare of an individual or group; and developing a support/referral process for interventions to address unhealthy lifestyle behaviors.[3]

Athletic Training Education

To qualify for certification as an AT, an individual must earn an undergraduate or graduate degree, having completed an accredited entry-level athletic training education program. Effective July 1, 2006, the recognized accrediting agency is the Commission on Accreditation of Athletic Training Education (CAATE), known formally as the Joint Review Committee on Educational Programs in Athletic Training (JRC-AT).[4] The Executive Committee for Education (ECE) of the NATA is responsible for matters pertaining to athletic training education.[5]

Using a competency-based approach, athletic training education programs are designed to provide an effective blend of classroom and clinical experience. Education content is based on cognitive (knowledge), psychomotor (skill), and affective competencies (professional behaviors) and clinical proficiencies (professional and practice-oriented outcomes).[4] Formal instruction must be provided to cover foundational behaviors of professional practice and professional competence in several content areas (**Box 1.1**).

BOX 1.1 Athletic Training Education—Formal Instruction Areas

NATA Athletic Training Education Competencies

- Evidence-based practice
- Prevention and health promotion
- Clinical examination and diagnosis
- Acute care of injuries and illnesses

- Therapeutic interventions
- Health care administration
- Psychosocial strategies and referral
- Professional development and responsibility

Completed under the supervision of a clinical instructor, the clinical education experience involves the acquisition and practice of the *Entry-Level Athletic Training Clinical Integration Proficiencies (CIP)*. The new CIPs require that students demonstrate the ability to examine and diagnose a patient, provide appropriate acute/emergent care, plan and implement appropriate therapeutic interventions, and make decisions pertaining to safe return to participation. This approach to student assessment better reflects the comprehensive nature of real patient care in a clinical environment.[5]

The ATC Credential

To earn the ATC Credential, an individual must complete a CAATE-accredited athletic training education program and pass the national certification examination administered by the BOC. Current and specific information regarding requirements for certification is available on the BOC Web site (www.bocatc.org).

The ATC credential holder must demonstrate continuing competence and requalify for certification.[2] Specifically, ATC credential holders must complete a predetermined number of continuing education units, including evidence-based practice and recertification in emergency cardiac care, within a specified time period. Continuing education programs provide an opportunity for athletic trainers to acquire new, innovative evidence-based skills and techniques and to learn about current research within the profession. Continuing education units may be accumulated in a variety of ways, such as attending workshops, seminars, conferences, and conventions; speaking at a clinical symposium; publishing professional articles; or enrolling in related correspondence or postgraduate education courses. Current standards of continuing education requirements are available on the BOC Web site (www.bocatc.org).

Standards of Professional Practice

Standards of professional practice are ethical responsibilities that guide one's actions and promote high standards of conduct and integrity to assure high-quality health care.[1] A certified athletic trainer should never compromise the health of any individual in the athletic trainer's care. Decisions made by the athletic trainer in rendering care must be based on sound medical consideration. Individuals should be informed of the risks for injury, be protected from injury whenever possible, and, if an injury occurs, receive expedient health care and rehabilitation. Participants have a right to confidentiality about their health status. Athletic trainers must be sensitive about dissemination of health information and honor the wishes of an individual not to make the information public.

The NATA has established the *Code of Ethics* and four basic ethical principles for athletic trainers to follow. These include the following[1]:

1. Members shall respect the rights, welfare, and dignity of all.

2. Members shall comply with the laws and regulations governing the practice of athletic training.

3. Members shall maintain and promote high standards in the provision of services.

4. Members shall not engage in any form of conduct that constitutes a conflict of interest or reflects adversely on the profession.

A copy of the *Code of Ethics* is available on the NATA Web site (www.nata.org).

In addition, the BOC publishes the *Standards of Professional Practice*.[2] This document serves as a tool for informing the public, candidates for certification, and ATC credential holders about the standards of professional conduct and disciplinary procedures imposed for the practice of athletic training. A copy of the *Standards* is available on the BOC Web site (www.bocatc.org).

State Regulation of the Athletic Trainer

Athletic trainers, through their state associations, have worked to secure recognition and establish some type of regulation concerning the practice of athletic training within their respective states. States regulate professions to protect the public from harm by unqualified individuals. Without some type of regulation, no legal foundation assures quality of care because no legal definition exists regarding what an athletic trainer can and cannot do.

Licensure is the strictest form of state regulation and, therefore, is the most effective means of protecting the public.[2] Licensure is necessary to protect the general public, to ensure public safety, to maintain minimum standards in the practice of athletic training, and to promote the highest degree of professional conduct on the part of the athletic trainer.[6,7] It is the permission of a governmental body for an individual to practice a profession.

Certification within a state differs from certification as an athletic trainer. Successful completion of the BOC requirements for certification does not automatically qualify an individual for state certification. State certification indicates that a person has the basic knowledge and skills required in the profession and has passed a state certification examination. Many states that offer certification recognize a successful passing score on the BOC examination as a criterion for granting state certification.

Registration, which is used in some states, means that an individual intending to practice athletic training within the state must register with a governmental agency. The state may or may not have educational prerequisites for registration; however, an individual can be removed from the registry for abuse, fraud, or harm to the public or patient. In Hawaii, athletic trainers are exempt from the licensure requirements of other professions. A specific scope of practice is defined in the **exemption** statute of the licensing requirement. Athletic trainers do not register with the state but are held to the standards of the scope of practice as defined in the statutes.

To date, 49 states and the District of Columbia require athletic trainers to meet specific standards of practice within the individual state.[2] These laws define the role of the athletic trainer and set the legal parameters under which the athletic trainer can operate within that state. As such, the laws delineate the specific clientele and services that can be provided in various work settings. For information regarding individual state licensure laws or an update on states regulating the practice of athletic training, contact the NATA Government Affairs Committee (www.nata.org).

Although standards vary, in most states, athletic trainers provide services to athletes or physically active individuals under the direct supervision of a physician licensed in that state. Most states accept the successful completion of the BOC examination as a basis for obtaining licensure, although there may or may not be any mechanism for assessing continued competency. Athletic trainers may be restricted in the services they provide in nontraditional settings or in states that do not have licensure laws. Being properly licensed and practicing within the established standards of practice are two of the strongest safeguards against litigation.

Work Settings

Historically, the common work setting for athletic trainers has been organized sports programs (i.e., professional, collegiate, and high school venues). In recent years, as the qualifications of the athletic trainer have evolved, work setting opportunities have expanded outside the athletic arena.

Clinical Settings

Today, one of the most popular work settings for athletic trainers is in clinics or in area hospitals. The athletic trainer is a vital member of a team composed of a variety of health care professionals. Under the direction of a physician, the athletic trainer provides services to a diverse patient population. Some work settings specialize in only sport-related injuries, but others deal in cardiac rehabilitation, exercise physiology, biomechanical analysis, or performance enhancement, or the athletic trainer may serve as a clinic administrator. In some states, direct billing or licensure standards may restrict the athletic trainer from providing certain services, such as initial patient evaluation or use of electrical modalities. The athletic trainer may work in the clinic in the morning hours and be subcontracted in the afternoon and evening to area high schools or colleges to provide on-site medical coverage.

Secondary Schools

The NATA has taken the position that secondary schools should provide a certified athletic trainer to address the health care needs of student athletes.[1] Furthermore, it is recommended that the athletic trainer be available both on-site and on a full-time basis. The American Academy of Family Physicians and the AMA support the need to provide appropriate health care to high school student athletes and the role of the athletic trainer as an integral part of a high school athletic program.[8,9]

In the secondary school setting, securing the services of an athletic trainer generally occurs in two ways: (1) the athletic trainer is an employee of the school system or, as mentioned previously, (2) the school system develops a contractual agreement with a local hospital or clinic to provide on-campus athletic training services. In some secondary schools, athletic trainers extend their services to include faculty and students outside the athletic program. In this capacity, the athletic trainer administers care for injuries sustained on school property and provides educational seminars on a variety of health-related topics, such as exercise programs, prevention of injury or illness during physical activity, and proper nutrition.

Colleges/Universities

The responsibilities of the athletic trainer in collegiate settings vary. In some institutions, the athletic trainer functions solely as a member of the athletic health care team. At others, the athletic trainer may be expected to take on additional responsibilities, such as teaching or working in the campus health center.

Professional Sports

Athletic trainers for professional sport teams typically are hired by a single sport team to perform athletic training services throughout the year. During the competitive season, the athletic trainer concentrates on traditional duties. During the off-season, the athletic trainer is involved primarily with developing and supervising rehabilitation and reconditioning programs.

Industrial/Occupational Settings

In the industrial and occupational setting, athletic trainers provide employees with in-house athletic training services. Working under the direction of a physician, the athletic trainer can perform injury assessment, management, and rehabilitation; develop wellness and fitness programs; and provide education and counseling for employees. This practice has proven to be beneficial for both the company and the employee. Companies that employ an athletic trainer report decreases in the "frequency, severity, and cost of workers' compensation claims for musculoskeletal disorders."[1] In addition, employee productivity has increased subsequent to a decrease in the number of lost or restricted workdays.[1]

Physician Practices

In the capacity of physician extender, athletic trainers perform an array of services. In a variety of physician practices (e.g., orthopedics, osteopathy, family practice, primary care, pediatrics, and occupational medicine), athletic trainers are involved in areas such as triage, patient education, rehabilitation, and exercise prescription. The use of athletic trainers in this capacity can improve the quality of care provided to patients as well as increase physician productivity and efficiency. The patient receives additional personal attention, yet the physician is afforded the opportunity to meet with more patients in relatively the same amount of time. In addition, the potential exists for increased revenue through billing and insurance reimbursement of athletic training services.

Other Employment Settings

Athletic trainers are finding employment in a wide array of other settings. For example, one could find employment in a corporate setting in sales, marketing, or administration that sells to the profession or in patient care. The performing arts provide opportunities in dance, theater, or the entertainment business (e.g., Disney, television/movie studio sets, professional dance troupes). Another opportunity for employment is in the military (e.g., military academies, training camps), law enforcement (e.g., FBI, sheriff departments, police departments, and fire departments), or the government (e.g., NASA, Pentagon). The Armed Forces Athletic Trainers' Society (AFATS) has over 100 members who work in governmental service.[10] The Clinical and Emerging Practices Athletic Trainers' Committee (CEPAT) says the possibilities are endless. For other ideas, visit the NATA Web site at www.nata.org, the AFATS Web site at http://afats.org/index1.htm, or the CEPAT Web site at www.nata.org/CEPAT.

> The *Role Delineation Study*, published by the BOC, defines the current entry-level knowledge, skills, and abilities of the certified athletic trainer and serves as a blueprint for development of the certification examination. The *Athletic Training Education Competencies*, published by the NATA ECE, defines the educational domains used in preparing entry-level athletic trainers.

TEAM APPROACH TO DELIVERY OF HEALTH CARE

> A member of a high school basketball team was seen by his family physician for an injury sustained during practice. The physician determined that the athlete should not participate in activity for 1 week. After 5 days, the athlete's parents call the school athletic trainer to give approval for their child to play. How should the athletic trainer respond to this situation?

As members of a health care team, athletic trainers work under the direction of a licensed physician and with a variety of other professionals. The team approach provides an effective means for ensuring quality health care for physically active individuals.

Team Physician

In an organized sport, such as interscholastic, intercollegiate, or professional athletic programs, a team physician may be hired or may volunteer his or her services to direct the primary sports medicine team. This individual supervises the various aspects of health care and is the final authority to determine the mental and physical fitness of athletes in organized programs.[11]

The team physician should have an unrestricted medical license and be an MD or DO. The individual should have a fundamental knowledge of on-field medical emergency care (e.g., concussion, cardiac emergencies, spinal injuries, heat-related illnesses), be trained in basic cardiopulmonary resuscitation and automated external defibrillator use, and have a working knowledge of musculoskeletal injuries, medical conditions, and psychological issues affecting the athlete.[11]

In an athletic program, the team physician should administer and review preseason physical examinations; review preseason conditioning programs; assess the quality, effectiveness, and maintenance of protective equipment; diagnose injuries; dispense medications; direct rehabilitation programs; educate the athletic staff regarding emergency policies, procedures, health care insurance coverage, and legal liability; and review all medical forms, policies, and procedures to ensure compliance with school and athletic association guidelines.[11] This individual also may serve as a valuable resource in terms of current therapeutic techniques; facilitate referrals to other medical specialists; and provide educational counseling to sport participants, parents, athletic trainers, coaches, and sport supervisors (**Box 1.2**).

In many high school and collegiate settings, financial constraints may prevent hiring a full-time team physician. Instead, several physicians may rotate the responsibility of being present at competitions and are paid a per-game stipend. Primary care physicians, orthopedists, and other specialists (e.g., osteopaths, internists, general surgeons, and pediatricians) who have a broad and thorough understanding of sports injuries may serve as team physicians. A physician should be present at competitions, particularly those involving high-risk sports, to assess emergency injury and treat any injury or illness.

Primary Care Physician

In some settings, particularly those outside the traditional athletic setting, the primary care or family physician assumes a key role in providing medical care to athletes and physically active individuals

BOX 1.2 **Duties of the Team Physician**

- Plan and organize the preparticipation examination (PPE)
- Review PPE results and determine readiness for sport/physical activity participation
- Review preseason conditioning programs
- Assess the quality, effectiveness, and maintenance of protective equipment
- Manage injuries on the field, particularly involving collision and contact sports
- Provide for follow-up medical management of injury and illness
- Coordinate rehabilitation and safe return to participation
- Dispense medications
- Facilitate referrals to other health care providers, including medical specialists, athletic trainers, and allied health professionals
- Provide educational counseling regarding nutrition, strength and conditioning, ergogenic aids, substance abuse, and other medical problems that could affect the athlete
- Provide for proper documentation and medical record keeping
- Protect confidentiality of medical history
- Review all medical forms, policies, and procedures to ensure compliance with school and athletic association guidelines
- Educate the staff on emergency policies, procedures, health care insurance coverage, and legal liability
- Provide in-service training on current therapeutic methods, problems, and techniques

of all ages. The services provided by the primary care physician can vary with the background and expertise of the individual. Services performed by a primary care physician can range from completing a PPE for a young athlete to counseling a middle-aged patient with multiple risk factors for coronary artery disease regarding the parameters for safely beginning an exercise program. In some settings, the primary care physician will assume the responsibility for clearing an individual to participate in activity.

The Coach or Sport Supervisor

A coach is responsible for teaching the skills and strategies of a sport. A sport supervisor may not necessarily be a coach but, instead, may be responsible for administering and supervising recreational sport activities or activity areas within health club facilities. Both individuals are responsible for encouraging appropriate behavior and developing an overall awareness of safety and injury prevention. For brevity, coaches and sport supervisors are jointly referred to as coaches.

In the absence of an athletic trainer, the coach must assume a more active role in providing health care to participants. As such, coaches should maintain current certification in emergency cardiac care (i.e., cardiopulmonary resuscitation and automated external defibrillator) and emergency first aid. Coaches should meet with their respective staff to develop an emergency action plan and should periodically practice implementing that plan. In the absence of an athletic trainer, coaches also are expected to evaluate the daily status of participants before any activity, properly fit and use quality safety equipment, teach proper skill development and technique, and constantly reinforce the importance of safety and injury prevention throughout the year.[1] In addition, the coach can be responsible for informing the participant of the risk of injury, the strategies for preventing injuries, and the actions to take if an injury is sustained.

Sport/Physical Activity Participant

Individual participants play an essential role in working with the athletic trainer to maximize injury prevention. It is the responsibility of the participant to adhere to prescribed guidelines for the activity. Such responsibilities could include maintaining an appropriate level of fitness, performing within the rules or guidelines of an activity, and maintaining and wearing safety equipment. In the event of an injury, the individual should know where to seek immediate health care and follow medical advice from the physician or athletic trainer. If participants understand and practice safety and preventive measures, the number of injuries or illnesses can be reduced significantly.

Physical Therapist

Physical therapists provide a unique and valuable resource in the overall rehabilitation of an individual. Physical therapists often supervise the rehabilitation of injured participants in a hospital setting, an industrial clinic, or a sports medicine clinic. In some cases, an athletic trainer and physical therapist will combine efforts in designing and implementing rehabilitative care.

Strength and Conditioning Specialist

The use of proper strength and conditioning to improve physical skills, athletic performance, and fitness is the purview of the strength and conditioning specialist. A collaborative effort between the strength and conditioning specialist and an athletic trainer can be advantageous in designing and implementing conditioning programs for injured as well as healthy individuals.

Exercise Physiologist

An exercise physiologist can provide information pertaining to the physiological mechanisms underlying physical activity. As such, the exercise physiologist can offer theoretical and practical suggestions regarding the analysis, improvement, and maintenance of health and fitness as well as the rehabilitation of heart disease and other chronic diseases and/or disabilities.[12]

Nutritionist

Nutritionists are concerned primarily with the role of proper dietary care in the prevention and treatment of illnesses but can provide valuable input regarding the specialized needs of athletes and physically active individuals. Examples of particular needs include diets for enhancing performance and preventing injury, effective weight management strategies (e.g., weight gain, loss, or maintenance), physical activity and diabetes, counseling with regard to disordered eating, and nutrient supplementation.

Biomechanist

Applying basic laws of physics in performing mechanical analyses of human movement, a biomechanist can offer practical insight for improving human performance as well as preventing injuries related to sport and physical activity. Information pertaining to kinematics (i.e., the study of spatial and temporal aspects of motion) can provide valuable information pertaining to injury prevention, whereas information regarding kinetics (i.e., the study of forces associated with motion) provides a basis for understanding injury mechanisms.

Emergency Medical Technician and Paramedic

There are several levels of emergency medical service (EMS) providers. Emergency medical responders provide out-of-hospital care in medical emergencies and may be the first to arrive on the scene. They have a limited scope of practice and have the least amount of comprehensive education, clinical experience, and clinical skills. The emergency medical technician (EMT) (replacing EMT-Basic) is the entry level of EMS. Procedures and skills permitted at this level are generally noninvasive and focus on control of bleeding, use of certain airways and ventilators with a bag valve mask, supplemental oxygen administration, and splinting (e.g., fractures and full spinal immobilization). Advanced EMT (replacing EMT-Intermediate 1985) allows for more invasive procedures, such as intravenous (IV) therapy and the use of multilumen airway devices (endotracheal intubation in some states), and provides for enhanced assessment skills. EMT-Paramedic (replacing EMT-Intermediate 1999 and EMT-Paramedic) is the highest level of EMT and as such is generally seen as the highest level of pre-hospital medical provider. In addition to the previously mentioned training and clinical skills, these individuals can provide fluid resuscitation, pharmaceutical administration, obtaining IV access, cardiac monitoring (continuous and 12-lead), and other advanced procedures and assessments.[13]

 The athletic trainer must follow the physician's orders. As such, the athletic trainer should not permit the athlete to return to play and should advise the parent that the family physician is the final authority for determining the athlete's return to play.

LEGAL CONSIDERATIONS

 As the athletic trainer at a high school, you have been asked by the athletic director to speak at the annual preseason meeting attended by the athletes and their parents. What topics should be addressed at this meeting?

Prevention of injuries and reducing further injury or harm are major responsibilities of athletic trainers. Even with the best possible care, accidents do happen, some of which may result in legal action against several parties, such as the athletic trainer, the team physician, or the activity supervisor. Legal action involving the practice of athletic training typically is tried under tort law. A **tort** is a civil wrong done to an individual, whereby the injured party seeks a remedy for damages suffered. Such wrongs may occur from an act of omission, whereby an individual fails to perform a legal duty, or from an act of commission, whereby an individual commits an act that is not one's act to perform or an act that is one's duty to perform but that is carried out with the wrong procedure, leading to injury or harm. In lawsuits, actions are measured against a standard of care provided by individuals who have a direct duty to provide care.

Standard of Care

Standard of care is measured by what another minimally competent individual educated and practicing in that profession would have done in the same or similar circumstance to protect an individual from harm or further harm. Standard of care is dictated by the profession's duty or **scope of care**, which outlines the role and responsibilities of an individual in that profession and delineates what should be learned in the professional preparation of that individual. Standard of care may be further delineated by state and federal statutes, publications for organized governing bodies, as well as directives or recommendations published by state athletic associations.[14] In athletic training, the ECE of the NATA has determined the best educational practices that reflect the profession's interdisciplinary nature and commitment to learning across the professional's lifespan. These practices define the educational competencies that students enrolled in a CAATE-accredited athletic training program must master.

By delineating the scope of care for entry-level athletic trainers, the BOC establishes the standard of care that the public can expect to receive from a certified athletic trainer. As such, an individual responsible for providing athletic training services is held to the standard of care expected of an individual holding the ATC credential. Therefore, in states with specific registration, certification, or licensure laws, valid BOC certification and registration or licensure is essential to protect oneself against litigation.

Clearance for Participation

The final authority to clear an individual for activity falls outside the scope of care of a certified athletic trainer. The final authority in measuring an individual's status for participation rests with the physician (e.g., team physician or primary care physician).[1]

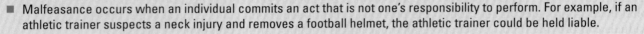

BOX 1.3 Definition of Negligent Torts

- Malfeasance occurs when an individual commits an act that is not one's responsibility to perform. For example, if an athletic trainer suspects a neck injury and removes a football helmet, the athletic trainer could be held liable.

- Misfeasance occurs when an individual commits an act that is one's responsibility to perform but either uses the wrong procedure or does the correct procedure in an improper manner. For example, if an athletic trainer suspects a neck injury and improperly secures the head and neck region to the rigid spine board, the athletic trainer could be held liable.

- Nonfeasance occurs when an individual fails to perform the legal duty of care. For example, if an athletic trainer suspects, or should have suspected, a neck injury and fails to use a rigid back board to stabilize the individual, the athletic trainer could be held liable.

- Malpractice occurs when an individual commits a negligent act while providing care.

- Gross negligence occurs when an individual has total disregard for the safety of others.

Negligence

Athletic trainers are expected to provide a duty of care to participants. Failure to provide this care can result in liability, or **negligence**. Negligent torts may occur as a result of **malfeasance**, **misfeasance**, **nonfeasance**, **malpractice**, or **gross negligence** (**Box 1.3**).

Although participants assume some risk, which is inherent in any physical activity, the individual does not assume the risk that a professional will breach the duty of care. To find an individual liable, the injured person must prove the following:[15]

1. There was a duty of care.

2. There was a breach of that duty.

3. There was harm (e.g., pain and suffering, permanent disability, or loss of wages).

4. The resulting harm was a direct cause from that breach of duty.

For example, if a spectator notices a large hole in the field before a game and a player steps into that hole and fractures an ankle, the spectator is not liable because that individual has no duty of care for the player. An athletic trainer or coach, however, does have a duty of care to check the field for hazards before competition. As such, the athletic trainer or coach could be held liable for the injury sustained by the participant.

Legal Liabilities

Athletic trainers and coaches can take several precautionary steps to limit the risk of litigation. These may involve the following:

- Informing the individual about the inherent risks of participation

- Foreseeing the potential for injury and correcting the situation before harm occurs

- Obtaining informed consent from the individual or guardian before participation in the sport/activity and before any treatment should an injury occur

- Using quality products and equipment that do not pose a threat to the individual

- Maintaining strict confidentiality of all medical records

Fortunately, the number of lawsuits brought against athletic trainers in the performance of their duties is small. Situations that can result in litigation are listed in **Box 1.4**.

BOX 1.4 Actions That Can Result in Litigation

- Failing to warn an individual about the risks involved in sport participation
- Treating an injured party without consent
- Failing to provide medical information concerning alternate treatments or the risks involved with the needed treatment
- Failing to provide safe facilities, fields, and equipment
- Being aware of a potentially dangerous situation and failing to do anything about it
- Failing to provide an adequate injury prevention program
- Allowing an injured or unfit player to participate, resulting in further injury or harm
- Failing to provide quality training, instruction, and supervision
- Using unsafe equipment
- Negligently moving an injured athlete before properly immobilizing the injured area
- Failing to employ qualified medical personnel
- Failing to have a written emergency action plan
- Failing to properly recognize an injury or illness (both immediate acute care and long-term treatment)
- Failing to immediately refer an injured party to the proper physician
- Failing to keep adequate records
- Treating an injury that did not occur within the school athletic environment

Failure to Warn

Athletic trainers should inform potential participants of the risks for injury during participation. Participants and parents of minor children should understand that risk for injury exists as well as the nature of that risk so that informed judgments can be made about participation. Understanding and comprehending the nature of the risk is determined by the participant's age, experience, and knowledge of pertinent information about the risk. An advanced gymnast, for example, knows and appreciates the risk of injury much more than a novice gymnast. Therefore, it is crucial to warn the novice of any inherent dangers in the activity and continually reinforce that information throughout the entire sport season. Warnings may be communicated at the preseason meeting with parents and participants; during prescreening, when the client is first introduced into the fitness or health facility; and by posting visible warning signs around equipment, requiring protective equipment, and discouraging dangerous techniques. (Other methods that may be used are discussed later in this chapter.)

Foreseeability of Harm

Another duty of care for athletic trainers and coaches is to recognize the potential for injury and then remove that danger before an injury occurs. **Foreseeability of harm** exists when danger is apparent or should have been apparent, resulting in an unreasonably unsafe condition. This potential for injury can be identified during regular inspections of gymnasiums, field areas, swimming pools, safety equipment, and athletic training facilities. For example, unpadded walls under basketball hoops, glass or potholes on playing fields, slippery floors near a whirlpool, exposed wiring, and failure to follow universal safety precautions against the spread of infectious diseases all pose a threat to safety. Unsafe conditions should be identified, reported in writing to appropriate personnel, restricted from use, and repaired or replaced as soon as possible.

Informed Consent

Informed consent implies that an injured party has been reasonably informed of the needed treatment, the possible alternate treatments, and the advantages and disadvantages of each course of action. Valid consent can be obtained only from one who is competent to grant it—that is, an adult who is physically and mentally competent or, in the case of children younger than 18 years, a parent. For minors, exceptions exist in emergency situations when parents are unavailable. Authorization to treat in the absence of the parent, or in the event the individual is physically unable to consent to treatment, should be obtained in writing before the beginning of participation. This consent may be obtained during preparticipation meetings as part of the documentation depicting consent to participate in that activity.

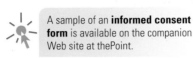

A sample of an **informed consent form** is available on the companion Web site at thePoint.

It is advisable to include an exclusionary clause on the consent form that identifies conditions that will not be treated by the athletic trainer (e.g., injuries not associated with direct participation in a sponsored activity). This can protect the athletic trainer from litigation when refusing to treat a particular injury. For example, suppose an individual is injured in a recreational bicycling accident and fails to seek immediate treatment from an emergency room or physician. Two days later, this individual reports to an athletic trainer with an infected, open wound. In this instance, the athletic trainer should immediately refer this individual to a physician for treatment. In most states, if the athletic trainer attempts to clean the wound and complications arise, the athletic trainer may be held liable for practicing medicine outside the scope of the athletic training profession.

Informed consent must be granted before any treatment. Athletic trainers must be sensitive to cultural and religious beliefs and practices as well—and honor those practices by providing appropriate care consistent with the wishes of the patient. For example, in some cultures, a woman may be taught not to undress or bare skin in the presence of a man other than her husband. Therefore, if a male athletic trainer is assigned to treat a woman with a thoracic injury and she does not feel comfortable, it is better to refer the patient to a female athletic trainer.

Failure to receive informed consent may constitute **battery**, which is any unpermitted or intentional contact with another individual without that individual's consent. Although many courts require that intent to harm be present in an allegation of battery, written documentation of informed consent should be obtained from an individual or parents of minor children before treatment to avoid litigation.

Refusing Help

Although the situation is rare, an injured participant may refuse emergency first aid for a variety of reasons, such as religious beliefs, cultural differences, avoidance of additional pain or discomfort, or the desire to be evaluated and treated by a more medically qualified individual. Regardless of the reason, a conscious and medically competent individual has the right to refuse treatment. An exemption to this standard may occur, however, when failure to move the injured party may result in an increased risk of further injury to the injured party or others in the vicinity of the accident. For example, during an organized bike race, if several bikers collide and fall down onto a busy road, it is appropriate to move any injured individuals off the road so as not to endanger those individuals and any approaching motorists. In this instance, it is best to have another employee summon EMS while the immediate care provider tries to persuade the injured party to accept immediate care until the ambulance arrives. It is helpful to have a witness to the event because, too often, an injured individual may initially refuse consent but later deny having done so.

Product Liability

Individuals often place a high degree of faith in the quality and safety of equipment used in sport and physical activity participation. Manufacturers have a duty of care to design, manufacture, and package safe equipment that will not cause injury to an individual when the equipment is used as intended. This is called an **implied warranty**. An **expressed warranty** is a written guarantee that the product is safe for use. In football, there is an implied warranty that the helmet can protect the head and brain from certain injuries if fitted and used properly. The National Operating Committee on Standards for Athletic Equipment (NOCSAE) has established minimum standards for football helmets to tolerate certain forces when applied to different areas of the helmet. Manufacturers and reconditioners of helmets place a visible expressed warranty on all helmets that meet NOCSAE standards. **Strict liability** makes the manufacturer liable for any and all defective or hazardous equipment that unduly threatens an individual's personal safety.

Any alteration or modification to protective equipment may negate the manufacturer's liability. It is essential that all involved parties understand the potential dangers associated with the use of equipment and that equipment should be used properly and for its intended purpose. For example, the practice of cutting down mouth guards to cover only the front teeth should be strongly prohibited. Furthermore, participants should be continually warned of the inherent dangers if equipment is used in a manner for which it was not intended.

Confidentiality

A major concern of all individuals involved in providing health care is the patient's right to privacy. If the individual is older than 18 years, release of any medical information must be acknowledged in writing by the participant. For individuals younger than 18 years, a parent or legal guardian must provide consent for the dissemination of this information. This permission should identify what, if any, information can be shared with someone other than the individual's physician. In many cases, schools and professional teams have participants give consent that all medical information can be shared between the athletic trainers and supervising physician. Information provided to others (e.g., coaches, parents, or supervisors) should be on a need-to-know basis only and given with the full knowledge and consent of the individual, supervising physician, and athletic trainer. Confidentiality extends to all medical records kept within the confines of the athletic training room, including the following:

- Consent-to-treat form
- Release-of-medical-information form
- Emergency information
- Treatment documentation, including injury report forms, medical referrals, physician evaluations, laboratory reports, surgical reports, and progress notes
- Living will
- Counseling

Legal Defenses

If the threat of litigation exists, many athletic trainers rely on certain conditions to strengthen their case. These include the individual's assumption of risk, Good Samaritan laws, and comparative negligence.

Assumption of Risk

Sport and exercise participants assume some inherent risks in their chosen activity. When individuals agree to participate in competitive activity, they should be informed of the risks of participation, testing, and physical activity and advised that participation is voluntary in nature. Many facilities require that each participant signs an expressed assumption-of-risk form. By signing the form, the individual acknowledges the material risks and that other injuries and even death are a possibility. The form also acknowledges that the individual has had an opportunity to ask questions and have them answered to one's complete satisfaction. Finally, the individual affirms a subjective understanding of the risks of participation in the activity and one's voluntary choice to participate, assuming all risks of injury or even death as a result of participation. These forms have successfully aided in the legal defense of individuals involved with providing health care. As stated previously, however, an individual does not assume the risk that a professional will breach the duty of care.

A sample of an **assumption-of-risk form** is available on the companion Web site at thePoint.

Good Samaritan Laws

Beginning in the early 1960s, several states enacted legislation to protect physicians or other recognized medical personnel from litigation as a result of emergency treatment provided to injured individuals at the scene of an accident. These laws, nicknamed "Good Samaritan" laws, were developed to encourage bystanders to assist others in need of emergency care by granting them immunity from potential litigation. Although the laws vary from state to state, immunity generally applies only when the person providing emergency first aid

1. acts during an emergency,

2. acts in good faith to help the victim,

3. acts without expected compensation, and

4. is not guilty of any malicious misconduct or gross negligence toward the injured party (i.e., does not deviate from acceptable first aid protocol).

Although Good Samaritan laws were intended to protect physicians and medical personnel, several states have expanded the language to include laypersons serving as emergency first aiders. These laws are easy to get around, however, and they should not be relied on by rescuers who erroneously believe the laws will protect them from litigation regardless of their actions. It is essential that sport and fitness coordinators be properly trained in emergency first aid and care of injuries if they are expected to supervise participants and render immediate first aid should a client or athlete sustain an injury during participation.

Comparative Negligence

When an injured person chooses to pursue litigation, several individuals, along with their employers, are named in the suit. These individuals may include the physicians, surgeons, athletic trainers, supervisors, and emergency personnel who provided medical services to the athlete. **Comparative negligence** refers to the relative degree of negligence on the part of the plaintiff and defendant, with damages awarded on a basis proportionate to each person's carelessness. For example, if an individual is found to be 30% at fault for one's own injury (contributory negligence) and the defendants to be 70% at fault, then on a $100,000 judgment, the defendants are responsible for $70,000 in damages and the individual (i.e., the plaintiff) assumes an equivalent of $30,000 in damages. The courts also weigh the relative degree of negligence on the part of each defendant and award payment of damages on a basis proportionate to each person's carelessness that leads to the eventual injury.

Preventing Litigation

All members of the sports medicine team should be aware of their duty of care consistent with current state law and should complete that duty of care within established policies and standards of practice. Several steps can reduce the risk of subsequent litigation and include performing regular inspections of athletic fields and facility design, performing safety checks of equipment and facilities, hiring qualified personnel, ensuring proper supervision and instruction, purchasing quality equipment, posting appropriate warning signs, maintaining accurate and complete health care records, and having a well-organized emergency action plan.

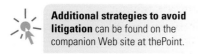 **Additional strategies to avoid litigation** can be found on the companion Web site at thePoint.

 During a preseason meeting for athletes and their parents, it would be appropriate for you, as the athletic trainer at a high school, to attend to the following: explanation of the risks involved in sport participation, completion of an assumption-of-risk form by the athlete and a parent, explanation of procedures for reporting injuries to the athletic trainer, obtaining written informed consent from the parents of minor children before participation, and obtaining emergency contact information.

SUMMARY

1. Sports medicine is a branch of medicine that applies medical and scientific knowledge to improve sport performance.

2. The NATA establishes standards for professionalism, education, research, and practice settings for athletic trainers. The NATA has played a critical role in the evolution of the skills and qualifications of the athletic trainer to a level that can be used in a variety of fields.

3. The BOC is responsible for awarding the ATC credential. As defined by the BOC, the major performance domains for the entry-level certified athletic trainer are prevention; clinical evaluation and diagnosis; immediate care; treatment, rehabilitation, and reconditioning; organization and administration; and professional responsibility.

4. Work settings for athletic trainers continue to expand as the qualifications of the athletic trainer increase. Work settings include, but are not limited to, secondary schools, colleges/universities, or professional athletic programs; sports medicine clinics; industrial/occupational settings; and physician practices.

5. Standards of professional practice are ethical judgments that guide a professional's actions and promote high standards of conduct and integrity.

6. For an athletic trainer, BOC certification and state licensure can help to meet one's duty of care in providing health care.

7. Decisions concerning whether an individual should participate in an activity should be made by the physician based on sound medical consideration and never compromise the health of the individual.

8. To find an individual liable, the injured person must prove duty of care, breach of that duty, harm caused by that breach, and harm as a direct cause of the breach of duty.

9. Steps to reduce the risk of injury and subsequent litigation should include obtaining informed consent; recognizing the potential for injury and correcting it; warning participants of the risk of injury; hiring qualified personnel; providing proper supervision and instruction; purchasing, fitting, and maintaining quality equipment; posting appropriate warning signs; maintaining accurate and complete health care records; protecting confidentiality of medical history; and having a well-organized emergency care system.

APPLICATION QUESTIONS

1. An athletic training student is preparing for the BOC examination. Would it be advantageous for the student to review the current edition of the *Role Delineation Study* prior to developing strategies for preparing to study for the examination? Explain your response.

2. Injury/illness prevention and wellness protection is one of the major domains of the athletic trainer. A local high school with an interscholastic athletic program cannot afford to hire an athletic trainer and has requested that you conduct a seminar for their coaching staff. The focus of the seminar would be strategies/policies that the coaches should implement in an effort to reduce the incidence and severity of injury (i.e., injury prevention). What areas would you address in speaking with the coaches? Why?

3. You are an athletic trainer at a high school. A 16-year-old football player sustained a compound fracture of the tibia and fibula in a game. The parents of the injured athlete are extremely concerned about the quality of care provided to their son and ask you if a team approach to health care delivery is preferable to a traditional doctor-to-patient approach. How would you respond to their question?

4. Is it appropriate for an athletic training department in an intercollegiate setting to use the same assumption-of-risk form for participants in every sport? Is it appropriate to include words such as *permanent physical impairment*, *paralysis*, and *death* on an assumption-of-risk form? Explain your response.

5. A first-year college athlete missed the preseason physical examination. The second day of preseason camp is the earliest an exam can be scheduled with the team physician. The coach insists that the athlete be allowed to participate during the first day of camp because the players will be doing only basic conditioning and technique drills. He states that no contact drills will be performed. Would you allow the athlete to participate? What implications exist concerning your legal responsibility to this athlete?

REFERENCES

1. National Athletic Trainers' Association. http://www.nata.org. Accessed July 20, 2015.
2. National Athletic Trainers' Association Board of Certification. http://www.bocatc.org. Accessed July 20, 2015.
3. National Athletic Trainers' Association Board of Certification. *Role Delineation Study/Practice Analysis*. 6th ed. Omaha, NE: National Athletic Trainers' Association Board of Certification; 2010.
4. Joint Review Committee on Educational Programs in Athletic Training. http://www.jrc-at.org. Accessed July 20, 2015.
5. National Athletic Trainers' Association Executive Committee for Education. http://www.nata.org/access-read/public/executive-committee-education-ece. Accessed July 20, 2015.
6. Rello MN. The importance of state regulation to the promulgation of the athletic training profession. *J Athl Train*. 1996;31(2):160–164.
7. Campbell D, Konin J. Regulation of athletic training. In: Konin J, ed. *Clinical Athletic Training*. Thorofare, NJ: Slack; 1997:23–32.
8. American Academy of Family Physicians. http://www.aafp.org/about/policies/all/sports-medicine-trainers.html. Accessed July 20, 2015.
9. American Medical Association. http://www.ama-assn.org/resources/doc/mss/x-pub/a13-handbook.pdf. Accessed July 20, 2015.
10. Wood I. Athletic trainers in the military and government. *NATA News*. 2012;24(10):26–27.
11. Herring SA, Kibler WB, Putukian M. Team physician consensus statement: 2013 update. *Med Sci Sports Exerc*. 2013;45(8):1618–1622.
12. American Society of Exercise Physiologists. http://www.asep.org. Accessed July 20, 2015.
13. National Registry of Emergency Medical Technicians'. https://www.nremt.org. Accessed July 20, 2015.
14. Quandt EF, Mitten MJ, Black JS. Legal liability in covering athletic events. *Sports Health*. 2009;1(1):84–90.
15. Connaughton D, Murphey M, Kaminski TW. Negligence liability. *Athl Ther Today*. 1999;4(1):50–51.

Preparticipation Examination

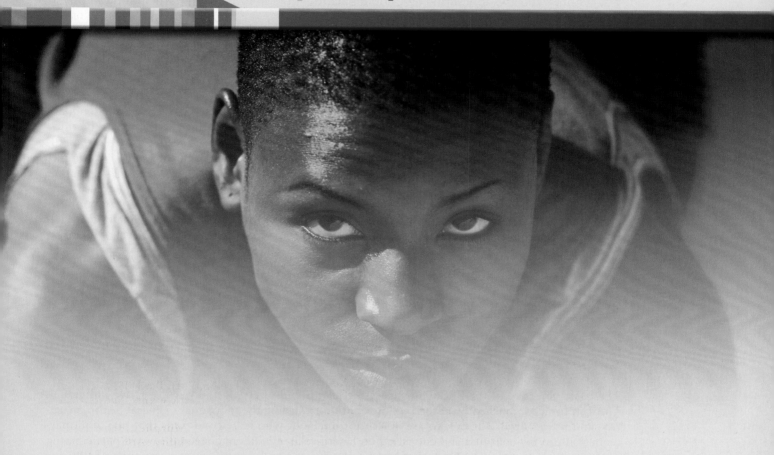

STUDENT OUTCOMES

1. Identify the goals and objectives of a preparticipation examination (PPE).
2. Design a PPE.
3. Identify the specific areas in a PPE that could be examined using a mass station screening process.
4. Identify follow-up questions intended to validate information on a medical history questionnaire.
5. Demonstrate the ability to take vital signs, and identify criteria used to denote abnormal pulse and blood pressure rates.
6. Explain the importance of completing a physical fitness profile as part of the PPE.
7. Demonstrate skinfold measurement at the various sites used to determine body composition.

8. Explain the criteria used to categorize hypermobility and hypomobility.

9. Describe specific methods of measuring strength, power, speed, cardiovascular endurance, agility, balance, and reaction time.

10. Identify specific conditions that could exclude an individual from participating in physical activity or sport.

INTRODUCTION

The preparticipation examination (PPE), often performed annually, is used to ensure an individual's health and safety while participating in physical activity or sport. Conducting a PPE can be time-consuming and sometimes costly, depending on assessment techniques utilized. However, the PPE is seen as an important information gathering tool to help health care providers identify and implement strategies to minimize risks associated with participation in physical activity.[1-3] This chapter examines the PPE process and, following an introduction of the general principles and goals of the PPE, presents information on organizing the PPE using a group format. This includes setting up the examination, gathering a medical history, and conducting the physical examination. Finally, the criteria used to determine if an individual should be allowed to participate, and at what level of intensity, are discussed.

GOALS OF THE PREPARTICIPATION EXAMINATION

? Why is it important to consider the age of the individual when conducting a PPE?

The basic objective of the PPE is to ensure the health and safety of a physically active individual. This can be accomplished by gathering information regarding the individual's general health, maturity, and fitness level. Those who are at risk for injury or who have conditions that may limit participation can be identified and counseled on health-related issues and steered toward participating in appropriate activities. Many states and sport governing bodies require some type of PPE for competitive athletes but differ greatly regarding specific requirements. It is highly recommended by the American Academy of Family Physicians, along with the American Academy of Pediatrics, the American College of Sports Medicine, the American Medical Society for Sports Medicine, the American Orthopaedic Society for Sports Medicine, the American Osteopathic Academy of Sports Medicine, and the National Athletic Trainers' Association to use a standardized and uniform national preparticipation history and physical examination form for medical screening in high schools and colleges.[2-5] Although the frequency and depth of PPEs may vary, most examinations share common goals (**Box 2.1**).

Because participants range in age from the very young to the very old, the focus of the PPE is dependent on the specific age group. For example, in the prepubescent child (i.e., 6 to 10 years of age), the focus may be on identifying previously undiagnosed congenital abnormalities. In the pubescent child (i.e., 11 to 15 years of age), the examination should center on maturation and establishing good health practices for safe participation. In the postpubescent or young adult group (i.e., 16 to 30 years of age), the history of previous injuries and sport-specific examinations are critical. For individuals with cardiovascular or pulmonary disease, the strenuousness of a sport is an additional consideration.

 A table showing the **classifications of sports based on strenuousness** can be found on the companion Web site at thePoint.

For the 16 to 30 years of age group, the more strenuous activities and those involving contact or collision sports may require a more extensive examination. Because the adult population (i.e., 30 to 65 years of age) has a high incidence of overuse injuries, these individuals need an examination based on the nature of the activity in which they intend to engage. The final group, those older than

---

BOX 2.1 Goals of the Preparticipation Examination

- Determine general health and current immunization status.

- Detect medical conditions that are not healed or may predispose the individual to injury or illness so that medical treatment can start before sport/activity participation.

- Identify behaviors posing a risk to health that may be corrected through informed counseling.

- Establish baseline parameters for determining when an injured individual may return to activity.

- Assess physical maturity.

- Evaluate level of physical fitness.

- Classify the individual as to readiness for participation.

- Recommend appropriate levels of participation for individuals with medical contraindications to exercise.

- Meet legal and insurance requirements related to participation in physical activity or sport.

---

65 years, often begins or increases activity to prevent a major medical illness. These individuals need an extensive examination based on individual needs, taking into consideration not only their physical needs but also any medications being taken and their possible side effects.

 Because age can be a factor that influences general health, maturity, and fitness level, it is essential that the focus of the PPE be altered to address issues or concerns specific to the age of the individual.

SETTING UP THE EXAMINATION

 A college soccer athlete has completed freshman year and is returning to begin the sophomore season. Describe a reevaluation examination for this athlete.

PPEs may be set up in a variety of ways. The organizational format depends on factors such as the level of activity (e.g., athlete in an organized competitive sport or individual in an exercise program), the community, the availability of personnel and facilities, the number of individuals being screened, and the personal preference of the evaluator.

Examination Format

Individual Format

The primary care physician (PCP) usually performs PPEs. Typically, the PCP is more knowledgeable about the individual's (and the family's) medical history, congenital or developmental deficiencies, immunization status, and recent injuries or illnesses that could limit participation in physical activity. A PPE administered by the PCP permits a closer clinician–patient relationship, and when the PPE is performed in the physician's office, a more thorough and comprehensive examination can be completed. The office setting provides greater privacy and a more optimal environment for counseling. The expense of the PPE is higher and the time commitment on the part of the physician is more significant; however, the cost can be covered by the family's medical insurance.

Group Format

Because some individuals may have a physician who does not understand the physical demands of a particular sport activity, organized competitive sport programs often use a group or station format to examine a large number of individuals during a limited span of time. A supervising or team physician and several different health care providers perform a series of examinations at different stations. Following the conclusion of the examination, the supervising/team physician determines the individual's readiness for sport participation. This format is more time efficient, reduces costs significantly, and allows athletic trainers and area medical specialists to be involved. This format has several disadvantages, however, including the organizational coordination needed to execute such a comprehensive examination, decreased privacy, brief and often impersonal time spent with each individual, difficulty in following up on any medical concerns that may arise, and inability to have essential communication with parents of those in early and middle adolescence after the examination. The athletic trainer can play a key role in minimizing several of the disadvantages associated with the group format PPE by carefully organizing and scheduling the implementation of the screenings. In consultation with and under the supervision of the physician, the athletic trainer can serve as the point person for facilitating referrals, developing and initiating rehabilitation programs, and following up with parents and other health care providers.[2,3]

Timing of the Examination

Ideally, a PPE is completed at least 6 weeks before the start of any physical activity. This allows for time to evaluate and correct minor problems, such as limited flexibility, muscle weakness, or minor illnesses. It also allows sufficient time for an individual with a potential medical problem to be referred to a specialist (e.g., cardiologist, neurologist, ophthalmologist). Although many high schools and colleges conduct PPEs during late July or early August for fall sports, PPEs also can be completed during the spring of the year, provided some mechanism exists to report and evaluate any injury or illness that may have occurred during the summer.

Frequency of the Examination

Although an annual complete physical examination is common, it probably is unnecessary unless there is a change in physician or records are not available. The American Academy of Family Physicians and other national medical groups recommend that an entry-level complete physical examination be performed, followed by a limited annual reevaluation. Many physicians also complete an entry-level examination at each level of participation (e.g., middle school, high school, and college). The entry-level examination is discussed in detail in this chapter. The reevaluation should focus on the medical history and a limited physical examination, including height, weight, blood pressure, pulse, visual acuity, cardiac auscultation, and examination of the skin.[2-4] Both the entry-level examination and the reevaluation should also include neurocognitive baseline assessment to assist with the recognition and treatment of potential concussions the patient may sustain during sports-related activities.[6,7]

 A complete PPE is not automatically required on an annual basis. The reevaluation of the soccer athlete should focus on the medical history and a limited physical examination, including height, weight, blood pressure, pulse, visual acuity, cardiac auscultation, examination of the skin, and neurocognitive baseline testing.

MEDICAL HISTORY

 Why should the PPE begin with the medical history?

A comprehensive medical history can identify a significant percentage of the problems affecting a physically active individual or sport participant. Typically, a written form is completed by the individual, answering in a yes/no format. To ensure accuracy, this information should be confirmed in person by the individual or the parents of minor children.

Questions in the medical history might explore current immunization status; past episodes of infectious diseases, loss of consciousness, recurrent headaches, musculoskeletal injuries, heat stroke, chest pains during or after exercise, seizures, breathing difficulties, disordered eating, and chronic medical problems; medication and drug use; allergies; heart murmurs or unusual heart palpitations; use of contact lenses, corrective lenses, dentures, prosthetic devices, or special equipment (e.g., pads, braces, neck rolls, eye guards); and family history of cardiac problems, vascular problems, sickle cell anemia, diabetes, high blood pressure, sudden death, or neurological problems. Underweight individuals can be questioned about weight loss, eating patterns, body image, and, in the case of females, menses dysfunction.

A sample medical history form and supplemental health history questionnaire for female participants are available on the companion Web site at thePoint.

When using a mass station screening approach, it is advisable to have the medical history station at the start of the examination. This station should have a knowledgeable clinician who can go through each questionnaire and ask detailed follow-up questions. The mass station affords the clinician an opportunity to cross-reference responses on the medical questionnaire. A "red flag" can be noted on specific responses. In health care, the term **red flag** is used to denote a potential problem or area of concern. When red flags are encountered, the health care provider should take extra caution to evaluate the information and determine an appropriate course of action. For example, a history of exercise-induced asthma should be pointed out to the clinician at the pulmonary station. This option allows a more knowledgeable clinician to conduct a thorough examination of the body system most affected by the condition.

 The medical history establishes a foundation. This information can reveal possible congenital, hereditary, or acquired conditions that may put the individual at risk for future problems. By beginning the PPE with the medical history, the information can be validated for accuracy during the actual examination.

THE PHYSICAL EXAMINATION

? Should a PPE be considered the equivalent of an annual medical examination?

The PPE is not intended to be all encompassing. Rather, it is intended to focus on the body systems that are of most concern to the individual depending on the activity or sport of choice. Particular attention should be paid to any areas of concern or red flags identified during the medical history.

Vital Signs

The PPE should establish the individual's baseline physiological parameters and vital statistics. Height and weight should be taken and compared to standard growth charts. Information such as pulse rate, blood pressure, and body temperature may be recorded at this station by an athletic trainer or other allied health professional (**Box 2.2**).

Pulse rate usually is taken at the carotid artery by doubling the pulse rate measured during a 30-second period. To further delineate potential cardiovascular problems, the pulse should be taken at the radial and femoral arteries to determine whether the heart rate and rhythm are regular. A weak or nonpalpable pulse at the femoral artery suggests coarctation of the aorta.[8] An irregular pulse raises suspicion for arrhythmia and requires an electrocardiographic (ECG) evaluation.[5]

Following proper guidelines is essential to ensure accurate readings when measuring blood pressure. It is important that a proper cuff size be used. The bladder should encircle the midarm and cover two-thirds of the length of the arm. For an obese arm, a wide cuff (15 cm) should be used. If the arm circumference exceeds 14 cm, a thigh cuff (18 cm wide) should be used. A pediatric cuff may be indicated for a very thin arm. The guidelines for obtaining accurate blood pressure measurements are listed in **Application Strategy 2.1**.

Individuals with abnormal heart rates or high blood pressure should be rechecked several times at 15- to 20-minute intervals, with the individual lying down between measurements to determine

BOX 2.2 Normal Vital Statistics

Pulse

Males	60–100 bpm
Females	60–100 bpm (may increase 10–15 bpm during pregnancy)
Children	120–140 bpm
Well-conditioned athletes	Can be 50 bpm or lower

Blood pressure

Adults	120/80 mg Hg
Children (age, 10 years)	105/70 mm Hg

if the high reading is accurate or caused by anxiety (e.g., white coat syndrome). If three consecutive readings are high, the individual should be identified as having hypertension (high blood pressure). **Table 2.1** shows hypertension standards by age in children, adolescents, and adults.[9]

Individuals with stage 2 hypertension should be further examined by a physician and restricted from high static activities and sports until the condition is controlled by lifestyle modification or drug therapy.[10] Mild-to-moderate hypertension in the absence of organ disease or heart disease does not preclude physical activity or sport participation, but this condition should be noted and evaluated on an individual basis. Following the start of an exercise or training program, individuals with hypertension should have their blood pressure checked every 2 to 4 months or more frequently, if indicated, to monitor the impact of exercise.

Body temperature is measured by a thermometer placed under the tongue, in the ear, or under the armpit. Average oral temperature usually is quoted as 37°C (98.6°F), but this can fluctuate considerably. During the early morning hours, temperature may fall to as low as 35.8°C (96.4°F), and in the later afternoon or evening, it may rise as high as 37.3°C (99.1°F). Rectal temperatures are higher than oral temperatures by an average of 0.4° to 0.5°C (0.7° to 0.9°F), although this, too, can be variable. In contrast, axillary temperatures are lower than oral temperatures by approximately 1°F but may take 5 to 10 minutes to register and generally are considered to be less accurate than other measurements.[11]

A glass or electronic thermometer may be used for oral temperatures. When using a glass thermometer, the thermometer must initially measure 35°C (96°F) or less. The clinician should insert the thermometer under the individual's tongue, instruct the individual to close the lips, and wait 3 to 5 minutes before removing and reading the temperature.[11] If using an electronic thermometer, a disposable cover should be placed carefully over the probe; a digital readout should appear in about 10 seconds. Some electronic thermometers beep when the temperature reaches its maximum.

Infrared tympanic thermometers measure infrared energy emitted by the tympanic membrane and provide a rapid, efficient, and noninvasive method of measuring body temperature. In this method, the external auditory canal must be free of cerumen. The probe is positioned in the canal so that the infrared beam is aimed at the tympanic membrane (if aimed elsewhere, the measurement is invalid). The digital temperature reading should appear in 2 to 3 seconds. This method measures core body temperature, which is higher than the normal oral temperature by approximately 0.8°C (1.4°F).[11]

General Medical Problems

When using the mass station format, general systemic problems should be investigated early in the process to allow for a follow-up evaluation of any red flags. Information about past surgeries or hospitalizations may lead to facts about a previous injury or an attempt to control a chronic disease. If a previous injury exists, it is necessary to determine if there has been adequate time for optimal healing and if rehabilitation must be completed before clearing the individual for participation.

APPLICATION STRATEGY 2.1

Measuring Blood Pressure

General Guidelines

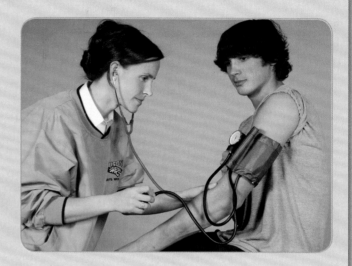

- No caffeine should be consumed during the hour before the reading; no smoking should be permitted 30 minutes before the reading.
- Take the measurement in a quiet, warm setting.
- Subject should sit quietly for 5 minutes, with the back supported and the arm supported at the level of the heart, before recording blood pressure.
- The air bladder should encircle and cover two-thirds of the length of the arm. If it does not, the bladder should be placed over the brachial artery. If the bladder is too short, misleadingly high readings can result.
- Manometer: Aneroid gauges should be calibrated every 6 months against a mercury manometer.

Technique

- Inflate the bladder quickly to about 200 mm Hg.
- Place the stethoscope over the brachial artery in the cubital fossa.
- Deflate the bladder by 3 mm Hg per second, and listen for the first soft beating sounds (systolic pressure).
- As pressure is reduced, the sound becomes louder and more distinct and then gradually disappears as blood is no longer constricted.
- The pressure at which the sound disappears is the diastolic pressure.
- If the sounds are weak, the patient should be asked to raise the arm and open and close the hand 5–10 times. Then, the clinician should reinflate the bladder quickly.
- Record blood pressure, patient position, arm, and cuff size.

Number of Readings and Sites

- Take at least two readings, separated by as much time as is practical. If readings vary by more than 5 mm Hg, take additional readings until two consecutive readings are close.
- If the initial values are elevated, obtain two other sets of readings at least 1 week apart.
- Initially, measure the pressure in both arms; if the pressures differ, use the arm with the higher pressure.
- If arm pressure is elevated, take the pressure in one leg (particularly in patients younger than 30 years).

Recurrent visits to a doctor and/or hospitalization for a chronic disease suggest a poorly controlled chronic condition, such as asthma, diabetes, hypertrophic cardiomyopathy, anemia, or a seizure disorder. General questions regarding these disorders should ascertain the presence, severity, frequency, and control of the condition.

The clinician also should be concerned about problems such as acute infection, malignancy, and progressive diseases (e.g., multiple sclerosis). Acute illnesses (e.g., gastritis, flu, fever, diarrhea, colds) tend to be self-limiting and usually require only temporary withdrawal from activity.

Inquiries should be made regarding the use of both prescription and over-the-counter medications. In some cases, medications can predispose an individual to certain conditions or illnesses. For example, the use of birth control pills or illicit drugs (e.g., anabolic steroids, amphetamines, cocaine) may lead to hypertension. In addition, the use of alcohol, tobacco, caffeine, ergogenic aids, or illegal substances should be identified through direct inquiry.

TABLE 2.1 Classification of Blood Pressure[a]

AGE AND PHASE	NORMAL (HIGH NORMAL)[b]	PREHYPERTENSIVE	STAGE 1 HYPERTENSION	STAGE 2 HYPERTENSION
6–9 years				
Systolic	104–110		122–129	≥129
Diastolic	68–72		70–85	≥85
10–12 years				
Systolic	111–116	N/A	126–133	≥133
Diastolic	73–75		82–89	≥89
13–15 years				
Systolic	117–120	N/A	136–143	≥143
Diastolic	75–78		86–91	≥91
16–18 years				
Systolic	<120	N/A	142–149	≥149
Diastolic	78–80		92–97	≥97
>18 years				
Systolic	<120	120–139	140–159	≥160
Diastolic	<80	80–89	90–99	≥100

[a]Definitions apply to people who are not taking antihypertensive drugs and are not acutely ill. When systolic and diastolic blood pressures fall into different categories, the higher category should be selected to classify blood pressure status. Blood pressure values are based on the average of two or more readings taken at each of two or more visits after the initial screening. For adults age 18 and older, optimal blood pressure is 120/80 mm Hg; prehypertension is blood pressure that is 120–139/80–89 mm Hg.[9]

[b]Data from the National High Blood Pressure Education Program Working Group on High Blood Pressure in Children and Adolescents. The fourth report on the diagnosis, evaluation, and treatment of high blood pressure in children and adolescents. *Pediatrics*. 2004;114(suppl 2):555–576.

Questions that should be asked regarding general medical conditions include the following:

1. Are you currently seeing a doctor for a medical problem?

2. Have you ever been diagnosed with a disease or been hospitalized overnight for a disease (e.g., diabetes, epilepsy, anemia, sickle cell anemia, mononucleosis, hepatitis)?

3. Have you ever been diagnosed with a progressive disease (e.g., muscular dystrophy, multiple sclerosis, tuberculosis)?

4. Have you ever been hospitalized for a chronic disease or illness?

5. Have you ever been told you have cancer?

6. Are you on any medications or allergic to any medications?

7. Have you ever had surgery?

8. Do you tend to bleed excessively?

9. Are you missing or have function of only one organ (e.g., eye, kidney, lung, testicle)?

If any of these questions receives a positive response, a plan must be in place to ensure appropriate follow-up assessment.

The Cardiovascular Examination

The cardiovascular examination should be completed in a quiet area so that outside noise does not interfere with auscultation of heart sounds. The physician should check for cardiac abnormalities to identify those individuals at risk for sudden death. Although the prevalence of cardiovascular disease in a young physically active population is low, it now appears that hypertrophic cardiomyopathy, the leading cause of sudden death, is relatively common (1:500 in the general population).[12]

The American Heart Association (AHA)[13] recommends that questions evaluating the cardiovascular system focus on a history of loss of consciousness, syncope or near syncope, dizziness, shortness of breath, heart palpitations, and chest pain during or after exercise, as well as heart problems and sudden death occurring in a family member younger than 50 years of age, which may indicate a predisposition to cardiac anomalies, such as a **prolonged QT syndrome**, **Marfan syndrome**, dilated cardiomyopathy, heart **arrhythmias**, or **mitral valve prolapse**.[8,10,14] Marfan syndrome should be suspected in an individual who is tall and has an arm span greater than height, long fingers and toes, pectus excavatum chest wall deformity, and a high-arched palate.

Questions that should be asked to participants include the following:

1. Have you ever experienced chest pain or discomfort in the chest, neck, jaw, or arms during or after exercise?

2. Have you ever experienced dizziness or passed out during or after exercise?

3. Have you ever experienced shortness of breath at rest or get tired more quickly than your friends with mild exercise?

4. Have you ever noticed rapid heart palpitations or felt like your heart "raced"?

5. Have you ever been told that you have high blood pressure or high cholesterol?

6. Have you ever been told that you have a heart murmur, an irregular heartbeat, or any heart disease?

7. Has anyone in your family had any heart problems, had a heart attack, or died suddenly before the age of 50 years?

8. Have you had a severe viral infection such as mononucleosis or myocarditis within the last month?

9. Has a physician ever restricted or denied your participation in sports for any heart problems?

10. Have any of your relatives had any of the following conditions: hypertrophic cardiomyopathy, dilated cardiomyopathy, Marfan syndrome, long QT syndrome, or significant heart arrhythmia?

If any of these questions receives a positive response, the individual should be fully evaluated by a cardiologist to determine the presence of conditions such as **hypertrophic cardiomyopathy**, conduction abnormalities, dysrhythmias, valvular problems, and coronary artery defects (**Box 2.3**). Assessment by a cardiologist will include a variety of techniques. For example, precordial auscultation in a supine and standing position can identify heart murmurs consistent with dynamic left ventricular outflow obstruction. Provocative maneuvers help to differentiate functional murmurs from pathologic murmurs. A decrease in venous return can be initiated by having an individual move from a squatting to a standing position while performing a **Valsalva maneuver**; venous return can be increased by having the individual take several deep inspirations, moving from a standing to a squatting position, or performing an isometric hand grip. Assessing the femoral artery pulses can exclude coarctation of the aorta.[5] General recommendations for murmurs requiring further evaluation before an individual can participate include the following:

- Any systolic murmur grade 3 through 6 in severity

- Any diastolic murmur

- Any murmur that gets louder with a Valsalva maneuver

BOX 2.3 Cardiovascular Red Flags Requiring Further Examination

- Chest pain during exertion
- Unusual fatigue or shortness of breath at rest or with mild exertion
- Dizziness or syncope with activity
- Breathing difficulty while lying down
- Ankle edema
- Heart palpitations or tachycardia
- Known heart murmur
- Abnormal heart rate or arrhythmia
- Uncontrolled hypertension
- Hypertrophic cardiomyopathy
- Congenital coronary artery anomalies
- Marfan syndrome or aortic coarctation
- Mitral valve prolapse
- Conduction abnormalities
- Arteriosclerotic coronary artery disease
- Anemia
- Enlarged spleen
- Dextrocardia (i.e., heart located on right side of chest)
- Family history of heart problems or sudden death

Hypertrophic cardiomyopathy is the most common cause of sudden death in young athletes, followed by congenital coronary artery anomalies, aortic rupture associated with Marfan syndrome, mitral valve prolapse, and cardiac conduction disorders. In the older physically active individual, arteriosclerosis is almost always the cause of sudden death. If any of these conditions are present, strenuous activity is precluded until an ECG or stress ECG is completed.

The Pulmonary Examination

The pulmonary examination may be done in conjunction with the cardiovascular examination. The physician auscultates for clear breath sounds and watches for symmetric movement of the diaphragm. A history of coughing spells or difficulty breathing may indicate exercise-induced bronchospasm. Although easily treated, this condition often goes undetected. In addition, up to 40% of athletes with environmental allergies or seasonal rhinitis experience exercise-induced bronchospasm, and up to 80% of asthmatics are similarly affected. Prolonged symptoms also may indicate possible congenital heart defects, cardiomyopathy, or valvular dysfunction.

The ears, nose, and mouth may be checked at this examination station as well. If any hearing problems are suspected, the individual should be referred to a specialist.

Questions that should be asked include the following:

1. Have you ever experienced excessive coughing during or after being physically active?

2. Have you ever experienced breathing difficulties or been told you have asthma, bronchitis, or allergies?

3. Have you ever had shortness of breath or heard unusual breath sounds during or after being physically active?

4. Have you ever had a collapsed lung?

If any abnormalities are found (e.g., wheezing, crackles, rhonchi, rubs, rales, abnormal inspiratory to expiratory ratio), appropriate lung function tests should be ordered. Patients who report with a history of asthma should have a peak expiratory flow (PEF) baseline assessment conducted.[2,3] The guidelines for performing an accurate PEF assessment test are listed in **Application Strategy 2.2**.[2,3,15] PEF is information gathered from the baseline assessment that can be used to determine the patient's participation status on a daily basis based on how the patient performs on daily PEF assessments as compared to baseline.[3] Concerns such as tuberculosis, uncontrolled asthma, exertional asthma, exercise-induced bronchospasm, pulmonary insufficiency resulting from a collapsed lung, or chronic bronchial asthma should be assessed by the physician and discussed with the individual (**Box 2.4**).[2,3]

The Musculoskeletal Examination

The musculoskeletal examination is critical to the physically active individual and the sport participant. A history of previous fractures, strains, tendinitis, sprains, and dislocations may suggest a

---

APPLICATION STRATEGY 2.2

Measuring Peak Expiratory Flow

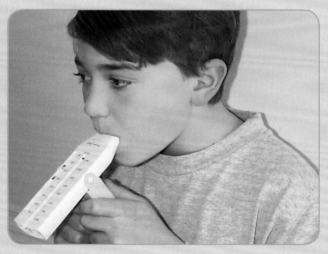

General Guidelines

- Patient should not consume food or beverages or otherwise have any foreign objects in mouth while taking test.
- If patient is taking daily medication to control condition, PEF should be administered after medication has been taken.

Technique

- Place a clean mouth piece on the peak flow meter.
- Slide all markers to bottom of peak flow meter.
- Instruct patient to stand upright.
- Instruct patient to hold peak flow meter upright and carefully as not to block the air vent.
- Ask patient to take a deep breath and fill lungs to capacity while placing lips around mouth piece. **Do not bite mouth piece or place tongue in tube.**
- Instruct patient to blow into peak flow meter quickly and as forcefully as possible.
- The marker will move to indicate the amount of air volume expelled: Make note of the number.
- Replace marker to bottom of peak flow meter and repeat for a total of three attempts.
- The highest number of the three attempts is the PEF number.
- Record the baseline PEF rate on the patient's PPE form.

Using Peak Expiratory Flow Baseline to Determine Daily Participation Status

- Prior to participation, repeat technique described for baseline assessment.
- If patient's PEF is above 80% of the baseline assessment, do not restrict participation.
- If patient's PEF is between 50% and 79% of baseline assessment, restrict from participation and initiate additional testing and/or treatment strategies.
- If patient's PEF is lower than 50% of baseline, implement emergency action plan for patients in respiratory distress.

BOX 2.4 Pulmonary Red Flags Requiring Further Examination

- Abnormal coughing
- Abnormal shortness of breath at rest or with minimal exertion
- Abnormal breath sounds (e.g., wheezing, rhonchi, rubs, rales)
- Abnormal or prolonged expiratory phase
- Asthma (uncontrolled or exertional)
- Exercise-induced bronchospasm
- Pneumothorax
- Pulmonary insufficiency
- Severe allergies

---

predisposition to injury recurrences or potential arthritis. Questions should focus on the nature of any injury sustained, when it occurred, who evaluated it, the duration of the treatment and rehabilitation, and if surgical intervention was necessary. Questions pertaining to the wearing of special protective equipment also may identify injuries or conditions that might otherwise have gone undetected. For example, the use of an ankle brace may indicate a chronic lateral ankle sprain, and the use of a neck roll may indicate previous neurological impairment of the cervical region.

Questions that might be asked include the following:

1. Have you ever sprained or dislocated a joint?

2. Have you had repeated backaches?

3. Have you ever strained (pulled) a muscle?

4. Have you ever fractured any bone?

5. Do you experience any persistent swelling of a joint or body region?

6. Have you ever experienced pain in any muscle or joint when you first wake up in the morning?

7. Have you ever been awakened at night because of pain in any joint or muscle?

8. Do you ever have pain during or after activity?

9. What special protective equipment do you use regularly?

The National Athletic Trainers' Association (NATA) advocates utilizing an orthopedic medical history in combination with a 90-second musculoskeletal screening for patients with no known or reported history of musculoskeletal injury (**Application Strategy 2.3**).[2,16] If red flags are noted, a more comprehensive examination of the specific body part should be completed (**Box 2.5**).

When determining whether an individual should be limited in activity, consideration must be given to the demands of the activity and to the needs of the individual. For example, limited range of motion or instability in the cervical or lumbar region may preclude the individual from participating in a collision or contact sport.

The Neurological Examination

The neurological examination need not be overly complicated. The assessment component of this examination should include pupillary examination and reaction to light (PEARL), cranial nerve assessment (**Table 2.2**), a brief sensorimotor examination of the upper and lower extremities (see **Application Strategy 2.3**), and testing of the deep tendon reflexes (**Table 2.3**).

APPLICATION STRATEGY 2.3

Musculoskeletal Examination

ATHLETIC TRAINER OBSERVES/ASSESSES	ACTION PERFORMED BY ATHLETE
Acromioclavicular joints: general habitus	Athlete faces the clinician as he or she:
Cervical spine motion	Looks at the ceiling, floor, over both shoulders, touches each ear to the respective shoulder
Trapezius strength	Shrugs the shoulders against resistance
Deltoid strength	Abducts the shoulders to 90° (resistance is applied at 90°)
Shoulder motion	Performs bilateral shoulder external and internal rotation, flexion, and extension
Elbow motion	Performs bilateral flexion and extension
Elbow and wrist motion	Places arms at sides, elbows at 90°; pronates and supinates wrists
Hand and finger motion, strength, and anomalies	Spreads fingers; makes a fist
Symmetry and knee effusions, ankle effusion	Tightens (contract) quadriceps; relaxes quadriceps
Hip, knee, and ankle motions	"Duck walks" away and toward clinician
Shoulder symmetry; scoliosis, level of inferior angle of the scapula	Athlete stands with his or her back to the clinician:
Scoliosis, hip motion, hamstrings tightness	Knees straight, touch toes (Adam's position)
Calf symmetry, leg strength	Raise upon toes, heels

BOX 2.5 Musculoskeletal Red Flags Requiring Further Examination

- Chronic joint or spinal instability
- Unhealed fracture, ligament, or muscular injury
- Muscle weakness
- Inflammation or infection of a joint
- Unusual hypomobility or hypermobility
- Growth or maturation disorders
- Symptomatic spondylolysis or spondylolisthesis
- Spear tackler's spine
- Herniated disk with spinal cord compression
- Repetitive stress disorders

TABLE 2.2 Cranial Nerve Assessment

CRANIAL NERVE	NAME	ASSESSMENT
I	Olfactory	Identify familiar odors (e.g., chocolate, coffee)
II	Optic	Test acuity—Snellen chart (blurring or double vision)
III	Oculomotor	Test papillary reaction to light Perform upward and downward gaze
IV	Trochlear	Perform downward and lateral gaze
V	Trigeminal	Touch face to note difference in sensation Clench teeth; push down on chin to separate jaws
VI	Abducens	Perform lateral and medial gaze
VII	Facial	Close eyes tight Smile and show the teeth
VIII	Vestibulocochlear (acoustic nerve)	Identify the sound of fingers snapping near the ear Balance and coordination (stand on one foot)
IX	Glossopharyngeal	Gag reflex; ability to swallow
X	Vagus	Gag reflex; ask the individual to swallow or say "Ahhh"
XI	Accessory	Resisted shoulder shrug
XII	Hypoglossal	Stick out the tongue

Patients who participate in activities that place them at a higher risk for sustaining concussions should undergo baseline assessment as part of the PPE.[7] In addition to the components of the neurological examination already presented, motor control and cognitive function as well as mental status should be assessed. Motor control is assessed through the Balance Error Scoring System (BESS) and involves evaluating a patient's ability to balance under three different conditions. Cognitive function is assessed through evaluating the patient's reaction time, ability to concentrate, and both working and delayed memory. Pen and paper as well as computerized

TABLE 2.3 Deep Tendon Reflex Testing

REFLEX	SITE OF STIMULATION	NORMAL RESPONSE	NERVE SEGMENT
Jaw	Mandible	Mouth closure	Cranial nerve V
Biceps	Biceps tendon	Biceps contraction	C5–C6
Brachioradialis	Brachioradialis tendon	Elbow flexion and/or pronation	C5–C6
Triceps	Triceps tendon	Elbow extension	C7–C8
Patellar	Quadriceps tendon	Knee extension	L3–L4
Medial hamstrings	Semimembranosus tendon	Knee flexion	L5–S1
Lateral hamstrings	Biceps femoris tendon	Knee flexion	S1–S2
Tibialis posterior	Tibialis posterior tendon behind medial malleolus	Plantar flexion with inversion	L4–L5
Achilles	Achilles tendon	Plantar flexion	S1–S2

programs provide tools for assessing a patient's cognitive functioning. Mental status involves assessing the patient's level of consciousness, ability to concentrate, identify where they are in time and space, and overall memory function. The Standardized Assessment of Concussion (SAC) is a useful tool for assessing mental status. Both the BESS and the SAC as well as other methods for assessing concussion are presented in detail in Chapter 20.

In the area of history, appropriately designed questions will give a clear indication if the individual is at risk for serious head or nerve injuries. The neurological history should include questions regarding past head injuries, loss of consciousness, amnesia, or seizures. A history of seizures requires detailed information concerning frequency, treatment, and whether adequate control has been achieved with prescribed medication. Any episodes of brachial plexus injuries (e.g., burners or stingers) or pinched nerves should be documented. A history of transient paresthesia, loss of sensation, or loss of motor function in any region of the body also should be noted. In addition, if an individual has a preexisting narrow cervical spinal canal, a straightened or reversed cervical lordotic curve, and a history of using a spear-tackling technique (**spear tackler's spine**), the individual should be fully evaluated by a neurosurgeon. A detailed examination of the neurological system, including cervical radiographs, may be warranted before considering participation.

Questions during this phase of the examination may include the following:

1. Have you ever had a head or neck injury?

2. Have you ever been knocked out, been unconscious, or been diagnosed with a concussion?

3. Do you have frequent or repeated headaches?

4. Have you ever had a seizure or been told you have epilepsy?

5. Have you ever had a burner, stinger, or one of your limbs feel numb or fall "asleep" during activity?

6. Have you ever experienced unexplained muscle weakness?

If problems such as recurrent concussions, headaches, or nerve palsies are identified, the individual should be seen by a specialist before being cleared for participation (**Box 2.6**). If seizure disorders are reported, the clinician should document the initial onset, frequency, and duration of the episodes; the use of medications to control the disorder; and whether the individual is informed of the condition and its side effects and predisposing factors.[16] Individuals with epilepsy should be discouraged from activities that may involve recurrent head trauma or the risk of falling, such as rock climbing, football, skiing, scuba diving, or parachuting.

BOX 2.6 Neurological Red Flags Requiring Further Examination

- More than one concussion
- Cervical spine instability
- Functional cervical spine stenosis
- History of frequent or repeated headaches
- History of seizures
- History of amnesia or tinnitus
- History of head injuries
- History of burners, stingers, or neurapraxia
- History of spinal cord shock or transient quadriplegia
- History of nerve palsy

The Eye Examination

A visual acuity is best tested using the Snellen or common eye chart (**Fig. 2.1**). The chart tests the individual's ability to clearly see letters based on a normalized scale. **Emmetropia**, or 20/20 vision, indicates that an individual can read the letters on the 20-ft line of the eye chart when standing 20 ft from the chart, indicating that the light rays are focused precisely on the retina. **Myopia**, or nearsightedness, occurs when the light rays are focused in front of the retina, making only those objects close to the eyes distinguishable. **Hypermetropia**, or farsightedness, occurs when the light rays are focused at a point behind the retina, making only those objects far from the eyes distinguishable. Vision should be assessed monocularly (one eye) and binocularly (both eyes). Individuals who wear corrective glasses or contact lenses should wear them at the time of the vision assessment.

In addition to assessing visual acuity, it may be appropriate to assess other aspects of vision. The presence of involuntary cyclical movement of the eyes (**nystagmus**) is noteworthy. Although it may be normal for an individual, the presence of nystagmus should be documented in the individual's medical file because it can provide valuable information in the event of head trauma. It also is important to note pupil size. Normally, the pupils are equal in size and shape; however, some individuals may have a congenital difference in pupil size (**anisocoria**). Again, this should be documented in case the individual sustains a head injury. In addition, in some situations, it is beneficial to have information regarding peripheral vision and depth perception.

Questions related to the eye examination might include the following:

1. Have you ever had problems with blurring or double vision?

2. Have you ever injured your eyes or the area around your eyes?

3. Do you wear glasses, contact lenses, or protective eyewear on a regular basis? What type?

4. Is your vision totally or partially impaired in either eye?

5. Are you color blind?

6. Do you have good peripheral vision?

If any of these questions receives a positive response, corrected vision is poorer than 20/50 (i.e., the individual can read at 20 ft what the average person can read at 50 ft), or no vision in one eye, the individual requires further evaluation by an ophthalmologist (**Box 2.7**). Individuals with sight in only one eye or with limited sight in both eyes may continue to participate in physical activities only if they are informed of the risks involved and understand the dangers associated with loss of depth perception and the potential for injury to the remaining good eye. These individuals should not participate in activities in which the eyes cannot

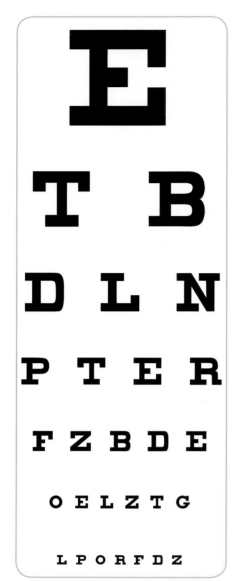

Figure 2.1. Snellen eye chart. Visual acuity is measured by the Snellen or common eye chart.

BOX 2.7 Ocular Red Flags Requiring Further Examination

- Corrected vision greater than 20/50
- Vision in one eye only
- Severely limited peripheral vision
- Severe myopia (i.e., nearsightedness)
- Retinal detachment or tear

be protected (e.g., boxing, wrestling, martial arts). An additional consent form specific to eye injuries that outlines the risks involved and the acceptance of those risks should be obtained from the individual.[11]

If glasses are worn, the lenses should be made of plastic, polycarbonate, or heat-treated (safety) glass to prevent them from shattering during activity. When possible, contact lenses should be of the soft type; the hard types often become dislodged, are associated more frequently with irritation from foreign bodies, and may shatter.

Myopia should be noted because such individuals tend to have retinal degeneration, which increases the possibility of retinal detachment. Individuals with retinal detachment may be excluded from contact sports. Those with a healed retinal tear may be allowed to participate in strenuous activity only after being examined and cleared by an ophthalmologist.

The Dental Examination

A dental examination usually is performed by a dentist. It is important to determine the number of teeth and the time of the last dental examination. This is critical because of the potential liability if teeth are avulsed (knocked out) during participation.

Questions that can be asked include the following:

1. When did you last see a dentist?

2. Have you ever had any problems with your teeth or gums?

3. Have you ever experienced bleeding gums after brushing or flossing your teeth?

4. Have you ever had any teeth knocked out, damaged, or extracted?

5. Do you wear dentures, crowns, or caps or have a partial plate?

6. Do you wear a mouth guard?

7. Do you smoke cigarettes or chew tobacco?

8. Have you ever had an injury to the jaw or face?

During an examination, the dentist can assess the gum condition and the presence of cavities. Dental appliance work should be checked to ensure it is in good condition. The importance of using properly fitted mouth guards as well as the safety and legal issues stemming from cutting down a mouth guard can be stressed. Dental red flags requiring further examination are listed in ▶ **Box 2.8**.

The Gastrointestinal Examination

This examination involves evaluating the digestive system, eating habits, and nutrition. During the physical examination, the patient should be supine, with the lower ribs exposed to the anterosuperior iliac spines. The clinician palpates for tenderness, masses, or **organomegaly** (i.e., enlarged organs) to ensure there is no inflammation of the liver (e.g., hepatitis or enlarged liver) or the spleen, especially for individuals involved in contact sports.

BOX 2.8 Dental Red Flags Requiring Further Examination

- Bleeding gums
- Lesions in the mouth
- Loose or displaced teeth
- Loose caps or crowns
- Dental appliances in poor condition

> **BOX 2.9** Gastrointestinal Red Flags Requiring Further Examination
>
> - Organomegaly (e.g., enlarged liver, spleen)
> - History of hepatitis or infectious mononucleosis
> - History of repeated episodes of diarrhea or constipation
> - History of gastritis or burning sensation in the stomach (ulcers)
> - Extreme tenderness over appendix, liver, or spleen
> - Suspicion of anorexia or bulimia

General questions about the gastrointestinal system may center on bouts of heartburn, indigestion, diarrhea, or constipation. Any positive responses to the questions should be further investigated (**Box 2.9**). Questions that may be asked include the following:

1. Do you eat regularly and have a balanced diet?

2. Do you skip meals?

3. Are there any food groups that you predominantly eat?

4. Do you view yourself as too thin, too fat, or just right?

5. Have you ever tried to control your weight? If so, how was this done?

6. Have you ever had excessive heartburn or indigestion?

7. Have you ever had an ulcer or vomited blood?

8. Have you ever been constipated or had diarrhea?

9. Have you ever had mononucleosis or hepatitis?

10. Do you have any food allergies or sensitivities?

For activities in which weight control is particularly important (e.g., gymnastics, ballet, crew, boxing, wrestling), it is advisable to investigate the individual's nutritional status to determine a tendency toward anorexia, bulimia, or disordered eating. This can be accomplished by having the individual record food intake for at least 3 days and then having the record analyzed by a nutritionist.

The Genitourinary Examination

Information gained at this station varies depending on the sex of the individual. For females, a complete menstrual history should be gathered. Any responses related to **oligomenorrhea** and **amenorrhea** necessitate further assessment and counseling about the increased risk of bone demineralization (osteopenia), stress fractures, and potential osteoporosis. Gynecologic symptoms that may need a further evaluation include **dysmenorrhea**, lower abdominal pain, unusual vaginal discharge, pain during urination, and use of birth control medication. Oral contraceptives may alter the pH of the vagina and increase the risk of pelvic inflammatory disease and hypertension. Discussion surrounding the use of birth control also may promote discussion of safe sexual practices, sexually transmitted diseases (STDs), and pregnancy.

Common questions that may be asked include the following:

1. Have you ever had problems with your kidneys or genitourinary organs?

2. Have you ever had a kidney or bladder infection?

3. Does it hurt to urinate?

4. Have you ever had an STD? If so, when? What medication was prescribed?

5. Have you noticed any skin lesions on the genitalia or any vaginal or penile discharge?

6. Have you ever been diagnosed as having sugar, albumin, or blood in the urine?

7. *Females:* Have you ever been or are you now pregnant? At what age did menarche occur? How many periods have you had during the last 6 months? When was your last menstrual period? What is the usual length of time between periods? Are the cycles fairly constant or irregular? Do you have a history of abnormal heavy bleeding (menorrhagia), scant bleeding, or intermittent bleeding?

8. *Males:* Are you missing a testicle, or do you have an undescended testicle? Have you ever had a history of testicular pain or a testicular abnormality, such as a hydrocele or varicocele?

As part of the physical examination, the kidney should be assessed by determining the presence of tenderness at the costovertebral angle. Generally, an individual with one kidney should be warned of the risks involved with participating in contact activities, especially if the remaining kidney is abnormally positioned or is diseased. Although not necessarily required in the PPE, a urinalysis should be performed if diabetes or kidney disease is suspected. Conditions such as albuminuria, hematuria, and hemoglobinuria can indicate problems with the urogenital system. These conditions do not preclude activity, but they should be evaluated. The individual should be informed of the potential dangers caused by these conditions. See **Box 2.10** for genitourinary red flags requiring further examination.

The Dermatological Examination

An examination of the skin can identify contagious lesions, such as herpes simplex (cold sores), molluscum contagiosum, tinea capitis or corporis, furuncles, impetigo, scabies, and secondary syphilis, which can preclude participation in sports. Skin infections that may be contagious to other participants should be identified and treated. In contrast, lesions such as warts, fungal infections, contact dermatitis, psoriasis, seborrhea, and nevi (birthmarks) require further evaluation but do not necessarily mean exclusion from participation. Early treatment typically is effective at managing these conditions.

Questions in this area might include the following:

1. Have you ever had problems with acne?

2. Have you ever had any skin rashes, itching, or scaling in areas covered by clothing, equipment, or footwear?

3. Do you have any unusual blemishes (e.g., warts, moles) that have changed in size or color over the past year?

BOX 2.10 Genitourinary Red Flags Requiring Further Examination

- One kidney or diseased kidney
- Absent or undescended testicle
- Hernia (femoral or inguinal)
- Pain with urination
- Possible exercise-induced amenorrhea or pregnancy
- Endometriosis and pelvic inflammatory disease
- Possible sexually transmitted disease
- Hematuria
- Albuminuria
- Hemoglobinuria
- Nephroptosis

BOX 2.11 Dermatological Red Flags Requiring Further Examination

- Herpes (e.g., simplex, gladiatorum)
- Impetigo
- Molluscum contagiosum
- Tinea capitis or corporis
- Furuncles
- Secondary syphilis
- Severe acne
- Dermatitis (e.g., contact, clothes)
- Warts
- Fungal infections
- Psoriasis

Any skin lesion associated with a contagious disease or STD warrants an immediate referral to a physician for treatment and appropriate counseling. Dermatological red flags that require further examination are identified in **Box 2.11**. Chapter 32 provides more detail and photographs of dermatological conditions.

The Examination for Heat Disorders

In activities that take place under conditions of high temperature, high humidity, or a combination of the two, a history should include questions about cramping, syncope, exhaustion, heat stroke, and sickle cell trait. Athletes who have sickle cell trait are at a higher risk of sustaining a sickling episode when dehydrated or participating in high heat stress conditions. A sickling episode may present similar to a patient experiencing a heat stress condition. Knowing that the patient has the condition will allow the athletic trainer to quickly recognize and manage the condition properly.[3] Questions concerning the use of medications are also important because certain medications can impair the body's ability to release heat (e.g., antihistamines) and place an individual at risk for heat illness (see Chapter 29). It also is advantageous to question the individual regarding regular caffeine consumption because excessive caffeine can increase the risk for heat disorders.

Specific questions related to heat disorders might include the following:

1. Have you ever suffered from heat illness or heat cramps?

2. Do you have sickle cell trait?

3. Have you ever participated in an activity in a high-temperature, high-humidity environment?

4. Have you ever passed out or become dizzy in the heat?

5. Do you have a heart problem, uncontrolled diabetes, hypertension, or poor eating habits?

6. Are you on any medications, such as diuretics, antihistamines, or β-blockers?

7. Do you drink more than two alcoholic or caffeinated beverages (e.g., cola, coffee, or tea) per day?

Individuals at a heightened risk of heat-related disorders include poorly acclimated or poorly conditioned individuals, children, overweight or large individuals, and those with excessive muscle mass. If an individual has a history of heat-related disorders or chronic illnesses, the condition should be investigated thoroughly (**Box 2.12**).

BOX 2.12 Heat-Related Red Flags Requiring Further Examination

■ Cardiac disease

■ Uncontrolled diabetes

■ Hypertension

■ Drug use (e.g., amphetamines, cocaine, hallucinogens, laxatives, narcotics)

■ Medication use (e.g., anticholinergics, diuretics, antihistamines, β-blockers)

■ Excessive muscle cramps during participation in heat

■ Heat exhaustion

■ Heat stroke

Laboratory Tests

The use of laboratory testing often is dictated by the focus of the PPE. Laboratory tests are not recommended by the American Academy of Pediatrics as part of a routine PPE, but decisions concerning the use of laboratory testing are at the discretion of the supervising physician and must be consistent with state law (if PPE regulation exists).

When used, the most frequently employed screening test has been the urine dipstick analysis for protein, glucose, and blood. Urine testing has not proven to be effective, however, at detecting renal disease among children. The costs involved, coupled with the low incidence of true renal pathology, do not bear out its use in the PPE.

Similarly, no evidence supports the routine use of blood work, such as **hemoglobin** and **hematocrit**, complete blood count, and blood chemistries. A few states, however, do require particular laboratory tests as a component of the PPE. If certain problems are suspected, information obtained from specific laboratory tests could be advantageous and, as such, should be ordered. For example, if concerns exist relative to the heart, an ECG or stress ECG may be necessary, but these tests should be reserved only for individuals with suggestive positive historical or clinical findings. In addition, drug screening must be performed in some institutions and at certain levels of competition.

A PPE focuses on general systemic conditions as well as on the cardiovascular, pulmonary, musculoskeletal, neurological, gastrointestinal, genitourinary, and dermatological systems, but it is not intended to be all encompassing. It is designed to determine an individual's readiness to participate in a specific sport or physical activity. As such, it should not be considered the equivalent of an annual medical examination.

THE PHYSICAL FITNESS PROFILE

Following completion of the physical examination, what advantages can be realized from assessing an individual's physical fitness level?

It is critical to assess the physical fitness status of an individual before the start of physical activity to determine whether the individual possesses the attributes, skills, and abilities necessary to meet the demands of the activity. Data from the examination can identify weaknesses that may hinder performance or predispose an individual to injury, and it establishes a baseline of data in the event that an injury is sustained.

A physical fitness profile can assess body composition; maturation and growth; flexibility, strength, power, and speed; agility, balance, and reaction time; and cardiovascular endurance. To be effective, the parameters of the test must be relevant and specific to the participant's selected activity. The test must be easy to perform, measure, and reproduce, and it must be inexpensive. The test should be standardized, controlled, and repeated during the program or season to assess improvement. Results should be explained to participants in a meaningful way so that the significance of those results can be understood.

Anthropometry and Body Composition

Anthropometry is used to determine an individuals' body type (i.e., **mesomorphic, endomorphic, ectomorphic**) and suitability for a desired activity, sport, or position played in that sport. Body composition provides detailed information regarding an individual's muscle, fat, and bone mass. The portion of total body weight that is composed of fat tissue is referred to as the percentage of body fat. The total body weight composed of nonfat or lean tissue, which includes muscles, tendons, bones, and connective tissue, is referred to as the lean body weight. Measurements of body composition can provide a reliable means of determining the amount of weight that an individual may safely gain or lose.

Hydrostatic weighting and skinfold measurement often are used to determine body fat measurements. Hydrostatic weighting is more accurate, but skinfold measurement is easier, faster, and nearly as reliable.

In performing skinfold measurements, seven to nine skinfold sites typically are used (**Application Strategy 2.4**), although many professionals believe that measurement at three sites is adequate (but a different three for males and females).[14] Most male and female athletes should fall between 12% and 17% body fat, although these percentages are only guidelines. Some male athletes may compete at 3% to 5%, whereas other male and female athletes perform very well at higher percentages. Generally, if the percentage of body fat is greater than the upper normal limit of 14% for males and 17% for females, the individual should be put on a weight-loss program or a weight training program to increase lean body mass, but this decision depends on the activity in which the individual wishes to participate. Additional methods of body composition measurement include girth measurements, bone diameter measurements, ultrasound measurement, arm radiograph measurement, and computed tomographic assessment of fat.

Maturation and Growth

Physical maturation refers to the developmental stage of an individual. In adolescents, growth spurts can affect participation in physical activity and may play a role in certain injuries. The growth spurt in girls usually occurs at about age 12; in boys, it occurs around age 14. For example, a growth spurt in a gymnast may adversely affect balance and flexibility, and a growth spurt in the bones of the foot may predispose a young individual to toe deformities if shoes are not repeatedly fitted to the growing foot. Pubertal growth accounts for 20% to 25% of final adult height, and pubertal weight gain accounts for 50% of ideal adult weight.

A common method of measuring maturation in males and females is the Tanner scale.[17] The five stages of this scale are based on pictorial standards of breast development and pubic hair for females and of genitalia and pubic hair for males. This assessment typically is conducted by a PCP in the privacy of an office and in the presence of a parent.

Flexibility

Flexibility is the total range of motion at a joint that occurs pain-free in each of the planes of motion. In most cases, less flexibility is better than too much; however, in certain activities (e.g., gymnastics or wrestling), excessive flexibility is a necessity. Several factors can limit flexibility and range of motion, such as the following:

- Bony block
- Joint adhesions
- Muscle tightness
- Tight skin or an inelastic, dense scar tissue
- Muscle bulk

APPLICATION STRATEGY 2.4

Standardized Description of Skinfold Sites and Procedures

SKINFOLD SITE	DESCRIPTION
Abdominal	Vertical fold; 2 cm on the right side of the umbilicus (see **Fig. A**)
Triceps	Vertical fold; on the posterior midline of the upper arm, halfway between the acromion and olecranon processes, with the arm held freely to the side of the body (see **Fig. B**)
Biceps	Vertical fold; on the anterior aspect of the arm over the belly of the biceps muscle, 1 cm
Chest/pectoral	Diagonal fold; one-half the distance between the anterior axillary line and the nipple (men) or one-third the distance between the anterior axillary line and the nipple (women)
Medial calf	Vertical fold; at the maximum circumference of the calf on the midline of its medial border
Midaxillary	Vertical fold; on midaxillary line at the level of the xiphoid process (An alternate method is a horizontal fold taken at the level of the xiphoid/sternal border in the midaxillary line.)
Subscapular	Diagonal fold (at a 45° angle); 1–2 cm below the inferior angle of the scapula
Suprailiac	Diagonal fold; in line with the natural angle of the iliac crest taken in the anterior axillary line immediately superior to the iliac crest
Thigh	Vertical fold; on the anterior midline of the thigh, midway between the proximal border of the patella and the inguinal crease (hip) (see **Fig. C**)

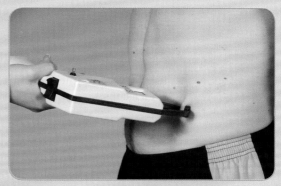

Figure A

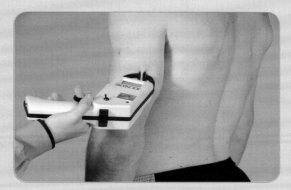

Figure B

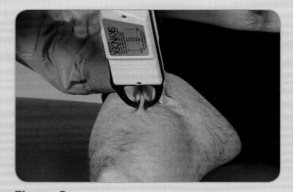

Figure C

General Guidelines

- All measurements should be made on the right side of the body.
- The caliper should be placed 1 cm away from the thumb and forefinger, perpendicular to the skinfold, and halfway between the crest and base of the fold.
- The pinch should be maintained while reading the caliper.
- Wait only 1–2 seconds before reading the caliper.
- Take duplicate measures at each site and test again if measurements are not within 1–2 mm.
- Rotate through measurement sites or allow time for skin to regain normal texture and thickness before retesting.

- Swelling

- Pain

- Presence of fat or other soft tissues that block normal motion

- Gender (females tend to be more flexible than males)

- Dominant limb tends to be less mobile than the nondominant limb

- Age (flexibility decreases with age)

- Race (Native Americans are more mobile than African Americans, who are more mobile than Caucasians.)

- Genetic makeup

Flexibility can be measured with a goniometer, flexometer, or tape measure. **Figure 2.2** provides an example of a goniometric measurement of knee flexion. Measurements should be taken to assess the flexibility of the hamstrings, quadriceps, gastrocnemius, shoulder, and low back. Hypermobility should be noted and recorded. Hypermobile traits include the following:

- Passive opposition of the thumb that can reach the flexor aspect of the forearm

- Passive hyperextension of the fingers so that they lie parallel with the extensor aspect of the forearm

- Ability to hyperextend the elbow at least 10°

- Ability to hyperextend the knee at least 10°

- Excessive passive dorsiflexion of the ankle and eversion of the foot

Laxity in one joint does not necessarily mean hypermobility in all joints or in all directions nor does it identify a pathologic state. Total range of motion can be related to genetic makeup or to the stresses placed on individual joints. Loose-jointed individuals tend to do poorly in strength events and are more susceptible to ligament sprains, dislocations, chronic back pain, disk prolapse, spondylolisthesis, pes planus, joint effusion, and tendinitis.[18] If strength and endurance are not at the appropriate level in hypermobile individuals, the joints cannot be supported and may become unstable and subject to injury. These individuals should avoid further stretching exercises and should support the joint through proper positioning, balance, and strengthening programs.

In contrast, tight-jointed or hypomobile individuals tend to be more susceptible to muscle strains, nerve pinch syndromes, and overstress tendinitis. If a person is hypomobile, mobilization or manipulation of the affected joint in the direction of tightness may be helpful. Tight supporting structures should be stretched, and active exercises be used to maintain the restored range of motion. It is important that these individuals retrain their kinesthetic sense so that the acquired range of motion can be maintained or improved.

Strength, Power, and Speed

Strength is the ability of a muscle or group of muscles to produce force in one maximal resistance (1 RM) effort, either statically or dynamically. The demands of a particular sport or activity dictate the level of strength that is needed to perform necessary skills. Strength measures can involve isometric, isotonic, or isokinetic testing through manual muscle testing, grip strength, sit-ups, push-ups, and pull-ups.

Power is the ability of a muscle to produce force in a given time (e.g., to move the body over a distance). Power activities can be measured by throwing a medicine ball, vertical jump and reach, single- or two-legged hop for distance, and stair

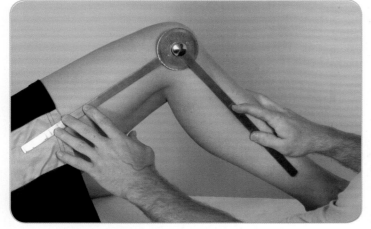

Figure 2.2. Use of a goniometer. The athletic trainer is using a goniometer to assess range of knee flexion.

climbing. As with strength, power measurement should be related to the activity in which the individual will be participating.

Speed is the ability to move body mass over time. It can be assessed by timed sprints (e.g., a 40-, 100-, or 400-m run).

Agility, Balance, and Reaction Time

Agility is the ability to change directions rapidly when moving at a high rate of speed. Balance is the body's coordinated neuromuscular response to maintain a defined position of equilibrium in response to changing visual, tactile, or kinesthetic stimuli. Agility and balance tests often are measured by time or accuracy (e.g., two correct out of three) and should be developed to be sport/activity-specific. Reaction time is measured by the ability to respond to a stimulus. Examples of agility, balance, and reaction tests include run-and-cut drills, carioca steps, shuttle runs, pivoting drills, front-to-back and side-to-side hops, figure-eight running drills, kicking a stationary or moving target, and beam-walking tests.

Cardiovascular Endurance

Cardiovascular endurance, commonly called aerobic capacity, is the body's ability to sustain submaximal exercise over an extended period, and it depends on the efficiency of the pulmonary and cardiovascular systems. Several tests may be used to assess cardiovascular endurance. The actual selection of tests should be dependent on the specific demands of the sport/activity. The Harvard step test is commonly used in a physical fitness profile. In this test, the individual is instructed to step up onto an 18-in platform using a four-step cadence "up-up-down-down" at a rate of about 30 times per minute (a metronome is used for cadence). Following 3.5 minutes at a pace of 2 seconds per step, the individual moves as fast as possible for 30 seconds (total time, 4 minutes). The individual then immediately sits down in a chair and relaxes for 3 minutes while the pulse is determined. The pulse is taken at 30, 60, 120, and 180 seconds after the exercise. The index formula for the pulse is[14]

$$\text{Index} = \frac{\text{duration of exercise (seconds)} \times 100}{2 \times \text{sum of any three pulse counts}}$$

The higher the index, the better the person's aerobic fitness. If the index is less than 65, the individual is not ready for strenuous activity. Other examples of common endurance tests include the 12-minute walk-run, 1.5-mile run, submaximal ergometer test, and a treadmill test. Although anaerobic fitness is not directly related to the cardiovascular system, if the proposed activity is primarily anaerobic, this measurement involves the ability to move large muscle groups for at least 1 minute but not more than 2 minutes.

 Testing the physical fitness of individuals before the start of participation in a program of physical activity or a sport can identify poorly conditioned individuals who may be at risk for certain injuries. By identifying deficits (i.e., excessive body fat percentage; hypermobile joints; or lack of flexibility, strength, power, agility, or endurance), individuals can be started on a corrective program to reduce the risk of injury during the program or season.

CLEARANCE FOR PARTICIPATION

 Can a physician totally exclude an individual from participation in a sport or physical activity?

Subsequent to the conclusion of the PPE, the physician must determine the level of participation based on conditions identified during the examination and knowledge regarding the physical demands of the physical activity. The physician must ask:

1. Will the condition increase the risk of injury to the individual or other participants?

2. Can participation be allowed if medication, rehabilitation, or protective bracing or padding is used? If so, can limited participation be allowed in the interim?

3. If clearance is denied for a particular activity, are there other activities in which the individual can participate safely?

Recent interpretations of the federal Rehabilitation Act and Americans with Disabilities Act have stated that individuals have the legal right to participate in any competitive sport regardless of a preexisting medical condition. For this reason, physicians cannot totally exclude an individual from participation but, rather, can recommend that the individual not participate because of a medical condition that increases the risk of further injury and/or death as a result of participation. In these situations, an exculpatory waiver may be used. An exculpatory waiver is based on the individual's assumption of risk and is a release signed by the individual or by the parent of an individual under the age of 18 years that releases the physician from liability of negligence.

Most physicians base their recommendations on the American Academy of Pediatrics Committee on Sports Medicine and Fitness guidelines including the risks of participation, the risk of acquiring a disease as a result of participation in the sport, and the severity of that disease. Other variables that must be considered include (1) advice of knowledgeable experts, (2) the current health status of the athlete, (3) sport in which the athlete participates, (4) the position played, (5) the level of competition, (6) the maturity of the competitor, (7) the relative size of the athlete (for collision/contact sports), (8) the availability of effective protective equipment that is acceptable to the athlete and/or sport governing body, (9) the availability and efficacy of treatment, (10) whether treatment (e.g., rehabilitation of an injury) has been completed, (11) whether the sport can be modified to allow safer participation, and (12) the ability of the athlete's parent(s) or guardian and coach to understand and to accept the risks involved in participation.[19] Potential dangers of associated training activities that lead to repetitive and/or excessive overload also should be considered. Under these guidelines, disqualifying conditions include carditis and fever.[19] Other conditions may allow participation with certain restrictions (e.g., medication, individual evaluation, consultation with a specialist, activity restriction). In general, any individual with only a solitary paired organ (e.g., an eye, kidney, testicle) should be individually evaluated to determine what protective equipment or appropriate activity may allow participation. Because of the complexities of the various medical conditions that may require further consultation with medical specialists, the reader should consult with the current "Medical Conditions and Sports Participation" as recommended by the American Academy of Pediatrics Council on Sports Medicine and Fitness.[19]

 Subsequent to interpretations of the Rehabilitation Act and Americans with Disabilities Act, a physician cannot totally exclude an individual from participation. The physician can only recommend that the individual not participate because of a medical condition that increases the risk of further injury and/or death as a result of participation.

SUMMARY

1. The basic objective of the PPE is to determine the general health and fitness level of a physically active individual to ensure safe participation in a particular sport/activity.

2. A medical history questionnaire should be completed before the PPE and should be validated for accuracy during the actual examination.

3. The physical examination involves assessing the vital signs; the general medical conditions; and cardiovascular, pulmonary, musculoskeletal, neurological, gastrointestinal, genitourinary, and dermatological systems. In addition, the eyes and teeth should be evaluated, and individuals at risk for heat-related illness should be identified.

4. The physical fitness of the individual should be assessed by measuring body composition, maturation, flexibility, strength, power, speed, agility, balance, reaction time, and cardiovascular endurance.

5. At the conclusion of the examination, the physician must ask:

- Will the abnormality increase the risk of injury to the individual or other participants?

- Can participation be allowed if medication, rehabilitation, or protective bracing or padding is used? If so, can limited participation be allowed in the interim?

- If clearance is denied for a particular activity, are there other activities in which the individual can safely participate?

APPLICATION QUESTIONS

1. You are the head athletic trainer at a university that participates in National Collegiate Athletic Association (NCAA) Division II athletics. In preparation for the upcoming year, you must organize PPEs for 75 new student athletes who will be participating in winter sports (i.e., basketball, swimming and diving, wrestling, gymnastics). Your goal is to administer the PPEs during the first week of the academic semester. What strategies and/or policies could you implement to ensure successful completion of that goal?

2. Should the PPE for high school athletes be performed by a family physician? What advantages or disadvantages does this practice entail? What other options are available?

3. You have been hired as the first athletic trainer at a college that participates in NCAA Division III athletics. Previously, the college contracted athletic training services through a local sports medicine center. One of your first administrative tasks is to develop a PPE form. Rather than create a form from scratch, you decide to review the forms used by other institutions. What criteria will you consider in determining how you can best use the existing forms to create a form for your institution?

4. You are an athletic trainer at a high school. In reviewing the history component of a student athlete's PPE, you have concerns about the accuracy of some of the information. What actions would you take in response to your concerns?

REFERENCES

1. Mayer F, Bonaventura K, Cassel M, et al. Medical results of preparticipation examination in adolescent athletes. *Br J Sports Med.* 2012;46(7):524–530.
2. Conley KM, Bolin DJ, Carek PJ, et al. National Athletic Trainers' Association position statement: preparticipation physical examinations and disqualifying conditions. *J Athl Train.* 2014;49(1):102–120.
3. Casa DJ, Guskiewicz KM, Anderson SA, et al. National Athletic Trainers' Association position statement: preventing sudden death in sports. *J Athl Train.* 2012;47(1):96–118.
4. Smith DM; American Academy of Family Physicians; Preparticipation Physical Evaluation Task Force. *Preparticipation Physical Evaluation.* 3rd ed. Minneapolis, MN: McGraw-Hill Healthcare; 2004.
5. Maron BJ, Douglas PS, Graham TP, et al. Task Force 1: preparticipation screening and diagnosis of cardiovascular disease in athletes. *J Am Coll Cardiol.* 2005;45(8):1322–1326.
6. King D, Brughelli M, Hume P, et al. Assessment, management and knowledge of sport-related concussion: systematic review. *Sports Med.* 2014;44(4):449–471.
7. Broglio SP, Cantu RC, Gioia GA, et al. National Athletic Trainers' Association position statement: management of sport concussion. *J Athl Train.* 2014;49(2):245–265.
8. Seto CK. Preparticipation cardiovascular screening. *Clin Sports Med.* 2003;22(1):23–35.
9. National Heart, Lung, and Blood Institute. *The Seventh Report of the Joint National Committee on Prevention, Detection, Evaluation, and Treatment of High Blood Pressure.* Washington, DC: National Heart, Lung, and Blood Institute; 2004.
10. Kaplan NM, Gidding SS, Pickering TG, et al. Task Force 5: systemic hypertension. *J Am Coll Cardiology.* 2005;45(8):1346–1348.
11. Bickley LS, Szilagyi PG. *Bates' Guide to Physical Examination and History Taking.* 9th ed. Philadelphia, PA: Lippincott Williams & Wilkins; 2007.

12. Maron BJ, Doerer JJ, Haas TS, et al. Sudden deaths in young competitive athletes: analysis of 1866 deaths in the United States, 1980–2006. *Circulation.* 2009;119(8):1085–1092.

13. Maron BJ, Thompson PD, Ackerman MJ, et al. Recommendations and considerations related to preparticipation screening for cardiovascular abnormalities in competitive athletes: 2007 update: a scientific statement from the American Heart Association Council on Nutrition, Physical Activity, and Metabolism: endorsed by the American College of Cardiology Foundation. *Circulation.* 2007;115(12):1643–1655.

14. American College of Sports Medicine. *ACSM's Guidelines for Exercise Testing and Prescription.* 8th ed. Baltimore, MD: Lippincott Williams & Wilkins; 2009.

15. Hadjiliadis D, Zieve D, Ogilvie I. How to use your peak flow meter. MedlinePlus. U.S. National Library of Medicine/National Institute of Health. http://www.nlm.nih.gov/medlineplus /ency/patientinstructions/000043.htm. Accessed January 9, 2014.

16. Carek PJ, Mainous AG III. A thorough yet efficient exam identifies most problems in school athletes. *J Fam Pract.* 2003;52(2):127–135.

17. Tanner JM. *Growth at Adolescence.* Oxford, United Kingdom: Blackwell Scientific; 1962.

18. Magee DJ. *Orthopedic Physical Assessment.* 5th ed. Philadelphia, PA: WB Saunders; 2008.

19. Rice SG; American Academy of Pediatrics Council on Sports Medicine and Fitness. Medical conditions affecting sports participation. *Pediatrics.* 2008;121(4):841–848.

3

Protective Equipment

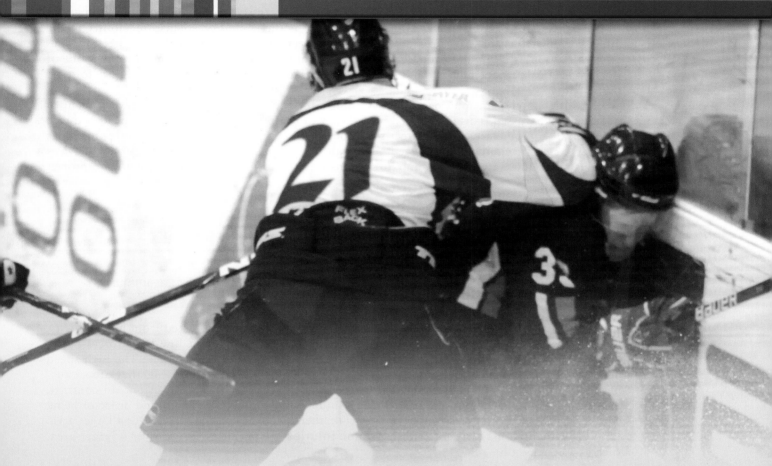

PhotoStock10 / Shutterstock.com

STUDENT OUTCOMES

1. Describe the forces that produce focal and diffuse injuries.

2. State the principles used to design protective equipment.

3. Identify the different types of soft and hard materials used to make protective pads.

4. Explain the athletic trainer's legal duty of care in selecting and fitting protective equipment.

5. List the agencies responsible for establishing material standards for protective devices.

6. Identify the information that should be documented to support an organization's legal duty to provide safe equipment.

7. Demonstrate proper selection and fitting of selected equipment (e.g., football helmets, mouth guards, and shoulder pads).

8. Identify and describe common protective equipment for the head and face, the torso, and the upper and lower body.

INTRODUCTION

Specialized equipment, when properly used, can protect a participant from accidental or routine injuries associated with a particular sport or physical activity, but limitations exist regarding the effectiveness of protective equipment. A natural outcome of wearing protective equipment is to feel more secure. Unfortunately, this often leads to more aggressive play, which can result in injury to the participant or an opponent. In many cases, it is the shared or sole responsibility of the athletic trainer to ensure that protective equipment meets minimum standards of protection, is in good condition, is clean and properly fitted, used routinely, and used as intended. This is one of the most critical responsibilities that an athletic trainer does to minimize the risk of injury to sport participants.

In this chapter, principles of protective equipment and materials used in the development of padding are discussed. This is followed by a review of protective equipment for the head and face and then of equipment used to protect the upper and lower body. When appropriate, guidelines for fitting specific equipment are listed. Although several commercial braces and support devices are illustrated, these are intended only to demonstrate the variety of products available to protect a body region.

PRINCIPLES OF PROTECTIVE EQUIPMENT

 What are the advantages of using high-density material in the protection of injuries?

In events involving impact and collisions, the participant must be protected from high-velocity, low-mass forces and from low-velocity, high-mass forces. High-velocity, low-mass forces occur, for example, when an individual is struck by a ball, puck, bat, or hockey stick. The high speed and low velocity of such an impact leads to forces being concentrated in a smaller area, causing **focal injuries** (i.e., injuries concentrated in a small area, such as a contusion). In contrast, an example of low-velocity, high-mass forces is an individual falling on the ground or ice or being checked into the sideboards of an ice hockey rink, thereby absorbing the forces over a larger area. Low-velocity, high-mass forces lead to **diffuse injuries** (i.e., injuries spread over a larger area, such as a concussion).

Sport-related and physical activity injuries can result from a variety of factors, including the following:

■ Illegal play

■ Poor technique

■ Inadequate conditioning

■ Poorly matched player levels

■ A previously injured area that is vulnerable to reinjury

■ Low tolerance of an individual to injury

■ Inability to adequately protect an area without restricting motion

■ Poor quality, maintenance, or cleanliness of protective equipment

Potential means by which equipment can protect an area from accidental or routine injuries associated with a particular activity are listed in **Box 3.1**. Equipment design extends beyond the physical protective properties to include size, comfort, style, tradition, and both initial and long-term maintenance costs. Individuals responsible for the selection and purchase of equipment should be less concerned about appearance, style, and cost, and be most concerned about the ability of the equipment to prevent injury.

> **BOX 3.1 Equipment Design Factors That Can Reduce Potential Injury**
>
> - Increase the impact area
> - Transfer or disperse the impact area to another body part
> - Limit the relative motion of a body part
> - Add mass to the body part to limit deformation and displacement
> - Reduce friction between contacting surfaces
> - Absorb energy
> - Resist the absorption of bacteria, fungi, and viruses

Materials Used

The design and selection of protective equipment is based on the optimal level of impact intensity afforded by the given thickness, density, and temperature of the energy-absorbing material. Soft, **low-density material** is light and comfortable to wear, but such material is effective only at low levels of impact intensity. Examples of low-density material include gauze padding, foam, neoprene, Sorbothane, felt, and moleskin. Low-density materials are useful in reducing friction and preventing blisters and abrasions. In contrast, firmer, **high-density material** of the same thickness tends to be less comfortable, offers less cushioning of low-level impact, but can absorb more energy by deformation. As such, it transfers less stress to an area at higher levels of impact intensity. Examples of high-density material include thermomoldable plastics, such as orthoplast and thermoplast, and casting materials, such as fiberglass and plaster. High-density materials are useful in protecting the patient from direct blows and focal injuries.

Another factor to consider in energy-absorbing material is **resilience** to impact forces. Highly resilient materials regain their shape after impact and are used over areas that are subject to repeated impacts. Nonresilient (or slow-recovery resilient) material offers the best protection and is used over areas subjected to one-time or occasional impacts. It is important to select equipment that will absorb an impact and disperse it before injury occurs to the underlying body part.

Soft Materials

Soft materials are light because of the incorporation of air into the material. Examples include gauze padding, neoprene, Sorbothane, felt, moleskin, and foam. Gauze padding comes in a variety of widths and thicknesses and is used as an absorbent or protective pad. Neoprene sleeves provide uniform compression, therapeutic warmth, and support for a chronic injury, such as a recurrent quadriceps or hamstring strain. The nylon-coated rubber material is comfortable and allows full mobility, better absorption of sweat, and less skin breakdown; it also provides the individual with proprioceptive feedback in the affected area. Sorbothane often is used for shoe insoles to absorb and dissipate impact forces during walking and running. Felt is made from matted wool fibers and pressed into several thicknesses, ranging from 0.25 to 1 in. Felt can absorb perspiration but, in doing so, has less of a tendency to move under stress. Typically, it is necessary to replace felt daily. Moleskin is a thin felt product with an adhesive bonding on one side that prevents any movement once applied to the skin. This product is used over friction spots to reduce skin irritation or blisters.

Foam, like felt, comes in a variety of thicknesses, ranging from 0.125 to 1 in, and ranges in density from a very soft, open-cell foam to a denser, closed-cell foam. **Open-cell foam** has cells that are connected to allow the passage of air from cell to cell. Similar to a sponge, this material can absorb fluids and is used to pad bony prominences or to protect the skin under hard edges of protective equipment or custom-fabricated pads. Open-cell foams deform quickly under stress; therefore, they do not have good shock-absorbing qualities. **Closed-cell foam** is used primarily for protection because air cannot pass from one cell to another. The material rebounds and returns to its original shape quickly, but it offers less cushioning at low levels of impact and is not as comfortable next to the skin.

To use the differing properties of foam effectively, many equipment designers layer materials of varying density. Air management pads combine open- and closed-cell foams encased in polyurethane or nylon to provide maximal shock absorption. Soft, lower density material is placed next to the skin and is covered by increasingly denser, closed-cell material away from the skin to absorb and disperse higher intensity blows. The pad is airtight, which prevents quick deformation of the foam so energy can be dissipated over the entire surface of the pad. Air management pads often are used in football shoulder pads, but they are more expensive and require extensive maintenance if the nylon covering is torn. If the covering tears, air can pass into the pads, reducing their effectiveness. The liners must then be patched or replaced. Nylon prevents the absorption of perspiration or water, which can help to avoid additional weight, and is easily cleaned with a weak bleach solution.

Some dense foams are thermomoldable; that is, when heated, they can be molded and shaped to fit any body part. When cooled, they retain their shape. These pads can be used repeatedly to immobilize a body structure, deflect an impact, and absorb shock. The pad is secured to the body part with elastic or nonelastic tape.

Hard Materials

Hard materials include thermomoldable plastics, such as orthoplast and thermoplast, and casting materials, such as fiberglass and plaster, which can be used to splint or protect an area. Thermoplastics are divided into two categories: plastic and rubber. The plastic group uses a polycaprolactone base with varying amounts of inorganic filler, resins, and elastomers to affect the memory, stiffness, and durability of the material. The plastic category tends to conform better than the rubber category and is more appropriate for small splints, such as on the hand. Plastics include materials such as Aquaplast Bluestripe (WFR/Aquaplast), Multiform I and II (Alimed), Orfit (North Coast Medical), and Orthoplast II (Johnson & Johnson). Rubberlike materials use a polyisoprene base and include Aquaplast Greenstrip (WFR/Aquaplast), Orthoplast (Johnson & Johnson), Synergy (Rolyan), and Ultraform Traditions (Sammons).

Most of these materials are heated while lying flat for about 1 minute at temperatures between 150° and 180°F. The material is then shaped for 3 to 4 minutes before returning to a hardened form. Minor changes can be made with a heat gun, but changes should never be performed while the splint is on the patient.

Casting materials, such as fiberglass and plaster, are used to splint a body part, but conditions such as macerations, ulcerations, infections, burns, blisters, rashes, and allergic contact dermatitis can result from extended use. Individuals often report that such casts itch, smell, and are difficult to keep dry. Fiberglass casts with a stockinette or cast padding can limit moisture, but they must be dried (usually with a hair dryer) to prevent maceration, odor, and itching. A new Gore-Tex liner developed for use under fiberglass repels water; permits evaporation; and allows bathing, swimming, sweating, and hydrotherapy without any special drying of the cast or skin. The liner comes in 2-in, 3-in, and 4-in widths and is applied directly to the skin. Fiberglass casting material is then applied over the liner. Although slightly more expensive than traditional casts, those incorporating this type of liner do not have to be changed as often because they stay more comfortable throughout the immobilization period.

Construction of Custom Pads and Protective Devices

In some settings, the athletic trainer has access to the soft and hard materials mentioned earlier in this chapter. These materials can be used in constructing a variety of custom pads or protective devices. Custom pads can be advantageous for several reasons, such as cost, design, and availability. In addition, custom pads can be designed to meet the needs of the individual. The athletic trainer should ensure that custom-made devices are constructed and fit properly. The athletic trainer assumes legal responsibility for use of any custom-made devices.

Rules Regarding Protective Pads

The National Federation of State High School Associations (NFSHSA) and the National Collegiate Athletic Association (NCAA) have specific rules regarding the use of soft and hard materials to protect a body area. The on-site referee must determine that specific fabricated pads are made of soft materials or meet the standards for hard materials established by the NFSHSA or NCAA. Hard, abrasive, or unyielding substances may be used on the hand, wrist, forearm, or elbow if the substance is covered on all exterior surfaces with no less than a 0.5-in thick, high-density, closed-cell polyurethane or a material of the same minimum thickness and similar physical properties. In addition, a written authorization form must be signed by a licensed medical physician that indicates the cast or splint is necessary to protect the body part. This form must be available to the referee before the start of competition. The referee must verify that the hard material is properly padded according to the guidelines and has the right to eject the player for using the cast or splint as a weapon.[1]

High-density materials, such as thermomoldable plastics and casting materials, can absorb more energy by deformation and, in doing so, transfer less stress to an injured area.

LIABILITY AND EQUIPMENT STANDARDS

During football practice, an athletic trainer notices that the quarterback is wearing a helmet with a two-point chin strap. What action or actions should be taken by the athletic trainer, and why?

Legal issues concerning protective equipment are a major concern for every athletic trainer and organized sport program. An organization's duty to ensure the proper use of protective equipment usually is a shared responsibility among the members of the athletics staff. For example, the head coach may be responsible for recommending specific equipment for that particular sport. The athletics director may be responsible for purchasing this recommended equipment. The equipment manager or athletic trainer may then be responsible for properly fitting the equipment based on the manufacturer's guidelines, instructing and warning the individual about proper use of the equipment, regularly inspecting the protective equipment, and keeping accurate records of any repair or reconditioning of the equipment.

Negligence and standard of care for the athletic trainer are discussed in broad terms in Chapter 1. When focusing on protective equipment, the athletic trainer has a duty to:

- Select the most appropriate equipment
- Properly fit the equipment to the individual
- Instruct the individual in proper care of the equipment
- Warn the individual of any danger in using the equipment inappropriately
- Supervise and monitor the proper use of all protective equipment

It is the duty of the manufacturer to design, manufacture, and package safe equipment that will not cause injury to an individual when the equipment is used as it was intended. To protect the sport participant from ineffective and poorly constructed athletic equipment, several agencies have developed standards of quality to ensure that equipment does not fail under normal athletic circumstances or contribute to injury. The National Operating Committee on Standards for Athletic Equipment (NOCSAE) sets the standards for football helmets to tolerate certain forces when applied to different areas of the helmet. Currently, baseball, softball, lacrosse helmets and face masks, and soccer shin guards also must be NOCSAE-certified. Other testing agencies for protective equipment include the American Society for Testing and Materials (ASTM) and the Hockey Equipment Certification Council (HECC) of the Canadian Standards Association (CSA). These agencies have established material standards for equipment such as protective eyewear (ASTM) and ice hockey helmets and face masks (HECC).

In addition to agencies that establish standards for the manufacture of equipment, athletic governing bodies establish rules for the mandatory use of specific protective equipment as well as rules governing special protective equipment. These governing bodies include the NFSHSA, the National Association of Intercollegiate Athletics (NAIA), the NCAA, and the U.S. Olympic Committee. For example, the NCAA requires football players to use a face mask and helmet with a secured, four-point chin strap. In addition, all players must wear helmets that carry a warning label regarding the risk of injury and a manufacturer's or reconditioner's certification indicating that the equipment meets the NOCSAE test standards.[1]

After equipment has been purchased, the manufacturer's informational materials, such as brochures and warranties used in the selection process, should be cataloged for reference in the event an injury occurs. This information can document the selection process and particular attributes of the chosen equipment. When an individual provides one's own protective equipment, the responsibilities of the athletic trainer do not change. The athletic trainer must ensure that the equipment meets safety standards and is fitted correctly, properly maintained and cleaned, and used appropriately. Athletic trainers and coaches should know the dangers involved in using sport equipment and have a duty to properly supervise its fitting and intended use. Athletes should not be allowed to wear or alter any equipment that may endanger the individual or other team members.

> The athletic trainer should remove from practice any athlete whose helmet does not have a four-point chin strap. Interscholastic and collegiate athletic governing bodies require that helmets be secured with a four-point chin strap. As such, the two-point strap does not meet minimum protection standards and should not be allowed on the helmet. If the individual were to sustain an injury while wearing an improper helmet, the athletic trainer could be considered negligent.

PROTECTIVE EQUIPMENT FOR THE HEAD AND FACE

> **?** A high school athletic trainer is concerned about a variety of oral injuries that have occurred on the school's basketball teams. What rationale can be used to convince the administration to purchase mouth guards for the teams?

Many head and facial injuries can be prevented with regular use of properly fitted helmets and facial protective devices, such as face guards, eyewear, ear wear, mouth guards, and throat protectors. Helmets in particular are required in football, ice hockey, men's lacrosse, baseball, softball, whitewater sports (kayaking), amateur boxing, and bicycling and must be fitted properly to disperse impact forces.

Football Helmets

Football helmets have been found to be useful in preventing injury to the face, scalp, and skull, but there is little conclusive evidence to support that football helmets prevent concussions.[2,3] Football helmet designs typically use a single or double air bladder, closed-cell padding, or a combination of the two. Air bladders are excellent at absorbing shock, but they must be inspected daily by the players to ensure that adequate inflation is maintained for a proper fit.

Helmet shells can be constructed of plastic or a polycarbonate alloy. Polycarbonate is a plastic used in making jet canopies and police riot gear; it is lightweight and both scratch- and impact-resistant. Helmets vary in life expectancy. Typically, the polycarbonate alloy shell has a 5-year warranty; the ABS plastic shell has a 2-year warranty. Manufacturer's guidelines should be followed with regard to the appropriate time for retiring a helmet.

Heat, as an environmental factor, can alter the effectiveness of shock absorption in the liner and some shell materials. As a result, materials compress more easily and absorb less shock at higher compared with lower temperatures. As part of the testing process, the NOCSAE exposes new helmets to temperatures of 100°F ($\pm$3°F) for no less than 4 hours and no longer than 24 hours. A standard drop test is also conducted, and shock measurements are taken to determine if the helmet meets an established high severity index and thereby meets the NOCSAE football helmet standard test.[4]

The NOCSAE mark on a helmet indicates that it meets the minimum impact standards and can tolerate forces applied to several different areas. In addition, the NOCSAE includes a warning label regarding the risk of injury on each helmet that states the following[4]:

NO HELMET CAN PREVENT ALL HEAD OR ANY NECK INJURIES A PLAYER MIGHT RECEIVE WHILE PARTICIPATING IN FOOTBALL.

DO NOT USE THIS HELMET TO BUTT, RAM OR SPEAR AN OPPOSING PLAYER. THIS IS IN VIOLATION OF THE FOOTBALL RULES AND SUCH USE CAN RESULT IN SEVERE HEAD OR NECK INJURIES, PARALYSIS OR DEATH TO YOU AND POSSIBLE INJURY TO YOUR OPPONENT.

This warning label must be clearly visible on the exterior shell of all new and reconditioned helmets. In addition, the athletic trainer should continually warn athletes of the risks involved in football and ensure that the helmet is properly used within the guidelines and rules of the game.

Manufacturer's guidelines should always be followed when fitting a football helmet. Before fitting, the individual should have a haircut in the style that will be worn during the athletics season and wet the head to simulate game conditions. **Application Strategy 3.1** lists the general steps in fitting a football helmet.

Once fitted, the helmet should be checked daily for proper fit, which can be altered by hair length, deterioration of internal padding, loss of air from cells, and spread of the face mask. This check is performed by inserting a tongue depressor between the pads and the face. When moved back and forth, a firm resistance should be felt. A snug-fitting helmet should not move in one direction when the head moves in another. In addition, the helmet should be checked weekly by the athletic trainer to ensure proper fit and compliance with safety standards (**Box 3.2**).

Each helmet should have the purchase date and tracking number engraved on the inside. Detailed records should be kept that identify the purchase date, use, reconditioning history, and certification seals. Each individual also should be instructed regarding the proper use, fit, and care of the helmet. In addition, each individual should sign a statement that confirms having read the NOCSAE seal and been informed of the risks of injury through improper use of the helmet or face mask when striking an opponent. This statement should be signed, dated, and kept as part of the individual's medical files.

Ice Hockey Helmets

Ice hockey helmets must absorb and disperse high-velocity, low-mass forces (e.g., being struck by a stick or puck) and low-velocity, high-mass forces (e.g., being checked into the sideboard or falling on the ice) (**Fig. 3.1**). As with football helmets, ice hockey helmets reduce head injuries; however, they do not prevent neck injuries caused by axial loading. The use of head protection with a face mask seems to have given many players a sense of invulnerability to injury. Studies have shown that the risk of spinal cord injury and, in particular, quadriplegia may be threefold greater in hockey than in American football.[5] The major mechanism of injury is head-first contact with the boards secondary to a push or a check from behind.

Ice hockey helmet standards are monitored by the ASTM and the HECC, and ice hockey helmets are required to carry the stamp of approval from the CSA. When properly fitted, the helmet should sit level on the head one to two finger widths above the eyebrows. There should be a maximum of two finger widths between the neck and chin strap. The face mask should fit properly in the J-clips, and the chin should rest in the chin cup.[6] Proper fit is achieved when a snug-fitting helmet does not move, slide, or rotate when the head is turned.

Batting Helmets

Batting helmets are now compulsory in baseball and softball and require the NOCSAE mark.[1] Most batting helmets are open-faced with a double ear-flap design and can protect the majority of the superolateral cranium but not the jaw or facial area. Although some studies claim that batting helmets fitted with face shields may prevent or reduce the severity of facial injuries to children, no rigorous data currently support such a claim.[7]

APPLICATION STRATEGY 3.1

Proper Fitting of a Football Helmet

1. The player should have a haircut in the style that will be worn during the competitive season and should wet the hair to simulate game conditions. Measure the circumference of the head above the ears using the tape measure supplied by the manufacturer. The suggested helmet size is listed on the reverse side of the tape.
2. Select the proper-sized shell and adjust the front and back sizers and jaw pads for a proper fit.
3. Inflate the air bladder by holding the bulb with an arch in the hose; to deflate, the hose is in a straight position.
4. Ensure that the helmet fits snugly around the player's head and covers the base of the skull but does not impinge the cervical spine when the neck is extended. The ear holes should match up with the external auditory ear canal.
5. Check that the four-point chin strap is of equal tension and length on both sides, placing the chin pad an equal distance from each side of the helmet (**Fig. A**).
6. Check that the face mask allows for a complete field of vision and the helmet is one to two finger widths above the eyebrows and extends two finger widths away from the forehead and nose (**Fig. B**).
7. Check that the helmet does not move when the athlete presses forward on the rear of the helmet and presses straight down on top of the helmet (**Fig. C**).
8. Check that the helmet does not slip when the athlete is asked to "bull" the neck while you grasp the face mask pulling left, then right (**Fig. D**).

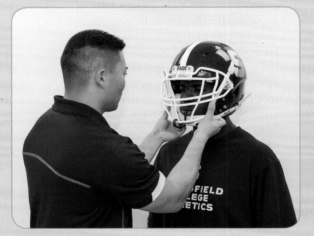

Figure A

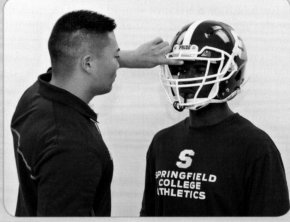

Figure B

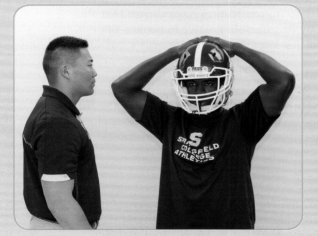

Figure C

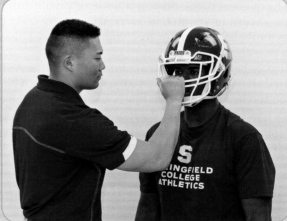

Figure D

- Check proper fit according to manufacturer's guidelines.

- Examine the shell for cracks, particularly around the holes. Replace the shell if any cracks are detected.

- Examine all mounting rivets, screws, Velcro, and snaps for breakage, sharp edges, and/or looseness. Repair or replace as necessary.

- Replace the face guard if bare metal is visible, has a broken weld, or is grossly misshapen.

- Examine and replace any parts that are damaged, such as jaw pads, sweatbands, nose snubbers, and chin straps.

- Examine the chin strap for proper shape and fit; inspect the hardware to see if it needs replacement.

- Inspect shell according to NOCSAE and the manufacturer's standards; only approved paints, waxes, decals, or cleaning agents are to be used on any helmet. Severe or delayed reaction to the substances may permanently damage the shell and affect its safety performance.

- If air- and fluid-filled helmets are used, and the team travels to a different altitude, recheck the fit prior to use.

It is best to have a thick layer of foam between the primary energy absorber and the head to allow the shell to move slightly and deform. This maximizes its ability to absorb missile kinetic energy from a ball or a bat and prevents excessive pressure on the cranium. The helmet should be snug enough that it does not move or fall off during batting and running bases.

Other Helmets

Lacrosse helmets are mandatory in the men's game and optional in the women's game. These helmets also are worn by field hockey goalies. The helmet is made of a highly resistant plastic or fiberglass shell and must meet NOCSAE standards. The helmet, wire face guard, and chin pad are secured with a four-point chin strap (**Fig. 3.2**). The helmet should not move in one direction when the head moves in another.

An effective bicycle helmet has a plastic or fiberglass, rigid shell with a chin strap, and an energy-absorbing foam liner. Regardless of the type, the helmet can provide substantial protection against injuries to the head and the upper and midface region. A stiffer shell results in better diffusion and resilience to impact. A firmer, dense foam liner is more effective at higher velocities, whereas less stiff foam provides more protection at lower velocities. Increasing the thickness of the liner may lead to a more effective level of protection, but the increased mass and weight of the helmet may make it more uncomfortable. Improved designs have produced helmets that are lightweight and aerodynamic, with an increase in the number of ventilation ports. Wearing a cycling helmet does not increase thermal discomfort to the head or body and has no additional impact on core temperature, head skin temperature, thermal sensation, heart rate, sweat rate, and overall perceived exertion.[8]

Although the rate of bicycle helmet usage has increased in the United States, at least one study has found that the overwhelming majority of children, adolescents, and their parents cannot properly fit a bicycle helmet. This increases the potential for exposure of the head's frontal region, which is the most common site of impact in bicycle head injuries.[9]

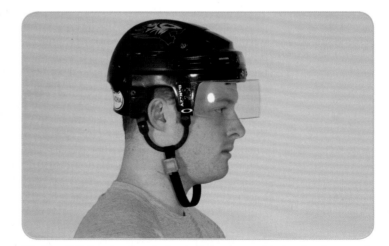

Figure 3.1. Ice hockey helmet. Helmets used in ice hockey must absorb and disperse high-velocity, low-mass forces (e.g., being hit by a high stick or a puck) and low-velocity, high-mass forces (e.g., being checked into the boards). Full face guards may be clear or wire mesh.

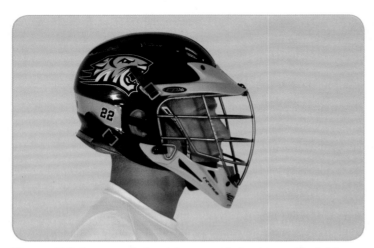

Figure 3.2. Lacrosse helmet. Lacrosse helmets provide full face and neck protection.

Common fitting errors include having the helmet rest too high on the forehead, improper strap position (failure of strap to make a "V" around the ear), and excessive front-to-back movement of the helmet.[9,10]

Bicycle helmet fitting should first begin with a properly conditioned helmet (i.e., certified by the Consumer Product Safety Commission, ASTM, American National Standards Institute, or CSA). The helmet should be less than 10 years old, and the plastic cover should be intact, with no visible cracks. When resting on the head, the following guidelines should be used to properly fit the helmet[9]:

- There should be space of less than two fingerbreadths in front of, and in the side of, the helmet.

- The helmet should rest two fingerbreadths above the eyebrows.

- The chin strap should form a "V" around the ear and clip below the ear.

- The helmet front should pull down over the forehead when the mouth is opened.

- Side-to-side, front-to-front, and rotational movement should be 1 in or less.

Face Guards

Face guards, which vary in size and style, protect and shield the facial region from flying projectiles. The NOCSAE has set standards for strength and deflection for football face guards worn at the high school and college levels. Football face guards are made of heavy-gauge, plastic-coated steel rod designed to withstand impacts from blunt surfaces, such as the turf or another player's knee or elbow. The effectiveness of a football face guard depends on the strength of the guard itself, the helmet attachments, and the four-point (or six-point) chin strap on the helmet. When properly fitted, the face mask should extend two finger widths away from the forehead and allow complete field of vision. No face protection should be less than two bars. If needed, eye shields made of Plexiglas or polycarbonate can be attached to the face mask.

Ice hockey face guards are made of clear plastic (polycarbonate), steel wire, or a combination of the two and must meet HECC and ASTM standards (see **Fig. 3.1**). Hockey face guards primarily prevent penetration of the hockey stick, but they also are effective against flying pucks and collisions with helmets, elbows, side boards, and the ice. The use of full-coverage face masks in amateur ice hockey has greatly reduced facial trauma. The use of a single chin strap, however, still allows the helmet to ride back on the head when a force is directed to the frontal region, thus exposing the chin to lacerations. The guard stands away from the nose approximately 1 to 1.5 in. If a wire mesh is used, the holes should be small enough to prevent penetration by a hockey stick.

Lacrosse face guards must meet NOCSAE standards. The wire mesh guard stands away from the face, but the four-point chin strap has a padded chin region in case the guard is driven back during a collision with another player (see **Fig. 3.2**). Face masks used by catchers and the home-plate umpire in baseball and softball should fit snugly to the cheeks and forehead but should not impair vision. These devices can be used by players in the field and must meet ASTM standards. Men's and women's fencing masks have an adjustable spring to prevent the mask from moving during competition.

Eyewear

Eye injuries are relatively common and almost always preventable if proper protective wear is used. There are three types of protective eyewear: goggles, face shields, and spectacles.

Goggles have several designs. One is the eyecup design seen in swimming, whereby the eye socket is completely covered. Goggles are made of hard, impact-resistant plastic that is watertight.

Because of the streamlined shape and design, contact lenses may be worn during competition when wearing these goggles. Vision may be slightly distorted; however, enhanced vision with the goggles could be a great advantage during flip turns. Another style of goggles can be worn over spectacles, such as ski goggles. These usually are well ventilated to allow air currents to minimize fogging. A third style of goggles is a sport goggle with a mask design. This type of goggle is relatively light-weight, may or may not include a shield, and is designed to withstand the forces generated by a ball traveling at significant speeds. After the introduction of mandatory protective eyewear in women's lacrosse, a 16% reduction in eye injuries occurred in the year immediately following the mandate.[11] Goggles worn for women's lacrosse must be ASTM-approved.[1]

Face shields are secondary protective devices that can be attached to specific helmets. Individuals who wear contact lenses often prefer the shield because there is less chance that a finger or hand can hit the eye. The shield can be tinted to reduce glare from the sun; however, the plastic can become scratched and may fog up in cold weather.

Spectacles (eyeglasses) contain the lenses, frame, and side shields commonly seen in industrial eye protective wear. The lenses should be 3-mm thick and be made from CR 39 plastic or polycarbonate, both of which can be incorporated with prescription lenses. CR 39 plastic lenses are less expensive, but they scratch more easily, often are thicker and heavier than polycarbonate, and are not impact resistant. In contrast, polycarbonate is lightweight, is scratch resistant, and can have an antifog and ultraviolet inhibitor incorporated into the lens. Of the clear materials developed for protective equipment, polycarbonate has the greatest impact resistance. A disadvantage of the polycarbonate is that static charges cause dust to cling to the lenses more readily than to glass lenses.

The frame should be constructed of a resilient plastic, with reinforced temples, hinges, and nose-piece. Adequate cushioning should protect the eyebrow and nasal bridge from sharp edges. Only polycarbonate eye protectors and eye frames that meet ASTM and parallel CSA standards offer enough protection for a sport participant. Approved eye guards protect the eye when impacted with a racquet ball traveling at 90 mph (40 m per second) or a racquet going 50 mph (22.2 m per second). Written acknowledgment that an eye guard meets standards can be found on the product package.

Regardless of the type of protection used, the lenses should be cleaned with warm, soapy water and rinsed with clean water, or a commercially available eyeglass cleaner should be used. A soft cloth is used to blot dry the lenses. A dry lens should never be wiped or rubbed because of the possibility of scratching the lens by moving foreign particles across the surface. The frames and elastic straps also may be cleaned with soap and water and air-dried. Lenses should be replaced when scratches affect vision or cracks appear at the edges. Protective eyewear always should be stored in a hard case to protect the polycarbonate lenses from being scratched.

Any individual with monocular vision should consult an ophthalmologist before participation in any sport or physical activity because of the resultant reduction of visual fields and depth perception. If a decision is made to participate, the individual should wear maximum eye protection during all practices and competitions. A sweatband should be worn to keep sweat out of the eye guard.

Although participants in physical activity often wear contact lenses because they improve peripheral vision and astigmatism and do not normally cloud during temperature changes, contact lenses do not protect against eye injury. Contact lenses come in two types: a hard or corneal type, which covers only the iris of the eye, and a soft or scleral type, which covers the entire front of the eye. Hard contact lenses often become dislodged and are more frequently associated with irritation from foreign bodies (e.g., corneal abrasions). Dust and other foreign matter may get underneath the lens and damage the cornea, or the cornea may be scratched while inserting or removing the lens.

Soft contact lenses can protect the eye from irritation by chlorine in pools. Although research has shown that pool water causes soft lenses to adhere to the cornea, reducing the risk of loss, wearing soft lenses while swimming is not recommended. Microorganisms found in pool water, especially *Acanthamoeba* sp., are responsible for a rare but serious corneal infection, *Acanthamoeba* keratitis. It is recommended that with or without contact lenses, goggles should always be worn in water to protect against foreign organisms and irritation from chlorine. Swimmers should wait 20 to 30 minutes after leaving the water before removing contact lenses or use saline drops if the lenses must be removed earlier. This allows time for the lenses to stop sticking to the cornea. Lenses should then be immediately disinfected. Removing the lenses too soon may cause corneal abrasions, leaving the cornea susceptible to infection.

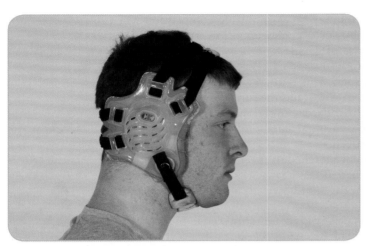

Figure 3.3. Ear protectors. Protective ear wear can prevent friction and trauma to the ear that may lead to permanent deformity.

Ear Wear

With the exception of boxing, wrestling, and water polo, few sports have specialized ear protection. Repeated friction and trauma to the ear can lead to a permanent deformity, called **hematoma auris** or cauliflower ear (see Chapter 20). For this reason, ear protection should be worn regularly in these sports. Proper fit is achieved when the chin strap is snug and the head gear does not move during contact with another player (**Fig. 3.3**). The protective ear cup should be deep enough so as not to compress the external ear. Ear protection should also be worn by those competing in the biathlon and other rifle competitions not to protect the outer ear but to protect hearing function.[1]

Mouth Guards

An intraoral, readily visible mouth guard is required in all interscholastic and intercollegiate football, ice hockey, field hockey, and men's and women's lacrosse. The American Dental Association has recommended requiring a mouth guard in acrobatics, basketball, bicycling, boxing, equestrian events, extreme sports, field events, field hockey, football, gymnastics, handball, ice hockey, in-line skating, lacrosse, martial arts, racquetball, rugby, shot putting, skateboarding, skiing, skydiving, soccer, softball, squash, surfing, volleyball, water polo, weight lifting, and wrestling.[12] The American Academy of Pediatric Dentistry recommends a properly fitted mouth guard for all children and adolescents participating in any contact or collision sport to lower the risk of orofacial injury.[13] The Academy of Sports Dentistry, although recommending the use of a properly fitted mouth guard in any contact or collision sport, highly recommends the use of a custom-fabricated mouth guard made over a dental cast and delivered under the supervision of a dentist.[14]

Properly fitted across the upper teeth, a mouth guard can absorb energy, disperse impact, cushion contact between the upper and lower teeth, and keep the upper lip away from the incisal edges of the teeth. This action significantly reduces dental and oral soft-tissue injuries and, to a lesser extent, jaw fractures, cerebral concussions, and temporomandibular joint injuries.[15,16] The practice of cutting down mouth guards to cover only the front four teeth invalidates the manufacturer's warranty, cannot prevent many dental injuries, and can lead to airway obstruction should the mouth guard become dislodged. Although some individuals may complain that use of a mouth guard adversely affects speech and breathing, a properly fitted mouth guard should not interfere with either function. The benefits of preventing oral injuries through the use of mouth guards far outweigh any disadvantages.

Three types of mouth guards are commonly available: type I (custom), type II ("boil and bite"), and type III (stock).[15] Stock or type III mouth guards are the least expensive and least protective. Stock mouth guards are designed for use without modification and in general are not recommended.[15] The most frequently used mouth guard is the type II guard. This "boil and bite" guard is thermally set and mouth-formed, with a firm outer shell fitted with a softer inner material. The guard is immersed in very warm water and then placed into the patient's mouth and molded in placed by the patient.[15] When properly fitted, the mouth-formed guard can virtually match the efficacy and comfort of the custom-made guard. This type of guard is readily available, is inexpensive, and has a loop strap for attachment to a face mask. The loop strap has two advantages: It prevents individuals from choking on the mouth guard, and it prevents the individual from losing the mouth guard when it is ejected from the mouth. These mouth guards often lack full extension into the labial and buccal vestibules. Therefore, they do not provide adequate protection against oral soft-tissue injuries. Furthermore, the thermoplastic inner material loses its elasticity at mouth temperature and may cause the protector to loosen.

The most effective type of mouth protector is the type I custom-fabricated protective mouth guard, which may be a pressure-formed, laminated type, or a vacuum-formed type. This protector is expensive and requires special training to obtain the best results. Individuals using this style of protection report that the mouth guard is more comfortable, does not interfere with breathing or speaking, permits more complete jaw closure, does not cause soft-tissue irritation, and causes less excess salivation.[17] Cost of the basic materials is higher than the thermally set mouth guards. The laminated mouth guard uses high heat and pressure to form the material, leading to less deformation of the material when worn for a long period of time. In addition, the mouth guard can be thickened in selected areas as needed and may have inserts added for additional wearer protection.[17] Vacuum-formed mouth guards, on the other hand, are less expensive and easier to design. A triple-layered, ethyl vinyl acetate material (thickness, 5 mm) makes for a sturdier and more protective mouth guard.[17] The fit of vacuum-formed mouth guards, however, can be compromised by an elastic memory because of the low heat used in their construction. After a few minutes of wearing the mouth guard, the warmth from the mouth can trigger the elastic memory, leading to adaptations in the design that make speaking and unrestricted breathing more difficult.

The recommended care of mouth guards is to thoroughly rinse the guard with water after each use and place it in a plastic mouth guard retainer box to air-dry. Periodically, the mouth guard should be soaked overnight in a weak bleach solution (i.e., 1 quart of water to 1 tablespoon of bleach).

Throat and Neck Protectors

Blows to the anterior throat can cause serious airway compromise as a result of a crushed larynx and/or upper trachea, edema of the glottic structures, vocal cord disarticulation, hemorrhage, or laryngospasm. The NCAA requires that catchers in baseball and softball wear a built-in or attachable throat guard on their mask.[1] Fencing masks and helmets used in field hockey, lacrosse, and ice hockey also provide anterior neck protectors to guard this vulnerable area.

Cervical neck rolls and collars are designed to limit excessive motion of the cervical spine and can be effective in reducing cervical hyperextension when compared to helmet and shoulder pads alone.[18] There is little evidence to support that neck rolls and collars decrease lateral cervical flexion, a common mechanism of brachial plexus traction injuries.[18] Several commercial collars can be added to the shoulder pads, including the Cowboy collar (McDavid), Longhorn neck roll, LaPorta collar, and numerous others of similar design.

The Cowboy collar is closed-cell, polyethylene foam that fits underneath the shoulder pads. This collar can be further reinforced by adding a plastic back plate along the posterior aspect of the support. The Longhorn neck roll is larger in diameter than conventional foam collars and can further restrict motion by attaching auxiliary pads over the collar at specific sites. The LaPorta collar is a more rigid, plastic shell secured directly to the shoulder pad arch. The helmet wedges into the collar, further restricting cervical motion. Cervical collars do not decrease axial loading on the cervical spine when the neck is flexed during a tackle.

 A properly fitted mouth guard will absorb energy, disperse impact, cushion the contact between the upper and lower teeth, and keep the upper lip away from the incisal edges of teeth. As such, a mouth guard will significantly reduce dental and oral soft-tissue injuries and, to a lesser extent, jaw fractures, cerebral concussion, and temporomandibular joint injuries.

PROTECTIVE EQUIPMENT FOR THE UPPER BODY

 How does use of a cantilevered system provide protection in football shoulder pads? Is this superior to flat shoulder pads?

In the upper body, special pads and braces often are used to protect the shoulder region, ribs, thorax, breasts, arms, elbows, wrists, and hands. Depending on the activity, special design modifications are needed to allow maximum protection while providing maximal performance.

Shoulder Protection

Shoulder pads should protect the soft- and bony-tissue structures in the shoulder, upper back, and chest. The external shell generally is made of a lightweight yet hard plastic. The inner lining may be composed of closed- or open-cell padding to absorb and disperse the shock; however, use of open-cell padding reduces peak impact forces compared with use of closed-cell pads.

Football shoulder pads are available in two general types: cantilevered and flat. A channel system, incorporated into both types, uses a series of long, thinner pads attached by Velcro in the shoulder pads. The pads can be individually fitted so that an air space exists at the acromioclavicular (AC) joint. The impact forces are placed entirely on the anterior and posterior aspect of the shoulder.

Cantilevered pads have a hard plastic bridge over the superior aspect of the shoulder to protect the AC joint. These bridges are lightweight, allow maximal range of motion at the shoulder, and can distribute the impact forces throughout the entire shoulder girdle. The cantilevers come in three types: inside, outside, and double. The inside cantilever fits under the arch of the pads and rests against the shoulder. It is more commonly used because it is less bulky than the outside cantilever, which sits on top of the pad outside of the arch. The outside cantilever is preferred by linemen, because it provides a larger blocking surface and more protection to the shoulder region. The double cantilever is a combination of the inside and outside cantilevers. It provides the greatest amount of protection but is not feasible for all players because of its bulk.

Flat shoulder pads are lightweight and provide less protection to the shoulder region but allow more glenohumeral joint motion. These pads often are used by quarterbacks and receivers, who must raise their arms above the head to throw or catch a pass. The flat pads often use a belt-buckle strapping to prevent pad displacement because the elastic webbing straps typically seen in most shoulder pads are inadequate to maintain proper positioning of the flat pads.

In addition to cantilevers, football shoulder pads consist of an arch, two sets of epaulets (shoulder flaps), shoulder cups, and anterior and posterior pads. The arch is shaped to fit the contour of the upper body. The epaulets extend from the edge of the arch and cover the shoulder cups to protect the top of the entire shoulder region. The shoulder cups attach to the arch, run under the epaulets, and should cover the entire deltoid. The anterior pads cover the pectoral muscles and protect the sternum and clavicles. The posterior pads cover the trapezius and protect the scapula and spine.

Football shoulder pads should be selected based on the player's position, body type, and medical history. Linemen need more protection against constant contact and require larger cantilevers. Quarterbacks, offensive backs, and receivers require smaller shoulder cups and flaps to allow greater range of motion in passing and catching. **Application Strategy 3.2** lists the general steps used in fitting football shoulder pads.

Elbow, Forearm, Wrist, and Hand Protection

The entire arm is subjected to compressive and shearing forces in a variety of sports, such as when blocking and tackling an opponent, deflecting projectiles, pushing opponents away to prevent collisions, or breaking a fall. Goalies and field players in many sports are required to have arm, elbow, wrist, and hand protection. In high school and collegiate play, however, no rigid material can be worn at the elbow or below unless covered on all sides by closed-cell foam padding.[1]

The use of a counterforce forearm brace may provide some relief for individuals with lateral and medial epicondylitis. These braces are designed to reduce tensile forces in the wrist flexors and extensors, particularly the extensor carpi radialis brevis. Although these braces may relieve pain on return to activity, debate continues about the effectiveness of counterforce forearm braces.[19] These braces should not be used for other causes of elbow pain, such as growth plate problems in children and adolescents or medial elbow instability in adults.

The forearm, wrist, and hand are especially vulnerable to external forces and often are neglected when considering protective equipment. In collision and contact sports, this area should be protected with specialized gloves and pads.

APPLICATION STRATEGY **3.2**

Fitting Football Shoulder Pads

1. Determine the chest girth measurement at the nipple line or measure the distance between shoulder tips. Select pads based on player position. Place the pads on the shoulders and tighten all straps and laces. The laces should be pulled together until touching. The straps should have equal tension and be as tight as functionally tolerable to ensure proper force distribution over the pads. Tension on the straps should prevent no more than two fingers from being inserted under the strap. The entire clavicle should be covered and protected by the pads. If the clavicles can be palpated without moving the pads, refit with a smaller pad (**Fig. A**).
2. Anterior view: The laces should be centered over the sternum with no gap between the two halves. There should be full coverage of the AC joint, clavicles, and pectoral muscles. Caps should cover the upper portion of the arch and entire deltoid muscle (**Fig. B**).
3. Posterior view: The entire scapula and trapezius should be covered with the lower pad arch extending below the inferior angle of the scapula to adequately protect the latissimus dorsi. The laces should be pulled tight and centered over the spine (**Fig. C**).
4. With the arms abducted, the neck opening should not be uncomfortable or pinch the neck. Finally, inspection should include the shoulder pads with the helmet and jersey in place to ensure that no impingement of the cervical region is present (**Fig. D**).

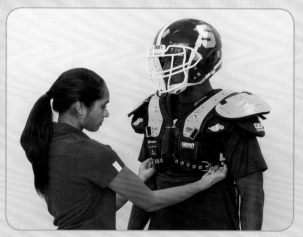

Figure A

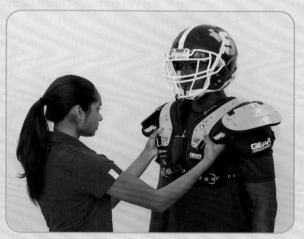

Figure B

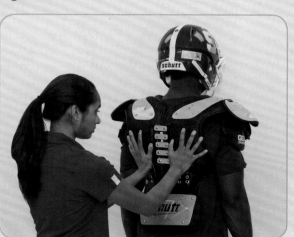

Figure C

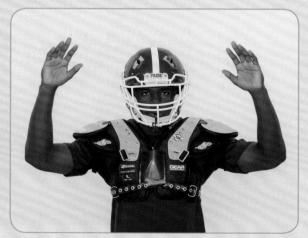

Figure D

Thorax, Rib, and Abdominal Protection

Many collision and contact sports require special protection of the thorax, rib, and abdominal areas. Commotio cordis, the second leading cause of sudden cardiac death in young athletes, is triggered by a blow from a small spherical fast moving object, such as a baseball or lacrosse ball, that strikes the athlete over the heart.[20] Although there are many commercially made wall protectors for use by youth lacrosse and baseball athletes, no chest wall protectors have been found to be effective in preventing commotio cordis.[20] Catchers in baseball and softball wear full thoracic and abdominal protectors to prevent high-speed blows from a bat or a ball. Individuals in fencing, and goalies in many sports, also wear full thoracic protectors (**Fig. 3.4A**). Quarterbacks and wide receivers in football may wear rib protectors composed of air-inflated, interconnected cylinders to absorb impact forces caused during tackling (**Fig. 3.4B**). These protectors should be fitted according to the manufacturer's instructions.

Sport Bras

Sport bras provide added support to prevent excessive vertical and horizontal breast motion during exercise. Although sport bras are designed to limit motion, few of those currently on the market actually do so, and as a result, many women continue to experience sore or tender breasts after exercise. Sport bras fall into two categories:

1. Bras made from nonelastic material with wide shoulder straps and wide bands under the breasts to provide upward support. Waist-length designs can prevent cutting in below the breasts.

2. Compressive bras that bind the breasts to the chest wall. Women with medium-sized breasts typically prefer this type.

Girls and women with small breasts may not need a special bra. Women with a size C cup or larger need a firm, supportive bra. The bra should have nonslip straps and no irritating seams or

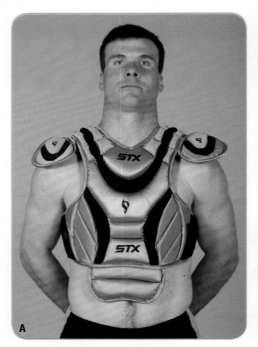 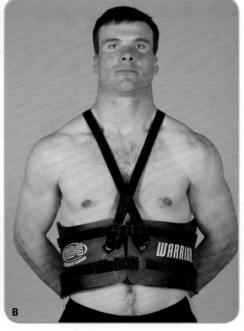

Figure 3.4. Chest and rib protection. A, Several sports require extensive chest protection (e.g., ice hockey). **B,** Rib protectors absorb impact forces caused during tackling.

fasteners next to the skin, and it should be firm and durable. Choice of fabric depends on the intensity of activity, support needs, sensitivity to fiber, and climatic and seasonal conditions. A cotton/polyester/Lycra fabric is a popular blend seen in sport bras. In hot weather, an additional outer layer of textured nylon mesh can promote natural cooling of the skin. In sports requiring significant overhead motion, bra straps should stretch to prevent the bra from riding up over the breasts. When overhead motion is not a significant part of the activity, nonstretch straps connected directly to a nonelastic cup are preferable.

Lumbar/Sacral Protection

Lumbar/sacral protection includes weight-training belts used during heavy weight lifting, abdominal binders, and other similar supportive devices (**Fig. 3.5**). Each should support the abdominal contents, stabilize the trunk, and prevent spinal deformity or injury during heavy lifting. Use of belts or binders may be beneficial in reducing spinal compression, stabilizing the spine, increasing motor unit recruitment in prime movers, and increasing exercise velocity.[21] The use of back belts to prevent occupational low back pain or to reduce lost work time because of occupational low back pain is not supported by the Canadian Centre for Occupational Health and Safety or by the U.S. National Institute for Occupational Safety and Health.[22,23] In contrast, the U.S. Occupational Safety and Health Administration's recent ergonomics regulation classified lumbar supports as personal protective equipment and suggested that they may prevent back injuries in certain industrial settings.[23]

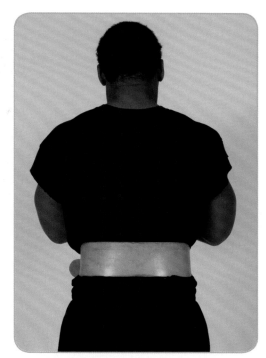

Figure 3.5. Lumbar/sacral protection. Abdominal binders support the abdominal contents, stabilize the trunk, and prevent spinal deformity or injury.

 Cantilevered pads have a hard plastic bridge over the superior aspect of the shoulder to protect the AC joint. These lightweight bridges allow maximal range of motion at the shoulder and can distribute the impact forces throughout the entire shoulder girdle. As such, they provide the greatest amount of protection to the shoulder region but are not feasible for all players because of their bulk.

PROTECTIVE EQUIPMENT FOR THE LOWER BODY

 A pitcher sustains a thigh contusion after being struck by a hard-driven baseball. What type of padding should be used to protect the thigh from another significant blow?

In the lower body, commercial braces commonly are used to protect the knee and ankle. In addition, special pads are used to protect bony- and soft-tissue structures in the hip and thigh region. Depending on the sport/activity, special design modifications are needed to allow maximum protection while providing maximal performance.

Hip and Buttock Protection

In collision and contact sports, the hip and buttock region require special pads, typically composed of hard polyethylene covered with layers of Ensolite to protect the iliac crest, sacrum, coccyx, and genital region. A girdle with special pockets can effectively hold the pads in place (**Fig. 3.6**). The male genital region is best protected by a protective cup placed in an athletic supporter.

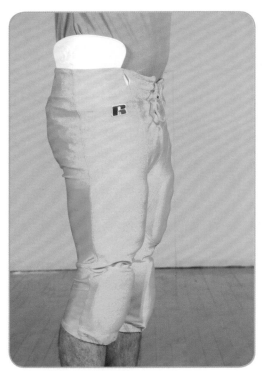

Figure 3.6. Hip protection. Girdle pads protect the gluteal and sacral area from high-velocity forces. Thigh pads can also be inserted to protect the quadriceps area.

Thigh Protection

Thigh and upper leg pads, such as those illustrated in **Figure 3.6**, slip into ready-made pockets in the girdle to prevent injury to the quadriceps area. Thigh pads should be placed over the quadriceps muscle group, approximately 6 to 7 in proximal to the patella. When using asymmetrical thigh pads, the larger flare should be placed on the lateral aspect of the thigh to avoid injury to the genitalia. In addition to thigh pads, neoprene sleeves can provide uniform compression, therapeutic warmth, and support for a quadriceps or hamstring strain.

Knee and Patella Protection

The knee is second only to the ankle and foot in incidence of injury. Knee pads can protect the area from impact during a collision or fall and, in wrestling, can protect the prepatellar and infrapatellar bursa from friction injuries. In football, knee pads reduce contusion and abrasions when falling on artificial turf.

Knee braces fall into three broad functional categories: prophylactic, functional, and rehabilitative. Prophylactic knee braces (PKBs) are designed to protect the medial collateral ligament by redirecting a lateral valgus force away from the joint itself to points more distal on the tibia and femur. Functional knee braces are widely used to provide proprioceptive feedback and to protect unstable anterior cruciate ligament (ACL) injuries or in postsurgical ACL repair or reconstruction (**Fig. 3.7A**). Rehabilitative braces provide immobilization at a selected angle after injury or surgery, permit controlled range of motion through predetermined arcs, and prevent accidental loading in non–weight-bearing patients (**Fig. 3.7B**).

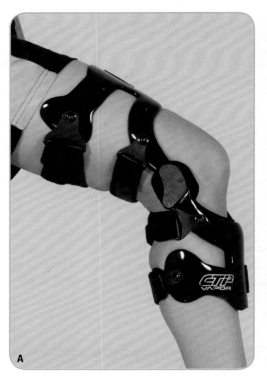
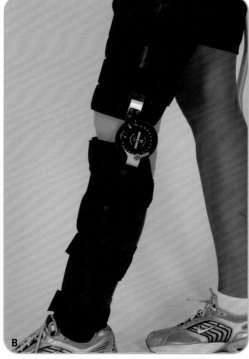

Figure 3.7. Knee braces. A, Functional knee braces control tibial translation and rotational stress relative to the femur and can provide extension limitations to protect the ACL. **B,** Rehabilitative braces provide absolute or relative immobilization following surgery.

Decisions to use any of the three major categories of knee braces should rest with the supervising physician or surgeon. Selection should be based on the projected objectives, needs of the participant relative to activity demands, cost-effectiveness, durability, fit, and comfort.

Prophylactic Knee Braces

Two general types of PKBs are the lateral and bilateral bar designs. The lateral bar PKBs are constructed with single, dual, or polycentric hinge designs. Each model has a knee hyperextension stop and is applied using a combination of neoprene wraps, Velcro straps, and/or adhesive tape. The bilateral bar PKB has a medial and lateral upright bar with biaxial hinges.

In a review of past studies between 1970 and 2006, results were inconclusive to advocate or discourage the use of PKBs in preventing knee ligament injuries in collegiate football players.[24] There is some evidence that the use of PKBs may be a contributing factor to injury.[24] As future innovations and design modifications are made in PKBs, benefits in injury prevention may become more cost-effective. Until then, clinicians should base decisions regarding PKB use on the individual needs of the athlete.

Functional Knee Braces

Functional knee braces, commonly called derotation or ACL braces, are designed to control tibial translation and rotational stress relative to the femur with a rigid, snug fit and extension limitations. There are two basic styles of ACL braces: hinge-post-strap and hinge-post-shell. Performance of either brace depends on the magnitude of anterior shear load and the internal torque applied across the tibiofemoral joint, and it may be affected by several factors, including the following:

- Technique of attachment

- Design of the brace, including hinge design; materials of fabrication; geometry of attachment interface; and mechanism of attachment

- Variables in attachment interface, including how the interface molds around the soft-tissue contours of the limb and how much displacement occurs between the rigid brace and the compliant soft tissues surrounding the distal femur and proximal tibia while loads are applied across the knee.

Derotation braces may be prescribed by a physician for individuals with a mild to moderate degree of instability who participate in activities with low or moderate load potential. Functional knee braces do not guarantee increased stability in those sports requiring cutting, pivoting, or other quick changes in direction. The braces also are used after surgical ACL reconstruction. No consensus exists in the literature relative to whether functional braces have any beneficial muscle activation or proprioceptive effects on the ACL-deficient or reconstructed limb.[25] It is suggested that patient satisfaction (e.g., symptom reduction or subjective improvement in function) may be positively related to proper fit and hinge alignment along with the maintenance of optimal muscle tone.[26,27]

Rehabilitative Braces

Rehabilitative braces come in two distinct designs: a straight immobilizer made of foam with two metal rods running down the side that is secured with Velcro to prevent all motion and a hinged brace that allows range of motion to be set by tightening a screw control. Early motion prevents joint adhesions from forming, enhances proprioception, and increases synovial nutrient flow to promote healing of cartilage and collagen tissue. The braces are lighter in weight, are adjustable for optimal fit, and can be easily removed and reapplied for wound inspection and rehabilitation. As the individual progresses through the rehabilitation program, the allowable range of motion can be adjusted periodically by the clinician. Rehabilitative braces are more effective in protecting against excessive flexion–extension than against anterior/posterior displacement.[27]

Patellofemoral Protection

Patella braces are designed to dissipate force, maintain patellar alignment, and improve patellar tracking. A horseshoe-type silicone or felt pad is sewn into an elastic or neoprene sleeve to relieve tension in recurring patellofemoral subluxation or dislocations. These braces relieve anterior knee pain syndrome.[28] An alternate brace for treating patellar pain is a strap worn over the infrapatellar tendon (**Fig. 3.8**).

Lower Leg Protection

Pads for the anterior tibial area should consist of a hard, deflective outer layer and an inner layer of thin foam. Velcro straps and stirrups help to stabilize the pad inside the sock. Many styles also incorporate padding or plastic shells over the ankle malleoli, which often are subject to repeated contusions. Several commercial designs are available.

Ankle and Foot Protection

Commercial ankle braces can be used to prevent or support a postinjury ankle sprain and come in three categories: lace-up brace, semirigid orthosis, or air-bladder brace (**Fig. 3.9**). A lace-up brace can limit all ankle motions, whereas a semirigid orthosis and air-bladder brace limit only inversion and eversion. Ankle braces have been compared with ankle taping. It is fairly well accepted that maximal loss in taping restriction for both inversion and eversion occurs after 20 minutes or more of exercise. Ankle braces are more effective in reducing ankle injuries, are easier for the wearer to apply independently, do not produce some of the skin irritation associated with adhesive tape, provide better comfort and fit, are more cost-effective, are comfortable to wear, and do not disrupt lower extremity dynamic balance.[29–32]

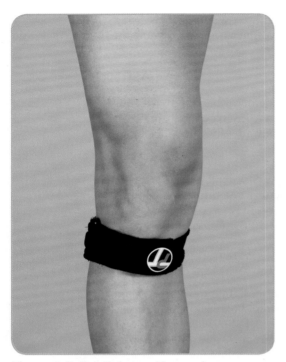

Figure 3.8. Patellofemoral brace. A strap worn over the infrapatellar ligament may relieve patellar pain.

Selection and fit of shoes also may affect injuries to the lower extremity. Shoes should adequately cushion impact forces and support and guide the foot during the stance and final push-off phase of running. In activities requiring repeated heel impact, additional heel cushioning should be present. Length should be sufficient to allow all toes to be fully extended. Individuals with toe abnormalities or bunions also may require a wider toe box. **Application Strategy 3.3** identifies factors when selecting and fitting athletic shoes.

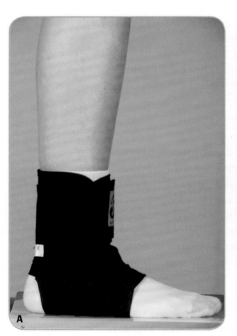
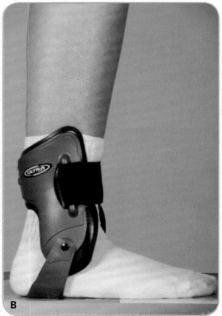
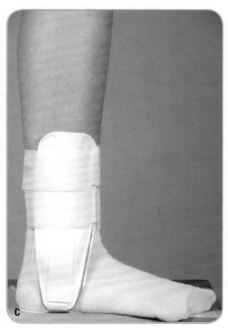

Figure 3.9. Ankle protectors. Commercial designs include the lace-up brace **(A)**, semirigid orthosis **(B)**, and air-bladder brace **(C)**.

APPLICATION STRATEGY 3.3

Factors in the Selection and Fit of Athletic Shoes

- Fit shoes toward late afternoon or evening, preferably after a workout, and wear socks typically worn during sport participation.
- Fit shoes to the longest toe of the largest foot, providing one thumb's width to the end of the toe box.
- The widest part of the shoe should coincide with the widest part of the foot. Eyelets should be at least 1 in apart with normal lacing. Women with big or wider feet should consider purchasing boy's or men's shoes.
- The sole of the shoe should provide moderate support but should not be too rigid. Sole tread typically comes in a horizontal bar (commonly used on asphalt or concrete) or waffle design (used on off-road terrain).
- The midsole may be composed of ethylene vinyl acetate (EVA), polyurethane, or preferably, a combination of the two. EVA provides good cushioning but will break down over time. Polyurethane has minimal compressibility and provides good durability and stability.
- A thermoplastic heel counter maintains its shape and firmness even in adverse weather conditions.
- Running shoes should position the heel at least 0.5 in above the outsole to minimize stretch on the Achilles tendon.
- While wearing the shoes, approximate athletic skills (walking, running, jumping, and changing directions).
- Individuals with specific conditions need special shoes, such as the following:
  - Runners with normal feet—more forefoot and toe flexibility
  - Overpronation—greater control on the medial side
  - Achilles tendonitis—a heel wedge of at least 15 mm
  - Court sports—added side-to-side stability
  - High, rigid arches—soft midsoles, curved lasts, and low or moderate hindfoot stability
  - Normal arches—firm midsole, semicurved lasts, and moderate hindfoot stability
  - Flexible low arch—very firm midsole, straight lasts, and strong hindfoot stability
- Walk in the newly purchased shoes for 2–3 days to allow them to adapt to the feet. Next, begin running or practicing in the shoes for about 25%–30% of the workout. To prevent blisters, gradually extend the length of time the shoes are worn.
- Avid runners should replace shoes every 3 months, recreational runners every 6 months.

In field sports, shoes may have a flat-sole, long-cleat, short-cleat, or multicleated design. The cleats should be properly positioned under the major weight-bearing joints of the foot and should not be felt through the sole of the shoe. Shoes with the longer, irregular cleats placed at the peripheral margin of the sole, with a number of smaller pointed cleats positioned in the middle of the sole, produce significantly higher torsional resistance and are associated with a significantly higher rate of ACL injury compared with shoes having flat cleats, screw-in cleats, or pivot disks.[33] When increased temperature is a factor, such as when playing on turf, only the flat-soled, basketball-style turf shoes are reported to have low-release coefficients at varying elevated temperatures.[34] This may lead to a lesser incidence of lower leg injuries. In individuals with arch problems, the shoe should include adequate forefoot, arch, and heel support. In all cases, individuals should select shoes based on the demands of the activity.

Specific foot conditions, such as fallen arches, pronated feet, or medial tibial stress syndrome, can be padded and supported with inner soles, semirigid orthotics, and rigid orthotics. Cushioning is a critical function of sport shoes with the midsole playing the most important role in attenuating impact shock.[35] Research has found that a 6.5-mm thick polymeric foam rubber material is more effective in absorbing heel-strike impact than a viscoelastic polymeric shoe insert.[36] Antishock heel lifts use a dense silicone mixture to cushion heel impact to relieve strain on the Achilles tendon, and heel cups reduce tissue shearing and shock in the calcaneal region. Other commercially available pads may be used to protect the forefoot region, bunions, and toes, or adhesive felt (moleskin), felt, and foam can be cut to construct similar pads.

Foot Orthotics

Orthotics are devices used in the treatment and prevention of foot and gait abnormalities and related conditions, such as plantar fasciitis, heel pain, shin splints, patellofemoral pain, and low back pain.

By changing the angle at which the foot strikes the surface, orthotics can make standing, walking, and running more comfortable and efficient. Orthotics are available in several forms and are constructed of a variety of materials. Foot orthotics fall into three broad categories: orthotics to change foot function, protective orthotics, and those that combine functional control and protection.

Foot orthotics can be rigid, soft, or semirigid. Rigid orthotics are designed to control motion. These orthotics are made from a firm material, such as plastic or carbon fiber, to increase their longevity and decrease the likelihood for changes in their shape. Most often, rigid orthotics are worn in dress or walking shoes. Soft orthotics assist in absorbing shock, improving balance, and relieving painful pressure sites. The use of soft, compressible materials in the construction of soft orthotics readily enables adjustment to changing weight-bearing forces. Eventually, however, the material breaks down; therefore, soft orthotics must be replaced regularly. Semirigid orthotics are used to provide for dynamic balance of the foot while walking or participating in sport and physical activity. This type of orthotic is constructed of layers of soft material that are reinforced with hard, rigid materials.

In addition to the proper selection of the appropriate type of orthotic, accurate fit is an essential component in the use of orthotics. As such, orthotics should be measured and fitted by a qualified medical professional.

 The pitcher's thigh should be protected with nonresilient padding made of high-density material, such as orthoplast or thermoplast. The padding should be layered with a soft material that has shock-absorbing qualities, such as closed-cell foam.

SUMMARY

1. Protective equipment is effective only when it is properly fitted and maintained, periodically cleaned and disinfected, and used as intended.

2. The sport participant must be protected from high-velocity, low-mass forces to prevent focal injuries and from low-velocity, high-mass forces to prevent diffuse injuries.

3. Design and selection of protective equipment is based on the following energy-absorbing material factors: thickness, density, resilience, and temperature.

4. The NOCSAE establishes standards for football, baseball, softball, and lacrosse helmets and face masks.

5. The HECC of the CSA establishes standards for ice hockey helmets and face masks.

6. The ASTM establishes standards for protective eyewear, ice hockey helmets and face masks, and other protective equipment.

7. The athletic trainer is ultimately responsible for knowing the rules and standards governing the selection and fitting of protective equipment for each sport.

APPLICATION QUESTIONS

1. A high school football coach has 50 sets of uniforms. The last student selected for the team is also the last student to receive a uniform. The available pants and shoulder pads are slightly large for the student. In addition, the helmet does not fit snugly. The coach does not anticipate that the student will see much playing time; he kept him on the team roster because the student is enthusiastic and a hard worker. As the school's athletic trainer, how would you respond to this situation? Is it acceptable for the student to practice in the uniform and safety equipment that was provided to him? Explain your response.

2. A high school basketball coach is concerned about the various oral injuries that have occurred on the school's basketball teams. The coach asks for your input in providing a rationale to convince the administration to contract with a local dentist to provide customized mouth guards for the teams. How would you respond? What recommendations might you consider in developing the rationale?

3. An athletic trainer for a college football team fits the place kicker with a football helmet that has a double bar face guard. However, the athletic trainer notices that the kicker has come to the practice field with a single bar face guard. The kicker insists that the double bar guard interferes with his vision during field-goal attempts. Should the athletic trainer permit the kicker to use the single bar face guard during practice? Why or why not?

4. A high school football player has been cleared to practice following rehabilitation for a cervical sprain. The school's athletic trainer makes alterations to the helmet and shoulder pads of the player as a prophylactic measure to reduce the potential for another future cervical sprain. The team physician is in support of the actions taken by the athletic trainer. Is the athletic trainer potentially liable if the athlete sustains an injury while wearing the altered equipment?

REFERENCES

1. Parsons JT. *2014–2015 NCAA Sports Medicine Handbook*. Indianapolis, IN: National Collegiate Athletic Association; 2014.

2. McCrory P, Meeuwisse W, Aubry M, et al. Consensus statement on concussion in sport: the 4th International Conference on Concussion in Sport, Zurich, November 2012. *J Athl Train*. 2013; 48(4):554–575.

3. Broglio SP, Cantu RC, Gioia GA, et al. National Athletic Trainers' Association position statement: management of sport concussion. *J Athl Train*. 2014;49(2):245–265.

4. National Operating Committee on Standards for Athletic Equipment. Standard performance specification for newly manufactured football helmets. http://www.nocsae.org. NOCSAE DOC (ND)002-13m13. Revised December 2013. Accessed July 23, 2015.

5. Banerjee R, Palumbo MA, Fadale PD. Catastrophic cervical spine injuries in the collision sport athlete, part 1: epidemiology, functional anatomy, and diagnosis. *Am J Sports Med*. 2004; 32(4):1077–1087.

6. Valovich McLeod TC. Proper fit and maintenance of ice-hockey helmets. *Athl Ther Today*. 2005; 10(6):54–57.

7. Nicholls RL, Elliott BC, Miller K. Impact injuries in baseball: prevalence, aetiology and the role of equipment performance. *Sports Med*. 2004; 34(1):17–25.

8. Sheffield-Moore M, Short KR, Kerr CG, et al. Thermoregulatory responses to cycling with and without a helmet. *Med Sci Sports Exerc*. 1997; 29(6):755–761.

9. Parkinson GW, Hike KE. Bicycle helmet assessment during well visits reveals severe shortcomings in condition and fit. *Pediatrics*. 2003; 112(2):320–323.

10. Wellbery C. Proper bicycle helmet fit reduces head injuries. *Am Fam Physician*. 2004;69(5): 1271.

11. Lincoln AE, Caswell SV, Almquist JL, et al. Effectiveness of the womens' lacrosse protective eyewear mandate in the reduction of eye injuries. *Am J Sports Med*. 2012;40(3):611–614.

12. American Dental Association. For the dental patient. The importance of using mouthguards. Tips for keeping your smile safe. *J Am Dent Assoc*. 2004;135(7):1061.

13. American Academy of Pediatric Dentistry. Journal of the American Academy of Pediatric Dentistry, Special Issue Reference Manual 1998– 1999, 20(1):23–24.

14. Academy of Sports Dentistry. Position statement: a properly fitted mouthguard. http:// www.academyforsportsdentistry.org/position -statement. Accessed January 23, 2015.

15. Tuna EB, Ozel E. Factors affecting sports-related orofacial injuries and the importance of mouthguards. *Sports Med*. 2014;44(6):777–783.

16. Desmarteau D. Recommendations for the use of mouthguards in contact sports: can they also reduce the incidence and severity of cerebral concussions? *Curr Sports Med Rep*. 2006;5(5): 268–271.

17. Croll TP, Castaldi CR. Custom sports mouth guard modified for orthodontic patients and children in the transitional dentition. *Pediatr Dent*. 2004;26(5):417–420.

18. Gorden JA, Straub SJ, Swanik CB, et al. Effects of football collars on cervical hyperextension and lateral flexion. *J Athl Train*. 2003;38(3): 209–215.

19. Kroslak M, Murrell AC. Tennis elbow counterforce bracing. *Techn Shoulder Elbow Surg*. 2007;8(2):75–79.

20. Maron BJ, Estes NA III. Commotio cordis. *N Engl J Med*. 2010;362(10):917–927.

21. Renfro GJ, Ebben WP. A review of the use of lifting belts. *Strength Cond J*. 2006;28(1):68–74.

22. Canadian Task Force on Preventive Health Care. Use of back belts to prevent occupational low-back pain. Recommendation statement from the Canadian Task Force on Preventive Health Care. *CMAJ*. 2003;169(3):213–214.

23. Occupational Safety and Health Administration. Ergonomic program: final rule. *Fed Register*. 2000;65(220):68261–68870.

24. Pietrosimone BG, Grindstaff TL, Linens SW, et al. A systematic review of prophylactic braces in the prevention of knee ligament injuries in collegiate football players. *J Athl Train*. 2008;43(4):409–415.

25. Birmingham TB, Bryant DM, Giffin JR, et al. A randomized controlled trial comparing the effectiveness of functional knee brace and neoprene sleeve use after anterior cruciate ligament reconstruction. *Am J Sports Med*. 2008;36(4):648–655.

26. Vandertuin JF, Grant JA. The role of functional knee braces in managing ACL injuries. *Athl Ther Today*. 2004;9(2):58–62.

27. Mallory N, Kelsberg G, Ketchell D, et al. Clinical inquiries. Does a knee brace decrease recurrent ACL injuries? *J Fam Pract*. 2003;52(10):803–804.

28. BenGal S, Lowe J, Mann G, et al. The role of the knee brace in the prevention of anterior knee pain syndrome. *Am J Sports Med*. 1997;25(1):118–122.

29. Hardy L, Huxel K, Brucker J, et al. Prophylactic ankle braces and star excursion balance measures in healthy volunteers. *J Athl Train*. 2008;43(4):347–351.

30. Osborne MD, Rizzo TD Jr. Prevention and treatment of ankle sprain in athletes. *Sports Med*. 2003;33(15):1145–1150.

31. Hume PA, Gerrard DF. Effectiveness of external ankle support. Bracing and taping in rugby union. *Sports Med*. 1998;25(5):285–312.

32. Thacker SB, Stroup DF, Branche CM, et al. The prevention of ankle sprains in sports. A systematic review of the literature. *Am J Sports Med*. 1999;27(6):753–760.

33. Lambson RB, Barnhill BS, Higgins RW. Football cleat design and its effect on anterior cruciate ligament injuries. A three-year prospective study. *Am J Sports Med*. 1996;24(2):155–159.

34. Torg JS, Stilwell G, Rogers K. The effect of ambient temperature on the shoe-surface interface release coefficient. *Am J Sports Med*. 1996;24(1):79–82.

35. Chiu HT, Shiang TY. Effects of insoles and additional shock absorption foam on the cushioning properties of sport shoes. *J Appl Biomech*. 2007;23(2):119–127.

36. Shiba N, Kitaoka HB, Cahalan TD, et al. Shock-absorbing effect of shoe insert materials commonly used in management of lower extremity disorders. *Clin Ortho Relat Res*. 1995;(310):130–136.

Protective Taping and Wrapping

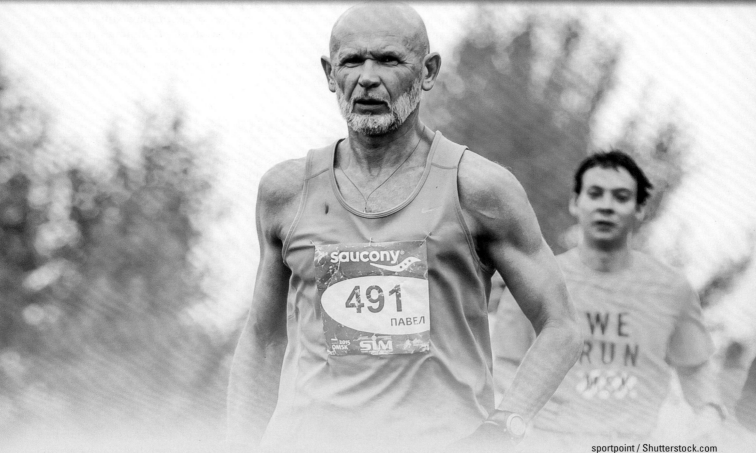

sportpoint / Shutterstock.com

STUDENT OUTCOMES

1. Identify uses of prophylactic tape and wraps in the management of musculoskeletal injuries.

2. Explain common principles used in the application of tape and wraps.

3. Identify characteristics of materials in protective taping and wrapping design.

4. Describe common taping and wrapping techniques used to prevent or reduce the risk of reinjury.

5. Differentiate between standard techniques for protective taping, McConnell taping, cohesive system taping, and Kinesio Taping techniques.

INTRODUCTION

Taping or wrapping a body part can provide support and prophylactic protection to prevent injury while allowing functional movement and is used extensively during rehabilitation to reduce the risk of reinjury. Providing support to an injured body part may allow for an early return to activity while controlling undesirable movement that may impede the healing process. No matter the technique utilized, each taping must be customized based on the particular patient and condition being treated.

In this chapter, the general principles of taping and wrapping are covered followed by information on the various types of tape and wrapping materials currently available. Techniques that serve as the building blocks common to many different types of taping applications are covered within this chapter. More recent taping techniques, such as cohesive taping systems and Kinesio Taping will also be discussed in more detail in the final section of this chapter.

PRINCIPLES OF TAPING AND WRAPPING

 As a prophylactic measure, a basketball player with a history of lateral ankle sprains is taped to reduce the risk of reinjury. What is the procedure for removing the tape?

Tape and wraps are devices used to:

1. Provide immediate first aid

2. Limit excessive joint movement

3. Support an injured body part

4. Provide compression

5. Provide proprioceptive feedback

6. Secure protective pads and dressings

7. Allow early resumption of activity

8. Reduce the chance of reinjury

There are two ways the application of tape assists in preventing reinjury of the tissues that stabilize joints. First, tape limits range of motion and provides additional external stabilization by acting as an external ligament. Second, tape enhances the stability of the joint through increasing joint **proprioception**. However, due to elongation and stretching, tape has been found to lose much of its supportive properties after about 20 minutes of activity.[1,2] Therefore, an injury must be fully evaluated to determine the pathology and severity and phase of healing to determine the appropriate technique and type of tape to utilize. Injured anatomical structures must be identified, and an appropriate therapeutic rehabilitation program should be developed to ensure a safe return to activity. Too often, a premature return to activity can lead to reinjury or a chronic injury. Although tape and wraps may allow the individual to resume early activity, their use should never take the place of a comprehensive rehabilitation program. Only those individuals who are participating in a supervised therapeutic exercise program should be taped or wrapped.

A rehabilitation program, as discussed in a later chapter, should focus on regaining full range of motion, proprioception, strength, endurance, and power in the injured body part while maintaining cardiovascular fitness. The individual should be able to complete, pain-free, all functional tests before being cleared for participation. In each phase of activity, the correct taping or wrapping technique should be selected and properly applied. It is also important to note that when improperly or poorly applied, a taping or wrapping technique can cause damage, including blisters or skin irritation, abnormal stress on body parts, and increased risk of injury to the region. Taping should not be applied if the injury assessment is not adequate or incomplete, the diagnosis is unknown, there is joint instability or a possible fracture, or if there is swelling or irritated skin.[3]

Tape and Wraps

With so many options available, selecting and purchasing taping products may be overwhelming. Factors such as color, width, strength, adherent properties, and tape quality go in to the decision-making process.

Makeup of Tape

Tape is described using four identifiers: *threads per square inch*, *tensile strength*, *composition, and adhesive mass.*[4]

◼ Threads per Square Inch

The number of vertical **threads per square inch** is referred to as warp, whereas horizontal threads per square inch are the woof. Less expensive, lighter tape contains 45 vertical fibers and 65 or fewer horizontal fibers per inch. Heavier tape contains 65 vertical fibers and 85 or more horizontal fibers.[3] Although tape is subjected to shear, tensile, flexure, and peel forces, ultimately, it is the tensile strength that is most important to consider.[5]

◼ Tensile Strength

Tensile strength is the measurement of how much tensile force a material can withstand before it fails. Manufacturers of athletic tape assess tensile strength in accordance with industry standards and report tensile strength as pounds per square inch. The higher the pounds per square inch, the stronger the tensile force or strength is of the tape.[4]

◼ Composition

Composition refers to the materials that are used to make the tape. In general, athletic tape is made primarily of cotton, synthetic fibers, or in combination.[4] Tape may be elastic or nonelastic. Elastic tape is used to hold protective pads and dressings in place, provide compression, give proprioceptive feedback, and provide support. One advantage of elastic tape is that it allows muscles to contract without impeding circulation or neurological function. The level of elasticity in tape varies from brand to brand—the more elastic the tape, the easier the application. Elastic tape should be stretched to between one-third and one-half of its elastic capability before application. If it is applied too tightly, the tape can restrict circulation and function of the body part, leading to increased pain or discomfort. Products come in a variety of widths and tensile strengths. A product must be selected according to the pathology of the injury and the desired effect. Nonelastic tape provides support to joints by restricting excessive motions.

The composition of tape may also be designed to produce tapes that are porous or nonporous. Porous tape, primarily made of synthetic fibers, allows heat and sweat to pass through minute openings in the tape, which allows the skin to remain cool while also permitting the tape itself to remain dry and to maintain its properties longer.[5] Nonporous tape, primarily made from cotton, makes the application more occlusive, thus increasing the potential for damage to the underlying skin from friction and retained heat. Nonporous tape will absorb the sweat and may result in decreased tape performance.[5] Like elastic tape, nonelastic tape comes in a variety of widths, primarily ranging from 0.5 to 3.0 in.

Tape may be bleached or unbleached. Bleached tape tends to be more aesthetically pleasing, but it is more expensive and does not offer better support compared with unbleached tape.[4] Nonelastic tape is more difficult to apply than elastic tape. The body's natural contours increase the potential for wrinkles and excessive pressure from friction on underlying tissues, which can lead to blisters or cuts under the tape if it is applied incorrectly. An effective, wrinkle-free, nonelastic taping technique requires extensive practice and patience.

◼ Adhesive Mass

The final identifier used to describe tape is **adhesive mass** or stickiness. Zinc oxide adhesive is utilized in making athletic tape and assists in keeping the tape in place. Some people may be allergic to the adhesive or other materials found within the tape, and it is important to always question the patient regarding allergies before applying tape.[1]

Types of Tape

Different types of tapes can be categorized based on overall tensile strength with underwrap being the absolute weakness moving to the nontearable tapes being the strongest.[5] It is important to note that tensile strength can vary within each category depending on the product. Known tensile strengths are presented in **Table 4.1**.

■ Underwrap

The only product found in the "weakest category" is underwrap, which is also referred to as pre-wrap. Prewrap is a pressed foam rubber. Prewrap has less than 1 lb of tensile strength and acts as a protective layer. In order to keep the prewrap in place, an adhesive spray needs to be applied to the skin first. The prewrap is then laid down, followed by the application of tape. Again, it is important to check with the patient to see if he or she has allergies to the chemicals contained within the spray.[1]

■ Stretch Tearable Tape

The second category is stretch tearable tape. Made out of cloth adhesive material that stretches, tearable tape is used to keep pads in place and stimulate proprioception but will do little to limit range of motion.[5] Termed "tearable" because the material can be ripped by hand, scissors are not needed to cut the tearable tape. Tensile strength of tearable tape varies and is a factor that should be considered in light of the goal of the taping technique selected.

■ Cohesive Tearable Tape

In the middle of the strength spectrum is cohesive or self-adhesive tearable tape. Made of synthetic material, cohesive tape is designed to adhere to itself, sweat-resistant, and breathable.[5] An advantage of cohesive tape is that the application of tape adherent sprays and underwrap can be eliminated. Tensile strength of cohesive tearable tape varies from product to product.

■ Athletic Tearable Tape

Many different manufacturers make the white tearable tape that is instantly recognizable as "athletic tape." Although the most common color is white, athletic tape comes in many different colors and is made out of cotton or synthetic fibers. Tensile strength varies by manufacturer, and different grades/strengths of tearable tape are offered within product lines. The use of spray tape adherent and prewrap is needed when using cotton athletic tape. All cotton athletic tape, regardless of the manufacturer, is nonporous. The combination of the underwrap and nonporous nature of cotton tape can result in the taping technique becoming wet as it absorbs the athlete's sweat. When wet, the material stretches and, in some ranges of motion, loses some of the stabilizing properties provided by the initial taping technique.[1,2,5,6] Synthetic athletic tape is porous and does not become wet and therefore can maintain much of the stabilizing properties provided by the initial taping technique.[6]

TABLE 4.1 Known Tensile Strength			
TEARABLE STRETCH	**COHESIVE TEARABLE**	**ATHLETIC TAPE**	**NONTEARABLE SPECIALTY TAPE**
		COACH[a] (36 psi)	
		ZONAS[a] (38 psi)	
PowerFAST[b] (23 psi)	PowerFlex[b] (23 psi)		
	PowerSpeed[b] (32 psi)		
	VictoryTape[b] (37 psi)		
	PowerTape[b] (41 psi)		

[a]COACH and ZONAS are trademark products of the Johnson & Johnson Sports Medicine. Data was collected from Andover Healthcare Department of Sports Medicine Education, Research, and Development.
[b]PowerFAST, PowerFlex, PowerSpeed, VictoryTape, and PowerTape are Andover Healthcare, Inc. products, and data on tensile strength was collected directly from Andover Healthcare Department of Sports Medicine Education, Research, and Development.

■ Nontearable Tape

Tape that cannot be torn with the fingers is classified as nontearable. Also known as specialty tape, there is a wide range of tape within this category such as moleskin, ELASTIKON, Leukotape, Jaystrap, and Kinesio tape. Nontearable tape has the strongest tensile strength.

Wraps

All cloth elastic wraps contain fibers that allow it to be stretched. Elastic wraps can be used to secure pads and dressings, provide compression and support, and give proprioceptive feedback. These wraps are typically secured in place with metal clips or tape. A special type of elastic wrap, called a **cohesive elastic bandage**, is composed of two layers of rayon separated by spandex and is designed to make the material adhere to itself eliminating the need for adhesive tape or metal clips to prevent slippage. Like stretch tape, elastic wrap should be stretched to between one-third and one-half of its elastic capability before application. If it is applied too tightly, the wrap can restrict circulation and function of the body part, leading to increased pain or discomfort. Products come in a variety of widths and tensile strengths. A product must be selected according to the pathology of the injury and the desired effect.

Application of Tape

The body part should be clean, dry, and free of hair before application. Hair should be removed with an electric shaver or disposable razor. Any minor open wounds, such as blisters or cuts, should be cleaned with normal saline and covered with a sterile dressing. Areas sensitive to friction, such as the Achilles tendon or dorsum of the foot, should be protected with a pad and lubricant. Petroleum jelly or a commercial skin lubricant may be applied to a gauze or foam pad.

Unless the specific technique being applied requires the body part being taped to be placed in a specific position, the body part is usually taped in a **functional position**. For example, when applying a hip spica, the patient is required to stand on a table with the hip and knee placed in slight flexion, which is a functional position for the hip. This position is accomplished by placing the patient's heel on a 1.5- to 2.0-in heel lift. Old tape cores wound with tape or a commercial taping block may be used. Tape rolls, even those of the appropriate height, compress and become unusable over time.

When the skin has been prepared appropriately, a light layer of tape adherent is sprayed onto the skin surface and allowed to dry. This provides a sticky surface permitting the tape to adhere better to the skin and provides a layer of protection for the skin. For individuals who are sensitive to tape, are taped on a daily basis, or are allergic to tape, a single layer of foam underwrap may be applied over the skin before tape application. It is critical that only one layer of underwrap be applied because several layers may increase sweating under the tape and, in doing so, compromise the effectiveness of the taping technique.

Proper positioning of the athletic trainer is as important as proper positioning of the patient. To avoid unnecessary low back stress, a table of an appropriate height should be used to prevent excessive bending at the waist. If it is necessary to reach above shoulder level, the athletic trainer should stand on a bench or the patient should be seated. When several dozen patients must be taped in a short amount of time, proper positioning is critical to prevent overtiring of the athletic trainer.

To avoid wrinkles in the tape, only a few inches of tape should be unrolled at one time. As the tape is guided around the contours of the body part, slight tension should be applied. In tearing the tape, the roll should be held in one hand and pinched between the thumb and index finger of each hand (**Fig. 4.1**). A quick push of the roll away from the body while

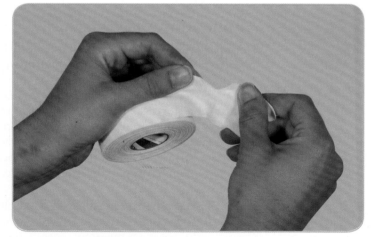

Figure 4.1. Tearing tape. Hold the tape roll in the dominant hand. Pinch the tear site with the index finger and thumb of both hands. Hold the nondominant hand still as the dominant hand pushes the roll quickly away from the body.

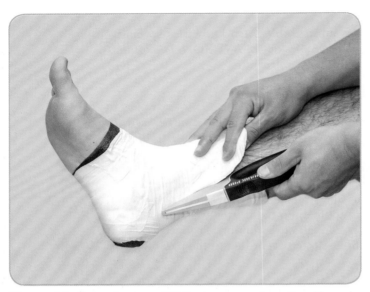

Figure 4.2. Removing tape. Lift the tape away from the skin and advance the scissors or tape cutters along the body's natural contours, avoiding sensitive tissues.

holding one hand still results in the tape ends being evenly torn.

In most taping techniques, each subsequent strip of tape should overlap the previous strip by one-half to one-third the width of the tape. The tape should be applied snugly but without impairing circulation. Circulation can be assessed by taking a pulse distal to the tape application, feeling for skin temperature, or blanching the nails to check capillary refill. Skin color and temperature should be the same bilaterally above and below the taping. Following the application of the tape, the patient should check the body part for support and function.

Removal of Tape

Because prolonged contact with the skin may cause tissue breakdown and bacteria formation, tape should be removed immediately after activity. The tip of the tape cutters or scissors can be dipped in a skin lubricant to facilitate removing the tape from the skin. The scissors or tape cutter should lift the tape up and away from the skin and then advance along the body's natural contours (**Fig. 4.2**). For example, with an injury to the lateral aspect of the ankle, the initial position of the tape cutter is the posteromedial aspect of the tape application. Next, the cutter is moved distally around the posteromedial malleolus, extending through the arch toward the toes. In this manner, the tape cutter or scissors does not place any undue pressure on sensitive, injured structures. In removing the tape, the skin must be stabilized while the tape is pulled in the direction of the natural hair growth. Tearing tape rapidly off the skin can lead to damaged skin, open wounds, and pain. Following the removal of the tape, the skin should be cleansed with a de-adhesive and then washed with soap and water and dried thoroughly. In addition, a skin moisturizer should be applied to prevent skin dryness and breakdown. **Application Strategy 4.1** summarizes application techniques for taping a body part.

The skin should be inspected regularly for signs of irritation, blisters, or infection, including areas that are red, dry, hot, and tender. These signs indicate a possible allergic reaction to the tape or tape adherent. If the skin cannot be protected from irritation, it may be necessary to fit the patient with an appropriate commercial brace rather than risk continued irritation.

Application of Wraps

The application of elastic wraps should begin with the body part in a position of maximum muscle contraction. This ensures that movement and circulation are not impaired during activity. A wrap should be started distal to the injury site and continue to the area proximal to the injury. This prevents any edema formation from settling in the distal digits and provides support against gravitational forces. The wrap should be stretched from one-half to one-third of its total elastic capability before application. Excessive stretching may constrict circulation, compress superficial nerves, and impair function. Each turn of the wrap should overlap at least one-half of the previous, underlying strip. The end of the wrap may be secured with elastic tape for added support. **Application Strategy 4.2** summarizes application techniques for wrapping a body part.

 Using a tape cutter dipped in a skin lubricant, the tape should be removed immediately after practice. The cutter should follow a path along the body's natural contours; because the injury is an inversion sprain, the cut should take place on the medial side of the ankle. During cutting, the tape should be lifted up and away from the skin. Removing the tape involves slowly pulling it in the direction of the natural hair growth. Following the removal, the skin should be cleansed and a skin moisturizer should be applied.

APPLICATION STRATEGY 4.1

Application Techniques for Taping a Body Part

Prior to Application

- First check with patient for allergies to any materials used in the taping technique.
- The body part should be clean, dry, and free of hair.
- Cover open wounds with a sterile dressing.
- Apply a lubricated pad over sensitive areas, such as the dorsum of the foot, Achilles tendon, or popliteal space.
- Spray a light layer of tape adherent onto the skin surface.
- For individuals sensitive or allergic to tape, or who must be taped on a daily basis, apply a single layer of foam underwrap.

During Application

- Use a table at an appropriate height to minimize the low back stress of the athletic trainer.
- Should it be necessary to reach above the shoulder level, the athletic trainer should stand on a bench or the patient should be seated.
- Place the body part to be taped in a position of function to ensure the desired result.
- If the hip and knee must be slightly flexed, place the heel on a 1.5- to 2.0-in heel lift.
- Unroll only a few inches of tape at one time as a way to prevent wrinkles.
- Guide the tape around the contours of the body part while applying slight tension.
- Each strip of tape should overlap the previous strip by one-half to one-third the width of the tape.
- When completed, check circulation.

After Participation in Activity

- Remove the tape immediately to prevent skin breakdown.
- Dip the tip of the tape cutters or scissors in a skin lubricant, lift the tape up away from the skin, and cut along the body's natural contours.
- Always cut on the side opposite the injury site.
- Remove the tape in the direction of the natural hair growth.
- Cleanse the skin with tape remover and then soap and water. Dry thoroughly.
- Apply a skin moisturizer to prevent dry skin.
- Inspect the skin regularly for signs of irritation, blisters, or infection.

APPLICATION STRATEGY 4.2

Application Techniques for Wrapping a Body Part

- Cover open wounds with a sterile dressing and secure with tape.
- Place the injured muscles in a shortened state but then have them maximally contracted.
- If the hip and knee must be slightly flexed, place the heel on a 1.5- to 2-in heel lift.
- Begin distal to the injured area and move in a proximal direction, lifting up against gravity.
- Stretch the wrap one-half to one-third of its total elastic capability prior to application.
- Overlap each turn of the wrap by at least one-half of the previous underlying strip.
- Secure the end of the wrap with elastic tape for added support.
- After participation, remove the wrap and wash it in a washing machine on a delicate cycle. If possible, hang the wrap to dry to prevent losing its elasticity.

COMMON TAPING AND WRAPPING TECHNIQUES

? An individual has sustained a mild thigh contusion. Immediate management of the injury includes maintaining compression on the injury throughout the remainder of the day. How should the compression be applied, and why?

The following taping and wrapping techniques are provided as a guide to application. When taping or wrapping a body part, it is appropriate to adapt the technique to the individual's needs.

Taping and Wrapping Techniques for the Lower Extremity

Great Toe Taping

This taping technique is used to limit motion at the 1st metatarsophalangeal joint. Preparation for this taping includes placing an adhesive dressing (e.g., Band-Aid) over the nail of the great toe for protective purposes. This technique begins with the placement of **anchor strips** on the great toe and at the midfoot (**Fig. 4.3A**). If prevention of hyperextension of the toe is desired, a strip of tape is applied from the distal anchor to the proximal anchor on the plantar surface of the foot (**Fig. 4.3B**). Additional supportive strips are applied until the base of the 1st metatarsal is covered (**Fig. 4.3C**).

This procedure is completed by reanchoring the strips at the great toe and midfoot (**Fig. 4.3D**). If the injury involves hyperflexion, the supportive tape strips run on the dorsum of the toe and foot. Occasionally, the patient may have both a hyperextension and a hyperflexion injury; in this case, the two tapings may be combined to limit motion in both directions. This technique is most often applied using cloth athletic tape. However, variations include using tearable elastic tape.

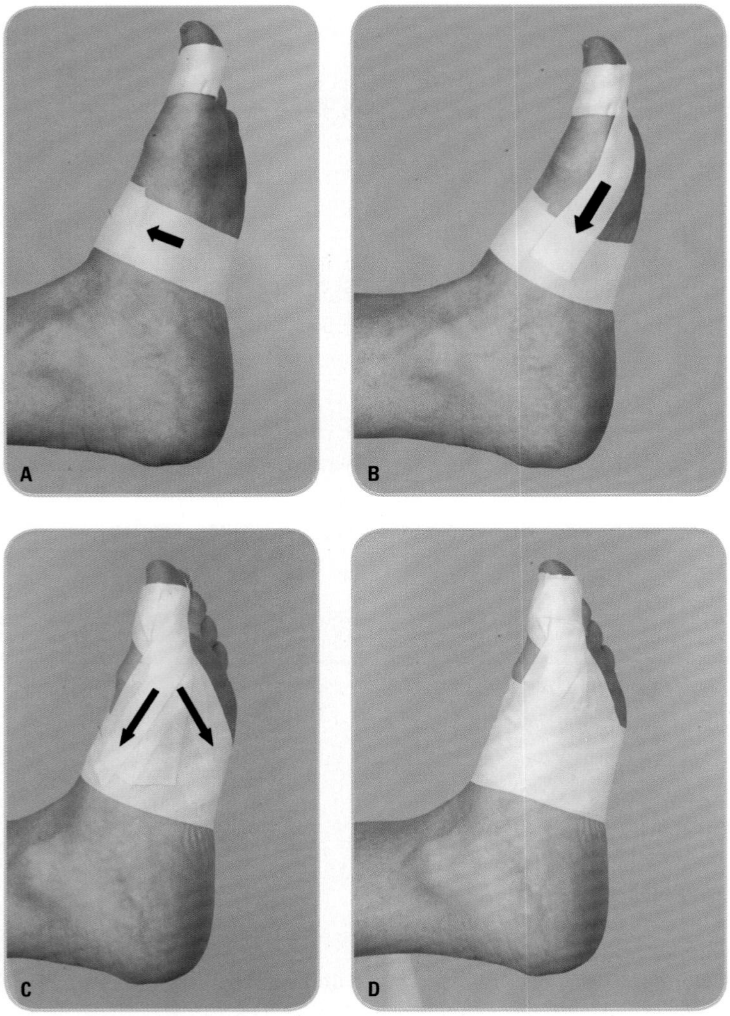

Arch Support

Arch support may be necessary in individuals with plantar fasciitis, high arches, fallen arches, or arch sprains and strains, or in those who run or jump excessively. Several techniques can be used to support the arches of the foot. In taping the arches, the patient's foot should be in a position of slight plantar flexion.

■ Arch Support: Technique 1

A simple arch support uses three to four circular strips of tape applied around the midfoot region. The first strip is anchored on the dorsum of the foot and encircles the lateral border of the foot. As the strip moves across the plantar aspect, the strip is secured under the 5th metatarsal with one hand while the other hand applies slight tension in an upward direction through the medial longitudinal arch (**Fig. 4.4A**). In this manner, tension is applied only through the arch area and does not constrict the blood vessels on the lateral aspect of the foot. Each subsequent strip overlaps the previous, underlying strip by one-half, until the entire arch is covered. In addition, by applying the strips from the distal to the proximal aspect of the foot,

Figure 4.3. Great toe taping. A, Apply anchors. **B,** Apply strip to plantar surface. **C,** Apply additional support strips. **D,** Apply anchors to close.

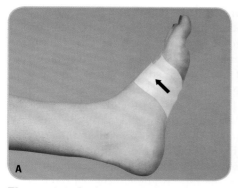 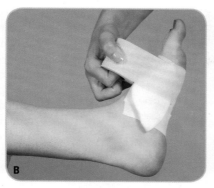 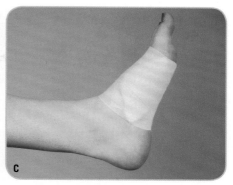

Figure 4.4. Arch support: Technique 1. A, Apply tape across the plantar aspect, secure under the 5th metatarsal, apply slight tension in an upward direction through the medial longitudinal arch (MLA). **B,** Apply overlapping strips until arch is covered. **C,** A pad can be applied under circular straps for additional support.

the exposed edges of the tape do not roll when socks are placed on the foot. An arch pad may be added to this technique for additional support (**Fig. 4.4B** and **C**). This technique is most often applied using cloth athletic tape. However, variations include using tearable elastic tape.

■ Arch Support: Technique 2

If additional support is required, an alternative X-arch technique may be applied. This technique can be particularly useful in providing support for the plantar fascia. An anchor strip is placed at the level of the distal metatarsal heads. Beginning at the base of the great toe, the tape is pulled along the medial aspect of the foot, around the heel, and angled across the arch to end at the starting point (**Fig. 4.5A**). The second strip begins at the base of the 5th metatarsal and then moves along the lateral aspect of the foot, around the heel, and angled across the arch, back to its point of origin (**Fig. 4.5B**). Alternating subsequent strips of tape, the same pattern is followed until the entire arch is covered. The technique is closed using the simple arch taping technique (**Fig. 4.5C**). An alternative closing technique is to use elastic tape. Special care should be taken when laying tape around the posterior aspect of the heel as blisters can easily form with this technique.

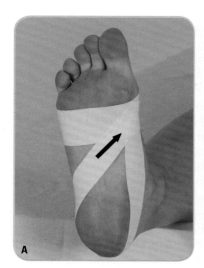 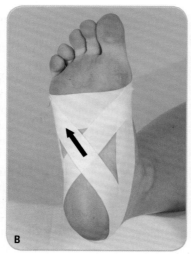 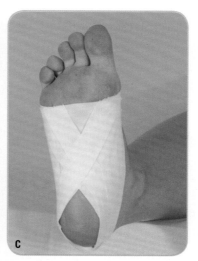

Figure 4.5. Arch support: Technique 2. X-pattern arch taping. **A,** Following placement of anchor, apply tape moving from the great toe, along the medial foot, around the heel, and angled back to starting point. **B,** The next strip begins at the 5th metatarsal, moves along the lateral foot, around the heel, and angled back to starting point. **C,** Finish using a simple arch taping.

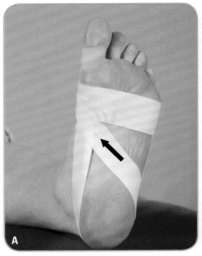
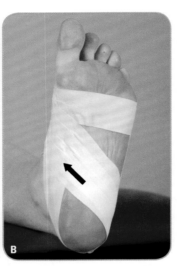

Figure 4.6. Arch support: Technique 3. Alternate arch support taping. **A,** Following placement of anchor, apply tape moving from the great toe, along the medial foot, around the heel, and angled back to starting point. **B,** Follow same pattern but angle toward the medial longitudinal arch (MLA) proximal to the previous strip. Finish using a simple arch taping.

■ Arch Support: Technique 3

This technique provides additional support to the medial longitudinal arch. This technique differs from the previous taping in the direction of pull of the support strips. Following the application of the distal anchor, the tape is pulled from the base of the great toe along the medial aspect of the foot, around the heel, and angled across the arch to end at the starting point (**Fig. 4.6A**). The next strip of tape initially follows the same pattern, but from underneath the foot, the tape is angled toward the medial longitudinal arch proximal to the previous strip (**Fig. 4.6B**). The process is repeated until the arch is covered. The technique is closed by applying a simple arch taping.

Metatarsal Arch Taping

This technique can be advantageous in the management of metatarsalgia and Morton neuroma (see Chapter 15). It is designed to provide support for the metatarsal arch. A teardrop-shaped felt pad is placed slightly proximal to the heads of the 2nd through 4th metatarsals (**Fig. 4.7A**). The pad is held in place by anchoring it with elastic tape (**Fig. 4.7B**). Caution must be taken to avoid applying the tape too tightly, resulting in restriction of normal foot movement.

Closed Basket Weave Ankle Taping

The closed basket weave technique is used to provide external support to ankle ligaments and joint proprioception during activity. Studies have shown that taping the ankle does reduce the risk of future sprains, although it is unclear whether the enhanced ability to detect inversion or eversion movements is a direct result of the taping.[1,7] Because most ankle sprains are caused by excessive inversion, this explanation focuses on providing support to the lateral ligaments. Adaptations can be made for eversion ankle sprains by neutralizing the pull of the stirrups for support.

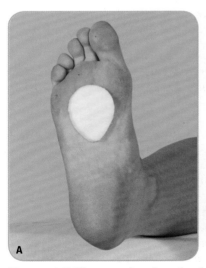
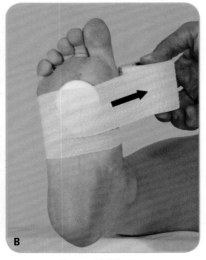

Figure 4.7. Metatarsal arch taping for metatarsalgia and Morton neuroma. A, Apply teardrop pad slightly proximal to the 2nd through 4th metatarsal heads. **B,** Anchor using elastic tape.

The lower leg and foot should be clean, dry, and free of hair. A gauze or foam pad with a lubricant should be applied to the dorsum of the ankle and Achilles tendon area. The patient is placed in a subtalar neutral position with the foot held at 90° flexion. A proximal anchor should be placed approximately 4 to 6 in above the ankle joint, distal to the belly of the gastrocnemius. The distal anchor is positioned so that it bisects the styloid process of the 5th metatarsal. Beginning on the medial aspect of the superior anchor, a **stirrup strip** is applied so that it runs down behind the medial malleolus, under the heel, and behind the lateral malleolus, then pulls up on the lateral aspect, and ends on the superior anchor (**Fig. 4.8A**).

Next, beginning on the medial aspect of the distal anchor, a horseshoe strip of tape is placed along the base of the 1st

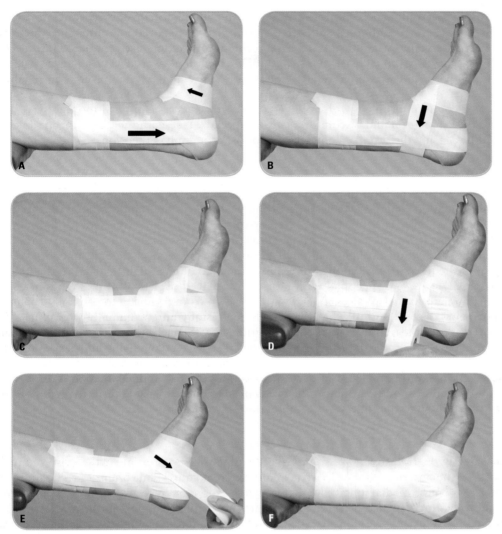

Figure 4.8. Closed basket weave ankle taping. A, Apply proximal and distal anchors; apply a stirrup strip. **B,** Apply a horseshoe strip. **C,** Continue to alternate stirrups and horseshoes. **D,** Apply figure eight. **E,** Apply heel locks. **F,** Close with horizontal anchor strips.

metatarsal and behind the heel, following the base of the 5th metatarsal, and ends on the lateral aspect of the distal anchor (**Fig. 4.8B**). The next stirrup overlaps the first by one-half to two-thirds of the previous underlying stirrup. A second horseshoe is applied, working again from medial to lateral, overlapping one-half to two-thirds of the previous underlying strip. This alternation continues until at least three stirrups and three horseshoes are in place (**Fig. 4.8C**).

The design of this technique gives the tape an appearance of a woven basket and increases the overall strength on the taping. A figure eight and heel locks are then applied (**Fig. 4.8D**). The figure eight starts on the lateral malleolus, crosses over the dorsum of the foot to the medial arch, follows under the foot and up on the lateral aspect of the foot, crosses over the top of the foot to the medial malleolus, and then continues behind the lateral malleolus and back to the starting point. The technique continues by initiating the application of the heel locks (**Fig. 4.8E**). The tape is directed over the dorsum of the foot and down the medial arch, angled back toward the heel as it crosses the bottom of the foot, and pulled up on the lateral aspect of the heel so that it runs behind the lateral malleolus and around the heel to the medial malleolus. From the medial malleolus, the tape is directed over the dorsum of the foot and down the lateral side, angled back toward the heel as it crosses the bottom of the foot, and pulled up on the medial aspect of the heel so that it moves behind the medial malleolus and around the heel to the lateral malleolus. Finally, the taping technique is closed from distal to proximal using horizontal anchor strips, which overlap one-half to two-thirds of the previous underlying strip (**Fig. 4.8F**). For additional support, a second figure eight and additional heel locks may be applied. There are many variations to this basic technique, including use of moleskin, ELASTIKON, and other specialty tapes to increase the strength of the technique as well as using fewer strips of tape when working with patients who have less severe injuries or who have completed their rehabilitation program.

The most common problem with applying tape is that it can be applied too tightly, resulting in constriction of circulation and discomfort. This is especially true with the distal anchor, but this can be avoided by placing the distal anchor on the foot without applying tension.

Achilles Tendon Taping

Taping of the Achilles tendon limits excessive dorsiflexion and, in doing so, reduces the tension placed on the tendon. The patient lies in a prone position on the taping table with the lower leg extended over the table. The foot is passively dorsiflexed to determine the spot of discomfort. This indicates the point to which motion is to be allowed while restricting any further, painful motion. The patient holds the foot in slight plantar flexion, and, using nonelastic tape, anchors are applied at the base of the metatarsals and 4 to 6 in above the ankle joint, slightly distal to the belly of the gastrocnemius (**Fig. 4.9A**). A heel pad with lubricant is placed over the Achilles tendon. Using 2-in elastic tape, three to five strips are applied in an X pattern from the distal to proximal anchor, forming a **checkrein** (**Fig. 4.9B** and **C**). The X is reanchored distally and proximally with nonelastic tape (**Fig. 4.9D**). The patient then moves to a seated position, and, using elastic tape, a figure eight and heel locks are applied (**Fig. 4.9E** and **F**). Caution should be taken to avoid applying added pressure over the irritated Achilles tendon area. In addition, a heel lift also may be placed in the shoe to limit dorsiflexion; however, lifts should be placed in both shoes to prevent any undue stress on other body parts. This technique can be modified to meet the needs of the patient by using different types of specialty tapes or using different types of tape in combination.

Taping for Medial Tibial Stress Syndrome

Often incorrectly referred to as *shin splints*, medial tibial stress syndrome (MTSS) is used to denote pain found on the anterior shin. MTSS has many different causes, but often, MTSS pain is directly related to stress on the medial longitudinal arch that is caused by hyperpronation.[8] Although rest has been found to be the best treatment for this condition, providing support to the medial longitudinal arch may help to alleviate symptoms (see **Fig. 4.6**). If the condition is related to tendinitis of the tibialis posterior muscle, taping the ankle to limit eversion may provide some relief as well (see **Fig. 4.8**). If you suspect the pain is due to periositis, the patient may find relief with the basic taping for anterior shin pain described in **Figure 4.10**. The purpose of this technique is to provide support to the muscles attaching on the anteromedial and anterolateral aspects of the lower leg and decrease stress being placed on the tibia. Stress fractures and compartment syndromes do not benefit from taping and actually may be aggravated by compression from the tape. Taping should not be attempted until the true source of the patient's pain is determined.

The patient stands on a table facing the athletic trainer. A heel lift is placed under the heel of the leg being taped to relax the muscles. Anchors are placed distally above the malleoli and proximally at the tibial tuberosity (**Fig. 4.10A**). Medial and lateral anchor strips are placed from distal to proximal, lifting up against gravity (**Fig. 4.10B**). These strips should follow the line of the malleoli. Tape is applied in an alternating oblique direction, forming an X over the anterior shin and working distal to proximal until the entire anterior shin is covered (**Fig. 4.10C**). Next, medial and lateral anchors are applied, followed by the placement of distal and proximal anchors (**Fig. 4.10D**).

Knee Hyperextension

This taping limits hyperextension of the knee and may be applied with elastic or nonelastic tape. With the patient standing on a table with the heel elevated, a superior anchor is placed at midthigh, encircling the entire thigh, and then an inferior anchor is applied 2 to 3 in below the tibial tuberosity (**Fig. 4.11A**). A gauze pad with lubricant is placed in the popliteal space, reducing the friction of the nerves and circulatory supply to the knee. From the inferior anchor, apply tape strips in an X pattern

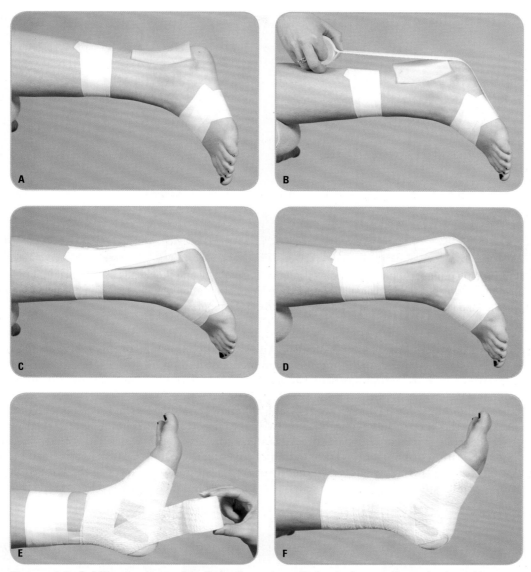

Figure 4.9. Achilles tendon taping. A, Apply anchors. **B,** Apply three to five strips in an X pattern from distal to proximal anchor. **C,** Form a checkrein. **D,** Reanchor the X distally and proximally. **E and F,** Apply a figure eight and heel locks.

over the gauze in the popliteal space. The X pattern should begin wide and should then narrow as the popliteal space is covered. The last strip runs perpendicular to the anchors (**Fig. 4.11B**). The technique is completed by applying two to three anchors on the lower leg and four to five anchors on the thigh, each overlapping one-half to two-thirds of the previous underlying strip (**Fig. 4.11C**). When completed, the taping should allow knee flexion and extension but should limit hyperextension.

Patellofemoral Taping: McConnell Technique

The term patellofemoral syndrome refers to a collection of biomechanical dysfunctions that result in pain in, around, and under the patellofemoral joint due to patellar misalignment. This technique is designed to be used in conjunction with a comprehensive therapeutic intervention program to treat patellofemoral pain by correcting patella alignment and strengthening muscles needed to control hip and knee motion.[9] It is not so much the application of the tape that corrects the alignment, but rather the technique allows the patient to exercise pain-free so he or she can utilize exercise to correct the alignment issues. The McConnell technique also provides a sustained stretch of tight lateral

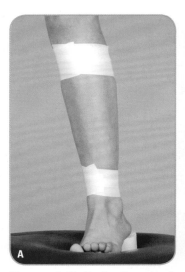
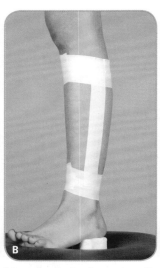
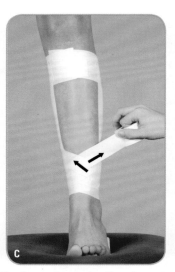
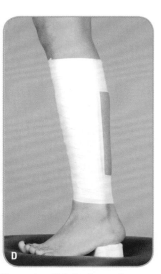

Figure 4.10. Taping for anterior shin pain. A, Apply anchor distally above the malleoli and proximally at the tibial tuberosity. **B,** Apply medial and lateral anchor strips distal to proximal. **C,** Apply strips in an alternating oblique direction, forming an X over the anterior shin. **D,** Apply medial and lateral anchors; apply distal and proximal anchors.

structures and improves lower limb mechanics. An essential component of this taping is an evaluation of the patella orientation, including the components of gliding, tilt, rotation, and anteroposterior orientation.[9] Pain reduction has been shown to occur as a result of an inferior shift in patellar displacement with proper application.[10]

The area should be shaved and clean, and tape adherent should be applied. The patient should be positioned with the knee in full extension. The two tapes used for this technique are specialty tapes, Fixomull and Leuko Sportstape (Beiersdorf Australia, Ltd, New South Wales, Australia). The initial step is the application of base strips (Fixomull tape) covering the patellar. This is performed by placing strips on the lateral condyle and extending them across the anterior aspect of the knee to the medial femoral condyle of the knee. For the remainder of the technique, the Leuko Sportstape is used.

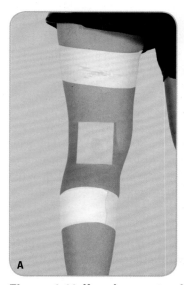
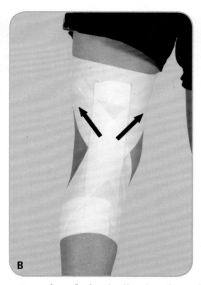
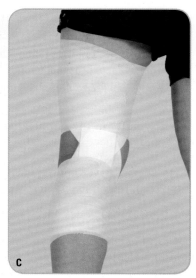

Figure 4.11. Knee hyperextension strapping. A, Apply distal and proximal anchors. **B,** From the inferior anchor, apply tape strips in an X pattern; pattern should begin wide and become narrow; the last strip should be perpendicular to the anchors. **C,** Apply two to three anchors on the lower leg and four to five anchors on the thigh.

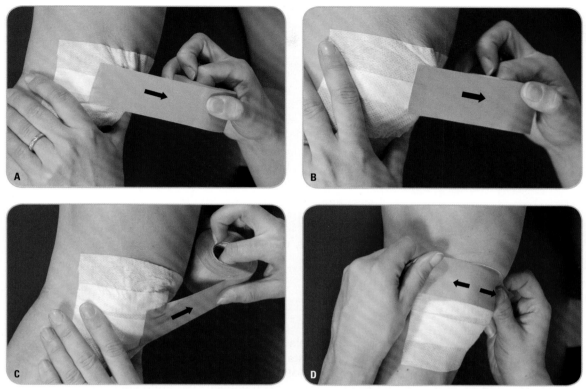

Figure 4.12. Patellofemoral taping using the McConnell technique. A, Lateral glide correction. **B,** Lateral tilt correction. **C,** External rotation correction. **D,** Anterior–posterior correction.

In correcting a lateral glide, the tape begins on the lateral border of the patella and is pulled medially (**Fig. 4.12A**). The soft tissue should be lifted over the medial femoral condyle toward the patella to provide more secure fixation. A lateral tilt correction is performed by placing the tape on the middle of the patella. The next step is to pull the tape medially to lift the lateral border (**Fig. 4.12B**). The soft tissue over the medial femoral condyle should be lifted toward the patella for more secure fixation. A correction of external rotation is completed by applying the tape to the middle of the inferior border of the patella. Rotating the inferior pole internally and the superior pole externally, the tape is pulled upward and medially (**Fig. 4.12C**). In correcting an anteroposterior condition, the middle of tape is placed on the superior half of the patella. The tape is attached equally on both sides, lifting the inferior pole (**Fig. 4.12D**).

The tape is worn by the patient throughout the day. Because the tape is likely to loosen, the patient should be instructed to tighten the strips as necessary.

Quadriceps and Hamstrings Wrap

A thigh strain may involve either the quadriceps or the hamstrings muscle group. This technique can be used to provide compression and/or support for either group. When applying a wrap to the hamstring, quadriceps, or groin muscle groups, the wrap is applied over compression shorts and under the outer garment. As such, you may want to instruct the patient to void his or her bladder prior to having the wrap applied.

If the quadriceps muscles are involved, the heel of the injured leg should be elevated 2 to 3 in on a taping block. With the thigh in a neutral position, an elastic wrap is placed on the anterior aspect of the midthigh distal to the painful site (**Fig. 4.13A**). The wrap is applied in an upward and lateral direction, encircling the thigh (**Fig. 4.13B**). Elastic tape is then applied over the wrap to provide additional support. For this technique, the 6-in wrap is used. Most often, a double-length wrap will be used.

Two techniques may be used if the injury is a hamstring strain. The first technique is appropriate when the strain is to the distal portion of the muscle group. The wrap is applied in a manner similar to

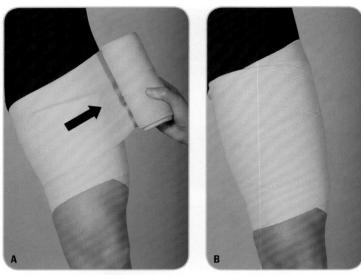

Figure 4.13. Quadriceps wrap. A, Place elastic wrap on the anterior midthigh distal to the painful site. **B,** Apply wrap in an upward and lateral direction, encircling the thigh.

the quadriceps wrap. It is directed in an upward and lateral manner, encircling the thigh, and elastic tape is then applied over the wrap to provide additional support. The second technique may be used when the injury occurs in the proximal portion of the muscle group. The wrap is placed on the posteromedial aspect of the thigh, and it encircles the thigh several times, pulling from a medial to lateral direction (**Fig. 4.14A**). The wrap is then pulled up across the greater trochanter, continues around the lower abdomen, is brought around the opposite iliac crest over the waist and gluteals, and then crosses the greater trochanter, ending back on the anterior thigh (**Fig. 4.14B**). The thigh is encircled again, moving in a medial to lateral direction. Repeating the same pattern, the wrap is then reinforced with elastic tape (**Fig. 4.14C**).

Quadriceps Contusion Wrap

This technique can be used to provide compression or protection for a quadriceps contusion. In the management of a contusion, if compression is desired, a felt pad of 0.5-in thickness should be placed over the injured site. The pad is secured by an elastic wrap (**Fig. 4.15A**). Beginning at a point distal to the injury, the wrap is applied in an upward and lateral direction, encircling the thigh (**Fig. 4.15B**). If the desired outcome is to protect the area during activity, a foam pad should be placed over the involved area. Following application of the elastic wrap, the wrap should be covered with elastic tape to provide additional support to the area.

Groin Wrap

The term groin strain may refer to damage of the muscle groups controlling hip flexion or hip adduction. When applying a wrap to support either of these muscle groups, it is important to pull the wrap in the same direction as the movement that is being supported. **Figure 4.16** depicts a groin wrap technique to support the hip adductor muscles, the muscles that are in the inside of the hip and move the thigh toward the midline of the body. When supporting the adductor muscles, the heel is elevated on a taping block, with the hip internally rotated. The wrap is then placed on the lateral aspect of the thigh and encircles the thigh in a medial direction to draw the thigh further into internal rotation (**Fig. 4.16A**). The wrap continues around the thigh, crossing over the greater trochanter and continuing across the lower abdomen, covering the iliac crest and around the waist and gluteals, and then crossing the greater trochanter and ending back on the thigh (**Fig. 4.16B**). Following the same pattern, the wrap is then reinforced with elastic tape (**Fig. 4.16C**).

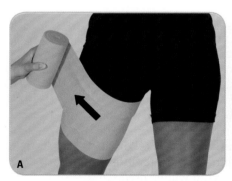
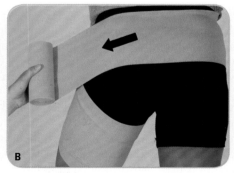
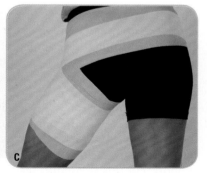

Figure 4.14. Hamstrings wrap. A, Encircle thigh several times, pulling from a medial to lateral direction. **B,** Pull wrap up across the greater trochanter, around the lower abdomen to the opposite iliac crest, over the waist and gluteals, cross the greater trochanter, and end on the anterior thigh. **C,** Repeat the pattern and reinforce with nonelastic tape.

Hip Contusion Wrap

This technique is designed to keep padding in place that is intended to prevent iliac crest contusion from reinjury. A protective pad should be placed over the iliac crest at the point where the contusion is located. The pad is secured by applying an elastic wrap in a **spica** pattern. The wrap starts at the distal aspect of the anterior thigh and moves over the top of the pad, around the waist, diagonally down toward the lateral thigh, and behind the thigh to the starting point (**Fig. 4.17A**). This pattern is repeated for the length of the wrap (**Fig. 4.17B and C**). Application of elastic tape over the wrap provides additional support.

Taping and Wrapping Techniques for the Upper Extremity

Shoulder Spica Wrap

This technique can be used to provide support and stabilization for the glenohumeral joint.

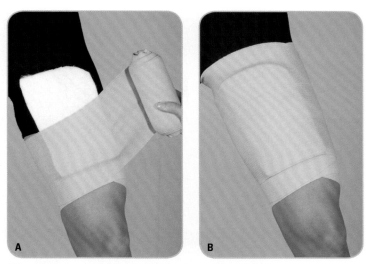

Figure 4.15. Quadriceps contusion wrap. A, Place a pad over the injured site. **B,** Distal to injury, apply elastic wrap in an upward and lateral direction encircling the thigh.

The patient should hold the injured arm in internal rotation. The technique begins by encircling the arm in a posterior-to-anterior direction at the midbiceps. Next, the anterior chest is crossed in the region of the pectoralis major (**Fig. 4.18A**). Wrapping in this direction maintains internal rotation of the glenohumeral joint and limits external rotation. The limitation of motion is determined by the amount of internal rotation in which the arm is placed initially. The wrap is brought under the opposite axilla, across the back, and over the acromion process in an anterior direction (**Fig. 4.18B**). The wrap is then continued through the axilla, around the arm, and again across the anterior chest (**Fig. 4.18C**). Finally, the wrap is secured with nonelastic tape (**Fig. 4.18D**).

Elbow Hyperextension

This technique is designed to restrict painful motion while permitting functional movement. The patient should be instructed to clench the fist and hold the elbow in slight flexion with the palm facing up. To determine the degree of flexion, the elbow should be extended to the point of discomfort and then slightly flexed from that point. Using either nonelastic or elastic tape, anchors are

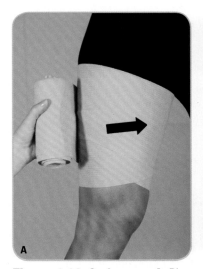
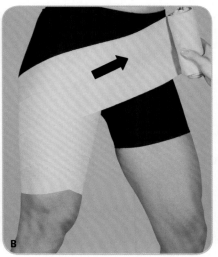
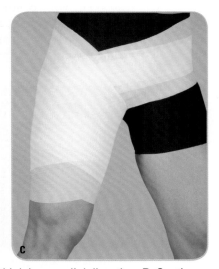

Figure 4.16. Groin wrap. A, Place wrap on the lateral thigh and encircle the thigh in a medial direction. **B,** Continue to wrap around the thigh, over the greater trochanter, across the lower abdomen, cover the iliac crest, around the waist and gluteals, cross the greater trochanter, and end on the thigh. **C,** Reinforce with elastic tape.

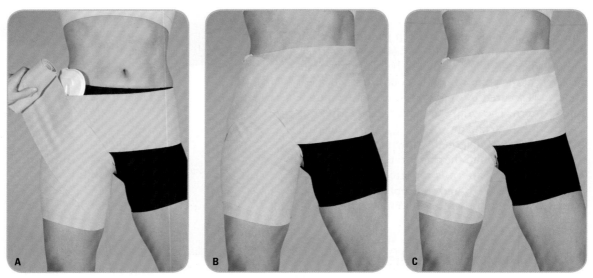

Figure 4.17. Hip contusion wrap. A, Place a protective pad over the iliac crest; apply elastic wrap in a spica pattern. **B,** Repeat the pattern. **C,** Reinforce with elastic tape.

applied to the midregion of the forearm and upper arm (**Fig. 4.19A**). After approximating the distance between the two anchors, two strips of tape (the same length as the distance between the anchors) are torn from the roll. A checkrein is constructed by placing these two pieces of tape back to back and then adding five or six additional pieces of tape over the template in an X fan shape (**Fig. 4.19B**). If additional strength is needed to prevent full extension, nontearable may be substituted to create the checkrein. The checkrein is then attached to the anchors by applying three or four additional anchors. The anchors should overlap each other by one-half to two-thirds. Using elastic tape or wrap,

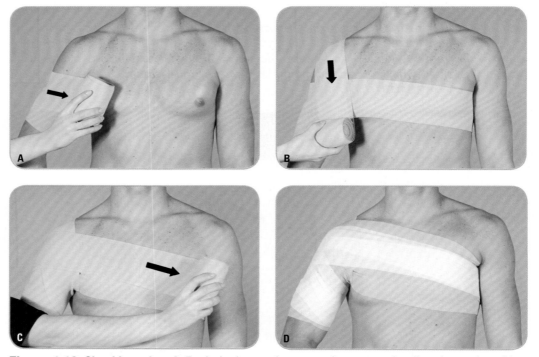

Figure 4.18. Shoulder spica. A, Encircle the arm in a posterior-to-anterior direction at the mid-biceps. **B,** Cross the anterior chest and bring the wrap under the opposite axilla, across the back, and over the acromion process. **C,** Continue to wrap through the axilla, around the arm, and again across the anterior chest. **D,** Reinforce with nonelastic tape.

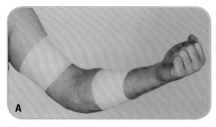
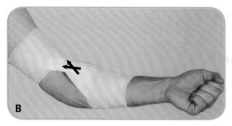
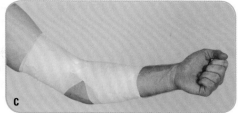

Figure 4.19. Elbow hyperextension. A, Apply anchors to the midregion of the forearm and the upper arm. **B,** Construct a checkrein in an X fan shape. **C,** Attach the checkrein by applying three to four additional anchors.

a figure eight then may be applied to further secure the taping and prevent slipping during activity (**Fig. 4.19C**). The radial pulse should be checked and monitored to determine if the tape is too tight.

Elbow Sprain Taping

The purpose of this taping is to provide support for the collateral ligaments of the elbow. The patient's arm is placed in a position of slight flexion. Anchors are applied to the midregion of the forearm and upper arm. If the injury is to the medial collateral ligament, three or four strips of nonelastic tape are placed over the ligament in an X pattern (**Fig. 4.20A**). If additional strength is needed, consider using tape with higher tensile strength such as nontearable tape. The strips are then secured above and below the joint with elastic tape (**Fig. 4.20B**). The cubital fossa should remain open. The same technique can be modified for injury to the lateral collateral ligaments by changing the location of the strips.

Wrist Taping

Hyperextension or hyperflexion of the wrist may damage the ligaments of the wrist. Taping can provide support and stability for the wrist.

■ Wrist Taping: Technique 1

For a mild sprain, three or four circular strips of tape may be applied to the wrist. The strips should be positioned from distal to proximal and should overlap the previous underlying strip by one-half to two-thirds the width of the tape (**Fig. 4.21**).

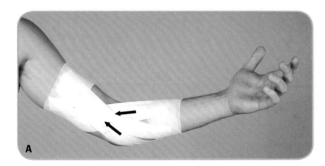

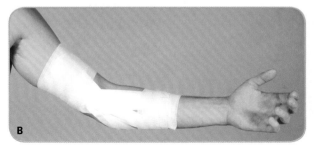

Figure 4.20. Elbow sprain taping. A, Apply anchors to the midregion of the forearm and upper arm. **B,** Place three to four strips of nonelastic tape over the ligament in an X pattern. Secure above and below the joint with elastic tape.

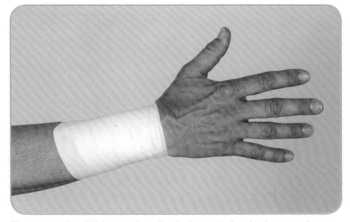

Figure 4.21. Wrist taping: Technique 1. Apply three to four circular strips of tape to the wrist.

■ Wrist Taping: Technique 2

This technique can help to limit painful wrist motion. The patient should be instructed to spread his or her fingers. The wrist is positioned in slight flexion or extension, depending on the injury. Anchor strips are placed around the wrist and at the heads of the metacarpals (**Fig. 4.22A**). If the intent is to limit hyperextension, three or four strips of tape are placed in an X pattern over the palmar aspect of the hand; if the intent is to limit hyperflexion, the X pattern is positioned over the dorsum of the hand (**Fig. 4.22B**). Next, using either elastic or nonelastic tape, a figure eight is applied around the wrist and hand (**Fig. 4.22C–E**). The figure eight should begin on the radial aspect of the proximal anchor, travel across the dorsum of the hand around the metacarpal heads and across the palm of the hand, and end on the ulnar side of the proximal anchor (**Fig. 4.22F**). As the tape is brought through the web space of the thumb and index finger, the tape should be crimped to prevent irritation of the skin.

Thumb Taping

Most thumb injuries occur when the thumb is hyperextended. Thumb taping is designed to provide support and limit extension of the first metacarpophalangeal joint. The thumb is placed in a position

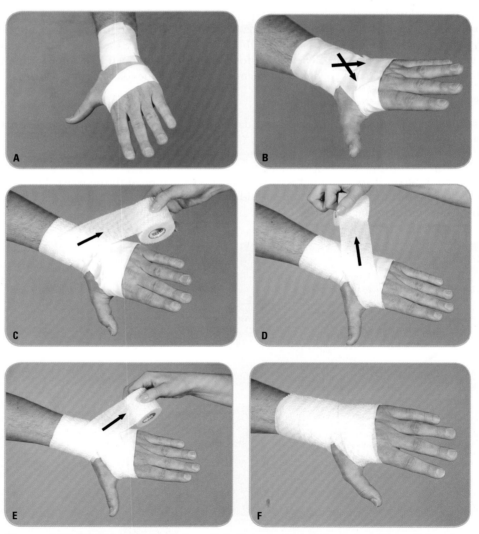

Figure 4.22. Wrist taping: Technique 2. A, Place anchor strips around the wrist and metacarpal heads. **B,** Place three to four tape strips in an X pattern over the palmar aspect or dorsum of the hand. **C–F,** Apply a figure eight beginning on the radial aspect of the proximal anchor.

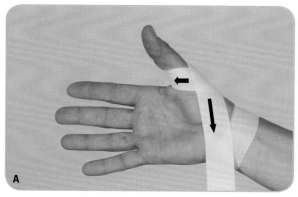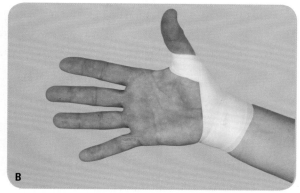

Figure 4.23. Thumb spica. A, Apply an anchor on the wrist; apply tape on the ulnar aspect of the proximal anchor and continue upward over the palmar aspect of the thenar eminence, cross over the MP joint, and encircle the thumb; this line of pull makes an X pattern. **B,** Apply three to four Xs; apply an anchor at the wrist to finish.

of slight flexion and adduction, and an anchor is placed on the wrist. Next, a strip of tape is applied, beginning on the ulnar aspect of the proximal anchor and continuing upward over the palmar aspect of the thenar eminence on the thumb, crossing over the metacarpophalangeal joint, and encircling the thumb (**Fig. 4.23A**). The strip is then reanchored on the dorsal aspect of the anchor. This line of pull makes an X pattern. Three or four X patterns should be applied before finishing the taping with additional anchors (**Fig. 4.23B**). Based on the direction of movement that causes the patient pain, this technique can be modified by placing the restraining strips so that the line of pull is in the opposite direction of the motion that causes pain.

Finger Taping Technique

Sprains of the interphalangeal joints occur frequently. Taping can assist in providing support for an unstable interphalangeal joint. "Buddy" taping for the fingers involves using an adjacent finger for support. Strips of narrow tape are applied around the proximal phalanx and distal phalanx of the two fingers, leaving the joints uncovered to permit limited flexion and extension of the fingers (**Fig. 4.24**).

If additional support for the medial and lateral collateral ligaments is needed, anchors can be placed just proximal and distal to the injured joint. Working from distal to proximal, two narrow strips of tape are applied in an X pattern over the collateral ligaments, followed by a longitudinal strip to connect the two anchors (**Fig. 4.25A and B**). A figure eight may be applied, using care not to impinge on the circulation. Because the blood supply is very superficial and easily compressed, capillary refill should be checked after taping.

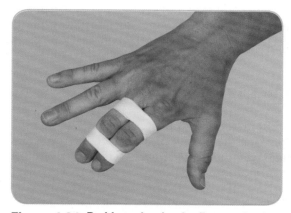

Figure 4.24. Buddy taping for the fingers. Apply narrow tape strips around the proximal and distal phalanx of two fingers.

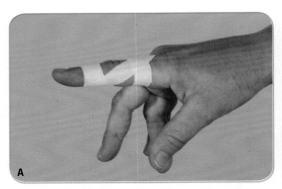
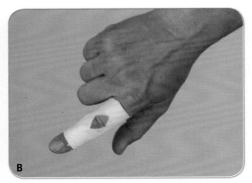

Figure 4.25. **Collateral ligament taping. A,** Apply anchors proximal and distal to the injured joint; working from distal to proximal, apply two narrow tape strips in an X pattern over the collateral ligaments. **B,** Apply a longitudinal strip to connect the two anchors.

A felt pad of 0.5-in thickness should be placed over the injured site. The wrap should begin distal to the injury site and be applied in an upward and lateral direction, encircling the thigh. This prevents any edema formation from settling in the distal digits and provides support against gravitational forces. The wrap should be stretched from one-half to one-third of its total elastic capability. Excessive stretching may constrict circulation, compress superficial nerves, and impair function. Each turn of the wrap should be overlapped by at least one-half of the previous, underlying strip.

POWERFLEX TAPING SYSTEM

Developed by Andover Healthcare, Inc, the PowerFlex Taping System was introduced in 2012 as an alternative to using the traditional combination of prewrap and cotton zinc oxide tape taping techniques.[11] All taping techniques previously described within this chapter can be applied using the PowerFlex Taping System (**Fig. 4.26A–F**), which includes PowerFlex, PowerTape, and VictoryTape. Because the PowerFlex line of products are cohesive, the need for using spray adherents and prewrap has been eliminated.[5] Using porous synthetic tape for both the underwrap and tape permits sweat to pass through the materials, decreasing or eliminating the need to reapply tape between bouts of exercise within the same day.[5] Using cohesive, synthetic tape as the underwrap in conjunction with basic cotton athletic tape has been found to be more effective in maintaining range-of-motion restrictions than the traditional prewrap and cotton zinc oxide tape combination.[12] When using both self-adherent or cohesive prewrap and tape, range-of-motion restrictions were maintained even after 30 minutes of exercise, whereas the traditional prewrap and cotton zinc oxide tape combination did not.[6] Most of the major tape manufacturers now offer cohesive tape products.

KINESIO TAPING

Developed by Japanese chiropractor Kenzo Kase, DC, in 1973, therapeutic taping has been used to support muscles by improving the quality of muscle contractions in weakened muscles, reduce muscle fatigue, reduce cramping and potential injury to muscle tissue, increase range of motion, and relieve pain.[13] Although it is uncertain how Kinesio Taping (KT) works, it is thought that when a muscle is inflamed, swollen, or stiff due to fatigue or injury, the interstitial space between the skin and underlying connective tissues become compressed, thereby compromising the flow of lymphatic fluid. This tissue compression can then stimulate pain receptors beneath the skin. The intent of KT application is to create convolutions in the skin to increase the interstitial space. These convolutions are created when the muscles and skin of the impacted area are stretched prior to the application of

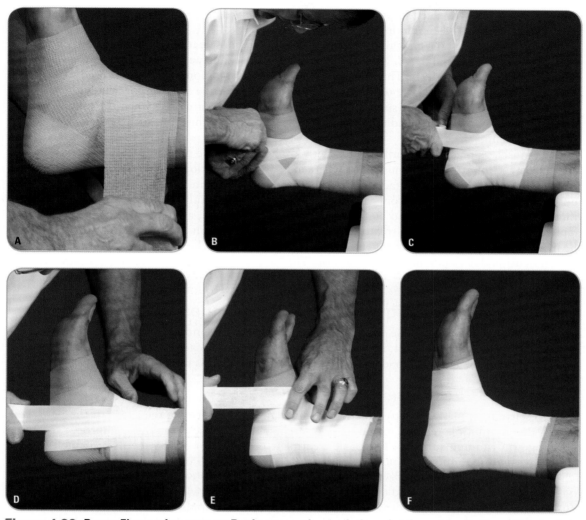

Figure 4.26. PowerFlex taping system: Basic prevention technique for the ankle. A, PowerFlex is directly applied to clean and dry ankle. Tape adherent spray and anchor strips are not needed. **B,** A series of heel locks secures the ankle joint in a neutral position. **C,** A series of figure eight strips are applied next. **D,** The basket weave technique begins by applying stirrups on the medial aspect of the ankle and ending on the lateral aspect. **E,** Alternating between applying horseshoe strips and stirrups. **F,** Finishing with anchor strips.

the tape. After the tape has been applied and the muscles return to a relaxed position, convolutions of the skin are formed, which increases the interstitial space, allowing for greater flow of lymphatic and venous fluids and thus less pain.[13,14] It is thought that the taping method can also inhibit muscles that may result in a muscle imbalance, enhance joint stability by increasing nutrition to the joint synovial fluid and hyaline cartilage, and increase range of motion by activating the neurological and circulatory systems.[13–16] Originally used primarily in sports medicine, it is currently being applied in other specialties, such as in orthopedics, traumatology, surgery of the motor system, neurology, oncology, and pediatrics.

Kinesio Tex Tape is designed to allow for a longitudinal stretch of 55% to 60% of its resting length but is not designed to stretch horizontally. The tape is made of a polymer elastic strand wrapped by 100% cotton fibers to permit the evaporation of body moisture. The material is latex-free, nonmedicated, quick-drying, and approximately the same weight and thickness of skin.[15,17] The tape is easy to apply, noninvasive, comfortable to wear, and can provide continued treatment for up to 3 to 5 days. KT can be used jointly with other treatment options such as ultrasound, electrical stimulation, hydrotherapeutic treatments, joint mobilization/joint mechanics, myofascial release, ice/heat, and intramuscular stimulation/trigger point.[18]

Application of the tape typically runs from one end of a muscle to the other. The strip of tape can be applied in the shape of a Y, I, X, fan, web, and donut. The shape is dependent on the size of the muscle and the desired effects. The Y technique is the most common shape and is used to surround a large muscle to either facilitate or inhibit muscle stimuli.[15] I strips are used for acute injury to limit edema and pain in small areas, such as the teres minor; X strips are used when the muscle's origin and insertion may change depending on the movement pattern of the joint, such as the biceps brachii or triceps brachii.[15,19]

The muscle is placed on gentle stretch with application of the tape at 10% of its resting static length.[20] For chronically weak muscles or where increased contraction is desired, the tape is stretched from the origin to insertion to facilitate muscle function. For acute muscle injury or overstretched muscles, the tape is stretched from the insertion to the origin to inhibit muscle function.[19] For optimal adherence, the skin should be free of oil or lotions, shaved, and dry. In general, anchors are applied at both margins of the treatment area approximately 2 in below the origin or 2 in above the insertion of the muscle using a 1- to 2-in width strip of tape. The anchors are applied to the skin without tension due to potential skin irritation. The base anchors are secured and the desired tension is applied.[21]

Kinesio Taping Techniques for Specific Injuries

Some common examples of the use of therapeutic taping are included in this section. Because KT certification programs exist, it is recommended that health care practitioners complete these programs to become more proficient and knowledgeable about this method of taping.

Medial Tibial Stress Syndrome

Prior to selecting a method of treatment, the clinician must determine the cause of the pain. Pain may be due to multiple reasons including poor arch support, muscle weakness, improper footwear, or changes in running surfaces. The basic treatment protocol for MTSS involves a single Y strip applied with no tension on the inferior base of the 5th metatarsal just proximal to the head of the 5th metatarsal. Apply light (15% to 25%) or paper-off tension as each strip passes over the medial longitudinal arch moving toward the origin of the tibialis anterior, with one strip on either side of the muscle belly (**Fig. 4.27A**). Additional horizontal Y strips are then applied. Place the base of a 2-in KT strip on the medial calf with no tension just inferior to the painful site. While securing the base with one hand, apply light-to-moderate tension (25% to 50%) to the tails as you pull the skin laterally across the tibial border surrounding the area of pain. Apply the last inch of the tails with no tension in a splayed pattern to limit tension on the skin (**Fig. 4.27B**).[15]

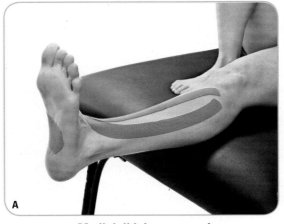
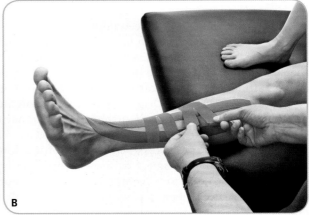

Figure 4.27. Medial tibial stress syndrome.

Quadriceps Strain

In the postacute phase with the patient supine, apply an I strip of 2-in KT just superior to the anterior superior iliac spine (ASIS) with no tension. Have the patient move into hip extension. Apply light (15% to 25%) or paper-off tension until the I strip reaches the involved injured area. Just prior to passing over the suspected hematoma area, increase tension using the space correction technique. Apply light-to-moderate tension (25% to 50% of available tension) over the painful site. Once beyond the painful site, reduce tension to light. Secure the final 2 to 3 in of tape with no tension and then initiate glue activation of the tape prior to any further patient movement (**Fig. 4.28**).[15]

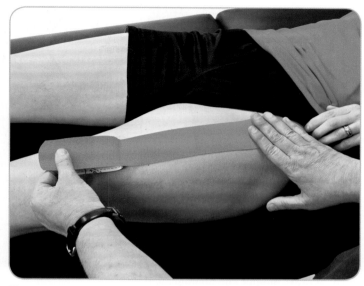

Figure 4.28. Quadriceps strain.

Patellar Tendinopathy

With the patient supine and the knee extended, the KT is measured and cut equal to the distance between the medial and lateral femoral condyles (**Fig. 4.29A**). The patient is then moved to a long-sitting position with the hip flexed at about 45°. Tear the paper backing of the tape in the middle third of the tape and place this section of the tape directly over the inferior pole of the patella (**Fig. 4.29B**). Apply a moderate tension (25% to 50%) with a downward pressure over the inferior pole of the patella. The patient then flexes the knee to about 90°, and the KT is positioned around the patella in the direction of the vastus lateralis and medialis with 15% to 25% tension (**Fig. 4.29C**).[15]

Rotator Cuff Impingement

This condition often refers to impingement of the supraspinatus, the long head of the biceps tendon, or the subacromial bursae under the coracoacromial arch. Begin by placing the base of a KT Y strip 2 in inferior to the greater tuberosity of the humerus with no tension. Ask the patient to move into shoulder adduction with the hand behind the back and to do lateral neck flexion to the opposite

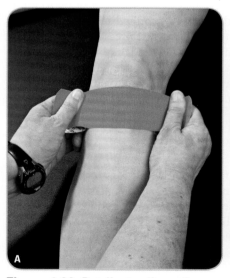
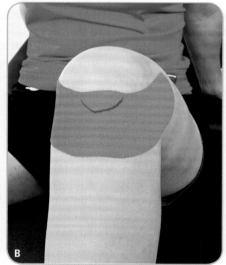
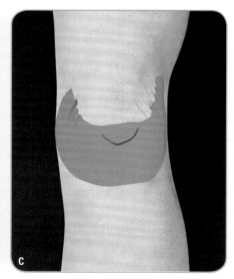

Figure 4.29. Patellar tendinopathy.

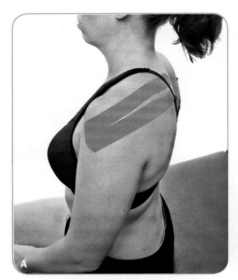
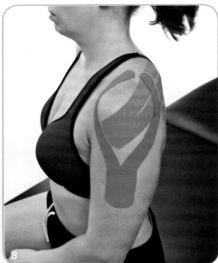
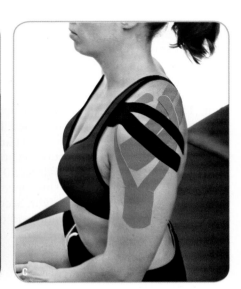

Figure 4.30. Rotator cuff impingement.

side. Apply light tension (15% to 25%) or paper-off tension to the Y strip. The superior tail should travel superior to the spine of the scapula, between the upper and middle trapezius muscles and end on the superior medial border of the scapula (**Fig. 4.30A**). The inferior tail should travel along the spine of the scapula with the final 1 to 2 in applied with no tension. Initiate glue activation of the tape prior to any patient movement.[15]

A second Y strip is applied over the deltoid muscle, moving from the insertion to the origin. Place the base of the KT Y strip 2 in inferior to the deltoid tuberosity with no tension. Both anterior and posterior tails are applied with light (15% to 25%) or paper-off tension. With the patient's arm abducted 90°, externally rotated, and in horizontal extension, apply the anterior tail around the outer border of the anterior deltoid to approximately the acromioclavicular (AC) joint with no tension on the final 2 in. With the arm remaining in abduction, move the arm into horizontal flexion with internal rotation. Apply the posterior tail along the outer border of the posterior deltoid to approximately the AC joint with no tension on the final 2 in (**Fig. 4.30B**).[15]

Finally, place the base of a 6- to 8-in Y strip on the anterior shoulder over the coracoid process with no tension. The base can be adjusted to place the cut of the Y just below the area of pain. While holding the base with one hand to ensure that no additional tension is applied to the base, apply moderate-to-severe tension (50% to 75%) to the tails while applying inward pressure over the area of pain with approximately half of the Y strip length. When half of the Y strip length is reached, slide the hand securing the base up to the point of end tension on the tape. Have the patient move into shoulder flexion with horizontal flexion and apply the remaining tails in a splayed out pattern to dissipate the created force with no tension. Initiate activation prior to any further movement by the patient (**Fig. 4.30C**).[15]

Erector Spinae Muscle Strain

Using an H technique, begin by having the patient move into flexion with rotation to the nonpainful side. Apply two I strips of KT with very light to moderate tension (15% to 25%) (**Fig. 4.31A**). Measure the third strip to extend approximately 2 in on either side of the previously applied strips. After removing about 2 in of the paper backing from one end of the I strip, apply light-to-moderate tension (15% to 25%) to secure the base and extend over the region of muscle spasm or pain. Do not add any inward tension. Slide the hand holding the base toward the middle of the back and hold no tension over the region of the transverse and spinous process. Have the patient move into rotation to assist with minimizing tension on the ends. While continuing to apply no pressure over the spinal

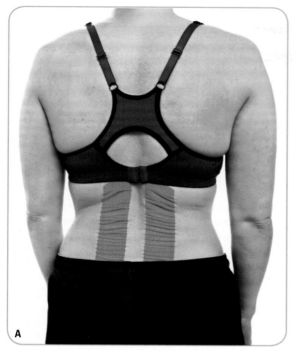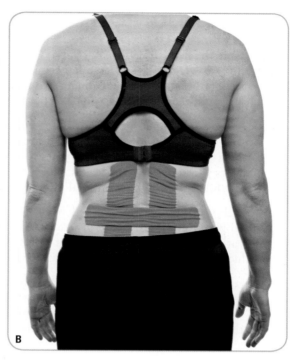

Figure 4.31. Erector spinae muscle strain.

column, use the other hand to apply another zone of light-to-moderate tension (15% to 25%) on the ipsilateral side. Secure the base with no tension (**Fig. 4.31B**). Initiate glue activation prior to any patient movement.[15]

SUMMARY

1. Taping and wrapping a body part provides support and protection while allowing functional movement. Tape and wraps may be used to provide immediate first aid, support an injured body part, or provide pain-free functional movement.

2. Taping products and techniques should be based on the needs of the patient. Patient needs can only be assessed by conducting a comprehensive orthopedic evaluation.

3. Used in conjunction with a comprehensive rehabilitation program, tape or wraps can allow for the early resumption of activity without the threat of reinjury.

4. When using tape, the skin should be inspected regularly for signs of irritation, blisters, or infection. In particular, skin that is red, dry, hot, and tender suggests an allergic reaction to the tape or tape adherent.

5. If the skin cannot be protected from irritation, it may be necessary to fit the patient with an appropriate brace rather than allow for continued irritation.

6. Tape types can be categorized based on strength: prewrap, tearable elastic, cohesive, basic athletic cloth tape, and specialty tape. Within each category, quality of tape is evaluated based on tensile strength and elongation properties.

7. Synthetic tape is porous, allowing sweat to escape from the patient, keeping the skin and tape dry. Cotton tape is nonporous and traps the sweat under the taping technique.

APPLICATION QUESTIONS

1. You are the head athletic trainer at a National Collegiate Athletic Association (NCAA) Division I university. During a professional seminar attended by your peers from other universities, one of the conference athletic trainers proposes mandatory ankle taping for football players for both practice and game situations. What are the pros and cons of this proposal?

2. You are responsible for submitting a budget request for athletic training supplies and must decide how much and what type of tape to order. What factors should you consider when making your decision? How can you make your supply budget stretch to meet the needs of the patients you serve? What policies might you put into place to decrease the amount of tape being used while still providing optimal injury prevention services for your patients?

3. A high school soccer player has been experiencing mild-to-moderate bilateral distal medial tibial pain during preseason practice. You suspect that the pain may be due to an overload on the athlete's arches. What different types of arch support and exercises might you suggest to reduce strain on the supporting structures?

4. As an interscholastic athletic trainer, a 16-year-old member of the girls varsity basketball team sustained two ankle sprains in the past two seasons. In both instances, return-to-play guidelines, as outlined by her family physician, included ankle taping for the remainder of the season. Prior to the start of her third year, her parents request a meeting with you to discuss taping versus bracing as an intervention for the prevention of another ankle sprain. What evidence-based research can you locate to support your recommendations as to what intervention you would recommend for this athlete?

5. An 18-year-old lacrosse player sustains a moderate ankle sprain at the end of practice. What options might you consider to provide compression to the injury site as part of the immediate management for this condition? What recommendations would you suggest to the athlete to care for this injury during the evening hours?

REFERENCES

1. Bandyopadhyay A, Mahapatra D. Taping in sports: a brief update. *J Hum Sport Exerc.* 2012;7(2):544–552.
2. Bragg RW, Macmohan JM, Overom EK, et al. Failure and fatigue characteristics of adhesive athletic tape. *Med Sci Sports Exerc.* 2002;34(3):403–410.
3. Mitchell L. Brace yourself taping essentials. *SportEX Dynamics.* 2006;7(1):16–20.
4. Schaeffer SL, Slusarski J, VanTeim V, et al. Tensile strength comparison of athletic tapes: assessed using ASTM D3759M-96, standard test method for tensile strength and elongation of pressure-sensitive tapes. *J Ind Technol.* 1999;16(1):2–6.
5. O'Neil R. [Personal Interview]. Vice-President CBI Health Quebec, Andover Healthcare, Inc. Sports Medicine Education, Research & Development. Salisbury MA. March 2015.
6. Purcell SB, Schuckman BE, Docherty CL, et al. Differences in ankle range of motion before and after exercise in 2 tape conditions. *Am J Sports Med.* 2009;37(2):383–389.
7. Verhagen EA, van Mechelen W, de Vente W. The effect of preventive measures on the incidence of ankle sprains. *Clin J Sport Med.* 2000;10(4):291–296.
8. Reshef N, Guelich DR. Medial tibial stress syndrome. *Clin Sports Med.* 2012;31(2):273–290.
9. McConnell J. The management of chondromalacia patella: a long term solution. *Aust J Physiother.* 1986;32(4):215–223.
10. Derasari A, Brindle TJ, Alter KE, et al. McConnell taping shifts the patella inferiorly in patients with patellofemoral pain: a dynamic magnetic resonance imaging study. *Phys Ther.* 2010;90(3):411–419.
11. Andover Healthcare, Inc. *PowerTape™ & VictoryTape™. New. Innovative. Different.* http://coflexnl.com/pdf/PowerTape%20Brochure.pdf. Accessed November 16, 2015.
12. Van Wagoner R, Docherty CL, Simon J. Self-adherent underwrap maintains range of motion restriction after exercise. *J Athl Train.* 2012;47(2):S71.
13. Kase K. *Illustrated Kinesio-Taping.* 4th ed. Tokyo, Japan: Ken'i-kai Information; 2003.
14. Kahonov L. Kinesio taping, part 1: an overview of its use in athletes. *Athl Ther Today.* 2007;12(3):17–18.
15. Kase K, Wallis J, Kase T. *Clinical Therapeutic Applications of the Kinesio Taping Method.* 2nd ed. Tokyo, Japan: Ken'i-kai; 2003.

16. Pope ML, Baker A, Grindstaff TL. Kinesio taping technique for patellar tendinopathy. *Athl Train Sports Health Care.* 2010;2(3):98–99.

17. Zajt-Kwiatkowska J, Rajkowska-Labon E, Skrobot W, et al. Application of Kinesio Taping® for treatment of sports injuries. *Medsportpress.* 2007;13(1):130–134.

18. Silverman RS. Q&A: the unique benefits of therapeutic taping. *Rehab Manag.* 2010; 23(6):26–29.

19. Kahanov L, Kaltenborn JM. Kinesio taping, part II: an overview of use with athletes. *Athl Ther Today.* 2007;12(4):5–7.

20. Halseth T, McChesney JW, Debeliso M, et al. The effects of Kinesio taping on proprioception at the ankle. *J Sports Sci Med.* 2004;3(1):1–7.

21. Osterhue DJ. The use of Kinesio™ taping in the management of traumatic patella dislocation. A case study. *Physiother Theory Pract.* 2004; 20(4):267–270.

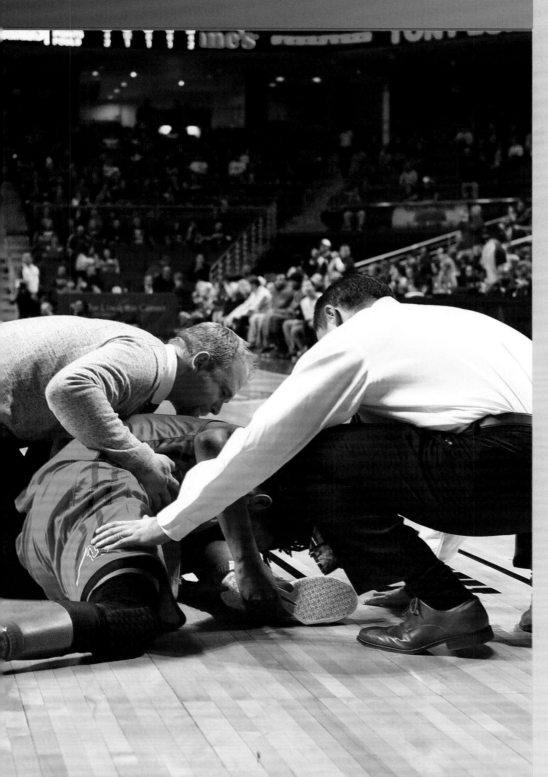

Clinical Examination and Diagnosis

Evidence-Based Health Care

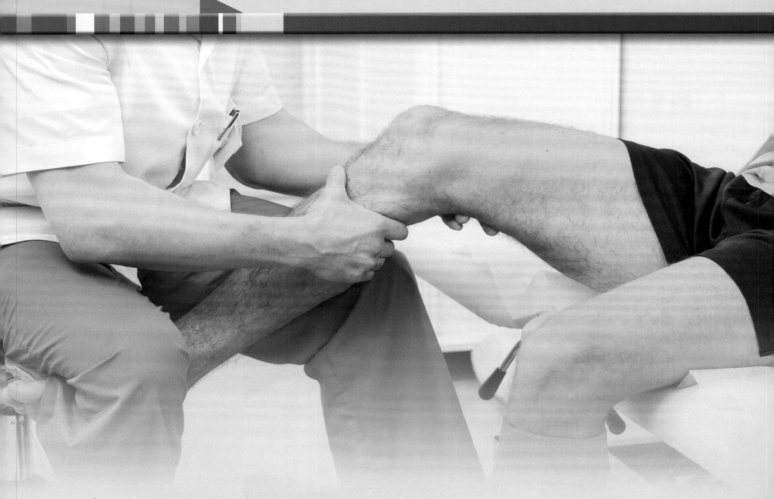

STUDENT OUTCOMES

1. Explain how to practice evidence-based health care.
2. Describe methods to search for health care–related evidence.
3. Recognize different methods to evaluate health care evidence.
4. Identify values used to assess the accuracy of diagnostic tests.
5. Identify values used to assess the effectiveness of clinical treatments.

INTRODUCTION

Evidence-based health care (EBHC) is part of a cultural shift in current health care practice that aims to provide patients with the best quality care by integrating the best evidence with clinical expertise and the individual patient's values and circumstances.[1] One reason for the need for EBHC is the volume of new information available to clinicians each day. Traditional sources of information such as textbooks and expert opinion are quickly outdated given the volume of new information available on a daily basis (>760,000 new biomedical articles were added to PubMed, a biomedical database, in 2014 alone).[2]

TYPES OF EVIDENCE

 An athletic trainer has a patient who recently tore her anterior cruciate ligament (ACL). The patient is asking what type of treatment would be best. What type of outcome evidence should the clinician use to provide treatment recommendations?

As health care providers try to determine the best quality care for patients, it is important to consider patient-oriented evidence as much, if not more, than disease-oriented evidence. Patient-oriented evidence or **patient-oriented evidence that matters (POEM)** provides information on areas about which patients would be most concerned (e.g., mobility, mortality, symptom improvement, health care cost, and quality of life). Typically, patient-oriented evidence provides a more holistic view of a patient's health status. **Disease-oriented evidence** is physiological information such as blood pressure and joint range of motion measures, or symptoms such as headache and nausea. Because disease-oriented evidence has traditionally been gathered by clinicians, it may also be referred to as **clinician-oriented evidence**. Changes in disease-oriented evidence may or may not have a significant impact on a patient's health status; therefore, its use when determining the best quality care for patients may be limited. Patient-oriented outcome measures are common forms of patient-oriented evidence. **Patient-oriented outcome measures** usually are self-reported questionnaires that patients complete throughout treatment to assess their quality of life. Generic patient-based outcome measures assess quality of life from a broad prospective, whereas specific disease or anatomical patient-based outcome measures assess quality of life from a narrower point of view. Examples of outcome measures are given in **Box 5.1**.

 The athletic trainer should seek out POEM to provide the best treatment advice for the patient with an ACL tear. Patient-oriented outcome measures would provide a broad quality of life assessment. Examples of patient-oriented evidence that could be used in this case would include Short Form 12 (SF-12) health survey questionnaire or the International Knee Document Committee (IKDC) Subjective Knee Form.

HOW TO PRACTICE EVIDENCE-BASED HEALTH CARE

 An athletic trainer has a patient who injured her knee. Which diagnostic tests would provide the athletic trainer with the most accurate diagnosis? What is the best treatment for this patient's condition? How can the athletic trainer quickly answer these questions?

There are five steps athletic trainers need to follow to practice EBHC: (1) Develop a clinical question; (2) search for the best evidence; (3) evaluate the evidence for validity, impact, and applicability; (4) integrate the evidence into the clinical decision; and (5) evaluate the efficiency and effectiveness of steps 1 to 4.

BOX 5.1 Examples of Patient-Based Outcome Measures

Generic Outcome Measures

INSTRUMENT	AVAILABLE AT
Quality of Well-Being (QWB)	https://hoap.ucsd.edu/qwb-info/
Short Form 36 Health Survey Questionnaire (SF-36)	https://www.optum.com/optum-outcomes/what-we-do.html
Short Form 12 Health Survey Questionnaire (SF-12)	https://www.optum.com/optum-outcomes/what-we-do.html

Disease-Specific Outcome Measures

INSTRUMENT	AVAILABLE AT
Hip Disability and Osteoarthritis Outcome Score (HOOS)	http://www.koos.nu/
Rheumatoid and Arthritis Outcome Score	http://www.koos.nu/

Anatomy-Specific Outcome Measures

INSTRUMENT	AVAILABLE AT
Foot and Ankle Outcome Score (FAOS)	http://www.koos.nu/
Disabilities of the Arm, Shoulder and Hand (DASH) Questionnaire	http://www.orthopaedicscore.com/scorepages/disabilities_of_arm_shoulder_hand_score_dash.html
International Knee Document Committee (IKDC) Subjective Knee Form	http://www.sportsmed.org/Research/IKDC_Forms/
Michigan Hand Outcome Questionnaire	http://www.orthopaedicscore.com/scorepages/Michigan_Hand_Outcome_Questionnaire.html
Oswestry Low Back Pain Score	http://www.orthopaedicscore.com/scorepages/oswestry_low_back_pain.html
Oxford Hip Score	http://www.orthopaedicscore.com/scorepages/oxford_hip_score.html

Developing a Clinical Question

Clinicians commonly use the **PICO** or **PICO/T** formats to develop their clinical questions for more effective evidence searches. PICO/T is an acronym:

- P = Patient/Problem
- I = Intervention/Variable of Interest
- C = Comparison
- O = Outcome
- T = Time

Comparison and Time are not always included in the clinical question; therefore, those terms are optional. Templates for and examples of different types of clinical questions are shown in **Box 5.2**.

BOX 5.2 PICO or PICO/T Clinical Question Templates

For an Intervention or Therapy

■ In ___(P)___ , what is the effect of ___(I)___ on ___(O)___ compared with ___(C)___ within ___(T)___?

Example: In patients with ankle sprains, what is the effect of cryotherapy on pain compared with electrical stimulation treatment?

For Etiology

■ Are ___(P)___ who have ___(I)___ at [increased/decreased] risk for/of ___(O)___ compared with ___(P)___ with/without ___(C)___ over ___(T)___?

Example: Are football players who have a family history of cardiovascular conditions at an increased risk for a cardiovascular condition compared with football players without a family history of cardiovascular conditions over a football season?

Diagnosis or Diagnostic Test

■ Are/Is ___(I)___ more accurate in diagnosing ___(P)___ compared with ___(C)___ for ___(O)___?

Example: Is the Lachman's test more accurate in diagnosing patients with knee injuries compared with the anterior drawer test for ACL tears?

Prevention

■ For ___(P)___ , does the use of ___(I)___ reduce the future risk of ___(O)___ compared with ___(C)___?

Example: For soccer players, does the use of ankle braces reduce the future risk of ankle sprains compared with ankle taping?

Prognosis/Predictions

■ Does ___(I)___ influence ___(O)___ in patients who have ___(P)___ over ___(T)___?

Example: Does the type of ACL graft used influence knee stability in patients who have ACL replacement surgery over 20 years?

Adapted from Melnyk B, Fineout-Overholt E. *Evidence-Based Practice in Nursing & Healthcare*. Philadelphia, PA: Lippincott Williams & Wilkins; 2005.

Searching the Literature

To efficiently search the literature, it is important to use appropriate evidence databases, which are collections of organized information. **Box 5.3** provides a list of the most common health care–related databases used by athletic trainers. Some databases contain only **filtered information**. Filtered information means that other clinicians and researchers have already searched the existing evidence, evaluated it, and synthesized a clinical recommendation. Examples of filtered information include clinical practice guidelines, critically appraised topics (CATs), Cochrane reviews, evidence-based synopses, meta-analysis, and systematic reviews (SRs). Other databases contain both filtered information and **unfiltered information**. Unfiltered information includes individual research studies and expert opinions. Busy clinicians will find that filtered information is a more efficient and effective means of quickly assessing information to inform their clinical practice.

Athletic trainers can improve the effectiveness of their evidence search by using appropriate **search terms**, which are words with precise meaning. If an athletic trainer has used the PICO/T format to develop the clinical question, then the athletic trainer can use the PICO/T terms as the search terms. Some databases, such as PubMed/MEDLINE, Cumulative Index of Nursing and Allied Health Literature (CINAHL), and SPORTDiscus, support the use of **Boolean terms** (e.g., "and,"

BOX 5.3 Relevant Evidence Databases for Athletic Trainers

Databases That Only Contain Filtered Information

Cochrane (http://www.cochrane.org)

Centre for Evidence-Based Physiotherapy: PEDro (http://www.pedro.org.au)

National Guideline Clearing House (http://www.guideline.gov)

TRIP (http://www.tripdatabase.com/)

Databases That Contain Both Filtered and Unfiltered Information

CINAHL (https://www.ebscohost.com/nursing/products/cinahl-databases)

EMBASE (https://www.elsevier.com/solutions/embase-biomedical-research)

PubMed/MEDLINE (http://www.ncbi.nlm.nih.gov/pubmed)

Clinical Queries (http://www.ncbi.nlm.nih.gov/pubmed/clinical)

SPORTDiscus (https://www.ebscohost.com/academic/sportdiscus-with-full-text)

"or," and "not"). In these databases, health care providers can focus their literature search by using the Boolean terms in addition to their search terms (see **Box 5.4**). Using **Medical Subject Heading (MeSH)** terms can also improve the effectiveness of one's search within the PubMed/MEDLINE databases. MeSH terms are the controlled medical vocabulary used by the U.S. National Library of Medicine in the PubMed/MEDLINE databases (see **Box 5.5** for examples).

Evaluate the Evidence

Once evidence related to the clinical question is obtained, it must be evaluated for impact (level of importance), reliability (how reproducible are the results), validity (do the results really represent what we think they represent), and applicability (how well does the evidence apply to the current clinical question). Larger quantities of strong evidence should have a greater impact on clinical decisions than smaller quantities of weaker evidence. The **hierarchy** or **level of evidence** (**Fig. 5.1**) can help clinicians decide which pieces of evidence are stronger or weaker than others. Filtered information tends to be stronger than unfiltered information; therefore, it appears higher on the evidence hierarchy. See **Box 5.6** for a description of each type of evidence. In addition to the type of evidence, studies that evaluate patient-oriented evidence are more meaningful than those that only report disease-oriented evidence. Finally, treatments that demonstrate a larger effect size are more meaningful. **Effect size** measures the difference in outcomes between the treatment and nontreatment groups. The larger the difference or effect size, the greater the impact the treatment will have.

Clinicians commonly use one of three scales to efficiently communicate the impact or strength of individual pieces of evidence and overall clinical recommendation. Those scales include the following:

- Strength of Recommendation Taxonomy (SORT) scale, which includes a 3-point, alphabetic scale (e.g., A, B, C) to score clinical recommendations, and a 3-point, numeric scale (e.g., 1, 2, 3) to score individual pieces of evidence (**Box 5.7**).[3]

- Oxford Centre for Evidence-Based Medicine (CEBM) 2011 Levels of Evidence, which uses a 5-point numeric scale to rate evidence, where level 1 is the strongest and level 5 is the weakest.[4]

- Grading of Recommendations Assessment, Development, and Evaluation (GRADE), which can be used to rate SRs and clinical guidelines. Clinicians use the GRADE scale to classify evidence as either "high," "moderate," "low," or "very low." Classifications are based on the quality of evidence, the likelihood of both desirable and undesirable effects, common patient values, and a judicious use of resources.[5]

BOX 5.4 Using Search and Boolean Terms to Streamline Evidence Searches

Example 1

To answer the following clinical question:

Is the <u>Lachman's test</u> more accurate in diagnosing <u>patients with knee injuries</u> compared with the <u>anterior drawer test</u> for <u>ACL tears</u>?

The following searches were done in the PubMed database (www.ncbi.nlm.gov/pubmed):

Term Used During a Search	Number of Articles Returned in a PubMed Search
Knee Injuries	26,265
ACL	17,419
Lachman	1,725
Anterior Drawer	705
Anterior Drawer **NOT** Ankle	547
Lachman **AND** Knee Injuries	480
Lachman **AND** Anterior Drawer	210
Lachman **AND** Anterior Drawer **AND** ACL	202
Lachman **AND** Anterior Drawer **AND** ACL **AND** Diagnosis	156

Notice how the PICO terms became the search terms and the addition of the Boolean terms "AND" and "NOT" decreased the number of results one would need to evaluate.

Example 2

To answer the following clinical question:

In <u>patients with ankle sprains</u>, what is the effect of <u>cryotherapy</u> on <u>pain</u> compared with <u>electrical stimulation treatment</u>?

The following searches were done in the PubMed database (www.ncbi.nlm.gov/pubmed):

Term Used During a Search	Number of Articles Returned in a PubMed Search
Ankle Sprain	13,956
Cryotherapy	24,527
Cryotherapy **OR** Cold Therapy	43,559
Electrical Stimulation	163,553
Pain	597,854
Cryotherapy **AND** Ankle Sprain	67
Cryotherapy **AND** Ankle Sprains **AND** Electrical Stimulation	4
Cryotherapy **AND** Ankle Sprains **AND** Pain	25

Notice how the PICO terms became the search terms and the addition of Boolean term "OR" increased the number of results, whereas the use of "AND" decreased the number of results one would need to evaluate.

BOX 5.5 Examples of MeSH Terms

Search Terms	MeSH Term Used by MEDLINE/PubMed
Ankle sprain	Ankle injuries
Chronic ankle sprain	Ankle injuries
Syndesmotic ankle sprain	Ankle injuries
MRI	Magnetic resonance imaging
Shoulder dislocation	Shoulder dislocation
Glenohumeral dislocation	Shoulder dislocation
Shoulder labral tear	Shoulder
Shoulder	Shoulder
Labral	*No related MeSH term*
Tear	Tear
	Lacerations

Athletic trainers can also use **appraisal scales** to assess the design of individual research studies. Appraisal scales are intended for specific types of research. Clinicians and researchers should only use preferred reporting items for systematic reviews and meta-analyses (PRIMAS) to assess meta-analyses and SRs, the Jadad and physiotherapy evidence database (PEDro) scales to evaluate randomized controlled trial (RCT), either QUADAS-2 or the Standards for Reporting Diagnostic Accuracy (STARD) statement to assess diagnostics studies, and Strengthening the Reporting of Observational Studies in Epidemiology (STROBE) to evaluate epidemiologic research.

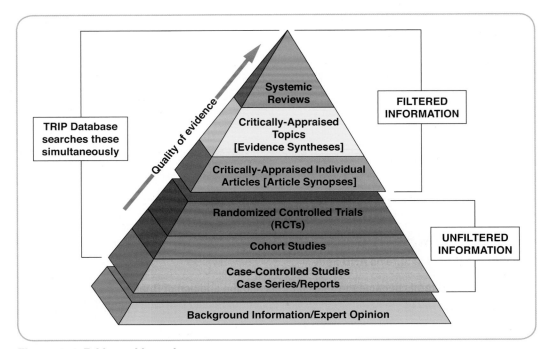

Figure 5.1. Evidence hierarchy.

BOX 5.6 Types of Evidence

Filtered

Meta-analysis	A study that pools results of two or more studies to obtain an overall answer to a question or interest[a]
Systematic review	A methodical review of the existing literature on a clearly described specific question. A description of how the evidence on the topic was found, including the databases, search terms, and inclusion and exclusion criteria, is included in the article.[a]
Critically appraised topic	A short summary of the best available evidence on an individual topic. Unlike in a systematic review, an exhaustive search of the literature was not completed.
Cochrane review	A systematic review created by a global independent network of health practitioners from over 120 countries[b]

Unfiltered

Randomized controlled (clinical) trial	A research study in which a group of patients is randomized into an experimental group and a control group. These groups are followed up for the outcomes of interest.[a]
All-or-none	Case series in which all of the patients experience the same outcome; for example, everyone one who wears an ankle brace does not sustain an ankle sprain.[c]
Cohort study	A research study in which two groups of patients, one that did receive the treatment/injury of interest and one that did not, are followed and an outcome of interested is measured[a]
Case-control	A research study in which two groups of patients, one that did receive the treatment/injury of interest and one that did not, are examined by looking back at existing records for an outcome of interest[a]
Case series	Describes characteristics of between two and five patients with an uncommon disease/injury or who have undergone a similar procedure[a]
Case report	Describes characteristics of a single patient with an uncommon disease/injury or who has undergone a unique treatment[a]
Controlled laboratory study	An in vitro or in vivo investigation in which one group receiving an experimental treatment is compared with one or more groups receiving no treatment or an alternate treatment. Laboratory studies that only include healthy people (no patients) are considered controlled laboratory studies.[a]
Descriptive laboratory study	An in vivo or in vitro study that describes characteristics such as anatomy, physiology, or kinesiology of a broad range of subjects or a specific group of interest[a]
Expert or consensus opinion	An idea that cannot be substantiated by direct evidence. It is a hypothesis based on related information.

[a]Hertel J. Keep it simple: study design nomenclature in research article abstracts [editorial]. *J Athl Train*. 2010;45(3):213–214.

[b]The Cochrane Collaboration. About us. http://www.cochrane.org/about-us. Accessed January 8, 2015.

[c]Merlin T, Weston A, Tooher R. Extending an evidence hierarchy to include topics other than treatment: revising the Australian 'levels of evidence.' *BMC Med Res Methodol*. 2009;9:34.

BOX 5.7 SORT Scale

Clinical Recommendation Subscale

Strength of Recommendation	Definition
A	Recommendation based on consistent and good-quality patient-oriented evidence[a]
B	Recommendation based on inconsistent or limited-quality patient-oriented evidence[a]
C	Recommendation based on consensus, usual practice, opinion, disease-oriented evidence,[a] or case series for studies of diagnosis, treatment, prevention, or screening

Individual Evidence Subscale

Strength of Study/ Evidence	Diagnosis	Treatment/Prevention/ Screening	Prognosis
Level 1— good quality	■ Validated clinical decision rule ■ SR/meta-analysis of high-quality studies ■ High-quality diagnostic cohort study[b]	■ SR/meta-analysis of RCTs with consistent findings ■ High-quality individual RCT[c] ■ All-or-none study[d]	■ SR/meta-analysis of good-quality cohort studies ■ Prospective cohort study with good follow-up
Level 2— limited-quality patient-oriented evidence	■ Unvalidated clinical decision rule ■ SR/meta-analysis of lower quality studies or studies with inconsistent findings ■ Lower quality diagnostic cohort study or diagnostic case-control study[d]	■ SR/meta-analysis of lower quality clinical trials or of studies with inconsistent findings ■ Lower quality clinical trial[c] ■ Cohort study ■ Case-control study	■ SR/meta-analysis of lower quality cohort studies or with inconsistent results ■ Retrospective cohort study or prospective cohort study with poor follow-up ■ Case-control study ■ Case series
Level 3— other evidence	Consensus guidelines, extrapolations from bench research, usual practice, opinion, disease-oriented, evidence (intermediate or physiological outcomes only), or case series for studies of diagnosis, treatment, prevention, or screening		

Consistency Across Studies

Consistent — Most studies found similar or at least coherent conclusions (coherence means that differences are explainable).

or

If high-quality and up-to-date systematic reviews or meta-analyses exist, they support the recommendation.

Inconsistent — Considerable variation among study findings and lack of coherence

or

If high-quality and up-to-date systematic reviews or meta-analyses exist, they do not find consistent evidence in favor of the recommendation.

[a]Patient-oriented evidence measures outcomes that matter to patients: morbidity, mortality, symptom improvement, cost reduction, and quality of life. Disease-oriented evidence measures intermediate, physiological, or surrogate end points that may or may not reflect improvements in patient outcomes (e.g., blood pressure, blood chemistry, physiological function, pathologic findings).

[b]High-quality diagnostic cohort study: cohort design, adequate size, adequate spectrum of patients, blinding, and a consistent, well-defined reference standard.

[c]High-quality RCT: allocation concealed, blinding if possible, intention-to-treat analysis, adequate statistical power, adequate follow-up (greater than 80%).

[d]In an all-or-none study, the treatment causes a dramatic change in outcomes, such as antibiotics for meningitis or surgery for appendicitis, which precludes study in a controlled trial.

RCT, randomized controlled trial; *SR,* systematic review.

From Ebell MH, Siwek J, Weiss BD, et al. Strength of recommendation taxonomy (SORT): a patient-centered approach to grading evidence in the medical literature. *Am Fam Physician.* 2004;69(3):548–556.

Reliability

The reliability of research results affects the impact evidence should have on clinical decisions. The **reliability** indicates how reproducible the results are when the measurement should be the same (e.g., measuring a patient's ankle dorsiflexion range of motion multiple times without treatment or a change in injury status should result in the same value). **Intrarater reliability** values determine the consistency of the measurements made by a single researcher or instrument (e.g., the same clinician measures ankle dorsiflexion multiple times), whereas the reliability of measurements made between several researchers or instruments is **interrater reliability** (e.g., clinician A and clinician B both measure a patient's ankle dorsiflexion). Interclass correlation coefficients (ICCs) are common statistical values used to report both intrarater and interrater reliability for continuous data (e.g., range of motion, force, and temperature). Kappa coefficients should be reported for categorical data (e.g., positive and negative diagnostic test results) and weighted kappa coefficients for ordinal data (e.g., manual muscle test or grades of edema).[6] ICC and kappa coefficient values fall on a scale of 0 to 1.0, with values closer to 1.0 indicating greater agreement or reliability within or between researchers and/or instruments. Typically, reliability values greater than 0.7 are acceptable.[7]

Validity

Besides study design and reliability of research results, the validity of results should be considered. **Validity** is the assurance that measurements represent what we think they represent (e.g., differences in weight scale results represent true changes in an individual's body weight, or changes in a patient-oriented outcome scale represent true changes to the patient's health status).

Diagnostic Accuracy

There are several statistics measures that may be used to assess **diagnostic accuracy**, that is, the ability of a diagnostic test/technique to discriminate between disease/injury and health. When assessing a diagnostic test, the results of the test are compared to those of a reference standard. **Reference standards** reflect the patient's true status, that is, injured or healthy. The results of the diagnostic test are compared to the reference standard in a 2 × 2 contingency table, and there are four possibilities: true positive, false positive, false negative, and true negative (see **Box 5.8**). **True positives** indicate individuals who have a positive diagnosis according to the diagnostic test and really have the injury according to the reference standard. **False positives** indicate individuals who have a positive diagnosis according to the diagnostic test but really do not have the injury according to the reference standard. **False negatives** indicate individuals who have a negative diagnosis according to the diagnostic test but really do have the injury according to the reference standard. **True negatives** indicate individuals who have a negative diagnosis according to the diagnostic test and really do not have the injury according to the reference standard.

The sensitivity and specificity of a diagnostic test can help clinicians determine which tests to use when there are several options. Sensitivity and specificity can be calculated from the contingency table values and are scaled from 0% to 100%, where 100% is perfect sensitivity or specificity (see **Box 5.8** for data regarding the Thessaly test for detecting meniscal tears in an ACL-deficient knee[8]). **Sensitivity** is the ability of the diagnostic test to detect an injury. When a clinician uses a diagnostic test with a high sensitivity, a negative test helps to rule out the injury. A mnemonic to help remember this relationship is with high sensitivity (*Sn*), a negative (*N*) test rules out (*out*) the injury, or *SnNout*.[1] Using the example for **Box 5.6**, the Thessaly test had a sensitivity of 79%, making it a useful test to rule in a meniscal tear in those patients with an ACL-deficient knee. **Specificity** is the ability of a diagnostic test to detect health. A mnemonic to help remember this relationship is with high specificity (*Sp*), a positive (*P*) test rules in (*in*) the injury, or *SpPin*.[1] Using the example for **Box 5.6**, the Thessaly test had a specificity of 41%, making it less useful at ruling out a meniscal tear in those patients with an ACL-deficient knee. Clinicians will find diagnostic tests with higher sensitivity and/or specificity more accurate and therefore more helpful when making clinical decisions.

The reciprocal of sensitivity and specificity are the false negative and false positive rates. The **false negative rate** is the *inability* of a diagnostic test to detect injury. The **false positive rate** is the *inability* of a diagnostic test to detect health. Sensitivity and specificity values are reported and used more often than the false negative and false positive rates.

BOX 5.8 Determining the Accuracy of Diagnostic Tests

Diagnostic Data Contingency Table[a]

		Reference Standard		
		Dx+	Dx−	Row Total
Thessaly Test (Diagnostic Test)	Dx+	True positives 31 (A)	False positives 24 (B)	55 (A + B)
	Dx−	False negatives 8 (C)	True negatives 17 (D)	25 (C + D)
	Column total	39 (A + C)	41 (B + D)	Grand total 80 (A + B + C + D)

[a]Adapted from Mirzatolooei F, Yekta Z, Bayazidchi M, et al. Validation of the Thessaly test for detecting meniscal tears in anterior cruciate deficient knees. *Knee*. 2010;17(3):221–223.

Formulas for Diagnostic Validity Measures

Term	Formula	Example
Diagnostic accuracy	(A + D) / N	(31 + 17) / 80 = 60%
Sensitivity	A / (A + C)	31 / (31 + 8) = 79%
Specificity	D / (B + D)	17 / (24 + 17) = 41%
False positive rate	B / (B + D) (1 − Specificity)	24 / (24 + 17) = 59% 1 − 0.41 = 0.59 = 59%
False negative rate	C / (A + C) (1 − Sensitivity)	8 / (31 + 8) = 21% 1 − 0.79 = 0.21 = 21%
Positive predictive value (PV+)	A / (A + B)	31 / (31 + 24) = 56%
Negative predictive value (PV−)	D / (C + D)	17 / (8 + 17) = 68%
Prevalence	(A + C) / N	(31 + 8) / 80 = 49%
Positive likelihood ratio (LR+)	Sensitivity / (1 − Specificity)	0.79 / (1 − 0.41) = 1.3
Negative likelihood ratio (LR−)	(1 − Sensitivity) / Specificity	(1 − 0.79) / 0.41 = 0.5

Predictive values can help clinicians determine whether a diagnostic test would be effective as a screening tool and can also be calculated from contingency table results (see **Box 5.8**). The **positive predictive value (PV+)** estimates how many people who have a positive test actually have the injury. The **negative predictive value (PV−)** estimates how many people who have a negative test are actually healthy. In the example in **Box 5.8**, the Thessaly test has a PV+ of 56% and PV− of 68%, meaning it would be a better tool for screening for a healthy meniscus than for an injured meniscus during a preseason physical exam.

The sensitivity, specificity, and predictive values for a diagnostic test are all influenced by the prevalence of the injury. **Prevalence** describes how common the injury is, that is, the number of injury cases in a given population. In the example in **Box 5.8**, 49% of the studied population had meniscal tears. If the prevalence of an injury is high, then the possibility of positive diagnostic test result by chance increases and results in higher sensitivity, specificity, and positive predictive values. If the prevalence of an injury is low, then the possibility of a positive diagnostic test by chance decreases, resulting in lower sensitivity and specificity values and high negative predictive values.

Likelihood Ratios

Likelihood ratios can help clinicians determine how likely it is that a patient does or doesn't have an injury based on the diagnostic test results. A **positive likelihood ratio (LR+)** tells a clinician how much more likely the patient is to have the condition if the diagnostic test is positive. **Negative likelihood ratios (LR−)** tell an athletic trainer how less likely the patient is to have the condition if the diagnostic test is negative. Based on the likelihood ratio of a diagnostic test, providers can view those test results as being unimportant and unhelpful to very important and helpful (**Fig. 5.2**). Unlike sensitivity, specificity, and prediction values, the prevalence of a condition will not influence the likelihood ratio results. Based on the scale presented in Figure 5.2 and the Thessaly test, LR+ of 1.3 and LR− of 0.5 (**Box 5.8**) has limited value to a clinician trying to rule in or rule out a meniscal injury in an ACL-deficient knee.

Probability of a Diagnosis

Clinicians start with a **pretest probability**, which is their hypothesis that a patient has an injury. Clinicians can use their past clinical experience, the patient's medical history, and signs and symptoms, as well as the prevalence of the injury, to estimate the pretest probability that a patient is injured. The clinician can then choose which diagnostic test(s) to use, based on each test's sensitivity and specificity values. The best tests would have demonstrated both high sensitivity and high specificity. Based on the diagnostic test result and the diagnostic test's likelihood ratios, the clinician can determine the **posttest probability** of the patient having the injury on a nomogram (**Fig. 5.3**). Using the Thessaly test example in **Box 5.8**, the pretest probability of a meniscal tear base on prevalence would be 49%. If a patient's Thessaly test was positive and based on the Thessaly test LR+ value of 1.3, the posttest probability of a meniscal tear would be approximately 56%. If a patient's Thessaly test was negative and based on the Thessaly test LR− value of 0.5, the posttest probability of a meniscal tear would be approximately 32%. If several diagnostic tests are used, then the posttest probability becomes the pretest probability for the second test, and so on.

Risk of Injury

Data from observational studies are used to determine the distribution of injury/disease in a population. The **incidence** of injury is the number of new injuries occurring during a set amount of time, whereas the **incidence rate (IR)** is the number of new cases during a set observation period (IR =

Negative Likelihood Ratios (LR−) value range				Postive Likelihood Ratios (LR+) value range		
0 to 0.1	0.1 to 0.2	0.2 to 0.5	0.5 to 2.0	2.0 to 5.0	5.0 to 10.0	>10.0
Test results are important and helpful	Test results are unimportant and unhelpful					Test results are important and helpful

Figure 5.2. Interpreting likelihood ratios.

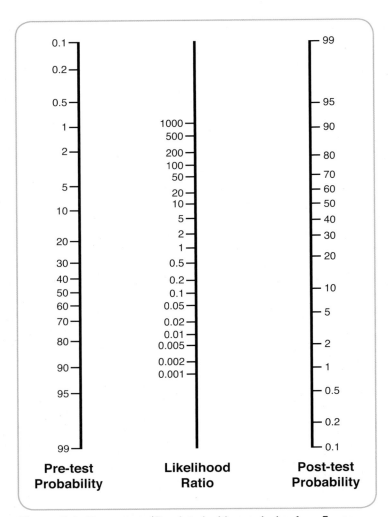

Figure 5.3. Nomogram. (Reprinted with permission from Fagan TJ. Letter to the editor: a nomogram for applying likelihood ratios. *N Engl J Med.* 1975;293:257. Copyright © [1975] Massachusetts Medical Society.)

number of new cases during / total person-time at risk). The total person-time at risk for sport injury IRs could be the number of practices and/or games in which athletes participated. The **prevalence (P)** is the total number of existing patients with the injury or disease at a given point of time (P = number of existing cases / total population at risk for injury or disease).

Treatment Effectiveness

To assess the effectiveness of a treatment or intervention, it is best to use an RCT, in which patients are randomly assigned to either a treatment or control (i.e., no treatment, or some other comparison) group. The researchers then need to define what a successful treatment outcome would be (e.g., patient returns to participation or patient reports pain reduction on a 5-point Likert scale of global effect). A 2 × 2 contingency table is again used to organize the treatment data (see **Box 5.9** for data regarding a comparison between foot orthoses and inserts on patellofemoral pain[9]). To assess the effectiveness, the athletic trainer looks at the number of unsuccessful or failed treatments. The treatment or **experimental event rate (EER)** is the number of adverse outcomes or unsuccessful treatments. In the example in **Box 5.9**, we can see that foot orthoses failed to reduce pain in 15% of the patients treated with orthoses. The **control event rate (CER)** is the number of adverse or unsuccessful outcomes in the control group. In the example in **Box 5.9**, we can see that 43% of the patients treated with inserts failed to have their pain reduced.

The EER and CER are used to calculate the relative risk of the treatment. The **relative risk (RR)** tells us how likely an adverse event or unsuccessful treatment will occur in the treatment group relative to the control group. In the example in **Box 5.9**, patients who received the foot orthoses were only 35% as likely to continue to experience knee pain compared to those treated with flat inserts.

Clinicians may find the relative risk reduction more helpful than the relative risk. The **relative risk reduction (RRR)** indicated the reduction in unsuccessful treatments relative to the control group. For the example presented in **Box 5.9**, patients who received orthoses were 65% less likely to have pain compared to those who received flat inserts. Because the RRR is a relative value, it does not provide any idea how large the treatment effect is; therefore, clinicians might find the absolute risk reduction more helpful. The **absolute risk reduction (ARR)** provides us with the actual difference in risk between the treatment and control group. For the example in **Box 5.9**, the ARR is 28%, indicating that orthoses reduced pain 28% more often than the flat inserts.

The **number needed to treat (NNT)** is helpful when determining whether a treatment is a good allocation of time and/or resources. The NNT indicates how many patients would need to receive the therapy to prevent one adverse or unsuccessful outcome. Positive values indicate that a treatment is helpful, and the closer the value is to 1, the more effective the treatment. In the treatment example in **Box 5.9**, the NNT for foot orthoses is 3.6, which is rounded to 4. This means that for every four patients with patellofemoral pain treated with orthoses, we should expect one patient to experience pain relief.

BOX 5.9 Determining the Effectiveness of Treatment

	Outcomes		
	Unsuccessful/Adverse	Success	Row Total
Foot orthoses (treatment group)	6 (A)	35 (B)	41 (A + B)
Flat inserts (control group)	17 (C)	23 (D)	40 (C + D)
Column total	23 (A + C)	58 (B + D)	Grand total 81 (A + B + C + D)

Term	Formula	Example
Experimental event rate (EER)	A / (A + B)	6 / (6 + 35) = 15%
Control event rate (CER)	C / (C + D)	17 / (17 + 23) = 43%
Relative risk (RR)	EER / CER	0.15 / 0.43 = 35%
Relative risk reduction (RRR)	(CER − EER) / CER	(0.43 − 0.15) / 0.43 = 65%
Absolute risk reduction (ARR)	CER − EER	0.43 − 0.15 = 28%
Number needed to treat (NNT)	1 / ARR	1 / 0.28 = 3.6
Absolute risk increase (ARI)	EER − CER	0.15 − 0.43 = −28%
Number needed to harm (NNH)	1 / ARI	1 / −0.28 = −3.6

To know how good a treatment is at preventing injury or assessing how harmful a treatment is (i.e., serious side effects or complications), clinicians should use the **absolute risk increase (ARI)** and **number needed to harm (NNH)**. The ARI provides clinicians with the actual increase in risk between the treatment and control groups, whereas the NNH tells a clinician how many patients need to receive the treatment for just one patient to experience a harmful treatment. For the example in **Box 5.9**, there is no increase in risk as indicated by a positive ARR and NNT and if erroneously calculated, both a negative ARI of −28% and negative NNH value of −3.6. This means the use of foot orthoses in patients with patellofemoral pain will not increase the number of patients who experience pain compared to those patients who receive flat inserts, and therefore, they will be harmed by the orthoses.

Integrating Evidence into Clinical Decisions

After a clinician has gathered all the information relative to the clinical question, the clinician must decide how to use that evidence. Remember that the purpose of EBHC is to provide the best possible care by integrating evidence with clinical experience and the individual patient's values and circumstances. Evidence should be assessed on the strength (evidence hierarchy), the types of outcomes measured (patient- versus disease-oriented), consistency of the results (all for, all against, or mixed results), and the applicability (evidence is from a similar population or the exact same treatment settings/dosage used). Clinical experience should influence how a clinician uses evidence but should not be an excuse to ignore the best available evidence. Finally, patients should provide input regarding the care they receive.

Pathology ↔ Impairment ↔ Functional Limitation ↔ Disability

• Pathology—disruption of physiology (tissue)

• Impairment—loss of function (e.g., ROM, strength)

• Functional Limitation—ADLs (e.g., walking, running, serving)

• Disability—inability to perform role (e.g., football player, dancer)

Figure 5.4. Nagi disablement model. *ADLs,* activities of daily living; *ROM,* range of motion.

Disability Models

Athletic trainers will find the models of disablement helpful when trying to understand how disease/injury and treatment affects a patient. The Nagi disablement model is a classic model that represents how disease/injury at a tissue level affects body systems, the whole person, as well as the person's role in society (**Fig. 5.4**).[10] Today, most health care professions are moving toward the World Health Organization's (WHO) International Classification of Functioning, Disability and Health (ICF) (**Fig. 5.5**).[11,12] Unlike the Nagi model, the ICF model takes into consideration how personal and environmental factors may also influence an individual's function, disability, and health. Changes in disease-oriented outcomes typically represent changes in Nagi's impairments or the WHO's body function or structure, whereas changes in patient-oriented outcomes represent changes in Nagi's functional limitations and disabilities or the WHO's activities and participation.

Evaluate the Efficiency and Effectiveness of Steps 1 to 4

The last step of EBHC is to reflect on and evaluate the EBHC process and identify ways the process can be more efficient and effective. Clinicians could ask themselves: (1) Was the clinical question well formulated? (2) Did we use the best databases? (3) Did we use the best search terms? (4) Could the search be streamlined by searching multiple databases or using multiple search terms in a single search? (5) Could we appraise the evidence? or (6) Could the evidence be integrated into the clinical

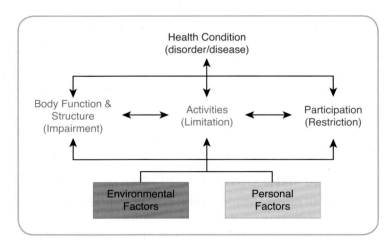

Figure 5.5. WHO's International Classification of Functioning, Disability, and Health Model. (From World Health Organization. *Towards a Common Language for Functioning, Disability and Health: ICF.* Geneva, Switzerland: World Health Organization; 2002.)

decision? Clinicians may find filtered information more helpful when speed is most important. Learning how to use Boolean terms effectively can reduce the reviewing of unrelated material after an evidence search. Becoming more familiar with EBHC-related terms, the hierarchy of evidence, and diagnostic and treatment statistics may improve one's ability to quickly appraise the evidence and determine its impact, reliability, and validity, as well as its applicability to the current clinical decision.

 The athletic trainer should develop two separate PICO/T questions: one to determine the accuracy of diagnostic tests to be considered and the second to assess the treatment being considered. Using one of the filtered databases should expedite the evidence search for both PICO/T questions. The athletic trainer will find that diagnostic tests with LR+ of greater than 10 and LR− of less than 0.1 will have the greatest impact on improving diagnostic accuracy. The use of multiple diagnostic tests can also improve the accuracy of the posttest probability of the diagnosis. The clinician can determine the effectiveness of treatment with the relative and the absolute risk rates, whereas NNT would help decide whether resources (e.g., cost, time, equipment) required for the treatment are worth the risk of an unsuccessful treatment.

SUMMARY

1. The purpose of EBHC is to integrate the best available evidence into clinical decisions while including patient values.

2. Patient-oriented evidence provides a broader view of health than disease- or clinician-oriented evidence.

3. There are five steps to practicing EBHC: (1) Ask a PICO/T question; (2) search health care–related databases; (3) evaluate the evidence for impact, reliability, validity, and applicability; (4) integrate the evidence into the clinical practice; and (5) evaluate the process and look for ways to become more efficient and effective.

4. The SORT, CEBM 2011 Levels of Evidence, and GRADE scales are used to rate evidence.

5. Diagnostic accuracy is dependent on the sensitivity, specificity, and prevalence of diagnostic tests. Positive and negative likelihood ratios of diagnostic tests help clinicians determine the probability of a diagnosis based on the results of the diagnostic tests.

6. The effectiveness of treatment can be determined by the NNT, RRR ARR, ARI, and NNH.

7. The disablement models help to explain the effects injury/disease can have on a person's role in society. Disease-oriented outcomes represent impairments, whereas patient-oriented outcomes represent a patient's activity and participation level.

APPLICATION QUESTIONS

1. You have been an athletic trainer for 20 years. Why is it important for you to practice EBHC?

2. You suspect a patient has lateral epicondylitis of the elbow. How would you determine which diagnostic tests would be most helpful in confirming the correct diagnosis?

3. You diagnose a patient with lateral epicondylitis of the elbow. How would you identify the most effective treatment for this patient?

REFERENCES

1. Straus SE, Richardsons WS, Glasziou P, et al. *Evidence-Based Medicine: How to Practice and Teach EBM*. 3rd ed. Edinburgh, Scotland: Elsevier Churchill Livingstone; 2005.
2. U.S. National Library of Medicine. Key MEDLINE® indicators. Published February 7, 2014. Updated December 14, 2014. http://www.nlm.nih.gov/bsd/bsd_key.html. Accessed January 14, 2015.
3. Ebell MH, Siwek J, Weiss BD, et al. Strength of recommendation taxonomy (SORT): a patient-centered approach to grading evidence in the medical literature. *Am Fam Physician*. 2004; 69(3):548–556.
4. Howick J, Chalmers I, Glasziou P, et al. The Oxford 2011 levels of evidence. http://www.cebm.net/index.aspx?o=5653. Accessed January 9, 2015.
5. Guyatt GH, Oxman AD, Vist GE, et al. GRADE: an emerging consensus on rating quality of evidence and strength of recommendations. *BMJ*. 2008;336(7650):924–926.
6. Sim J, Wright CC. The kappa statistic in reliability studies: use, interpretation, and sample size requirements. *Phys Ther*. 2005;85(3): 257–268.
7. Fitzpatrick R, Davey C, Buxton M, et al. Evaluating patient-based outcome measures for use in clinical trials: a review. *Health Technol Assess*. 1998;2(14):1–74.
8. Mirzatolooei F, Yekta Z, Bayazidchi M, et al. Validation of the Thessaly test for detecting meniscal tears in anterior cruciate deficient knees. *Knee*. 2010;17(3):221–223.
9. Collins N, Crossley K, Beller E, et al. Foot orthoses and physiotherapy in the treatment of patellofemoral pain syndrome: randomised clinical trial. *BMJ*. 2008;337:a1735.
10. Nagi S. Some conceptual issues in disability and rehabilitation. In: Sussman M, ed. *Sociology and Rehabilitation*. Washington, DC: American Sociological Association; 1965:100–113.
11. World Health Organization. *Towards a Common Language for Functioning, Disability and Health: ICF*. Geneva, Switzerland: World Health Organization; 2002.
12. Snyder AR, Parsons JT, Valovich McLeod TC, et al. Using disablement models and clinical outcomes assessment to enable evidence-based athletic training practice, part I: disablement models. *J Athl Train*. 2008;43(4):428–436.

6

Clinical Assessment and Diagnosis

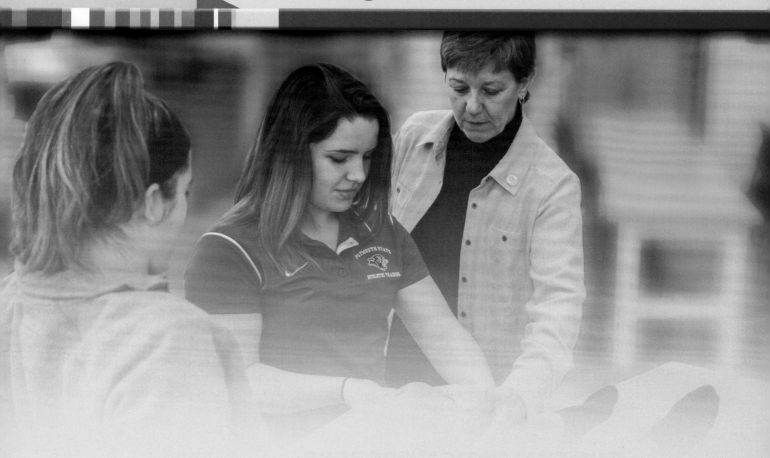

STUDENT OUTCOMES

1. Differentiate between the history of the injury, observation and inspection, palpation, and special tests (HOPS) injury assessment format; the subjective evaluation, objective evaluation, assessment, and plan (SOAP) note format used to assess and manage musculoskeletal injuries; and the history and physical examination model used to assess for general medical conditions.

2. Explain the general components of the history portion of the assessment process.

3. Differentiate the types of pain as indicators of potential pathologies.

4. Describe the processes involved in the visual observation and inspection of an ill or injured patient.

5. Describe the basic principles that direct the palpation component of the assessment process.

6. Identify the various types of tests included during a physical examination.

7. Describe how range of motion (ROM), goniometry, and manual muscle testing are similar yet different with regard to testing procedures and purpose.

8. Explain how the assessment process differs based on purpose for conducting assessment.

9. Describe testing techniques used by medical specialists in diagnosing an injury.

10. List the reasons for maintaining clear, accurate, and up-to-date medical documentation of services provided.

INTRODUCTION

One of the major performance domains for the athletic trainer is clinical assessment and diagnosis. Using standardized clinical practices, the athletic trainer makes decisions relative to the nature and severity of an injury or illness. Because the assessment process involves searching for atypical or dysfunctional anatomy, physiology, or biomechanics, a strong understanding of each content area in conjunction with the knowledge of how to conduct a thorough evaluation is essential for an accurate clinical assessment. A poor assessment can have a devastating effect on the proper treatment and development of appropriate rehabilitation protocols.

This chapter begins with a description of the assessment process. The process has two main steps: the history and the physical examination. Both the history portion and the physical examination have several subcomponents that may or may not be used, depending on the situation and purpose for which the assessment is being conducted. When working with healthy individuals who have orthopedic complaints with no underlying medical issues, the assessment process follows a more narrow sequence called HOPS/HIPS (history, observations/inspection, palpation, and special tests). When assessing a patient for the purposes of developing a complex therapeutic intervention program, a subjective evaluation, objective evaluation, assessment, and plan (SOAP) sequence is followed. For patients who present with broader general medical issues, the history and physical examination (HPE) becomes more complex and lengthy. A table comparing these different assessment formats is presented in **Table 6.1**.

THE EVALUATION PROCESS

 A 15-year-old male ice hockey athlete enters the athletic training clinic complaining of hip pain. What additional information is needed to make a clinical diagnosis and devise a plan of treatment? What steps need to be taken in order to obtain the needed information?

The purpose of the evaluation process is to determine which tissues have been damaged and the extent or severity of the damage so that appropriate treatment can be rendered. The evaluation process involves gathering information from multiple sources: the patient, the physical examination, and diagnostic testing. The clinician looks for diagnostic signs and symptoms obtained through the evaluation process and interprets the information to help determine the type and extent of the injury. A **diagnostic sign** is an objective, measurable, physical finding regarding an individual's condition. A sign is what the clinician hears, feels, sees, or smells when assessing the patient. For example, a swollen knee is a diagnostic sign. A **symptom** is information provided by the patient regarding his or her perception of the problem. Examples of these subjective feelings include blurred vision, ringing in the ears, sharp stinging pain, locking or catching within the knee joint, weakness, and inability to move a body part. Obtaining information about symptoms can determine if the individual has an acute injury, resulting from a specific event (**macrotrauma**) leading to a sudden onset of symptoms, or a chronic injury, characterized by a slow, insidious onset of symptoms (**microtrauma**) that culminates in a painful inflammatory condition. Another important source of information is the opposite, healthy paired limb or organ.

TABLE 6.1 Comparison of Assessment Models

HOPS/HIPS	SOAP	HPE
Primary use: orthopedic assessment	Primary use: therapeutic intervention plan	Primary use: medical assessment

History
■ Chief complaint
  • Onset/MOI
  • Symptoms
  • Signs
  • Dysfunction
  • Training/working conditions
  • Recurrent condition
  • Previous treatment
  • Disabilities resulting from injury or illness
■ Related medical history
  • Past injury/illness
  • Family history
  • Medical conditions
	Subjective
	■ Includes all information obtained in the history portion of the HOPS/HIPS format
	■ Pain rating scales and other standardized patient outcome measures utilized more frequently in this format.
		History
		■ History of present illness: includes all information obtained in the history portion of the HOPS/HIPS format
		■ Past medical history
		■ Past surgical history
		■ Medications
		■ Allergies and reactions
		■ Social history
		■ Family history
		■ Review of systems

Inspection, Palpation, and Special Tests
■ Observation and analysis of overall appearance, body symmetry, swelling, deformity, discoloration, bleeding, deformity, general motor function, balance, gait, and posture
■ Palpation and analysis of overall skin temperature and moisture, tone, tenderness, crepitus, deformity, swelling, and pulse
■ Findings from range of motion, MMT, neurological testing, joint stress testing, and other special tests to assess for specific pathologies
	Objective
	■ Includes all information obtained in the inspection, palpation, and special tests section of HOPS/HIPS
	■ Information more frequently recorded using objective measures such as goniometry, grading scales, and other standardized patient outcome measures.
	■ Includes information obtained from other providers such as physician notes, results from imaging studies, or records documenting prior treatment/progress
	■ When used with providing daily treatments, type, duration, and frequency of treatment is also included.
		Physical Examination
		■ All information included with the HOPS/HIPS and SOAP note format is included as needed.
		■ Overall appearance
		■ Vital sign assessment
		■ HEENT examination
		■ Cardiac auscultation
		■ Respiratory auscultation and percussion
		■ Abdominal auscultation and percussion
		■ Gross motor function screening
		■ Neurological screening
		■ Laboratory diagnostics as needed
		  • Blood work
		  • Imaging
		  • Urinalysis

At the conclusion of the HOPS/HIPS format, the clinician should be able to identify potential clinical diagnoses and initiate appropriate management strategies.	**Assessment** ■ The clinical diagnosis is entered in the assessment section when completing an initial evaluation. For example: grade 2 ATFL sprain. ■ When the clinician is evaluating a patient frequently to determine how the patient is responding to treatment, the assessment should indicate the patient's progress. For example: Patient is responding to treatment and progressing appropriately toward meeting goals. ■ Problems list	**Assessment** ■ Differential diagnoses ■ Problems list ■ Treatment plan
	Plan ■ Short-term goals ■ Long-term goals ■ Treatment plan	

ATFL, anterior talofibular ligament; *MOI*, mechanism of injury.

From Kettenbach G. *Writing Patient/Client Notes: Ensuring Accuracy in Documentation.* 4th ed. Philadelphia, PA: FA Davis; 2009; Bickley LS, Szilagyi PG. *Bates' Guide to Physical Examination and History Taking.* Philadelphia, PA: Lippincott Williams & Wilkins; 2007; Magee DJ. *Orthopedic Physical Assessment.* 5th ed. Philadelphia, PA: Elsevier Saunders; 2008.

For example, if an injury occurs to one of the extremities, the results of individual tests performed on the noninjured body part can be compared with those for the injured body part. This process is referred to as **bilateral comparison**. Differences can indicate the level and severity of injury. The baseline of information gathered on the noninjured body part also can be used as a reference point to determine when the injured body part has been rehabilitated and, as such, when to allow a return to full participation in an activity. Under most circumstances, an assessment of the noninjured body part should precede an assessment of the injured body part. In some acute injuries, such as fractures or dislocations, an assessment of the noninjured body part is not necessary.

The injury evaluation process must include several key components—namely, taking a history of the current condition, visually inspecting the area for noticeable abnormalities, physically palpating the region for abnormalities, and completing functional and stress tests. Although several evaluation models may be used, each follows a consistent, sequential order to ensure that an essential component is not omitted without sufficient reason to do so. Two popular evaluation methods use for assessing patients with orthopedic conditions are the HOPS format and the SOAP note format. Each has its advantages, but the SOAP note format is much more inclusive of the entire injury management process. A third method, the HPE, is utilized when assessing patients for general medical complaints.

The HOPS Format

The HOPS format is often followed when evaluating the initial injury and forms the basis of the initial injury report. The HOPS format is easy to use and follows a basic, consistent format. Information obtained in the *history* is then verified during *observation*, *palpation*, and *special tests*. As the clinician moves through the sequence, information is obtained that either helps to support or eliminate potential pathologies until the final clinical diagnosis is made. Both subjective and objective information are obtained through this sequence and help the clinician in recognizing and identifying problems contributing to the condition. The HOPS format focuses on the evaluation component of injury management and excludes the rehabilitation process.

History

The *subjective* evaluation (i.e., history of the injury) includes the primary complaint (also known as the chief complaint or current complaint), mechanism of injury (MOI), characteristics of the symptoms, and pertinent medical history. This information comes from the patient and reflects his or her attitude, mental condition, and perceived physical state.

Observation, Palpation, and Special Tests

The *objective* evaluation utilizes measurable findings relative to the patient's condition. Observations are made to detect signs that may suggest certain pathologies. Palpation is used to assess areas of tenderness and abnormalities in the surface anatomy. Special tests include a wide range of clinical assessment techniques such as ROM testing, testing for joint instability, the balance error scoring system, and test for specific pathologies. Although the history may sometimes elicit inconsistent information depending on how questions are posed and the ability of the patient to accurately respond to questions, objective information should remain consistent relative to the patient's recovery process. This information can be measured repeatedly to track progress from the initial evaluation through the final clearance for discharge and a return to participation in a sport or other physical activity.

The SOAP Note Format

The **SOAP** note format is actually a method of documenting findings and provides a structured sequence for the clinician to follow when completing the evaluation process.[1] The SOAP format utilizes a problem-oriented approach and advanced sequence structure for decision making and problem solving in the management and rehabilitation phase. SOAP notes can also be tailored to use during an initial intake or during follow-up evaluations. SOAP notes document patient care and serve as a vehicle of communication between the on-site clinicians and other health care professionals.

These notes are intended to provide information concerning the ongoing status and tolerance of a patient and, in doing so, to avoid duplication of services by health care providers.

Subjective Portion

The **subjective** evaluation includes all information obtained through the history portion of the process. When used during the initial intake of a new patient, the subjective portion is very similar to that used in the HOPS format. When using the SOAP note format for follow-up evaluations with patients who have been receiving ongoing treatment or participating in ongoing rehabilitation programs, the subjective portion provides the clinician opportunity to document the patient's progress using the patient's own words, that is, "I have less pain now than I did 2 days ago."

Objective Portion

The objective evaluation includes information obtained through observation, inspection, palpation, and special testing, just as in the HOPS format. However, results of diagnostics testing as well as notes from other health care providers are also included. For example, if the patient had imaging studies performed and the results were known, the results would be included under objective findings. When used with follow-up evaluations of patients who have been receiving ongoing treatments, the clinician documents the activities and treatments the patient completed during the session as well as the results from any tests (e.g., ROM) performed during the session in the objective portion of the SOAP note.

Two additional components are found in the SOAP note format that is not included within the HOPS format: assessment and planning.

Assessment

Following the objective evaluation, the clinician analyzes and assesses the patient's status and prognosis. Although a definitive diagnosis may not be known, the clinician can indicate his or her clinical or working diagnosis. The suspected site of injury, involved structures, and severity of damage are identified and documented as problems to be addressed during treatment. Subsequent to having made an assessment, both long-term and short-term goals are established based on the problems list generated. Long-term goals should reflect the anticipated status of the patient after a period of rehabilitation and might include pain-free ROM; bilateral strength, power, and muscular endurance; cardiovascular endurance; and a return to full functional status. Short-term goals are developed to outline the expected progress within days of the initial injury and might include immediate protection of the injured area and control of inflammation, hemorrhage, muscle spasm, or pain. When making an assessment for follow-up evaluations of patients who have been receiving ongoing treatments, assessment focuses on the patient's progress and response to treatment. Long-term goals are updated only when patient is being fully assessed again. Short-term goals are updated with each progress note. Progress notes may be written daily, weekly, or biweekly to document progress.

Plan

The final section of the note lists the therapeutic modalities and exercises, educational consultations, and functional activities used to achieve the documented goals. The action plan should include the following information:

- The immediate treatment given to the injured or ill individual
- If referral is needed, where is the patient being referred and for what purpose
- The frequency and duration of treatments, therapeutic modalities, and exercises
- Evaluation standards to determine progress toward the goals
- Ongoing patient education
- Criteria for discharge

As the short-term goals are achieved and updated, a periodic "in-house review" of the patient's records permits health care providers to evaluate joint ROM; flexibility; muscular strength, power, and endurance; balance or proprioception; and functional status. In addition, these reviews allow health care providers to discuss the continuity of documentation, the efficacy of treatment, the average time to discharge, and other parameters that may reflect quality of care. When it is determined that the patient can be discharged and cleared for participation, a discharge note should be written to close the file. All information included within the file is confidential and cannot be released to anyone without written approval from the patient.

In a clinical setting, SOAP notes are the sole means of documenting the services provided to the patient. All clinicians have an ethical responsibility to keep accurate and factual records. This information verifies specific services rendered and evaluates the progress of the patient as well as the efficacy of the treatment plan. Insurance companies use this information to determine if services are being appropriately rendered and qualify for reimbursement. More importantly, this comprehensive record-keeping system can minimize the ever-present threat of malpractice and litigation. In general, the primary error in writing SOAP notes is the error of omission, whereby clinicians fail to adequately document the nature and extent of care provided to the patient. Formal documentation and the regular review of records can reduce this threat and can minimize the likelihood that inappropriate or inadequate care is being rendered to a patient.[1]

The History and Physical Examination Format

In addition to being able to perform comprehensive clinical assessments of patients with orthopedic conditions, athletic trainers also see patients who present with common illnesses and general medical conditions. Athletic trainers need to be able to recognize and differentiate among conditions in order to determine if referral is warranted and, if so, how quickly (urgency) and to which specialist. Athletic trainers working as physician extenders in the private medical practice or hospital setting may only use the HPE format when assessing patients.

History

Consistent with histories taken in the HOPS and SOAP note model, history taking within the HPE also focuses on obtaining subjective information from the patient. However, the amount and type of information solicited is much more in-depth and, in addition to history of current complaint, may include the following: past medical history, past surgical history, family medical history, social history, allergies and reactions, and medications. Often, much of the extended history information is obtained through questionnaires the patient completes prior to seeing the clinician. The clinician should review the forms and clarify with the patient any information that has not been included or needs to be discussed in greater depth. **Review of systems** (ROS) is also included as part of the history. When conducting an ROS history, the clinician poses questions to the patient that targets every system within the body in an attempt to screen for potential problems that may impact the patient's overall health. Sample questions used to conduct an ROS are presented in **Table 6.2**.

Physical Examination

The physical examination (PE) seeks to obtain objective information about the patient's current health status and potential causes of the reason for seeking assistance. Like HOPS, the PE includes observation of the patient's overall appearance, movements, responses, and reactions. Palpation and special tests are also included within the PE but are not individual categories of the PE but rather are used to gather information about different aspects of the patient's health. See **Table 6.1** for a list of components included under the PE. At the conclusion of the examination process, the clinician will make an assessment or clinical diagnosis, identify problems, and develop a plan for meeting the patient's needs. When conducting an evaluation of patient with a general medical condition, the plan will often include referral to another health care provider who specializes in the treatment of a specific illness or medical condition.[2]

Each component of the subjective and objective assessments are described in detail in the following sections and are repeated throughout each chapter on the various body regions.

TABLE 6.2 Review of Systems

SYSTEM	SAMPLE QUESTIONS
General	Have you noticed that your clothes are fitting differently now? What is your energy level like?
Skin	Have you been experiencing any skin irritations or changes in skin color, freckles, or moles?
HEENT (head)	Have you been experiencing headache or dizziness?
HEENT (eyes)	Have you had any trouble seeing lately?
HEENT (ears)	Have you noticed a ringing in your ears or having a more difficult time hearing people speak?
HEENT (nose/sinus)	Have you had a running nose, nosebleeds, or a sense of being stuffed up?
HEENT (throat)	Has your throat been sore lately or have you experienced any toothaches or bleeding gums?
Lymphatic	Have you noticed any lumps or tenderness in your neck or groin?
Respiratory	Have you experienced any wheezing, shortness of breath, feeling winded, or coughing up phlegm?
Cardiovascular	Do you ever feel as though your heart is racing or experience pain in your chest, arms, or jaw?
Gastrointestinal	Do you have stomachaches, heartburn, or nausea? Any trouble with bowels?
Urinary	Any trouble with urination?
Peripheral vascular	Do your feet and hands ever feel inappropriately cold? Do you have problems with leg or feet cramping or swelling?
Musculoskeletal	Do you have pain, stiffness, or aching in any of your joints? Do you have difficulty walking, getting up from or into chairs, beds, cars? Have you experienced joints that are swollen and warm?
Hematologic	Have you noticed that you bruise easily or have difficulty stopping a cut from bleeding?
Endocrine	Have you noticed that you often feel thirsty or sweat excessively? Are you more sensitive to heat and cold than you used to be?
Neurological	Do you ever experience a pins and needles sensation anywhere in your body? How about changes in memory, concentration, or orientation? Has anyone told you that it is becoming more difficult to understand you?
Psychiatric	Have you noticed any change in your mood? Do you feel anxious or nervous, depressed or blue?
Genital	Females: Has there been a change in the frequency, flow, or consistency of your period? Have you noticed any vaginal discharge, irritation, or smell? Have you noticed any lumps in your breast or discharge? Males: Have you noticed any penal discharge, irritation, masses, or pain?

From Bickley LS, Szilagyi PG. *Bates' Guide to Physical Examination and History Taking.* Philadelphia, PA: Lippincott Williams & Wilkins; 2007.

In order to develop a list of differential diagnoses and come to a clinical diagnosis, the clinician will need to obtain both subjective and objective information from the patient. An easy way to remember the proper sequence is HOPS: History, Observation/inspection, Palpation, and Special Tests. During the history-taking portion of the evaluation, the clinician allows the patient to state in his or her own words (subjective) the MOI and the onset and characteristics of symptoms he or she is experiencing. During the observation and inspection phase, the clinician will look for signs that might provide clues into what injury or illness the patient might have. Next, the clinician will palpate, looking for areas of tenderness or abnormalities. Information gathered during the history, observation/inspection, and palpation will direct the clinician in the next step of the process: special tests. There are many different kinds of special tests, and the clinician should select only those tests needed to help reject or support possible diagnosis that were considered based on information obtained in the history, observation, and palpation portion of the exam.

HISTORY OF THE INJURY

 A female high school long jumper sustains an ankle injury during practice and immediately reports to the athletic training room. What questions should be asked to identify the cause and extent of this injury?

Obtaining an accurate and complete history of the injury can be the most important step of the clinical assessment process. A complete history includes information regarding the primary complaint, cause or mechanism of the injury, characteristics of the symptoms, and any related medical history that may have a bearing on the specific condition. This information can provide potential reasons for the symptoms and can identify injured structures before initiating the PE. An individual's medical history file can be an excellent resource for identifying past injuries, subsequent rehabilitation programs, and any factors that may predispose the individual to further injury. Specific to collegiate athletes, the National Collegiate Athletic Association (NCAA) has identified primary components that should be in an intercollegiate athlete's medical record and readily accessible to the athletic trainer (**Box 6.1**).[3]

History taking involves asking appropriate questions, but it also requires establishing a professional and comfortable atmosphere. When taking a history, the athletic trainer should introduce himself or herself to the patient and address the patient by name. The athletic trainer should present with a competent manner, listen attentively, and maintain eye contact in an effort to establish rapport with the injured individual. Ideally, this encourages the individual to respond more accurately to questions and instructions.

Often, an unacknowledged obstacle to the evaluation process is the sociocultural dynamics that may exist between the patient and clinician that can hinder communication. It is important for all clinicians to understand and respect each cultural group's attitudes, beliefs, and values as related to health and illness. If English is a second language to the patient, it may be necessary to locate an interpreter. If an interpreter is used, it is important to speak to the client, not to the interpreter. It also may be necessary to speak slower, not louder, and to refrain from using slang terms or jargon. To ensure understanding, the patient should be asked to repeat the instructions.

When communicating with older clients, a skilled interviewer must consider other issues that may impact the effectiveness of history taking. The client's education and socioeconomic status may affect his or her vocabulary, self-expression, ability to comprehend, and ability to conceptualize questions asked by the interviewer.[4] Elderly individuals tend to view the world concretely, think in absolute terms, and may be confused by complicated questions. These individuals also may present with some anxiety if they perceive that the clinician is dismissing the magnitude of their complaints or becoming impatient with the length of time that patients take to answer a question. In addition, patients who may have hearing loss might feel uncomfortable asking the interviewer to repeat information.[4] A skilled clinician takes note of the patient's comfort level by recognizing not only verbal expression but also any emotion behind the expression, such as hidden fears, beliefs, or expectations. Patience, respect, rapport, structure, and reflecting on important information are all useful in conducting a comprehensive medical history.

The history begins by gathering general information, such as the individual's name, sex, age, date of birth, occupation, and activity in which the individual was participating when the injury occurred. Notes regarding body size, body type, and general physical condition also are appropriate.

Although information provided by the individual is subjective, it should still be gathered and recorded as quantitatively as possible. The individual should be asked to quantify the severity of pain using a pain rating scale, of which there are many types. The Visual Analogue Scale (VAS) and the Numerical Rating Scale (NRS) are generic pain rating scales that are simple to use; easy to administer, complete, and score; and have been found to be valid and reliable measures of pain.[5] The patient is asked to rate his or her severity of pain using a graph, number, or image that is placed within a continuum anchored by two opposing descriptions of pain severity. Examples of VAS and NRS are shown in **Box 6.2**. Pain rating scales should only be used to record a patient's pain level throughout the length of treatment or rehabilitation process and be compared to baseline or prior scores in order to generate data points indicating how well the patient is progressing. The patient also can be asked

BOX 6.1 National Collegiate Athletic Association Guideline 1b: Medical Evaluations, Immunizations, and Records

The following primary components should be included in the athlete's medical record:

1. History of injuries, illnesses, new medications or allergies, pregnancies, and operations, whether sustained during the competitive season or off-season

2. Referrals for and feedback from consultation, treatment, or rehabilitation with subsequent care and clearances

3. Comprehensive entry-year health-status questionnaires and an updated health-status questionnaire each year thereafter, including information on the following:

   ■ Illnesses suffered (acute and chronic); athletic and nonathletic hospitalization

   ■ Surgery

   ■ Allergies, including hypersensitivity to drugs, foods, and insect bites/stings

   ■ Medications taken on a regular basis

   ■ Conditioning status

   ■ Musculoskeletal injuries (previous and current)

   ■ Cerebral concussions or episodes involving a loss of consciousness

   ■ Syncope or near syncope with exercise

   ■ Exercise-induced asthma or bronchospasm

   ■ Loss of paired organs

   ■ Heat-related illness

   ■ Cardiac conditions and family history of cardiac disease, including sudden death in a family member younger than 50 years and Marfan syndrome

   ■ Menstrual history

   ■ Exposure to tuberculosis

4. Immunization records, including the following:

   ■ Measles, mumps, rubella (MMR)

   ■ Hepatitis B

   ■ Diphtheria, tetanus, and boosters when appropriate

   ■ Meningitis

5. Written permission signed by the student athlete or by the parent if the athlete is younger than 18 years that authorizes the release of medical information to others, specifically what information may be released and to whom

Adapted from Parsons JT, ed. *2014–2015 NCAA Sports Medicine Handbook.* Indianapolis, IN: National Collegiate Athletic Association; 2014.

to quantify the length of time the pain lasts. In using such measures, the progress of the injury can be determined. If the individual reports that pain begins immediately after activity and lasts for 3 or 4 hours, a baseline of information has been established. As the individual undergoes treatment and rehabilitation for the injury, a comparison with the baseline information can determine if the condition is getting better, worse, or remains the same. Pain rating scales should not be used to compare a patient's perceived level of pain to that reported by other patients.

Although the intent of taking a history is to narrow the possibilities of conditions causing the injury, the history should always be taken with an open mind. If too few factors are considered,

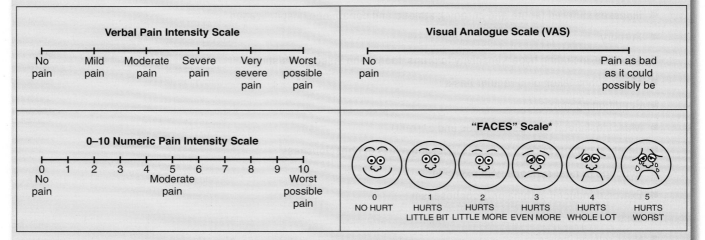

From Hawker GA, Mian S, Kendzerska T, et al. Measures of adult pain. Visual Analog Scale for Pain (VAS Pain), Numeric Rating Scale for Pain (NRS Pain), McGill Pain Questionnaire (MPQ), Short-Form McGill Pain Questionnaire (SF-MPQ), Chronic Pain Grade Scale (CPGS), Short Form-36 Bodily Pain Scale (SF-36 BPS), and Measure of Intermittent and Constant Osteoarthritis Pain (ICOAP). *Arthritis Care Res.* 2011;63(suppl 11):S240–S252.

the athletic trainer may reach premature conclusions and fail to adequately address the severity of the injury. It is essential to document in writing the information obtained during the history.

Primary Complaint

The reason the patient is seeking assistance may be multilayered. Although the patient's primary complaint may be pain or dysfunction, your goal is to determine the cause of his or her pain or dysfunction. The starting point is to learn as much as you can from the patient about his or her perception of the current injury or the patient's *primary complaint*. Questions should be phrased to allow the individual to describe the current nature, location, and onset of the condition.[2] The following questions could be asked:

- How can I help you today? What seems to be the problem?

- Do you have pain or discomfort? If so, where? Describe how it feels. What increases your pain? What decreases your pain?

- When did the injury occur? Or if a general medical issue, when did the symptoms begin?

- What activities or motions are weak or painful?

It is important to realize that the individual may not wish to carry on a lengthy discussion about the injury or may trivialize the extent of pain or disability. The clinician must be patient and keep the questions simple and open-ended. It is advantageous to pay close attention to words and gestures used by the patient to describe the condition because these may provide clues to the quality and intensity of the symptoms.

Mechanism of Injury

After identifying the primary complaint, the next step is to determine the MOI. When assessing a patient who has sustained an injury, the MOI is probably the most important information gained in the history. For an acute injury, questions that might be asked to determine MOI include the following:

■ How did the injury occur? What did you do? How did you do it?

■ Did you fall? If so, how did you land?

■ Were you struck by an object or another individual? If so, in what position was the involved body part, and in what direction was the force?

For chronic injuries or conditions, potential questions to determine MOI may include the following:

■ How long has the injury been a problem?

■ Do you remember a specific incident that initiated or provoked the current problem?

■ Have there been recent changes in running surface, shoes, equipment, techniques, or conditioning modes?

■ What activities make the condition feel better? What activities make the condition feel worse?

It is important to visualize the manner in which the injury occurred as a way to identify possible injured structures. However, analyzing the mechanics of injury to the human body is complicated by several factors. First, potentially injurious forces applied to the body act at different angles, over different surface areas, and over different periods of time. Second, the human body is composed of many different types of tissue, which respond differently to applied forces. Finally, injury to the human body is not an all-or-nothing phenomenon; that is, injuries range in severity. The skilled clinician needs to be able to connect information gained in the history about the MOI with how different types of mechanical load affect anatomical structures in order to safely and effectively conduct the rest of the evaluation. Injury mechanisms and how tissues respond to specific types of mechanical load is described in depth in Chapter 10.

Characteristics of the Symptoms

The primary complaint must be explored in detail to discover the evolution of symptoms, including the location, onset, severity, frequency, duration, and limitations caused by the pain or disability.[2] The individual's pain perception can indicate which structures may be injured. There are two categories of pain: somatic and visceral.

Somatic pain arises from the skin, ligaments, muscles, bones, and joints and is the most common type of pain encountered in musculoskeletal injuries. It is classified into two major types: *deep* and *superficial*. Deep somatic pain is described as diffuse or nagging, as if intense pressure is being exerted on the structures, and may be complicated by stabbing pain. Deep somatic pain is longer lasting and usually indicates significant tissue damage to bone, internal joint structures, or muscles. Superficial somatic pain results from injury to the epidermis or dermis and usually is a sharp, prickly type of pain that tends to be brief.

Visceral pain results from disease or injury to an organ in the thoracic or abdominal cavity, such as compression, tension, or distention of the viscera. Similar to deep somatic pain, it is perceived as deeply located, nagging, and pressing, and it often is accompanied by nausea and vomiting. *Referred pain* is a type of visceral pain that travels along the same nerve pathways as somatic pain. It is perceived by the brain as being somatic in origin. In other words, the injury is in one region, but the brain considers it in another. For example, **referred pain** occurs when an individual has a heart attack and feels pain in the chest, left arm, and, sometimes, the neck. **Figure 6.1** illustrates cutaneous areas where pain from visceral organs can be referred.

Pain can travel up or down the length of any nerve and be referred to another region. An individual with a low back problem may feel the pain down the gluteal region and into the back of the leg. If a nerve is injured, pain or a change in sensation, such as a numbing or burning sensation, can be felt along the length of the nerve.

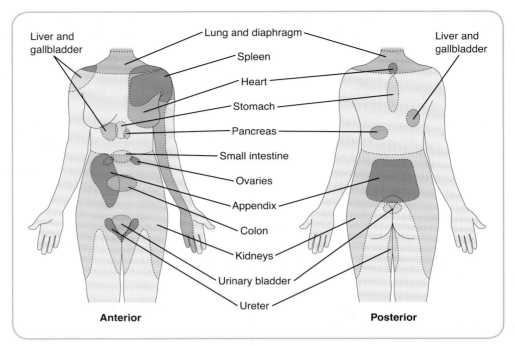

Figure 6.1. Referred pain. Certain visceral organs can refer pain to specific cutaneous areas. If all special tests are negative yet the individual continues to feel pain at a specific site, it may be referred pain.

In assessing the injury, the clinician should ask detailed questions about the location, onset, nature, severity, frequency, and duration of the pain. For example, the following questions should be asked:

- Where is the pain?

- Can you point to a specific painful spot?

- Is the pain limited to that area, or does it radiate into other parts of the leg or foot?

- Can you describe the pain (e.g., dull, sharp, or aching)?

- What decreases or increases the intensity and/or type of pain you are experiencing?

In chronic conditions, the following questions should be asked:

- When does the pain begin (e.g., when you get out of bed, while sitting, while walking, during exercise, or at night)?

- How long does the pain last?

- Is the pain worse before, during, or after activity?

- What activities aggravate or alleviate the symptoms?

- Does the pain wake you up at night?

- How long has the condition been present?

- Has the pain changed or stayed the same?

- In the past, what medications, treatments, or exercise programs have improved the situation?

If *pain is localized*, it suggests that limited bony or soft-tissue structures may be involved. *Diffuse pain* around the entire joint may indicate inflammation of the joint capsule or injury to several structures. If *pain radiates* into other areas of the limb or body, it may be traveling up or down the length of a nerve. These responses also can determine if the condition is disabling enough to require referral to a physician. **Table 6.3** provides more detailed information regarding pain characteristics and probable causes.

TABLE 6.3 Pain Characteristics and Possible Causes

CHARACTERISTICS	POSSIBLE CAUSES
Morning pain with stiffness that improves with activity	Chronic inflammation with edema, or arthritis
Pain increasing as the day progresses	Increased congestion in a joint
Sharp, stabbing pain during activity	Acute injury, such as ligament sprain or muscular strain
Dull, aching pain aggravated by muscle contraction	Chronic muscular strain
Pain that subsides during activity	Chronic condition or inflammation
Pain on activity relieved by rest	Soft-tissue damage
Pain not affected by rest or activity	Injury to bone
Night pain	Compression of a nerve or bursa
Dull, aching, and hard to localize; aggravated by passive stretching of the muscle and resisted muscle contractions	Muscular pain
Deeply located, nagging, and very localized	Bone pain
Sharp, burning, or numbing sensation that may run the length of the nerve	Nerve pain
Aching over a large area that may be referred to another area of the body	Vascular pain

In assessing the primary complaint of an acute injury, it also is important to determine if the individual experienced other unusual sounds/sensations at the time of injury. Sometimes, patients will report "feeling" a pop or snap that was not heard. Specifically, the following questions should be asked:

■ Did you hear anything?

■ Did you feel anything?

The report of particular sounds and feelings at the time of injury can provide valuable input regarding the type of injury and the structures involved. Hearing a "pop" is characteristic of a rupture to a ligament or tendon, and hearing a snapping or cracking sound may suggest a fracture. Unusual feelings can be presented in a variety of ways. For example, having sustained a tear to the anterior cruciate ligament, an individual may report a feeling of the knee giving way. Following a rupture of the Achilles tendon, an individual may report a feeling of being shot or kicked in the lower leg. In future chapters, signs and symptoms that are unique to specific injuries and conditions will be discussed.

Disability Resulting from the Injury

The clinician should attempt to determine the limitations experienced by the individual because of pain, weakness, or disability from the injury. Questions should not be limited to sport and physical activity but, rather, should determine if the injury has affected the individual's job, school, or daily activities. **Activities of daily living (ADLs)** are actions that most people perform without thinking, such as combing one's hair, brushing one's teeth, and walking up or down stairs. A skilled clinician will be able to apply his or her knowledge of functional anatomy to identify structures that might be potentially damaged based on the patient's ability or inability to perform ADLs pain-free.

Related Medical History

Information should be obtained regarding other problems or conditions that might have affected the current injury. Information documented on patient's preparticipation examination or medical clearance forms may provide baseline data that can be used to verify past childhood diseases; allergies; cardiac, respiratory, vascular, musculoskeletal, or neurological problems; use of contact lenses, dentures, or prosthetic devices; and past episodes of infectious diseases, loss of consciousness, recurrent headaches, heat stroke, seizures, eating disorders, or chronic medical problems.[2] Previous musculoskeletal injuries or congenital abnormalities may place additional stress on joints and may predispose the individual to certain injuries. In some situations, it may be appropriate to ask if the individual is taking any medication. The type, frequency, dosage, and effect of a medication may mask some injury symptoms.

 In attempting to determine the cause and extent of injury, the female long jumper should be asked questions pertaining to the following: primary complaint (i.e., what, when, and how questions), MOI (i.e., position of the ankle at the time of injury and the direction of force), characteristics of symptoms (i.e., nature, location, severity, and disability), unusual sensation (i.e., sounds and feelings), related medical history, and past injuries/treatment.

OBSERVATION AND INSPECTION

? A detailed history of the injury has been gathered from the long jumper. The information suggests she has inverted her right ankle and sprain one or more of the lateral ligaments. In the continued assessment of this individual, an observation and inspection should be performed. What observable factors might indicate the seriousness of the injury?

The objective evaluation during an injury assessment begins with observation and inspection. Although explained as a separate step, observation begins the moment the injured person is seen, and it continues throughout the assessment. **Observation** refers to the visual analysis of overall appearance, symmetry, general motor function, posture, and gait. **Inspection** refers to factors seen at the actual injury site, such as swelling, redness, ecchymosis, cuts, or scars.

Observation

Often, the athletic trainer observes the individual sustaining an injury and will quickly form a list of potential injuries based on the witnessed MOI. In many instances, however, the individual comes to the sideline, office, athletic training room, or clinic complaining of pain or discomfort. The specifics of what the athletic trainer needs to attend to will depend on how the patient presents on first glance. Patients with acute injury or illness usually present differently than those with chronic conditions or illnesses. The athletic trainer should immediately assess the individual's state of consciousness and body language, which may indicate pain, disability, fracture, dislocation, or other conditions. It also is important to note the individual's general posture, willingness and ability to move, ease of motion, and overall attitude in order to determine the severity of the condition and the urgency of the situation. Evaluation and management of acute injury and illnesses will be specifically addressed in Chapter 7.

General observations may focus on the patient's estimated age, physical condition, and personal hygiene. Potential questions to address in the observation include the following:

- Does the individual appear to be healthy? Is skin color and moisture appropriate for environment? Is there any obvious discoloration, swelling, bleeding, deformity, or limited ROM present?

- Is the individual's weight appropriate for height, or is the individual underweight or overweight? Is the individual's weight appropriate for the type and level of sport/physical activity participation? Could this be a contributing factor in his or her injury?

- Is the individual's speech slurred, hoarse, loud, soft, incoherent, slow, fast, or hesitant?

- How is the individual's breathing pattern, depth, and quality?

- Is the individual's hearing impaired? Is the individual's hearing better through one ear?

- Is the individual oriented to the surroundings or disoriented and unaware of time or place?

- Does the individual seem to be hesitant or avoid eye contact?

By observing these factors, the skilled clinician can more accurately document the patient's characteristics both quickly and accurately.[6]

Symmetry and Appearance

The body should be scanned visually to detect **congenital** (i.e., existing at birth) or functional problems that may be a contributing factor. This includes observing any abnormalities in the spinal curves, general symmetry of the various body parts, and general posture of the body from anterior, lateral, and posterior views.

If it is not **contraindicated**, the clinician should observe the normal swing of the individual's arms and legs during walking. By standing behind, in front, and to the side of the individual, an observation from all angles is permitted. A shoulder injury may be evident in a limited arm swing or by holding the arm close to the body in a splinted position. A lower extremity injury may produce a noticeable limp, or **antalgic gait**. Running on a treadmill can show functional problems that may have contributed to a lower extremity injury. Postural and gait assessment will be discussed in depth in a later chapter.

Motor Function

Many clinicians begin observation using a scan examination to assess general motor function. This examination rules out injury at other joints that may be overlooked because of intense pain or discomfort at the primary site of injury. In addition, pain in one area can be referred from another area. Assessing motor function should only be conducted after fracture, dislocation, or spinal injury has safely been ruled out. To assess gross motor function, observe the injured person performing gross motor movements of the neck, trunk, and extremities by asking the individual to do the following:

- Extend, flex, laterally flex, and rotate the neck.

- Bend forward to touch the toes.

- Stand and rotate the trunk to the right and left.

- Bring the palms together above the head and then behind the back.

- Perform straight leg raises in hip flexion, extension, and abduction.

- Flex the knees.

- Walk on the heels and toes.

Any hesitation by the patient to move a body part or favoring one side over the other should be noted.

Inspection of the Injury Site

Using discretion in safeguarding the person's privacy, the injured area should be fully exposed. This may require the removal of protective equipment and clothing.

The localized injury site should be inspected for any deformity, swelling (i.e., edema or joint effusion), discoloration (e.g., redness, pallor, or ecchymosis), signs of infection (i.e., redness, swelling, pus, red streaks, or swollen **lymph nodes**), scars that might indicate previous surgery, and general skin condition (e.g., oily, dry, blotchy with red spots, sores, or hives). Swelling inside the joint is called localized intra-articular swelling, or **joint effusion**, and this swelling makes the joint appear enlarged, red, and puffy. The amount of swelling should be measured in a quantifiable manner using girth measurements (**Application Strategy 6.1**). **Ecchymosis** is the superficial discoloration of tissue indicative of injury. **Keloids**, which are scars that form at a wound but grow beyond its boundaries, may indicate a previous injury. This condition is more common in individuals with dark skin, and it is particularly important to note if surgery may be indicated. The injured area should be compared to the opposite side if possible. This **bilateral comparison** helps to establish normal parameters for the individual.

APPLICATION STRATEGY 6.1

Taking Girth Measurements

1. Identify the joint line using prominent bony landmarks. The individual should be non–weight-bearing.
2. Using a marked tongue depressor or tape measure, make incremental marks (e.g., 2 in, 4 in, and 6 in) from the joint line. (Do not use a cloth tape measure because they tend to stretch.)
3. Encircle the body part with the measuring tape, making sure not to fold or twist the tape (**Fig. A**). If measuring ankle girth, use a figure eight technique by positioning the tape across the malleoli proximally and around the navicular and base of the 5th metatarsal distally (**Fig. B**).
4. Take three measurements and record the average.
5. Repeat these steps for the noninjured body part and record all findings.
6. Increased girth at the joint line indicates joint swelling. Increased girth over a muscle mass indicates hypertrophy; decreased girth indicates atrophy.

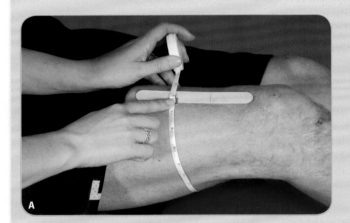 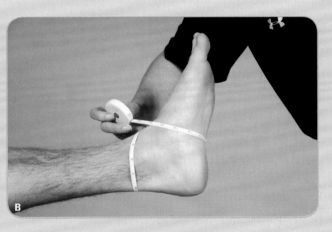

 Observable factors relative to the injured site that might indicate the seriousness of the injury sustained by the female long jumper include deformity, swelling, discoloration, and signs of previous injury. It is important to perform a bilateral inspection of the injury site as well as of the surrounding area. In addition, observation of general presentation, including the presence of guarding or antalgic gait, will provide important information concerning the nature of the injury.

PALPATION

? Inspection of the patient's ankle revealed mild swelling on the anterolateral aspect of the ankle. Otherwise, no abnormal findings were evident. Observation of the patient, however, suggests guarding and hesitation to walk. Based on the information provided concerning the patient's condition, explain how palpation can be utilized to help determine the extent and severity of the injury.

Informed consent must be granted before making physical contact with a patient. If the patient is younger than 18 years, permission must be granted by the parent or guardian. In some cultures and religions, the act of physically touching an exposed body part may present certain moral and ethical issues. Likewise, some patients may feel uncomfortable being touched by a health care provider of the opposite gender. If a same-gender clinician is not available, the evaluation should be observed by a third party (e.g., another clinician, parent, or guardian).

Bilateral palpation of paired anatomical structures can detect eight physical findings:

1. Temperature

2. Swelling

3. Point tenderness

4. Crepitus

5. Deformity

6. Muscle spasm

7. Cutaneous sensation

8. Pulse

The clinician should have clean, warm hands. Latex examination gloves should be worn as a precaution against disease and infection. Palpation should begin with gentle, circular pressure, followed by gradual, deeper pressure, and it should be initiated on structures away from the site of injury and progress toward the injured area. Palpating the most painful area last avoids any carryover of pain into noninjured areas.

Skin temperature should be noted when the fingers first touch the skin. Increased temperature at the injury site could indicate inflammation or infection, whereas decreased temperature could indicate a reduction in circulation.

The presence of localized or diffuse swelling can be determined through palpation of the injured area. In addition, palpation should assess differences in the density or "feel" of soft tissues that may indicate muscle spasm, hemorrhage, scarring, myositis ossificans, or other conditions.

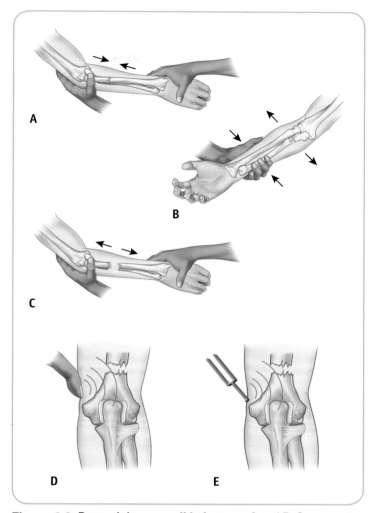

Figure 6.2. Determining a possible fracture. A and **B**, Compression (axial and circular). **C**, Distraction. **D**, Percussion. **E**, Vibration.

Point tenderness and crepitus may indicate inflammation when felt over a tendon, bursa, or joint capsule. It is important to note any trigger points that may be found in muscle and, when palpated, may refer pain to another site.

Palpation of the bones and bony landmarks can determine the possibility of fractures, crepitus, or loose bony or cartilaginous fragments. Possible fractures can be assessed with percussion, vibrations through use of a tuning fork, compression, and distraction (**Fig. 6.2**). The region should be immobilized if test results indicate a possible fracture.

Cutaneous sensation can be tested by running the fingers along both sides of the body part and asking the patient if it feels the same on both sides. This technique can determine possible nerve involvement, particularly if the individual has numbness or tingling in the limb.

Peripheral pulses should be taken distal to an injury to rule out damage to a major artery. Common sites are the radial pulse at the wrist and the dorsalis pedis pulse on the dorsum of the foot (**Fig. 6.3**).

 Palpation of bony and soft-tissue structures will provide information pertaining to several physical findings, including temperature, swelling, point tenderness, crepitus, deformity, muscle spasm, cutaneous sensation, and pulse. It is important to perform a bilateral palpation of key anatomical structures of the foot, ankle, and lower leg.

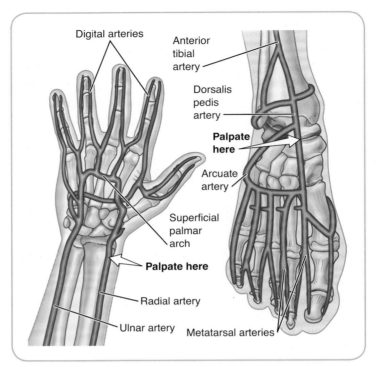

Figure 6.3. Peripheral pulses. The pulse can be taken at the radial pulse in the wrist **(A)** or at the dorsalis pedis on the dorsum of the foot **(B)**.

PHYSICAL EXAMINATION TESTS

> **?** The palpation component of the assessment of the patient's ankle confirms the presence of fever and swelling over the anterolateral aspect of the ankle. Palpation also reveals point tenderness in the area of the anterior talofibular ligament. Otherwise, no abnormal findings were present. How should testing proceed to determine the integrity of the soft-tissue structures and the extent and severity of injury?

This portion of the examination may require the clinician to use many different types of "special test" in order to help confirm or rule out a potential diagnosis. The tests are grouped by category: (1) ROM and functional testing, (2) stress tests, (3) special tests, (4) neurological testing, and (5) activity-specific functional testing. The specific tests needed and the order in which the tests are performed will be guided by the information gained through the history, inspection, and palpation portions of the assessment process. General principles regarding the PE are discussed in this chapter; more extensive explanations are provided in the individual joint chapters.

Range of Motion and Functional Tests

Functional tests identify the patient's ability to move a body part through the ROM actively passively and against resistance. The purpose of conducting ROM and functional testing is to determine which type of tissue has been damaged based on when the patient experiences pain. Contractile tissue such as muscles and tendons are assessed using active and resistive ROM. Inert tissues, such as joint capsules, ligaments, bones, cartilage and such, are assessed using passive range of motion. By looking at how the body responds to the various ROM testing will assist the clinician in identifying where the source of the pain is located. Once the source of pain has been identified, a treatment program can be designed to target the pain source and address the underlying problem causing the pain.[7] As with all tests, the noninjured side should be evaluated first to establish **normative data**. All motions common to each joint should be tested. Occasionally, it also may be necessary to test the joints proximal and distal to the injury to rule out any referred pain. Active and passive range of motion can be measured subjectively by the clinician "eyeballing" how much ROM occurs at the injured joint and comparing with the ROM found at the comparative noninjured joint. The motion is then documented as either full or limited. If pain is present, the motion is also documented as painful. If pain is not present, the test is documented as being painless. Active and passive range of motion can also be objectively measured using a **goniometer** to measure the actual degrees of motion that occur at the injured joint.[8]

Active Range of Motion

Active range of motion (AROM) is joint motion performed voluntarily by the individual through muscular contraction. Unless contraindicated, AROM should always be performed before **passive range of motion (PROM)**. The AROM indicates the individual's willingness and ability to move the injured body part.[8] Active movement determines possible damage to contractile tissue (i.e., muscle, muscle–tendon junction, tendon, and tendon–periosteal union)[7] and measures muscle function and movement coordination.

Measurement of all motions, except rotation, starts with the body in anatomical position. For rotation, the starting body position is midway between internal (medial) and external (lateral) rotation. The starting position is measured as 0°.

It is important to assess the individual's willingness to perform a movement, the fluidity of movement, and the extent of movement (joint ROM). If symptoms are present, their location in the arc of movement should be noted. Any increase in intensity or quality of symptoms also should be noted. Limitations in motion may result from pain, swelling, muscle spasm, muscle tightness, joint contractures, nerve damage, or mechanical blocks, such as a loose body. If the individual has pain or other symptoms with movement, it can be difficult to determine if the joint, muscle, or both are injured. It is important to assess the following[8]:

- The point during the motion at which pain begins

- The presence of pain in a limited ROM (i.e., painful arc)

- The type of pain and if it is associated with the primary complaint

Anticipated painful movements should be performed last to avoid any carryover of pain from testing one motion to the next. Findings from AROM alone are not adequate to help the clinician determine the source of the patient's pain.[9] The clinician should make note of all motions that cause pain as well as where the pain was located and compare findings with information gathered through the PROM and resisted range of motion portions of the examination.

Passive Range of Motion

In **passive movement**, the injured limb or body part is moved by the clinician through the ROM with no assistance from the injured individual (**Fig. 6.4**). As PROM is performed, the individual

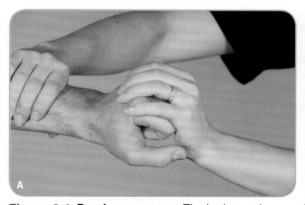
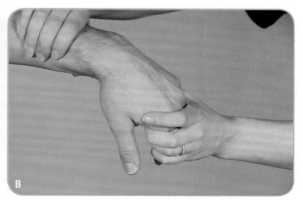

Figure 6.4. Passive movement. The body part is moved through the ROM with no assistance from the injured individual. Any limitation of movement or presence of pain is documented. **A,** Starting position. **B,** End position.

TABLE 6.4 Normal and Abnormal Joint End Feels

END FEEL	STRUCTURE	EXAMPLE
Normal End Feel Sensations (Physiological)		
Soft	Soft-tissue approximation	Elbow flexion (contact between soft tissue of the forearm and anterior arm)
Firm	Muscular stretch Capsular stretch Ligamentous stretch	Hip extension (passive stretch of iliopsoas muscle) External rotation at the shoulder (passive stretch of anterior glenohumeral joint capsule) Forearm supination (tension in the palmar radioulnar ligament of the inferior radioulnar joint, interosseous membrane, oblique cord)
Hard	Bone to bone	Elbow extension (contact between olecranon process and olecranon fossa)
Abnormal End Feel Sensations (Pathological)		
Soft	Occurs sooner or later in the ROM than is usual or in a joint that normally has a firm or hard end feel; feels boggy	Soft-tissue edema Synovitis Ligamentous stretch or tear
Firm	Occurs sooner or later in the ROM than is usual or in a joint that normally has a soft or hard end feel	Increased muscular tonus Capsular, muscular, ligamentous shortening
Hard	Occurs sooner or later in the ROM than is usual or in a joint that normally has a soft or firm end feel; a bony grating or bony block is felt	Chondromalacia Osteoarthritis Loose bodies in joint Myositis ossificans Fracture
Empty	No end feel, because the end of the ROM is never reached because of pain; no resistance is felt except for the patient's protective muscle splinting or muscle spasm	Acute joint inflammation Bursitis Fracture Psychogenic in origin

From Cyriax JH. *Cyriax's Illustrated Manual of Orthopaedic Medicine.* 2nd ed. Oxford, United Kingdom: Butterworth-Heinemann; 1993; Norkin CC, White DJ. *Measurement of Joint Motion: A Guide to Goniometry.* 4th ed. Philadelphia, PA: FA Davis; 2009; Cyriax J. *Textbook of Orthopaedic Medicine, Volume One: Diagnosis of Soft Tissue Lesions.* 8th ed. London, United Kingdom: Baillière Tindall; 1982; Kendall FP, McCreary EK, Provance PG, et al. *Muscles: Testing and Function with Posture and Pain.* 5th ed. Baltimore, MD: Lippincott Williams & Wilkins; 2005.

should be positioned to allow the muscles to be in a relaxed state. The PROM distinguishes injury to contractile tissues from injury to noncontractile or inert tissues (i.e., bone, ligament, bursae, joint capsule, fascia, dura mater, and nerve roots).[9] Again, any potentially painful motions should be performed last to avoid any carryover of pain from one motion to the next.

A gentle overpressure should be applied at the end of the ROM to determine **end feel**.[8] Overpressure is repeated several times to determine whether an increase in pain occurs, which could signify damage to noncontractile joint structures. Different end feels can assist the clinician in identifying the type of disorder present. Three normal end feel sensations (i.e., soft, firm, and hard) and four abnormal end feel sensations (i.e., soft, firm, hard, and empty) exist (**Table 6.4**).

Differences in ROM between active and passive movements can result from muscle spasm, muscle deficiency, neurological deficit, contractures, or pain. If pain occurs before the end of the available ROM, it may indicate an acute injury. Stretching and manipulation of the joint are contraindicated. If pain occurs simultaneously at the end of the ROM, a subacute injury may be present, and a mild stretching program may be started cautiously. If no pain is felt as the available

TABLE 6.5 Interpreting Range of Motion Findings

AROM[a]	PROM[a]	TISSUE TYPE INJURED
Pain is elicited during concentric contraction of muscle (active contraction).	Pain is elicited when tissue is stretched (passive stretch).	Contractile
Pain is elicited with both eccentric and concentric contraction.	Pain is elicited with all passive motions.	Inert

[a]Through the full range of motion.

From Cyriax JH. *Cyriax's Illustrated Manual of Orthopaedic Medicine.* 2nd ed. Oxford, United Kingdom: Butterworth-Heinemann; 1993; Norkin CC, White DJ. *Measurement of Joint Motion: A Guide to Goniometry.* 4th ed. Philadelphia, PA: FA Davis; 2009; Cyriax J. *Textbook of Orthopaedic Medicine, Volume One: Diagnosis of Soft Tissue Lesions.* 8th ed. London, United Kingdom: Baillière Tindall; 1982.

ROM is stretched, a chronic injury is present. An appropriate treatment and rehabilitation program should be initiated immediately. Interpreting the findings from ROM testing is presented in **Table 6.5**

Accessory movements are movements within the joint that accompany traditional AROM and PROM but cannot be performed voluntarily by the individual. Joint play motions occur within the joint but only as a response to an outside force and not as a result of any voluntary movement. Joint play motions allow the joint capsule to "give" so that bones can move to absorb an external force. These movements include distraction, sliding, compression, rolling, and spinning of joint surfaces. Joint play movements aid the healing process, relieve pain, reduce disability, and restore the full normal ROM. If joint play movement is absent or decreased, this movement must be restored before functional voluntary movement can be accomplished fully.[10]

The presence of accessory movement can be determined by manipulating the joint in a position of least strain, called the **loose packed** or **resting position** (**Table 6.6**). The resting position is the position in the ROM in which the joint is under the least amount of stress. It is also the position in which the joint capsule has its greatest capacity. The advantage of testing accessory movements in the loose packed position is that the joint surface contact areas are reduced, proper joint lubrication is enhanced, and friction and erosion in the joints are decreased.

In contrast, a **close packed position** is the position in which two joint surfaces fit precisely together. In this position, the ligaments and joint capsule are maximally taut (**Table 6.7**). The joint surfaces are maximally compressed and cannot be separated by distractive forces nor can accessory movements occur. Therefore, if a bone or ligament is injured, pain increases as the joint moves into the close packed position. If swelling is present within the joint, the close packed position cannot be achieved.

Resisted Range of Motion and Manual Muscle Testing[8,11]

Resisted range of motion (RROM) and manual testing can assess muscle strength/weakness. RROM testing is performed by applying an overload pressure in a stationary or static position (sometimes referred to as a **break test**) or dynamically throughout the full ROM. RROM testing allows the clinician to determine the presence of muscle weakness within a group of muscles performing the same task. For example, when testing resisted knee flexion, the patient describes pain and demonstrates weakness. The clinician is able to state that weakness was present with knee flexion but will be unable to state in which of the three hamstring muscles the lesion is located that caused the weakness. In contrast, manual muscle testing (MMT) guidelines require the clinician to place the body part in a very specific position in order to isolate one single muscle as much as possible in order to test only that one muscle. For example, to perform an MMT of the biceps femoris, which is one of the three flexors of the knee, the patient lies prone with the knee flexed between 50° and 70°. The hip is in slight lateral rotation, and the leg slightly externally rotated while the clinician applies resistance. Differences and similarities in RROM and MMT are described in the following discussion.

TABLE 6.6 Loose Packed Position of Selected Joints

JOINT(S)	POSITION
Glenohumeral	55° abduction, 30° horizontal adduction
Elbow (ulnohumeral)	70° elbow flexion, 10° forearm supination
Radiohumeral	Full extension, full forearm supination
Proximal radioulnar	70° elbow flexion, 35° supination
Distal radioulnar	10° forearm supination
Wrist (radiocarpal)	Neutral with slight ulnar deviation
Carpometacarpal	Midway between abduction–adduction and flexion–extension
Metacarpophalangeal	Slight flexion
Interphalangeal	Slight flexion
Hip	30° flexion, 30° abduction, slight lateral rotation
Knee	25° flexion
Ankle (talocrural)	10° plantar flexion, midway between maximum inversion and eversion
Subtalar	Midway between extremes of inversion and eversion
Tarsometatarsal	Midway between extremes of range of motion
Metatarsophalangeal	Neutral
Interphalangeal	Slight flexion

■ Resisted Range of Motion

RROM testing follows PROM and is done prior to MMT. Testing resistance throughout the full ROM offers two advantages: First, a better overall assessment of weakness can be determined, and second, a painful arc of motion can be located, which might otherwise go undetected if the test is only performed in the midrange. To perform RROM throughout the full ROM, have the patient place the limb in the elongated position. The clinician stabilizes proximal to the joint and applies an accommodating resistance to the distal aspect of the limb. The patient is instructed to move the body part through the requested ROM while the clinician applies enough pressure to make the patient work but not so much as to prevent motion from occurring. RROM may also be tested in a static position through the use of a break test.

In performing a break test, overload pressure is applied with the joint in a neutral position to relax joint structures and reduce joint stress. The muscles are more effectively stressed in this position but do not allow the clinician to discover where within the ROM the weakness occurs. Performing RROM in a static position is also easily confused with performing an MMT. When performing a break test, the limb is stabilized proximal to the joint to prevent other motions from compensating for weakness in the involved muscle. Resistance is provided distally on the bone to which the muscle or muscle group attaches; resistance should not be distal to a second joint. In a fixed position, the individual is asked to elicit a maximal contraction while the body part is stabilized to prevent little or no joint movement. Presence of pain and/or weakness during RROM is an indication that MMT should be performed to determine the exact muscle that is injured.

■ Manual Muscle Testing

MMT procedures require that before resistance can be applied, the patient first should be able to demonstrate the ability to contract the muscle, move the joint through full ROM with gravity

TABLE 6.7 Close Packed Positions of Selected Joints

JOINT(S)	POSITION
Glenohumeral	Abduction and lateral rotation
Elbow (ulnohumeral)	Extension
Radiohumeral	Elbow flexed 90°, 5° forearm supination
Proximal radioulnar	5° forearm supination
Distal radioulnar	5° forearm supination
Wrist (radiocarpal)	Extension with radial deviation
Metacarpophalangeal (fingers)	Full flexion
Metacarpophalangeal (thumb)	Full opposition
Interphalangeal	Full extension
Hip	Full extension, medial rotation and abduction
Knee	Full extension, lateral rotation of tibia
Ankle (talocrural)	Maximum dorsiflexion
Subtalar	Full supination
Midtarsal	Full supination
Tarsometatarsal	Full supination
Metatarsophalangeal	Full extension
Interphalangeal	Full extension

eliminated and move the joint through full ROM against gravity.[11] If a patient can complete AROM and demonstrates weakness or pain during RROM, MMT is indicated. When performing MMT, the body segment is placed in a specific position to isolate the muscle or muscle group. Slight variations in positioning will impact how well a specific muscle is isolated, so it is important when performing MMT to test the body part as depicted in your reference material.[11] As with the break test, the patient is asked to perform an isometric contraction while the clinician applies resistance in an attempt to "break" the contraction. A standardized grading system can be used to measure muscle contraction (**Table 6.8**).[11]

Goniometry

The available AROM and PROM can be measured objectively using a goniometer (**Fig. 6.5**). The goniometer is a protractor with two rigid arms that intersect at a hinge joint. It is used to measure both joint position and available joint motion, and it can determine when the individual has regained normal motion at a joint.[8] The arms of the goniometer measure 0° to 180° of motion, or 0° to 360° of motion. The axis of the goniometer is aligned with the axis of the joint. The moving arm is aligned with specific landmarks on the moving body part. The stationary arm is aligned with specific landmarks on the nonmoving body part. Each joint has established landmarks for aligning the axis, moving arm, and nonmoving. To ensure that the measurements are valid and reliable, it is important that the clinician utilizes the established protocols for measuring ROM that are found in published reference materials.

TABLE 6.8 Grading System for Manual Muscle Testing

NUMERIC	VERBAL	CLINICAL FINDINGS
5	Normal	Complete ROM against gravity with maximal overload
4	Good	Complete ROM against gravity with moderate overload
3+	Fair +	Complete ROM against gravity with minimal overload
3	Fair	Complete ROM against gravity with no overload
3−	Fair −	Some, but not complete, ROM against gravity
2+	Poor +	Initiates motion against gravity
2	Poor	Complete ROM with some assistance and gravity eliminated
2−	Poor −	Initiates motion if gravity is eliminated
1	Trace	Evidence of slight muscular contraction; no joint motion
0	Zero	No muscle contraction palpated

From Kendall FP, McCreary EK, Provance PG, et al. *Muscles: Testing and Function with Posture and Pain.* 5th ed. Baltimore, MD: Lippincott Williams & Wilkins; 2005.

The normal ROM for selected joints is listed in **Table 6.9** and in the individual joint chapters. Age and gender may influence ROM. Women in their teens and early 20s tend to have a greater ROM in all planes compared with men. ROM decreases after 20 years in both genders, with the decrease occurring to a greater extent in women.

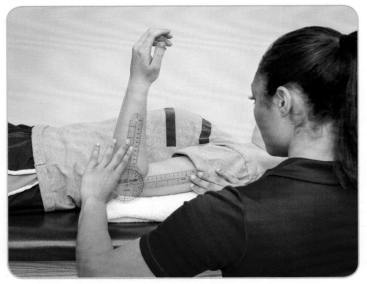

Figure 6.5. Goniometry measurement at the elbow. In the anatomical position, the elbow is flexed. The goniometer axis is placed over the lateral epicondyle of the humerus. To accommodate using a goniometer that ranges from 0° to 180°, the stationary arm is held parallel to the longitudinal axis of the radius, pointing toward the styloid process of the radius. The moving arm is held parallel to the longitudinal axis of the humerus, pointing toward the tip of the acromion process. The ROM is measured at the site where the pointer intersects the scale.

Stress Tests

Each body segment has a series of tests to assess joint function and integrity of joint structures. These tests assess the integrity of noncontractile tissues (e.g., ligaments, intra-articular structures, and the joint capsule). Stress tests occur in a single plane and are graded according to severity. Specifically, sprains of ligamentous tissue generally are graded on a three-degree scale after a specific stress is applied to a ligament to test its laxity (**Table 6.10**). **Laxity** describes the amount of "give" within a joint's supportive tissue. **Instability** refers to a joint's inability to function under the stresses encountered during functional activities.

Ligamentous testing should be done bilaterally and compared with baseline measures. It is essential to perform a test at the proper angle because a seemingly minor change in the joint angle can significantly alter the laxity of the tissue being stressed. In some instances, it may be appropriate to perform ligamentous stress testing before any other testing. During a stress test, it is important that the patient be able to relax the involved area because muscle guarding could interfere with the effectiveness of testing. If functional testing causes pain, the patient may find it more difficult to maintain a

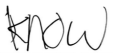

TABLE 6.9 Normal Ranges of Motion at Selected Joints (No Changes)

JOINT	MOTION	RANGE OF MOTION	JOINT	MOTION	RANGE OF MOTION
Cervical	Flexion	0°–80°	Digits 2–5	Flexion	0°–90°
	Extension	0°–70°	MCP	Extension	0°–45°
	Lateral flexion	0°–45°		Abduction	0°–20°
	Rotation	0°–80°			
Lumbar	Forward flexion	0°–60°	PIP	Flexion	0°–100°
	Extension	0°–35°	DIP	Flexion	0°–90°
	Lateral flexion	0°–20°	Hip	Flexion	0°–120
	Rotation	0°–50°		Extension	0°–30°
Shoulder	Flexion	0°–180°		Abduction	0°–40°
	Extension	0°–60°		Adduction	0°–30°
	Abduction	0°–180°		Internal rotation	0°–40°
	Internal rotation	0°–70°	Knee	External rotation	0°–50°
	External rotation	0°–90°		Flexion	0°–135°
	Horizontal abduction–adduction	0°–130°		Extension	0°–15°
Elbow	Flexion	0°–150°		Medial rotation with knee flexed	0°–25°
	Extension	0°–10°		Lateral rotation with knee flexed	0°–35°
Forearm	Pronation	0°–80°	Ankle	Dorsiflexion	0°–20°
	Supination	0°–80°		Plantar flexion	0°–50°
Wrist	Flexion	0°–80°		Pronation	0°–30°
	Extension	0°–70°	Subtalar	Supination	0°–50°
	Ulnar deviation	0°–30°		Inversion	0°–5°
	Radial deviation	0°–20°		Eversion	0°–5°
Thumb			Toes		
CMC	Abduction	0°–70°	1st MTP	Flexion	0°–45°
	Flexion	0°–15°		Extension	0°–75°
	Extension	0°–20°	1st IP	Flexion	0°–90°
	Opposition	Tip of thumb to tip of 5th finger	2nd to 5th MTP	Flexion	0°–40°
MCP	Flexion	0°–50°		Extension	0°–40°
IP	Flexion	0°–80°	PIP	Flexion	0°–35°
			DIP	Flexion	0°–30°
				Extension	0°–60°

CMC, carpometacarpal; *DIP*, distal interphalangeal; *IP*, interphalangeal; *MCP*, metacarpophalangeal; *MTP*, metatarsophalangeal; *PIP*, posterior interphalangeal.

From Lesser JM, Hughes SV, Jemelka JR, et al. Compiling a complete medical history: challenges and strategies for taking a comprehensive history in the elderly. *Geriatrics*. 2005;60(11):22–25.

relaxed position. As such, if a ligamentous injury is suspected, initiating testing with stress tests may be advantageous.

Figure 6.6 demonstrates a **valgus** stress test on the elbow joint to assess the integrity of the medial collateral ligaments. During an on-site assessment, tests to determine a possible fracture and major ligament damage at a joint should always be performed before moving an individual who is injured. Only the specific tests deemed to be necessary for the specific injury should be used. Because of the wide variety of stress tests, each is discussed within subsequent chapters.

TABLE 6.10 Grading System for Ligamentous Laxity

GRADE	LIGAMENTOUS END FEEL	DAMAGE
I	Firm (normal)	Slight stretching of the ligament with little or no tearing of the fibers. Pain is present, but the degree of stability roughly compares with that of the opposite extremity.
II	Soft	Partial tearing of the fibers. The joint line "opens up" significantly when compared with the opposite side.
III	Empty	Complete tearing of the ligament. The motion is restricted by other joint structures, such as tendons.

Special Tests

Special tests have been developed for specific body parts or areas as a means of detecting injury or related pathology. In general, special tests occur across planes and are not graded. For example, Speed's test is used as a technique for assessing pathology related to biceps tendon, and Thompson test is used to assess potential rupture of the Achilles tendon.

Neurological Testing

A segmental nerve is the portion of a nerve that originates in the spinal cord and is referred to as a nerve root. Most nerve roots share two components:

1. A **somatic** portion, which innervates a series of skeletal muscles and provides sensory input from the skin, fascia, muscles, and joints

2. A **visceral** component, which is part of the autonomic nervous system

The autonomic system supplies the blood vessels, dura mater, periosteum, ligaments, and intervertebral disks, among many other structures.

Nerves commonly are injured by tensile or compressive forces, and these injuries are reflected in both motor and sensory deficits. The motor component of a segmental nerve is tested using a **myotome**, a group of muscles primarily innervated by a single nerve root. The sensory component is tested using a **dermatome**, an area of skin supplied by a single nerve root. An injury to a segmental nerve root often affects more than one peripheral nerve and does not demonstrate the same motor loss or sensory deficit as an injury to a single peripheral nerve. Dermatomes, myotomes, and reflexes are used to assess the integrity of the central nervous system (CNS). Peripheral nerves are assessed using MMT and noting cutaneous sensory changes in peripheral nerve patterns. Neurological testing is only necessary in orthopedic injuries when an individual complains of numbness, tingling, or a burning sensation or suffers from unexplained muscular weakness.

Dermatomes

The sensitivity of a dermatome can be assessed by touching a patient with a cotton ball, paper clip, the pads of the fingers, or opposite ends of a cotton-tipped applicator. In doing so, the clinician should ask the individual about the sensations being experienced. It is important to determine the nature of the sensation (e.g., a sharp or dull sensation)

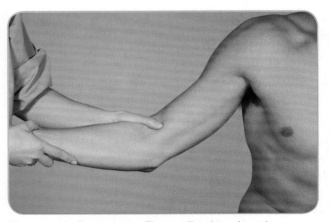

Figure 6.6. Stress tests. The application of a valgus stress on the elbow joint can assess the integrity of the joint medial collateral ligaments.

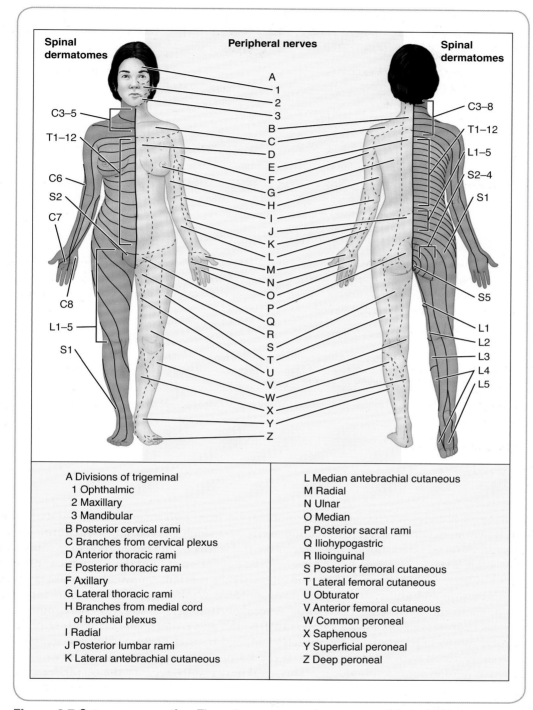

Spinal dermatomes | **Peripheral nerves** | **Spinal dermatomes**

C3–5
T1–12
C6
S2
C7
C8
L1–5
S1

C3–8
T1–12
L1–5
S2–4
S1
S5
L1
L2
L3
L4
L5

A
1
2
3
B
C
D
E
F
G
H
I
J
K
L
M
N
O
P
Q
R
S
T
U
V
W
X
Y
Z

A Divisions of trigeminal
 1 Ophthalmic
 2 Maxillary
 3 Mandibular
B Posterior cervical rami
C Branches from cervical plexus
D Anterior thoracic rami
E Posterior thoracic rami
F Axillary
G Lateral thoracic rami
H Branches from medial cord
  of brachial plexus
I Radial
J Posterior lumbar rami
K Lateral antebrachial cutaneous

L Median antebrachial cutaneous
M Radial
N Ulnar
O Median
P Posterior sacral rami
Q Iliohypogastric
R Ilioinguinal
S Posterior femoral cutaneous
T Lateral femoral cutaneous
U Obturator
V Anterior femoral cutaneous
W Common peroneal
X Saphenous
Y Superficial peroneal
Z Deep peroneal

Figure 6.7. Cutaneous sensation. The cutaneous sensation patterns of the spinal nerve dermatomes differ from the patterns innervated by the peripheral nerves.

and to assess whether the same sensation was experienced in testing the uninjured body segment. Abnormal responses may be decreased tactile sensation (**hypoesthesia**), excessive tactile sensation (**hyperesthesia**), or loss of sensation (**anesthesia**). **Paresthesia** is another abnormal sensation characterized by a numb, tingling, or burning sensation. **Figure 6.7** illustrates dermatome patterns for the segmental nerves.

TABLE 6.11 Myotomes Used to Test Selected Nerve Root Segments

NERVE ROOT SEGMENT	ACTION TESTED
C1–C2	Neck flexion[a]
C3	Neck lateral flexion[a]
C4	Shoulder elevation
C5	Shoulder abduction
C6	Elbow flexion and wrist extension
C7	Elbow extension and wrist flexion
C8	Thumb extension and ulnar deviation
T1	Intrinsic muscles of the hand (finer abduction and adduction)
L1–L2	Hip flexion
L3	Knee extension
L4	Ankle dorsiflexion
L5	Toe extension
S1	Ankle plantar flexion, foot eversion, hip extension
S2	Knee flexion

[a]These myotomes should not be performed in an individual with a suspected cervical fracture or dislocation because they may cause serious damage or possibly death.

Myotomes

The majority of muscles receive segmental innervation from two or more nerve roots. Selected motions, however, may be innervated predominantly by a single nerve root (**myotome**). Resisted muscle testing of a selected motion can determine the status of the nerve root that supplies the myotome (**Table 6.11**). In assessing nerve integrity, the patient must hold the isometric muscle contraction for at least 5 seconds while the clinician resists the motion. A normal response is a strong muscle contraction and ability to withstand resistance.[11] Weakness in the myotome indicates a possible injury to the spinal cord nerve root. A weakened muscle contraction may indicate partial paralysis (**paresis**) of the muscles innervated by the nerve root being tested. In a peripheral nerve injury, complete paralysis of the muscles supplied by that nerve occurs. For example, the L3 myotome is tested with knee extension. If the L3 nerve root is damaged at its origin in the spine, a weak muscle contraction occurs. This weakness results because the quadriceps receives innervation from the L2 and L4 segmental nerves. If, however, the peripheral femoral nerve, which contains segments of L2, L3, and L4, is damaged proximal to the quadriceps muscle, the muscle cannot receive any nerve impulses; therefore, it is unable to contract and execute a knee extension.

Reflexes

Damage to the CNS can be detected by stimulation of the deep tendon reflexes (DTRs) (**Table 6.12**). Reflex testing is limited, however, because not all nerve roots have a DTR. The most familiar DTR is the patellar, or knee jerk, reflex elicited by striking the patellar tendon with a reflex hammer, causing a rapid contraction of the quadriceps muscle (**Fig. 6.8**). DTRs tend to be diminished or absent if the specific nerve root being tested is damaged. Exaggerated, distorted, or absent reflexes indicate

TABLE 6.12 Deep Tendon Reflexes

REFLEX LEVEL	STIMULATION SITE	NORMAL RESPONSE	SEGMENTAL
Jaw	Mandible	Mouth closes	Cranial nerve V
Biceps	Biceps tendon	Biceps contraction	C5–C6
Brachioradialis	Brachioradialis tendon or just distal to the musculotendinous junction	Flexion of elbow and/or pronation of forearm	C5–C6
Triceps	Distal triceps tendon just superior to olecranon process	Elbow extension/muscle contraction	C7–C8
Patella	Patellar tendon	Leg extension	L3–L4
Medial hamstrings	Semimembranosus tendon	Knee flexion/muscle contraction	L5, S1
Lateral hamstrings	Biceps femoris tendon	Knee flexion/muscle contraction	S1–S2
Tibialis posterior	Tibialis posterior tendon behind medial malleolus	Plantar flexion of foot with inversion	L4–L5
Achilles	Achilles tendon	Plantar flexion of foot	S1–S2

degeneration or injury in specific regions of the nervous system. This may be demonstrated before other signs are apparent. Abnormal DTRs are not clinically relevant, however, unless they are found with sensory or motor abnormalities.

Superficial reflexes are reflexes provoked by superficial stroking, usually with a moderately sharp object that does not break the skin (**Table 6.13**). This action produces a reflex muscle contraction. For example, the normal response when testing the upper abdominal reflex is for the umbilicus to move up and toward the areas being stroked; this reflex represents segmental level T7 through T9. An absence of a superficial reflex indicates a lesion in the cerebral cortex of the brain (upper motor neuron lesion).

Pathological reflexes (**Table 6.14**) can indicate upper motor neuron lesions if bilateral or lower motor neuron lesions if unilateral. The presence of the reflex often serves as a sign of some pathologic condition.

Peripheral Nerve Testing

Motor function in peripheral nerves is assessed by resisted MMT throughout the full ROM. Sensory deficits are assessed in a manner identical to that of dermatome testing, except the cutaneous patterns differ (**Fig. 6.7**). Special compression tests also may be used on nerves close to the skin surface, such as the ulnar and median nerves. For example, the Tinel sign test is performed by tapping the skin directly over a superficial nerve. A positive sign, indicating irritation or compression of the nerve, results in a tingling sensation traveling into the muscles and skin supplied by the nerve.

Activity-Specific Functional Testing

Before permitting an individual to return to sport and physical activity after an injury, the individual's condition must be fully evaluated so that the risk of reinjury is minimal. Prior to starting the functional return to play testing sequence, the patient should have full pain-free ROM, have no active inflammation or acute swelling present, and demonstrate preinjury strength and ROM. Activity-specific tests involve the performance of active movements typical of those executed by the individual during sport or activity participation. The initial assessment should involve assessing the patient's walking gait, ability to perform double- and single-leg hopping, and ability to run in a

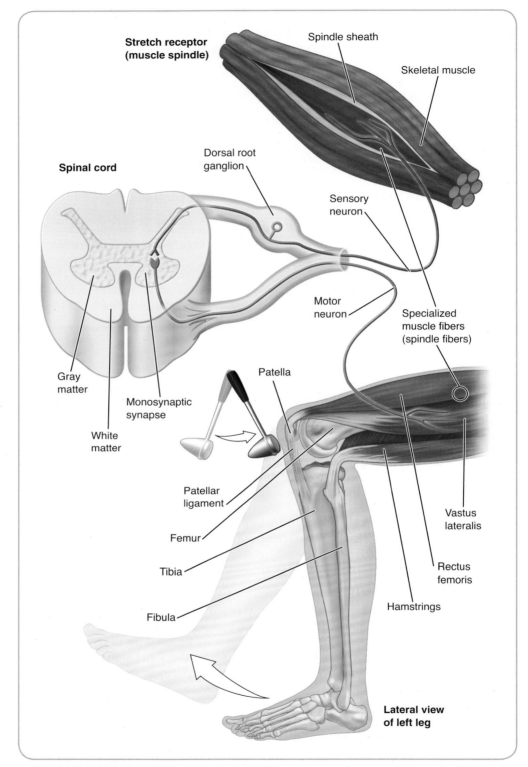

Figure 6.8. Reflexes. Reflexes can indicate the presence of nerve root damage. The most familiar stretch reflex is the knee jerk, or patellar reflex, performed by tapping the patellar tendon with a reflex hammer, causing involuntary knee extension.

TABLE 6.13 Superficial Reflexes

REFLEX	NORMAL RESPONSE	SEGMENTAL LEVEL
Upper abdominal	Umbilicus moves up and toward area being stroked	T7–T9
Lower abdominal	Umbilicus moves down and toward area being stroked	T11–T1
Cremasteric	Scrotum elevates	T12, L1
Plantar	Flexion of toes	S1–S2
Gluteal	Skin tenses in the gluteal area	L4–L5, S1–S3
Anal	Anal sphincter muscles contract	S2–S4

straight line, figure eight, and Z and S patterns at one-fourth, one-half, three-fourth, and full speed without pain or instability. These movements should assess strength, agility, flexibility, joint stability, endurance, coordination, and balance. Once the patient has successfully completed the initial phase of functional testing, activity-specific skills can be introduced to an increasing, more challengingly levels until gamelike situations are replicated. Any individual who has been discharged from rehabilitation also should be cleared by a physician for participation.

 The testing component of an assessment should include special tests to rule out possibility of fracture before beginning ROM and MMT. However, because a sprain of the anterior talofibular ligament is suspected based on the MOI and location of swelling, fever, and point tenderness, joint stability stress testing is most appropriate to perform at this point. Depending on the findings, additional tests that may be considered are ROM, MMT, neurological, and functional assessment. Based on those findings, activity-specific functional testing may or may not be appropriate.

TABLE 6.14 Pathological Reflexes[a]

REFLEX	ELICITATION	POSITIVE RESPONSE	PATHOLOGY
Babinski[b]	Stroke lateral aspect of sole of foot.	Extension of big toe; fanning of four small toes Test is normal in newborns.	Pyramidal tract lesion Organic hemiplegia
Chaddock	Stroke lateral side of foot beneath lateral malleolus.	Same response as previous	Pyramidal tract lesion
Oppenheim	Stroke anteromedial tibial surface.	Same response as previous	Pyramidal tract lesion
Gordon	Squeeze calf muscle firmly.	Same response as previous	Pyramidal tract lesion
Brudzinski	Passive flexion of one lower limb	Similar movement occurs in opposite limb.	Meningitis
Hoffman (digital)[c]	"Flicking" of terminal phalanx of index, middle, or ring finger	Reflex flexion of distal phalanx of thumb and of distal phalanx of index or middle finger (whichever one was not "flicked")	Increased irritability of sensory nerve in tetany Pyramidal tract lesion

[a]A bilateral positive response indicates an upper motor neuron lesion. A unilateral positive response may indicate a lower motor neuron lesion.
[b]The test is most commonly performed in the lower limb.
[c]The test is most commonly performed in the upper limb.

BOX 6.3 Laboratory Blood Testing

- Red blood cell count determines the approximate number of circulating red blood cells (erythrocytes). A decreased count indicates possible anemia, chronic infection, internal hemorrhage, certain types of cancers, or deficiencies in iron, vitamin B12, or folic acid.

- White blood cell count determines the approximate number of circulating white blood cells (leukocytes). A decreased count indicates an inability to fight infections.

- Hemoglobin gives the red color to erythrocytes. It transports oxygen to the tissues and carries away the carbon dioxide. A decreased count indicates possible anemia or carbon monoxide poisoning.

- Hematocrit measures the volume of erythrocytes packed by centrifugation in a given volume of blood and is expressed as a percentage. A decreased value indicates anemia.

- Platelets aid in blood clotting. A decreased value indicates decreased clotting ability, internal bleeding, or a possible bleeding disorder.

LABORATORY TESTS

 In assessing an injury, what special laboratory tests and imaging techniques can be used by the athletic trainer to reach an accurate diagnosis?

A variety of laboratory tests can be used in the assessment of an injury and illness (**Box 6.3**). For example, if an individual has a grossly swollen knee, the physician may draw fluid out of the joint with a hypodermic needle to examine the synovial fluid (**Table 6.15**). If the individual reports a sore throat, lethargy, and fever, a throat culture and blood test may be ordered. A complete blood count (CBC) can address several factors; however, other common factors that are tested include hemoglobin, hematocrit, and iron levels. An individual who has blood in the urine likewise requires a urinalysis. Common factors assessed in this laboratory test include pH, glucose, and bacteria (**Table 6.16**).

Radiography

The most common imaging technique is radiography, or the X-ray (**Fig. 6.9**). A radiograph provides an image of certain body structures and can rule out fractures, infections, and **neoplasms**. The image is formed when a minute amount of radiation passes through the body to expose sensitive film placed on the other side. The ability to penetrate tissues depends on the tissue composition and mass. For example, bones (calcium) restrict rays from passing through; therefore, these images appear white on the film. Lungs or other air-filled structures, however, allow most X-rays to pass through, resulting in the images appearing black. Soft tissues (e.g., heart, kidneys, or liver), allow varying degrees

---

TABLE 6.15 Synovial Fluid Classifications

TYPE	APPEARANCE	SIGNIFICANCE
Group 1	Clear yellow	Noninflammatory state, no trauma
Group 2[a]	Cloudy	Inflammatory, arthritis, excludes most patients with osteoarthritis
Group 3	Thick exudate, brownish	Septic arthritis; occasionally seen in gout
Group 4	Hemorrhagic	Trauma, bleeding disorders, tumors, fractures

[a]Inflammatory fluids clot and should be collected in heparin-containing tubes. All group 2 or 3 fluids should be cultured if the diagnosis is uncertain.

TABLE 6.16 Normal Ranges for Selected Blood Variables in Adults

LABORATORY TEST	MEN	GENDER NEUTRAL	WOMEN
Hemoglobin (g/dL)	13–18		12–16
Hematocrit (%)	42–52		37–48
Red blood cell count (10^{12}/L)	4.5–6.5		3.9–5.6
White blood cell count		4.3–10.8 (10^9/L)	
Platelet count		150–350 (10^9/L)	
Iron, total (μg/dL)		50–100	

of penetration and are difficult to identify on the radiograph. Images are preserved on sheets of film. As film quality and electronic technology have advanced, better imaging has been achieved, and the dose of radiation to the patient has been decreased. The use of radiographs is contraindicated on the thyroid gland, pregnant abdomen, and reproductive organs. If the information gained outweighs the risk, however, these areas can be shielded with a lead drape.

Some forms of radiographs use radiopaque dyes that are absorbed by the tissues, allowing them to be visualized by radiographic examination. A **myelogram** uses an opaque dye that is introduced into the spinal canal through a lumbar puncture. The patient is placed in a tilted position, allowing the dye to flow to different levels of the spinal cord. In viewing the contrasts, physicians can identify pathologies of the spinal canal (e.g., tumors, nerve root compression, and disk disease). Another form of radiographic testing is the **arthrogram**. Again, an opaque dye, air, or a combination of the two is injected into a joint space. The visual study of the joint can detect capsular tissue tears and articular cartilage lesions.

Computed Tomography

A computed tomography (CT) scan is a form of radiography that produces a three-dimensional, cross-sectional picture of a body part (**Fig. 6.10**). This test is used to reveal abnormalities in bone, fat, and soft tissue and is excellent at detecting tendinous and ligamentous injuries in varying joint positions. Scanners use a beam of light across a "slice" or layer of the body. A special receptor located opposite the beam detects the number of rays passing through the body. The tube emitting the beams of light rotates around the body, and thousands of readings are taken by the receptors. The computer determines the density of the underlying tissues based on the absorption of X-rays by the body, allowing more precision in viewing soft tissues. The computer records the data, analyzes the receptor readings, and calculates the absorption of the light beams at thousands of different points. This information is then converted into a

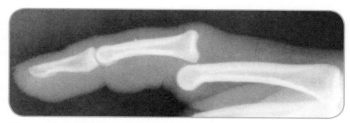

Figure 6.9. Radiography. Bone absorbs the X-rays and, therefore, appears white on the radiograph. This radiograph demonstrates a dorsal dislocation of the proximal interphalangeal joint.

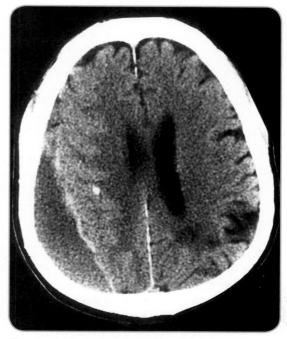

Figure 6.10. Computed tomography. A male patient reported increased sleepiness and a change in personality 3 weeks after falling and striking his head. The cranial CT scan demonstrates a chronic subdural hematoma.

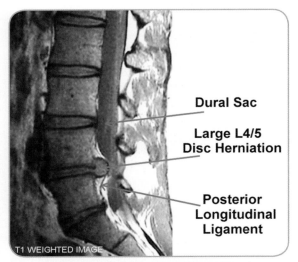

Figure 6.11. Magnetic resonance imaging. This magnetic resonance image depicts a large L4–L5 disk herniation.

two-dimensional image, or slice, of the body and is displayed on a video screen and/or radiographic film. These slices can be obtained at varying positions and thicknesses, allowing the radiologist or physician to study the area and its surroundings. A CT scan is relatively safe because the patient is exposed to little radiation during the procedure. A CT scan also yields highly detailed results.

Magnetic Resonance Imaging

Magnetic resonance imaging (MRI) is an excellent tool for visualizing the CNS, spine, and musculoskeletal and cardiovascular systems (**Fig. 6.11**). One of its assets is the ability to provide soft-tissue differentiation (e.g., ligamentous disruption, such as an anterior cruciate ligament tear). It also is used to demonstrate space-occupying lesions in the brain (e.g., tumor or hematoma) and joint damage (e.g., meniscal tears or osteochondral fractures) as well as to view blood vessels and blood flow without the use of a contrast medium (e.g., cardiac function). In many cases, the MRI has replaced myelography and arthrography.

Images are obtained by placing the patient in an MRI tube that produces the magnetic field. This causes the body's hydrogen nuclei to align with the magnetic axis. The tissues are then bombarded by radio waves, which causes the nuclei to resonate as they absorb the energy. When the energy from the radio waves ceases, the nuclei return to their state of equilibrium by releasing energy, which is then detected by the MRI unit and transformed by a computer into visible images.

Radionuclide Scintigraphy (Bone Scan)

A bone scan is used to detect stress fractures of the long bones and vertebrae, degenerative diseases, infections, or tumors of the bone. A **radionucleotide** material, technetium-99m, is injected into a vein and is slowly absorbed by areas of bone undergoing remodeling. Several hours after the injection, the patient is placed under a recording device that scans radioactive signals and records the images on film. In some scans, active images are recorded on videotape. A total body scan or even a localized scan can take close to an hour. Any areas subject to stress (e.g., fractures or increases of metabolic activity, such as bone marrow centers or tumors) show as areas of greatest uptake and appear darker on the film (**Fig. 6.12**). Bone scans may be clinically correlated to plain-film radiographs or other diagnostic tests. No special preparation is needed before the bone scan, and the risk to the patient is minimal. The body excretes the radioactive material over a 24-hour period.

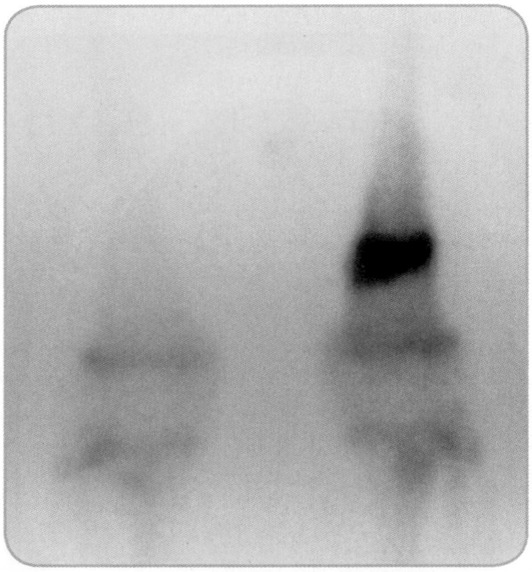

Ultrasonic Imaging

Sonography, as it sometimes is called, uses sound waves to view the various internal organs and certain soft-tissue structures, such as tendons. The energy produced is similar to that used during therapeutic ultrasound treatments but has a frequency of less than 0.8 MHz. Although it commonly is used to monitor the development of the fetus during pregnancy, it also is used to view tendons and for other soft-tissue imaging. Similar to a sonar device on a submarine, a piezoelectric crystal is used to convert electrical pulses into vibrations that penetrate the body structures. The sound waves are reflected away from the tissues and create a two-dimensional image of the subcutaneous structures.

Figure 6.12. Radionuclide scintigraphy. Bone scans can detect stress fractures long before the fracture becomes visible on traditional radiographs. This individual had increased his daily run from 5 to 8 miles per day and included hill climbing over the past few months. He reported increasing pain in his thigh. The bone scan showed increased density in a transverse line, indicating medial periosteal reaction.

Electromyography

Certain muscular conditions can be detected using electromyography. This diagnostic tool consists of a thin electrode needle that is inserted into the muscle to determine the level of muscular contraction following an electrical stimulation. Motor unit potentials can be observed on an oscilloscope screen or recorded on an electromyogram. Electromyography is used to detect denervated muscles, nerve root compression injuries, and other muscle diseases.

 In some cases, a definitive diagnosis requires laboratory tests or imaging techniques. In the majority of cases, these tests can only be ordered by a physician or appropriately licensed medical specialist. It is essential that athletic trainers be aware of their duty of care that is consistent with current state law.

DOCUMENTATION

? Why is it so critical that athletic trainers document their actions while caring for each patient?

Athletic trainers are required to maintain medical records in accordance with state and federal regulatory agencies.[12] Specifically, clinicians should conform to the Health Insurance Portability and Accountability Act (HIPAA) guidelines and when working in schools systems, the Federal Educational Rights Privacy Act (FERPA) guidelines.[12] Part of medical records is the report that documents the findings of the evaluation process and the subsequent treatment provided. Maintaining clear and accurately scribed injury reports and SOAP notes serve several purposes: (1) to enhance communication among those providing care for the patient by storing all pertinent information in a centralized document, (2) to facilitate continuity of care by decreasing the chance of replication of services or risk of assuming services are being provided when they are not, and (3) to provide evidence of services provided for purposes of billing and legal protections.

When documenting the evaluation process and the subsequent treatment provided, the clinician should adhere to eight basic principles. **First**, use correct medical terminology so that you convey the precise structure, location, pathology, condition, or process under examination. **Second**, use only standardized and accepted medical abbreviations. Medical abbreviations are widely used in medical documentation to decrease time spent on writing notes. However, a downfall of using abbreviations is that information may not be accurately conveyed due to differences in interpretations. A list of commonly used and accepted medical abbreviations is provided in **Table 6.17**. **Third**, use correct punctuation. Periods, dashes, and slashes have specific meaning in medical documents (refer to **Table 6.17**), and the skilled clinician should be aware of how punctuation use is different when writing medical notes than when writing narratives. **Fourth**, strive to be as accurate as possible. **Fifth**, while maintaining accuracy, also strive for brevity. Although using anatomical/medical terms and abbreviations will aid in being brief, it is important to record information that is most pertinent. For example, when describing the MOI for an ankle sprain, a brief yet accurate description is as follows: *Patient inverted R ankle upon landing.* The longer version is as follows: *Patient was playing basketball and attempting to rebound an opponent's ball. Upon landing, the patient inverted her right ankle which she described as "rolling inward."* **Sixth**, write (or type) legibly with an instrument that cannot be erased or removed. If the revision is needed, the clinician simply draws one line (or strike out) through the original word or phrase and clearly writes in the new information so that both the original and revised information is visible. The clinician should sign and date when the revision was made. **Seventh**, documents should be completed and filed at the time services are rendered. And **eighth**, the clinician needs to sign and date each note in a manner that clearly identifies who created the note/provided services.

 Clear and accurate injury reports and SOAP notes in a centralized document can enhance communication between health care providers decreasing the chance of replication of services or assuming that services are being provided when they are not and can provide evidence of services provided for purposes of billing and legal protections.

TABLE 6.17 Common Abbreviations and Symbols Used in Medical Documentation

<	Less than		EENT	Eyes, ears, nose, throat
>	Greater than		ELOP	Estimated length of program
↑	Increase		EMS	Emergency medical services
↓	Decrease		EMT	Emergency medical technician
Δ	Change		EOA	Examine, opinion, and advice; esophageal obturator airway
abnor.	Abnormal		ES	Electrical stimulation
AC	Acute; before meals; acromioclavicular		EV	Eversion
ADL	Activities of daily living		exam.	Examination
ant.	Anterior		FH	Family history
ante	Before		FROM	Full range of movement
A&O	Alert & oriented		FWB	Full weight bearing
AOAP	As often as possible		Fx	Fracture
AP	Anterior–posterior; assessment and plans		G1–4	Grades 1–4
AROM	Active range of motion		GA	General appearance
ASAP	As soon as possible		HA	Headache
AT	Athletic training; athletic trainer		H/O	History of
B	Bilateral		HP	Hot pack
BID or bid	Twice daily		H&P	History and physical
c	With		HPI	History of present illness
CC	Chief complaint; chronic complainer		ht.	Height; heart
ck.	Check		HTN	Hypertension
C/O	Complained of; complaints; under care of		Hx	History
CP	Cerebral palsy; chest pain; chronic pain		IC	Individual counseling
CPR	Cardiopulmonary resuscitation		IN	Inversion
CWI	Crutch walking instruction		IPPA	Inspection, percussion, palpation, and auscultation
D	Day		L	Left; liter
d/c, DC	Discharged; discontinue; decrease		LAT	Lateral
DF	Dorsiflexion		LBP	Low back pain
DOB	Date of birth		LE	Lower extremity
DTR	Deep tendon reflexes		LOM	Limitation of motion
DVT	Deep vein thrombosis		MAEEW	Moves all extremities equally well
Dx	Diagnosis		MEDS	Medication
E	Edema		mm	Muscle; millimeter; mucous membrane

(continued)

TABLE 6.17 Common Abbreviations and Symbols Used in Medical Documentation *(continued)*

MMT	Manual muscle test		PT	Point tender
MOD	Moderate		PWB	Partial weight bearing
N	Normal; never; no; not		Px	Physical examination; pneumothorax
NC	Neurological check; no complaints; not completed		qd	Once daily
NEG	Negative		qid	Four times daily
NKA	No known allergies		R	Right
NP	No pain; not pregnant; not present		rehab	Rehabilitation
NPO	Nothing by mouth		R/O	Rule out
NPT	Normal pressure and temperature		ROM	Range of motion
NSA	No significant abnormality		RROM	Resisted range of motion
NSAID	Nonsteroidal anti-inflammatory drug		RTP	Return to play
NT	Not tried		Rx	Therapy; drug; medication; treatment; take
NWB	Non–weight-bearing		s	Without
O	Objective finding; oral; open; obvious; often; other		SLR	Straight leg raises
OH	Occupational history		stat	Immediately
ORIF	Open reduction/internal fixation		STG	Short-term goals
p	After		Sx	Signs, symptom
P&A	Percussion and auscultation		T	Temperature
PA	Posterior–anterior; physician assistant; presents again		TENS	Transcutaneous electrical nerve stimulation
PE	Physical examination		tid	Three times daily
PF	Plantar flexion		TTWB	Toe touch weight bearing
PH	Past history; poor health		UE	Upper extremity
PMH	Past medical history		UK	Unknown
PNF	Proprioceptive neuromuscular facilitation		US	Ultrasound
PNS	Peripheral nervous system		w	White; with
PPPBL	Peripheral pulses palpable both legs		WBAT	Weight bearing as tolerated
pre-op	Preoperative		whp	Whirlpool
PRE	Progressive resistive exercise		WNL	Within normal limits
prn	As needed		W/O	Without
prog.	Prognosis		y.o.	Year old
PROM	Passive range of motion		1tive	Positive

SUMMARY

1. In an injury assessment, a problem-solving process incorporates subjective and objective information that is reliable, accurate, and measurable.

2. The HOPS format includes history, observation and inspection, palpation, and special tests.

3. A more popular method of injury management is the SOAP note format, which assesses the individual's status and prognosis and establishes short- and long-term goals for recovery. The format outlines the treatment plan, such as the frequency and duration of treatments, rehabilitation exercises, ongoing patient education, evaluation standards to determine progress, and criteria for discharge.

4. When evaluating patients who present with symptoms suggestive of a general medical condition, the assessment process is divided into the history and physical examination.

5. The subjective information gathered during the history taking should include the primary complaint, the MOI, characteristics of the symptoms, disabilities resulting from the injury, and related medical history.

6. The objective assessment should include observation and inspection, bony and soft-tissue palpation, functional tests, stress tests for specific joints or structures, neurological testing, and activity-specific functional tests.

7. ROM testing includes assessing active, passive, and resistive motions and is used to gather information about the amount of motion present and the presence of pain.

8. ROM can be objectively measured using a goniometer. Specific landmarks are utilized to measure each specific ROM and thus are considered reliable methods of obtaining objective measurements of motion.

9. MMT is used to assess the strength of a specific muscle by isolating the muscle and requiring the muscle to meet a specific resistance. MMT is graded based on a scale of 0 to 5.

10. Special tests denote any given number of tests that are used to assess for the presence of absence of a specific pathology.

11. The use of a variety of laboratory tests and imaging techniques can be instrumental in establishing an accurate diagnosis of an injury or illness. In the majority of cases, these tests can only be ordered by a physician or appropriately licensed medical specialist.

APPLICATION QUESTIONS

1. You have been a high school athletic trainer for 5 years. Effective this year, the school hired a second athletic trainer on a part-time basis (i.e., working 20 to 25 hours per week). It has been your practice to use the HOPS method when performing and documenting an injury assessment. The new athletic trainer prefers to use the SOAP method and asks permission to continue to use that format. Describe the benefits and challenges to adopting this request.

2. As the host interscholastic athletic trainer, a member of the visiting lacrosse team sustains a knee injury during the first half of the game. In gathering a history of the injury on the field, what questions, if any, would be appropriate to ask regarding any previous history of injury to the same knee? What value is there in asking these questions?

3. A 15-year-old soccer player sustains an ankle injury. The MOI and observable signs suggest a mild inversion ankle sprain. Where would you begin palpating for point tenderness to determine the extent and severity of injury without causing additional pain?

4. While working as a physician extender, you routinely forget to complete the ROS portion of the history. Create a list of questions that will allow you to assess all systems required within the ROS process.

5. As a high school athletic trainer, you have a student athlete that has sustained a significant ankle injury that warrants an X-ray. How would you proceed?

REFERENCES

1. Kettenbach G. *Writing Patient/Client Notes: Ensuring Accuracy in Documentation*. 4th ed. Philadelphia, PA: FA Davis; 2009.
2. Bickley LS, Szilagyi PG. *Bates' Guide to Physical Examination and History Taking*. Philadelphia, PA: Lippincott Williams & Wilkins; 2007.
3. Parsons JT, ed. *2014-2015 NCAA Sports Medicine Handbook*. Indianapolis, IN: National Collegiate Athletic Association; 2014.
4. Lesser JM, Hughes SV, Jemelka JR, et al. Compiling a complete medical history: challenges and strategies for taking a comprehensive history in the elderly. *Geriatrics*. 2005;60(11):22–25.
5. Hawker GA, Mian S, Kendzerska T, et al. Measures of adult pain. Visual Analog Scale for Pain (VAS Pain), Numeric Rating Scale for Pain (NRS Pain), McGill Pain Questionnaire (MPQ), Short-Form McGill Pain Questionnaire (SF-MPQ), Chronic Pain Grade Scale (CPGS), Short Form-36 Bodily Pain Scale (SF-36 BPS), and Measure of Intermittent and Constant Osteoarthritis Pain (ICOAP). *Arthritis Care Res*. 2011;63(suppl 11):S240–S252.
6. Documenting general observations. *Nursing*. 2006;36(2):25.
7. Cyriax JH. *Cyriax's Illustrated Manual of Orthopaedic Medicine*. 2nd ed. Oxford, United Kingdom: Butterworth-Heinemann; 1993.
8. Norkin CC, White DJ. *Measurement of Joint Motion: A Guide to Goniometry*. 4th ed. Philadelphia, PA: FA Davis; 2009.
9. Cyriax J. *Textbook of Orthopaedic Medicine, Volume One: Diagnosis of Soft Tissue Lesions*. 8th ed. London, United Kingdom: Baillière Tindall; 1982.
10. Magee DJ. *Orthopedic Physical Assessment*. 5th ed. Philadelphia, PA: Elsevier Saunders; 2008.
11. Kendall FP, McCreary EK, Provance PG, et al. *Muscles: Testing and Function with Posture and Pain*. 5th ed. Baltimore, MD: Lippincott Williams & Wilkins; 2005.
12. National Athletic Trainers' Association. *Athletic Training Services: An Overview of Skills and Services Performed by Certified Athletic Trainers*. Dallas, TX: National Athletic Trainers' Association; 2010.

7

Acute Injuries: Assessment and Disposition

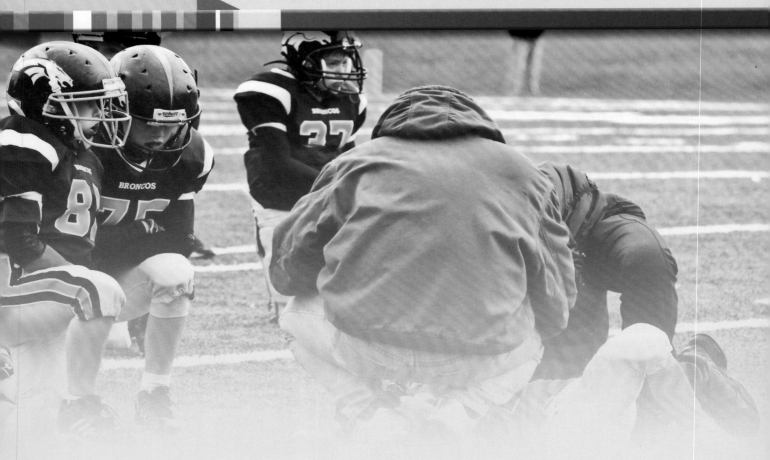

SUSAN LEGGETT / Shutterstock.com

STUDENT OUTCOMES

1. Identify planning strategies designed to prevent the incidence and severity of acute injury and enhance an effective and appropriate response.

2. Design a venue-specific emergency action protocol.

3. Define triage and explain the importance of triage when assessing acute injuries.

4. Delineate between a primary and secondary survey.

5. List the primary questions asked during the history portion of an on-field assessment of a patient with an acute injury.

6. Describe the components of an on-site inspection and palpation.

7. Compare how muscle and joint function is assessed on field as compared to how muscle and joint function is assessed in nonacute, off-field situations.

8. Explain how to conduct an on-field neurological examination.

9. List the components of a vital sign assessment and identify normal findings.

10. Identify the signs and symptoms of acute fracture and management strategies.

11. Describe proper procedures for removal of protective equipment.

12. Explain different procedures for transporting the patient from the site of injury.

13. Identify patients who are experiencing conditions that may result in sudden death in sports, and explain the appropriate acute response.

INTRODUCTION

No other act in athletic training gets the heart racing as much as being called out to the scene of an acute injury where there is the potential of finding a patient in a life-threatening situation. Upon arriving at the scene, the athletic trainer needs to assess the situation, evaluate the patient, determine the type and extent of injury that has been sustained, and provide immediate appropriate care. In an acute injury situation, the presence of life-threatening conditions should be established or ruled out, followed by conditions that may develop into life-threatening conditions if not properly addressed in a timely manner. Next, orthopedic injuries should be addressed in order of severity: fractures, dislocations, grade 3 strains and sprains, significant open wounds, etc. Within this chapter, strategies for preventing and preparing for emergency situations and minimizing the extent of injury are presented. Assessment methods for evaluating patients with acute injury are then discussed followed by strategies to remove patients from the injury site. Finally, this chapter provides a review of the leading causes of sudden death in sports along with the recognition and acute management of these conditions.

THE EMERGENCY ACTION PLAN

 A gymnast slipped off the springboard on an approach to a vault and collided full force into the horse. As the on-site athletic trainer, you observe the gymnast lying motionless on the floor. Based on this information, is it appropriate to activate the institution's emergency medical plan?

Administrators, medical directors, athletic trainers, and coaches all have shared responsibilities to ensure that the athlete's short- and long-term health is protected.[1] The majority of the responsibility falls on the supervising physician and athletic trainer; however, each person has differing levels of responsibility in meeting this goal. The Inter-Association Consensus Statement on Best Practices for Sports Medicine Management for Secondary Schools and Colleges recommends using a concept referred to as athlete-centered medicine when designing policies and procedures for the prevention of injury and provision of health care.[1] The recommendations put forth in the consensus statement are presented in **Box 7.1**. A primary consideration is the inclusion of a well-written emergency action plan.

Although the rate of catastrophic injury in sports is low, the more prepared and better practiced the athletic trainer and sports medicine team is in responding, the more successful the response will be.[2] The **emergency action plan** (EAP) serves as a blue print on how to respond to emergency situations. The EAP should be a written document that is comprehensive yet flexible enough to adapt to any emergency situation at any activity venue. The plan should identify the following general principles[3]:

- The personnel, with their qualifications, needed to perform responsibilities in executing the plan

- Equipment needed to carry out the tasks required in the event of an emergency

- The mechanism of communication to the emergency care providers and the mode of transportation for the patient

- The facilities to which the patient will be taken, including how and when those facilities will be notified in advance of the scheduled event or contest

> ### BOX 7.1 Best Practices in Planning to Prevent or Decrease the Incidence and Severity of Acute Injury
>
> - Establish and define the relationships among all involved parties.
> - Develop a chain of command regarding provision of health care and medical decision making, with the supervising physician as the final authority.
> - Establish a safe practice and playing environment by monitoring environmental risk factors.
> - Develop and implement an EAP.
> - Plan and train for emergencies during competition and practice sessions.
> - Determine which venues and activity settings require the on-site presence of the athletic trainer and team physician and which sites require that they be available.
> - Provide appropriate health care during events, and ensure an adequate number of athletic trainers for the number of sport participants.
> - Establish criteria for safe return-to-practice and play and implement the return-to-play (RTP) process.
>
> Adapted from Courson R, Goldenberg M, Adams KG, et al. Inter-association consensus statement on best practices for sports medicine management for secondary schools and colleges. *J Athl Train.* 2014;49(1):128–137.

- Documentation verifying the implementation and evaluation of the emergency plan, actions taken during the emergency, evaluation of the emergency response, and institutional personnel training
- Documentation of an annual review and rehearsal of the emergency plan and notations indicating whether the emergency plan was modified and, if so, how the plan was changed

Every institution/facility should have an emergency response team. The team should be composed of athletic training personnel, personnel responsible for the overall health and safety of students (e.g., campus police/safety), and the campus medical director. The designated emergency response team should meet with representatives from local **emergency medical service** (EMS) agencies and emergency departments to discuss, develop, and evaluate the facility's emergency plan. As part of this process, individual responsibilities and protocols for an emergency situation should be determined. In developing the emergency medical plan, it is important to recognize that in any given situation, the members of the emergency response team can vary. For example, a physician may or may not be on site, the athletic trainer may be working alone or part of an on-site staff, and emergency medical technicians may be present at an event or available only if summoned. The following questions should be addressed relative to each event:

- What emergency equipment must be available on site?
- What equipment will be provided by the local EMS agency (e.g., spine board and splints) if in attendance at an event?
- Who will be responsible for ensuring that the emergency equipment is operational?
- What type of communication will be used to contact emergency personnel? Who will activate the facility's emergency medical plan?
- Who will assess the injured individual on site, and under what circumstances will a local EMS agency be called to the site?
- If a physician is present, what are the responsibilities of other medical personnel (e.g., athletic trainer and emergency medical technician)?
- If a physician is not present and the athletic trainer is evaluating the situation, what are the responsibilities of emergency medical technicians responding to the situation?

■ If it becomes necessary to stabilize and transport an individual to a medical facility, who will direct the stabilization and what protocol will be followed for the removal of protective equipment?

■ Who will supervise other participants if the athletic trainer is assessing and providing care to an injured individual?

■ Who will be responsible for the proper disposal of items and equipment exposed to blood or other bodily fluids?

A written emergency protocol should be developed for each activity site to address these questions (**Box 7.2**). The emergency response team should practice the emergency plan through regular

---

BOX 7.2 Sample Venue-Specific Emergency Protocol

Springfield University Emergency Protocol for Potter Field

1. **Call 555 to notify campus security** to activate **EMS**.

   ■ **Instruct** personnel to "report to and meet at, as we have an injured student-athlete in need of emergency medical treatment."

   ■ **Location:** Springfield University Potter Field

   ■ **Directions:** Street entrance (gate off of Wilbraham Avenue). Cross street: Alden Street.

2. **Provide necessary information to dispatch officer:**

   ■ Name, address, telephone number of caller

   ■ Number of victims; condition of victims

   ■ First aid treatment initiated

   ■ Specific location of patient as needed to locate scene

   ■ Other information as requested by dispatcher

3. **Provide appropriate emergency care** until arrival of EMS personnel.

4. **On arrival of EMS personnel:**

   ■ Provide pertinent information (method of injury, vital signs, treatment rendered, medical history).

   ■ Assist with emergency care as needed.

5. **Note:** Athlete should be accompanied by member of coaching staff, residence life staff, or other university representative.

   ■ Athletic training staff cannot leave the venue without another health care provider present in order to accompany the athlete to the emergency department. A staff member should accompany the student-athlete to hospital.

   ■ Notify the director of athletic training health care services of any action taken.

   ■ Complete and enter information in patient's medical chart upon return to the main athletic training facility.

6. **Emergency hand signals**

   ■ **Activate EMS:** Make large circular motion overhead.

   ■ **Need AED/O$_2$ emergency jump kit:** Tap self on chest several times with overexaggerated motions.

   ■ **Need splint kit:** Tap self twice with open hand on either arm or leg to indicate location of fracture dislocation.

   ■ **Need stretcher:** supinated hands in front of body or waist level

Adapted from Andersen JC, Courson RW, Kleiner DM, et al. National Athletic Trainers' Association position statement: emergency planning in athletics. *J Athl Train.* 2002;37(1):99–104.

educational workshops and training exercises. The use of interactive or simulation practice exercises can better prepare individuals to assume their roles in rendering emergency care.

 Although the condition of the gymnast may eventually warrant activation of the institution's emergency medical plan, there is not sufficient information at this point to activate the plan. The athlete may be unconscious or may be self-assessing his level of pain prior to moving. It is important that the athletic trainer assess the athlete's condition to determine whether activation of the emergency medical plan is necessary.

ASSESSING EMERGENT CONDITIONS

 In assessing the condition of the injured gymnast, what sequential process can be used to determine if the central nervous system (CNS) and/or cardiorespiratory systems are critically injured? What conditions warrant activation of the emergency medical plan, including summoning the local EMS agency?

Injuries or conditions that impair, or that have the potential to impair, vital function of the CNS and cardiorespiratory system are considered to be emergency situations. In responding to an on-field or on-site injury, the initial assessment performed by the athletic trainer is intended to rule out any life-threatening conditions. The **primary survey** determines the level of responsiveness and assesses the airway, breathing, and circulation. If at any time during the assessment conditions exist that are an immediate threat to life, or if "red flags" are noted (**Box 7.3**), the assessment process should be terminated and the emergency medical plan should be activated.

Occasionally, situations can occur in which more than one individual is injured. **Triage** refers to the rapid assessment of all injured patients followed by a return to the most seriously injured to provide immediate treatment.

BOX 7.3 Red Flags Indicating a Serious Emergency Resulting in Activation of the Emergency Medical Plan

- Unconscious
- Loss of consciousness in the presence of head trauma
- Respiratory distress, failure, or airway obstruction
- No pulse
- *Severe* chest or abdominal pains
- Excessive arterial bleeding
- Severe heat illness (core rectal temperature greater than 102°F)
- Severe shock
- Suspected spinal injury
- Fractures involving several ribs, the femur, or pelvis
- Severe hypoglycemia
- Collapse in response to sickling episode (sickling collapse)
- Extreme ranges deviating from normal blood pressure, pulse, or respiration rates

Once it has been determined that a life-threatening condition does not exist, a secondary survey is performed to identify the type and extent of any injury and the immediate **disposition** of the condition. Decisions must be made regarding the on-field management of the injury (e.g., controlling bleeding or immobilizing a possible fracture or dislocation), the safest method of transportation from the field (e.g., manual conveyance, stretcher, or spine board), and the need for rapid referral of the individual for further medical care.

On-Site History

Regardless of the setting (e.g., on-site or athletic training clinic), assessment protocols should contain the same basic components. During an on-field (on-site) assessment, the athletic trainer should assume a position close to the injured individual. One hand should be placed on the forehead of the injured individual to stabilize the head and neck to prevent any unnecessary movement. The history of the injury can be obtained from the individual or, if the individual is unconscious, from bystanders who may have witnessed the injury. Questions should be open-ended to allow the person to provide as much information as possible about the injury. The athletic trainer should listen attentively for clues that may indicate the nature of the injury. On-site history taking should be relatively brief as compared to a more comprehensive clinical evaluation. Critical areas of information include the following:

- **The location and type of pain.** The site of the injury should be identified; it is important to be aware that several areas may be injured. Sharp intense pain may be associated with a fracture, whereas throbbing pain may indicate ligamentous injury.

- **The presence of abnormal neurological signs.** The presence of any tingling, numbness, or loss of sensation should be noted, and nerve involvement should be suspected.

- **The mechanism of injury.** The position of the injured body part at the point of impact and the direction of force should be identified.

- **Associated sounds.** A report of hearing a "snap" or a "pop" may indicate a fracture or rupture of a ligament or tendon.

- **A history of the injury.** A preexisting condition or injury may have exacerbated the current injury or may complicate the injury assessment. Depending on the urgency of the situation and the severity of the current injury, a history that involves seeking information about past injury to same area may or may not be needed.

The history part of the evaluation will enable the athletic trainer to determine the possibility of an associated head or spinal injury, to rule out injury to other body areas, and, if necessary, to calm the individual. If the individual cannot open his or her eyes on verbal command or does not demonstrate withdrawal from painful stimulus, a serious red flag injury exists. **Application Strategy 7.1** lists several questions used to determine a history of the injury and to assess the level of responsiveness.

On-Site Observation and Inspection

In an on-site evaluation, observation begins while watching the athlete participating. An alert athletic trainer may witness how the forces were applied, which body part sustained contact, and the athlete's immediate response to the blow. For example, an athlete slides head first into the boards during a hockey game and remains motionless on the ice. From this scenario, the clinician immediately suspects a cervical spinal cord injury even before taking a history or arriving at the side of the injured athlete. When the mechanism of injury has not been witnessed, the initial observation is often conducted as you approach the injured individual and, therefore, occurs prior to the history taking. Critical areas to observe include the following:

- **The surrounding environment.** Note any equipment or apparatus that may have contributed to the injury.

- **How the patient responded to the blow.** Was there immediate deformity or dysfunction apparent? Notice if the patient attempted to utilize the body part but was unsuccessful. Athletes who fall to the ground without placing arms out to break the fall may already be unconscious or have neurological impairment.

APPLICATION STRATEGY 7.1

Determining the History of Injury and Level of Responsiveness

Stabilize the head and neck. Do not move the individual unnecessarily until a spinal injury is ruled out. If nonresponsive,

1. Call the person's name loudly and gently tap the sternum or touch the arm. If there is no response, rap the sternum more forcibly with a knuckle or pinch the soft tissue in the armpit (axillary fold). Note if a withdrawal from the painful stimulus occurs. If no response, immediately initiate EMS and begin the primary survey.
2. If ABC are adequate, gather a history of the injury. If you did not see what happened, question other players, supervisors, officials, and bystanders. Ask:
   - What happened?
   - Did you see the individual get hit, or did the individual just collapse?
   - How long has the individual been unresponsive?
   - Did the individual become unresponsive suddenly or deteriorate gradually?
   - If it was gradual, did anyone talk to the individual before you arrived?
   - What did the person say? Was it coherent? Did the person moan, groan, or mumble?
   - Has this ever happened before to this individual?

If conscious, ask:

1. What happened? Note if the individual is alert and aware of his or her surroundings or has any short- or long-term memory loss. If the individual is lying down, determine if the person was knocked down, fell, or rolled voluntarily into that position.
2. Are you in pain? Where is the pain? Is it localized, or does it radiate into other areas?
3. Did you hear any sounds or any unusual sensations when the injury occurred?
4. Have you ever injured this body part before or experienced a similar injury?
5. Do you have a headache? Are you experiencing any nausea? Are you dizzy? Can you see clearly?
6. Are you taking any medication (e.g., prescription, over the counter, or vitamins)?

It is important to avoid leading the individual. Instead, the individual should be encouraged to describe what happened, and the clinician should listen attentively for clues to the nature of the injury.

- **Body position.** The position of the individual (e.g., prone, supine, or side lying) should be observed. The appearance of a gross deformity in one of the limbs should be noted. In severe brain injuries, a neurological sign called "posturing" of the extremities can occur (**Fig. 7.1**). **Decerebrate rigidity** is characterized by an extension of all four extremities. **Decorticate rigidity** is characterized by an extension of the legs and marked flexion in the elbows, wrists, and fingers.

- **Movement of the individual.** An individual holding an injured body part and expressing pain indicates consciousness as well as an intact CNS and cardiovascular system. If the individual is not moving or is having a seizure, possible systemic, psychological, or neurological dysfunction should be suspected.

- **The level of responsiveness.** Sometimes referred to the "shake and shout" stage, the clinician tries to arouse the unconscious individual by touching or gently tapping (without moving the head or neck) and by shouting into each ear. This action will determine whether the person is alert, restless, lethargic, or nonresponsive. There are several different ways to assess and document level of responsiveness. From a basic first aid perspective, the mnemonic AVPU (alert, voice, pain, unresponsive) is used.[4] EMSs utilize A/OX4, whereas emergency departments and neurological may depend on the Glasgow Coma Scale.[5] Comparisons of these scales are presented in **Table 7.1**.

- **The primary survey.** The "ABC technique" should be employed to ensure an open *Airway*, adequate *Breathing*, and *Circulation*.

- **Inspection for head trauma.** The pupils of the eyes should be observed, noting a normal appearance, dilation, or constriction. The presence of unequal pupils (**anisocoria**) (**Fig. 7.2**) may

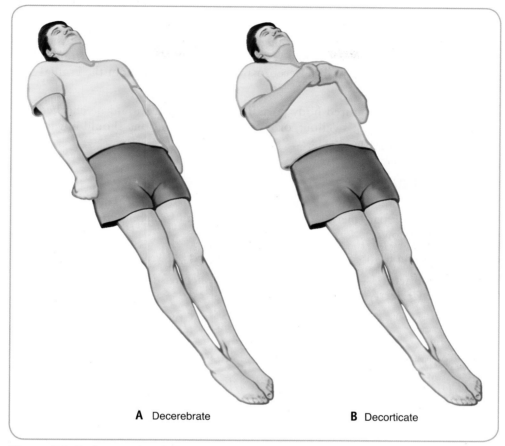

A Decerebrate   **B** Decorticate

Figure 7.1. Body posturing. A, Decerebrate rigidity is characterized by extension in all four extremities. **B,** Decorticate rigidity is characterized by the extension of the legs and flexion of the elbows, wrist, and fingers. Both conditions indicate a severe brain injury.

TABLE 7.1 Scales for Assessing Level of Responsiveness

NAME	PURPOSE OF SCALE	CRITERIA/SCORING		
AVPU	Simple and quick way to measure patient's responsiveness, thus indicating level of consciousness; based on four criteria	**Alert (A):** fully awake and spontaneously engages **Voice (V):** appears "out of it" and needs verbal prompts to respond; may grunt, moan, or slightly move limb in response to questions **Pain (P):** does not respond to voice but will respond to painful stimulus **Unresponsive (U):** no eye, voice, or motor response to painful stimulus		
A/OX4	Alert and oriented in four areas: name, location, time, and event. For each area correctly identified, 1 point is awarded.	1. Does the patient know his or her name? 2. Does the patient know where he or she is? 3. Does the patient know the time? 4. Does the patient know what happened or what is happening?		
Glasgow Coma Scale (GCS)[5]	Assesses function in three spheres and awards points based on response; can be used to obtain baseline information for comparison with future tests. Points are awarded based on response.	**Eye Opening** 4 = spontaneously 3 = to voice stimulus 2 = to painful stimulus 1 = do not open 1 = no response	**Verbal Response** 5 = normal conversation 4 = disoriented conversation 3 = words, not coherent 2 = no words, just sound 2 = decerebrate posture	**Motor Response** 6 = normal response 5 = localizes to pain 4 = withdrawals to pain 3 = decorticate posture 1 = no response
Comparison of AVPU and GCS[6]		A = GCS 15 V = GCS 12	P = GCS 8	U = GCS 3

indicate the presence of bleeding within the brain. The facial area and the area behind the ears should be inspected for any redness or ecchymosis. Ecchymosis under the eye (**raccoon eyes**) or behind the ear (**Battle sign**) suggests the presence of a fracture of the bones of the face and skull (**Fig. 7.3**). The presence of any clear fluid or bloody discharge from the ears or nose should be noted; this fluid could be cerebrospinal fluid leaking from the cranial area as a result of a skull fracture.

- **Inspection of the injured body part.** The injured area should be checked for joint alignment, redness, ecchymosis, swelling, or cuts. These observations should always be compared to the uninjured body part.

On-Site Palpation

The palpation should include a general head-to-toe assessment. This is done using a gentle, squeezing motion to palpate methodically down the trunk of the body to the fingers and toes. Palpation includes the following:

- **Bony palpation**
- **Possible fractures**—detected with palpation, percussion, vibration, compression, and distraction (see **Fig. 6.2**)

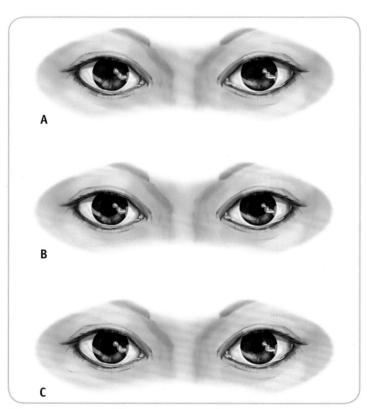

Figure 7.2. Assessing pupil size and reaction. A, Pinpoint is commonly observed in poisonings, brainstem dysfunction, and opiate use. **B,** Dilated but reactive is seen in the dark or occasionally after seizures. Fixed and dilated is associated with brainstem herniation secondary to increased cranial pressure (ICP) (e.g., severe cranial injury). **C,** One dilated and fixed may indicate ipsilateral uncal herniation with oculomotor (cranial nerve III) compression or a subdural or epidural hematoma. Note that anisocoria (unequal pupil size) is a normal variant.

- **Crepitus**—associated with fracture, swelling, or inflammation
- **Soft-tissue palpation**
- **Swelling**—may indicate diffuse hemorrhage or inflammation in a muscle, ligament, bursa, or joint capsule
- **Deformity**—an indentation may indicate a rupture in a musculotendinous unit; a protruding, firm bulge may indicate a joint dislocation, ruptured bursa, muscle spasm, or hematoma.
- **Skin temperature**
- Normally, the skin is dry, but certain conditions, such as cold, shock, or fever, can alter surface blood vessels.
- Skin temperature is assessed by placing the back of the hand against the individual's forehead or by palpating appendages bilaterally.

On-Site Functional Testing

When not contraindicated, the athletic trainer should identify the individual's willingness to move the injured body part. For a lower extremity injury, this should be expanded to include the willingness to bear weight. Movement is contraindicated, however, in the presence of a possible head or spinal injury, fracture, dislocation, or muscle/tendon rupture. Functional testing includes the following:

- **Active range of motion (ROM).** The individual is asked to move the injured body part through the available ROM. The quantity and quality of movement in the absence of pain should be noted.

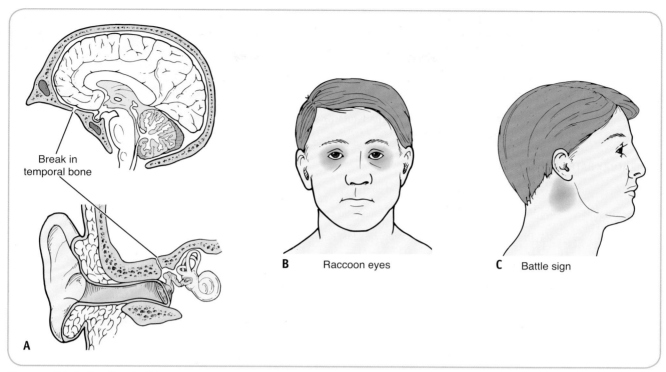

Figure 7.3. A, Basilar skull fractures in the temporal bone can cause cerebrospinal fluid (CSF) to leak from the nose or ear. **B,** Periorbital ecchymosis, called raccoon's eyes, may result from a facial fracture or basilar skull fracture. **C,** Battle sign over the mastoid process is also a sign of basilar fracture but may not become apparent until several days following the injury. There may be bloody drainage from the ear immediately following the fracture.

■ **Weight bearing.** If the individual successfully completes active, passive, and resisted motion ROMs, walking may be permitted. If the individual is unable to perform these tests, however, or if critical signs and symptoms are apparent, removal from the area should be performed in a non–weight-bearing manner.

On-Site Stress Testing

Testing for ligamentous integrity is performed before any muscle guarding or swelling occurs that may obscure the extent of injury. Typically, only single-plane tests are performed, the results of which are then compared with the noninjured limb.

On-Site Neurological Testing

Neurological testing is critical to prevent a catastrophic injury. Although listed as a separate testing phase, neurological testing, if warranted, may be performed earlier in the evaluation. Critical areas to include are as follows:

■ **Cutaneous sensation.** This can be done by running the fingernails along both sides of the injured individual's arms and legs to determine if the same feeling is experienced on both sides of the body part. Pain perception also can be tested by applying a sharp and a dull point to the skin; the ability of the individual to distinguish the difference should be noted.

■ **Motor function.** A cranial nerve assessment (see Chapter 20) should be completed. In addition, the ability of the individual to wiggle the fingers and toes on both the hands and the feet should be assessed, and a bilateral comparison of grip strength should be performed.

■ **Reflexes.** Damage to the CNS can be detected by stimulation of the deep tendon reflexes (DTRs). Exaggerated, distorted, or absent reflexes indicate injury in specific regions of the nervous system.

TABLE 7.2 Abnormal Vital Signs and Possible Causes

PULSE

Rapid, weak	Shock, internal hemorrhage, hypoglycemia, heat exhaustion, or hyperventilation
Rapid, bounding	Heat stroke, fright, fever, hypertension, apprehension, hyperglycemia, or normal exertion
Slow, bounding	Skull fracture, stroke, drug use (barbiturates and narcotics), certain cardiac problems, or some poisons
No pulse	Blocked artery, low blood pressure, or cardiac arrest

RESPIRATORY RATE AND QUALITY

Shallow breathing	Shock, heat exhaustion, insulin shock, chest injury, or cardiac problems
Irregular breathing	Airway obstruction, chest injury, diabetic coma, asthma, or cardiac problems
Rapid, deep	Diabetic coma, hyperventilation, or some lung diseases
Frothy blood	Lung damage, such as a puncture wound to the lung from a fractured rib or other penetrating object
Slowed breathing	Stroke, head injury, chest injury, or use of certain drugs
Wheezing	Asthma
Crowing	Spasms of the larynx
Apnea	Hypoxia (lack of oxygen), congestive heart failure, or head injuries
No breathing	Cardiac arrest, poisoning, drug abuse, drowning, head injury, or intrathoracic injuries, with death imminent if action is not taken to correct condition

BLOOD PRESSURE

Systolic <100 mm Hg	Hypotension caused by shock, hemorrhage, heart attack, internal injury, or poor nutrition
Systolic >140 mm Hg	Hypertension caused by certain medications, oral contraceptives, anabolic steroids, amphetamines, chronic alcohol use, and obesity

SKIN TEMPERATURE

Dry, cool	Exposure to cold or cervical, thoracic, or lumbar spine injuries
Cool, clammy	Shock, internal hemorrhage, trauma, anxiety, or heat exhaustion
Hot, dry	Disease, infection, high fever, heat stroke, or overexposure to environmental heat
Hot, moist	High fever
Isolated hot spot	Localized infection
Cold appendage	Circulatory problem
"Goose pimples"	Chills, communicable disease, exposure to cold, pain, or fear

SKIN COLOR

Red	Embarrassment, fever, hypertension, heat stroke, carbon monoxide poisoning, diabetic coma, alcohol abuse, infectious disease, inflammation, or allergy
White or ashen	Emotional stress (e.g., fright or anger), anemia, shock, heart attack, hypotension, heat exhaustion, insulin shock, or insufficient circulation
Blue or cyanotic	Heart failure, some severe respiratory disorders, and some poisoning; in dark-skinned individuals, a bluish cast can be seen in the mucous membranes (mouth, tongue, and inner eyelids), lips, and nail beds
Yellow	Liver disease or jaundice

(continued)

TABLE 7.2 Abnormal Vital Signs and Possible Causes *(continued)*	
PUPILS	
Constricted	Individual is using an opiate-based drug or has ingested a poison.
Unequal	Head injury or stroke
Dilated	Shock, hemorrhage, heat stroke, use of a stimulant drug, coma, cardiac arrest, or death

However, DTRs are not normally assessed during evaluation of acute, on-field injuries. Pathologic reflexes (see **Table 6.14**) can indicate upper motor neuron lesions if bilateral or lower motor neuron lesions if unilateral. The presence of the reflex often serves as a sign of some pathologic condition.

Vital Signs

When warranted, the vital signs should be assessed to establish a baseline of information. Vital signs indicate the status of the cardiovascular system and the CNS and include pulse, respiratory rate and quality, blood pressure, and temperature. Although not specifically cited as vital signs, skin color, pupillary response to light, and eye movement also may be assessed to determine neurological function. Abnormal vital signs indicate a serious injury or illness (**Table 7.2**).

Pulse

Factors such as age, gender, aerobic physical condition, degree of physical exertion, medications or chemical substances being taken, blood loss, and stress can influence pulse rate and volume. Pulse usually is taken at the carotid artery because a pulse at that site is not normally obstructed by clothing, equipment, or strappings. Normal adult resting rates range from 60 to 100 beats per minute; for children, the normal resting range is from 120 to 140 beats per minute. Aerobically conditioned athletes may have a pulse rate as low as 40 beats per minute. The pulse rate is assessed by counting the carotid pulse rate for a 30-second period and then doubling it. An assessment of pulse volume, which reflects the sensation of the contraction (e.g., strong/weak), also is important.

Respiration

An individual's breathing rate also varies with gender and age. It averages from 10 to 25 breaths per minute in an adult and from 20 to 25 breaths per minute in a child. The breathing rate is assessed by counting the number of respirations in a 30-second period and then doubling it. The character of the respiration (e.g., rapid, shallow, deep, gasping, or labored) should be noted as well. In addition to assessing the rate of respirations, it may be useful to measure the quality and effectiveness of the patient's respirations. As a person inhales, oxygen is pulled into the lungs to oxygenate the blood. **Blood oxygen levels** or oxygen saturation (SpO_2) is a measurement of the amount of oxygen in the blood. SpO_2 levels are measured using a pulse oximeter (**Fig. 7.4**). The pulse oximeter is placed on the finger and measures the saturation peripherally; the measurement is referred to as the SpO_2 level. Normal SpO_2 levels are between 95 and 100. SpO_2 levels between 95 and 90 are considered low, and the patient

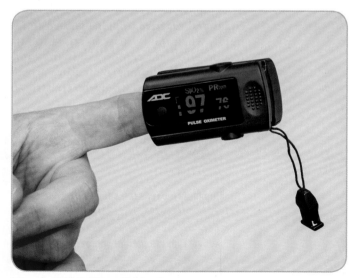

Figure 7.4. Pulse oximeter.

would benefit from having oxygen administered.[7] Readings less than 90 is considered hypoxemia, and oxygen should be administered. Levels below 80 may impair brain and heart function; therefore, EMS should be activated and oxygen administered immediately.

Blood Pressure

Blood pressure is the pressure or tension of the blood within the systemic arteries, generally considered to be the aorta. As one of the most important vital signs, blood pressure reflects the effectiveness of the circulatory system. Changes in blood pressure are very significant. **Systolic blood pressure** is measured when the left ventricle contracts and expels blood into the aorta. It is approximately 120 mm Hg for a healthy adult and 125 to 140 mm Hg for healthy children aged 10 to 18 years. **Diastolic blood pressure** is the residual pressure in the aorta between heartbeats and averages 70 to 80 mm Hg in healthy adults and 80 to 90 mm Hg in healthy children aged 10 to 18 years. Blood pressure may be affected by gender, weight, race, lifestyle, and diet. Blood pressure is measured in the brachial artery with a sphygmomanometer and a stethoscope (see **Application Strategy 2.1**).

Temperature

Core temperature can be measured by a thermometer placed under the tongue, in the ear, or armpit or rectum. Average oral temperature usually is quoted at 37°C (98.6°F), but this can fluctuate considerably. During the early morning hours, it may fall as low as 35.8°C (96.4°F), and during the later afternoon or evening hours, it may rise as high as 37.3°C (99.1°F). Rectal temperatures are higher than oral temperatures by an average of 0.4° to 0.5°C (0.7° to 0.9°F). This is important to remember when assessing a patient with heat illness. Using oral temperature to assess for heat illness may provide inadequate information to determine appropriate treatment.[8] In contrast, axillary temperatures are lower than oral temperatures by approximately 1°F.[9]

Skin Color

Skin color can indicate abnormal blood flow and a low blood oxygen concentration in a particular body part or area. Three colors commonly are used to describe light-skinned individuals: red, white or ashen, and blue. The colors and their potential indications also can be seen in **Table 7.2**. In dark-skinned individuals, skin pigments mask cyanosis; however, a bluish cast can be seen in mucous membranes (e.g., mouth, tongue, and inner eyelids), the lips, and nail beds. Fever in these individuals can be seen by a red flush at the tips of the ears.

Pupils

The pupils are extremely responsive to situations affecting the CNS. The mnemonic PEARL (pupils equal and reactive to light) is used to identify pupil assessment (**Table 7.3**). The rapid constriction of pupils when the eyes are exposed to intense light is called the **pupillary light reflex**. The pupillary response to light can be assessed by holding a hand over one eye and then moving the hand away quickly, or by shining light from a penlight into one eye and then observing the pupil's reaction. A normal response would be constriction with the light shining in the eye and dilation as the light

TABLE 7.3 Using the Mnemonic PEARL to Assess the Pupils	
LETTER	**ASSESSMENT**
P	Pupils: Are pupils the same shape?
E	Are the pupils equal to one another?
A	Active: Can the patient smoothly track an object with both pupils?
RL	React to light: (pupillary light reflex). When a light is shone on the pupil, does it respond appropriately?

is removed. The pupillary reaction is classified as brisk (normal), sluggish, nonreactive, or fixed. The eyes may appear normal, constricted, unequal, or dilated.

Eye movement is tested by asking the individual to focus on a single object. An individual experiencing **diplopia** sees two images instead of one. This condition is attributed to failure of the external eye muscles to work in a coordinated manner. The tracking ability of the eyes can be assessed by asking the individual to follow the clinician's fingers as they move through the six cardinal fields of vision. The individual's depth perception can be assessed by placing a finger several inches in front of the individual and then asking the person to reach out and touch the finger. This assessment should be repeated several times, with the clinician's finger in several different locations.

 The athletic trainer should assess the scene and perform a primary survey of the gymnast. The gymnast is conscious and can relate to you what happened and where the pain is located. Inspection and palpation reveal no gross deformity, whereas assessing the integrity of the joint structures found negative results. All vital signs were normal, but the patient did have difficulty with eye tracking and exhibited sensitivity to light. The patient may have sustained a concussion and should be more specifically assessed for the presence of a possible concussion. What action(s) should you do next?

DISPOSITION

? Depending on the severity of findings in any acute injury, what options for treatment does the athletic trainer have?

Information gathered during the assessment must be analyzed, and decisions should be made based on the best interests of the injured individual. It is especially important to determine whether the situation can be handled on site or whether a referral to a physician is warranted. As a general rule, the individual should always be referred to the nearest trauma center or emergency clinic if any life-threatening situation is present, if the injury results in a loss of normal function, or if no improvement is seen in injury status after a reasonable amount of time. Examples of these injuries are provided in **Box 7.3**. Other conditions that are not necessarily life threatening but are serious enough to warrant referral to a physician for immediate care include the following:

- Eye injuries

- Dental injuries in which a tooth has been knocked loose or out

- Minor or simple fractures

- Lacerations that might require suturing

- Injuries in which a functional deficit is noticeable

- Loss of normal sensation or diminished or absent reflexes

- Noticeable muscular weakness in the extremities

- Any injury if you are uncertain about its severity or nature

 Information gathered through the injury assessment will determine what course of action should be taken by the athletic trainer. An injured patient may be treated on site, monitored for changes in signs and symptoms, or referred to the emergency department. Conditions such as altered level of consciousness, impaired CNS function, or life-threatening bleeding warrant activation of EMS.

APPLICATION STRATEGY **7.2**

Management Algorithm for Bone Injuries

1. Remove clothing and jewelry from around the injury site. (Cut clothing away with scissors to avoid moving the injured area.)
2. Check distal pulse and sensation. If either is abnormal, activate.
3. Cover all wounds, including open fractures, with sterile dressings and secure them.
4. Do not attempt to push bone ends back underneath the skin.
5. Pad the splint to prevent local pressure.
6. Apply minimal in-line traction and maintain it until the splint is in place and secured.
7. Immobilize the joints above and below the fracture site.
8. Splint in the position found if:

   - Pain increases with gentle traction or the limb resists positioning.
   - The fracture is severely angulated.
   - Do not straighten unless it is absolutely necessary to incorporate the limb into the splint; move as little as possible.
   - Splint firmly but do not impair circulation.
   - Recheck distal pulse and sensation after applying splint.
   - Check vital signs, treat for shock, and transport to medical facility.

MANAGEMENT OF BONE INJURIES

 What signs and symptoms indicate that a possible fracture is present? What standard of care is necessary to treat this potentially serious injury?

Possible fractures can be detected with palpation, percussion, use of a tuning fork (vibrations), compression, and distraction (see **Fig. 6.2**). Palpation can detect deformity, crepitus, swelling, or increased pain at the fracture site. Percussion uses a tapping motion of the finger over a bony structure. A tuning fork works in the same manner; vibrations travel through the bone and cause increased pain at a fracture site. Compression is performed by gently compressing the distal end of the bone toward the proximal end or by encircling the body part (e.g., a foot or a hand) and gently squeezing, thereby compressing the heads of the bones together. Again, if a fracture is present, pain increases at the fracture site. Distraction employs a tensile force, whereby the application of traction to both ends of the fractured bone helps to relieve pain.

A suspected fracture should be splinted before the individual is moved to avoid damage to surrounding ligaments, tendons, blood vessels, and nerves. **Application Strategy 7.2** explains the immediate management of fractures.

 Signs and symptoms indicating a possible fracture include deformity, crepitus, swelling, or increased pain at the fracture site. The joint above and below the suspected fracture site should be immobilized in an appropriate splint.

EQUIPMENT CONSIDERATIONS

 In sports such as football, ice hockey, and lacrosse, equipment may hinder a full assessment of an injury. What can be done to expose the area without causing additional pain to the athlete?

One of the primary concerns during an on-site assessment of an injured individual is that of equipment. If the injured body part cannot be adequately inspected with protective gear in place, the next option is to use palpation to check for the presence of deformity, point tenderness, fever, swelling, and crepitus. To protect both you and the patient, gloves should be worn when palpating areas that cannot be visually inspected first. Protective equipment can be removed but should be done so in a manner that causes the least amount of movement. Often, clothing and straps must be cut in order to remove the equipment and access the injury site.

When dealing with potentially life-threatening injuries, such as traumatic spinal cord injury, helmets and shoulder pads create potential barriers to providing appropriate care. The 2015 Task Force on the Appropriate Prehospital Management of the Spine-Injured Athlete developed 14 recommendations for health care providers when dealing with on-field management of athletes with potential spinal cord injury.[10] All 14 recommendations are listed in **Box 7.4**. However, the actual consensus statement should be read in its entirety to ensure in-depth understanding.

BOX 7.4 The Task Force on the Appropriate Prehospital Management of the Spine-Injured Athlete: 2015 Recommendations

Recommendation 1: It is essential that each athletic program have an EAP developed in conjunction with local EMS.

Recommendation 2: It is essential that sports medicine teams conduct a "time out" before athletic events to ensure EAPs are reviewed and to plan the options with the personnel and equipment available for that event.

Recommendation 3: Proper assessment and management of the spine-injured athlete-patient will result in activation of the EAP in accordance with the level or severity of the injury.

Recommendation 4: Protective athletic equipment *may* be removed prior to transport to an emergency facility for an athlete-patient with suspected cervical spine instability.

Recommendation 5: Equipment removal should be performed by at least three rescuers trained and experienced with equipment removal at the earliest possible time. If fewer than three people are present, the equipment should be removed at the earliest possible time after enough trained individuals arrive on the scene.

Recommendation 6: Athletic protective equipment varies by sport and activity, and styles of equipment differ within a sport or activity. Therefore, it is essential that the sports medical team be familiar with the types of protective equipment specific to the sport and associated techniques for removal of the equipment.

Recommendation 7: A rigid cervical stabilization device should be applied to spine-injured athlete-patients prior to transport.

Recommendation 8: Spine-injured athlete-patients should be transported using a rigid immobilization device.

Recommendation 9: Techniques employed to move the spine-injured athlete-patient from the field to the transportation vehicle should minimize spinal motion.

Recommendation 10: It is essential that a transportation plan be developed prior to the start of any athletic practice or competition.

Recommendation 11: Spine-injured athlete-patients should be transported to a hospital that can deliver immediate, definitive care for these types of injuries.

Recommendation 12: It is essential that prevention of spine injuries in athletics be a priority and requires collaboration between the medical team, coaching staff, and athletes.

Recommendation 13: The medical team must have a strong working knowledge of current research as well as national and local regulations to ensure up-to-date care is provided to the spine-injured athlete-patient.

Recommendation 14: It is essential that future research continue to investigate the efficacy of devices used to provide SMR.

Adapted from National Athletic Trainers' Association. Appropriate prehospital management of the spine-injured athlete. Update from 1998 document. Retrieved from http://www.nata.org/sites/default/files/Executive-Summary-Spine-Injury-updated.pdf. Accessed November 17, 2015.

The Task Force advocates for **removal of protective equipment** *prior* to transporting the athlete to the emergency department; in other words, the equipment comes off on the field. Removal of helmets and shoulder pads is recommended in order to provide immediate access to the airway and chest in the event cardiopulmonary resuscitation (CPR), automated external defibrillator (AED), or the administration of oxygen is needed. Guidelines for the removal of any piece of protective equipment should be defined within the emergency medical plan.

Helmet Removal

Only qualified medical personnel with training in equipment removal should attempt to remove equipment.[10] Three trained individuals are needed to carry out the task. One individual maintains in-line stabilization of the head, neck, and helmet while another person cuts the chin strap. Next, while one assistant continues to maintain stabilization of the chin and back of the neck, the other individual removes any accessible internal helmet padding, such as cheek pads. In removing the pads, a flat object, such as a tongue depressor or the flat edge of tape scissors, can be slid between the helmet and the pad. A slight turn of the inserted object causes the pad to unsnap from the helmet. If an air cell–padding system is present, the system should be deflated by releasing the air at the external port with an inflation needle or a large gauge hypodermic needle. The helmet should then be slid off the occiput with slight forward rotation of the helmet. If the helmet does not move with this action, slight traction can be applied to the helmet as it is carefully rocked anteriorly and posteriorly, with great care being taken not to move the head and neck unit. The helmet should not be spread apart by the ear holes because this only serves to tighten the helmet on the forehead and occiput region.[10] **Application Strategy 7.3** demonstrates the basic steps in the removal of a football helmet.

Shoulder Pad Removal

Shoulder pads *may be removed* in the presence of a suspected spinal cord injury, respiratory distress, and/or cardiac distress. The chest is exposed by cutting the shirt from the neck to the waist and from the midline to the end of each arm sleeve. Next, all straps securing the shoulder pads to the arms are cut, the laces or straps over the sternum are cut, and the two halves of the shoulder pads are spread apart. All accessories, such as neck rolls or collars, are then cut and/or removed. One individual maintains cervical stabilization in a cephalad direction by placing his or her forearms on the athlete's chest while manually stabilizing the chin and occiput. Assistants should be positioned on each side of the athlete with their hands placed directly against the skin in the thoracic region of the back. Additional support should be provided at other strategic locations down the body as deemed appropriate for the size of the patient. While the patient is lifted, the individual in charge of the head/shoulder stabilization should remove the helmet and then immediately remove the shoulder pads by spreading apart the front panels and pulling them around the head. Next, the remaining jersey and any other accessories are removed, and the patient is lowered, with appropriate immobilization being continued.[11] Guidelines for removing shoulder pads are presented in **Application Strategy 7.3**.

Protective equipment should be removed prior to transporting the athlete to the emergency department. This is recommended in order to provide immediate access to the airway and chest in the event CPR, AED, or the administration of oxygen is needed.

MOVING THE INJURED PARTICIPANT

What criteria should be used to determine whether an injured individual should be allowed to walk off the field or site of the injury? What is the safest method for transporting an individual with a lower extremity injury?

Once the extent and severity of the injury have been determined, a decision must be made regarding how to safely remove the individual from the area. Possible methods include ambulatory assistance, manual conveyance, and transport by a stretcher or spine board.

APPLICATION STRATEGY 7.3

Removal of Protective Equipment

1. One individual maintains in-line stabilization of the head, neck, and helmet to minimize cervical spine movement. This can be accomplished by applying an in-traction force through the patient's chin and occiput, in a cephalad direction, making sure to maintain the athlete's position. Cut the jersey from the neck to the waist and from the midline to the end of each sleeve. Cut all straps used to secure the pads to the torso and arms (**Fig. A**). Attempting to unbuckle the straps may cause unnecessary movement. Cut the laces over the sternum and then cut and/or remove any accessory such as a neck roll or collar.

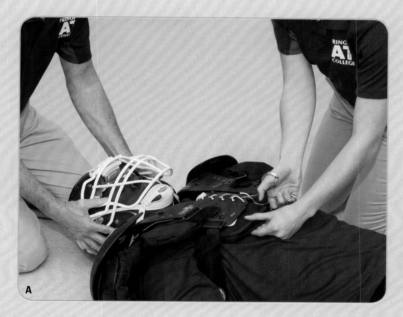

2. Another individual cuts the chin strap. A flat object is slid between the helmet and cheek pad. The object is then to be twisted to unsnap and separate the cheek pad from the helmet. Repeat on the other side and remove both cheek pads (**Fig. B**). If an air cell–padding system is present, deflate the system by releasing the air at the external port with an inflation needle or large gauge hypodermic needle.

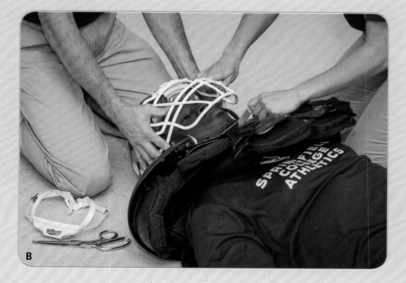

(continued)

3. The captain, the in-charge responder, maintains cervical stabilization in a cephalad direction by placing his or her forearms on the patient's chest while holding the chin and occiput (**Fig. C**).

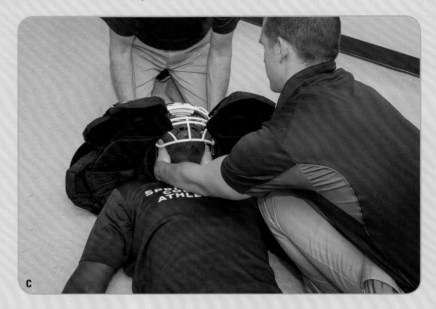

C

4. Slide the helmet off the occiput with a slight forward rotation of the helmet. If the helmet does not move, slight traction can be applied to the helmet and a gentle anterior and posterior maneuver may be applied, although the head/neck unit must not be allowed to move (**Fig. D**).

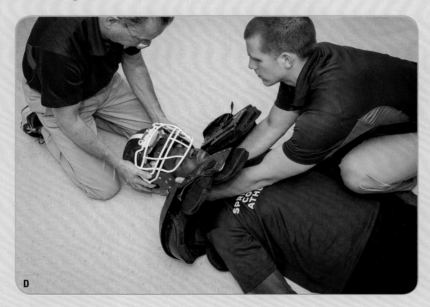

D

(continued)

APPLICATION STRATEGY 7.3 *(continued)*

5. Assistants on either side of the patient place their hands directly under the thoracic region of the back. Additional support is placed down the body as deemed appropriate based on the size of the patient. While the patient is lifted, the individual in charge of head/shoulder stabilization should remove the helmet (if not already done) and then immediately remove the shoulder pads by spreading apart the front panels and pulling them around the head (**Fig. E**).

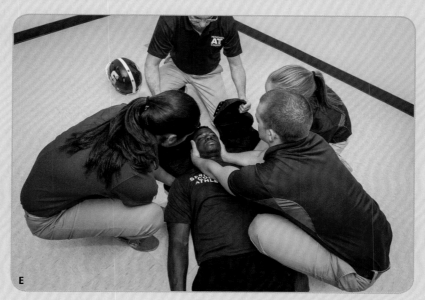

E

6. In-line stabilization is maintained while the athlete is prepared for movement onto a scoop stretcher (**Fig. F**).

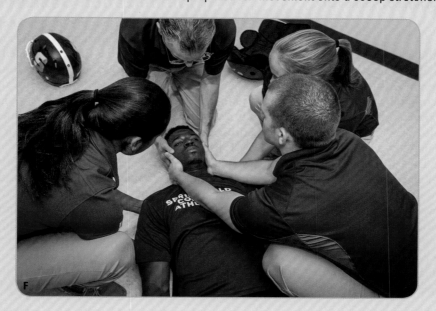

F

Adapted from: Kleiner DM, Almquist JL, Bailes J, et al. *Prehospital Care of the Spine-Injured Athlete: A Document from the Inter-Association Task Force for Appropriate Care of the Spine-Injured Athlete*. Dallas, TX: Inter-Association Task Force for Appropriate Care of the Spine-Injured Athlete; 2001.

Ambulatory Assistance

Ambulatory assistance is used to aid an injured individual who is able to walk. This implies that the injury is minor and no further harm will occur if the individual is ambulatory. In performing this technique, two individuals of equal or near equal height should support both sides of the individual. The injured individual drapes his or her arms across the shoulders of the assistants while the arms of the assistants encircle the injured person's back. This position enables the assistants to escort the individual to an appropriate area for further evaluation and treatment.

Manual Conveyance

If the individual is unable to walk or the distance is too great to walk, manual conveyance should be used. The individual continues to drape his or her arms across the assistants' shoulders while one arm of each assistant is placed behind the individual's back and the other arm is placed under the individual's thigh. Both assistants lift the legs up, placing the individual in a seated position. The individual is then carried to an appropriate area (**Fig. 7.5**). Again, it is essential that the injury be fully evaluated before moving the individual in this manner.

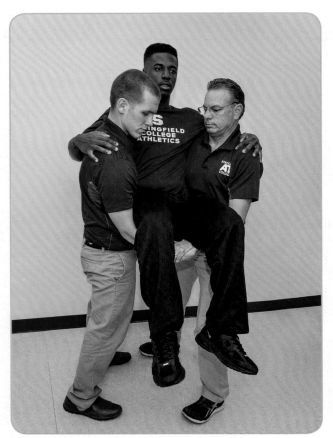

Figure 7.5. **Manual conveyance: chair carry.**

Transport by Rigid Immobilization Device

When dealing with a potential spinal cord injury, the **goal is spinal motion restriction (SMR)** and not immobilization of the spine. SMR is intended to prevent further injury to the spine by reducing as much motion as possible.[10] The Task Force on the Appropriate Prehospital Management of the Spine-Injured Athlete recommends the following criteria when considering using SMR: (1) blunt trauma with altered level of consciousness, (2) spinal pain or tenderness, (3) neurological complaint (e.g., numbness or motor weakness), and (4) anatomical deformity of the spine. SMR is also recommended when there is a high-energy mechanism of injury and with any of the following: (1) drug or alcohol intoxication, (2) inability to communicate, and (3) a distracting injury.[10]

Due to the potentially harmful effects of being placed on the traditional long spine board for prolonged periods of time, it is recommended that alternative rigid immobilization devices be considered in place of the long spine board, such as a vacuum mattress or scoop stretcher.[10,12] Best practices now recommend using an 8-person team to lift the supine athlete onto the immobilization device.[10] Guidelines for using a scoop stretcher to lift a supine patient from the field can be seen in **Application Strategy 7.4**. Log rolls may be used to position the athlete onto the scoop stretcher spine board when the patient is found in a prone position. Once the patient is secured on the rigid immobilization device, the stretcher is raised to waist level. The individual should be carried feet first so that the captain, or person at the patient's head, can constantly monitor the individual's condition.

 Patients who are able to walk should be assisted off the field using an ambulatory assist. For those who are unable to bear weight on the lower extremities, manual conveyance may be used to carry them off the field. Patients who have a suspected spinal cord injury, fracture, or other condition where they need to be quickly removed from the field should be transported using a scoop stretcher or vacuum mattress.

APPLICATION STRATEGY 7.4

Transporting an Injured Individual on a Scoop Stretcher

Unless ruled out, assume the presence of a spinal injury.

1. The captain of the response team maintains manual in-line stabilization. A second member of the response team applies a rigid cervical collar to the patient as soon as possible. Manual in-line stabilization is maintained until the patient has been stabilized on the scoop stretcher and a head immobilization device has been applied (**Fig. A**).

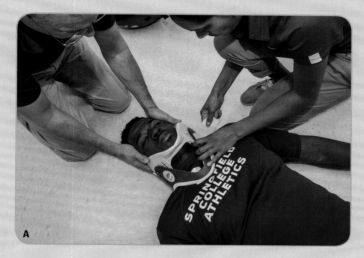

2. The scoop stretcher is placed beside the patient to determine the appropriate length. The scoop stretcher is then extended to accommodate the height of patient. The scoop is unlatched at the top and bottom and separated into two sides. One side is placed on either side of the patient (**Fig. B**).

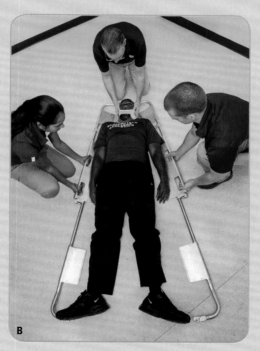

(continued)

3. The top latch is then secured, and the two sides are drawn together until the bottom latch is secured and the patient is resting on top of the stretcher.
4. The patient's body is first secured to the scoop stretcher followed by using a head immobilization device to secure the head to stretcher. All voids should be filled with soft material, such as towels. Straps are then tightened (**Fig. C**).

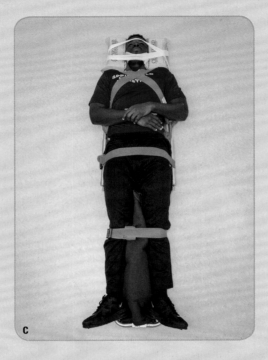

C

PREVENTING SUDDEN DEATH IN ATHLETICS

 A high school field hockey player suddenly collapses on the turf during practice. No known contact occurred with any other player or equipment. What immediate actions should you take? What possible conditions may lead to sudden death in sport?

In order to prevent sudden death in athletics, one must be able recognize when a potential sudden death event is occurring and know the appropriate response to either prevent the event or minimize the extent of damage. There are a variety of causes of sudden death in sport activities. Many of the strategies already addressed in Chapter 2 (Preparticipation Examination) and earlier in this chapter ("The Emergency Action Plan" section) are intended to help prevent or minimize the risk. Within this section, brief focus will be on the 10 conditions covered in the National Athletic Trainers' Association (NATA) position statement on preventing sudden death in athletics[10] from an early recognition and emergency medical response perspective. More in-depth information on each condition is provided in later chapters.

Asthma

Athletes who have a history of asthma should be monitored for signs of acute asthma exacerbation. **Mild acute asthma exacerbation** (or asthma attack) occurs when the patient has mild **dyspnea** during activity. They may experience wheezing or coughing. The patient's peak expiratory flow

(PEF) is equal or greater than 70% of the baseline (determined during preparticipation examination). Patients experiencing a mild asthma attack should be removed from activity and directed to self-administer short-acting β_2-agonist medication. Known as rescue inhalers, a commonly used bronchodilator medication is albuterol.

A patient experiencing a **moderate acute asthma exacerbation** presents with more pronounced wheezing, coughing, decreased ability to speak, inability to continue participation, and a PEF that is between 40% and 69% of the baseline. Patients experiencing a moderate asthma attack should be removed from activity and the environment triggering the attack. The patient is directed to use the rescue inhaler and should be monitored. If SpO_2 levels are below 95%, oxygen should be administered. If the patient does not respond relatively quickly after three bronchodilator treatments, refer to the nearest health center for more advanced treatment.

Severe acute asthma exacerbation is experienced with a PEF of less than 40% of baseline. The patient may be unable to speak and coughs frequently. Activity is impossible. In some cases, the patient may be drowsy, confused, or cyanotic. Administer the rescue inhaler and oxygen and either activate EMS or refer the patient to the nearest health care facility.[13,14]

Catastrophic Brain Injuries

A blow to the head may result in a focal brain injury such as a hematoma, cerebral contusion, or intracranial bleeding or in a diffuse brain injury such as cerebral concussion, diffuse cerebral swelling, or diffuse axonal injury.[15] Second impact syndrome (SIS), a type of diffuse brain injury, is precipitated by an earlier event where a patient sustains a concussion which is unresolved. If, while in this postconcussive state, the patient receives a second blow to the head, SIS may result. Diffuse cerebral swelling and brainstem herniation occurs.[16] This cascade of events can occur in 3 to 5 minutes from the time the patient receives the blow.[17] Although diffuse brain injuries and focal brain injuries will not present exactly the same, there are several red flags indicative of traumatic brain injury that necessitate immediate and accurate response to prevent death from occurring (**Table 7.4**).

The first step in providing appropriate care is recognizing that the patient has sustained a traumatic brain injury and immediate activation of the EAP and summoning EMS is imperative. For patients with a Glasgow Coma Scale of less than 9 and an SpO_2 level of less than 90%, supplemental oxygen should be administered while waiting for EMS to arrive.[18] Otherwise, maintain an open airway, monitor level of consciousness and the ABC, assess all vital signs, and treat for shock.

TABLE 7.4 Red Flags Indicating Presence of Traumatic Brain Injury	
SYSTEM	**FINDING**[a]
LOC	1. AVPU less than "A" 2. GCS <9 3. Initial loss of consciousness following by lucid period followed by a gradual decline in mental status 4. Gradual decline in mental status, LOC 5. Coma 6. Convulsions
Reflex	(+) Babinski (+) Oppenheim
Blood pressure	Rising blood pressure
Pulse	Rapid, weak or falling pulse
Respiration	Irregular or abnormal breathing patterns
PEARL	Pupils unequal, inability to track or react to light

[a]All findings need to be present to suspect presence of TBI.

LOC, level of consciousness.

Cervical Spine Injuries

There are seven cervical vertebrae and eight cervical nerve roots extending from the upper most region of the spinal cord. Nerve roots C1–C4 control a person's ability to breathe as well as the bladder/bowel functions and use of the limbs. If this portion of the spinal cord is damaged, the person may become quadriplegic and need assistance in breathing. In some cases, if care is not rendered quickly, the damage may result in death. If the spinal cord is damaged between C5 and C8, the person will be able to breathe on his or her own but will have decreased function of portions of the arms and/or legs. Injury to the cervical spinal cord should be suspected when the athlete is unconscious or has an altered level of consciousness, presents with bilateral neurological symptoms or dysfunction such as diminished dermatome response, weakness during myotome testing, and poor reflexes.

Athletes who complain of unprovoked neck pain or who are tender upon palpation of the cervical vertebrae should be treated for a potential spinal cord injury. The EAP should be implemented and EMS activated at once. In-line stabilization of the cervical region should be administered without applying traction.[13] Access to the airway and chest should be provided, and the patient should be stabilized and transported as described previously in this chapter.[10]

Diabetes Mellitus

The definition, cause, and pathophysiology of diabetes are discussed in great detail later in this text. From an acute recognition and treatment perspective, it is important to know that mild hypoglycemia can be treated on site; however, severe hypoglycemia may lead to unconsciousness and death and is considered a medical emergency that requires the immediate activation of EMS.[10] Signs and symptoms of hypoglycemia include increased heart rate, sweating, palpitations, hunger, nervousness, headache, trembling, dizziness, or, in severe cases, unconsciousness.[10] A blood sugar level between 60 and 70 mg per dL is considered mild hypoglycemia.

Because glucose levels in the blood are low compared to high levels of insulin, treatment focuses on getting 10 to 15 g of a fast-acting carbohydrate into the system quickly. This can be found in 4 oz (½ cup) of juice or regular soda, 1 tablespoon of honey or corn syrup, 2 tablespoons of raisins, 4 packets or 4 teaspoons of sugar, and four or five saltine crackers.[19] Chocolates, which contain a high level of fat, should not be used for treating a hypoglycemic reaction because the fat interferes with the absorption of sugar. After initial recovery, the individual should wait 15 minutes and check the blood sugar level. If the level is still less than 70 mg per dL or no meter is available and the individual still has symptoms, another 10 to 15 g of carbohydrates should be administered. Blood testing and treatment should be repeated until the blood glucose level has normalized. Even when the blood glucose level has returned to normal, however, physical performance and judgment may still be impaired, or the individual may relapse if the quick sugar influx is rapidly depleted. After the symptoms resolve, the individual should be instructed to have a good meal as soon as possible to increase carbohydrates in the body.

Blood glucose levels below 40 mg per dL is considered severe hypoglycemia, and EMS should be activated.[10] If the person is unconscious or unable to swallow, the individual should be rolled on his or her side so close attention can be given to the airway so that saliva drains out of the mouth, not into the throat. Sugar or honey should be placed under the tongue because it is absorbed through the mucous membrane. Patient's ABC, level of consciousness, and vitals should be monitored while waiting for EMS to arrive.[10]

Exertional Heat Stroke

Exertional heat stroke (EHS) is among the top three causes of death in sports and occurs more often during the hotter months.[10] EHS is identified through the presence of two criteria, core body temperature of greater than 104° to 105°F and CNS dysfunction (**Table 7.5**). Because successful treatment requires that the core body temperature be dropped to 102°F within 30 minutes of collapse, it is essential to obtain an accurate measurement of the core temperature via rectal or ingestible thermometers. The longer the length of time the core temperature remains above 105°F, the greater the risk of death and permanent damage. EMS should be activated as soon as EHS is suspected. The patient should be immersed in cold (35°F) moving water. A rectal probe or ingestible thermometer should be in place to monitor core temperature during the cooling process.

TABLE 7.5 Central Nervous System Dysfunction and Signs/Symptoms Associated with Exertional Heat Stress

CNS DYSFUNCTION	ADDITIONAL SIGNS AND SYMPTOMS
Disorientation	Core body temperature greater than 104°F
Confusion	Dehydration
Dizziness	Hot, sweaty skin as opposed to the dry skin that is a manifestation of classical EHS
Vomiting	Hypotension
Diarrhea	Hyperventilation
Loss of balance	
Staggering	
Irritability	
Irrational or unusual behavior	
Apathy, aggressiveness	
Hysteria, delirium	
Collapse, loss of consciousness, coma	

Adapted from National Athletic Trainers' Association. Appropriate prehospital management of the spine-injured athlete. Update from 1998 document. Retrieved from http://www.nata.org/sites/default/files/Executive-Summary-Spine-Injury-updated.pdf. Accessed November 17, 2015.

The patient should not be removed from the cold water immersion until the core temperature reaches 102°F. At this point, the patient should be transported via EMS to the nearest medical center. If cold water immersion is not an option, the patient should be covered in cold wet towels and have cold water continuously poured onto the towels. Fans may be used to assist in the cooling process.[10]

Exertional Sickling

Exertional sickling occurs in athletes who have *sickle cell trait*. **Exertional sickling** is when a red blood cell (RBC) changes shape from round to sickle or half-moon shape. The sickled RBCs clump together, in essence causing a log jam in the small blood vessels, leading to decreased blood flow and a break down in the muscle tissue and death.[20] If proper intervention and treatment strategies are not employed, exertional sickling may result in death. Exertional sickling is often confused with exertional heat cramps, and comparisons of the two are presented in **Table 7.6**. Exertional sickling should be suspected if the patient has sickle cell trait and shows signs of fatigue, difficulty breathing, leg or low back pain, and leg or low back cramps.[20] The patient should be immediately removed

TABLE 7.6 How Exertional Hat Cramping Differs from Exertional Sickling

EXERTIONAL CRAMPING	EXERTIONAL SICKLING
Muscle twinge prior to onset of cramping	No muscle twinging prior to cramping
Extremely painful muscle cramping	Muscle cramping present, limited pain
Athlete "hobbles to ground" due to cramps	Athlete "drops to ground" due to weakness
Muscular cramps visible, athlete in obvious pain	Musculature appears normal, athlete will be relatively quiet.

from activity, administered high flow oxygen at 15 L per minute using a nonrebreather face mask and the EAP should be activated.[10] Continue administering oxygen and monitoring vitals until EMS arrives on the scene.

Lightning Injury

Most injuries from lightning can be prevented by having a lightning policy in place and following it. In the event a patient is struck by lightning, quick action is needed to save lives. Patients who have been struck by lightning are safe to touch but precaution should be taken to ensure the safety of the athletic trainer who is providing care. If multiple persons have been struck, triage patients and assist those with no cardiac activity first. In other words, those who appear to be dead should be treated first. Most deaths from lightning strikes are the result of cardiac arrest; therefore, it is essential to start CPR and utilize an AED if indicated. EMS should be activated immediately. Monitor the patients until EMS arrives.

Sudden Cardiac Arrest

There are multiple underlying reasons, as well as specific traumatic causes, which might result in sudden cardiac death during athletics. These factors will be examined fully in later chapters. However, it is important to be able to recognize when sudden cardiac arrest (SCA) has occurred, one must respond appropriately. SCA should be *suspected* in any patient who collapses and is unresponsive. An assessment of the patient's ABC should be conducted and AED shock applied if indicated. The EAP should be initiated immediately. CPR and an AED should be provided and utilized as indicated, and the patient's vital signs should be continually monitored until EMS arrives.

 The high school field hockey player who suddenly collapsed on the turf during practice may have suffered from SCA. Immediately initiate the EAP and begin CPR. Apply an AED shock if indicated and continue treatment until the EMS arrives.

SUMMARY

1. In consultation with the supervising physician and local EMS agencies, the athletic trainer should coordinate the development of an emergency plan. The purpose of this plan is to ensure rapid and complete emergency care to an injured individual. The plan should be evaluated annually and should be practiced by all parties on a regular basis.

2. In an emergency injury assessment, the presence of a head or spinal cord injury should be assumed. As such, the head and neck should be stabilized before proceeding. The assessment of all injuries, no matter how minor, should include a primary injury assessment to determine the level of responsiveness and to assess the ABC. A secondary assessment determines the presence of moderate to severe injuries.

3. As a general rule, an individual should always be referred to the nearest trauma center or emergency clinic if any life-threatening situation is present or if the injury results in a loss of normal function.

4. The secondary assessment should follow a logical progression to elicit important information in order to determine the appropriate response. The sequence includes history, palpation, and special.

5. The use of a variety of laboratory tests and imaging techniques can be instrumental in establishing an accurate diagnosis of an injury or illness. In the majority of cases, these tests can only be ordered by a physician or appropriately licensed medical specialist.

6. In the presence of suspected fracture, the area should be immobilized and referred for evaluation by a physician.

7. Protective equipment should be removed if equipment impairs your ability to properly assess the patient or inhibits the ability to provide proper care, as in the case of head or neck injury.

8. When dealing with suspected cervical spine injury, manual in-line stabilization is applied and a cervical collar is utilized. The patient should be secured to a rigid splint and transported to a medical facility. A long spine board should be used only as a last resort.

9. Sudden death in athletics can be prevented by the ability to quickly recognize conditions leading to sudden death and providing the appropriate response immediately. Early activation of the EMS is an essential component of providing appropriate care.

APPLICATION QUESTIONS

1. As the first full-time athletic trainer at a coeducational high school that fields 16 interscholastic teams, the athletic director has instructed you to form a committee to develop an EAP for use at the various venues of the facility. When looking at potential committee members, who would you most likely want on this committee and would each of these individuals be critical in developing the school's EAP?

2. What information should be included with the EAP? How should the plan be adapted for each of the different venues where activities take place? What information should be provided to the dispatcher once the EAP has been initiated?

3. How does the assessment of an acute on-field injury differ from conducted on a patient who complains of long-term pain and discomfort with no known cause. How do you go about ruling out life-threatening conditions during the on-field assessment? If no life-threatening conditions are present, what is your order of exclusion or triage?

4. How can vital signs assist you in assessing the presence of nonorthopedic injury? Why is it important to include a vital sign assessment? What other diagnostic information can be obtained through clinical examination during an on-field or sideline evaluation?

5. You suspect a men's lacrosse player has sustained a cervical spine injury. How should this injury be managed on field?

REFERENCES

1. Courson R, Goldenberg M, Adams KG, et al. Inter-association consensus statement on best practices for sports medicine management for secondary schools and colleges. *J Athl Train*. 2014;49(1):128–137.
2. Courson R (2012, March 22). NATA offers guidelines for emergency action planning in athletics. http://www.nata.org/News%20Release/nata-offers-guidelines-emergency-planning-athletics. Published March 22, 2012. Accessed September 25, 2015.
3. Andersen JC, Courson RW, Kleiner DM, et al. National Athletic Trainers' Association position statement: emergency planning in athletics. *J Athl Train*. 2002;37(1):99–104.
4. Jevon P. Neurological assessment. Part 1—assessing level of consciousness. *Nurs Times*. 2008;104(27):26–27.
5. Teasdale G, Allen D, Brennan P, et al. The Glasgow Coma Scale: an update after 40 years. *Nurs Times*. 2014;110:12–16.
6. Kelly CA, Upex A, Bateman DN. Comparison of consciousness level assessment in the poisoned patient using the alert/verbal/painful/unresponsive scale and the Glasgow Coma Scale. *Ann Emerg Med*. 2005;44(2):108–113.
7. World Health Organization. *Pulse Oximetry Training Manual*. Geneva, Switzerland: World Health Organization; 2011.
8. Casa D, DeMartini JK, Bengeron MF, et al. National Athletic Trainers' Association position statement: exertional heat illness. *J Athl Train*. 2015;50(9):986–1000.
9. Bickley LS, Szilagyi PG. *Bates' Guide to Physical Examination and History Taking*.

9th ed. Philadelphia, PA: Lippincott Williams & Wilkins; 2007.

10. National Athletic Trainers' Association. Appropriate prehospital management of the spine-injured athlete. Update from 1998 document. http://www.nata.org/sites/default/files/Executive -Summary-Spine-Injury-updated.pdf. Accessed November 17, 2015.

11. Kleiner DM, Almquist JL, Bailes J, et al. *Prehospital Care of the Spine-Injured Athlete: A Document from the Inter-Association Task Force for Appropriate Care of the Spine-Injured Athlete*. Dallas, TX: Inter-Association Task Force for Appropriate Care of the Spine-Injured Athlete; 2001.

12. Del Rossi G, Rechtine GR, Conrad BP, et al. Are scoop stretchers suitable for use on spine-injured patients? *Am J Emerg Med*. 2010;28(7):751–756.

13. Casa DJ, Guskiewicz KM, Anderson SA, et al. National Athletic Trainers' Association position statement: preventing sudden death in sports. *J Athl Train*. 2012;47(1):96–118.

14. Pollart SM, Compton RM, Elward KS. Management of acute asthma exacerbations. *Am Fam Physician*. 2011;84(1):40–47.

15. Jordan BD. The clinical spectrum of sport-related traumatic brain injury. *Nat Rev Neurol*. 2013; 9(4):222–230.

16. Bey T, Ostick B. Second impact syndrome. *West J Emerg Med*. 2009;10(1):6–10.

17. Kolb JJ. How a cautious approach to TBI patients may help reduce the incidents of second impact syndrome. *JEMS*. 2014;39(1):3–7.

18. Dewall J. The ABCs of TBI. Evidence-based guidelines for adult traumatic brain injury care. *JEMS*. 2010;35(4):54–61.

19. American Diabetes Association. Diabetes basics. http://www.diabetes.org/diabetes-basics/. Accessed October 1, 2015.

20. National Athletic Trainers' Association. Consensus statement: sickle cell trait and the athlete. http://www.nata.org/sites/default/files/ SickleCellTraitAndTheAthlete.pdf. Accessed October 3, 2015.

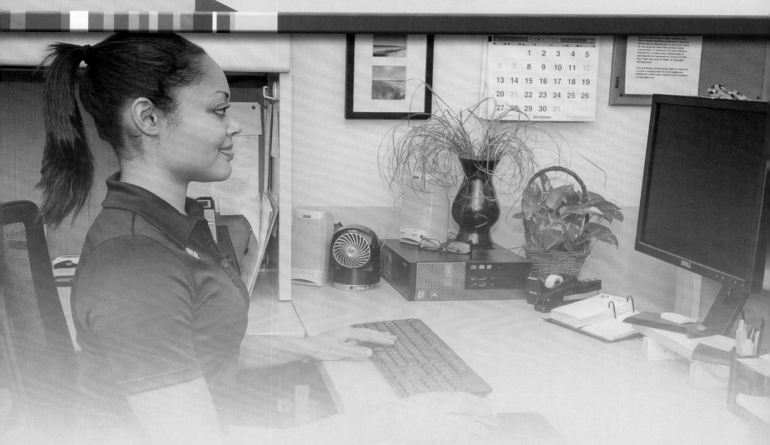

CHAPTER

8

Assessment of Body Alignment Posture and Gait

STUDENT OUTCOMES

1. Describe somatotyping and identify the three basic somatotypes.

2. List the key components of a static postural assessment.

3. Identify normal and abnormal postural findings.

4. Describe cross syndrome in relation to faulty posture.

5. Explain the kinematics of the hip, knee, lower leg, ankle, and foot and identify the muscles that are responsible for coordinated and smooth gait.

6. Define the gait cycle and its phases.

7. Differentiate normal parameters of gait including base width, step length, stride length, lateral pelvic shift, vertical pelvic shift, and pelvic rotation.

8. Identify differential diagnosis of antalgic gait.

189

INTRODUCTION

The evaluation of a patient's body alignment, posture, and gait, along with a solid health history, can provide the practitioner with valuable insight into the patient's pathology or potential pitfalls. This is especially true when assessing chronic injuries or during the preparticipation examination. This chapter begins with describing somatotyping and an examination of different body types followed by an overview of posture. Key terminology needed to understand the importance of optimal posture in maintaining normal function is presented. Information on how to conduct a postural assessment, identify normal and faulty posture, and interpret findings is included. The second half of this chapter focuses on the principles of gait and gait assessment.

SOMATOTYPING

Prior to beginning an assessment of posture or gait, it is important to note the overall body appearance. Although body typing provides a general appearance, it can be helpful to identify normative values for each individual patient. Somatotyping taxonomy was developed in the 1940s, by American psychologist William Herbert Sheldon, to categorize the human body according to the relative contribution of three fundamental elements. Somatotypes are named after the three germ layers of embryonic development: the endoderm (develops into the digestive tract), the mesoderm (becomes muscle, heart, and blood vessels), and the ectoderm (forms the skin and nervous system) (**Fig. 8.1**).[1]

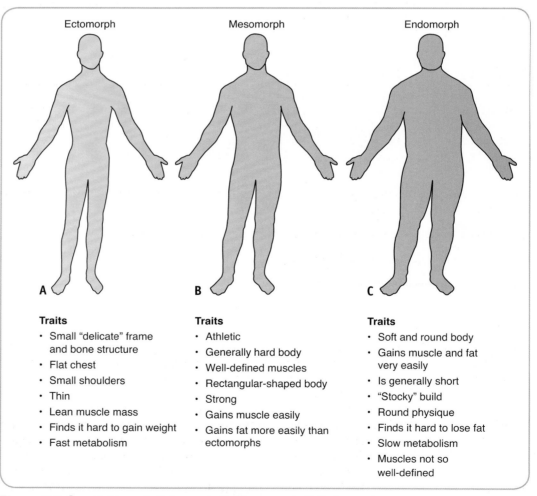

Ectomorph	Mesomorph	Endomorph
A	B	C

Traits
- Small "delicate" frame and bone structure
- Flat chest
- Small shoulders
- Thin
- Lean muscle mass
- Finds it hard to gain weight
- Fast metabolism

Traits
- Athletic
- Generally hard body
- Well-defined muscles
- Rectangular-shaped body
- Strong
- Gains muscle easily
- Gains fat more easily than ectomorphs

Traits
- Soft and round body
- Gains muscle and fat very easily
- Is generally short
- "Stocky" build
- Round physique
- Finds it hard to lose fat
- Slow metabolism
- Muscles not so well-defined

Figure 8.1. Somatotypes. A, Ectomorph. **B,** Mesomorph. **C,** Endomorph.

Ectomorph

An ectomorph is a typical lean individual. Ectomorphs have a light build with small joints and lean muscle. Usually, ectomorphs have long thin limbs with stringy muscles. Shoulders tend to be thin with little width.

Mesomorph

A mesomorph has a large bone structure, large muscles, and a naturally athletic physique. Mesomorphs find it quite easy to gain and lose weight. They are naturally strong and build muscle mass quickly.

Endomorph

The endomorph body type is solid and generally soft. Endomorphs have a tendency to gain weight very easily. Endomorphs are usually of a shorter build with thick arms and legs. Muscles are strong, especially the upper legs.

Mixed Body Type

Very often, people cannot be easily classed as one of the three main body types. Although there are some people who are purely ectomorphs, endomorphs, or mesomorphs with little or no characteristics of the other body types, very frequently, people fall into mixed categories, such as ecto-mesomorphs or endo-mesomorphs, where largely, they are like the mesomorph but with traits of the ectomorph (such as small joints or a trim waist) or traits of the endomorph (such as a tendency to gain fat easily).

ASSESSMENT OF POSTURE

> **?** A 21-year-old male lacrosse player presents with long-term pain in the thoracic region. He cannot identify when his pain began or describe a specific cause or mechanism of injury. No indications of acute injury are found during inspection and palpation. How might the patient's posture factor into his current symptoms?

Regardless of the injury, evaluating the patient from head to toe is an important aspect of the assessment process. Posture control serves three main purposes:

1. Antigravity function: maintaining an erect posture and keeping eyes level

2. Maintenance of equilibrium and balance

3. Providing mechanical support for motion

Optimal Posture

Optimal posture implies balanced dissemination of body mass around the center of gravity where the compression forces on spinal disks is balanced by ligamentous tension and with minimal energy expenditure from postural muscles.[2] Joint range of motion (ROM) and muscle length and strength also play a major role in achieving optimal posture.[3]

When the body is in an upright position, the line of gravity passes anterior to the spinal column (**Fig. 8.2**). To maintain body position, this moment must be counteracted by tension in the back muscles. Other forces impacting optimal posture include body weight, tension in the spinal ligaments and paraspinal muscles, intra-abdominal pressure, and any applied external loads. When the body is upright, the major form of loading on the spine is axial, and the lumbar spine supports the weight of the body segments above it. When the paraspinal muscles are fatigued, there are increased levels of co-contraction, which also help to stiffen the spine and increase spinal stability.[4]

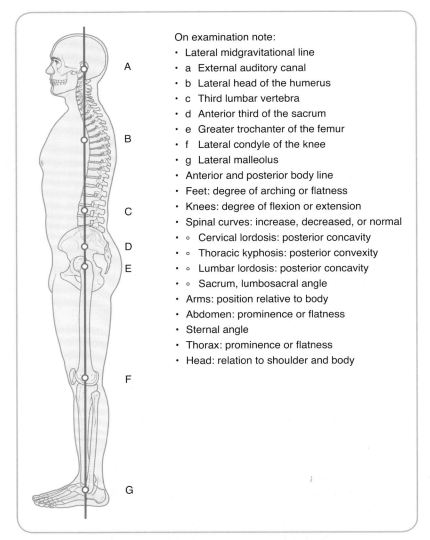

On examination note:
- Lateral midgravitational line
- a External auditory canal
- b Lateral head of the humerus
- c Third lumbar vertebra
- d Anterior third of the sacrum
- e Greater trochanter of the femur
- f Lateral condyle of the knee
- g Lateral malleolus
- Anterior and posterior body line
- Feet: degree of arching or flatness
- Knees: degree of flexion or extension
- Spinal curves: increase, decreased, or normal
  - ◦ Cervical lordosis: posterior concavity
  - ◦ Thoracic kyphosis: posterior convexity
  - ◦ Lumbar lordosis: posterior concavity
  - ◦ Sacrum, lumbosacral angle
- Arms: position relative to body
- Abdomen: prominence or flatness
- Sternal angle
- Thorax: prominence or flatness
- Head: relation to shoulder and body

Figure 8.2. Lateral view of normal posture with midgravitational line.
The line of gravity for the head and trunk passes anterior to the spinal column during upright standing. The moment arm for head/trunk weight at any given vertebral joint is the perpendicular distance between the line of gravity and the spinal column.

Optimal posture depends on maintaining normal body structure and function. As such, posture is a result of habit: Good habits result in good posture, whereas poor habits result in poor or faulty posture. Maintaining optimal posture is important in achieving pain-free, efficient body movement and motion. Failure to maintain an optimal posture often results in discomfort, pain, and dysfunction. Because posture is impacted by both the structure and function of the musculoskeletal system, examination of posture is conducted using three different assessments: (1) examination of alignment in standing, (2) tests for flexibility and muscle length, and (3) tests for muscle strength.[3]

Examination in Standing: Alignment

A quick head-to-foot visual scan by the practitioner can detect significant asymmetries in posture that will assist in identifying the cause of the patient's symptoms. For example, the patient who presents with forward head position where the ear lobes are anterior to the shoulders often also complains of neck pain. Shoulder asymmetries in height are frequently observed in unilateral overhead throwing athletes, whereas anterior shoulder position is common in patients with

APPLICATION STRATEGY 8.1

Postural Assessment Checklist

Anterior View

- Are the head and neck in the midline of the body? Is the nose centered? Does the jaw appear normal?
- Is the slope of the shoulder muscles bilaterally equal? (The level of the shoulder on the dominant side usually is lower than the nondominant side.)
- Do both shoulders have a well-rounded deltoid musculature with no prominent bony structures?
- Are any scars or muscular atrophy present in the arms?
- Is the space between the arms and body the same on both sides?
- Are both hands held in the same position?
- Does the rib cage look symmetrical with no bony protrusions?
- Are the folds of the waist at the same height?
- Are the kneecaps level and facing forward? Are the knees straight and the heads of the fibula level?
- Are the distal bony prominences of the lower leg bilaterally level?
- Are arches present on both feet? When standing in a comfortable position, do the feet angle equally?

Lateral View

- Can an imaginary, straight plumb line be drawn from the ear through the middle of the shoulder, hip, knee, and ankle?
- Does the back have any excessive curves?
- Are the elbows held near full extension?
- Do the chest, back, and abdominal muscles have good tone with no obvious chest deformities?
- Does the pelvis appear to be level?
- Are the knees straight, flexed, or hyperextended? (Normal is a position of slight flexion.)

Posterior View

- Are the head and neck centered? Is there any abnormal prominence of bony structures or muscle atrophy?
- Are the scapula at the same height and resting at the same angle? Are both scapulas lying flat against the rib cage?
- Does the spine appear to be straight?
- Is there any atrophy in the muscle groups of the shoulder and arm?
- Is the posterior side of the elbow at the same height bilaterally? Is the space between the body and elbow the same on both sides?
- Do the ribs protrude?
- Are the waist folds level? Are the posterior gluteal folds level?
- Are the skin creases on the posterior knee level?
- Do both Achilles tendons descend straight to the floor? Are the heels straight, angled in (varus), or angled out (valgus)?

chronic impingement syndrome. **Application Strategy 8.1** provides details of the key features used to conduct a postural assessment from the anterior, lateral, and posterior views.

When assessing postural alignment, you should view from the anterior, posterior, and lateral views. From the **anterior view**, a straight line, perpendicular to the floor, should intersect the forehead, nose, manubrium, and umbilicus pubis and have an even spacing between the feet. Parallel lines to the floor should be used to assess the shoulders and hips. If the shoulders are equal and parallel to the floor, this would indicate symmetry between the right and left shoulders. In addition, the patient should be viewed at the anterior superior iliac spine (ASIS) level to assess if the pelvis is equal indicating symmetrical pelvic height (**Fig. 8.3**). The **posterior view** provides the practitioner with similar information as the anterior view with slightly different kinematic checkpoints. The perpendicular line should proceed from the occiput, straight down the spine to the sacrum. Feet should be equal distance from center and should be parallel. In addition, when examining the patient from a posterior

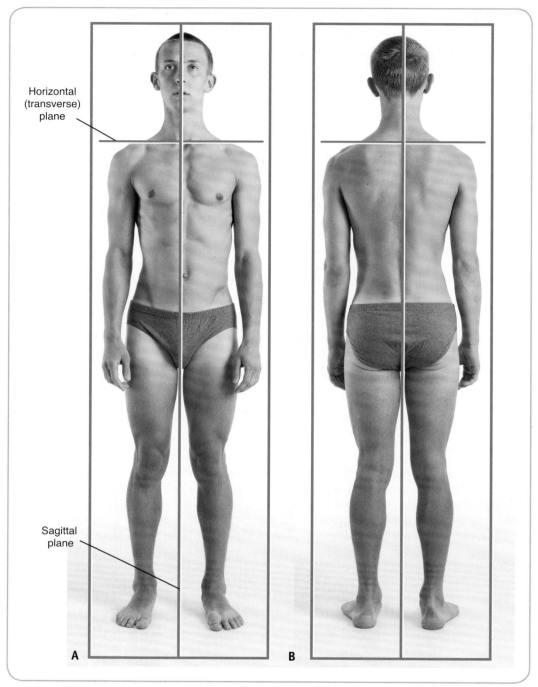

Horizontal (transverse) plane

Sagittal plane

A   B

Figure 8.3. Postural assessment. Front (**A**) and back (**B**) views with midsagittal and horizontal (transverse) plane.

view, the presence of any dark areas of skin pigmentation, such as café au lait spots, should be noted because this could indicate a possible collagen disease or abnormal growth of neural tissues (neurofibromatosis). The lower lumbar spine and sacrum should be observed for tufts of hair (Faun's beard), indicating possible spina bifida occulta. From the **lateral view**, the joints should look stacked. The ears should be directly over the shoulders. The anterior aspect of the shoulders should be in alignment with the greater trochanter. The head, ear, shoulder, and hip should all be in a straight line to the midtarsal area on the foot. The head, pelvis, and spine are in a neutral position (**Fig. 8.4**).

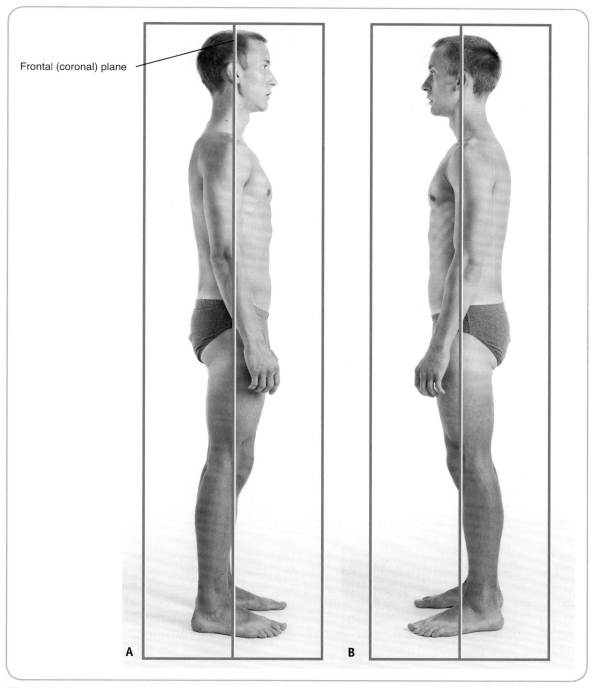

Frontal (coronal) plane

A   B

Figure 8.4. Postural assessment. Right and left side views with frontal (coronal) midline.

Deviations from Norm

As the clinician assesses postural alignment, it is common to view deviations. Postural deviations may result from mechanical stress derived from lateral spinal muscle imbalances or from sustaining repeated impact forces.[3] Often, these same forces result in back pain and/or injury. Excessive spinal curvatures can be congenital or acquired through weight training or sports participation. The most common deviations are lordosis, swayback, flat back, and kyphosis. These deviations can be observed from a lateral view. The one common deviation that can be viewed from the posterior view is scoliosis.

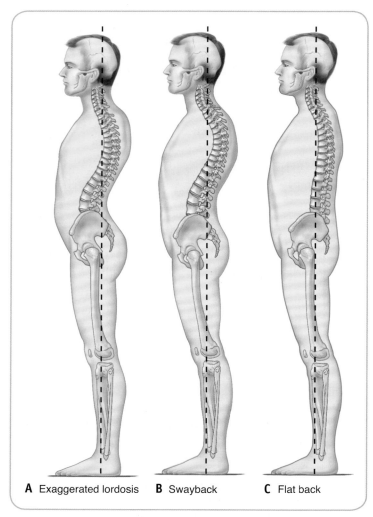

A Exaggerated lordosis **B** Swayback **C** Flat back

Figure 8.5. Lumbar anomalies. A, Lordosis. **B,** Swayback. **C,** Flat back.

■ Lordosis

Lordosis increases the anterior lumbar curve from neutral when compared to normal or optimal posture. This increased anterior lumbar curve will cause the pelvis to move into an anterior tilt position (see **Fig. 16.13**). The rotations will cause the ASIS to move inferiorly and the ischial tuberosity to move superiorly. Lordosis is often associated with weakened abdominal muscles in combination with tight muscles, especially the hip flexors, tensor fasciae latae, and deep lumbar extensors. Normally, the pelvic angle is approximately 30° (see **Fig. 8.2**). With excessive lordosis, this angle can increase to 40° and can be accompanied by a mobile spine and anterior pelvic tilt (**Fig. 8.5A**). Other causes of lordosis include congenital spinal deformity, such as bilateral congenital hip dislocation, spondylolisthesis, compensatory action resulting from another deformity (e.g., kyphosis), hip flexion contractures, poor postural habits, and overtraining in sports requiring repeated lumbar hyperextension (e.g., gymnastics, figure skating, football linemen, javelin throwing, or swimming the butterfly stroke). Because lordosis places added compressive stress on the posterior elements of the spine, low back pain is a common symptom predisposing many individuals to low back injuries.

■ Swayback

Swayback is a decrease of the anterior lumbar curve and increase in the posterior thoracic curve from neutral. This position causes the head and superior aspect to the femur to shift anterior in order to compensate for the posterior position. An individual with a swayback deformity (**Fig. 8.5B**) presents with an increased lordotic curve and kyphosis. This condition often results from weakness in the lower abdominals, lower thoracic extensors, hip flexors, compensatory tight hip extensors, lower lumbar extensors, and upper abdominals. The deformity results as the spine bends back sharply at the lumbosacral angle.[5] Subsequently, the entire pelvis shifts anteriorly, causing the hips to move into extension. For the center of gravity to remain in its normal position, the thoracic spine flexes on the lumbar spine, increasing the lumbar and thoracic curves.

■ Flat Back

Flat back is a decreased anterior lumbar curve. This curve typically causes the pelvis to rotate into the posterior pelvic rotation (see **Fig. 16.13**). With posterior pelvic rotation, the ASIS moves superiorly and the ischial tuberosity moves inferiorly. The term flat back refers to a relative decrease in lumbar lordosis (20°), which shifts the center of gravity anterior to the lumbar spine and hips (**Fig. 8.5C**).[3] The condition may result from the use of Harrington rods in the treatment of scoliosis, degenerative disk disease involving multiple levels of the spine, ankylosing spondylitis, and postlaminectomy syndrome compression fractures, most commonly caused by osteoporosis.

The most common clinical sign is the tendency to lean forward when walking or standing. In an effort to bring the body into better alignment, the low back, buttocks, and posterior thigh muscles are recruited to tilt the pelvis. This action causes these muscles to fatigue more quickly, leading to aching and pain. The body also may compensate by exhibiting increased hip and knee flexion. If hip flexion is accentuated, however, a hip flexion contracture may occur. Treatment involves strengthening the gluteal, low back, abdominal, and hamstring musculature.

■ Kyphosis

Kyphosis (**Fig. 8.6A**) is an increase in the posterior thoracic curve from neutral. This curvature will most likely cause an anterior head position, an increase in lordosis, and an anterior pelvic rotation. The cause of kyphosis can be congenital, idiopathic (unknown), or secondary to osteoporosis. Congenital kyphosis arises from deficits in the formation of either the vertebral bodies or the anterior and posterior vertebral elements. Idiopathic kyphosis, also known as **Scheuermann disease** or osteochondritis of the spine, is present in about 7% of the population and involves the development of one or more wedge-shaped vertebrae in the thoracic or lumbar regions through abnormal behavior of the epiphyseal plate.[6] The individual typically has a round-shouldered appearance, with or without back pain. Weight lifters, gymnasts, and football linemen, who overdevelop the pectoral muscles, also are prone to this condition. In addition, it may be caused by overtraining with the butterfly stroke, hence the nickname "swimmer's back."

■ Scoliosis

Scoliosis is a lateral curvature in the thoracic spine. The lateral curvature could cause bilateral asymmetries of the shoulder or pelvic area when viewing the patient from the anterior or posterior view.

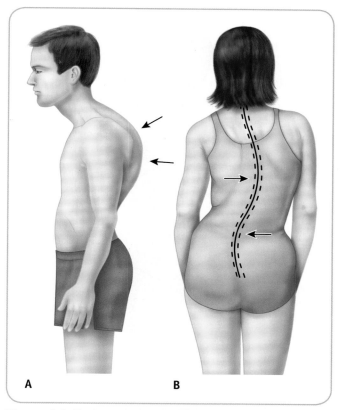

Figure 8.6. Faulty alignments of the thoracic region include kyphosis (A) and scoliosis (B).

Scoliosis is found in 2% to 3% of the population (**Fig. 8.6B**).[6] The lateral deformity, coupled with rotational deformity of the involved vertebrae, may range from mild to severe. Scoliosis may appear as either a C- or an S-shaped curve involving the thoracic spine, lumbar spine, or both. Scoliosis can be structural or nonstructural. Structural scoliosis involves an inflexible curvature that persists with lateral bending of the spine. Nonstructural scoliosis curves are flexible and are corrected with lateral bending. Although congenital abnormalities, certain cancers, and leg length discrepancy may lead to scoliosis, approximately 70% to 90% of all cases are idiopathic. Idiopathic scoliosis most commonly is diagnosed between the ages of 10 and 13 years but can be seen at any age and is more common in females.[6]

Symptoms associated with scoliosis vary with the severity of the condition. Mild cases (curvature <20°) usually are asymptomatic and self-limiting. If scoliosis presents during childhood, reassessment should occur every 3 to 4 months until the adolescent has skeletally matured. Active treatment is not necessary as long as the curve is nonprogressive. If the individual is skeletally immature and the curve is moderate (20° to 45°) and progressive, bracing is necessary. In many instances, the treatment allows enough time out of the brace for daily participation in sport and physical activity. In general, relatively unrestricted physical activity is recommended for almost all adolescents with scoliosis. Mild-to-moderate cases can be treated with strength, flexibility, and general fitness activities. Severe scoliosis, which is characterized by extreme lateral deviation and localized rotation of the spine, can be painful and deforming, and it may require surgery (fusion with spinal instrumentation).[6]

■ Cross Syndrome

There are two commonly seen postural syndromes whose characteristics have been described by Janda[7] from observation:

■ Upper cross syndrome (UCS), also referred to as shoulder cross syndrome or proximal

■ Lower cross syndrome (LCS), also referred to as pelvic cross syndrome or distal

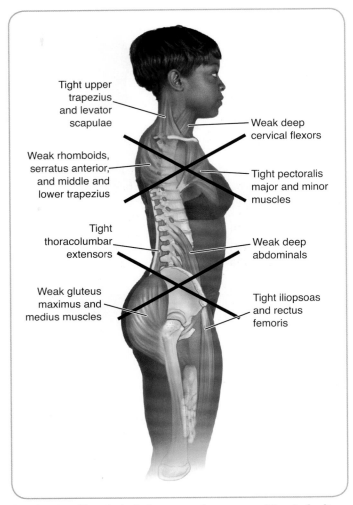

Figure 8.7. Muscle imbalance syndromes resulting in faulty posture include upper cross syndrome and lower cross syndrome.

Labels in figure:
- Tight upper trapezius and levator scapulae
- Weak deep cervical flexors
- Weak rhomboids, serratus anterior, and middle and lower trapezius
- Tight pectoralis major and minor muscles
- Tight thoracolumbar extensors
- Weak deep abdominals
- Weak gluteus maximus and medius muscles
- Tight iliopsoas and rectus femoris

In **upper cross syndrome**, tightness of the upper trapezius and levator scapula on the dorsal side crosses with tightness of the pectoralis major and minor (**Fig. 8.7**). Weakness of the deep cervical flexors ventrally crosses with weakness of the middle and lower trapezius. This pattern of imbalance creates joint dysfunction, particularly at the atlanto-occipital joint, C4–C5 segment, cervicothoracic joint, glenohumeral joint, and T4–T5 segment. Janda[7] noted that these focal areas of stress within the spine correspond to transitional zones in which neighboring vertebrae change in morphology. Specific postural changes are seen in UCS, including forward head posture, increased cervical lordosis and thoracic kyphosis, elevated and protracted shoulders, and rotation or abduction and winging of the scapulae. These postural changes decrease glenohumeral stability as the glenoid fossa becomes more vertical due to serratus anterior weakness leading to abduction, rotation, and winging of the scapulae. This loss of stability requires the levator scapula and upper trapezius to increase activation to maintain glenohumeral centration.[7]

Lower crossed syndrome, tightness of the thoracolumbar extensors on the dorsal side, crosses with tightness of the iliopsoas and rectus femoris. Weakness of the deep abdominal muscles ventrally crosses with weakness of the gluteus maximus and medius (see **Fig. 8.7**). This pattern of imbalance creates joint dysfunction, particularly at the L4–L5 and L5–S1 segments, sacroiliac (SI) joint, and hip joint. Specific postural changes seen in LCS include anterior pelvic tilt, increased lumbar lordosis, lateral lumbar shift, lateral leg rotation, and knee hyperextension. If the lordosis is deep and short, then imbalance is predominantly in the pelvic muscles; if the lordosis is shallow and extends into the thoracic area, then imbalance predominates in the trunk muscles.[7]

Assessing Flexibility and Muscle Length and Strength

Good posture and good body mechanics are linked. Good body mechanics depend on proper body alignment and muscle function such as strength, length, flexibility, and balance.[3] When considering body mechanics, the more flexibility present, there is less stability. The less flexible, the more stable the structure becomes. Therefore, assessing flexibility and muscle length and strength provides the clinician with potential causes of why faulty posture may be present and why the patient is experiencing pain or dysfunction. Assessing flexibility and muscle length and strength will be discussed in Chapters 14 to 22 in relation to specific parts of the body and specific pathologies.

 The lacrosse player appears to have normal posture except for a slight forward head position, mild increase in cervical lordosis, and thoracic kyphosis. This patient appears to have UCS, which would result in thoracic pain of unknown origin. Further testing revealed the patient has shortened and tight pectoral muscles. This patient will benefit from a program to strengthen the posterior thoracic muscles, lengthen the anterior thoracic muscles, and improve scapulothoracic rhythm as well as working on normal head positioning.

THE GAIT CYCLE

? A 26-year-old female patient presents with a history of recurrent and growing pain in her right hip but cannot identify an acute mechanism of injury. The patient began adding running to her exercise program about a year ago and feels that might have something to do with her pain. Inspection and palpation results are normal. How will conducting a gait assessment assist the clinician in determining the cause of the patient's pain?

Despite variation in individual gait patterns, enough commonality exists in human gaits that one can describe the typical gait cycle. Assessment of gait can provide the clinician clues regarding a patient's impairment and subsequent dysfunction. Postinjury, the clinician often uses gait training in the rehabilitation program for patients with lower extremity injury. In order to be able to teach a patient proper gait function, an understanding of the normal gait cycle is required. The gait cycle requires a set of coordinated, sequential joint actions of the lower extremity. This section describes the kinematics of the hip, knee, lower leg, ankle, and foot and identifies the muscles that are responsible for specific movements and potential causes of dysfunction.

Kinematics of the Lower Leg, Ankle, and Foot

Toe Flexion and Extension

Several muscles contribute to flexion of the second through fifth toes. These include the flexor digitorum longus, flexor digitorum brevis, quadratus plantae, lumbricals, and interossei. The flexor hallucis longus and brevis produce flexion of the hallux. Conversely, the extensor hallucis longus, extensor digitorum longus, and extensor digitorum brevis are responsible for extension and overextension of the toes.

Dorsiflexion and Plantar Flexion

Motion at the ankle occurs primarily in the sagittal plane, with ankle flexion and extension being termed dorsiflexion and plantar flexion, respectively (**Fig. 8.8A**). The medial and lateral malleoli serve as pulleys to channel the tendons of the leg muscles either posterior or anterior to the axis of rotation and, in doing so, enable their contributions to either plantar flexion or dorsiflexion. Muscles with tendons passing anterior to the malleoli (i.e., the tibialis anterior, extensor digitorum longus, and peroneus tertius) are dorsiflexors. Those with tendinous attachments running posterior to the malleoli contribute to plantar flexion. The major plantar flexors are the soleus, gastrocnemius, plantaris, and flexor hallucis longus, with assistance being provided by the peroneal longus and brevis and by the tibialis posterior.

Inversion and Eversion

Rotations of the foot in the medial and lateral directions are termed inversion and eversion, respectively (**Fig. 8.8B**). These movements occur primarily at the

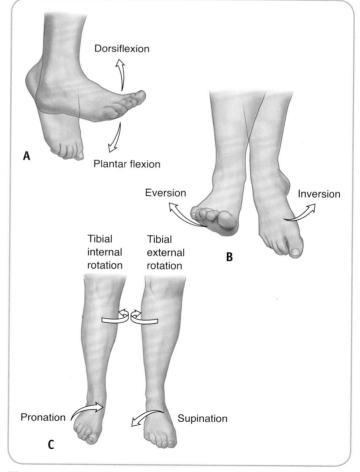

Figure 8.8. Motions of the foot and ankle. A, Dorsiflexion and plantar flexion. **B,** Eversion and inversion. **C,** Supination of the subtalar joint results in external rotation of the tibia; pronation is linked with internal rotation of the tibia.

subtalar joint, with secondary contributions from gliding movements at the intertarsal and tarso-metatarsal joints. The tibialis posterior is the major inverter, with the tibialis anterior providing a minor contribution. The peroneus longus and brevis, with tendons passing behind the lateral malleolus, are primarily responsible for eversion, with assistance being provided by the peroneus tertius.

Pronation and Supination

The lower extremity moves through a cyclical sequence of movements during gait. Among these, the action at the subtalar joint during weight bearing has the most significant implications for lower extremity injury potential. During heel contact, the hindfoot typically is somewhat inverted. As the foot rolls forward and the forefoot initially contacts the ground, the foot is plantar-flexed. This combination of calcaneal inversion, foot adduction, and plantar flexion is known as supination. During weight bearing at midstance, both calcaneal eversion and foot abduction tend to occur as the foot moves into dorsiflexion; these movements are known collectively as pronation. Supination of the subtalar joint also results in external rotation of the tibia, with pronation being linked to internal tibial rotation (**Fig. 8.8C**).

Although a normal amount of pronation is useful in reducing the peak forces sustained during impact, excessive or prolonged pronation can lead to several overuse injuries, including stress fractures of the second metatarsal and irritation of the sesamoid bones, plantar fasciitis, Achilles tendinitis, and medial tibial stress syndrome.[8] Normal walking gait typically involves approximately 6° to 8° pronation.

Kinetics of the Lower Leg, Ankle, and Foot

The lower extremity sustains not only the weight of the body but also the weight of any carried loads and the forces of foot impacts during gait as well. Because force is what ultimately causes injury, understanding the kinetic aspects of lower leg, ankle, and foot function is an important foundation for understanding injury mechanisms.

Forces Commonly Sustained by the Lower Leg, Ankle, and Foot

During training, the bones of the lower extremity are subjected to a complex array of loading patterns, including tension, compression, bending, and torsion. During running, the foot sustains impact forces that can reach two- to threefold body weight, and the magnitudes of the forces increase with gait speed. Running-related injuries occur in 40% to 50% of runners annually, with cavus feet and leg length inequality being documented risk factors.[9]

Foot Deformation During Gait

The structures of the foot are anatomically linked, with approximately 50% of body weight distributed through the subtalar joint to the calcaneus, and the remaining 50% channeled through the transverse tarsal joints to the forefoot.[10] Plantar pressure distribution is affected by gender, shoe type, support surface, and fatigue as well as by individual foot conformation and gait characteristics.[2,11,12]

If the foot were a more rigid structure, each impact with the support surface would generate extremely large forces of short duration through the skeletal system. Because the foot is composed of numerous bones that are connected by flexible ligaments and are restrained by flexible tendons, it deforms with each ground contact. In doing so, it absorbs much of the shock and transmits a much smaller force of longer duration up through the skeletal system.

The process of foot deformation during weight bearing results in the storage of mechanical energy in the stretched tendons, ligaments, and plantar fasciae. As the tibia rotates forward over the talus during gait, additional energy is stored in the gastrocnemius and soleus as they develop eccentric tension. During the push-off phase, the stored energy in all these elastic structures is released, contributing to the force of push-off and actually reducing the metabolic energy cost of walking or running.

Kinetics of the Knee

Because the knee is positioned between the body's two longest bony levers (i.e., the femur and the tibia), the potential for torque and force development at the knee is significant. The key role played by the knee during weight bearing makes the knee subject to large forces during the gait cycle.

Forces at the Tibiofemoral Joints

Weight bearing and tension development in muscles crossing the knee are the predominant forces acting at the tibiofemoral joints, with both contributing to joint compression. The medial compartment sustains the majority of the load during stance, with compressive force at the joint reaching an estimated threefold body weight during the stance phase of gait, increasing to around three- to sixfold body weight during stair climbing.[13,14] Comparison of front and back squat exercises shows significantly higher knee compressive forces during the back squat as compared to the front squat, with shear forces at the knee during squat exercises being small and posteriorly directed.[15] During sport participation, knee forces undoubtedly are large, although quantitative estimates are lacking. Tension in the knee extensors also increases lateral stability of the knee, with tension in the knee flexors contributing to medial stability.

Forces at the Patellofemoral Joint

Compressive force at the patellofemoral joint has been found to be half the body weight during normal walking gait, increasing up to eightfold body weight during stair climbing.[14] During stair climbing, there is an increase in patellofemoral pressure, lateral force distribution, and lateral patellar tilt.[16]

Knee Motion During the Gait

During midstance of normal gait, the knee is flexed to approximately 20°, internally rotated approximately 5°, and slightly abducted. Knee motion during the swing phase includes approximately 70° of flexion, 15° of external rotation, and 5° of adduction.

Patellofemoral Joint Motion

During movements of knee flexion and extension, the patella glides in the trochlear groove, primarily in a vertical direction, with an excursion of as much as 8 cm. When the knee is fully extended, the inferior pole of the patella rests on the distal portion of the femoral shaft, just proximal to the femoral groove. During flexion, the patella makes initial contact with the groove at 10° to 20° of flexion, and it becomes seated within the groove as the knee approaches 20° to 30°. In this position, the lateral border of the trochlea is prominent, forming a barrier against lateral displacement of the patella. The inferior border of the patella tilts upward and medially during knee flexion, with the contact area increasingly shifted superiorly on the medial and lateral facets of the posterior patella.[17,18] The patella also undergoes medial and lateral displacement as the tibia is rotated laterally and medially, respectively, with the center of the patella following a circular path during knee flexion/extension.[19]

Kinematics and Major Muscle Actions of the Hip

Because the hip is a ball-and-socket joint, the femur can move in all planes of motion. However, the massive muscles crossing the hip tend to limit ROM particularly in the posterior direction.

Flexion

The major hip flexors are the iliacus and psoas major, which because of their common attachment at the femur are referred to jointly as the iliopsoas. Four other muscles cross the anterior aspect of the hip to contribute to hip flexion—namely, the pectineus, the rectus femoris, the sartorius, and the tensor fascia latae. Because the rectus femoris is a two-joint muscle that is active during both hip flexion and knee extension, it functions more effectively as a hip flexor when the knee is in flexion, as occurs when a person kicks a ball. The sartorius also is a two-joint muscle. Crossing from the ASIS to the medial surface of the proximal tibia just below the tuberosity, the sartorius is the longest muscle in the body.

Extension

The hip extensors are the gluteus maximus and the three hamstrings—namely, the biceps femoris, the semitendinosus, and the semimembranosus. The gluteus maximus usually is active only when the hip is in flexion, as occurs during stair climbing or cycling, or when extension at the hip is resisted. The nickname "hamstrings" derives from the prominent tendons of the three muscles, which are readily palpable on the posterior aspect of the knee. The hamstrings cross both the hip and the knee, contributing to hip extension and knee flexion.

Abduction

The gluteus medius is the major abductor at the hip, with assistance from the gluteus minimus. The hip abductors are active in stabilizing the pelvis during single-leg support of the body and during the support phase of walking and running. For example, when body weight is supported by the right foot during walking, the right hip abductors contract isometrically and eccentrically to prevent the left side of the pelvis from being pulled downward by the weight of the swinging left leg. This allows the left leg to move freely through the swing phase without scuffing the toes. If the hip abductors are too weak to perform this function, lateral pelvic tilt occurs with every step.

Adduction

The hip adductors include the adductor longus, adductor brevis, and adductor magnus. These muscles are active during the swing phase of gait, bringing the foot beneath the body's center of gravity for placement during the support phase. The relatively weak gracilis assists with hip adduction. The hip adductors also contribute to flexion and internal rotation at the hip, especially when the femur is externally rotated. Strength and flexibility deficits in the hip adductors have been linked to increased risk of injury among ice hockey and soccer players.[20]

Medial and Lateral Rotation of the Femur

Although several muscles contribute to lateral rotation of the femur, six function solely as lateral rotators. These six muscles are the piriformis, gemellus superior, gemellus inferior, obturator internus, obturator externus, and quadratus femoris. The femur of the swinging leg rotates laterally to accommodate the lateral rotation of the pelvis during the stride.

The major medial rotator of the femur is the gluteus minimus, with assistance from the tensor fascia latae, semitendinosus, semimembranosus, gluteus medius, and the four adductor muscles. The medial rotators are relatively weak; their estimated strength is approximately one-third that of the lateral rotators.

Kinetics of the Hip

Forces at the Hip During Standing

The hip is a major weight-bearing joint that is subject to extremely high loads during sport participation. During upright standing, with weight evenly distributed on both legs, the weight supported at each hip is half the weight of the body segments above the hip. The total load on each hip in this situation is greater than the weight that is being supported, however, because tension in the large, strong hip muscles further adds to compression at the joint.

Forces at the Hip During Gait

Compression on the hip is approximately the same as body weight during the swing phase of normal walking gait but increases up to three- to sixfold the body weight during the stance phase.[21]

Body weight, impact forces translated upward through the skeleton from the foot, and muscle tension contribute to this compressive load. Walking or running increases the forces on the hip. Use of a crutch or a cane on the side opposite an injured lower limb serves to more evenly distribute the load between the legs throughout the gait cycle. It is better to use no assistive device than to use a crutch or a cane on the same side as the lower extremity injury because this actually increases joint forces on the injured side.[20]

> The hip and lower extremity is part of a kinetic chain that transfers forces from the ground to body. Each joint within this chain is a link that must function smoothly and effectively to produce an efficient and pain-free gait. By performing a gait assessment, the clinician will be able to determine if the patient has normal muscle and joint function of each link in the kinetic chain that are responsible for walking and running. If dysfunction is found, the location and type of dysfunction will assist the clinician in determining if it is the related to or even the cause of the patient's hip pain.

GAIT ASSESSMENT

> **?** The 26-year-old female patient presented with a history of recurrent and growing pain in her right hip but could not identify an acute mechanism of injury. The patient began adding running to her exercise program about a year ago and feels that might have something to do with her pain. How will the athletic trainer determine what is a normal gait for this patient and, if the gait is altered, what factors could contribute to her pathology?

The gait cycle (**Fig. 8.9**) begins with a period of single-leg support in which body weight is supported by one leg while the other leg swings forward. The swing phase can be divided into the initial swing, midswing, and terminal swing. The period of double support begins with the contact of the swing leg with the ground or floor. As body weight transfers from the support leg to the swing leg, the swing leg undergoes a loading response and becomes the new support leg. A new period of single support then begins as the swing leg loses ground contact. The time during which body weight is balanced over the support leg is referred to as midstance. As the body's center of gravity shifts forward, the terminal stance phase of the support leg coincides with the terminal swing phase of the opposite leg.

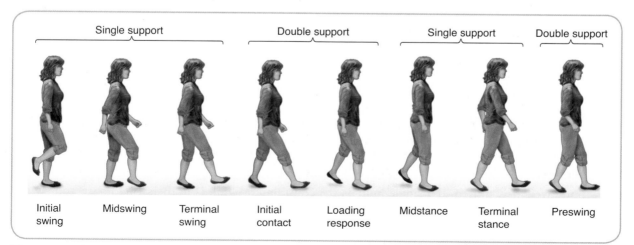

Figure 8.9. Gait. The gait cycle consists of alternating periods of single-leg support and double-leg support.

TABLE 8.1 Gait Terminology

TERM	DEFINITION
Arm swing	Amplitude and frequency with which the arm is moved during gait
Cadence	How fast one walks: number of steps per minute
Foot angle	Angle between line from heel to second toe and line of direction
Forward lean	Leading with torso in front of pelvis
Forward pelvis	Leading with pelvis in front of torso
Pelvic list	Up and down motion of pelvis
Pelvic sway	Side-to-side motion of pelvis
Stance phase	Time spent in weight bearing or in contact with the ground
Step	Sequence of events from a specific point in the gait on one extremity to the same point in the opposite extremity
Step length	Distance traveled between the initial contacts of the right and left foot
Step width	Distance between the points of contact of both feet
Stride	Two sequential steps
Stride length	Linear distance covered in one stride
Stride time	Time required to complete a single stride
Torso swing	Rotational movement of torso

Differences in running gait have been documented based on both gender and age. Among recreational runners, females appear to have greater hip adduction, hip internal rotation, and knee abduction compared to males.[8] A study of elite master sprinters showed an age-related decline in running speed related to reduction in stride length and increase in ground contact time.[9]

The lower extremity is dedicated to the task of weight bearing and ambulation or stance and swing. The health of all aspects of the lower extremity is critical to normal and efficient activities of daily living. Because pathology that affects the lower extremity often provides the practitioner with a visual clue, it is critical to understand normal and abnormal patterns of ambulation so that the athletic trainer can recognize and treat pathologies quickly. Specific terminology used to describe the components of the gait assessment is presented in **Table 8.1**.

There are two phases to normal walking cycle: stance phase and swing phase. Stance phase is when the foot is on the ground. Swing phase is when the foot is moving forward. Sixty percent of the normal cycle is spent in stance phase (25% of which is spent in double stance) and 40% in swing phase. Each phase is then divided into its smaller components in the following section.

Basic Gait Cycle

The gait cycle is composed of two phases, with eight components (**Fig. 8.10**).

Stance Phase

Body weight is shifted to a single limb as the contralateral limb is in the swing phase and swings through. Subcomponents of this include the following:

- Initial contact (heel strike)
    - The mechanical goals of the heel strike are to lower the forefoot to the ground, continue deceleration (reverse forward swing), and to preserve the longitudinal arch of the foot.

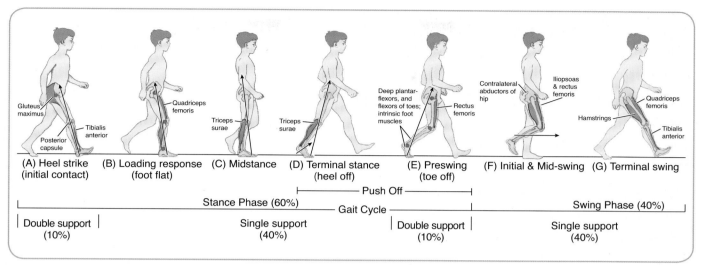

Figure 8.10. Gait cycle: Stance and swing phase. The activity of one limb between two repeated events of walking. Eight phases are typically described, two of which have been combined in **(F)** for simplification.

- Loading response (flat foot)

- Midstance

- Terminal stance (heel off)

- Preswing phase (toe off): Preswing coincides with initial contact of opposite limb and is the only point in the gait cycle where double limb support occurs. The primary function of this phase of gait is to position the limb in preparation for the swing.

Swing Phase

Swing phase is composed of the initial swing (acceleration), midswing, and terminal swing (deceleration).

- Initial swing starts as the foot is lifted from contact with the ground and continues until the foot of the moving limb is aligned with the foot of the nonmoving limb.

- Midswing is a continuation of the initial swing, moving the foot from parallel with the foot of nonmoving limb forward into almost full knee extension.

- Terminal swing occurs when the knee is in full extension and initial contact is about to happen.

Assessing Gait

The patient is instructed to wear clothing such as midthigh length shorts and a loose but not overly large fitting shirt that will allow the clinician to observe muscle and joint function of the lower extremity. Socks and shoes should not been worn during initial assessment. However, the assessment can be repeated later with the patient wearing shoes for comparison of findings. Identify a walking path that is free from obstacles and long enough to allow the patient to assume a normal walking pace before having to turn around. The athletic trainer will need to observe the patient from an anterior and posterior view as well as a lateral view (right and left). The athletic trainer may need to ask the patient to walk back and forth for several minutes while focusing on different parts of the gait. At times, the athletic trainer may need to kneel down to get the correct perspective of foot motion. **Table 8.2** is a checklist that can be used during gait assessment.

Observe the following normative findings:

a. The width of the normal base (step width) measures from 2 to 4 in and the normal step is from heel to heel. Note if the patient is walking with a wider base. This may indicate a possible pathology. Patients usually widen their base if they are on an unstable surface or feel dizzy, such as a patient

TABLE 8.2 Checklist for Gait Assessment

ITEM	FINDINGS: ANTERIOR VIEW	FINDINGS: POSTERIOR VIEW	FINDINGS: LATERAL VIEW
Initial contact			
Loading response			
Midstance			
Terminal stance			
Preswing			
Initial swing			
Midswing			
Terminal swing			
Stride length			
Step length			
Stride width			
Pelvic list			
Pelvic sway			
Torso movement			
Arm swing			
Weight-bearing sequence			
Non–weight-bearing sequence			
Cadence			
Circle if present; indicate right/left.	Gluteus maximus gait	Stiff knee gait	Calcaneal gait
	Trendelenburg gait	Steppage or drop foot gait	
	Psoatic gait	Short leg gait	

Los Amigos Research & Education Center. *Observational Gait Analysis-Revised.* Downey, CA: Los Amigos Research & Education Center; 2013.

who sustained a concussion. A patient could also widen the normal base of support if he or she is suffering from a decreased sensation in the sole of the foot. Normal step length is approximately 15 in. Step length can be affected by muscle contraction, walking on an unstable surface, or other balance and neuromuscular control pathologies. Step width and step length is depicted in **Figure 8.11**.

b. Center of gravity: The body's center of gravity lies 2 in in front of the second sacral vertebra. In normal gait, the body oscillates no more than 2 in in a vertical direction. A smooth pattern of gait as the body advances forward indicates controlled vertical oscillations.

c. The knee should remain flexed during all components of the stance phase except for initial contact to prevent the excessive vertical displacement of the center of gravity.

d. The pelvis and truck shift laterally approximately 1 in to the weight-bearing side during gait to center the weight over the hip.

e. The average length of a step is approximately 15 in, and the average adult walks at a cadence of approximately 90 to 120 steps per minute.

f. During the swing phase, the pelvis rotates 40° forward, whereas the hip joint on the opposite extremity acts as the fulcrum for rotation.

Assessing Gait in Elderly Patients

When assessing gait in elderly patients or patients with neurocognitive deficits, additional precautions are needed. Begin the evaluation with a general neuro-logical test looking at cranial nerve function (including visual fields and acuity) and cerebellar function (heel to shin, Romberg) and assess the peripheral nervous systems. Pay particular attention to normal/abnormal foot sensation, proprioception (great toe position sense, 10-g monofilament, vibratory), and overall muscle function. The athletic trainer should also look for musculoskeletal abnormalities and de-formities, particularly of the foot and lower extremities and the spine.

Standing and balance

- Observe how the patient rises. Do they need to use their arms to push off, or do you notice any balance problems in rising from the chair? When they stand, is it done with or without support? Ask the patient to stand with his or her eyes closed and turn 360°.

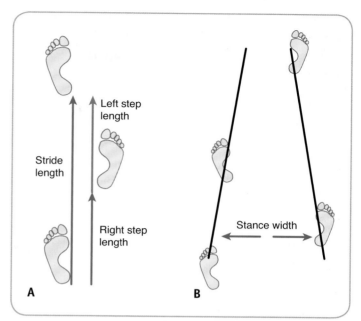

Figure 8.11. Stride length and stance width. A, One stride length is equal to the sum of on right and left step length. **B, Stance width.** The effect of acceleration on stance width is gradual reduction as the individual gets upright and into his or her stride.

Walking

- Observe how the patient begins to walk (i.e., hesitancy or multiple attempts). Notice the step height for both feet, foot clearance (looking for foot drop), step symmetry between right and left sides, and the speed of the gait.

- Look for signs of path deviation and the need to use adaptive equipment to maintain a straight path. Observe the posture and trunk for evidence of swaying, flexion, arm swing, and stability.

- Assess tandem and heel-walking gaits.

Endurance

- Observe the patient for any signs of fatigue or for comorbid problems that compromise walking.

The Timed Get Up and Go Test (TGUAGT) is one of the most commonly used tests to assess healthy adults for risk of falling through assessment of gait and balance.[22] The TGUAGT begins by observing the patient rising from the chair to a standing position. The patient walks at his or her usual pace 3 m (approximately 10 ft), turns around, walks back to the chair, and sits down. Patients are allowed to use their walking assists, such as canes, if normally used in everyday life. However, pa-tients are instructed *not* to use their arms as an assist in rising from the chair. Performing this test in less than 20 seconds indicates that the individual is independent for transfers and mobility, whereas times greater than 30 seconds suggests increased risk for falls and dependence.[22]

Causes of Altered Gait Patterns

Most altered gait patterns occur during the stance phase as the patient responds to pain or dysfunc-tion. When a patient alters his or her gait to alleviate pain, the patient is said to walk with an **anta-lgic gait**, or limp. The patient will remain on the involved extremity for as short a time as possible. Additional causes for altering gait, such as nerve damage, are presented in **Table 8.3.**

TABLE 8.3 Abnormal Gait Patterns

TERM	DESCRIPTION	CAUSE
Stiff knee or hip gait	The patient will lift the knee of the involved side higher than normal to clear the ground due to knee or hip stiffness.	Associated with stiffness, laxity, or pain in knee or hip
Equine gait	The patient will bear weight primarily on the lateral edge of foot with no heel strike on initial contact.	Associated with congenital condition where Achilles tendon is shortened
Trendelenburg gait	The patient will thrust the thorax laterally to keep the center of gravity over the weight-bearing leg.	Associated weak gluteus medius muscle
Psoatic limp	The patient will have difficulty swinging leg through, and trunk movement is exaggerated.	Associated with hip conditions such as Legg-Calvé-Perthes disease. Look for this in adolescent patients.
Quadriceps gait	The patient will use trunk to swing leg forward and push off with toes instead of flexing and extending at knee.	Associated with injury to quadriceps muscle
Short leg gait	The patient will shift from side to side.	Associated with leg length difference due to skeletal shortening of one leg
Drop foot gait	The patient will lift knee higher to allow the foot to clear ground. Foot often slaps when it lands on ground.	Associated with weak dorsiflexors or anterior compartment syndrome

Initial Contact

If the patient is complaining of foot pain, it could be a result of heel pathology, such as a heel spur or a calcaneal fat pad contusion. To relieve the pain, the patient might try to hop onto the involved foot in an attempt to avoid heel strike completely or may attempt to strike with the midfoot or on the toes. The knee is normally extended during initial contact. If the patient is unable to extend the knee, it could be a result of weak quadriceps, an extension lag from a past injury, acute inflammation, or patellofemoral pathology.

Loading Response

The dorsiflexors of the foot permit the foot to move in to plantar flexion through eccentric elongation so that the foot flattens smoothly on the ground. Patients with weak or nonfunctioning dorsiflexors may slap the foot down after heel strike (**drop foot**) instead of letting it land smoothly. Patients who suffer from posterior tibial tendinopathy will also struggle with the foot flat stage as the muscle is eccentrically loaded to decelerate the foot. The patient will have pain and shift his or her weight to the lateral aspect of the foot.

Midstance

During the midstance phase, weight is normally borne evenly on all aspects of the foot. Patients with rigid pes planus, pes cavus, or subtalar arthritis may develop pain when walking on uneven ground. Pain may appear on the medial aspect of the lower leg or foot for a patient who has pes planus. Patients who have pes cavus may have pain on the lateral aspect of the foot or lower leg due to the weight bearing being shifted in a lateral direction. Patients who suffer from fallen transverse arches of the forefoot may develop painful calluses over the metatarsal heads. During midstance, if the gluteus medius muscles are weak, the patient will tend to lurch forward to the involved side to place the center of gravity over the hip.

Preswing

Patients with turf toe or **hallux rigidus** of the metatarsophalangeal joint may be unwilling or unable to hyperextend the metatarsophalangeal joint of the great toe. The lack of great toe extension may force the patient to push off from the lateral side of his or her forefoot. This shift in gait will eventually lead to pain and dysfunction. **Metatarsalgia** or **interdigital neuromas** could also cause the patient to not want to toe off leading to a lateral shift to compensate.

Acceleration

The dorsiflexors of the ankle are active during the entire swing phase by shortening the extremity so that it can clear the ground by holding the ankle in a neutral position. If the patient suffers from drop foot, this will cause the patient to hip the hike in order to assist with having the foot clear the ground. The knee also serves to shorten the extremity with maximum knee flexion approximately 65°. Patients who cannot obtain an adequate amount of flexion to allow the foot to clear the ground will have a shorten stride length or will lean the torso to the opposite site in an attempt to elevate the hip.

Midswing

If the ankle dorsiflexors are not working to keep the ankle in neutral, the tip of the toe will scrap the ground and produce a character shoe scrape. To compensate, the patient may flex his or her hip excessively to bend the knee, permitting the foot to clear the ground. This gait is referred to as the **steppage gait** and may be due to paralysis of the anterior tibial and fibular muscles and is seen in lesions of the lower motor neuron, such as multiple neuritis, lesions of the anterior motor horn cells, and lesions of the cauda equina.

Deceleration

The hamstring muscles contract to slow down the leg just prior to heel strike. This deceleration allows the heel to strike the ground in a controlled manner. If the hamstrings are weak or injured, the initial contact may be excessively harsh, causing thickening of the heel pad.

Although gait assessment is an essential tool for the practitioner, it is only part of the diagnostic process. It is critical to match the findings of the gait assessment to the history obtained from the patient. Realize that not every deviation from the norm is relevant to the patient's pathology.

 Gait assessment reveals on initial contact that the patient has very limited heel strike and that initial contact is being made on the lateral aspect of the midfoot on the same limb as her painful hip. During the swing phase, the patient does not fully extend the knee and walks with a forward lean. The clinician concludes the patient has a shortened Achilles tendon and tight hamstrings as well as tight hip flexors, which is resulting in poor running biomechanics. These factors may be placing additional stress on her hip.

SUMMARY

1. Prior to beginning an assessment of posture or gait, it is important to note the overall body appearance. Somatotyping categorizes the human body according to the three types: endomorph, mesomorph, and ectomorph.

2. Although there are some people who are purely ectomorphs, endomorphs, or mesomorphs with little or no characteristics of the other body types, very frequently, people fall into mixed categories, such as ecto-mesomorphs or endo-mesomorphs.

3. Optimal posture implies balanced dissemination of body mass around the center of gravity, where the compression forces on spinal disks are balanced by ligamentous tension and with minimal energy expenditure from postural muscles. Joint ROM and muscle length and strength also play a major role in achieving optimal posture.

4. Assessment of posture involves comparing alignment between the left and right and anterior and posterior aspects of the body along the line of the center of gravity. Observations made

from the anterior, posterior, and lateral aspect will assist the clinician in detecting deviations from optimal posture positions.

5. Postural deviations may result from mechanical stress derived from lateral spinal muscle imbalances or from sustaining repeated impact forces. Often, these same forces result in back pain and/or injury. Excessive spinal curvatures can be congenital or acquired through weight training or sports participation.

6. The most common deviations are lordosis, swayback, flat back, and kyphosis.

7. Muscular imbalances developed through excessive or incorrect training techniques, overuse, and repetitive motion can lead to cross syndrome, a common cause of faulty posture.

8. Assessment of gait can provide the clinician clues regarding a patient's impairment and subsequent dysfunction. Postinjury, the clinician often utilizes gait training in the rehabilitation program for patients with lower extremity injury.

9. The gait cycle requires a set of coordinated, sequential joint actions of the lower extremity. Each joint within the lower extremity functions like a link in a chain. Each link must work efficiently in order for smooth and efficient gait to occur. Dysfunction can be caused by muscular imbalances, injury, improper tissue healing, injury, and swelling.

10. The gait is divided into two sections: stance phase and swing phase. The stance phase is further divided into the initial contact, loading response, midstance, and terminal stance. The swing phase is further divided into the preswing, midswing, and terminal swing.

11. Gait is assessed from the lateral, anterior, and posterior aspect to detect quality of gait.

12. Most altered gait patterns occur during the stance phase as the patient responds to pain or dysfunction. When a patient alters his or her gait to elevate pain, the patient is said to walk with an antalgic gait, or limp. Gait patterns are also altered due to dysfunction, such as a weak gluteus medius muscle.

13. When assessing gait in elderly patients, additional testing is done prior to gait analysis to determine if assessment is appropriate and safe to perform.

APPLICATION QUESTIONS

1. It's peewee football season and the coaches are trying to determine how to match up players safely. Using somatotyping terminology and concepts, describe what considerations should be examined when setting up pairings.

2. A 25-year-old information technologist complains of nagging, constant pain in the midthoracic region with no history of trauma or illness. How might this person's job contribute to his pain?

3. As part of the preparticipation screening process, all student athletes will be screened for posture. Describe the most efficient way to set up the postural assessment screening station and identify the materials needed for the station to run smoothly.

4. What injuries might a 16-year-old male football athlete with a flat back be at higher risk of sustaining than his counterpart who has normal posture?

5. Your postural assessment suggests that your 18-year-old patient has swayback. In order to determine the cause of the condition, which muscles will you assess and why?

6. Your patient presents with a history of tibial stress fractures over a 6-year period, corresponding with when she began running regularly. Analysis of running routine, surface, footwear, and diet does not help to identify a cause for the recurrent stress fractures. What information might

be gathered through a combined postural and gait assessment that may help you in identifying a potential cause of her recurrent stress fractures?

7. How might a patient with repetitive hamstring strain present during a gait assessment during a time of noninjury?

REFERENCES

1. Hollin CR. *Psychology and Crime: An Introduction to Criminological Psychology*. 2nd ed. East Sussex, United Kingdom: Routledge; 2013.

2. Bischof JE, Abbey AN, Chuckpaiwong B, et al. Three-dimensional ankle kinematics and kinetics during running in women. *Gait Posture*. 2010;31(4):502–505.

3. Kendall FP, McCreary EK, Provance PG, et al. *Muscles: Testing and Function with Posture and Pain*. 5th ed. Philadelphia, PA: Lippincott Williams & Wilkins; 2005.

4. Grondin DE, Potvin JR. Effects of trunk muscle fatigue and load timing on spinal responses during sudden hand loading. *J Electromyogr Kinesiol*. 2009;19(4):e237–e245.

5. McGregor AH, Hukins DW. Lower limb involvement in spinal function and low back pain. *J Back Musculoskelet Rehabil*. 2009;22(4):219–222.

6. Schiller JR, Eberson CP. Spinal deformity and athletics. *Sports Med Arthrosc*. 2008;16(1):26–31.

7. Janda V. Muscles and motor control in low back pain—assessment and management. In: Twomey L, ed. *Physical Therapy of the Low Back*. New York, NY: Churchill Livingstone; 1987.

8. Ferber R, Davis IM, Williams DS III. Gender differences in lower extremity mechanics during running. *Clin Biomech (Bristol, Avon)*. 2003;18(4):350–357.

9. O'Connor KM, Hamill J. The role of selected extrinsic foot muscles during running. *Clin Biomech (Bristol, Avon)*. 2004;19(1):71–77.

10. Fukuchi RK, Duarte M. Comparison of three-dimensional lower extremity running kinematics of young adult and elderly runners. *J Sports Sci*. 2008;26(13):1447–1454.

11. Fields KB, Sykes JC, Walker KM, et al. Prevention of running injuries. *Curr Sports Med Rep*. 2010;9(3):176–182.

12. Mendelsohn FA, Warren MP. Anorexia, bulimia, and the female athlete triad: evaluation and management. *Endocrinol Metab Clin North Am*. 2010;39(1):155–167.

13. Winby CR, Lloyd DG, Besier TF, et al. Muscle and external load contribution to knee joint contact loads during normal gait. *J Biomech*. 2009;42(14):2294–2300.

14. Costigan PA, Deluzio KJ, Wyss UP. Knee and hip kinetics during normal stair climbing. *Gait Posture*. 2002;16(1):31–37.

15. Gullett JC, Tillman MD, Gutierrez GM, et al. A biomechanical comparison of back and front squats in healthy trained individuals. *J Strength Cond Res*. 2009;23(1):284–292.

16. Goudakos IG, König C, Schöttle PB, et al. Stair climbing results in more challenging patellofemoral contact mechanics and kinematics than walking at early knee flexion under physiological-like quadriceps loading. *J Biomech*. 2009;42(15):2590–2596.

17. Nakagawa S, Kadoya Y, Kobayashi A, et al. Kinematics of the patella in deep flexion. Analysis with magnetic resonance imaging. *J Bone Joint Surg Am*. 2003;85(7):1238–1242.

18. Moro-oka T, Matsuda S, Miura H, et al. Patellar tracking and patellofemoral geometry in deep knee flexion. *Clin Orthop Relat Res*. 2002;(394):161–168.

19. Iranpour F, Merican AM, Baena FR, et al. Patellofemoral joint kinematics: the circular path of the patella around the trochlear axis. *J Orthop Res*. 2010;28(5):589–594.

20. Chan GN, Smith AW, Kirtley C, et al. Changes in knee moments with contralateral versus ipsilateral cane usage in females with knee osteoarthritis. *Clin Biomech (Bristol, Avon)*. 2005;20(4):396–404.

21. Steinke H, Hammer N, Slowik V, et al. Novel insights into the sacroiliac joint ligaments. *Spine (Phila Pa 1976)*. 2010;35(3):257–263.

22. Herman T, Giladi N, Hausdorff JM. Properties of the "timed up and go" test: more than meets the eye. *Gerontology*. 2011;57(3):203–210.

Psychosocial Intervention and Patient Care

STUDENT OUTCOMES

1. Describe the prevalence of psychological disorders in the United States.

2. Explain the role of the athletic trainer in assessing a patient exhibiting signs and symptoms of psychological distress.

3. Identify common signs and symptoms of psychological distress.

4. Demonstrate patient-centered counseling skills used in motivational interviewing to build a strong relationship with the patient.

5. Identify the key elements for achieving cultural competence and how the LEARN model can be used to enhance communication to better understand the worldview of the patient.

6. Describe the decision-making model and the two alternatives to possible interventions that may occur when a patient exhibits psychological distress.

7. Identify different methods used to facilitate change in identified behaviors in a patient.

8. Describe the elements that a practitioner might use in motivational interviewing.

9. Explain when and how to make a referral for a patient exhibiting psychological distress and identify potential licensed mental health professionals that could be contacted to assist.

10. Describe the affective cycle of injury and what indicators are used to demonstrate a successful recovery.

11. Describe effective intervention strategies used for help seeking and rehabilitation intervention.

INTRODUCTION

Psychological factors can enhance or inhibit an individual's success in sport participation. As such, knowledge of the physical, psychological, emotional, social, and performance factors that affect an individual is essential for the health care practitioner. An understanding of each component and their interrelationships are necessary to effectively treat the whole person.

In this chapter, psychosocial factors associated with an individual's health and well-being, sport performance, and injury will be presented. The role of the athletic trainer in facilitating help seeking by the patient using a decision-making process to help the athlete will also be discussed.

THE PREVALENCE OF PSYCHOLOGICAL DISORDERS

? Jim, a 19-year-old, highly competitive wrestler, has come into the athletic training room early in the morning wanting to talk with you. Jim looks like he did not sleep well last night, appears disheveled, and out of sorts. After cordial greetings, you ask how you can be of assistance today. Jim reports that he has been under a lot of stress lately with trying to make weight for the upcoming season. He has had disrupted sleep, missed several early morning classes, and has had difficulty keeping up with his homework. He is feeling challenged about having to lose weight, yet his coach insists that he will be able to excel in the new weight class. What concerns about Jim's presentation and situation comes to mind that warrants further assessment?

The World Health Organization (WHO) defines health as "physical, mental, and social well-being" and contends that historically, psychological (mental) well-being has not received much attention.[1] Statistics show mental disorders to be the number one cause of disability in the United States.[2] Healthy People 2010[3] identified the top 10 health indicators, showing substance abuse ranking fourth and mental illness ranking sixth. It is estimated that 26.2% of people older than 18 years old in the United States suffer from a mental illness in any given year, with 45% meeting the criteria for two or more psychological disorders; this translates into over 57.7 million adults.[4] The Substance Abuse and Mental Health Services Administration (SAMHSA)[5] reports 10.7% of adolescents suffers from a diagnosable mental illness each year in the United States, with 977,000 adolescents (38%) receiving treatment for depression.

The prevalence of mental illnesses is expected to increase globally and affect both males and females, across all socioeconomic groups, ages, races, and ethnic groups. Mental health and behavioral disorders account for nearly one-fourth of disability in the world.[6] As such, all health care providers will encounter individuals experiencing mental health concerns.

Psychological Concerns and Athletes

There is a small body of research about psychological disorders in athletes. Study findings have been mixed, with some showing athletes as having a higher risk for psychological concerns, whereas other studies show the prevalence of psychological disorders to be the same for athletes and nonathletes. However, there seems to be agreement among most researchers that athletes experience a greater degree of stress related to the additional demands of their sport, risk of injury, and expectations for success. Although mental health help seeking for psychological concerns is low in the general population, athletes appear less likely to seek help for psychological problems. Barriers identified with mental health help-seeking include not being able to distinguish between normative stress and distress; negative attitudes about professional help-seeking; personal characteristics of the individual experiencing distress; stigma about mental illness; and practical concerns related to finances, lack of transportation, and time.[7]

The risk of injury, being injured, rehabilitation demands, and career-ending injuries have unique stressors specific to sports. These stressors can have a psychological effect on the individual, resulting in psychological distress.[8,9] The Team Physician consensus statement and the National Athletic Trainers' Association (NATA) consensus statement recommend that athletic trainers know how to monitor injured athletes for changes in behavior, signs of psychological distress, and suicidal behavior associated with injury.[10–12]

Substance abuse and high-risk drinking have been shown to be higher for athletes than nonathletes, with athletes drinking greater quantities of alcohol and engaging in binge drinking more often than nonathletes.[13] Studies have shown that athletes engage in gambling and are more likely to have gambling problems. These gambling problems seem to persist into adulthood.[14] Research shows college student athletes engage in a wide range of risky behaviors, including excessive alcohol use, unprotected sex, drinking and driving, and using illegal substances.[15] Athletic trainers report being prepared for psychological distress related to injury and less prepared for noninjury mental health concerns.[16]

Identifying Psychological Distress

Treating the whole person includes the ability to assess psychological well-being. This critical component can be done by taking a comprehensive medical history and assessing for signs and symptoms of psychological distress. In addition to a formal assessment, it is recommended that practitioners note any changes in behavior, affect, or cognition, and if these changes appear to come on gradually or suddenly. Psychological distress can be associated with a patient's internal state (i.e., psychological/emotional) and external stressors (i.e., sociological, cultural, contextual).[12] Common signs and symptoms of psychological distress are listed in **Box 9.1**.

BOX 9.1 Common Signs and Symptoms of Psychological Distress

Any change in behavior or the continued presence of signs and symptoms of psychological distress may warrant a referral to a licensed mental health professional. Beware of the following:

- Social withdrawal
- Emotional outbursts, such as agitation or irritability
- Excessive worry
- Changes in sleep patterns
- Change in appetite
- Denying the seriousness or extent of injury
- Signs and symptoms of depression
- Signs and symptoms of anxiety
- Lack in commitment or motivation to one's sport or rehabilitation
- Poor focus, concentration, or judgment
- Unconfirmed reports of pain
- Change in mood or inappropriate affect
- Suicidal thoughts

Jim has come into the athletic training room to discuss personal issues. It is evident that Jim feels comfortable talking with you. To help facilitate the discussion, it is important for you to employ helping skills to develop a relationship with Jim while assessing for red flags associated with psychological distress.

ROLE OF THE ATHLETIC TRAINER: THE PSYCHOSOCIAL DOMAIN

? Jim shares with you that he is homesick for his family and friends. In high school, he was popular and outgoing. Wrestling has been his life. He won the state title at the 180-lb weight class and received a full scholarship to wrestle at the university. His family is delighted that Jim is the first to go to college and is grateful that he is wrestling for such a prestigious university. Jim reports feeling pressured to succeed in sports and academics to please his parents.

For many individuals, the development and maintenance of a physically fit body provides a focal point for social and economic success as well as being essential to their identity as a physically active person. When participation in sport or physical activity is central to one's lifestyle, experiencing psychological distress or sustaining an injury can negatively impact an active lifestyle and overall well-being. Therefore, practitioners must know how to identify distress, provide education and support, and know when and how to refer patients with psychological concerns to the appropriate licensed mental health professionals.

Athletic trainers are considered second-level helpers for psychosocial concerns. Psychologists, psychiatrists, licensed counselors, and licensed independent clinical social workers are considered professional helpers, because they are trained and licensed to diagnose and treat psychological distress and disorders. Second-level helpers consist of health care practitioners who work in a wide range of allied health care fields providing direct patient care but who are not educated nor trained to provide mental health services.[17] The role of the athletic trainer, as a second-level helper and that which is consistent with the Role Delineation Competencies, is to be able to identify psychological distress and provide education, support, and make referrals when appropriate to mental health professionals. The NATA developed a consensus statement to guide the education of athletic trainers when working with athletes with psychological concerns.[10]

Helping Skills

Helping is defined as "assisting patients in exploring feelings, gaining insight, and making positive change in their lives."[18] Building a helping relationship is essential for effective helping. Using traditional patient-centered helper skills have been shown to be effective with establishing a working relationship with patients.[17,19] The OARS patient-centered counseling skills framework used in motivational interviewing has been shown to be effective for building the relationship as well as with facilitating change.[19] OARS stands for

- Open-ended questions

- Affirming

- Reflecting

- Summarizing

Open-ended questions are used to open the conversation and to allow the patient room to share his or her thoughts and feelings. An example of an open-ended question is "Tell me about your sleeping habits." *Affirming* patients is critical; that is, letting them know that they are doing a good job, that they are courageous, and so forth. It is important to remember that sharing personal challenges and struggles is not easy. *Reflections* are statements used to repeat or state back information to the patient to demonstrate that you, the helper, understand the meaning of what has been shared. A reflection could be a rephrase of what was heard or it could be a paraphrase with the addition of information from you about a hunch.

An example of this might be "I hear you say that you do not sleep well for several nights before a big match. I wonder if you are feeling some prematch performance anxiety." Finally, it is important to *summarize* what you have talked about to ensure that you and the patient are on the same page. It is often helpful to summarize the discussion prior to moving toward action. Use of these microskills by health care practitioners is effective when working with patients in health care settings, especially when time is limited.[20]

Cultural Competence

Cultural competence is the ability to embrace another person's worldview by "learning new patterns of behavior and effectively applying them in appropriate settings."[21(p3)] There are five key elements for achieving cultural competence: (1) value diversity, (2) having the capacity for cultural self-assessment, (3) being aware of the inherent dynamics when cultures interact, (4) institutionalizing cultural knowledge, and (5) developing appropriate adaptations for service delivery.[21] A recent study found that athletic trainers reported a high level of cultural competence, although this was not evidenced in how the athletic trainers delivered care.[22] Schlabach and Peer[23] believe that cultural competence is a foundational behavior for all athletic trainers. They contend that athletic trainers need to demonstrate that they embrace diversity and be knowledgeable and willing to serve all individuals in the global community.

The LEARN model was introduced in 1983 by Berlin and Fowkes[24] for assisting health care practitioners to enhance communication and better understand the worldview of a patient who may be culturally different from themselves. LEARN stands for

- Listen

- Elicit

- Acknowledge

- Recommend

- Negotiate

Listening requires that athletic trainers employ active listening skills. *Elicit* refers to using open-ended questions to gain general information about the patient's worldview. Next, it is important for the athletic trainer to *acknowledge* and discuss cultural similarities and differences with the patient. Intervention strategies need to integrate the patient's perspective or worldview about health, disease, and the health care system. Finally, the helper offers *recommendations* while keeping in mind that all intervention strategies are most effective when *negotiated* with the patient. The LEARN model is a collaborative effort between the athletic trainer and patient to assist with identifying culturally appropriate interventions. It is recommended that all athletic training education programs include multicultural training for entry-level practitioners, especially where athletic trainers provide services in a multitude of employment settings with patients across the lifespan that encompass many and varied diverse peoples.[25]

 You can empathize with Jim's concerns about succeeding in wrestling and in academics. As you ask open-ended questions and allow Jim to express his thoughts and feelings, you want to affirm that what Jim is feeling is normal for competitive athletes. As you listen to Jim's story, what have you learned about Jim's worldview?

THE DECISION-MAKING MODEL

? During your discussion, you have learned the following: Jim is concerned about a decrease in academic performance, is feeling homesick and misses his family and friends, is feeling pressured by the coach's decision to perform at a lower weight class, and feels stress associated with family expectations for success. You have noted a number of red flags that have concerned you about Jim and would like to consult with a mental health professional to develop effective strategies to work with Jim. Identify a mental health professional for a confidential consultation about how best to proceed with Jim.

The decision-making model (DMM), developed by Bacon and Anderson,[26] is a protocol to assist health care practitioners with identifying red flags associated with psychological distress and determining if these signs and symptoms warrant an emergency intervention, although unlikely, or the more typical planned intervention. Most patients exhibiting psychological distress will fall under a planned intervention. The DMM (**Fig. 9.1**) provides a guide for the athletic trainer to assess red flags that may signal psychological distress and help determine the patient's readiness for help seeking. Knowing a patient's level of readiness allows the athletic trainer to select effective strategies to facilitate readiness for change and/or help seeking.

Preliminary Assessment

The preliminary assessment begins when the practitioner encounters a patient who exhibits or self-reports signs and symptoms of psychological distress. These signs and symptoms may become apparent while taking a medical history or observed by the practitioner during the assessment. Using effective helping skills will aid in developing rapport with the patient and will facilitate the gathering of pertinent information. Other forms of data collection include direct observation, information from medical and educational records, and from key informants, when appropriate. This preliminary assessment is used to identify red flags; that is, signs and symptoms of psychological distress. Gourlay and Barnum[12] suggest identifying signs and symptoms in four domains: behavioral, cognitive, emotional/psychological, and medical/physical and to inquire about prior psychological distress, psychotropic medications, substance abuse, and prior hospitalizations. Examples of common signs and symptoms associated with stress can be seen in **Table 9.1**.

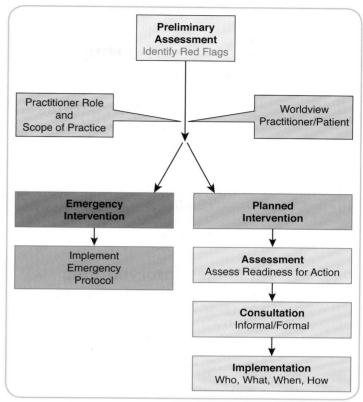

Figure 9.1. The decision-making model. (From Bacon VL, Anderson MK. *The Athletic Trainer's Role in Facilitating Healthy Behavior Change: The Psychosocial Domain.* Bridgewater, MA: Bridgewater State College; 2007. Reprinted with permission.)

TABLE 9.1 Common Signs and Symptoms Associated with Stress	
COGNITIVE	**PHYSICAL**
Confusion in thinking	Excessive sweating
Difficulty making decisions	Feeling dizzy
Decrease in concentration	Increased heart rate
Memory dysfunction	Elevated blood pressure
Poor judgment	Rapid breathing
Lowered academic performance	Increased symptoms of anxiety
EMOTIONAL	**BEHAVIORAL**
Emotional shock	Changes in behavior patterns
Feelings of anger, grief, loss, or depression	Changes in eating
Feeling overwhelmed	Withdrawal or isolative behavior
Decreased personal hygiene	Less attention to presentation
Presents with flattened affect	
Displays inappropriate and/or excessive affect	

From Bacon VL, Anderson MK. *The Athletic Trainer's Role in Facilitating Healthy Behavior Change: The Psychosocial Domain.* Bridgewater, MA: Bridgewater State College; 2007.

It is important to be mindful of the practitioner's role when working with patients exhibiting psychological distress, to adhere to the scope of practice listed in the Board of Certification (BOC) Role Delineation Study and licensing guidelines, as well as to demonstrate cultural competence as previously described. It is recommended that athletic trainers consult with a licensed mental health professional when working with patients with a psychological distress or disorder for guidance throughout the process.

Emergency Interventions

The emergency intervention protocol is implemented when presented signs and symptoms warrant immediate attention. Some examples of situations or conditions necessitating immediate attention include (1) a risk of suicide as assessed by a licensed mental health professional, (2) child or elder abuse where the patient is currently at risk, or (3) psychotic disorders where the patient may not be able to adequately care for himself or herself. Every institution, agency, school, or health care facility should have a protocol in place to address both medical and psychological emergencies. It is important for practitioners to be familiar with the established protocol as well as which mental health professional to contact for consultation or for making a referral.

Planned Interventions

Once it is determined that the athlete is not experiencing severe psychological distress and is not in danger of harming himself or herself or others, the athletic trainer may proceed with a planned intervention. It is important to use good helping skills and be culturally sensitive while building rapport and developing an effective helping relationship. The planned intervention entails three components:

- An assessment of readiness for action, which is typically mental health help seeking

- A selection and implementation of effective strategies that are consistent with the level of readiness

- A consultation/referral with a licensed mental health professional

Assessment

An essential factor in facilitating change is the practitioner's ability to assess the patient's level of readiness for any behavior, particularly one's readiness for change. The stages of change, also known as the transtheoretical model, was developed in 1982 by Prochaska, Norcosse, and DiClemente to help promote behavior change. The basic premise of the model, described in *Changing for Good*,[27] is that change is a process with predictable stages. There are specific processes that are effective at promoting change in each stage. Stages are not necessarily completed in order, and difficulties may be encountered in any of the stages. The five stages include the following:

- Precontemplation

- Contemplation

- Preparation

- Action

- Maintenance that leads to termination

Learning how to assess readiness for change will assist with determining what strategies have been shown to be effective for facilitating change. More specifically, the practitioner will assess patient's readiness for help seeking, that is, addressing the patient's psychological concerns with a licensed mental health professional. The authors list nine methods to facilitate a change with regard to an identified behavior, called change processes, and their intended use[27]:

1. Consciousness raising: to increase information about the self and the problem

2. Social liberation: to increase social alternatives for behaviors that are problematic

3. Emotional arousal: to experience and express feelings about one's problems and solutions

4. Self-reevaluation: to assess feelings and thoughts about the self with respect to a problem

5. Commitment: to choose to make a commitment to act, or believe in one's ability to change

6. Countering: to substitute alternatives for problem behaviors

7. Environment control: to avoid stimuli that elicit problem behaviors

8. Reward: to reward one's self, or being rewarded by others, for making change

9. Helping relationships: for enlisting the help of someone who cares

Implementation

The implementation of strategies by the athletic trainer to facilitate mental health help seeking requires the athletic trainer to continue to employ effective communication skills and to work within his or her role and professional boundaries. Using effective strategies can play a significant role in patient motivation, especially with rehabilitation adherence and with positive health outcomes.[28]

Motivational interviewing (MI) is a method used by many practitioners to enhance a patient's motivation to change. The elements of MI encompass the practitioner's ability to[20]

- Work in collaboration with the patient

- Listen for change talk used or not used by the patient

- Listen for language from the patient about wanting to maintain the "status quo"

- Think about resistance from the patient as being related to one or more of the following factors:

  - A lack of agreement between the practitioner and patient

  - Little to no collaboration

  - Low empathy from the practitioner

  - Little patient autonomy

When using MI, there are four basic principles to guide the practitioner while conversing with the patients: (1) Express empathy, (2) develop discrepancy, (3) roll with resistance (avoid arguing), and (4) support self-efficacy. MI is often used in conjunction with change theory, because MI has been shown to be effective with facilitating motivation for change for the different stages of change.[20]

Consultation and Referrals to Licensed Mental Health Professionals

An important competency for athletic trainers is the ability to identify psychological distress and to know how to make a referral for psychological concerns as well as to select and recommend appropriate mental health professionals. Estimates about the prevalence of mental illness are high and expected to increase. Current estimates show 19% of adults (43 million) and 60% of children and adolescents have a diagnosable mental disorder necessitating a mental health intervention. What is also known is that a central factor preventing those in need of mental health services from taking action continues to be not seeking professional help.[10] Knowing how to assess for readiness for change will assist with determining what strategies will help facilitate change in the patient's readiness for mental health help seeking, that is, addressing their psychological concerns with a licensed mental health professional.

Licensed Mental Health Professionals

There are several types of mental health professionals available to athletic trainers for referrals. Each profession has unique education and clinical training that must comply with state licensing requirements. It is important to be familiar with the different professions and to make certain that the mental health professional holds a valid license to practice.

◼ Psychiatrist

Psychiatrists are licensed medical doctors who are educated and trained to provide mental health services. Formal education and training entails completing a 4-year undergraduate degree, 4 years of medical school, and then completing an internship and residency for a minimum of 3 years. Psychiatrists are trained to diagnose and treat mental illness, including the ability to prescribe psychotropic medicine. Psychiatrists work in a variety of settings, such as private practice, mental health centers, and hospitals.

◼ Psychologist

Psychologists are mental health professionals who have completed an approved clinical or counseling degree, which consists of an undergraduate degree, a master's degree, and an approved doctoral program (120 credit hours). In addition to their formal education, they complete a mental health practicum, a 1-year predoctoral internship, and 1 to 2 years of postdoctoral training. Psychologists are trained to conduct psychological testing to assist in the prevention, assessment, diagnosis, and treatment of mental disorders. Licensed psychologists work in a variety of settings, including private practice, mental health centers, hospitals, government settings, and in applied research.

◼ Social Worker

Social workers are mental health professionals who are educated and trained to work with patients and who provide a wide variety of services. A bachelor's degree in social work is the minimum standard and prepares professionals for entry-level positions. A master's degree in social work is required in order to provide direct clinical mental health services. Licensed independent clinical social workers (LICSWs) are trained and licensed to provide direct mental health care, supervision, and the administration of health care programs. LICSWs complete 60 credit hours of education at the master's level, a practicum, an internship, and 2 years of postdegree experience. LICSWs work in a wide range of employment settings.

◼ Professional Counselor

Professional counselors are prepared for work in schools, colleges, community mental health settings, and private practice. Each type of counselor has different education and training requirements. Licensed professional counselors are educated and trained to provide therapy, have completed minimum of 60 credit hours of formal education at the master's degree level, a practicum, an internship, and 2 years of postdegree experience.

◼ Marriage and Family Therapist

Marriage and family therapists provide direct mental health services similar to professional counselors. They complete a 60 credit hours master's degree program, a practicum and an internship, as well as 2 years of postdegree experience. Licensed marriage and family therapists provide assessment and treatment using a family systems perspective with individuals, families, and groups. They work in a variety of practice settings, including private practice, community mental health centers, and hospitals.

◼ Sport Psychologist/Sport Performance Consultant

Sport psychologists and sport performance consultants are trained to work with athletes to achieve optimal performance. Whereas a sport psychologist often has completed the education, training, and is licensed to practice as a mental health professional, a sport performance consultant is not trained to diagnose and treat mental health issues. It is important to ascertain whether a sport psychologist holds a state-approved psychologist license. Some sport psychologists and sport performance consultants are certified with the Association for the Advancement of Applied Sports Psychology. Although this certification is good to have, it is not required.

 Individuals that could be consulted to help with strategies for Jim include a psychologist, social worker, or professional counselor. These individuals are educated and trained to assess and treat patients with a mental illness or disorder.

INJURY AND REHABILITATION

> **?** Riley, a female distance runner, is diagnosed with plantar fasciitis a week before an Olympic qualifying race. She has been training for this race and a potential spot on the Olympic team for the past 3 years. The injury will prevent her from competing at her desired level for approximately 1 month, eliminating any chance of a position on the Olympic team. How might this patient react to the inability to race competitively? What impact will this reaction have on her rehabilitation? How can the athletic trainer provide education, guidance, and support to help this person cope with the physical, psychological, and emotional effects of being injured and completing a successful injury rehabilitation plan?

Sports injury is a potential risk for all athletes and physically active individuals. Athletic trainers are well equipped to conduct an assessment of an injury and to make decisions about the medical needs of the injured patient. In addition to treating the physical injury, recovery and rehabilitation involves an understanding of an injured patient's psychological response to being injured as well as knowledge about psychological factors associated with rehabilitation and recovery.

Understanding the Impact of Injury

A number of theories have been offered that provide a framework for understanding the impact of injury on a physically active individual. Although each model looks at the impact of injury somewhat differently, they all contend that psychosocial factors are complex and need to be given consideration. In 1986, Feltz[8] suggested there are three potential psychological effects of injury: (1) emotional trauma of the injury, (2) psychological factors associated with rehabilitation and recovery, and (3) the psychological impact of the injury on an individual's future with respect to continuing to be physically active or involved in sports. Evidence-based practices recommend a psychosocial approach when addressing injury rehabilitation with athletes.[29]

The stage perspective by Kübler-Ross[30] suggests that there are stages of grieving through which an individual progresses when confronted with loss. Kübler-Ross[30] identified the following stages: (1) disbelief, denial, and isolation; (2) anger; (3) bargaining; (4) depression; and (5) acceptance. Although this model has some intuitive appeal, the stereotypic linear pattern of distinct emotional responses has not stood up to empirical scrutiny.[31] Furthermore, if an individual reacts to injury in stages, then practitioners should be able to predict a patient's progress during rehabilitation; however, this rarely is the case for injured individuals.

The affective cycle of injury has had great appeal, because this model identifies four quadrants impacted when an individual has sustained an injury: physical well-being, emotional well-being, social well-being, and self-concept.[32] Heil's model is holistic in nature. He contends that these quadrants are interrelated and may be a source of stress for the patient. Heil's model depicts the process of rehabilitation and recovery that begins with distress and then moves to denial and finally to determined coping for those who recover psychologically.

Heil identified 10 indicators of successful recovery[33]:

1. Know the game: being educated about the rehabilitation process

2. Goal-directed thinking: setting realistic short-term and long-term goals

3. Focused attention: the ability to focus, which is helpful with sport performance and rehabilitation

4. Controlled emotional intensity: the ability to channel emotions

5. Precise skill execution: using good form with body building and with rehabilitation exercises

6. Training intensity: understanding training principles for conditioning and rehabilitation; that is adequate load without overloading, which can lead to reinjury

7. Performance over pain: the ability to cope with pain and use pain management techniques

8. Calculated risk taking: effective decision making for optimal performance and injury prevention

9. Mental toughness: the ability to remain positive and determined

10. Self-actualization: the ability to grow from successes and challenges

Regardless of the framework used, it is important for the practitioner to understand the psychosocial factors associated with injury and recovery as well as to monitor the injured individual's level of stress for signs and symptoms of psychological distress.

Injury, Rehabilitation, and Recovery

A collaborative team approach to injury rehabilitation has been shown to have a positive influence on rehabilitation outcomes.[29] It is essential that the athletic trainer involve the patient in all phases of treatment as well as to provide education about the many challenges the injured person will face during the rehabilitation process. Injured individuals may experience a plethora of thoughts and emotions (e.g., fear, isolation, disruption in identity, loss of income, or potential scholarships), which left untreated, may lead to psycho-socio-emotional difficulties (**Table 9.2**). It is important for the injured individual to experience a steady rate of recovery in order to reduce the patent's frustration and enhance the patient's belief in the ability to achieve a successful outcome.

Strategies to Facilitate and Enhance Coping Skills Postinjury

A number of strategies can be employed by the practitioner to assist athletes and physically active individuals cope more effectively with injury. Several strategies have shown to be effective in assisting athletes through the recovery process, such as education, goal setting, social support, and the use of mental skills during rehabilitation.[33,34] These strategies assist the injured individual to negotiate challenges, maintain his or her motivation, and regain his or her confidence. Research has found that when athletic trainers are skilled with employing mental skills and maintain a positive attitude about the rehabilitation process, athletes' recovery rates and adherence with rehabilitation are improved.[35,36]

Education

It is imperative that the clinician inform the injured patient about the injury and recovery process. This includes sharing information about the treatment plan, intended goals, and any side effects or sensations that may be experienced along the way. Educating the patient helps him or her understand the rehabilitation process, avoid surprises, and, hopefully, reduce anxiety associated with the recovery and rehabilitation process.[37] Stiller-Ostrowski, Gould, and Covassin[38] state that injured athletes report good communication skills as being very important for having a good rapport with athletic trainers, which is also associated with favorable rehabilitation outcomes.

TABLE 9.2 Signs and Symptoms of Anxiety in Rehabilitation	
CATEGORY	**SIGNS AND SYMPTOMS**
Physical	Muscle tension and bracing; short, choppy breathing; decreased coordination; fatigue; rushed speech; minor secondary injuries or nagging illness with recurrent physical complaints; and sleeping problems
Cognitive	Excessive negativity and overly self-critical statements of low confidence in rehabilitation, extreme thinking and unrealistic expectations, and very narrow focus
Emotional	Anger, depression, irritability, moodiness, and impatience
Social	Decreased communication, social withdrawal, intolerance, and abruptness with others
Performance	Overall decline in motivation and enjoyment in rehabilitation, loss of interest in sports and other activities, nervousness and physical tension during therapy, trying too hard in therapy or "giving up" in response to obstacles and setbacks, and decrease in school or work performance

Goal Setting

Goal setting is an effective strategy shown to increase motivation during the recovery program. This practice helps to guide the individual's efforts by providing a sense of control that may enhance motivation, persistence, and commitment, and thus facilitates the incorporation of new strategies to improve performance. Individuals who set specific personal goals exhibit an increase in self-efficacy; that is, they feel empowered and experience greater satisfaction with the rehabilitation and recovery process.[9,39]

Gould[39] suggests the following guidelines for setting goals for improved effectiveness:

- Set measurable goals.
- Goals should be moderately difficult yet realistic.
- Set both short-term and long-term goals.
- Have both process and performance goals.
- Set goals for specific program.
- Make the goals positive.

Goal setting is best accomplished when patients have a strong working relationship and work collaboratively toward rehabilitation goals. Goals should be written to include a target date and should be monitored by the athletic trainer, as well as evaluated. **Box 9.2** provides guidelines for establishing goals for rehabilitation.

Social Support

Social support has been extensively researched and has been found to play a significant role with rehabilitation and recovery for athletes and is seen as a central factor in the rehabilitation process.[40,41] Social support encompasses listening, emotional support, assistance, and reality confirmation.[42] Social support comes from key individuals in the patient's family, circle of friends, teammates, coaches, and athletic trainers. A strong positive correlation has been found between the athletic trainer's positive beliefs about recovery and the injured athlete's positive beliefs about his or

---

BOX 9.2 Guidelines to Goal Setting

Goals should be:

- **Specific and measurable.** The patient must know exactly what to do and be able to determine if gains are made.
- **Stated in positive versus negative language.** Knowing what to do guides behavior, whereas knowing what to avoid creates a focus on errors without providing a constructive alternative.
- **Challenging but realistic.** Overly difficult goals set up the individual for failure and pose a threat to the individual. The lower the individual's self-confidence, the more important success becomes and the greater the importance of setting attainable goals.
- **Established on a timetable for completion.** This allows a check on progress and an evaluation of whether realistic goals have been set.
- **Integrated as short-, intermediate-, and long-term goals.** A comprehensive program links daily activities with expectations for specific competitions as well as for season and career goals.
- **Personalized and internalized.** The patient must embrace goals as his or her own, not as something from the outside.
- **Monitored and evaluated.** Feedback must be provided to assess goals, and the goals should be modified based on progress.
- **Linked to life goals.** This identifies sport and rehabilitation as learning experiences in life, and it helps the individual put sport/physical activity in a broader perspective. This is especially important for individuals whose return to sport/activity is doubtful.

her own recovery process.[41] It is imperative that athletic trainers help secure a supportive network for the athlete to reduce potential isolation and increase rehabilitation outcomes.

Mental Skills Techniques

Mental skills techniques have been successful for enhancing performance as well as with facilitating recovery from injury. Specifically, the use of relaxation, imagery, and positive self-talk have been shown to facilitate the recovery process and to increase adherence rates.[33] Athletes can learn and practice these skills and strategies and employ them as needed.

■ Relaxation

Relaxation is an effective technique to help reduce pain and the effects of anxiety. Once an individual has learned deep relaxation skills, he or she can use these skills to reduce and often remove localized tension associated with injury as well as to facilitate recovery from fatigue.[43] Relaxation techniques can help reduce tension, slow breathing, and lower heart rate, all of which are important techniques that can extend over the course of one's life. Two general methods of relaxation training exist; namely, mind to muscle and muscle to mind. Mind to muscle is accomplished with the aid of meditation and/or imagery techniques. Muscle to mind involves breathing exercises and progressive relaxation, the active contraction of various muscles. Relaxation techniques are most effective when practiced and learned during times of low demand; that is, out of season. A review of the literature by Williams[43] shows that individuals with an internal locus of control who maintain a positive outlook appear to be more successful with learning and applying relaxation techniques (**Table 9.3**).

■ Imagery

Imagery has long been used in the physical training process to enhance performance. It involves the mental practice of a skill before the actual physical performance of the skill. In the rehabilitation process, imagery can be used to mentally practice the skills or processes that will expedite and promote a safe return to activity, such as envisioning healing, soothing (i.e., pain management), or performance (i.e., proper technique of an exercise). Imagery can be enhanced by preceding it with relaxation exercises, such as passive or progressive relaxation. These relaxation techniques can

TABLE 9.3 Relaxation Techniques	
TECHNIQUE	**EXAMPLES**
Pain Reduction	
Deep breathing	Emphasize slow, deep, rhythmic breathing.
Muscle relaxation	Passive or progressive relaxation
Meditation	Repetitive focusing on mantra or breathing
Therapeutic massage	Manual manipulation of muscles, tendons, and ligaments
Pain Focusing	
External focus	Listening to relaxing or inspiring music, watching a movie, or playing chess
Soothing imagery	Generating calming images (e.g., lying on a beach or floating in space)
Neutral imaginings	Imagining playing chess or building a model airplane
Rhythmic cognitive activity	Saying the alphabet backward or meditating
Pain acknowledgment	Giving pain a "hot" color, such as red, and then changing it to a less painful "cool" color, such as blue
Dramatic coping	Seeing pain as being part of an epic challenge to overcome insurmountable odds
Situational assessment	Evaluating the causes of pain to take steps to reduce it

reduce anxiety and the physical manifestations of pain and can increase the vividness and control in imagery. Mental imagery can serve to motivate the individual to realize that this technique can facilitate his or her performance on return to activity.[44]

■ Positive Self-talk

Control over one's cognition has been shown to directly impact a person's self-confidence.[45] Injured individuals often express negative thoughts and feelings about the injury, which in turn, can lead to low self-esteem and low self-confidence. Negative thinking leads to negative feelings and ultimately to unproductive behavior (e.g., poor performance, poor recovery). The negative thoughts can be redirected into positive thoughts that direct and motivate the individual to succeed with his or her rehabilitation.

> The distance runner will not be able to try out for a position on the next Olympic team. Clearly, her emotional and psychological state will have a direct impact on the success or failure of the therapeutic exercise program. Goal setting and mental skills training can be beneficial in addressing psychological influences that may inhibit the program. If progress is inhibited for several days because of suspected psychological issues, the athletic trainer should consult with a licensed mental health professional.

SUMMARY

1. Statistics show mental disorders to be the number one cause of disability in the United States.

2. Athletes experience a greater degree of stress related to the additional demands of their sport, risk of injury, and expectations for success.

3. Psychological distress can be associated with a patient's internal state (i.e., psychological/emotional) and external stressors (i.e., sociological, cultural, contextual).

4. Athletic trainers are considered second-level helpers for psychosocial concerns.

5. The OARS patient-centered counseling skills used in MI stands for open-ended questions, affirming, reflecting, and summarizing.

6. The five key elements for achieving cultural competence are to (1) value diversity, (2) have the capacity for cultural self-assessment, (3) be aware of the inherent dynamics when cultures interact, (4) institutionalize cultural knowledge, and (5) develop appropriate adaptations for service delivery.

7. The LEARN model can assist practitioners to enhance communication and to better understand the worldview of a patient who may be culturally different from themselves. LEARN stands for listen, elicit, acknowledge, recommend, and negotiate.

8. The DMM is a protocol to assist with identifying red flags associated with psychological distress and determining if these signs and symptoms warrant an emergency or planned intervention.

9. During the preliminary assessment, red flags denoting possible psychological distress should be noted in four domains: behavioral, cognitive, emotional/psychological, and medical/physical.

10. Situations or conditions necessitating an emergency intervention include (1) a risk of suicide as assessed by a licensed mental health professional, (2) a child or elder abuse where the patient is currently at risk, or (3) psychotic disorders where the patient may not be able to adequately care for himself or herself.

11. Planned intervention entails the assessment of readiness for action, typically help seeking, the selection and implementation of effective strategies consistent with the level of readiness, and consultation/referral with a licensed mental health professional.

12. The stages of change, also known as the transtheoretical model, include the stages of precontemplation, contemplation, preparation, action, and maintenance that leads to termination.

13. When using MI, the practitioner should express empathy, develop discrepancy, roll with resistance (avoid arguing), and support self-efficacy.

14. Mental health professionals that may be consulted for psychosocial issues include psychiatrists, psychologists, social workers, professional counselors, marriage and family therapists, or sport psychologists.

15. The affective cycle of injury, developed by Heil, identifies four quadrants impacted when an individual has sustained an injury: physical well-being, emotional well-being, social well-being, and self-concept. These factors may stem from the emotional trauma of the injury, the psychological factors associated with rehabilitation and recovery, and the psychological impact of the injury on an individual's future with respect to continuing to be physically active or involved in sports.

16. Strategies that may facilitate and enhance coping skills postinjury include education, goal setting, social support, and mental skills techniques encompassing relaxation techniques, imagery, and positive self-talk.

APPLICATION QUESTIONS

1. When doing a formal assessment, why is it important to note changes in behavior, affect, and cognition?

2. Explain the role of a second-level helper, and how it differs from the role of a mental health professional?

3. Describe in detail the OARS patient-centered counseling skills.

4. In the opening scenario of this chapter, Jim, the collegiate wrestler, is Latino. Apply the LEARN model to demonstrate your cultural competence.

5. Identify and describe the steps of the planned intervention using the DMM protocol that you would use with Jim the wrestler.

6. Create an MI dialogue demonstrating the elements of MI when working to facilitate help seeking with Jim.

7. Describe the training and credentials of two mental health professionals.

8. Identify and describe the strategies that you would employ with Riley, the female distance runner, to facilitate and enhance coping postinjury.

REFERENCES

1. World Health Organization. *Mental Health Action Plan 2013-2020*. Geneva, Switzerland: World Health Organization; 2013.

2. Substance Abuse and Mental Health Services Administration. *Achieving the Promise: Transforming Mental Health Care in America, Executive Summary*. Rockville, MD: President's New Freedom Commission on Mental Health; 2003.

3. U.S. Department of Health and Human Services. *Healthy People 2010: Understanding and Improving Health*. 2nd ed. Washington, DC: U.S. Government Printing Office; 2000.

4. National Institute of Mental Health. The numbers count: mental disorders in America. http://www.nimh.nih.gov/health/publications. Accessed March 4, 2011.

5. Substance Abuse and Mental Health Services Administration. *Behavioral Health Barometer, United States, 2014*. Rockville, MD: Substance Abuse and Mental Health Services Administration; 2014.

6. Institute of Health Metrics and Evaluation. *The Global Burden of Disease 2010*. Washington, DC: Lancet; 2010.

7. Gulliver A, Griffiths K, Christensen H. Barriers and facilitators to mental health help-seeking for

young elite athletes: a qualitative study. *BMC Psychiatry.* 2012;12:157.

8. Feltz DL. The psychology of sport injuries. In: Vinger PF, Hoerner EF, eds. *Sports Injuries: The Unthwarted Epidemic.* 2nd ed. Littleton, MA: PSG Publishing; 1986:336–344.

9. American College of Sports Medicine, American Academy of Family Physicians, American Academy of Orthopaedic Surgeons, et al. Psychological issues related to injury in athletes and the team physician: a consensus statement. *Med Sci Sports Exerc.* 2006;38(11):2030–2034.

10. Neal TL, Diamond AB, Goldman S, et al. Inter-association recommendations for developing a plan to recognize and refer student-athletes with psychological concerns at the collegiate level: an executive summary of a consensus statement. *J Athl Train.* 2013;48(5):716–720.

11. Henderson JC. Suicide in sport: athletes at risk. In: Pargman D, ed. *Psychological Bases of Sport Injuries.* 3rd ed. Morgantown, WV: Fitness Information Technology; 2007:267–285.

12. Gourlay L, Barnum M. Recognizing psychological disorders, part 1: overview. *Athl Ther Today.* 2010;15(6):15–18.

13. Brenner J, Swanik K. High-risk drinking characteristics in collegiate athletes. *J Am Coll Health.* 2007;56(3):267–272.

14. Weiss SM, Loubier SL. Gambling habits of athletes and nonathletes classified as disordered gamblers. *J Psychol.* 2010;144(6):507–521.

15. Centers for Disease Control and Prevention. *Excessive Alcohol Use: Addressing a Leading Risk for Death, Chronic Disease, and Injury.* Atlanta, GA: Centers for Disease Control and Prevention; 2011.

16. Biviano GM. *Athletic Trainers' Comfort and Competence in Addressing Psychological Issues of Athletes* [master's thesis]. San Jose, CA: San Jose State University Press. http://scholarworks.sjsu.edu/etd_theses/3801/. Accessed July 24, 2015.

17. Egan G, Owen JJ, Reese RJ. *The Skilled Helper: A Problem-Management and Opportunity-Development Approach to Helping.* 10th ed. Belmont, CA: Thomas/Brooks Cole; 2013.

18. Hill CE. *Helping Skills: Facilitating Exploration, Insight and Action.* 3rd ed. Washington, DC: American Psychological Association; 2009.

19. Miller WR, Moyers TB. Eight stages of learning motivational interviewing. *J Teach Addict.* 2006;5(1):3–17.

20. Rollnick S, Miller WR, Butler CC. *Motivational Interviewing in Health Care: Helping Patients Change Behavior.* New York, NY: Guilford Press; 2008.

21. King MA, Sims A, Osher D. How is cultural competence integrated in education? http://cep.air.org/cultural/Q_integrated.htm. Accessed February 20, 2011.

22. Marra J, Covassin T, Shingles RR, et al. Assessment of certified athletic trainers' level of cultural competence in the delivery of health care. *J Athl Train.* 2010;45(4):380–385.

23. Schlabach GA, Peer KS. *Professional Ethics in Athletic Training.* St. Louis, MO: Mosby Elsevier; 2008.

24. Berlin EA, Fowkes WC Jr. A teaching framework for cross-cultural health care. Application in family practice. *West J Med.* 1983;139(6):934–938.

25. Geisler PR. Multiculturalism and athletic training education: implications for educational and professional progress. *J Athl Train.* 2003;38(2):141–151.

26. Bacon VL, Anderson MK. *The Athletic Trainer's Role in Facilitating Healthy Behavior Change: The Psychosocial Domain.* Bridgewater, MA: Bridgewater State College; 2007.

27. Prochaska JO, Norcross JC, DiClemente CC. *Changing for Good.* New York, NY: Harper Collins Publishing; 1994.

28. Levensky E, Forcehimes A, O'Donohue W, et al. Motivational interviewing: an evidence-based approach to counseling helps patients follow treatment recommendations. *Am J Nurs.* 2007;107(10):50–58.

29. Podlog L, Heil J, Schulte S. Psychosocial factors in sports injury rehabilitation and return to play. *Phys Med Rehabil Clin N Am.* 2014;25(4):915–930.

30. Kübler-Ross E. *On Death and Dying: What the Dying Have to Teach Doctors, Nurses, Their Own Families.* New York, NY: MacMillan; 1969.

31. Wagman D, Khelifa M. Psychological issues in sport injury rehabilitation: current knowledge and practice. *J Athl Train.* 1996;31(3):257–261.

32. Heil J. *Psychology of Sport Injury.* Champaign, IL: Human Kinetics; 1993.

33. O'Connor EO, Heil J, Harmer P, et al. Injury. In: Taylor J, Wilson G, eds. *Applying Sport Psychology: Four Perspectives.* Champaign, IL: Human Kinetics; 2005:187–206.

34. Brown C. Injuries: The psychology of recovery and rehab. In: Murphy SM, ed. *Sport Psychology Interventions.* Champaign, IL: Human Kinetics; 2005:215–235.

35. Tracey J. Inside the clinic: health professionals' role in their clients' psychological rehabilitation. *J Sport Rehab.* 2008;17(4):413–431.

36. Hamson-Utley JJ, Martin S, Walters J. Athletic trainers' and physical therapists' perceptions of the effectiveness of psychological skills within sport injury rehabilitation programs. *J Athl Train.* 2008;43(3):258–264.

37. Fisher LA, Wrisberg CA. What athletic training students want to know about sport psychology. *Athl Ther Today.* 2006;11(3):32–33.

38. Stiller-Ostrowski JL, Gould DR, Covassin T. An evaluation of an educational intervention in psychology of injury for athletic training students. *J Athl Train.* 2009;44(5):482–489.

39. Gould D. Goal setting for peak performance. In: William JM, ed. *Applied Sport Psychology: Personal Growth to Peak Performance*. 6th ed. New York, NY: McGraw-Hill; 2010:201–220.

40. Williams RA, Appaneal RN. Social support and sport injury. *Athl Ther Today*. 2010;15(4):46–49.

41. Bone JB, Fry MD. The influence of injured athletes' perceptions of social support from ATCs on their beliefs about rehabilitation. *J Sport Rehabil*. 2006;15(2):156–167.

42. Richman JM, Rosenfeld LB, Hardy CJ. The social support survey: a validation study of a clinical measure of the social support process. *Res Soc Work Pract*. 1993;3(3):288–311.

43. Williams JM. Relaxation and energizing techniques for regulation of arousal. In: Williams JM, ed. *Applied Sport Psychology: Personal Growth to Peak Performance*. 6th ed. New York, NY: McGraw-Hill; 2010:247–266.

44. Monsma E, Mensch J, Farroll J. Keeping your head in the game: sport-specific imagery and anxiety among injured athletes. *J Athl Train*. 2009;44(4):410–417.

45. Krane V, Williams JM. Psychological characteristics of peak performance. In: Williams JM, ed. *Applied Sport Psychology: Personal Growth to Peak Performance*. 6th ed. New York, NY: McGraw-Hill; 2010:169–188.

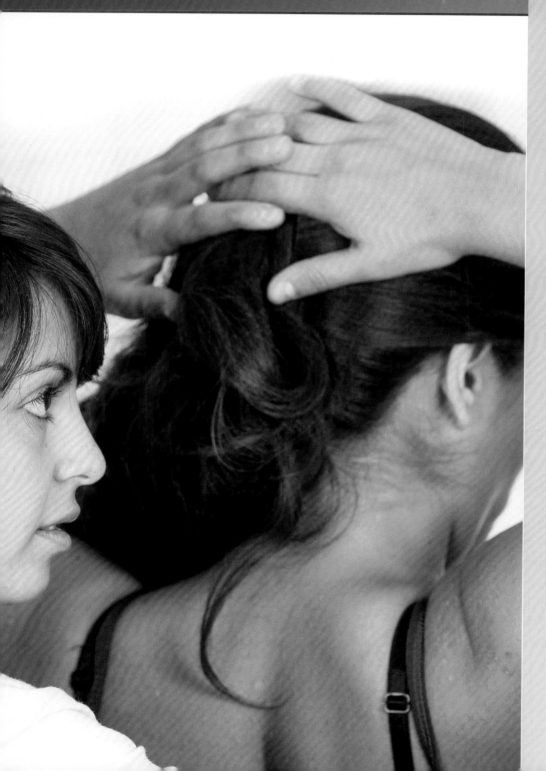

Therapeutic Interventions

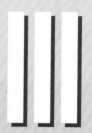

Tissue Healing and Wound Care

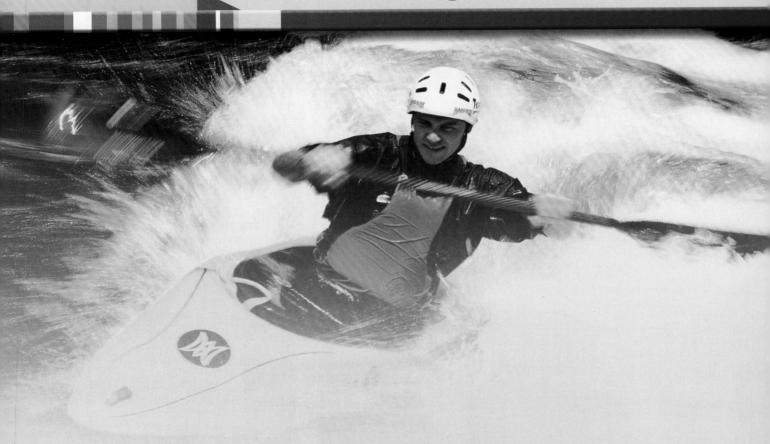

STUDENT OUTCOMES

1. Describe the major mechanical forces that produce injury to biological tissues; namely, compression, tension, shear, stress, strain, bending, and torsion.

2. Explain the effect of the material constituents and structural organization of the skin, tendons, ligaments, muscles, and bone on their ability to withstand the mechanical loads to which each is subjected.

3. List common injuries of the skin, muscles, tendons, joints, and bone.

4. Describe the processes by which tissue healing occurs in the skin, tendons, muscles, ligaments, and bone.

5. Explain wound care for both superficial and deep soft-tissue injuries.

6. Describe the appropriate immediate management of bone injuries.

7. Explain the mechanisms by which nerves are injured and the processes by which nerves can heal.

8. Describe the types of altered sensations that can result from a nerve injury.

9. Describe the appropriate immediate management of nerve injuries.

10. Explain the neurological basis of pain, including factors that mediate pain.

INTRODUCTION

Human movement during sport and exercise typically is faster and produces greater force than activities of daily living. As a result, the potential for injury also is heightened. Understanding the different ways in which forces act on the body is necessary to comprehend techniques to prevent injuries. Likewise, knowing the material and structural properties of the skin, tendons, muscles, ligaments, bones, and nerves can lay a foundation for understanding the response of these tissues to applied forces can facilitate an individual's safe return to sport participation.

This chapter begins with a general discussion of injury mechanisms, including descriptions of force and torque as well as their effects. This is followed by sections on soft tissues, bones, and nerves, addressing the mechanical characteristics of these tissues, the classification of injuries, processes by which the specific tissues heal, and general wound care for these injuries. A more detailed explanation of wound care for specific injuries is discussed in individual chapters.

INJURY MECHANISMS

 When the human body sustains force, the potential exists to strengthen body tissues or to injure them. A previously sedentary, middle-aged adult wants to initiate a running program as a way to improve his cardiovascular fitness. What advice should be provided to this individual for reducing the risk of sustaining a mechanical stress–related injury? Why?

Analyzing the mechanics of injuries to the human body is complicated by several factors. First, potentially injurious forces applied to the body act at different angles, over different surface areas, and over different periods of time. Second, the human body is composed of many different types of tissue, which respond differently to applied forces. Finally, injury to the human body is not an all-or-nothing phenomenon; that is, injuries range in severity. This section introduces the types of mechanical loading that can cause injury and describes the basic mechanical responses of biological tissues to these forms of loading.

Force and Its Effects

Force may be thought of as a push or a pull acting on a body. A multitude of forces act on our bodies routinely during the day. The forces of gravity and friction enable us to move about in predictable ways when muscles produce internal forces. During participation in sports and physical activities, force is applied to sticks, balls, bats, racquets, clubs, and other objects. Force is absorbed from impact with the ground or floor, the object used, in contact sports, and even other participants.

When a force acts, two potential effects on the target object exist. The first is acceleration, or change in velocity, and the second is deformation, or change in shape. For example, when a racquetball is struck with a racquet, the ball is both accelerated (i.e., put in motion in the direction of the racquet swing) and deformed (i.e., flattened on the side that is struck). The greater the stiffness of the material to which a force is applied, the greater the likelihood that the deformation will be too small to be easily seen. The more elastic the material to which a force is applied, the greater the likelihood that the deformation will be temporary, with the material springing back to regain its original shape.

When tissues sustain a force, two primary factors dictate whether injury occurs—namely, the size, or magnitude, of the force and the material properties of the involved tissues (**Box 10.1**).

BOX 10.1 Factors Affecting the Likelihood of Injury

■ Size or magnitude of the force

■ The force's moment arm, which determines the amount of torque generated

■ Direction in which the force is applied (i.e., axial torque generated compression, tensile, or shear force)

■ Material properties of the tissues affected and their ability to sustain strain

■ Area over which the force is applied

■ Magnitude of stress produced by the force

A load-deformation curve demonstrates the deformation of a structure in response to progressive loading or force application. If a load is relatively small, the response of the structure is elastic. As such, when the load is removed, the material will return to its original size and shape. Within the elastic region of the load-deformation curve, the greater the stiffness of the material, the steeper the slope of the line becomes. Therefore, greater stiffness translates to less deformation in response to a given load. If a load exceeds the material's **yield point**, or **elastic limit**, however, the response of the structure is plastic. In this situation, when the load is removed, some amount of deformation will remain. Loads exceeding the ultimate failure point on the load-deformation curve result in mechanical failure of the structure, which translates into the fracturing of bone or rupturing of soft tissues.

The direction of an applied force also has important implications for injury potential. Many tissues are **anisotropic**, meaning that the structure is stronger in resisting force from certain directions compared to others. The anatomical design of many of the joints of the human body also means they are more susceptible to injury from a given direction. For example, lateral ankle sprains are much more common than medial ankle sprains because of the bony configuration and ligamentous support on the medial side. Consequently, when discussing injury mechanisms, force commonly is categorized according to the direction from which the force acts on the affected structure.

Force acting along the long axis of a structure is termed **axial force**. In fencing, when an opponent is touched with the foil, the foil is loaded axially. When the human body is in an upright standing position, body weight creates axial loads on the femur and tibia.

Axial loading that produces a squeezing or crushing effect is termed **compressive force**, or compression (**Fig. 10.1A**). The weight of the human body constantly produces compression on the bones that support it. The 5th lumbar vertebra must support the weight of the head, trunk, and arms when the body is erect, producing compression on the intervertebral disk below it. When a football player is sandwiched between two opposing players, the force acting on that player is compressive. In the absence of sufficient padding, compressive forces often result in bruises or contusions.

Axial loading in the direction opposite that of compression is called **tensile force**, or tension (**Fig. 10.1B**). Tension is a pulling force that tends to stretch the object to which it is applied. Muscle contraction produces tensile force on the attached bone, enabling movement of that bone. When the foot and ankle are inverted, the tensile forces applied to the lateral ligaments may result in an ankle sprain.

Whereas compressive and tensile forces are directed, respectively, toward and away from an object, a third category of force, termed **shear force**, acts parallel or tangent to a plane passing through the object (**Fig. 10.1C**). Shear force tends to cause one part of the object to slide or displace with respect to another part of the object. For example, shear forces acting on the spine can cause spondylolisthesis, a condition involving anterior slippage of a vertebra with respect to the vertebra below it.

When the human body sustains force, another important factor related to the likelihood of injury is the magnitude of the stress produced by that force. Mechanical **stress** is defined as force divided by the surface area over which the force is applied (**Fig. 10.2**). When a given force is distributed over a large area, the resulting stress is less than if the force were distributed over a smaller area. Alternatively, if a force is concentrated over a small area, the mechanical stress is relatively high. A high magnitude of stress, rather than a high magnitude of force, is what tends to result in injury to

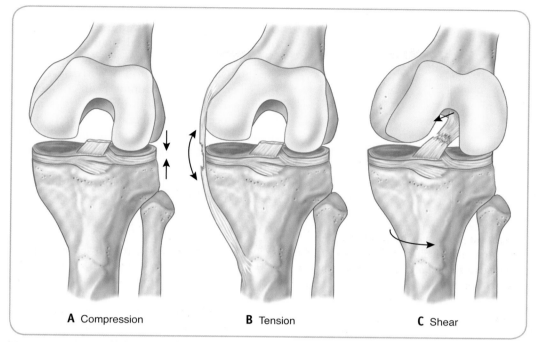

A Compression   **B** Tension   **C** Shear

Figure 10.1. Mechanisms of injury. Compression **(A)** and tension **(B)** are directed along the longitudinal axis of a structure, whereas shear **(C)** acts parallel to a surface.

biological tissues. One of the reasons that participants in contact sports wear pads is because a pad dissipates force across its entire area, thereby reducing the stress acting on the player.

Strain may be thought of as the amount of deformation an object undergoes in response to an applied force. Application of compressive force to an object produces shortening and widening of the structure, whereas tensile force produces lengthening and narrowing of the structure. Shear results in internal changes in the structure on which the force is acting. The ultimate strength of biological tissues determines the amount of strain that a structure can withstand without fracturing or rupturing.

Injury to biological tissues can result from a single traumatic force of relatively large magnitude or from repeated forces of relatively smaller magnitude. When a single force produces an injury, the injury is called an **acute injury** and the causative force is termed a **macrotrauma**. An acute injury, such as a ruptured anterior cruciate ligament or a fractured humerus, is characterized by a definitive moment of onset followed by a relatively predictable process of healing. When repeated or chronic loading over a period of time produces an injury, that injury is called a **chronic injury** or **stress injury**, and the causative mechanism is termed **microtrauma**. A chronic injury, such as glenohumeral bursitis or a metatarsal stress fracture, develops and worsens gradually over time, typically culminating in a threshold episode in which pain and inflammation become evident. Chronic injuries may persist for months or years.

Many tissues, including tendons, ligaments, muscles, and bones, tend to respond to gradually increased mechanical stress by becoming larger and stronger. According to the basic principle

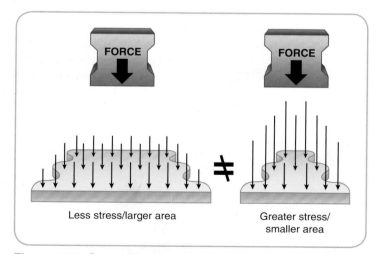

Figure 10.2. Stress. The stress produced by a force depends on the area over which the force is spread. For example, the stress sustained by the superficial tissues of the arm would be lower than that with the force distributed directly over a small, bony landmark. The risk of injury increases when force is sustained over smaller areas.

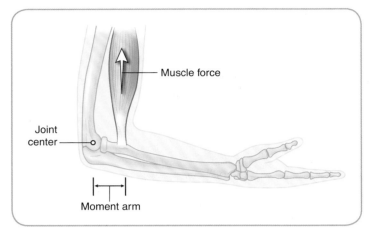

Figure 10.3. Movement and torque. Torque is the product of the magnitude of muscle force and the muscle's moment arm (perpendicular distance of the muscle's line of action to the axis of rotation at the joint center).

of overload, when stressed at tolerable levels, the tissues of the body will adapt and improve their function. Accordingly, in designing an exercise program, it is important to ensure a gradual increase in the intensity and duration of activities. For example, when a runner's training protocol incorporates progressively increasing mileage, it is important that this occur in a deliberate and carefully planned manner so that the body can adapt to the increased mechanical stress and, thereby, prevent a potential injury. Overuse syndromes and stress fractures result from the body's inability to adapt to an increased training regimen.

Torque and Its Effects

When a swinging door is opened, a hand applies force to the door, causing it to rotate about its hinges. Two factors influence whether the door will swing in response to the force. One factor is the force's **magnitude**. Equally important, however, is the force's **moment arm**, which is the perpendicular distance from the force's line of action to the axis of rotation. The product of a force and its moment arm is called **torque**, or moment. Torque may be thought of as a rotary force. It is the amount of torque acting on an object that determines whether a rotating body, such as a door, will move.

In the human body, torque produces rotation of a body segment about a joint. When a muscle develops tension, it produces torque at the joint that it crosses. The amount of torque produced is the product of muscle force and the muscle's moment arm with respect to the joint center (**Fig. 10.3**). For example, the torque produced by the biceps brachii is the product of the tension developed by the muscle and the distance between its attachment on the radius and the center of rotation at the elbow.

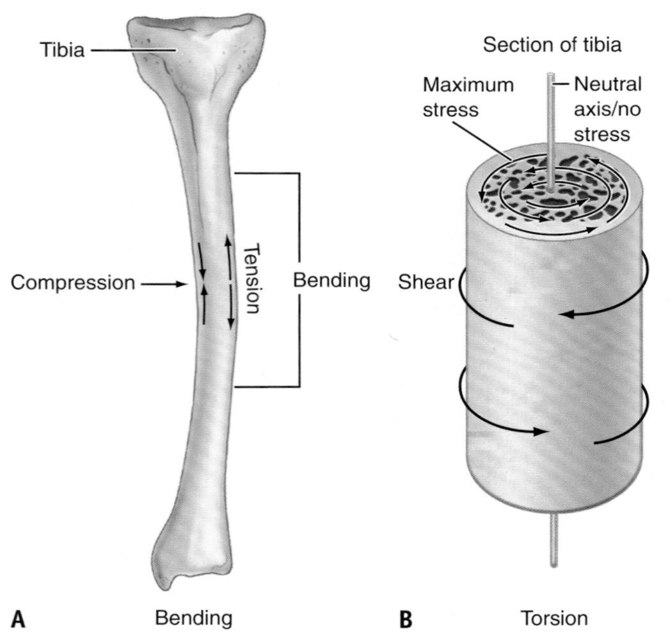

Excessive torque can produce injury. Such torque usually is generated by forces external to the body rather than by the muscles. The simultaneous application of forces from opposite directions at different points along a structure, such as a long bone, generates a torque known as a **bending moment**, which can cause bending and, ultimately, fracture of the bone. For example, if a football player's leg is anchored to the ground and the player is tackled on that leg from the front while being pushed into the tackle from behind, a bending moment is created on the leg. When bending is present, the structure is loaded in tension on one side and in compression on the opposite side (**Fig. 10.4A**). Because bone is stronger in resisting compression compared with tension, the side of the bone loaded in tension will fracture if the bending moment is sufficiently large.

The application of torque about the long axis of a structure such as a long bone can cause **torsion**, or twisting of the structure (**Fig. 10.4B**). Torsion results in the creation of shear stress throughout the structure. This often is seen in skiing accidents in

Figure 10.4. Bone injury mechanisms. A, Bones loaded in bending are subject to compression on one side and tension on the other. **B,** Bones loaded in torsion develop internal shear stress, with maximal stress at the periphery.

which one boot and ski are firmly planted as the skier rotates during a fall. The result is a torsion load that can cause a spiral fracture of the tibia.

 According to the overload principle, the body, when stressed at tolerable limits, will adapt and improve its function. As such, the runner should be advised to incorporate gradual and progressive increases in mileage and time so that the body can adapt to the new training and, thereby, reduce the likelihood of injury.

SOFT-TISSUE INJURIES

? Two weeks into a new running program, a previously sedentary, middle-aged man reports a dull, diffuse pain along the distal third of the posteromedial border of the tibia of his lower left leg. He indicates that 5 days ago, he began experiencing pain while running, but it did not restrict his performance. He reports that for the past 2 days, however, the pain has increased with continued activity and as such has restricted his performance. Based on this information, what actions, if any, should be taken with regard to this patient? Why?

The skin, tendons, muscles, and ligaments are soft (nonbony) tissues that behave in characteristic ways when subjected to different forms of loading. The anatomical structure and material composition influence the mechanical behavior of each tissue.

Anatomical Properties of Soft Tissue

The major building block of the skin, tendons, and ligaments is collagen, a protein that is strong in resisting tension. Collagen fibers have a wavy configuration in a tissue that is not under tension (**Fig. 10.5**). This enables collagenous tissues, which are inelastic, to stretch slightly under tensile loading as these fibers straighten. As such, collagen fibers provide strength and flexibility to tissues, but they are relatively inelastic. Elastin, another protein substance, provides added elasticity to some connective tissue structures.

The Skin

The integumentary system comprises the skin, hair, nails, and glands of the skin and is the largest organ in the body. It provides protection and sensation, regulates fluid balance and temperature, and produces vitamins (e.g., vitamin D) and immune system components. The skin is composed of three regions. The outer region, known as the epidermis, has multiple layers containing the pigment melanin, along with the hair, nails, sebaceous glands, and sweat glands (**Fig. 10.6**). The outer surface, made up of dead epithelial cells, is replaced every 3 to 4 weeks by new cells pushed up from the dermis. The dermis is the largest portion of the skin and provides both strength and structure. It contains

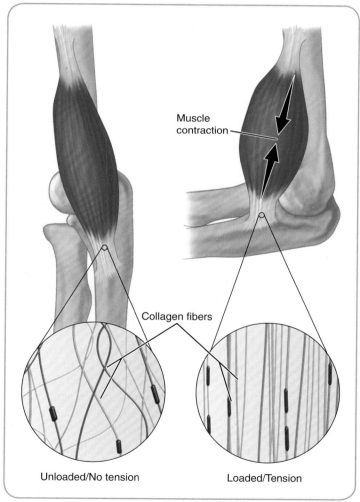

Figure 10.5. Collagen fibers. Collagen fibers have a wavy configuration when unloaded and a straightened configuration when loaded in tension.

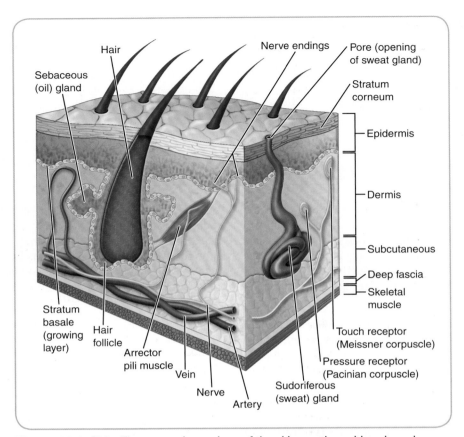

Figure 10.6. Skin. The two major regions of the skin are the epidermis and the dermis.

blood vessels, nerve endings, hair follicles, sebaceous glands, and sweat glands and is beneath the epidermis. The dermis is composed of dense, irregular connective tissue, which is characterized by a loose, multidirectional arrangement of collagen fibers. This fiber arrangement enables resistance to multidirectional loads, including compression, tension, and shear. This type of tissue also forms fascia, which are fibrous sheets of connective tissue that surround muscles. Dense, irregular connective tissue also covers internal structures, such as the liver, lymph nodes, and testes, as well as bones, cartilage, and nerves. The innermost layer of skin is the subcutaneous or hypodermal layer. The primary tissue is adipose, which provides cushioning between the skin layers, muscles, and bones and is instrumental in regulating body temperature because of its insulating properties.

Elastic fibers and reticular fibers are other components of the skin. Elastic fibers provide the skin with some elasticity. Reticular fibers are composed of a type of collagen known as reticulin. These fibers function like collagen fibers but are much thinner, and they provide support for internal structures, such as the lymph nodes, spleen, bone marrow, and liver.

Tendons, Aponeuroses, and Muscles

Tendons connect muscles to bones. They are composed of dense, regular connective tissue that consists of tightly packed bundles of unidirectional collagen fibers (**Fig. 10.7**). The collagen fibers are arranged in a parallel pattern, enabling resistance to high, unidirectional tensile loads when the attached muscle contracts. By virtue of their collagenous composition, tendons are about twice as strong as the muscles to which they attach.

The aponeuroses are another set of structures formed by dense, regular connective tissue. These are strong, flat, sheetlike tissues that attach muscles to other muscles or bones.

Muscle is a highly organized structure that can

- Be stretched or increased in length (extensibility)

- Return to normal length after lengthening or shortening takes place (elasticity)

- Respond to a stimulus (irritability)

- Develop tension

A sheath known as the endomysium surrounds each muscle cell, or fiber. Small numbers of fibers are bound up into fascicles by a dense connective tissue sheath called the perimysium. A muscle is composed of several fascicles surrounded by the epimysium (**Fig. 10.8**).

The structure and composition of muscles enable it to function in a **viscoelastic** fashion, that is, with both elasticity and time-dependent extensibility. **Extensibility** is the ability to be stretched or increase in length, whereas **elasticity** is the ability to return to normal length after either lengthening or shortening has taken place. The viscoelastic aspect of muscle extensibility enables muscle to stretch to greater lengths over time in response to a sustained tensile force. This means that a static stretch maintained for 30 seconds is more effective than a series of short, ballistic stretches for increasing muscle length.

Another of muscle's characteristic properties, **irritability**, is the ability to respond to a stimulus. Stimuli affecting muscles can be either electrochemical, such as an action potential from the attaching nerve, or mechanical, such as an external blow to the muscle.

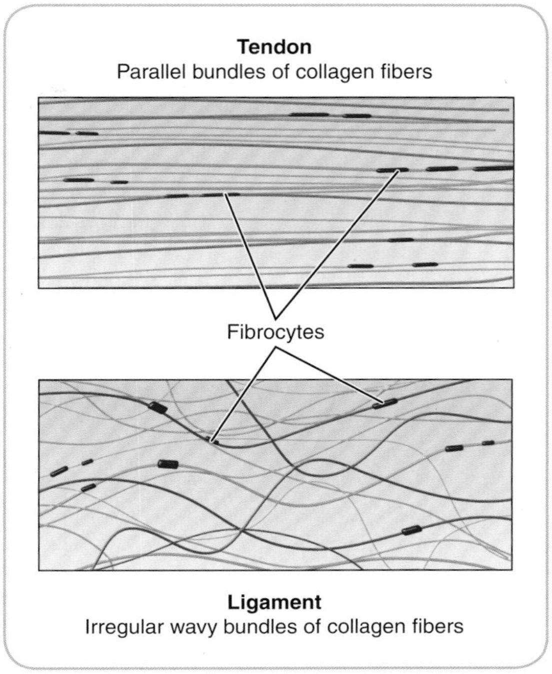

Figure 10.7. Collagen arrangements in tendon and ligament tissue. The arrangement of collagen in tendons and ligaments differs, producing differences in their ability to resist tensile loads.

If the stimulus is of sufficient magnitude, muscle responds by developing tension. The ability to develop **tension** is a property unique to muscle. Although some sources refer to this ability as contractility, a muscle may or may not shorten when tension is developed. For example, isometric "contraction" involves no joint movement and no change in muscle length, and eccentric "contraction" actually involves lengthening of the muscle developing tension. Only when a muscle develops tension concentrically does it also shorten. When a stimulated muscle develops tension, the amount of tension present is the same throughout the muscle and tendon and at the site of the tendon attachment to bone.

Joint Capsule and Ligaments

A joint capsule is a membrane that encloses a joint. It functions to hold the bones firmly in place. The outer portion of the capsule is fibrous and composed primarily of collagen. The inner lining of the capsule consists of a synovial membrane, which secretes a clear, slightly yellow liquid, called synovial fluid that provides lubrication inside the articular capsule at synovial joints. (Joints are explained in more detail later in this chapter.)

Ligaments connect bone to bone. Similar to tendons, they are composed of dense, regular connective tissue that consists of tightly packed bundles of unidirectional collagen fibers. In ligaments, however, the parallel collagen fibers also are interwoven. This arrangement is well suited to ligament function, not only by providing resistance to large tensile loads along the long axis of the ligament but also by providing resistance to smaller tensile loads from other directions.

Ligaments contain more elastin than tendons and, as such, are somewhat more elastic. This is critical from a functional standpoint, because ligaments are connected at both ends to bones, whereas tendons attach on one end to muscle, a tissue with some elasticity.

Bursa

Bursae are membranous sacs that contain small amounts of synovial fluid and serve to reduce friction. Common sites for bursa are in the tissues where friction develops, including the area between tendons and bones, tendons and skin, and ligaments and bones.

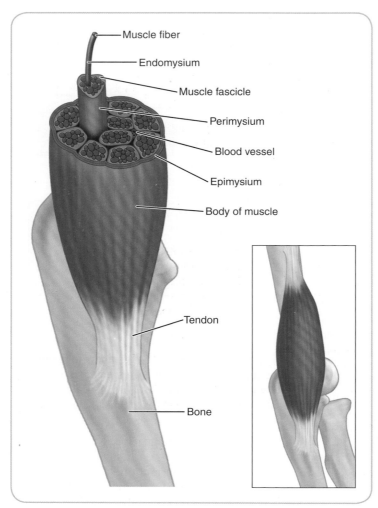

Figure 10.8. Muscle tissue. Skeletal muscle is composed of muscle cells, connective tissue, blood vessels, and nerves.

Anatomical Properties of Joints

A joint is the site at which two bones connect. The study of joints is called **arthrology**. Joints can be classified by structure, function, or the number of axes present that permit motion.

Classification of Joints

The structural classification of joints focuses on the material binding the bones together. In this case, joints are classified as fibrous, cartilaginous, or synovial. Functionally, joints are classified as synarthrodial (i.e., immovable joints), amphiarthrodial (i.e., slightly movable joints), or diarthrodial (i.e., freely movable joints). Human movement often is described in three dimensions based on a system of planes and axes. Based on movement potential, joints are classified as nonaxial (i.e., slipping movements only because the joint has no axis around which movement can occur), uniaxial (i.e., movement in one plane), biaxial (i.e., movement in two planes), or multiaxial (i.e., movement in or around three planes).

■ Fibrous Joints

The fibrous joints of the bones are held together by fibrous tissue. The amount of movement at a fibrous joint (**synarthrosis**) depends on the length of the fibers uniting the bones. A fibrous joint can absorb shock, but it permits little or no movement of the articulating bones. **Sutures**, which are seen only in the skull, involve irregularly grooved, articulating bone sheets tightly bound by fibers that are continuous with the periosteum. **Syndesmoses** are joints that are joined by dense fibrous tissue that permit extremely limited motion. The tissue may be a ligament or a fibrous membrane (e.g., the inferior tibiofibular joint or the interosseous membrane between the interosseous borders of the radius and ulna). A unique joint, the **gomphosis** joint, is found between a tooth and the bone in its alveolus (socket) where the fibrous tissue of the periodontal ligament firmly anchors the tooth.

■ Cartilaginous Joints

The cartilaginous joints (amphiarthroses) unite bones by either hyaline cartilage or fibrocartilage. The sternocostal joints and the epiphyseal plates before ossification are examples of a primary cartilaginous joint, or a **synchondrosis**, whereby the articulating bones are held together by a thin layer of hyaline cartilage. In a secondary cartilaginous joint, the articular surfaces of the bones are covered with hyaline cartilage, which in turn is fused to an intervening pad, or plate, of fibrous tissue or fibrocartilage. These are strong, slightly movable joints designed for strength and shock absorption. Examples of secondary cartilaginous joints are the pubic symphysis (**symphyses**), intervertebral joints, and the manubriosternal joint (between the manubrium and the body of the sternum).

■ Synovial Joints

From a functional perspective, synovial joints (**diarthroses**) are the most common and most important type of joint. They normally provide free movement between the articulating bone surfaces.

Freely movable joints predominantly are seen in the limbs, whereas immovable and slightly movable joints largely are restricted to the axial skeleton. Diarthrodial joints are classified according to their shape, which dictates the type and range of motion permitted. The classifications are as follows:

- **Plane.** The articulating surfaces are nearly flat, and the only movement permitted is nonaxial gliding or short slipping movement. Examples include the intermetatarsal, intercarpal, and facet joints of the vertebrae.

- **Hinge.** One articulating bone surface is concave, and the other is convex. Strong collateral ligaments restrict motion to a single plane (uniaxial). Hinge joints permit flexion and extension only and can be seen at the elbow and the interphalangeal joints.

- **Pivot.** A rounded or conical end of one bone rotates within a sleeve or ring composed of bone (and, possibly, ligaments), allowing the uniaxial rotation of one bone around its own long axis or against another. The atlantoaxial joint and both the proximal and distal radioulnar joints are examples of this type of joint.

- **Condyloid.** The oval (ellipsoidal) articular surface of one bone fits into a reciprocal concavity of another. These biaxial joints permit all angular motions, namely, flexion, extension, abduction, adduction, and circumduction. The key characteristic of these joints is that both articulating surfaces are oval. The radiocarpal (wrist) joint and the metacarpophalangeal (knuckle) joints are typical condyloid joints.

- **Saddle.** These biaxial joints resemble a condyloid joint; however, saddle joints allow greater freedom of movement. Each articular surface has both concave and convex areas; that is, it is shaped like a saddle. The carpometacarpal joint of the thumb is an example of this type of joint.

- **Ball-and-socket.** The spherical or hemispherical head of one bone articulates with the cuplike socket of another. These joints are multiaxial and the most freely moving synovial joints in that they permit universal movement in all axes and planes, including rotation. Examples include the shoulder and hip joints.

General Structure of Synovial Joints

Diarthrodial joints are distinguished by five features (**Fig. 10.9**):

1. **Articular cartilage.** Glassy-smooth hyaline cartilage covers the ends of the bony surfaces. These cushions absorb compression placed on the joint and thereby protect the bone ends from being crushed. The cartilage has no nerves or blood vessels; it is nourished by the synovial fluid covering its free surface. The nutrients in the synovial fluid come from the capillaries in the synovial membrane.

2. **Joint (synovial) cavity.** Unique to synovial joints, the joint cavity is filled with synovial fluid.

3. **Articular capsule.** The joint cavity is enclosed by a double-layered capsule. The external layer is a tough, flexible, fibrous capsule that is continuous with the periosteum of the articulating bones. The capsule functions to help hold the bones of the joint in place. The inner layer is a synovial membrane composed of loose connective tissue, which covers all internal joint surfaces that are not hyaline cartilage. The synovial membrane produces synovial fluid that lubricates the joint.

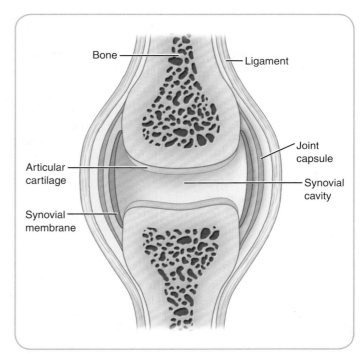

Figure 10.9. Joint capsule. Synovial joints have articular cartilage, a joint (synovial) cavity, an articular capsule, a synovial membrane, synovial fluid, and reinforcing ligaments.

4. **Synovial fluid.** A small amount of synovial fluid occupies all free spaces within the joint capsule. This fluid is derived largely by filtration from blood flowing through the capillaries in the synovial membrane. Synovial fluid has a viscous, egg white consistency because of its content of hyaluronic acid secreted by cells in the synovial membrane, but it thins and becomes less viscous as it warms during joint activity. Synovial fluid also is found within the articular cartilages, providing a slippery, weight-bearing film that reduces friction between the cartilages. In a weeping action, the fluid is forced from the cartilages when a joint is compressed. As pressure on the joint is relieved, the synovial fluid seeps back into the articular cartilages like water into a sponge. Synovial fluid also contains phagocytic cells that clear the joint cavity of microbes and cellular debris.

5. **Reinforcing ligaments.** Synovial joints are reinforced by a number of ligaments. More commonly, the ligaments are intrinsic, or capsular; that is, they are thickened parts of the fibrous capsule. In some cases, ligaments may remain distinct and are found outside the capsule (extracapsular) or deep to it (intracapsular). Because intracapsular ligaments are covered with synovial membrane, they do not actually lie within the joint cavity (extrasynovial).

Some synovial joints have other distinguishing features besides those listed previously. **Articular disks** are present in some synovial joints where the articulating surfaces are incongruous (e.g., the articular disk of the wrist joint). These fibrocartilaginous pads help to protect and hold the bones together. In some joints, they are attached to only one of the bones (e.g., the menisci in the knee). Articular disks have no nerves except at the attached margins. Some synovial joints have a fibrocartilaginous ring, called a **labrum**, which deepens the articular surface of one of the bones (e.g., the acetabular labrum in the hip joint). In other synovial joints, a tendon passes within the capsule of the joint (e.g., the long head of the biceps brachii muscle runs within the shoulder joint capsule).

Classification of Skin Injuries

Forces applied to the body in different ways and from different directions result in different types of injury. Because the skin is the body's first layer of defense against injury, it is the most frequently injured body tissue.

Abrasions are common, such as minor skin injuries caused by shear when the skin is scraped with sufficient force, usually in one direction, against a rough surface. The greater the applied force, the more layers of skin are scraped away.

Blisters are minor skin injuries caused by repeated application of shear in one or more directions, as happens when a shoe rubs back and forth against the foot. The result is the formation of a pocket of fluid between the epidermis and dermis as fluid migrates to the site of injury.

Skin bruises are injuries resulting from compression sustained during a blow. Damage to the underlying capillaries causes the accumulation of blood within the skin.

Incisions, lacerations, avulsions, and punctures are breaks in the skin resulting from injury. An incision is a clean cut produced by the application of a tensile force to the skin as it is stretched along a sharp edge. A laceration is an irregular tear in the skin that typically results from a combination of tension and shear. An avulsion is a severe laceration that results in the complete separation of the skin from the underlying tissues. A puncture wound results when a sharp, cylindrical object penetrates the skin and underlying tissues with tensile loading.

Classification of Muscle/Tendon Injuries

Muscle contusions result from a direct compressive force sustained from a heavy external blow, such as an opponent's knee. These acute direct muscle injuries may not lead to any structural damage to the muscle itself and vary in severity in accordance with the contact force, the contraction state of the affected muscle at the moment of injury, and the area and depth over which blood vessels are ruptured (**Box 10.2**). **Ecchymosis**, or tissue discoloration, may be present if the hemorrhage is superficial. As blood and lymph flow into the damaged area in a diffuse or circumscribed (**hematoma**) manner, swelling occurs, which can compress muscle fibers causing pain and loss of motion. The most frequently injured muscles are the rectus femoris and vastus intermedius, which lie next to the

BOX 10.2 Signs and Symptoms of Contusions

- Mechanism is an acute direct compressive force from a heavy external blow.
- Pain is localized over the injury site.
- Ecchymosis may be present if the hemorrhage is superficial.
- Bleeding and lymph flow may be diffuse or circumscribed (hematoma) which can limit range of motion.
- Swelling may compress nerves, leading to pain and temporary paralysis.

femur and have limited space for movement when exposed to a direct blow. Complications of contusions may involve acute compartment syndrome, active bleeding, or large hematomas.

Muscle contusions are rated in accordance with the extent to which associated joint range of motion is impaired (**Table 10.1**). A first-degree contusion causes little or no restriction in the range of movement, a second-degree contusion causes a noticeable reduction in range of motion, and a third-degree contusion causes severe restriction of motion. With a third-degree contusion, the fascia surrounding the muscle may be ruptured, causing swollen muscle tissues to protrude.

Traumatic injury to muscles and tendons, termed **strains**, are indirect injuries, that is, stretch induced caused by sudden forced lengthening over the viscoelastic limits of muscles during a powerful contraction. The likelihood of strains depends on the magnitude of the force and the structure's cross-sectional area. The greater the cross-sectional area of a muscle, the greater its strength, meaning it can produce more force and translate that force to the attached tendon. In a similar manner, the larger the cross-sectional area of the tendon, the greater the force it can withstand. The increased cross-sectional area translates to reduced stress. Because tendons are stronger than their attached muscle, the muscle portion of the musculotendinous unit almost always ruptures first. This area is associated with a biomechanically weak point because the muscle cross-sectional area is smallest. The injury can produce rupturing of tissue and subsequent hemorrhage and swelling (**Box 10.3**). A tendon begins to develop tears when it is stretched approximately 8% to 10% beyond its normal length.[1] The highly vascular paratenon is susceptible to inflammation, more commonly at the tendon's bony attachment.

The terminology and classification of muscle injuries in sport is in flux. In 2013, the Munich Consensus Statement was published reclassifying traditional grading of muscle injuries based on functional or structural disorders.[2] However, the recommendations have not been universally accepted. For athletic trainers, the traditional grading system is currently being followed. Strains are

TABLE 10.1 Classifications of Contusions

	FIRST DEGREE	SECOND DEGREE	THIRD DEGREE
Damage to tissue	Superficial tissues are crushed.	Superficial and some deep tissues are crushed.	Deeper tissues are crushed (fascia surrounding muscle may rupture, allowing swollen tissues to protrude).
Weakness	None	Mild to moderate	Moderate to severe
Muscle spasm	None	None	Possible
Loss of function	Mild	Moderate	Severe
Ecchymosis	Mild	Moderate	Severe
Swelling	Mild	Moderate	Severe
Range of motion	No restriction	Decreased	Significantly decreased because of swelling

---

BOX 10.3 Signs and Symptoms of Strains and Sprains

Strains

- History of acute onset is present.
- Mechanism of injury results from overstretch or overload.
- Pain is localized over the injury site, which tends to be at or near a musculotendinous junction.
- Discoloration, in severe cases, is caused by blood pooling distal to the site of trauma.
- If moderate, muscle weakness is evident.

Sprains

- History of acute onset is present.
- Mechanism of injury may result from overstretch or overload.
- Pain is localized over the injury site.
- Joint instability is detectable, if assessed before joint effusion.
- If severe, injury may result in subluxation or dislocation of the joint.

---

graded by the extent of anatomical damage as first, second, and third degree (**Table 10.2**). First-degree strains involve only microtearing of the collagen fibers anywhere along the muscle-tendon-bone unit, although most injuries are located at the muscle–tendon junction. These partial tears have a maximum diameter of less than a muscle fascicle/bundle tear and are characterized by mild pain and local tenderness but may present with no readily observable symptoms and no loss of function. Second-degree or moderate injuries involve muscle tears greater than a muscle fascicle/bundle and are characterized by moderate pain, muscle weakness, and some loss of function. A simultaneous injury to the external perimysium, which may serve as an intramuscular barrier function in case of bleeding, may also be used to differentiate a moderate from a minor partial muscle tear. The majority of partial muscle tears heal without scar formation, whereas greater muscle tears can result in a fibrous scar.[2]

TABLE 10.2 Classifications of Strains

	FIRST DEGREE	SECOND DEGREE	THIRD DEGREE
Tears to muscle	< A muscle fascicle/ bundle	> A muscle fascicle/ bundle	Most or all muscle fibers are torn (rupture) or a tendinous avulsion is seen.
Weakness	Mild	Moderate to severe (reflex inhibition)	Moderate to severe
Muscle spasm	Mild	Moderate to severe	Moderate to severe
Loss of function	Mild	Moderate to severe	Severe (reflex inhibition)
Swelling	Mild	Moderate to severe	Moderate to severe
Palpable defect	No	No	Yes (if early)
Pain on contraction	Mild	Moderate to severe	None to mild
Pain with stretching	Yes	Yes	No
Range of motion	Decreased	Decreased on swelling	May increase or decrease depending on swelling

Third-degree injuries produce a major loss of tissue continuity that results in a significant loss of function or movement. Total muscle tears where the continuity of the whole muscle is disrupted are rare. More frequently, a *subtotal* muscle tear or tendinous avulsion is seen. Clinical experience shows that injuries involving more than 50% of the muscle diameter (subtotal tears) usually have a similar healing time compared with complete tears.[2] Tendinous avulsions are included here because they mean biomechanically that a total tear of the proximal or distal attachment of the muscle has occurred. The most frequently involved locations are the proximal rectus femoris, the proximal hamstrings, the proximal adductor longus, and the distal semitendinosus.[2] In third-degree injuries, tearing of muscle tissue can damage small blood vessels, which may present as swelling and ecchymosis, particularly if the damage is superficial rather than deep. Severe pain may be followed by decreased pain attributed to nerve separation.

Two muscle conditions related to overexertion include *fatigue-induced muscle disorders* and *delayed-onset muscle soreness (DOMS)*. Muscle fatigue is known to predispose an individual to injury. Fatigued muscles absorb less energy in the early stages of stretch as compared to nonfatigued muscles and have increased stiffness, which can also predispose an individual to subsequent injury.[3] DOMS occurs several hours after unaccustomed deceleration movement (eccentric contractions), whereas fatigue-induced muscle disorders occur during activity. DOMS has characteristic acute inflammatory pain with stiff, weak muscles and pain at rest and usually resolves within 1 week. Fatigue-induced muscle disorders are characterized by an aching, circumscribed firmness, dull ache to stabbing pain that increases with activity. If unrecognized, the pain can persist for a longer period of time and lead to structural injuries such as partial tears.[2]

Although typically not associated with injury, muscle **cramps** and **spasms** are painful involuntary muscle contractions common in sport. A cramp is a painful, involuntary contraction that may be **clonic**, with alternating contraction and relaxation, or **tonic**, with continued contraction over a period of time. Cramps appear to be brought on by a biochemical imbalance, sometimes associated with muscle fatigue. Exercise-associated muscle cramps (EAMCs) are a common condition experienced by recreational and competitive athletes. Despite their commonality and prevalence, their cause remains unknown. Theories for the cause of EAMC are primarily based on anecdotal and observational studies rather than sound experimental evidence. Without a clear cause, treatments and prevention strategies for EAMC are often unsuccessful.[4] A muscle spasm is an involuntary contraction of short duration caused by a reflex action that can be biochemically derived or initiated by a mechanical blow to a nerve or muscle.

Myositis and **fasciitis** refer, respectively, to inflammation of a muscle's connective tissues and inflammation of the sheaths of fascia surrounding portions of muscle. These are chronic conditions that develop over time as the result of repeated body movements that irritate these tissues.

Tendinopathy refers to any tendon pathology. Because tendons lack a good blood supply, many tendons lack a direct inflammatory response (**tendinitis**). Instead, degenerative changes result (**tendinosis**). Although both conditions may be present simultaneously, tendinosis is far more common than tendinitis. Because neither of these two conditions can be verified without histopathological examination, the term tendinopathy is preferred.[1] Tendinopathy is characterized by pain and swelling with tendon movement (**Box 10.4**).

BOX 10.4 Signs and Symptoms of Tendinopathy

- History of chronic onset is present.
- Mechanism of injury is caused by overuse or by repetitive overstretching or overload.
- Pain exists throughout the length of the tendon and increases during palpation.
- Swelling may be minor to major, and thickening of the tendon may be present.
- Crepitus may be present.
- Pain occurs at the extremes of motion during passive and active ranges of motion.
- Pain increases during stretching and resisted range of motion; strength decreases with pain.

Tenosynovitis denotes inflammation of the synovial sheath surrounding a tendon and is common in the hands and feet. Tenosynovitis may be acute or chronic. Acute tenosynovitis is characterized by a grating sound (crepitus) with movement, inflammation, and local swelling. Chronic tenosynovitis has the additional symptom of nodule formation in the tendon sheath. Not all tendons are encased in a synovial sheath. Some tendons have a peritendinous layer of thick tissue around the tendon. Inflammation of these tendons is called **peritendinitis**. Long-term tendinopathy can lead to the accumulation of mineral deposits resembling bone in the affected tissues, a process known as **ectopic calcification**. Accumulation of mineral deposits in muscle is known as myositis ossificans. A common site for this condition is the quadriceps region. The muscle typically is very tender, and as the ossificans develops, a hardened mass can be palpated within the muscle mass. In tendons, the condition is called **calcific tendinopathy**.

Overuse injuries may result from intrinsic factors (e.g., a malalignment of limbs, muscular imbalances, other anatomical factors) or extrinsic factors (e.g., training errors, faulty technique, incorrect surfaces and equipment, poor environmental conditions). In general, overuse injuries are classified in four stages based on pain and dysfunction:

Stage 1: pain after activity only

Stage 2: pain during activity that does not restrict performance

Stage 3: pain during activity that restricts performance

Stage 4: chronic, unremitting pain even at rest

Joint Injury Classifications

Sprains are acute traumatic injury to ligaments. Abnormally high tensile forces produce a stretching or tearing of tissues that compromise the ability of the ligament to stabilize the joint. The tissue tearing also results in the flow of blood and lymph into the damaged area, producing swelling and restricting range of motion.

Sprains are categorized as first, second, and third degree (**Table 10.3**). First-degree sprains involve only microtearing of the collagen fibers. Signs and symptoms include mild discomfort, mild point tenderness, minimal or no swelling, and minimal or no loss of function. Second-degree injuries involve tearing of nearly half the ligament fibers, which results in a moderate loss of function and detectable joint instability. They are characterized by moderate pain, moderate swelling, and ecchymosis. Third-degree sprains produce a major loss of tissue continuity that results in a significant loss of function, severe instability, and severe pain.

TABLE 10.3 Classifications of Sprains

	FIRST DEGREE	SECOND DEGREE	THIRD DEGREE
Damage to ligament	Few fibers of ligament are torn.	Nearly half of fibers are torn.	All ligament fibers are torn (rupture).
Distraction with	<5-mm distraction	5–10-mm distraction	>10-mm distraction stress tests
Weakness	Mild	Mild to moderate	Mild to moderate
Muscle spasm	None	None to minor	None to minor
Loss of function	Mild	Moderate to severe	Severe (instability)
Swelling	Mild	Moderate	Moderate to severe
Pain on contraction	None	None	None
Pain with stretching	Yes	Yes	No
Range of motion	Decreased	Decreased on swelling; dislocation or subluxation possible	May increase or decrease depending on swelling; dislocation or subluxation possible

A dislocation is a traumatic injury that occurs when the bones that comprise a joint are forced beyond their normal position, resulting in the displacement of one joint surface on another. A partial or incomplete dislocation is called a **subluxation**. The resultant damage includes rupturing of the joint capsule and ligaments as well as potential tearing of surrounding muscle–tendon units. In addition, many acute dislocations have an associated fracture or nerve injury. Signs and symptoms associated with a dislocation include pain, swelling, point tenderness, deformity, and loss of limb function.

Because of extensive stretching of the connective tissues surrounding a joint associated with a traumatic dislocation, susceptibility to chronic or recurrent dislocations is increased. Less force is required to sustain a recurrent dislocation. Whereas recurrent dislocations may be less painful, the subsequent damage to joint structures can be extensive and may lead to chronic joint problems. The most common sites for dislocations are the fingers and the glenohumeral joint of the shoulder.

Osteoarthritis is a type of arthritis attributed to the degeneration of the articular cartilage in a joint. Individuals with osteoarthritis experience pain and limited movement at the involved joint. Osteoarthritis has no definitive cause; rather, it is attributed to a combination of factors, including stresses sustained during certain types of physical activity, joint trauma, and the aging process. It is one of the leading causes of disability among American adults. It should be noted, however, that physical activity is being promoted as a potential strategy for managing arthritis.[5]

Bursitis involves irritation of one or more bursae. It may be acute or chronic, depending on whether it is brought on by a single traumatic compression or by repeated compressions associated with overuse of the joint. Local swelling of a bursa can be very pronounced, particularly at the olecranon bursa of the elbow and the prepatellar bursa of the knee. An inflamed bursa is typically swollen, point tender, and can be warm to the touch.

 The runner's symptoms suggest a stage 3 overuse injury. He should be advised to stop running until a complete assessment can be performed. Because the pain is only present on the left leg, the assessment should include attention to both intrinsic and extrinsic factors that could contribute to injury.

SOFT-TISSUE HEALING

? An assessment of the middle-aged male runner suggests a possible lower leg strain. Clearly, identification of the type of injury is advantageous in making decisions concerning management, but identification is only part of the process. Why is an understanding of the healing of soft tissue essential in determining the management of injury?

The reparative process for injured soft tissues involves a complex series of interrelated physical and chemical activities. Because the normal healing process takes place in a regular and predictable fashion, knowledge of the various signs and symptoms exhibited at the injury site is essential for monitoring the progress of healing. Ultimately, this information is critical to decisions regarding appropriate rehabilitation and return to play decisions.

Healing of soft tissues is a three-phase process involving inflammation, proliferation, and maturation. Although it is useful to discuss the healing phenomenon in terms of these different stages, it should be recognized that these processes usually overlap, both spatially and temporally, within injured tissues.

Inflammatory Phase (Days 0 to 6)

The familiar symptoms of inflammation have long been recognized and, in fact, were documented by early Greek and Roman physicians as rubor (redness), calor (local heat), tumor (swelling), dolor (pain), and, in severe cases, functio laesa (loss of function). Although inflammation can be produced by an adverse response to chemical, thermal, and infectious agents, the focus of this explanation is the characteristic course of the inflammatory response following injury.

Depending on the nature of the causative forces, inflammation can be acute or chronic. Acute inflammatory response is of relatively brief duration and involves a characteristic hemodynamic activity that generates **exudate**, a plasmalike fluid that exudes out of tissue or its capillaries and is composed of protein and granular leukocytes (white blood cells). Alternatively, chronic inflammatory response is of prolonged duration and is characterized by the presence of nongranular leukocytes and the production of scar tissue.

The beginning of the acute inflammatory phase involves the activation of three mechanisms that act to stop blood loss from the wound. The first mechanism involves local vasoconstriction that lasts from a few seconds to as long as 10 minutes. Larger blood vessels constrict in response to signals from neurotransmitters, and the capillaries and smaller arterioles and venules constrict because of the influence of serotonin and catecholamines released from the platelets and serum during injury. The resulting reduction in the volume of blood flow in the region promotes increased blood viscosity or resistance to the flow, which further reduces blood loss at the injury site.

A second response to the loss of blood is the platelet reaction. The platelet reaction provokes clotting as individual cells irreversibly combine with each other and with fibrin to form a mechanical plug that occludes the end of a ruptured blood vessel. As the fibrin forms the blood clot or scab, this covering mechanism on the skin surface protects the underlying tissues from harmful bacterial invasion. The platelets also produce an array of chemical mediators that play significant roles in the inflammatory and proliferation phases of healing. These mediators include serotonin, adrenaline, noradrenaline, and histamine, all of which are primary agents in the inflammatory response. The enzyme adenosine triphosphatase, which is central in supplying the energy needed for healing, also is found in platelets.

The third response is the activation of the coagulation cascade. A cascade is a heightened physiological response consisting of several different, interrelated processes. Fibrinogen molecules are converted into fibrin for clot formation through two different pathways. The extrinsic pathway is activated by thromboplastin, which is released from damaged tissue. The intrinsic pathway, inside the blood vessels, is enabled by the interaction between platelets and the Hageman factor. Both paths result in the formation of prothrombin activator, which converts prothrombin into thrombin.

Following vasoconstriction, vasodilation is brought on by a local axon reflex and the complement and kinin cascades. In the complement cascade, approximately 20 proteins that normally circulate in the blood in the inactive form become active to promote a variety of activities essential for healing. One process activated is the attraction of neutrophils and macrophages to rid the injury site of debris and infectious agents through **phagocytosis**. As the flow of blood to the injured area slows, these cells are redistributed to the periphery, where they begin to adhere to the endothelial lining. The movement of a neutrophil from the circulation into tissue is called **diapedesis**. Mast cells and basophils also are stimulated to release histamine, further promoting vasodilation. The kinin cascade provokes the conversion of the inactive enzyme kallikrein to the activated bradykinin in both blood and tissue. Bradykinin promotes vasodilation and increases permeability of the blood vessel wall, contributing to the formation of tissue exudate.

In addition, increased blood flow to the region causes swelling. Blood from the broken vessels and damaged tissues forms a hematoma, which in combination with necrotic tissue, forms the **zone of primary injury**.

Approximately 1 hour postinjury, swelling, or **edema**, occurs as the vascular walls become more permeable, and increased pressure within the vessels forces a plasma exudate out into the interstitial tissues (**Fig. 10.10**). This increased permeability or porosity of the blood vessel walls typically exists for only a few minutes in cases of mild trauma, with a return to normal permeability in 20 to 30 minutes. More severe trauma can result in a prolonged state of increased permeability and, sometimes, in delayed onset of increased permeability, with swelling not becoming apparent until sometime after the original injury. The tissue exudate provides a critically important part of the body's defense, both by diluting toxins present in the wound and by enabling delivery of the cells that remove damaged tissue and enable reconstruction.

The complement and kinin cascades act to speed the arrival of reparative cells in the exudate. **Mast cells** are connective tissue cells that carry heparin, which prolongs clotting, and histamine.

Platelets and basophil leukocytes also transport histamine, which serves as a vasodilator and increases blood vessel permeability. The leukocytes release enzymes that interact with phospholipids in the cell membranes to produce arachidonic acid. Arachidonic acid activates further inflammation of the affected cells through the production of chemical mediators, including prostaglandins and leukotrienes. Bradykinin, a major plasma protease present during inflammation, increases vessel permeability and stimulates nerve endings to cause pain. This chain of chemical activity produces the **zone of secondary injury**, which includes all the tissues affected by inflammation, edema, and hypoxia. After the debris and waste products from the damaged tissues are ingested through phagocytosis, the leukocytes reenter the bloodstream, and the acute inflammatory reaction subsides.

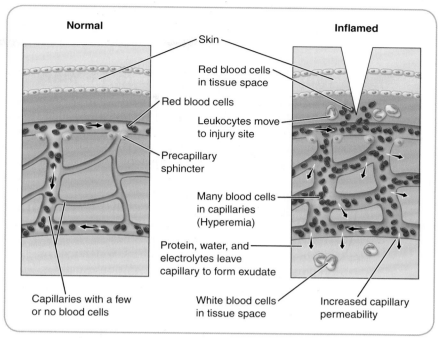

Figure 10.10. Acute inflammatory process. Edema forms when histochemical agents open the pores in the vascular walls, allowing plasma to migrate into the interstitial space.

The Proliferative Phase (Days 3 to 21)

The proliferative phase involves repair and regeneration of the injured tissue and takes place from approximately 3 days following the injury through the next 3 to 6 weeks, overlapping the later part of the inflammatory phase. The proliferative processes include the development of new blood vessels (angiogenesis), fibrous tissue formation (fibroplasia), generation of new epithelial tissue (reepithelialization), and wound contraction.

This stage begins when the size of the hematoma is sufficiently diminished to allow room for the growth of new tissue. Although the skin has the ability to regenerate new skin tissue, the other soft tissues replace damaged cells with scar tissue.

Healing through scar formation begins with the accumulation of exuded fluid containing a large concentration of protein and damaged cellular tissues. This accumulation forms the foundation for a highly vascularized mass of immature connective tissues that include fibroblasts, which are capable of generating collagen. The fibroblasts begin to produce immature collagen through the process known as fibroplasia.

Fibroplasia and angiogenesis are interdependent processes, with the deposition of the new connective tissue matrix fueled by nutrients from the blood supply and the newly forming blood vessels reliant on mechanical support and protection from the matrix. The developing connective tissue at the wound site is primarily types I and III collagen, cells, blood vessels, and a matrix containing glycoproteins and proteoglycans. Type III collagen is particularly useful at this stage because of its ability to rapidly form cross-links that contribute to stabilization at the wound site. Fibroblasts are chemically drawn to the region that secretes the collagen. The enzymatic reactions involved in collagen production are dependent on specific concentrations of oxygen, ascorbate, ferrous ions, and lactate within the microenvironment of the wound.

Fibroblasts also produce attachment factors that promote angiogenesis by helping the growing vessels attach to basement membrane collagen. The primary driving force for angiogenesis, however, comes from the platelet response and the hypoxic wound environment. New vessel formation begins with the activation of enzymes by a potent growth factor, which acts on the existing vessels to dissolve their basement membranes and liberate endothelial cells. These cells are then chemically drawn to hypoxic sites within a wound, where they fuse and form new vessels.

Other characteristics of the proliferation stage include an increase in the number of blood vessels present, increased water content in the injury zone, and reepithelialization at the surface caused by epithelial cells migrating from the periphery and toward the center of the wound.

Maturation Phase (Up to 1+ Year)

The final phase of soft-tissue wound repair is known as the maturation, or remodeling, phase. This period involves maturation of the newly formed tissue into scar tissue. The associated processes include decreased fibroblast activity, increased organization of the extracellular matrix, decreased tissue water content, reduced vascularity, and a return to normal histochemical activity. In soft tissue, these processes begin approximately 3 weeks postinjury, overlapping the proliferative phase. Types I and III collagen continue to increase, replacing immature collagen and resulting in contraction of the wound.

Although the epithelium typically has regenerated completely by 3 to 4 weeks postinjury, the tensile strength of the wound at this time is only approximately 25% of normal.[6] After several more months, strength may still be as much as 30% below the preinjury level.[7] This is partly because of the orientation of the collagen fibers, which tends to be more vertical during this period of time than in normal tissue, where their orientation usually is horizontal. The collagen turnover rate in a newly healed scar also is very high, so failure to provide appropriate support for the wound site can result in a larger scar. Excessive scar tissue is called keloid tissue.

Because scar tissue is fibrous, inelastic, and nonvascular, it is less strong and less functional than the original tissues. In addition, the development of the scar typically causes the wound to shrink, resulting in decreased flexibility of the affected tissues following the injury. This explains why someone, such as a person with paraplegia who has a healed pressure sore from a wheelchair seat in poor condition, can easily redevelop breakdown in the same area if the pressure stresses reoccur in that same area.[8]

Remodeling continues for a year or more as collagen fibers become oriented along the lines of mechanical stress to which the tissue usually is subjected. The tensile strength of scar tissue may continue to increase for as long as 2 years postinjury. **Box 10.5** summarizes the three stages of the healing process. **Figure 10.11** demonstrates the injury healing timeline schematic.

Muscle fibers are permanent cells that do not reproduce or proliferate in response to either injury or training. Reserve cells in the basement membrane of each muscle fiber, however, are able to regenerate muscle fiber following injury. Severe muscle injury can result in scarring or the formation of **adhesions** within the muscle, which inhibits the potential for fiber regeneration from the reserve cells. Consequently, following severe injury, muscle may regain only approximately 70% of its preinjury strength.[9]

Because tendons and ligaments have few reparative cells, healing of these structures is a slow process that can take more than a year. Regeneration is enhanced by proximity to other soft tissues that can assist with supplying the chemical mediators and building blocks required. For this reason, isolated ligaments, such as the anterior cruciate, have poor chances for healing.[10] If tendons and ligaments undergo abnormally high tensile stress before scar formation is complete, the newly forming tissues can be elongated. If this occurs in ligaments, joint instability may result.

Because tendons, ligaments, and muscles **hypertrophy** and **atrophy** in response to levels of mechanical stress, complete immobilization of the injury leads to atrophy, loss of strength, and a decreased rate of healing in these tissues. The amount of atrophy generally is proportional to the time of immobilization. As such, although immobilization may be necessary to protect the injured tissues during the early stages of recovery, strengthening exercises should be implemented as soon as appropriate during rehabilitation of the injury. Increased risk for reinjury exists as long as the strength of affected tissues is less than the preinjury level.

The Role of Growth Factors

Growth factors are proteins that play crucial roles during all three phases of the healing process. Their functions include attracting cells to the wound, stimulating their proliferation, and directing the deposition of the extracellular matrix.

BOX 10.5 Phases of Soft-Tissue Wound Healing

Inflammation (0–6 Days)

- Vasoconstriction promotes increased blood viscosity (thickness), reducing blood loss through bleeding.
- The platelet reaction initiates clotting and releases growth factors that attract reparative cells to the site.
- The coagulation cascade affects clot formation.
- The complement and kinin cascades provoke vasodilation and increase blood vessel wall permeability, facilitating the migration of neutrophils and macrophages in plasma exudate to cleanse the site through phagocytosis.

Proliferation (3–21 Days)

- Fibroblasts produce a supportive network of types I and III collagen.
- The platelet response and hypoxic wound environment stimulate angiogenesis.
- Epithelial cells migrate from the periphery toward the center of the wound to enact reepithelialization.

Maturation (Up to 1+ Years)

- Fibroblast activity decreases and habitual loading produces increased organization of the extracellular matrix.
- A return to normal histochemical activity allows for reduced vascularity and water content.
- Types I and III collagen continue to proliferate, replacing immature collagen precursors and resulting in contracture of the wound.
- Scar tissue formation results in decreased size and flexibility of the involved tissues.
- Remodeling causes collagen fiber alignment along lines of habitual stress, with tensile strength increasing for up to 2 years postinjury.

First discovered in the granules of platelets, platelet-derived growth factor (PDGF) also is released from macrophages, endothelial cells, vascular smooth cells, and fibroblasts. The presence of PDGF is one of the most important factors in the success of the first two stages of healing. PDGF acts as a chemical attractant for fibroblasts, neutrophils, and macrophages and also promotes the replication of fibroblasts and vascular smooth muscle cells. It also activates macrophages and stimulates fibroblasts to secrete types I and III collagen.

Another important growth factor, transforming growth factor–β, is actually a group of several different proteins with similar structural and chemical properties. Transforming growth factor–β is produced by platelets, macrophages, bone cells, monocytes, and lymphocytes and is capable of both stimulating and inhibiting fibroblasts. Transforming growth factor–β also stimulates angiogenesis and accelerates collagen deposition.

Another group of proteins with a common high affinity for heparin is called basic fibroblast growth factor. The platelet-derived enzyme heparinase chemically separates this factor from heparin. Basic fibroblast growth factor stimulates proliferation of endothelial cells and is distributed in endothelial cells, macrophages, and fibroblasts. It is critically important in angiogenesis, releasing the basement membrane–degrading enzymes that separate endothelial cells before new vessel formation.

Two closely related growth factors are epidermal growth factor and transforming growth factor–α. Both originate from transmembrane proteins, and both act on the epidermal growth factor receptor. Whereas both of these growth factors facilitate the development of granulation tissue, transforming growth factor–α also regulates angiogenesis and promotes epidermal regrowth.[11]

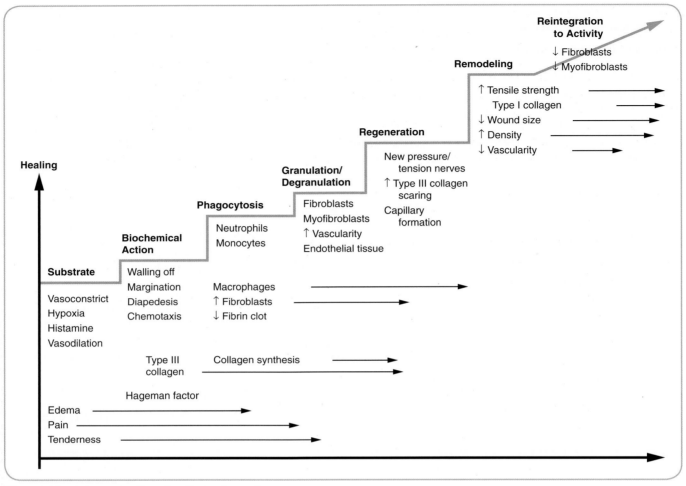

Figure 10.11. Injury healing timeline schematic.

 Fortunately, the normal healing process takes place in a regular and predictable fashion. Knowledge of the various signs and symptoms exhibited at the injury site from the time of injury and its subsequent progression is essential for monitoring the progress of healing and for making appropriate decisions regarding management of the injury. If the runner's condition is not managed properly, it could result in both delayed and less-than-optimal healing, exacerbation of the condition, and development of additional injuries.

SOFT-TISSUE WOUND CARE MANAGEMENT

? The initial management of the runner's condition involves reducing pain and inflammation. Describe a strategy for accomplishing this goal.

Soft-tissue injuries may involve open wounds (e.g., abrasions, blisters, lacerations, and puncture wounds) or closed wounds (e.g., contusion, muscle tears, sprains, and bursitis). This section explains the immediate care of both broad categories of soft-tissue injuries.

Care of Open Soft-Tissue Injuries

In providing wound care for open soft-tissue injuries, it is critical to follow universal precautions and infection control standards (**Box 10.6**). Wound care includes the use of effective cleansers to control bacteria that may lead to infection. Discussion must also include whether these cleaners are toxic to healthy cells. One study comparing the bactericidal effectiveness and cytotoxicity to human fibroblast cells of four common cleansers (i.e., Cinder Suds, Nitrotan, hydrogen peroxide, and Betadine) at various dilutions determined that only Betadine was effective against bacteria and not harmful to human fibroblast cells at a 1:10 dilution of the commercially purchased solution.[12] In addition to using safety equipment, disinfecting equipment and materials used during wound care, and properly discarding contaminated materials, several steps in general wound care should be followed:

- If possible, wash hands before beginning treatment.

- Apply gloves.

- Apply direct pressure to the wound with sterile gauze or a nonstick material.

- Cleanse the wound and the area around the wound (at least twice the size of the wound) with normal saline or potable tap water.[13]

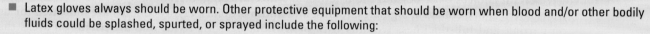

BOX 10.6 General Guidelines for Preventing the Spread of Bloodborne Pathogens

- Latex gloves always should be worn. Other protective equipment that should be worn when blood and/or other bodily fluids could be splashed, spurted, or sprayed include the following:

  Eyewear/face guards

  Masks and/or protective guards

  Gowns or aprons

- Following any exposure to potentially infectious material, immediately wash and disinfect hands and other skin surfaces.

- Clean large spills of bodily fluids and bloodborne pathogens by flooding the contaminated area with disinfectant prior to removing the spill. Following removal, the area should be disinfected again and thoroughly scrubbed.

- Disinfect all horizontal surfaces (i.e., treatment tables, taping tables, work space, and floors) regularly, after each use, and immediately after spills or soiling occurs. Use a scrubbing process.

- Disinfect with a cleaning solution of 1:10 to 1:100 solution (bleach to water). Caution should be used when using this solution near therapeutic modalities or skin because of the caustic and corrosive properties of bleach. The solution must be mixed daily to be effective.

- Soiled linens and towels should be separated from regular laundry, handled with gloves, and placed in a leak-proof bag that is visibly designated for biohazard items.

- All items should be washed with detergent and water for 25 minutes at a minimum of 71°C (160°F). Disinfectant solution such as chlorine bleach can provide an extra margin of safety in low-temperature washing and transporting laundry inside and outside health care facilities.

- All disposable contaminated products (e.g., gauze, paper towels, cotton) should be handled with gloves and placed in leak-proof biohazard bags.

- Sharps containers should be readily available, leak-proof, puncture-resistant, red in color, and visibly designated with a biohazard sign. Reusable sharps, such as pointed scissors or tweezers, should be sterilized after each use.

- Disposal of contaminated items and sharps containers should be in compliance with OSHA standards.

OSHA, Occupational Safety and Health Administration.

- Dress and bandage the wound site securely for continued activity.

- Creams or ointments may or may not be used with occlusive dressings. If used, dressings should be covered beyond their borders with underwrap and elastic adhesive tape where possible.

- Change dressings as necessary and look for signs of infection (i.e., local heat, swelling, redness, pain, pus, and elevated body temperature).

- Maintain a moist wound environment for optimal healing.[13]

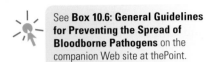

See **Box 10.6: General Guidelines for Preventing the Spread of Bloodborne Pathogens** on the companion Web site at thePoint.

Wounds must be covered with an appropriate dressing. Proper dressings have several essential functions in that they (1) should absorb the wound exudate, (2) should not stick to the wound surface, (3) should not create a new injury to the patient (e.g., through allergy or macerations of the surrounding skin), and (4) should support the injured part.[14] The decision about what type of dressing to use depends on the location, size, type/depth of wound, amount of drainage/exudate expected, presence of infection, need for debridement, and expected frequency and difficulty in dressing change, costs, and patient comfort.[8]

Common gauze dressings are relatively inexpensive, but they must be changed frequently, which increases its cost factor. Dry gauze prevents contamination, but it can lock in exudate and does not keep the wound moist. Wet gauze strips are used to pack wounds with tunnels or fistulas to aid in drainage. Nonadherent gauze, such as Telfa and Xeroform, absorbs some drainage or allows drainage through it but prevents any outer gauze dressing from adhering to the wound or sutures/staples and, thereby, prevents further injury when the dressing is removed.[8]

Several choices exist beyond the traditional gauze dressing, including hydrocolloids, hydrogels, transparent films, collagen, alginates, foams, and antimicrobials. Hydrocolloids are indicated for use on partial- and full-thickness wounds with or without necrotic tissue and are useful on areas that require contouring, such as the heels or ears. Hydrogel dressings, made commonly with a glycoprotein base, hydrate to contribute to bulk absorbency and act as a semipermeable membrane to water vapor and for gas exchange. A hydrogel membrane, Xenaderm, which was developed and manufactured in New Zealand, is absorbent to 7 times its own weight in plasma, is semipermeable to allow water vapor loss and gas exchange, and is translucent so that the progress of the wound can be observed.[14] Hydrogel dressings may be used on wounds with necrotic tissue, such as minor burns or tissue damaged by radiation. Transparent films are used on partial-thickness wounds with little or no exudate, on wounds with necrosis, or as a primary or secondary dressing over lacerations, abrasions, and second-degree burns. Collagen dressings typically are indicated for pressure ulcers, venous ulcers, surgical wounds, diabetic ulcers, abrasions, second-degree burns, and traumatic wounds, but they usually require a secondary dressing. Alginates are seaweed derivatives similar in nature to hydrogels but often manufactured in sheet or fiber forms that hydrate and act as semipermeable barriers to water vapor.[14] Alginates are indicated for wounds with moderate-to-heavy exudate, such as overinfected wounds, diabetic ulcers, and pressure ulcers, and also require a secondary dressing. Foam dressings have small, open cells capable of holding fluids. The area of the dressing directly over the wound is nonadherent (for easy removal) and is available with an adhesive border that can act as a bacterial barrier. Antimicrobial dressings are indicated for wounds that would benefit from topical antimicrobial agents. These dressings reduce the risk of infection in wounds, sites with percutaneous lines, and surgical incisions.[15] In all cases, regardless of the dressing selected, a moist—not wet—environment is best to ensure adequate healing.[16]

Individuals who have diabetes, wound contamination with a foreign material, a wound length greater than 2 in (5 cm), and wounds on the lower extremity increase the risk factors for wound infection.[17] Sutures may be necessary if the laceration exposes the full dermis. The so-called "golden period" of laceration care that necessitated suture application within 6 to 10 hours from the time of the initial injury to reduce the risk of infection appears to not be as important as previously thought. Improvements in irrigation and decontamination of open wounds have led to successful healing in lacerations older than 12 hours on a variety of sites.[17]

Application Strategy 10.1 explains the basic care for common skin injuries. It is assumed that the clinician is already gloved. These techniques can be adapted for use with other open wounds as well.

APPLICATION STRATEGY 10.1

Care of Open Wounds

Abrasions

1. Clean and remove visible contaminants with a fluid flush using water and sweeps of gauze.
2. Clean the wound site and area around the wound with normal saline or potable tap water.
3. Dress and bandage the wound securely for continued play.
4. For dirty abrasions, or when it has been at least 5 years since a tetanus booster, refer for medical care.

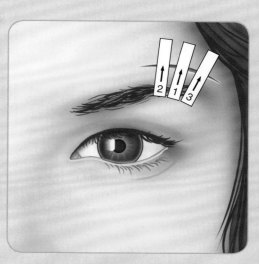

Blisters

1. Clean both the wound site and the area around the wound with normal saline or potable tap water.
2. If a blister isn't too painful, try to keep it intact. Unbroken skin over a blister provides a natural barrier to bacteria and decreases the risk of infection.
3. Cover the area with a topical triple antibiotic and a dry, sterile dressing. Do *not* aspirate a blood-filled blister unless it will open during activity possibly leading to infection.
4. If the blister is large and subject to continued compression, use a small, sterile needle to aspirate the clear fluid, or incise the skin of clear blisters according to physician protocol.
5. Once the fluid is removed, cleanse the area again with normal saline or potable tap water.
6. Pad the nontender skin around the blister with an adhesive, soft-foam material (donut pad), New-Skin, or 2nd Skin.
7. Dress and bandage the wound site securely for continued play.

Incisions and Lacerations

1. Clean both the wound site and the area around the wound with normal saline or potable tap water.
2. Spray tape adherent on a cotton-tipped applicator and apply above and below the wound.
3. Beginning in the middle of the wound, bring the edges together, and secure the Steri-Strips below the wound. Lift up and secure above the wound. Make sure the edges of the wound are well approximated.
4. Apply a second Steri-Strip in a similar manner immediately adjacent to one side of the original strip. Apply a third strip on the other side. Alternate sides until the entire wound is covered.
5. Dress the wound with an occlusive or nonstick sterile dressing.
6. Individuals who have diabetes, wound contamination with a foreign material, a wound length greater than 2 in (5 cm), and wounds on the lower extremity increase the risk factors for wound infection.[18]
7. Sutures may be desirable for any depth of laceration. At least one study has shown that in a large number of lacerations older than 12 hours, DERMABOND may be used on facial lacerations. Any wound open to the full thickness of the dermis should be sutured as soon as possible.
8. Refer for medical care if it has been more than 5 years since a tetanus booster or if signs of infection appear.

Care of Closed Soft-Tissue Injuries

Closed wound care focuses on immediately reducing inflammation, pain, and secondary hypoxia. Several initial steps should be followed in providing general acute care:

■ Apply crushed ice packs for 30 minutes directly to the skin as quickly as possible following the injury (40 minutes for a large muscle mass, such as the quadriceps). Do not place a towel or elastic wrap (dry or wet) between the crushed ice pack and skin, because this will reduce the effectiveness of the treatment.

See **Application Strategy 10.2: Care of Closed Wounds** on the companion Web site at thePoint for information regarding the basic care of closed soft-tissue injuries after the acute protocol has been followed. Because the severity of injuries can range from mild to severe, these guidelines are provided as a general guide. Each injury must be assessed and treated on an individual basis.

- Apply the crushed ice cold pack for 30 minutes. Elevate the body part at least 10 to 12 in above the level of the heart.

- Following the initial ice treatment, remove the ice pack, apply a compression wrap, and continue elevation.

- Reapply the crushed ice pack every 2 hours (every hour if the individual is active between applications, such as walking on crutches or showering) until bedtime.

- Instruct the individual to wear the compression wrap throughout the night.

Application Strategy 10.2 provides greater detail in caring for a variety of closed wounds.

> An accepted strategy for managing the runner's pain and inflammation is the application of cold to the area. Cold, ideally in the form of a crushed ice pack, should be applied directly to the site and surrounding area for 30 minutes and then reapplied every 2 hours throughout the day.

BONE INJURIES

? Following a period of rehabilitation, including abstaining from running for a period of 3 weeks, the runner is symptom-free. He is given clearance from his physician to resume his running program with some modifications (i.e., a more gradual increase in time and intensity of running sessions). Within 4 weeks, however, he returns complaining of localized pain in the same area (i.e., posteromedial tibia approximately 3 in proximal to the ankle joint). The pain has been present for 1 week and is particularly noticeable during weight-bearing activities. What injury should be suspected? What are the implications for the individual's continued training?

In keeping with its material constituents and structural organization, bone behaves predictably in response to stress. The composition and structure of bone make it strong for its relatively light weight.

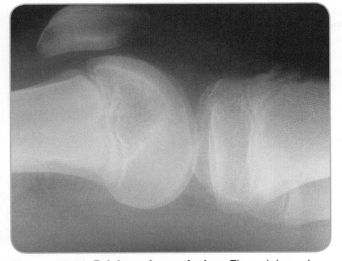

Figure 10.12. Epiphyseal growth plate. The epiphyseal plates of the femur and tibia are visible in this radiograph. Note that the individual has a mild irregularity of the tibial tubercle characteristic of Osgood-Schlatter disease.

Anatomical Properties of Bone

The primary constituents of bone are calcium carbonate, calcium phosphate, collagen, and water. The minerals, making up 60% to 70% of bone weight, provide stiffness and strength in resisting compression. Collagen provides bone with some degree of flexibility and strength in resisting tension. Aging causes a progressive loss of collagen and an increase in bone brittleness. As such, the bones of children are more pliable than those of adults.

Longitudinal bone growth continues only as long as the bone's epiphyseal plates, or growth plates, continue to exist (**Fig. 10.12**). Epiphyseal plates are cartilaginous disks near the ends of the long bones. Longitudinal bone growth takes place on the diaphysis (central) side of the plates. During or shortly after adolescence, the plate disappears and the bone fuses, terminating longitudinal growth. Most epiphyses close by age 18 years, but some may be present until approximately age 25 years.

Although the most rapid bone growth occurs before adulthood, bones continue to grow in diameter

APPLICATION STRATEGY 10.2

Care of Closed Wounds

Contusions

For superficial contusions:

1. Pad with soft (open-cell) material next to the skin and denser (closed-cell) material as an external covering.
2. Cut a hole that matches the contused area in the soft material, or keep it solid.
3. Secure the pad with elastic athletic tape or an elastic wrap.
4. Following play, and periodically during the next few days, apply ice with the limb in a lengthened position, compression, and elevation to the site.
5. Repeat until pain and swelling are gone.

For deep contusions, determine disability after temporary paralysis subsides:

1. In moderate and severe cases, follow acute protocol for at least 24 hours with the muscle in a stretched position.
2. If an antalgic gait is present, fit for crutches and instruct the athlete to use a partial or non–weight-bearing gait.
3. Seek medical advice for complications.

Muscle Injuries

1. Rest the affected area and avoid any activity that may cause pain or lead to further degeneration or tearing of the tendon.
2. Ice with a compression wrap to the muscle belly or tendon to help decrease inflammation.
3. Maintain soft-tissue and joint integrity and mobility through passive movements within pain limits, specific to the muscle involved to prevent joint stiffness.
4. Do gentle isomeric muscle contractions performed intermittently and at a low intensity to avoid pain. Muscle setting may be done in a shortened position to maintain mobility of the actin–myosin filaments without stressing the injured tissue.
5. Gradually resume activity at a lower intensity than you maintained before your symptoms began. Substitute a different activity from the type of activity that caused the initial injury.
6. Use nonsteroidal anti-inflammatory drugs (as directed) and encourage regeneration of the injured muscle tendon through progressive strengthening exercises, monitoring any flare-up of the initial symptoms.
7. Resume low-intensity functional activities that do not exacerbate the condition.

Ligament Sprains

Mild Injury

1. Use protective device (brace) or athletic tape to limit joint laxity and motion at end range.
2. If ice is applied immediately before return, use a mild warm-up before allowing return to play.
3. Heat may be applied when swelling has subsided, and palpable pain upon movement is minimal.

Moderate-to-severe cases are treated by acute care protocol and referred for medical care:

1. In a neutral stable position, follow general guidelines for ice application and immobilize, if necessary.
2. Modify daily activity, sport activity level, or equipment.

Dislocations

1. Splint using standard first aid procedures and refer for medical care.
2. Assess the distal pulse, sensation, and movement; treat for shock and activate emergency action plan (EAP).

Bursitis

Mild Cases

1. Pad (donut pad) the area surrounding the bursitis.
2. Apply heat after 72 hours; continue to pad until pain-free.

(continued)

APPLICATION STRATEGY **10.2** *(continued)*

Moderate-to-Severe Cases

1. Limit movement by placing a compression pad over the bursa using a compression wrap.
2. Immobilize, if necessary, and modify daily activities.
3. Apply heat when pain and inflammation are under control.

Infected Bursa

1. Immobilize the joint and apply hot packs.
2. Refer to a physician for medical care. Antibiotics may be prescribed.

throughout most of a person's lifespan. The internal layer of the periosteum builds new, concentric layers of bone tissue on top of the existing ones. At the same time, bone is resorbed or eliminated around the sides of the medullary cavity so that the diameter of the cavity is continually enlarged. The bone cells that form new bone tissue are called **osteoblasts**, and those that resorb bone are known as **osteoclasts**. In healthy adult bone, the activity of osteoblasts and osteoclasts, referred to as bone turnover, is largely balanced. The total amount of bone remains approximately constant until women reach 40 years and men reach 60 years, when a gradual decline in bone mass begins. As such, physically active individuals past these ages may be at increased risk for bone fractures; however, regular participation in weight-bearing exercise has been shown to be effective in reducing age-related bone loss.

Regardless of age, some bones are more susceptible to fracture as a result of their internal composition. Bone tissue is categorized as either **cortical**, if the porosity is low (with 5% to 30% nonmineralized tissue), or **cancellous**, if the porosity is high (with 30% to >90% of nonmineralized tissue) (**Fig. 10.13**). Most human bones have outer shells of cortical bone, with cancellous bone underneath. Cortical bone is stiffer, which means that it can withstand greater stress but less strain than cancellous bone; however, cancellous bone has the advantage of being spongier than cortical bone, which means that it can undergo more strain before fracturing. The mineralization of cancellous bone varies with the individual's age and with the location of the bone in the body. Both cortical and cancellous bone is anisotropic. As such, they exhibit different strengths and stiffness in response to forces applied from different directions. Bone is strongest in resisting compressive stress and weakest in resisting shear stress.

Bone size and shape also influence the likelihood of fracture. The direction and magnitude of the forces to which they are habitually subjected largely determine the shape and size of the bone. The direction in which new bone tissue forms is in response

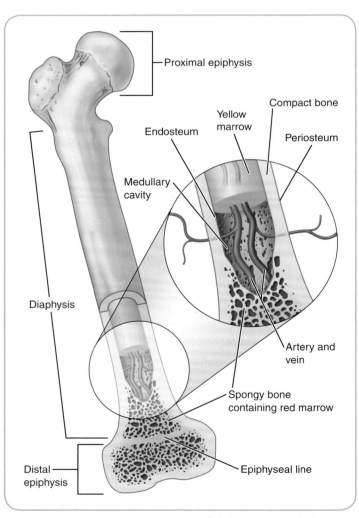

Figure 10.13. Bone macrostructure. Epiphyseal growth lines are found at both ends of the bone. Cortical bone surrounds the cancellous bone and the medullary cavity. Cancellous bone is more porous than cortical bone.

to the adaptation required in resisting encountered loads, particularly in regions of high stress, such as the femoral neck. The mineralization and girth of bone increases in response to increased levels of stress. For example, the bones of the dominant arm of tennis players and professional baseball players have been found to be larger and stronger than the bones of their nondominant arms.[18–20]

Classification of Bone Injuries

A **fracture** is a disruption in the continuity of a bone (**Fig. 10.14**). Signs of fracture include swelling and bruising (discoloration), deformity or shortening of the limb, point tenderness, grating or crepitus, guarding or disability, and exposed bone ends.

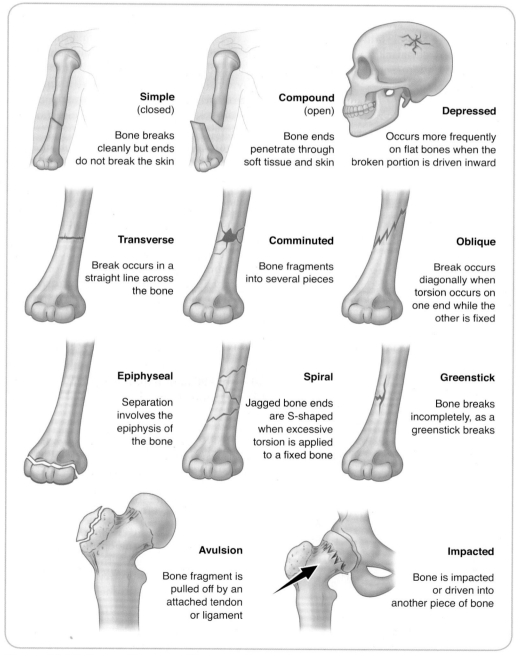

Figure 10.14. Types of fractures. The type of fracture sustained is dependent on the type of mechanical load that causes the injury.

The type of fracture that is sustained depends on the type of mechanical loading that caused it as well as on the health and maturity of the bone at the time of injury. Fractures are considered to be closed when the bone ends remain intact within the surrounding soft tissues and to be open, or compound, when one or both bone ends protrude from the skin.

Excessive torsional and bending loads, as exemplified by tibial fractures resulting from skiing accidents, often produce spiral fractures of the long bones. Such fractures are the result of a combined loading pattern of shear and tension, producing failure at an oblique angle to the long axis of the bone.

Because bone is stronger in resisting compression than in resisting tension and shear, acute compression fractures of bone are rare. Under combined loading, however, a fracture resulting from a torsional load may be affected by the presence of a compressive load. An **impacted** fracture is one in which the opposite sides of the fracture are compressed together. Fractures that result in depression of bone fragments into the underlying tissues are termed **depressed**.

Because the bones of children contain relatively larger amounts of collagen compared with adult bones, they are more flexible and more resistant to fracture under day-to-day loading than adult bones are. Consequently, **greenstick** fractures, or incomplete fractures, are more common in children than in adults. A greenstick fracture is an incomplete fracture typically caused by bending or torsional loads.

Avulsions are another type of fracture caused by tensile loading that involve a tendon or ligament pulling a small chip of bone away from the rest of the bone. Explosive throwing and jumping movements may result in avulsion fractures. When loading is very rapid, a fracture is more likely to be **comminuted**, meaning that it contains multiple fragments.

Stress fractures result from repeated, low-magnitude forces. Stress fractures differ from acute fractures in that they can worsen over time, beginning as a small disruption in the continuity of the outer layers of cortical bone and ending as a complete cortical fracture, with possible displacement of the bone ends. Stress fractures of the metatarsals, femoral neck, and pubis have been reported among runners when bone growth is exceeded by bone breakdown from repetitive stress. Stress fractures of the pars interarticularis region of the lumbar vertebrae occur with higher-than-normal frequencies among football linemen and female gymnasts.

Osteopenia, a condition of reduced bone mineral density, predisposes an individual to all types of fractures but particularly to stress fractures. The condition is found primarily among adolescent female athletes, especially distance runners, who are amenorrheic. Although **amenorrhea** among this group is not well understood, it appears to be related to a low percentage of body fat and/or high training mileage. The link between the cessation of menses and osteopenia also is not well understood. Possible contributing factors include hyperactivity of osteoclasts, hypoactivity of osteoblasts, hormonal factors, and insufficiencies of dietary calcium or other minerals or low caloric intake.

Classification of Epiphyseal Injuries

The bones of children and adolescents are vulnerable to epiphyseal injuries, including injuries to the cartilaginous epiphyseal plate, articular cartilage, and apophysis. The apophyses are sites of tendon attachments to bone, where bone shape is influenced by the tensile loads to which these sites are subjected. Both acute and repetitive loading can injure the growth plate, potentially resulting in premature closure of the epiphyseal junction and termination of bone growth. Little League elbow, for example, is a stress injury to the medial epicondylar epiphysis of the humerus. Salter[21] has categorized acute epiphyseal injuries into five distinct types (**Fig. 10.15**):

Type I: a complete separation of the epiphysis from the metaphysis with no fracture to the bone

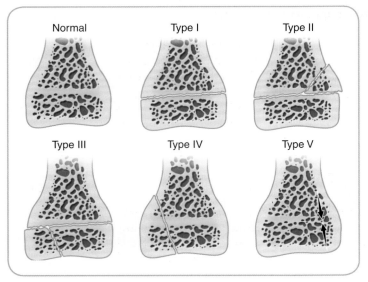

Figure 10.15. Epiphyseal injuries. Five distinct types of injuries involve the epiphysis.

Type II: a separation of the epiphysis and a small portion of the metaphysis

Type III: a fracture of the epiphysis

Type IV: a fracture of a part of the epiphysis and metaphysis

Type V: a compression of the epiphysis without fracture, resulting in compromised epiphyseal function

Another category of epiphyseal injuries is referred to collectively as osteochondrosis. **Osteochondrosis** results from the disruption of blood supply to an epiphysis, with associated tissue necrosis and potential deformation of the epiphysis. Because the cause of the condition is poorly understood, it typically is termed idiopathic osteochondrosis. Osteochondroses most commonly occur between the ages of 3 and 10 years and are more prevalent among boys than girls.[20] Specific disease names have been given to sites where osteochondrosis is common, such as Legg-Calvé-Perthes disease, which is osteochondrosis of the femoral head.

The apophyses also are subject to osteochondrosis, particularly among children and adolescents. These conditions, referred to as **apophysitis**, may be idiopathic; however, they can be associated with traumatic avulsion-type fractures. Common sites for apophysitis are the calcaneus (i.e., Sever disease) and the tibial tubercle at the site of the patellar tendon attachment (i.e., Osgood-Schlatter disease).

Bony Tissue Healing

Healing of acute bone fractures is a three-phase process, as is soft-tissue healing. The acute inflammatory phase lasts approximately 4 days. The formation of a hematoma in the medullary canal and surrounding tissues causes damage to the periosteum and the surrounding soft tissues. The ensuing inflammatory response involves vasodilation, edema formation, and histochemical changes associated with soft-tissue inflammation.

During repair and regeneration, osteoclasts resorb damaged bone tissues, whereas osteoblasts build new bone. Between the fractured bone ends, a fibrous, vascularized tissue, known as a **callus**, is formed (**Fig. 10.16**). The callus contains weak, immature bone tissue that strengthens with time through bone remodeling. The process of callus formation is known as endochondral bone healing. An alternative process, known as direct bone healing, can occur when the fractured bone ends are immobilized in direct contact with one another. This enables new, interwoven bone tissue to be deposited without the formation of a callus. Unless a fracture is fixed by metal plates, screens, or rods, healing normally takes place through the endochondral process. Because noninvasive treatment generally is preferred, a fixation device is only implanted when it appears unlikely that the fracture will heal acceptably without one.

Maturation and remodeling of bone tissue involves osteoblast activity on the concave side of the fracture, which is loaded in compression, and osteoclast activity on the convex side of the fracture, which is loaded in tension. The process continues until normal shape is restored and bone strength is commensurate with the loads to which the bone is routinely subjected.

Because stress fractures continue to worsen as long as the site is overloaded, it is important to recognize these injuries as early as possible. Elimination or reduction of the repetitive mechanical stress causing the fracture is the primary factor necessary for healing. This allows for a gradual restoration of the proper balance of osteoblast and osteoclast activity in the bone.

Management of Bone Injuries

Possible fractures can be detected with palpation, radiographs and magnetic resonance imaging, percussion, compression, and distraction (see **Fig. 6.2**). Palpation can detect deformity, crepitus, swelling, or increased pain at the fracture site. Compression is performed by gently compressing the distal end of the bone toward the proximal end or by encircling the body part (e.g., a foot or a hand) and gently squeezing, thereby compressing the heads of the bones together. Again, if a fracture is present, pain increases at the fracture site. Distraction employs a tensile force, whereby the application of traction to both ends of the fractured bone helps to relieve pain.

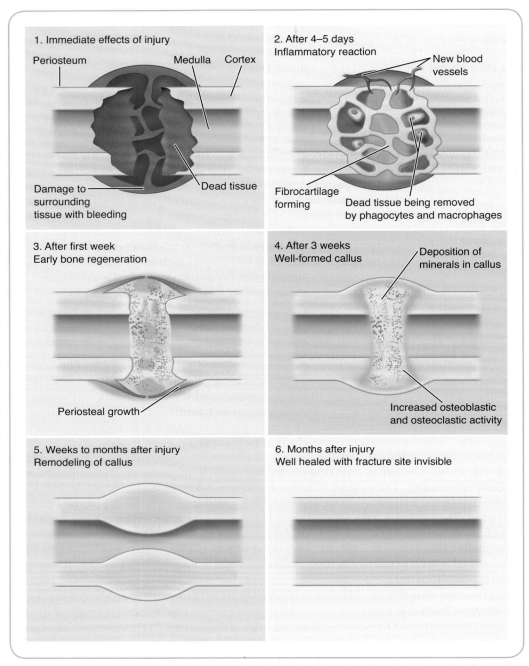

Figure 10.16. **Bone healing.** The process of endochondral bone healing involves callus formation.

A suspected fracture should be splinted before the individual is moved to avoid damage to surrounding ligaments, tendons, blood vessels, and nerves. **Application Strategy 10.3** explains the immediate management of fractures.

 Pain localized over a bone that is particularly painful during weight-bearing activities is a classic symptom of a stress injury. The runner should be referred to a physician for further evaluation. In addition, he should be advised to stop running and to reduce weight-bearing activities through cross-training.

APPLICATION STRATEGY 10.3

Management Algorithm for Bone Injuries

1. Remove clothing and jewelry from around the injury site. (Cut clothing away with scissors to avoid moving the injured area.)
2. Check distal pulse and sensation. If either is abnormal, activate EAP.
3. Cover all wounds, including open fractures, with sterile dressings, and secure them.
4. Do not attempt to push bone ends back underneath the skin.
5. Pad the splint to prevent local pressure.
6. Immobilize the joints above and below the fracture site.
7. Splint in the position found if
   - Pain increases with gentle traction or the limb resists positioning.
   - The fracture is severely angulated.
   - Do not straighten unless it is absolutely necessary to incorporate the limb into the splint; move as little as possible.
   - Splint firmly but do not impair circulation.
   - Recheck distal pulse and sensation after applying splint.
   - Check vital signs, treat for shock, and transport to medical facility.

NERVE INJURIES

 The runner is diagnosed with a tibial stress fracture. If the runner had continued his running program rather than seeking medical attention, would he have been susceptible to a nerve injury?

The nervous system is divided into the central nervous system, consisting of the brain and spinal cord, and the peripheral nervous system, which includes 12 pairs of cranial nerves and 31 pairs of spinal nerves, along with their branches (**Fig. 10.17**). The human body has 8 pairs of cervical spinal nerves (C1 through C8), 12 pairs of thoracic nerves (T1 through T12), 5 pairs of lumbar nerves (L1 through L5), 5 pairs of sacral nerves (S1 through S5), and 1 pair of tiny coccygeal nerves (designated C0). Injuries to any of these nerves can be devastating to the individual, potentially resulting in temporary or even permanent disability.

Anatomical Properties of Nerves

Each spinal nerve is formed from anterior and posterior roots on the spinal cord that unite at the intervertebral foramen. The posterior branches are the **afferent (sensory) nerves** that transmit information from sensory receptors in the skin, tendons, ligaments, and muscles to the central nervous system. The anterior branches are the **efferent (motor) nerves** that transmit control signals to the muscles. The nerve fibers are heavily vascularized and are encased in a multilayered, segmental protective sheath called the myelin sheath. Myelin protects and electrically insulates fibers from one another, and it increases the speed of transmission of nerve impulses. Myelinated fibers (axons bearing a myelin sheath) conduct nerve impulses rapidly, whereas unmyelinated fibers tend to conduct impulses quite slowly.

Classification of Nerve Injuries

Tensile or compressive forces most commonly injure nerves. Tensile injuries are more likely to occur during severe, high-speed accidents, such as automobile accidents or impact collisions in contact sports. When a nerve is loaded in tension, the nerve fibers tend to rupture before the surrounding connective tissue sheath. Because the nerve roots on the spinal cord are not protected by connective

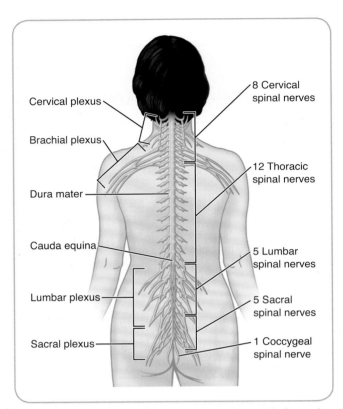

Figure 10.17. Spinal nerves. Each spinal nerve is formed from anterior and posterior roots on the spinal cord. The posterior branches are afferent nerves; the anterior branches are efferent nerves.

tissue, they are particularly susceptible to tensile injury, especially in response to stretching of the brachial plexus or cervical nerve roots.

Nerve injuries caused by tensile forces typically are graded in three levels. Grade I injuries represent **neurapraxia**, the mildest lesion. A neurapraxia is a localized conduction block that causes temporary loss of sensation and/or motor function from selective de-myelination of the axon sheath without true axonal disruption. Recovery usually occurs within days to a few weeks. Grade II injuries are called **axonotmesis injuries**, which produce significant motor and mild sensory deficits that last at least 2 weeks. Axonotmesis disrupts the axon and myelin sheath but leaves the epineurium intact. The epineurium is the connective tissue that encapsulates the nerve trunk and binds the fascicles together. Axonal regrowth occurs at a rate of 1 to 2 mm per day; full or normal function usually is restored. Grade III injuries represent **neurotmesis injuries**, which disrupt the endoneurium. These severe injuries have a poor prognosis, with motor and sensory deficits persisting for up to 1 year. Surgical intervention often is necessary to avoid poor or imperfect regeneration.

Compressive injuries of nerves are more complex because their severity depends on the magnitude and duration of loading and on whether the applied pressure is direct or indirect. Because nerve function is highly dependent on oxygen provided by the associated blood vessels, damage to the blood supply caused by a compressive injury results in damage to the nerve.

Nerve injuries can result in a range of afferent symptoms, from severe pain to a complete loss of sensation. Terms used to describe altered sensations include **hypoesthesia** (a reduction in sensation), **hyperesthesia** (heightened sensation), and **paresthesia** (a sense of numbness, prickling, or tingling). Pinching of a nerve can result in a sharp wave of pain that is transmitted through a body segment. Irritation or inflammation of a nerve can result in chronic pain along the nerve's course, known as **neuralgia**.

Nerve Healing

When a nerve is completely severed, healing does not occur, and loss of function typically is permanent. Unless such injuries are repaired surgically, random regrowth of the nerve occurs, resulting in the formation of a **neuroma**, or nerve tumor.

When nerve fibers are ruptured in a tensile injury but the surrounding myelin sheath remains intact, it sometimes is possible for a nerve to regenerate along the pathway provided by the sheath. Such regeneration is relatively slow, however, proceeding at a rate of less than 1 mm per day, or approximately 2.5 cm per month.

Management of Nerve Injuries

If nerves are injured, cutaneous sensation or muscle movement may become impaired. Neurological testing is explained and demonstrated in Chapter 6. Sensation is assessed by touching the person with a cotton ball, paper clip, pads of the fingers, fingernails, or a neurological hammer to determine if the individual can differentiate between sharp and dull. It also is important to determine if the sensation feels the same on the injured body segment as it does on the uninjured body segment.

APPLICATION STRATEGY 10.4

Management of Nerve Injuries

Mild Cases: Rest the Extremity

1. Ice, transcutaneous electrical nerve stimulation, ultrasound, and nonsteroidal anti-inflammatory drugs may be used to address persistent pain and tenderness.
2. Use protective padding or bracing to decrease repetitive compression or excessive tension forces.
3. Athlete may participate when motor and sensory nerve function returns to normal.

Moderate-to-severe cases need to be referred to a physician. After appropriate acute care protocol:

1. Perform neural flossing of neural tissues, beginning away from the site of the lesion and applying only gentle movement or tensile loads across the injured nerve.
2. Include strengthening exercises of the injured region and carefully monitor proper technique.
3. Instruct the athlete on appropriate posture, muscle tension, and joint stability.
4. Correct any biomechanical factors that may have contributed to the injury.
5. Do not allow a return to activity until the athlete is asymptomatic.

The motor component can be tested with manual muscle testing. In testing a myotome, a normal response is a strong muscle contraction. A weakened muscle contraction may indicate partial paralysis of the muscles innervated by the nerve root being tested. A peripheral nerve injury results in complete paralysis of the muscles supplied by that nerve. If a muscle tear is present, a weakened muscle contraction is accompanied by pain.

It is critical that a possible nerve injury be identified and the individual referred immediately to a physician for advanced evaluation and care. For this reason, **Application Strategy 10.4** explains only basic principles used in the management of nerve injuries.

 See **Application Strategy 10.4: Management of Nerve Injuries** on the companion Web site at thePoint for basic principles used in the management of nerve injuries.

 Nerve injuries typically are the result of tension or compression forces. As such, the runner was not likely to sustain a nerve injury. If left untreated, however, a stress fracture can become an acute fracture. The fractured ends of the bones and the swelling associated with an acute fracture pose a possible danger to nerves in the involved area.

PAIN

 An observation of two individuals involved in rehabilitation programs for similar lower leg injuries reveals different patient responses. One patient avoids exercises because of excessive pain; the other patient performs workouts without complaint. What variables may explain the different responses?

Pain is a negative sensory and emotional experience associated with actual or potential tissue damage. It also is a universal symptom common to most injuries. An individual's perception of pain is influenced by various physical, chemical, social, and psychological factors.

The Neurological Basis of Pain

Pain can originate from somatic, visceral, and psychogenic sources. Somatic pain originates in the skin as well as internal structures of the musculoskeletal system. Visceral pain, which often is diffuse or referred rather than localized to the problem site, originates from the internal organs. Psychogenic pain involves no apparent physical cause of the pain, although the sensation of pain is felt.

The stimulation of specialized afferent nerve endings, called **nociceptors**, produces the pain sensation. The name *nociceptor* is derived from the word noxious, meaning physically harmful or destructive. Nociceptors are prevalent in the skin, meninges, periosteum, teeth, and some internal organs.

In most acute injuries, pain is initiated by **mechanosensitive** nociceptors responding to the traumatic force that caused the injury. In chronic injuries and during the early stages of healing of acute injuries, pain persists because of the activation of **chemosensitive** nociceptors. Bradykinin, serotonin, histamines, and prostaglandins are all chemicals transported to the injury site during inflammation, which activate the chemosensitive nociceptors. Thermal extremes also can stimulate other specialized nociceptors to produce pain.

Two types of afferent nerves transmit the sensation of pain to the spinal cord. Small diameter, slow transmission, unmyelinated C fibers transmit low-level pain that might be described as dull or aching. Sharp, piercing types of pain are transmitted by larger, faster, and more thinly myelinated A fibers. Pain can be transmitted along both types of afferent nerves from somatic and visceral sources. Activity involving A and C fibers from the visceral organs also can provoke autonomic responses, such as changes in blood pressure, heart rate, and respiration.

Afferent nerves carrying pain impulses, along with those transporting sensations such as touch, temperature, and proprioception, articulate with the spinal cord through the substantia gelatinosa of the cord's dorsal horn. Specialized T cells then transmit impulses from all the afferent fibers up the spinal cord to the brain, with each T cell carrying a single impulse. Within the brain, the pain impulses are transmitted to the thalamus (primarily to its ventral posterior lateral nucleus) as well as to the somatosensory cortex, where pain is perceived.

According to the gate control theory of pain proposed by Melzack and Wall,[22] the substantia gelatinosa acts as a gatekeeper by allowing either a pain response or one of the other afferent sensations to be transported by each T cell. This theory is substantiated by the observation that increased sensory input can reduce the sensation of pain. For example, extreme cold often can numb pain. Because hundreds or thousands of "gates" are in operation, however, added sensory input more commonly reduces rather than eliminates the feeling of pain, because pain impulses get through to some of the T cells.

Factors That Mediate Pain

Some brain cells have the ability to produce narcotic-like, pain-killing compounds known as opioid peptides, which include β-endorphin and methionine enkephalin. Both compounds work by blocking neural receptor sites that transmit pain. Several different sites in the brain produce endorphins. Stressors such as physical exercise, mental stress, and electrical stimulation provoke the release of endorphins into the cerebrospinal fluid. A phenomenon called runner's high, which is a feeling of euphoria that occurs among long-distance runners, has been attributed to endorphin release. The brainstem and the pituitary gland produce enkephalins. Enkephalins block pain neurotransmitters in the dorsal horn of the spinal cord.

The central nervous system also imposes a set of **cognitive** (i.e., the quality of knowing or perceiving) and **affective** (i.e., pertaining to feelings or a mental state) filters on both the perception of pain and the subsequent expression of perceived pain. Social and cultural factors can powerfully influence the level of pain tolerance. For example, in American society, it is much more acceptable for females than males to express feelings of pain. Individual personality and a state of mental preoccupation also can be significant modifiers of pain.

Referred and Radiating Pain

Referred pain is perceived at a location that is remote from the site of the tissues actually causing the pain. A proposed explanation for referred pain begins with the fact that neurons carrying pain impulses split into several branches within the spinal cord. Although some of these branches connect with other pain-transmitting fibers, some also connect with afferent nerve pathways from the skin. This cross-branching can cause the brain to misinterpret the true location of the pain. In some instances, referred pain behaves in a logical and predictable fashion. Pain from internal organs typically is projected outward to corresponding **dermatomes** of the skin. For example, heart attacks can produce a sensation of pain in the superior thoracic wall and medial aspect of the left arm.

In most cases, the affected internal organ and corresponding dermatome receive innervation from the same spinal nerve roots.

Referred pain should not be confused with radiating pain, which is pain that is felt both at its source and along a nerve. Pinching of the sciatic nerve at its root may cause pain that radiates along the nerve's course down the posterior aspect of the leg.

 Differences in pain perception and tolerance can be caused by differences in chemical, social, and psychological influences as well as by differences in the severity of the original injury and the progression of the healing process.

SUMMARY

1. When a force acts, two effects occur on the target tissue: acceleration, or change in velocity, and deformation, or change in shape.

2. Two factors determine if injury occurs to a tissue: the magnitude of the force, and the material properties of the tissues involved.

3. Biological tissues are strongest in resisting the form of loading to which they most commonly are subjected.

4. Force exceeding a structure's yield point causes rupture or fracture.

5. Most common mechanisms of injury include compressive force from axial loading, which compresses or crushes an object; tensile force from tension or traction on an object; and shearing force, which acts parallel or tangent to a plane passing through the object.

6. In tendons, the collagen fibers are arranged in a parallel pattern, enabling resistance to high, unidirectional tensile loads when the attached muscle contracts.

7. In ligaments, the collagen fibers are largely parallel but also interwoven, providing resistance to large tensile loads along the long axis of the ligament and to smaller tensile loads from other directions.

8. The viscoelastic aspect of muscle extensibility enables muscles to stretch to greater lengths over time in response to a sustained tensile force.

9. Injury to soft tissue and joints can be acute or chronic. Muscle tears and sprains are common acute injuries associated with participation in sports and physical activities. Tendinitis and osteoarthritis are common chronic or overuse injuries.

10. Wound healing entails three overlapping phases: inflammation, proliferation, and maturation (remodeling). During the inflammatory phase, blood loss is curtailed, clotting takes place, and histochemical cascades promote coagulation, vasodilation, and attraction of specialized cells to rid the wound site of foreign or infectious agents. The proliferative phase includes angiogenesis, fibroplasia, reepithelialization, and wound contraction. The maturation phase involves remodeling of the newly formed tissue.

11. Growth factors are proteins that attract cells to the wound, stimulate their proliferation, and direct the deposition of the extracellular matrix.

12. The mineralization and girth of bone increases in response to increased levels of stress.

13. Because bone is stronger in resisting compressive forces than in resisting both tension and shear forces, acute compression fractures are rare. Most fractures occur on the side of the bone placed in tension.

14. Maturation of bone tissue involves osteoblast activity on the concave side of the fracture, which is loaded in compression, and osteoclast activity on the convex side of the fracture, which is loaded in tension.

15. Nerve injuries caused by tensile forces are graded in three levels: neurapraxia injury, with temporary loss of sensation or motor function; axonotmesis injury, with significant motor and sensory deficits that last at least 2 weeks; and neurotmesis injury, with significant motor and sensory deficits persisting for up to 1 year.

16. Pain associated with injury is transmitted by specialized afferent nerve endings called nociceptors. Mechanosensitive nociceptors respond to traumatic forces that cause the injury. Chemosensitive nociceptors respond to chronic injuries and are activated during the early stages of healing in acute injuries.

17. Pain is transmitted along two types of afferent nerves: small diameter, slow transmission, unmyelinated C fibers, which transmit low-level pain, and larger, faster, and finely myelinated A fibers, which transmit sharp, piercing types of pain.

18. Afferent nerves carry nerve impulses to the spinal cord through the substantia gelatinosa of the cord's dorsal horn up to the thalamus as well as to the somatosensory cortex, where pain is perceived.

19. Stressors, such as physical exercise, mental stress, and electrical stimulation, provoke the release of endorphins into the cerebrospinal fluid and can mediate the perception of pain.

APPLICATION QUESTIONS

1. An individual falls on an outstretched arm and sustains an elbow injury. How might you distinguish between a sprain and a muscular injury?

2. A 13-year-old female gymnast complains of foot pain that has been present for the past 2 weeks and continues to get worse, even after rest. The primary pain is the distal area of the 2nd metatarsal. The gymnast does not recall a specific acute mechanism of injury. What injury might you suspect? How could you assess this injury to confirm your course of action? What type of mechanical loading would most likely be associated with this injury?

3. A sedentary 60-year-old woman wants to begin a weight-bearing exercise program. What precautions should be taken to prevent any injury? Why?

4. A middle school athlete has groin pain but does not recall an injury. He is unable to balance on one leg. What type of pain might the athlete be experiencing? What would your course of action entail? *Second degree Sprain*

5. A middle-aged runner training for a first marathon overhead a statement concerning a surge of endorphin release resulting in a "runner's high." How would you respond?

6. A 16-year-old male sustains a mild ankle sprain during practice. Explain your initial acute management of the condition. What would you suggest that the athlete do during the evening and weekend hours to prevent further inflammation and pain?

REFERENCES

1. Sharma P, Maffulli N. Tendon injury and tendinopathy: healing and repair. *J Bone Joint Surg Am.* 2005;87(1):187–202.
2. Mueller-Wohlfahrt HW, Haensel L, Mithoefer K, et al. Terminology and classification of muscle injuries in sport: the Munich consensus statement. *Br J Sports Med.* 2013;47(6):342–350.
3. Garrett WE Jr. Muscle strain injuries. *Am J Sports Med.* 1996;24(6 suppl):S2–S8.
4. Miller KC, Stone MS, Huxel KC, et al. Exercise-associated muscle cramps: causes, treatment, and prevention. *Sports Health.* 2010;2(4): 279–283.
5. National Center for Chronic Disease Prevention and Health Promotion. Physical activity: the arthritis pain reliever. http://www.cdc.gov /arthritis/interventions/physical/pdf/general /howtoguide.pdf. Accessed January 27, 2015.

6. Wong ME, Hollinger JO, Pinero GJ. Integrated processes responsible for soft tissue healing. *Oral Surg Oral Med Oral Pathol Oral Radiol Endod.* 1996;82(5):475–492.

7. Orgill D, Demling RH. Current concepts and approaches to wound healing. *Crit Care Med.* 1988;16(9):899–908.

8. Harvey C. Wound healing. *Orthop Nurs.* 2005; 24(2):143–157.

9. Standish WB, Curwin S, Mandel S. *Tendinitis: Its Etiology and Treatment.* New York, NY: Oxford University Press; 2000.

10. Hefti F, Stoll TM. Healing of ligaments and tendons. *Orthopade.* 1995;24(3):237–245.

11. Rappolee DA, Mark D, Banda MJ, et al. Wound macrophages express TGF-alpha and other growth factors in vivo: analysis by mRNA phenotyping. *Science.* 1988;241:708–712.

12. Rabenberg VS, Ingersoll CD, Sandrey MA, et al. The bactericidal and cytotoxic effects of antimicrobial wound cleansers. *J Athl Train.* 2002; 37(1):51–54.

13. Korting HC, Schöllmann C, White RJ. Management of minor acute cutaneous wounds: importance of wound healing in a moist environment. *J Eur Acad Dermatol Venereol.* 2011;25(2):130–137.

14. McEwan C. Wound cleansing and dressing. *Am J Clin Dermatol.* 2000;1(1):57–62.

15. Mendez-Eastman S. Wound dressing categories. *Plast Surg Nurs.* 2005;25(2):95–99.

16. Reiman P. Wound care management update. *Dermatology.* 2005;26(9):34.

17. Quinn JV, Polevoi SK, Kohn MA. Traumatic lacerations: what are the risks for infection and has the 'golden period' of laceration care disappeared? *Emerg Med J.* 2014;31(2):96–100.

18. Jones HH, Priest JD, Hayes WC, et al. Humeral hypertrophy in response to exercise. *J Bone Joint Surg Am.* 1977;59:204–208.

19. Watson RC. Bone growth and physical activity. In: Mazess RB, ed. *International Conference on Bone Measurements.* DHEW Pub No. NIH 75-1083. Washington, DC: Department of Health, Education, & Welfare; 1973:380–385.

20. Greene DA, Naughton GA. Adaptive skeletal responses to mechanical loading during adolescence. *Sports Med.* 2006;36(9):723–732.

21. Salter RB. *Textbook of Disorders and Injuries of the Musculoskeletal System.* Baltimore, MD: Lippincott Williams & Wilkins; 1999.

22. Melzack R, Wall PD. Pain mechanisms: a new theory. *Science.* 1965;150(3699):971–979.

Therapeutic Medications

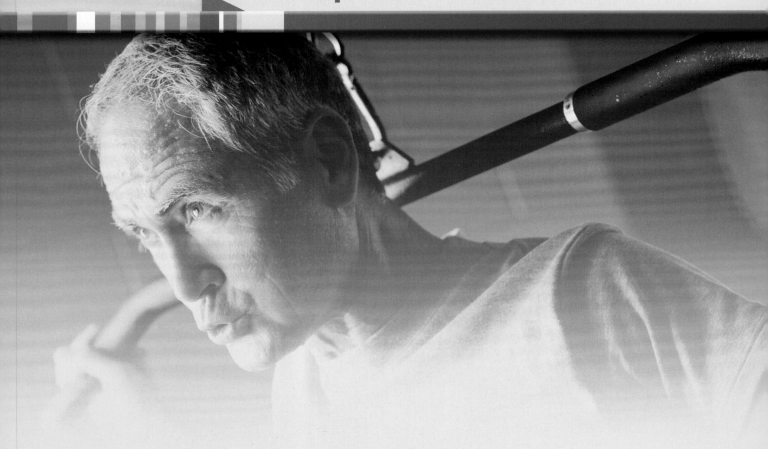

STUDENT OUTCOMES

1. Define the term pharmacokinetics.

2. List the five major principles associated with pharmacokinetics.

3. Describe the two common routes of drug administration—namely, enteral and parenteral.

4. Explain the factors that affect a drug's absorption rate in crossing cell membranes.

5. Explain the distribution, metabolization, and excretion of drugs from the body.

6. Describe the factors that influence the therapeutic effects produced by a drug.

7. Explain the importance of potentially dangerous drug interactions.

8. State the adverse side effects of common therapeutic medications.

9. Describe the process of naming drugs.

10. List the general guidelines for documentation and storage of therapeutic medications.

11. Describe the use of the Epocrates and other reference tools to access information regarding common therapeutic medications.

12. Identify the common therapeutic medications used to treat soft-tissue injuries.

13. Describe the uses and adverse effects of common performance-enhancing substances.

14. Describe the methods of drug testing.

INTRODUCTION

In 2014, the National Collegiate Athletic Association (NCAA) initiated a Student-Athlete Substance Use Study with the Executive Summary released in August 2014. Sixty percent of NCAA schools participated, with findings based on a spring 2013 NCAA-administered survey of approximately 21,000 student athletes. Excessive drinking is down significantly among student athletes. Overall, about 80% of student athletes reported alcohol use in the past year, which is similar to the rate seen in studies of similarly aged nonathletes. Alcohol excluded, student athletes are much less likely to engage in social drug use than other college students. For example, 22% of student athletes claim to have used marijuana in the past year versus about 33% of college students generally. Self-reported substance use is highest among Division III student athletes. Across virtually every social drug (including alcohol, tobacco, and marijuana) Division III student athletes reported higher usage rates than seen among student athletes in Divisions I and II. Substance use is generally higher among male student athletes. Although similar percentages of male and female student athletes report using alcohol, men use other social and ergogenic substances at higher rates than women. Student athletes in lacrosse report substance use rates that are notably higher than in other sports. Men's lacrosse players indicated the highest attention deficit hyperactivity disorder (ADHD) medication use, including 20% who reported using without a prescription. Of the student athletes surveyed, 9% reported using ADHD medication without a prescription. Overall use of ADHD medication, either with or without a prescription, was reported by 16% of student athletes. Nearly one-quarter of student athletes reported using prescription pain medication. Approximately 23% of student athletes reported using pain medication in the past year. Interestingly, 60% of student athletes see drug testing as a deterrent and support its use at the collegiate, professional, and Olympic level.[1]

This chapter examines the process of a drug's journey through the body. It begins with a discussion of pharmacokinetics and is followed by information regarding factors that contribute to the therapeutic effect of a drug, drug interactions, drug reactions, guidelines for use of therapeutic medications, and common medications used in the management of sports injuries. With the exception of nonsteroidal anti-inflammatory drugs (NSAIDs/cyclooxygenase [COX]-2 selective inhibitors) only over-the-counter (OTC) therapeutic medications are presented. Finally, information is presented concerning performance-enhancing substances (i.e., ergogenic aids) and drug testing.

PHARMACOKINETICS

 Why might an individual be given an enteric-coated medication?

A **drug** is a chemical agent that affects living processes. The effects can be beneficial or harmful. A drug is effective only when it reaches a particular site and interacts at the cellular level. This interaction may result in the reduction or enhancement of chemical processes in the body. This interaction can help to restore an impaired body function or prevent a disease process from occurring. The effects can be local, systemic, or both. Some medications result in only a local effect, as occurs when ulcer drugs block the production of stomach acid. Other medications, such as oral decongestants, produce both positive and negative effects throughout the body (i.e., systemically), even though the desired effect is to open

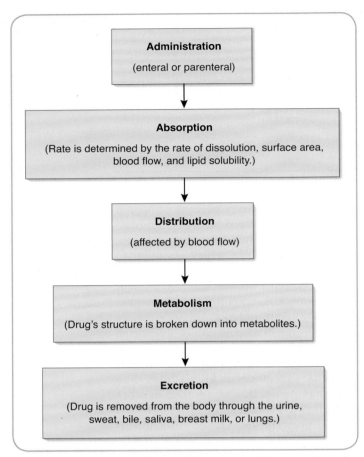

Administration

(enteral or parenteral)

Absorption

(Rate is determined by the rate of dissolution, surface area, blood flow, and lipid solubility.)

Distribution

(affected by blood flow)

Metabolism

(Drug's structure is broken down into metabolites.)

Excretion

(Drug is removed from the body through the urine, sweat, bile, saliva, breast milk, or lungs.)

Figure 11.1. Pharmacokinetics. Movement of the drug through the body involves five steps—namely, administration, absorption, distribution, metabolism, and excretion.

the nasal passages. Undesirable or negative effects are characterized as side effects of the medication.

Pharmacokinetics is the study of the movement of a drug through the body to produce the desired effects. Movement of the drug through the body involves five steps (**Fig. 11.1**):

1. Administration

2. Absorption

3. Distribution

4. Metabolism

5. Excretion

Each step can affect the concentration of a drug when it reaches the desired target. The amount of a drug's concentration when it reaches the target site within a certain time frame is referred to as the **bioavailability** of a drug. The bioavailability of a drug is influenced by two of the pharmacokinetic processes—namely, the route of drug administration and absorption. When the drug reaches the target site, the drug–receptor interaction either facilitates or inhibits a sequence of biological changes that ultimately alters the function of the cell, tissue, or organ. Drugs that facilitate or produce a change are called **agonists**; drugs that inhibit or block effects are **antagonists**.

Drug Administration

The means by which a drug is administered often determines its **absorption rate**. The absorption rate is the amount of time that it takes to move into the tissues to produce a therapeutic effect. Two general routes of drug administration exist—namely, enteral and parenteral. Each route is further divided into subroutes.

Enteral Route

Enteral routes (i.e., oral, sublingual, or rectal) use the gastrointestinal (GI) tract for entry into the body. These are the most commonly used routes for drug administration. Medications that use enteral routes are combined with substances called **vehicles** that facilitate entry into the body. These vehicles include tablets, capsules, liquids, powders, suppositories, enteric-coated preparations, and sustained-release preparations.

Enteric-coated preparations are drugs that are covered by acid-resistant materials (e.g., fatty acids, waxes, and shellac) that protect the drug from the acid and pepsin in the stomach. The drug passes through the stomach and is dissolved in the intestine, preventing stomach and duodenal irritation. An enteric-coated medication, such as Ecotrin aspirin, may be used if an individual has GI sensitivity to aspirin. Other enteric medications also are available.

Sustained-release preparations are capsules or tablets filled with tiny spheres that contain the drug. These spheres are coated and designed to dissolve at variable rates. Sustained-release preparations can reduce the number of daily doses and provide a relatively steady drug level for an extended period of time (i.e., usually 8 to 24 hours). Short-acting medications, such as antihistamines and decongestants, are offered as sustained-release preparations.

Oral medications are absorbed within the stomach, small intestine, or large intestine and can enter the bloodstream within 30 minutes after ingestion. Drugs placed under the tongue

TABLE 11.1 Enteral Routes of Drug Administration

ROUTE OF ADMINISTRATION	ADVANTAGES	DISADVANTAGES
Oral	Easy and convenient to administer Relatively inexpensive Usually safe Avoids sudden increases in plasma levels	Rates of absorption vary Difficult to control concentrations Must undergo initial liver metabolism (first-pass effect) Requires patient compliance May cause local stomach and duodenal irritation
Sublingual	Rapid onset	Must be absorbed by oral mucosa
Rectal	Alternative to oral medications Used for unconscious patients or in those who have trouble holding down foods or liquids	Can be poorly and incompletely absorbed May cause rectal irritation

(i.e., sublingual route) are quickly absorbed through the oral mucosa into the venous system that drains the mouth region. This allows the medication to avoid initial metabolism in the liver. Nitroglycerin tablets are the most commonly used sublingual medication. This route also is used when drugs, such as those in smokeless tobacco, are placed in the **buccal** region of the mouth (i.e., the space between the lip and gum). Suppositories and enemas are examples of drugs that enter the body through the rectal route; this route is used in individuals who have trouble holding down foods or liquids and in unconscious patients. **Table 11.1** lists advantages and disadvantages of enteral routes for drug administration.

Parenteral Route

Parenteral routes do not use the GI tract as entry to the body but, rather, use other methods, both invasive and noninvasive. Invasive avenues include intravenous, intra-arterial, intramuscular, and subcutaneous injections, whereas noninvasive percutaneous methods include inhalation, topical, and transdermal application.

Intravenous and intra-arterial injections put the drug directly into the bloodstream, where it is instantaneously absorbed. Drugs used for anesthesia before surgery and fluids given through an intravenous drip are examples of these routes. Pain medications often are injected intramuscularly, whereas local anesthetics and insulin are injected subcutaneously. Drugs that are given through intramuscular or subcutaneous means are absorbed at variable rates (i.e., rapid and slow) through capillary walls.

Inhaled drugs are rapidly absorbed through the lungs or sinus passages and should not irritate the nasal cavity, bronchial tubes, or lungs. Bronchial inhalers for exercise-induced bronchial spasms are an example of an inhaled drug.

Antibiotic, antifungal, and anesthetic ointments are applied topically. They penetrate the superficial layers of the skin and underlying tissue, but they do not provide deep skin penetration. Unlike inhaled and topical drugs, drugs administered with a transdermal patch provide a more controlled, slow release of medication into the body. Similar to topical medications, transdermal drugs must be capable of penetrating the skin. Examples include nicotine patches, medicated patches for motion sickness, and drugs used in iontophoresis. **Table 11.2** lists advantages and disadvantages of parenteral routes of drug administration.

Drug Absorption

Drug absorption is the movement of a drug from its site of administration into the blood. The rate of absorption determines the onset of the effect of the drug (i.e., the amount of absorption determines the intensity of the effects). Several factors affect the absorption rate of drugs, including the rate of dissolution, surface area, blood flow, and lipid solubility.

TABLE 11.2 Parenteral Routes of Drug Administration

ROUTE OF ADMINISTRATION	ADVANTAGES	DISADVANTAGES
Intravenous/intra-arterial	Instantaneous/complete absorption Rapid onset (10–15 seconds) Controlled dosage Allows administration of large volumes of fluid	Irreversible once in body Can overload the body with fluids Relatively expensive
Intramuscular/subcutaneous	Complete absorption Controlled dosage	Inconvenient Can produce local soreness
Inhalation	Quick absorption Rapid onset (58 seconds)	Patient compliance Can produce tissue irritation
Topical	Local effects Noninvasive Easy to administer Relatively safe	Only effective in treating outer layers of skin Can produce skin irritation
Transdermal	Local effects Noninvasive Easy to administer Relatively safe	Must be capable of passing through dermal layers of skin Can produce skin irritation Fat/sweat can affect absorption rates.

Factors Affecting Drug Absorption

The dissolution rate of a drug refers to the length of time that it takes for a drug to dissolve. The more rapidly a drug dissolves, the faster the onset of effects. As such, a liquid medication typically has a more rapid onset of effects compared with an enteric-coated preparation that dissolves more slowly.

The surface area in which a tablet or capsule dissolves plays a major role in its absorption rate—that is, the larger the surface area, the faster the absorption rate. For example, most oral medications are absorbed in the small intestine, which has a larger surface area than the stomach. Drugs that are inhaled are absorbed into the lungs, which also have a large surface area.

The blood flow in an area also influences the absorption rate. A drug is absorbed more rapidly when administered in areas of high blood flow. As such, drugs administered intravenously are absorbed more quickly than drugs administered orally.

A drug must pass through various cell membranes to reach the blood. Membranes that surround cells are called cytoplasmic membranes and are composed primarily of a double layer of phospholipids, or simple fats. The **blood–brain barrier** also is composed of highly phospholipid materials. Drugs that are lipid-soluble have the ability to cross cell membranes readily and enter the blood quickly; therefore, they are absorbed more quickly than other drugs. When it enters the blood, a drug is carried throughout the body to the target sites. This concept of **lipid solubility** explains the difference between water- and fat-soluble vitamin absorption. Fat-soluble vitamins are absorbed better than water-soluble vitamins and can accumulate in the body as a result of their increased ability to cross cell membranes.

Crossing Cell Membranes

For a drug to reach the target site, it must cross the cell membrane using one of three methods. First, a drug can cross via channels and pores; however, drugs are small enough in chemical structure for entry into the membrane by this method. Second, a drug may cross cell membranes via a transport system that uses natural body chemicals as carriers to move the drugs from one side of the membrane to the other. These body chemicals are extremely selective regarding which drugs they carry; as a result, few drugs cross cell membranes using the transport system. The most common method of crossing cell membranes is through direct penetration. As mentioned, cell membranes are phospholipids. A drug that crosses cell membranes through penetration must be lipid-soluble and have the ability to dissolve into the lipid membrane. These drugs move from an area of high lipid concentration to an area of low lipid concentration.

Drug Distribution

Following absorption, a drug is distributed throughout the body and may be influenced by several factors. In the same manner that blood flow affects the rate and amount of drug absorption, it also affects drug distribution. For example, blood flow to the heart, kidneys, liver, and brain is much greater than blood flow to the muscles or skin. Because tissue normally is well perfused, regional blood flow rarely is a limiting factor in drug distribution.

Exiting the Vascular System

Following distribution of a drug to a target site, it must be capable of exiting the vascular system and entering the cell membrane via a transport system or through lipid solubility. Most drugs leave the blood at the capillary beds, providing little or no resistance to the drug's exit. In the brain, a drug must pass from the blood through the blood–brain barrier. It must be lipid-soluble to cross the barrier in significant quantities; however, some drugs do not exit the blood. A drug that binds to proteins, particularly albumin, cannot leave the blood, because the albumin molecule is too large. Therefore, the drug never gets distributed to target sites and remains in the blood. Only free-floating (unbound) drug molecules can exit the blood to produce a therapeutic effect.

Receptorless Drugs

For most drugs to exert a therapeutic effect, absorption and distribution must occur at a **receptor**, or target site. A receptor is a functional macromolecule in a cell to which a drug binds to produce its effects; however, some drugs do not need to attach to a receptor to produce a therapeutic effect. These drugs produce their effects by acting through physical or chemical interactions. An example of a receptorless drug is an antacid, which decreases gastric acidity by direct chemical reaction with stomach acids. Antiseptics also are receptorless, because their effects are produced by direct physical and chemical reactions with the skin.

Drug Metabolism

Drug metabolism, or biotransformation, is the enzymatic alteration of the structure of a drug, whereby the original drug is broken down into **metabolites**. Most drug metabolism takes place in the liver via hepatic enzymes. This is called the **first-pass effect**. Metabolism in the liver can increase or decrease the therapeutic action as well as the toxicity of a drug. Many drugs are given by nonoral routes to avoid the first-pass effect, avoiding the loss of effectiveness once it has been metabolized. Not all drugs are metabolized, however. For example, aminoglycoside antibiotics (e.g., gentamicin) are excreted in the urine almost unchanged. Because the body does not have a mechanism to break down the drug, toxicity can occur with these types of medications. Drugs that are highly lipid-soluble often cannot be excreted by the kidneys. During metabolism, however, the liver can convert drugs into less lipid-soluble compounds, which can accelerate renal drug excretion. Drug metabolism also can inactivate a drug.

Many drug metabolites have the same effect as the original medication. As such, medications may be active before metabolization, after metabolization, or both. Some medications are specifically designed to become active after being metabolized; others become inactive and ineffective once metabolized. Drugs that are inactivated by the liver cannot be taken orally.

Metabolism also can be affected by the condition of the liver and other medications. Individuals with hepatic diseases may metabolize drugs slower or faster than a healthy individual does. Alcohol, cigarette smoking, and other medications may affect enzymes that speed or slow metabolism of specific medications.

Drug Excretion

Drug excretion is the process by which a drug is removed from the body through the urine, sweat, bile, saliva, breast milk, or lungs. There are two types of drug excretion—namely, renal (kidney) and

> **BOX 11.1** **Examples of the Pharmacokinetic Process**
>
> **Ibuprofen (e.g., Motrin)**
>
> - Administered orally
> - Quickly absorbed in the GI tract
> - Once in the blood, highly bound to plasma proteins (90%–99%)
> - Effects are due to the inhibitory actions on COXs, which are involved in the synthesis of prostaglandins.
> - Extensively metabolized in the liver and little is excreted unchanged
>
> **Acetaminophen (e.g., Tylenol)**
>
> - Administered orally
> - Quickly absorbed in the upper GI tract
> - Once in the blood, 20%–50% binds to plasma proteins; the remaining portion is left free floating.
> - Free-floating acetaminophen exits the blood and exerts therapeutic effects.
> - Metabolized in the liver
> - Excreted via the kidneys

hepatic (liver)—with most drugs excreted in the urine by the kidneys. The rate at which a drug is excreted is significantly determined by the quantity and frequency of the drug dosage. As with metabolism, kidney and liver function is very important to the ability of the body to excrete the medication and/or metabolites at the proper rate. Individuals with reduced kidney function are at risk for toxicity from many medications and must either avoid certain medications or use lower dosages. Ibuprofen is an example of a medication excreted by the kidneys. Some medications (i.e., diuretics) may increase excretion, resulting in the need to alter dosage. **Box 11.1** provides two examples of the pharmacokinetic process.

 Enteric-coated medications are used to prevent stomach and duodenal irritation. The individual may have GI sensitivity to a certain medication.

FACTORS CONTRIBUTING TO THE THERAPEUTIC EFFECT OF A DRUG

 What factors contribute to the therapeutic effect of a drug during the pharmacokinetic process? Does taking more medication increase its effectiveness?

Subsequent to absorption and distribution in the body, various factors contribute to the therapeutic effects of a drug. These include blood plasma levels, therapeutic range, half-life, dose response, and potency.

Blood Plasma Levels

In most cases, a direct correlation exists between the therapeutic and toxic response of a drug and the concentration level of a drug in the blood plasma. As a result, drug dosing objectives (i.e., frequency and quantity of the drug to be taken) often are referred to in terms of achieving specific blood plasma levels. There are two basic drug plasma levels:

1. **Minimum effective concentration** (MEC) refers to the minimum concentration that must be present for the drug to be effective.
2. **Toxic concentrations** reflect drug levels in blood plasma that are too high and, therefore, increase the risk of toxic effects.

Therapeutic Range

The range between the MEC and the toxic concentration is referred to as the **therapeutic range** of a drug. The objective of drug dosing is to maintain plasma levels within the therapeutic range. The wider this range, the safer the drug. For example, because acetaminophen has a toxic concentration range that is 30-fold greater than the MEC, it is considered to be a safe drug. In comparison, lithium has a much narrower toxic concentration range of only threefold greater than the MEC and, therefore, is not considered to be as safe a drug.[2,3]

Medications with a very narrow therapeutic range often require monitoring of blood levels. The asthmatic medication theophylline, for example, is a drug with a narrow therapeutic range. If the dose is too low, the patient runs the risk of an asthma attack; if the dose is too high, the extreme result can be arrhythmias or convulsions. A slight alteration in the dose or a change in absorption, distribution, metabolism, or excretion can easily result in the blood level falling below, or rising above, the therapeutic range of the drug.

Dosing Intervals and Plasma Concentrations

Drug concentrations in the blood rise during metabolism and decline during excretion. Because an adequate response to a drug cannot occur until plasma levels meet the MEC, a latency period occurs between the time of drug administration and the onset of effects. The extent of this delay is determined by the absorption rate. Because injected drugs are absorbed and enter the blood rapidly, they produce more rapid effects. In contrast, drugs that are taken orally usually require approximately 30 minutes before the onset of effects is noted. Time-release medications are examples of drugs that maintain an average plasma level over a period of time. As a result, the effects of time-release medications do not decline before the next dose. The effects continue throughout the dosing schedule. As long as plasma levels remain above the MEC, the therapeutic response continues. Once plasma levels drop below the MEC, however, the therapeutic response gradually diminishes. As metabolism continues, drug levels decline until excretion eliminates the drug from the body.

Maximal Efficacy

Maximal efficacy is the dose at which a response occurs and continues to increase in magnitude before reaching a plateau or threshold. Once the response reaches the threshold, the increase in response does not continue, even if more medication is given. Maximal efficacy serves as an index for the maximal response that a drug can produce. This explains why taking more than the recommended dose of a drug does not produce increased effects. In fact, taking more than the recommended dose can lead to toxicity.

Half-life

The time required for the amount of a drug in the body to reduce by 50% is called the drug's **half-life**. Half-lives can be as short as a few minutes or as long as a week. The longer the half-life of a drug, the slower it leaves the body. For example, acetaminophen has a half-life of 2 hours. Therefore, every 2 hours, 50% of the acetaminophen in the body is excreted. As such, 2 hours after ingesting 200 mg, approximately 100 mg remain, and after another 2 hours, 50 mg remain. If acetaminophen is administered with repeated doses over a period of time, it accumulates in the blood and reaches a threshold. This threshold declines if the dosing is diminished or discontinued.

It must be noted that not all drugs have a half-life. For example, alcohol is excreted by the body at a constant rate regardless of the amount present. One aspirin tablet generally is 5 g or 325 mg, with a half-life of approximately

See **Half-life of Aspirin,** available on the companion Web site at thePoint.

3.15 hours. Although the half-life of a drug depends on its volume distribution as well as its clearance, a single aspirin can remain in the body for several hours after ingestion.

Potency

When comparing two similar drugs, the drug that is more potent requires a lower dosage to produce the same effects. Potency serves as an index for the amount of drug that can be administered to elicit a desired response; it is not synonymous with maximal efficacy. Achieving pain relief with acetaminophen requires a higher dosage than that with morphine, because morphine is much more potent than acetaminophen, requiring less dosage to elicit a given response. The more potent medication, however, is not necessarily the best medication. A variety of factors must be considered, such as side effects, dosing, other available medications, and the patient's specific health factors.

For a drug to exert a therapeutic effect, it must reach a certain blood plasma level. This level is considered to be the therapeutic range, or the range between minimal effective concentration and toxic concentration. Maximal efficacy is the maximal response of a drug, no matter how much more of the drug is taken. Some drugs are more potent than others. A drug that requires a lower dosage for desired effects is more potent than a similar drug that requires a higher dosage.

DRUG INTERACTIONS

Why is drug interaction a major consideration in the pharmacokinetic process?

It is not unusual for an individual to use two or more drugs simultaneously, leading to the potential for a **drug interaction**, which refers to the ability of one drug to alter the effects of another drug. Such an interaction may intensify (synergistic action) or reduce (inhibit) the effects of the drug. In some cases, a drug interaction may become life threatening. Individual response to a drug interaction can be influenced by several factors, many of which alter pharmacokinetic processes (i.e., absorption, distribution, metabolism, and excretion). These factors include the following:

- Genetics and age
- Current illness or disease
- Quantity of drug ingested
- Duration of the drug therapy
- Time interval between taking two or more drugs
- Which drug is taken first

For example, if an individual is taking a muscle relaxant for a low back spasm and drinks alcohol, the depressant effects of both the muscle relaxant and the alcohol intensify, leading to increased drowsiness. In contrast, if two stimulants are combined, such as a nasal decongestant and caffeine, an increased central nervous system (CNS) stimulation effect may result in nervousness, heart palpitations, and even insomnia. Some drugs, such as the H_2-antagonist cimetidine (e.g., Tagamet), which is used to promote stomach ulcer healing by suppressing secretion of gastric acid, can reduce the hepatic (liver) metabolism of many drugs. Taken with NSAIDs, Tagamet may intensify the side effects of the NSAIDs.

Although most medications are not affected by food, drug interactions with food also may occur. Some drugs (e.g., tetracycline antibiotics) should not be taken with milk or milk products, because calcium combines with the medication and inactivates it. Other medications, such as NSAIDs, should be taken with food or plenty of fluids to reduce stomach irritation. Some antifungal medications require food to increase absorption of the medication. As such, it is always important to ask the physician or pharmacist for instructions on taking a medication.

Individuals often find themselves taking more than one drug at a time. Drug interaction refers to the ability of one drug to alter the effects of another drug. The resultant interaction could intensify or reduce the effects of a drug. Drug interactions can alter pharmacokinetic processes (i.e., absorption, distribution, metabolism, and excretion). In some cases, drug interaction may become life threatening.

ADVERSE DRUG REACTIONS

? A college athlete takes a medication prescribed by a physician. The athlete develops hives and problems with his breathing. What condition might the athlete be experiencing, and what is the appropriate management of this condition?

Prescription and OTC medications have the potential to produce adverse reactions. Adverse drug reactions range from mild to severe. Mild reactions are associated with side effects such as drowsiness, nausea, and an upset stomach. These reactions often are temporary and can be tolerated for short periods of time. If the reactions do not dissipate in a few days, a physician should be contacted immediately. About 80% of all allergic drug reactions are caused from β-lactam antibiotics, NSAIDs, and sulfonamides.[2]

 Severe reactions are life threatening and are characterized by respiratory depression, rash (e.g., hives or urticaria), allergic reactions (e.g., anaphylaxis), and shock. If a severe reaction occurs, activate the emergency action plan.

Adverse drug reactions often are immediate and may be local or systemic. Local reactions are isolated to a limited area and often are associated with topical medications. Systemic reactions affect the entire body, such as heart palpitations and acute bronchospasm. Adverse drug reactions that do not occur immediately usually are associated with long-term use of a drug, such as GI irritation from long-term use of some NSAIDs.

Certain drugs, such as tetracycline, sulfa drugs, and even NSAIDs, may make an individual more susceptible to ultraviolet rays from the sun, resulting in a decreased exposure interval needed to develop a sunburn, rash, or allergy to the sun. These reactions can occur with the first dose or up to 1 week after taking the medication. Aspirin and other NSAIDs cause urticarial in approximately 1% of the population.[2] Other drugs may increase an individual's risk of heat illness or dehydration. Diuretics also can lead to dehydration in an exercising individual. Before participation in physical activity, it is important to know if a medication increases the risk of sun sensitivity, heat illness, or other complications. This information is available from a pharmacist.

Unlike prescription medications, most OTC medication labels identify the risk of adverse drug reactions; however, a physician or pharmacist should be consulted before taking two or more drugs simultaneously. Depending on the severity of the adverse reaction, the individual should be taken to the nearest medical facility. Most adverse reactions subside once the medication is discontinued.

 The athlete is having a severe, adverse reaction to the medication. Management of this condition includes checking and monitoring vital signs, treating for shock, and initiating the emergency action plan.

DRUG NAMES

? Are there differences in the effectiveness of brand name and generic drugs?

The U.S. Food and Drug Administration (FDA) is responsible for supervising the manufacturing, labeling, and distribution of chemical substances, including therapeutic medications. Drugs are classified either as prescription or as nonprescription/OTC products. Prescription medications must be prescribed by a licensed practitioner and generally are dispensed by pharmacists. OTC drugs, which can

---

BOX 11.2 Information Found on Medication Containers

Prescription Medication Container	**Over-the-Counter Medication Container**

Prescription Medication Container

- Patient name
- Pharmacy name, address, and telephone number
- Name of medication
- Dose information and directions for use
- Number of refills (if any)
- Warnings for use (if any)
- Date prescription filled
- Practitioner who prescribed the medication
- Additional information depending on individual state laws

Over-the-Counter Medication Container

- Product name
- Manufacturer name and address
- Net contents
- Directions for safe and effective use
- Name of habit-forming drugs
- Cautions and warnings
- Name and quantity of active ingredients

---

be purchased directly by the consumer, usually are used to treat minor problems. Unlike prescription medication, containers holding OTC medication provide a variety of critical information (**Box 11.2**).

Every medication has a chemical, generic, and brand name. The **chemical name** describes the actual scientific compound; because of the complexity of chemical names, they are seldom used. The **generic name** is considered to be a drug's official name and is preferred over brand names for general use. **Trade names**, or **brand names**, are specific names used by the individual manufacturer. They are created by drug companies for ease of use by consumers and physicians, and they generally are shorter than the generic name, are capitalized, or carry the registered trademark symbol (®). In addition, generic drugs can appear under more than one trade name. For example, the common OTC medication acetaminophen can be identified with the following names:

Chemical name	49-hydroxyacetanilide
Generic name	acetaminophen
Trade or brand name	Tylenol; Panadol

Generally, the OTC products are of lower strength than their respective prescription counterparts. Use of doses higher than those indicated on OTC medication labels is not wise unless prescribed by a physician or other licensed practitioner, because this increases the risk of side effects and adverse reactions. In most cases, the prescription generic drug is therapeutically equivalent to, but is less expensive than, the primary brand-name drug.

Drugs differ not by generic or brand names but, rather, by the route of administration and the rate and extent of absorption. Drug names are used for written and verbal communication and for verifying the contents of drug containers.

 In most cases, a generic drug provides the same therapeutic effects as the brand-name equivalent. The generic form usually is less expensive.

GUIDELINES FOR THE USE OF THERAPEUTIC MEDICATIONS

 A college basketball team is preparing to take a 4-day, out-of-state trip for a tournament. Some of the athletes are taking prescription medications. What instructions should be provided to the athletes traveling with prescription medications?

State laws vary tremendously regarding who can prescribe, administer, and dispense medications; therefore, legal ramifications also vary. In general, prescription medications can be prescribed only by a licensed practitioner and dispensed only by a registered pharmacist. Depending on state regulations, only authorized persons (e.g., nurses, physician assistants, or physicians) can administer medications. **Administration of medication** is defined as providing one dose of a medication to a patient. **Drug dispensing** is defined as providing more than one individual dose.

Certified athletic trainers cannot administer or dispense prescription medications, nor should they be assigned duties that may put them in a situation to do so. Physicians cannot delegate the duties associated with prescription drug control or dispensing to certified athletic trainers. These duties extend beyond the role delineation and employment requirements of a certified athletic trainer and put the athletic trainer at risk for legal liability.[3]

Using Over-the-Counter Medications

Depending on state regulations, athletic trainers may be authorized to administer OTC medications. Before providing someone with an individual dose, however, the athletic trainer should have reason for doing so based on a written protocol developed in concert with the supervising team physician. These drug protocols should be part of the athletic training policy and procedures manual and should be readily available and used as a reference when administering any OTC medication. The drug protocols should include the following:

- Identification of the medical condition

- Screening questions that should be asked to identify the potential for any adverse effects

- General signs and symptoms of the condition

- Suggested treatment

- Suggested OTC medication

- Banned substance note

- Approval signature/date of the supervising physician

- Documentation for rescue inhalers (albuterol, Flovent, etc.)

- ADHD/attention deficit disorder (ADD) documentation from supervising physician on file

Before administering an OTC medication, it is important to determine if the individual is allergic to any type of medication (e.g., aspirin, sulfa drugs, and penicillin). The response should be noted and documented. When furnishing medication, both written and oral directions for the use of the medication should be provided to the individual. Following administration of medication, the athletic trainer should keep a written record, or "medication log," of the transaction, including the date, name of the individual, sport/activity, name of the medication, manufacturer, dosage, lot number (if available), expiration date of the medication, reason for administering the medication, and signature of the person administering the drug.[3] All drug distribution records should be maintained in accordance with appropriate legal guidelines.

See **Example of a Drug Protocol**, available on the companion Web site at thePoint, for an example of developing a drug protocol for a specific condition.

In addition, the athletic trainer should follow up with the individual to make sure that the medication is working and that the individual is following the appropriate drug dosing regimen. This is especially important when taking antibiotic and antifungal agents. Incomplete therapy can result in developing a resistance to the medication or a recurrence of the infection. Even though an individual may be feeling fine, the infection is not necessarily gone. The entire course of the prescribed treatment must be completed. **Box 11.3** lists tips for proper use of medications.

Poison Control Plan

In addition to having drug protocols developed and implemented, it is equally important to have a poison control plan that is readily available at all times. This plan should be part of the athletic training policies and procedures manual. Poison control centers are available in every state and can be

---

BOX 11.3 Tips for Proper Use of Medications

- Use only as directed.
- Keep medication in the original container; do not alter the label.
- Do not use if the container has been tampered with.
- Do not use the medication if discolored or if the expiration date has passed.
- Measuring spoons or cups should be used when measuring liquid medication.
- Never share your medication with another person.
- When directed, oral medications should be taken with food.
- If a corticosteroid is injected into a joint, do not stress the joint too soon following the injection because pain will be masked.
- If an overdose occurs, immediately contact the nearest poison control center and transport the patient to the nearest medical facility.

---

contacted through the local health department. Proper procedures and protocols should be discussed for various poison situations. These procedures should be developed in written form, posted in the athletic training facility, and practiced on a regular basis. **Box 11.4** lists information that should be provided over the phone to the poison control center if a potential medical poisoning occurs.

Traveling with Medications

It is important to plan ahead when traveling to ensure that an adequate supply of a particular medication is available in case of emergency (**Box 11.5**). If an individual forgets a medication or if a medication is depleted, it is not easy to obtain a refill. Each state has specific rules and regulations concerning the prescription and refill of medications. Physicians usually cannot prescribe medications from state to state, nor can pharmacists fill out-of-state prescriptions. If an individual needs prescription medication while traveling, seeking assistance from the host team physician may be warranted. Another solution is to have the individual's personal physician call the host team physician to discuss the situation. In either case, prescription medications should remain in the original containers and be kept either by the individual or by the athletic trainer.

Storing Medications

All prescription and OTC medications should be kept in the original container and stored in a locked cabinet or other secure place. They should be kept away from heat, direct light, dampness, and

---

BOX 11.4 Steps for the Management of a Medication Poison Situation

- Call the nearest poison control center.
- Provide the poison control center with the following information:
  - Your name and location
  - Name, age, and approximate weight of the person who has taken the medication
  - Name and dosage of the medication
  - Approximate time the medication was taken
  - Any signs and symptoms of the patient, including vital signs
- Proceed with the directions provided by the poison control center.

BOX 11.5 Tips for Traveling with Prescription Medications

■ Medications should not be placed in checked luggage.

■ Take a copy of any written prescriptions.

■ Plan ahead and make sure there is a source of medication while traveling.

■ Keep medications in the original container for identification purposes.

■ A large-enough supply should be taken to cover emergency situations.

■ Keep medications in a safe and secure location.

freezing temperatures. A dry environment with temperatures between 15° and 31.7°C (59° to 86°F) is suggested.[4] All stocked medications should be examined at regular intervals, and expired medications should be discarded. If medications are kept in athletic training, emergency, or travel kits, they should be routinely inspected for medication quality and security. When stocking medications, it is important to avoid overstocking. Overstocking often is determined by the quantity of expired medications in stock and by the quantity of medications in stock relative to the amount actually used during a given period. Overstocking wastes both medication and money.

Resources on Medications

The Physician's Desk Reference is no longer used since prescription medications change on a frequent basis. Physicians currently use Epocrates to access the most current diagnostic and treatment information in an online format. Medication can be reference for harmful interactions, pill identification, and ICD-9 codes.[5] The Food and Nutrition Information Center (fnic.nal.usda.gov) is an Internet source for drug information and provides consumer guidelines for drug use. A current list of banned substances can be retrieved from the NCAA (www.ncaa.org), United States Olympic Committee (USOC; www.teamusa.org), and Drug Free Sport (www.drugfreesport.com) Web sites.

 In preparing to take a 4-day, out-of-state trip for a college basketball tournament, the athletes taking prescription medications should be provided with the following instructions: Ensure an ample supply of medication for the entire trip, do not place medication in checked luggage, take a copy of your written prescription, keep medications in a safe and secure location, and keep medications in their original containers.

COMMON MEDICATIONS USED TO TREAT SPORT-RELATED INJURIES

 Following a head-first slide into second base, a softball player sustains an abrasion to the left forearm. What is the treatment for this injury, and what medication should be used as part of the treatment protocol?

A variety of different types of medications are used to treat soft-tissue injuries in sports. The more common medications include **analgesics** and **antipyretics**, NSAIDs, corticosteroids, anesthetics, antiseptics, topical antibiotics, and antifungal agents.

Analgesics and Antipyretics

Two of the more common analgesic–antipyretic medications are acetaminophen (e.g., Tylenol) and aspirin. Acetaminophen inhibits the synthesis of prostaglandins in the CNS but does not inhibit their synthesis in peripheral tissues. As a result, it acts as an analgesic and reduces fever, but it has no anti-inflammatory or antiplatelet (i.e., anticlotting) properties. Because it does not cause GI irritation, acetaminophen often is used as a replacement for aspirin. Overdosage of this medication can lead to liver damage and death.

Aspirin (i.e., acetylsalicylic acid) is a commonly used analgesic, antipyretic, and anti-inflammatory medication. Unfortunately, its use can lead to GI bleeding, nausea, vomiting, and development of gastric ulcers. In high doses, **tinnitus** and dizziness may result. Regardless of the circumstances, most practitioners prefer that no individual younger than 18 years receive aspirin. If aspirin is used in a child younger than age 18 years during chickenpox or influenza, the risk of **Reye syndrome** increases. This is a severe disorder characterized by recurrent vomiting that begins a week after onset of the condition, from which the child either recovers rapidly or lapses into a coma, with the possibility of death. Individuals who are intolerant to aspirin, particularly asthmatics, may have an anaphylactic reaction to it. In addition, because aspirin prolongs blood clotting time, it should not be used by individuals who engage in contact sports.

Nonsteroidal Anti-inflammatory Drugs

NSAIDs are aspirin-like drugs that suppress inflammation and pain, produce analgesia, and reduce fever. They are among the most commonly used drugs in the treatment of soft-tissue injuries and are distributed as both OTC and prescription medications. Use of OTC NSAIDs can, at times, be high. In a recent study, nearly 75% of high school football players who were surveyed reported using OTC NSAIDs daily without adult supervision.[6–8]

NSAIDs were developed in an attempt to decrease the GI and hemorrhagic effects produced by aspirin. Most NSAIDs produce the same effects as aspirin but without many of the side effects. Individuals may respond differently to various types of NSAIDs, which differ chemically and pharmacokinetically based on their duration of action, potency level, OTC and prescription status, and dosing regimen.

Therapeutic Effects

NSAIDs interfere with the biosynthesis of prostaglandins and other related compounds by inhibiting COX, an enzyme responsible for the synthesis of prostaglandins. Prostaglandins are lipid-like compounds produced by almost every living cell, with the exception of red blood cells (RBCs). Under normal conditions, these lipid-like compounds regulate cell function. During inflammation of a soft tissue, increased prostaglandin activity seems to mediate inflammation by increasing blood flow, capillary permeability, and the permeability effects of histamine and bradykinin. Because NSAIDs inhibit prostaglandin activity, they reduce inflammation and pain. The anti-inflammatory effects of NSAIDs result from the inhibition of COX-2. The adverse GI reactions are caused by inhibition of COX-1. One NSAID (e.g., celecoxib) appear to inhibit the COX-2 enzyme without inhibiting the COX-1 enzyme. The more traditional NSAIDs (e.g., naproxen and ibuprofen) reduce pain and inflammation by blocking COX-2, but unlike celecoxib, they also inhibit COX-1. This inhibition of COX-1 can lead to stomach irritation and ulcers.[2,3]

NSAIDs provide analgesia without sedation or the euphoria that often is associated with narcotic analgesics, such as morphine, meperidine (e.g., Demerol), codeine, and oxycodone (e.g., Percodan and Tylox). Narcotic analgesics containing propoxyphene (e.g., Darvon and Darvocet) were banned in 2010. Narcotic analgesics have the potential to produce physical dependence and tolerance; nonnarcotic analgesics, such as NSAIDs, do not normally produce dependence.

NSAIDs may reduce fever without reducing normal body temperature. The hypothalamus has a set point that determines body temperature; if this set point is elevated by fever-promoting substances (e.g., endogenous pyrogens), fever develops. NSAIDs inhibit prostaglandins and, as a result, lower the set point of the hypothalamus and reduce fever. In addition, NSAIDs have some antiplatelet (i.e., anticlotting) properties. In contrast to the strong antiplatelet properties of aspirin, however, the effects of NSAIDs are much lower in intensity. They are considered to be safe when used to treat acute soft-tissue injuries.

Adverse Effects

Side effects of NSAIDs can include GI irritation, increase in blood pressure, renal impairment, hypersensitivity reactions (e.g., asthma, urticaria, and rhinitis), and toxicity. Other side effects can be seen in **Box 11.6**. NSAIDs should be taken with food, milk, or a glass of water to decrease the risk of

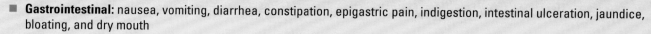

BOX 11.6 General Adverse Reactions to Nonsteroidal Anti-inflammatory Drugs

- **Gastrointestinal:** nausea, vomiting, diarrhea, constipation, epigastric pain, indigestion, intestinal ulceration, jaundice, bloating, and dry mouth

- **Central nervous system:** dizziness, anxiety, light-headedness, vertigo, headache, drowsiness, insomnia, depression, and psychic disturbances

- **Cardiovascular:** congestive heart failure, decreased or increased blood pressure, and cardiac arrhythmias

- **Renal:** hematuria, cystitis, elevated blood urea nitrogen, polyuria, dysuria, oliguria, and acute renal failure in those with impaired renal function

- **The senses:** visual disturbances, blurred or diminished vision, diplopia, swollen or irritated eyes, photophobia, reversible loss of color vision, tinnitus, taste change, and rhinitis

- **Skin:** rash, erythema, irritation, skin eruptions, exfoliative dermatitis, Stevens-Johnson syndrome, ecchymosis, and purpura

- **Metabolic/endocrinological:** decreased appetite, weight increase or decrease, hyperglycemia, hypoglycemia, flushing, sweating, menstrual disorders, and vaginal bleeding

- **Other:** thirst, fever, chills, and vaginitis

Adapted from Roach S. *Pharmacology for Health Professionals.* Philadelphia, PA: Lippincott Williams & Wilkins; 2005; with permission.

GI irritation. Alcohol should never be taken with NSAIDs, because it increases the risk of GI irritation and development of gastric ulcers. In the elderly, NSAIDs should be used cautiously, because the risk of serious ulcer disease in adults older than 65 years is increased with higher doses of NSAIDs.

The risk of renal impairment is relatively low with most NSAIDs. Signs of renal impairment include reduced urine output and rapid increase in serum creatinine and blood urea nitrogen. Signs and symptoms of a hypersensitive reaction or toxicity include dyspnea, rapid and irregular heartbeat, hematuria, upper abdominal tenderness, and jaundice. If any of these signs and symptoms develop, immediate medical attention is required.

Use and Availability

NSAIDs are used to treat mild-to-moderate pain associated with joints, muscles, and headaches. In addition, they often are used to treat inflammation associated with rheumatoid arthritis, tendinitis, and bursitis conditions. They are not, however, effective for the relief of severe pain.

NSAIDs are available in both OTC and prescription strengths and are routinely taken orally. Prescription strength NSAIDs can be prescribed only by a licensed practitioner. These NSAIDs are prescribed on a case-by-case basis and should not be shared among individuals with similar soft-tissue injuries or conditions. Sharing medication is not recommended, because individuals respond differently to the same medication. Non-prescription NSAIDs include ibuprofen (e.g., Advil, Motrin, and Motrin IB), ketoprofen (e.g., Orudis KT and Actron), and naproxen sodium (e.g., Aleve).

Pain relief usually is noted within 30 minutes after ingestion and lasts for several hours, depending on the dosage and duration of the particular NSAID. Both OTC and prescription products should be used only for short-term (i.e., 10 days maximum) treatment of inflammation and pain associated with soft-tissue injuries. When used as an antipyretic, NSAIDs should be used for only 3 days.[2] If pain, inflammation, or fever does not subside or increases within these time periods, consult a physician immediately. Ketorolac is an NSAID that can be injected intramuscularly (i.e., Toradol) and carries the same indications and risks as other NSAID medications.

As with most medications, and as mentioned previously, NSAIDs should not be used in combination with alcohol. A physician or pharmacist should be consulted before combining NSAIDs with other medications.

See **Common Nonsteroidal Anti-inflammatory Medications**, available on the companion Web site at thePoint, for a listing of the common NSAIDs used in treating soft-tissue injuries among sport participants.

Corticosteroids

Corticosteroids are steroid hormones that are produced naturally within the adrenal cortex but that also can be produced synthetically. They are powerful drugs that affect nearly the entire body.

Therapeutic Effects

Corticosteroids are lipid-soluble and block the body's natural response to inflammation by inhibiting the synthesis of chemical mediators (e.g., prostaglandins, leukotrienes, and histamine). As a result, swelling, warmth, redness, and pain associated with inflammation are decreased. The manner in which corticosteroids suppress inflammation, however, is much broader in scope than the manner in which NSAIDs do so. Corticosteroids inhibit prostaglandin synthesis, as do NSAIDs, but corticosteroids also act in several other ways to decrease inflammation.

Adverse Effects

Side effects of corticosteroids, which often resemble those of the condition for which they are prescribed to treat, include itching, burning, dry skin, and fluid retention. Side effects that are rare include an increase or decrease in appetite, dizziness, restlessness, facial or body hair growth, GI irritation, menstrual irregularities, and optic pain. Most of these side effects disappear soon after the medication is discontinued. Because oral NSAIDs and corticosteroids have similar effects on the GI tract, concurrent use severely increases the risk of GI irritation and ulceration. In addition, chronic use of corticosteroids can suppress the body's immune system, making the user more susceptible to infection.

Availability and Use

Corticosteroids are indicated for skin disorders, nasal inflammation, rheumatic disorders (e.g., bursitis, arthritis, and tendinitis), and skin infections. They are administered through oral and nasal inhalation, intra-articular injection, subcutaneous injection, intravenous injection, topically, and orally.

Corticosteroids should not be used by individuals who are infected with HIV or have AIDS, heart disease, hypertension, diabetes, gastritis, peptic ulcers, lupus, or other infections (e.g., bronchitis or flu). By reducing inflammation and pain, corticosteroids also may delay exercise-induced pain, placing an individual at increased risk for further injury. Corticosteroids are not banned by the NCAA, but the USOC bans all types, with the exception of most topical (e.g., ear, eye, and skin) agents. The USOC allows inhaled, local, or intra-articular injections if written permission is provided.[9,10]

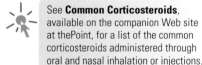
See **Common Corticosteroids**, available on the companion Web site at thePoint, for a list of the common corticosteroids administered through oral and nasal inhalation or injections.

Local Anesthetics

Anesthetics, frequently called "pain killers," inhibit the activity of sensory nerve receptors in the skin. Under normal conditions, the skin does not respond well to aspirin or other oral analgesics. When irritated, the same sensory nerve endings in the skin can lead to **pruritus** from a weak stimulation or to skin pain from a strong stimulation. The skin responds more readily to topical medications. Local anesthetics are categorized by route of administration and may be injectable, topical, or sprayed. Injectable anesthetics are prescription medications that can be administered only by a licensed professional (i.e., physician, physician assistant, nurse practitioner, or nurse).

Injectable Anesthetics

In the treatment of sports-related injuries, injectable anesthetics most commonly are used for **infiltrative anesthesia**, a process that produces numbness by interfering with nerve function in a localized, subcutaneous, soft-tissue area. Infiltrative anesthesia commonly is used for the treatment of soft-tissue injuries, such as hip pointers and turf toe. In addition, they are used as an anesthetic before minor surgical procedures, such as suturing or aspiration of bursal or joint fluid. They are classified by the duration of action—namely, short-, intermediate-, and long-term action. Side effects are minimal when used as directed. Large quantities of the drugs must be absorbed to produce any associated side effects, such as tremors, drowsiness, hypotension, or hypersensitivity and anaphylactic reactions.

Topical Anesthetics

Topical anesthetics are OTC and prescription medications that are applied to the skin. Topical anesthetics or analgesics often are used to relieve pain associated with musculoskeletal injury (e.g., strains, sprains, tendinitis, and bursitis). When used for these purposes, topical medications are called **counterirritants**. These medications stimulate nerve endings in the skin that respond to pain and to warm and cold sensations, which in theory distracts the user from the original pain or itching. Essentially, these products irritate the skin to relieve pain and itching. Counterirritants come in various forms, including lotions, rubs, liniments, and creams. Popular examples include Ben-Gay, Mineral Ice, Flexall 454, Menthol, Cramergesic, and Icy Hot. The FDA suggests that these drugs are safe when applied three to four times per day, but they are not suggested for long-term use. If pain persists after 7 days, a physician should be consulted immediately.

In addition to the counterirritant properties, topical anesthetics can further be classified according to whether they reduce itching, pain, or both. Most topical anesthetics are easily identified in their brand names by the suffix "-caine" (e.g., Americaine, Lanacane, Xylocaine, and Solarcaine).

Spray Anesthetics

In addition to creams, lotions, and liniments, a few spray anesthetics are on the market (e.g., aerofreeze, ethyl chloride, and fluoromethane). These products temporarily freeze the skin in an effort to decrease pain; however, the duration of action is quite limited and lasts for only approximately 1 minute. These products are not recommended for use, because the freezing action can damage the skin and delay healing.

Adverse Effects

Topical anesthetics are relatively safe when used as directed. Common side effects are limited to skin irritation (e.g., rashes or hives). These normally disappear once use of the product is stopped. Systemic absorption can occur if large amounts of these products are used over a large surface area or if used on deep wounds. Systemic absorption is toxic and may produce convulsions and paralysis of the CNS.

Individuals who are allergic to aspirin should not use methyl salicylate products, because the body may absorb the salicylate, the major ingredient in aspirin. In addition, products that produce warm sensations should never be used in combination with a heating pad or occlusive dressing. This may increase systemic absorption and result in skin and muscle necrosis. These products should never be used before exercise in hot, humid conditions or immediately following exercise. Application is appropriate after the body cools down. The NCAA and USOC permit the use of topical anesthetics; the NCAA also permits intra-articular injections of local anesthesia when medically justified.[9,10]

Muscle Relaxants

Unlike local anesthetics that inhibit sensory nerve receptors in the skin and subcutaneous tissue, muscle relaxants actually block afferent messages that travel from the muscles to the brain. Skeletal muscle relaxants are classified as either central or direct acting. Central agents exert their effects within the spinal cord, whereas direct-acting muscle relaxants affect the skeletal muscle cell. Both types are available by prescription only. Muscle relaxants prescribed for muscle spasms associated with musculoskeletal injury are central acting. They decrease local pain, spasm, and tenderness and, in doing so, allow increased range of motion. Examples of common muscle relaxants are chlorzoxazone (e.g., Parafon Forte and Muscol), cyclobenzaprine (e.g., Flexeril), diazepam (e.g., Valium), methocarbamol (e.g., Robaxin), and orphenadrine (e.g., Norflex). These drugs often are used in combination with rest and physical therapy (e.g., thermotherapy, cryotherapy, and electrotherapy) to relieve pain from acute muscle spasms associated with musculoskeletal conditions. Because central-acting muscle relaxants produce their effects by acting on the CNS, they often produce a general depression of CNS functions. As a result, common side effects include dizziness, drowsiness, and sedation. Muscle relaxants are not banned by either the NCAA or the USOC; however, they may be prohibited by international federations of certain sports.

See **Common Muscle Relaxant Medications,** found on the companion Web site at thePoint, for a list of the common muscle relaxants and their possible side effects.

Topical Antibiotics

Antibiotics are substances that kill disease-producing bacteria and are used to prevent and treat infections. Two basic types of bacteria cause most skin infections, namely, *Streptococcus* and *Staphylococcus*. Because it is difficult to predict which type of bacteria may be producing a skin infection, most topical antibiotics contain several active ingredients that treat both organisms; when purchasing, use triple antibiotic. Topical antibiotics are used on small open wounds, such as abrasions, and can be purchased as creams, ointments, or powders. Bacitracin, Neosporin, Neomycin, and Polysporin are examples of OTC topical antibiotics. These products are not designed to be used on deep wounds, because internal absorption of some of these antibiotics can be toxic. Topical antibiotics should be used in small amounts, generally three times daily, and for not more than 1 week.[2] Topical antibiotics are not banned by the NCAA or USOC.

See **Common Topical Antibiotics**, found on the companion Web site at thePoint, for a list of the common topical antibiotics and their possible side effects.

Oral Antibiotics

In the event of infection, oral antibiotics may be needed to treat infection or cellulitis. Selecting and administering oral antibiotics in a prudent manner is necessary due to the increase in antimicrobial resistance. Identifying the specific antigen allows the practitioner to prescribe first-choice medications needed to treat the infection. For the treatment of cellulitis caused by *Streptococcus* or *Staphylococcus*, cephalexin, erythromycin, or co-trimoxazole (if methicillin-resistant *Staphylococcus aureus* [MRSA] is present) may be used to treat the infection.

Antiseptics and Disinfectants

The terms antiseptic and disinfectant sometimes are used interchangeably, but they are not the same. **Antiseptics** are applied to living tissue to stop growth of microorganisms or destroy bacteria on contact and prevent infection. They are most appropriate in the cleansing and treatment of large, open skin wounds and come in sprays, powders, and swab-on liquids. Isopropyl alcohol, Betadine, and tincture of iodine are common OTC antiseptics. Antiseptics are for external use only and are not banned by the NCAA or USOC.

Disinfectants are chemical agents applied to nonliving objects. They most commonly are used to disinfect surgical instruments and cleanse medical equipment and facilities. Common disinfectants used in athletic training are alcohol products, Whizzer, and Iso-Quin. The companion Web site at thePoint provides information about disinfecting techniques used in the athletic training room to prevent the spread of infectious diseases related to bloodborne pathogens.

Antifungal Agents

Tolnaftate (e.g., Tinactin), miconazole nitrate (e.g., Micatin), and clotrimazole (e.g., Lotrimin and Mycelex) are agents that treat infections caused by fungal cells. In humans, fungal cells are either molds or yeasts. Tinea pedis, tinea cruris, and tinea corporis are caused by fungal molds, whereas candidiasis and moniliasis are caused by fungal yeasts. Products used to treat fungal molds usually are applied twice daily, with symptoms disappearing within a few days of initial treatment. Following disappearance of symptoms, the molds often can still be found within skin cracks and nail beds. For this reason, physicians suggest regular, continued application of antifungal agents as part of a preventive protocol. Before applying antifungal agents, the infected area should be cleansed thoroughly with mild soap and water. If the infection does not clear within 1 week (e.g., tinea cruris) or 1 month (e.g., tinea pedis and corporis), another antifungal agent should be used or a physician should be consulted.

See **Common Antifungal Agents**, found on the companion Web site at thePoint, for a list of these agents and their possible side effects.

Historically, drugs used to treat vaginal yeast infections were by prescription only, but a variety of antiyeast agents can now be purchased over the counter. Examples include clotrimazole (e.g., Gyne-Lotrimin, Mycelex-7), miconazole nitrate (e.g., Monistat), and tioconazole (e.g., Vagistat-1). Oral medications (e.g., Diflucan) are available as a prescription medication and can also be used to treat vaginal yeast infections. Approximately 25% of females of childbearing age will develop a yeast infection. Predisposing factors include pregnancy, obesity, diabetes, debilitation, and the use of certain drugs (e.g., oral contraceptives and systemic antibiotics). Depending on the product, it should be used once daily for 1 to 14 days. If a course of treatment does not resolve the problem, the possibility exists that some other microorganism is present, and a physician should be consulted immediately.

Antifungal agents are relatively safe when used as directed. Some can be toxic if they are absorbed systemically and, as such, should be for external use only. Side effects usually resemble a worsening of the condition being treated, including increased redness, irritation, and itching. These products are not banned by the NCAA or USOC.

> Treatment for the softball player who sustained an abrasion to the left forearm should include initiating proper first aid care for an open wound using universal precautions, cleaning the abrasion with sterile saline, and applying a topical triple antibiotic (e.g., Bacitracin, Neosporin) keeping the wound clean and covered.

PERFORMANCE-ENHANCING SUBSTANCES (ERGOGENIC AIDS)

 Ephedrine is found in many OTC sinus and cold medications. What adverse effects are associated with the use of ephedrine?

Ergogenic aids are substances taken in nonpharmacological doses specifically to enhance energy production, energy use, or recovery to provide a competitive edge. A substance is considered to be performance-enhancing if it benefits sport participation by increasing strength, power, speed, or endurance or by altering body weight or composition. Even substances that change behavior, arousal level, and/or perception of pain should be considered as performance-enhancing.[16] Some substances are legal and may be a part of one's normal diet (e.g., caffeine, alcohol, and tobacco). Taken in excess, however, even these substances can produce adverse effects in a healthy individual.

Caffeine

Coffee, tea, chocolate, and energy drinks are common beverages and foods found in the American diet. Each contains caffeine—the most widely abused drug in the world. Caffeine is a low-level CNS stimulant that increases alertness and feelings of well-being. It is used as a stimulant in fatigue states (e.g., Vivarin and NoDoz), in combination with analgesic compounds (e.g., Excedrin and Anacin), and in diet pills. Caffeine also is found in many new products, including energy drinks, sport gels, and alcoholic beverages.

Caffeine is rapidly absorbed, with peak levels being achieved in 30 to 60 minutes and a half-life of 3.5 hours.[11] Caffeine stimulates the secretion of adrenaline (epinephrine) and, except in the renal afferent artery, causes vasoconstriction. This response could produce a number of secondary metabolic changes that could promote an ergogenic action, such as enhancing the contractility of skeletal and cardiac muscle and assisting in fat metabolism.[12] Therefore, caffeine is considered to be an ergogenic aid for prolonged endurance exercise activities in doses of approximately 3 to 6 mg per kg body mass.[13] Ergogenic dose effects are found at approximately half the banned dose level, which equals three cups of coffee or six to eight caffeinated soft drinks.[14] Many individuals take caffeine in pill form.

When used in large doses (15 to 30 mg per kg), caffeine overdose may lead to agitation, delirium, seizures, dyspnea, cardiac arrhythmia, myoclonus, nausea, vomiting, hyperglycemia, and hypokalemia. With lower doses of caffeine, such as those via coffee consumption, adverse reactions may include tachycardia, palpitations, insomnia, restlessness, nervousness, tremor, headache, abdominal pain, nausea, vomiting, diarrhea, and diuresis.[15] Caffeine is considered by the NCAA and International Olympic Committee (IOC) to be a "restricted or controlled drug" when urine levels exceed 15 and 12 μg per mL, respectively.[14] Similar to most stimulants, caffeine does produce tolerance and can be addictive, with users experiencing withdrawal symptoms on cessation of use.

Tobacco

Tobacco is a low-level CNS stimulant and is widely used in the United States. Nicotine is the stimulating chemical and addictive substance in the product. Methods of consumption include cigarettes, cigars, and smokeless tobacco (i.e., loose-leaf tobacco [chewing], moist or dry powdered tobacco [snuff or "dipping"], and compressed tobacco ["plug"]). Nicotine is absorbed in the lungs when using cigarettes and cigars and through the oral mucosa when using smokeless tobacco.

Initially, small doses of nicotine stimulate, and large doses depress, the autonomic ganglia and myoneural junctions. The amount of nicotine in tobacco products varies widely. On average, one cigarette contains 1 mg of nicotine, and a pinch of smokeless tobacco contains 35 mg. Contrary to popular belief, smokeless tobacco is not a safe alternative to cigarette smoking, because the nicotine is more swiftly absorbed into the bloodstream, resulting in a more immediate stimulant effect.

Major League Baseball imposed a ban on the use of smokeless tobacco products in the minor leagues, and the NCAA has an all-sport ban on the use of smokeless tobacco during NCAA practices and games. The use of smokeless tobacco by adults has slowly declined since the late 1990s and rapidly declined in adolescents and teens during this same time period.[16] Side effects associated with the use of smokeless tobacco are similar to those of other products that contain nicotine, including feelings of well-being, increased heart rate, increased blood pressure, and addiction.[17] The use of smokeless tobacco also can lead to **halitosis**, permanently discolored teeth, oral abrasions, periodontal bone disease, tooth loss, and **leukoplakia**. Leukoplakia is a disease of the mouth characterized by white patches and oral lesions on the cheeks, gums, and/or tongue, which can lead to oral cancer.

Alcohol

Alcohol is the most abused recreational drug in the United States, and it is the number one drug of choice among intercollegiate athletes.[1] Alcohol is involved in more than one-third of the deaths attributed to unintentional injury, homicide, and suicide, which together account for 76% of mortality in the 15- to 19-year-old age group. More than half (58%) of 12th-grade students and one-fifth (20%) of 8th-grade students report having been drunk at least once in their life.[18]

When ingested, alcohol is rapidly absorbed, unaltered, into the body. Most absorption takes place in the stomach and small intestine. Absorption rates depend on several factors:

- Type and concentration of the alcohol

- The rate at which the beverage is consumed

- Current stomach contents

- Factors influencing the emptying of the stomach (e.g., levels of carbonated beverages, food, and emotional state)

- Body weight

- Gastric motility

Alcohol is metabolized at a constant rate, typically 1 oz of alcohol per hour. This equals one 12-oz beer (excluding lagers and malt liqueurs), 2.5 oz of wine, or 1 oz of distilled spirits. The rate of metabolism is related to the actions of liver enzymes, which can vary between individuals. Factors influencing these enzymes include age, menstrual cycle, heredity, race, liver disease, and previous experience with alcohol consumption.[19,20]

Alcohol is lipid-soluble. As such, it quickly crosses the blood–brain barrier and instantly acts as a CNS depressant. Alcohol is distributed unmodified throughout body fluids, tissues, and organs. The majority of alcohol is metabolized in the liver (90%), with the remainder being excreted through urine, sweat, and one's breath.

Unlike other ergogenic aids, alcohol rarely is used as such. In a 1982 American College of Sports Medicine Position Statement on alcohol use in sports, it was found that

1. Alcohol in small (i.e., 1.5 to 2.0 oz) to moderate (i.e., 3 to 4 oz) amounts has negative effects on psychomotor skills, including reaction times, hand–eye coordination, accuracy, balance, and complex coordination.

2. Alcohol has little or no benefit regarding energy metabolism or oxygen consumption.

3. Alcohol does not improve muscular work capacity and may decrease performance levels as well as impair temperature regulation during prolonged exercise in cold environments.

Therefore, it has been concluded that alcohol lacks ergogenic properties for the majority of sport-related activities. Alcohol may be an ergogenic aid in some aiming sports; however, no conclusive evidence has appeared to support this theory. Alcohol is considered to be an NCAA-banned substance in riflery but not in other NCAA sports.

Marijuana

Marijuana is a naturally occurring cannabinoid that contains the active ingredient δ9-tetrahydrocannabinol (THC). Marijuana is considered an illegal drug in all states except Colorado, Alaska, Oregon, and Washington, where the drug may be taken recreationally as a euphoriant. Medically, marijuana has been used as an antiemetic agent in conjunction with chemotherapy for patients with cancer and for lowering intraocular pressure in patients with glaucoma.

The active ingredient THC primarily affects the CNS and cardiovascular system. Adverse effects to the CNS include impaired motor coordination, decreased short-term memory, difficulty concentrating, and decline in work performance. Adverse effects to the cardiovascular system include tachycardia and changes in blood pressure (e.g., systolic blood pressure increases in a supine position and decreases in a standing position). The effects depend on the route, dose, setting, and previous experience of the user. Adverse effects on sport and physical activity performance include reduction of maximal exercise performance, with premature achievement of maximal volume of oxygen uptake (VO_{2max}), and no appreciable effect on tidal volume, arterial blood pressure, or carboxyhemoglobin compared to controls. Marijuana can inhibit sweating, leading to an increase in core body temperature.

Marijuana is not banned by the IOC but is considered a prohibited street drug by the NCAA; marijuana is tested by the NCAA. Because of its high lipid solubility, marijuana can be detected for up to 2 to 4 weeks by drug testing.

Diuretics

Diuretics, commonly known as "water pills," help to rid the body of unneeded water and salt through the urine, allowing the heart to pump blood more freely. In general, diuretics are used to treat high blood pressure, heart failure, kidney and liver problems, and glaucoma. Diuretics are categorized as follows:

- Carbonic anhydrase inhibitors
- Loop diuretics
- Osmotic diuretics
- Potassium-sparing diuretics
- Thiazides and related diuretics

Carbonic anhydrase inhibitors prevent the action of carbonic anhydrase, an enzyme that produces free hydrogen ions, which are then traded for sodium ions in the kidney tubules. As a result, sodium, potassium, bicarbonate, and water are excreted in the urine. Carbonic anhydrase inhibitors (e.g., acetazolamide and methazolamide) often are used to treat glaucoma, because these agents can decrease the production of aqueous humor in the eye, which in turn decreases intraocular pressure.

Loop diuretics (e.g., furosemide and ethacrynic) are more powerful. These agents are especially useful during emergencies, such as in the treatment of edema associated with chronic heart failure, cirrhosis of the liver, and renal disease.

Osmotic diuretics (e.g., mannitol and urea) are used to promote diuresis in the prevention and treatment of the oliguric phase (i.e., low urine production) of acute renal failure. These agents also are used to reduce cerebral edema as well as intraocular pressure before and after eye surgery.

Potassium-sparing diuretics work in two ways. First, certain medications (e.g., triamterene and amiloride) depress the reabsorption of sodium in the kidney tubules and, in doing so, increase sodium and water excretion. Second, they depress the excretion of potassium, hence the name potassium-sparing. For example, spironolactone, another potassium-sparing diuretic, acts on the hormone aldosterone, which enhances the reabsorption of sodium in the distal tubules of the kidney. When this action is blocked, sodium (but not potassium) and water are excreted. Potassium-sparing diuretics are used in the treatment of chronic heart failure and hypertension.

Thiazides and related diuretics inhibit the reabsorption of sodium and chloride, leading to moderate increases in the excretion of sodium, chloride, and water. They often are used in long-term treatment of hypertension, edema caused by chronic heart failure, hepatic cirrhosis, corticosteroid and estrogen therapy, and renal dysfunction.

Use of diuretics should be closely monitored by a physician. Abuse of diuretics can impair thermoregulation; exacerbate exercise-related dehydration; decrease stroke volume; increase arrhythmia; cause a reflex increase in total peripheral resistance, which may decrease muscle blood flow; and contribute to electrolyte depletion.[21] In addition, adverse reactions may involve fever, rash, photosensitivity, blurred vision, nausea, vomiting, headaches, vertigo, and diarrhea.[3]

Anabolic-Androgenic Steroids

Anabolic-androgenic steroids include more than 30 natural and synthetically made derivatives of testosterone. They most commonly are used to stimulate growth and accelerate weight gain. When naturally secreted from the pituitary gland (men, 4 to 10 mg per day; women, 1 mg per day), testosterone produces secondary sex characteristics. Tetrahydrogestrinone (THG) has received considerable media attention as a performance-enhancing substance. Although difficult to detect, there have been various reports of its use by high-profile athletes in several sports, including track and field, football, tennis, and baseball. After developing a way to detect THG in the urine following the 2004 Olympics, the FDA, Major League Baseball, and the World Anti-Doping Agency have banned this substance.[22]

Physiologically, anabolic steroids promote rapid synthesis of protein in the body by binding to androgen receptors at the cellular level, stimulating the production of ribonucleic acid, which in turn increases the synthesis of protein. In healthy individuals who do not exercise, steroids increase appetite and feelings of well-being but have no effect on muscle size or strength. Among individuals who are involved in high-intensity training, anabolic steroids can increase body weight, lean body mass, and muscle size as well as strength[23]; however, anabolic steroids provide little benefit in terms of aerobic capacity. Other adverse effects include bouts of uncontrolled anger and explosive behavior, increased appetite and sexual desires, and a lowered tolerance to pain.[24,25] Short- and long-term physical effects, such as those listed in **Box 11.7**, are dependent on the type of steroid used, the frequency of use, and the age of initiation.[26] Some of these effects are irreversible even after discontinuation of steroid use.

Anabolic steroids most commonly are used in 6- to 12-week cycles with pyramid or stacking techniques.[26] The term stacking denotes the simultaneous use of two or more types of anabolic

---

BOX 11.7 Physical Effects of Anabolic Steroid Use

Short Term	Long Term
Acne	Cardiovascular disease
Gynecomastia	Liver disease
Male pattern baldness	Testicular atrophy
Enhanced facial and body hair growth	Impotence/sterility
Menstrual irregularities	Decrease in sperm
Decreased breast development in women	Enlargement of clitoris
Deepening of the voice	Uterine atrophy
Increased risk of muscle strains/ruptures	Early closure of physis in children (shorter adult height)

steroids, which could include both oral and intramuscular injections, and the pattern of increasing a dose through a cycle is referred to as pyramiding. An individual using the pyramid technique begins with a lower daily dose, then moves to a higher dose in the middle of a cycle, and then ends with a lower dose at the end of a cycle. Pyramiding may lead to doses 10- to 40-fold greater than those used for medical indications. A common belief is that pyramiding and stacking maximize steroid receptor binding and minimize toxic side effects. These benefits have not been substantiated scientifically, but this has not appreciably influenced dosing patterns.

Human Growth Hormone

Human growth hormone (hGH) is a popular antiaging drug and commonly is used to enhance muscular strength and growth as well as for its musculoskeletal healing properties. hGH is used in growth hormone–deficient children (to stimulate skeletal and soft-tissue growth), growth hormone–deficient adults, the elderly, children with chronic renal failure, and children with large cutaneous burns (to accelerate wound healing). It also is used to increase lean body mass and decrease fat in patients postoperatively and is approved for treatment of wasting syndrome secondary to HIV infection.[11]

In its natural form, hGH is secreted from the anterior pituitary gland and mediates a plethora of metabolic and growth processes, with effects on the majority of body tissues. The hormone increases protein synthesis by enhancing uptake and transport of amino acids. Synthetic or recombinant hGH is administered intramuscularly or subcutaneously, with a typical dose being 0.30 mg per kg per week.[27]

The most common side effect of hGH is **acromegaly**, a condition described as gigantism and characterized by costal and mandibular growth; vertebral, phalangeal, and frontal bone overgrowth; widening of joint spaces; accelerated osteoarthritis; and soft-tissue swelling. As little as a twofold increase in recommended dosage may result in acromegaly, which leaves a narrow therapeutic window. The risk of acromegaly is significant for individuals consuming up to 20 mg per day. Other side effects include hypertension, hyperglycemia, glycosuria, diabetes, arthritis, menstrual irregularities, vision loss, sleep apnea, ventricular hypertrophy, myopathies, and characteristic coarsening of bones in the face, hands, and feet.[11,15]

In the athletic environment, hGH often is used in combination with various testosterone derivatives and is extremely difficult to detect in routine urine drug tests. Therefore, it is becoming increasingly popular among athletes. Efforts are being made, however, to develop a noninvasive technique to detect the use of hGH. Testosterone and hGH are not banned by the NCAA if prescribed by a physician.

Amphetamines

Amphetamines are powerful CNS stimulants that are banned by the NCAA and IOC. They are used for therapeutic purposes to treat a variety of conditions, such as refractory obesity, narcolepsy, ADD, and severe depression. Sport participants may use amphetamines to mask fatigue and pain and to improve certain mental tasks.[28,29]

Classified as sympathomimetics, amphetamines influence involuntary actions of the CNS (i.e., heart rate and blood pressure). Most users take amphetamines orally, but injectable and inhaled forms (e.g., cocaine and crack) also are available. Serious side effects include a lowered threshold for arrhythmias and provocation of angina, which may lead to sudden cardiac death, stroke, tremors, insomnia, psychosis, psychological addiction, and rhabdomyolysis. Little evidence suggests that many sport participants use amphetamines, but evidence does clearly indicate the use of less potent amphetamine-like products, such as ephedrine. Amphetamines are readily detected by urine tests because both unchanged amphetamines and metabolites appear in the urine.

Ephedra

Derived from the ancient Chinese herb ephedra, or ma huang, the ephedrine alkaloids (e.g., pseudoephedrine, norephedrine, methylephedrine, methylpseudoephedrine, and norpseudoephedrine) can have powerful effects on the body. Ephedra is a CNS stimulant that increases serum levels of norepinephrine and can, directly or indirectly, increase blood pressure, heart rate, cardiac output, and peripheral vascular resistance.[22] Traditionally used as a bronchodilator and nasal decongestant, ephedra is found in many OTC sinus and cold medications. It is used therapeutically to treat chronic postural hypotension, enuresis, and narcolepsy. Ephedra in dietary supplements was banned by the FDA in 2004.

Side effects of ephedra can be life threatening, because it increases heat production and body temperature and, as such, increases the risk of heat illness, especially in warm environments. Mild adverse effects include heart palpitations and irregular heartbeats, dizziness, headache, insomnia, nervousness, and skin flushing or tingling. Moderate to severe adverse reactions include tachycardia, life-threatening arrhythmias, hypertension, stroke, seizures, and death.[30] Recently, ephedra has been shown to be ergogenic for anaerobic exercise, especially when taken with caffeine; however, the potential for toxicity is high.[31] It is important to note that synthetic ephedrine derivatives are used to produce the street drugs ecstasy and methamphetamine, which are used as stimulants. Ephedra is banned by the IOC, NCAA, Major League Baseball, NASCAR, and the National Football League.

Blood Doping and Erythropoietin

The primary purpose of blood doping and use of erythropoietin is to stimulate the production of RBCs so that more oxygen is available for use during long-distance aerobic activities (e.g., cycling) to enhance oxygen-carrying capacity and skeletal muscle performance. Before the increased popularity of erythropoietin, two techniques were used to produce the desired effects of blood doping:

1. Homologous transfusions use blood from another person or donor and transfuse it into the identified individual. Two major concerns with this procedure are the compatibility of the transfusion between the donor and recipient and the risk of contracting HIV and hepatitis.

2. Autologous transfusions remove blood from the individual, freeze the blood, and reinfuse the blood several weeks later, after the recipient's body has had ample time to make new RBCs. Following the transfusion, the recipient has an increased concentration of RBCs.

Transfusions can improve performance during endurance exercises by increasing hemoglobin concentration, which leads to increased maximal oxygen consumption and total exercise time as well as improved tolerance in some extreme environmental conditions.[11] The IOC bans blood doping, but enforcement is limited by the lack of effective techniques for detection.

Intravenous use of recombinant human erythropoietin stimulates RBC production within days, and effects can be seen for as long as 3 to 4 weeks. Erythropoietin is used therapeutically in several conditions, including anemia secondary to end-stage renal disease; anemia secondary to prematurity, multiple myeloma, and cancer; and AIDS treated with zidovudine. Its use also increases the yield of autologous blood donors both safely and effectively over a 21-day period and can reduce the need for transfusions in patients undergoing hip replacement. Miscalculations in dosing and dehydration may result in a hematocrit level as high as 80% and can cause severe hyperviscosity leading to encephalopathy, stroke, seizures, and tissue hypoxia.[22] Rapid clotting also may lead to pulmonary embolism, myocardial infarction, and peripheral clot formation (i.e., vascular thrombosis). In addition, intravenous use increases other inherent risks (e.g., infection with hepatitis, infection with HIV, and endocarditis).

The prevalence of erythropoietin use is unknown. Various media reports concerning its use among athletes have appeared, but no scientific reports indicate its prevalence. According to the position statement of the American College of Sports Medicine on "The Use of Blood Doping as an Ergogenic Aid," any blood-doping procedure used to enhance athletic performance is unethical and unfair and exposes the individual to serious health risks.[32] Darbepoetin, a related substance, causes similar effects and was detected during the 2002 Winter Olympics in cross-country skiers, who subsequently were disqualified. Because recombinant human erythropoietin and darbepoetin can now be detected, newer strategies to evade detection and boost performance are likely to be used in the near future.

Creatine

Creatine is a nonessential dietary element found in protein-rich sources, such as meat and fish. It is the most widely used and marketed nonsteroidal, nonstimulant ergogenic aid in young athletes, and it has been reported to be used in 41% of 219 Division I intercollegiate athletes.[33] It is synthesized primarily in the liver and is stored predominantly in skeletal muscle. Hydrolysis of muscle phosphocreatine results in rapid production of adenosine triphosphate (ATP), which is needed for muscle contraction. As muscle stores of phosphocreatine become depleted, performance decreases. Oral creatine supplementation can increase muscle phosphocreatine stores by 6% to 8% and, in doing so, causes faster regeneration of ATP. This can result in shorter recovery periods and increased energy for repeated bouts of exercise. Increased muscle creatine also buffers the lactic acid produced during exercise, delaying muscle fatigue and soreness.[14] In anaerobic exercise, creatine depletion is a limiting factor.[34]

The total daily requirement of creatine is 2 g per day, approximately half of which comes from in vivo production and the other half from dietary sources.[34] Supplemental dosing varies. One method involves ingesting loading doses of 20 g daily, divided in four doses, for 5 to 10 days, followed by a maintenance dose of 5 g per day. Another method eliminates the loading phase and involves ingesting 3 g per day. Lower doses take longer to reach the desired intramuscular creatine levels.[33]

Creatine purports to be a safe ergogenic aid in adults. The adverse effects are few and dose-dependent, including weight gain and GI distress (e.g., nausea, bloating, cramping, and diarrhea). Although increased muscle cramping originally was thought to be a side effect of creatine use, recent studies with college football players showed that creatine supplementation did not appear to increase the incidence or injury or cramping and, when combined with resistance and anaerobic training, may positively affect cell hydration status and enhance performance variables further than the augmentation that is seen with training alone.[35,36] No other serious long-term, detrimental effects in the absence of other nutritional supplements have been consistently documented.[37] Several areas of concern, however, include the potential for renal damage in those with preexisting renal dysfunction, rhabdomyolysis, cardiovascular impact if the creatine is taken up by the myocardium, increased risk of heat illness because of potential dehydration, and increased risk of exertional compartment syndrome as a result of fluid retention that may accompany loading doses of the substance.[38] In the most recent position statement on creatine use, the American College of Sports Medicine discouraged creatine use in people younger than 18 years of age because of unknown potential adverse health effects.[38]

 Even though ephedrine is found in many OTC sinus and cold medications, adverse effects are associated with its use. The mild adverse effects of ephedrine include heart palpitations and irregular heartbeats, dizziness, headache, insomnia, nervousness, and skin flushing or tingling. Moderate-to-severe adverse reactions to ephedrine include tachycardia, life-threatening arrhythmias, hypertension, stroke, seizures, and death. Combining caffeine with ephedra greatly increases the severity of side effects.

DRUG TESTING

In 1965, Beckett developed the first chromatographic drug testing procedures for the Tour of Britain cycling competition. Three years later, the IOC drug testing program was implemented during the 1968 Summer Olympic Games. Following the lead of the IOC, the NCAA began drug testing at championship events in 1986. The intent of drug testing programs is threefold:

1. Drug testing discovers those individuals who may be experiencing problems.

2. Testing is performed to screen participants for evidence of drug use/abuse.

3. Drug testing protects individuals from injury or from causing injury to others.

Various drug testing methods (e.g., urine tests, blood tests, human hair tests, and radioimmunoassay) are available. Urine testing is the method of choice. It is noninvasive, and large volumes of urine can be collected easily. Analysis for the presence of drugs and their metabolites is usually seen in high concentrations in the urine. Two disadvantages of urine testing are the ease of tampering with the sample and the potentially humiliating experience for the individual.

Current drug testing uses gas chromatography/mass spectrometry (GC/MS). Factors influencing test accuracy include individual urine output/volume, urine pH, dosage, timing and formulation of used substances, occasional or chronic substance use, substances taken simultaneously, variability of testing equipment, individual metabolism, recent trauma, and shock. Although GC/MS may approach 100% accuracy, individuals have attempted to avoid detection using several methods:

- **Masking agents.** Diuretics often are used to counteract steroid-induced fluid retention and reduce the concentration of banned substances.[39]

- **Determination of drug half-life.** If drug testing is announced, individuals can determine the length of time during which a specific drug can be detected in the urine.

- **Substitution of urine.** Several methods can be used to substitute "clean" urine (e.g., self-catheterization and innovative "delivery systems"). In efforts to eliminate this problem, collection is conducted under constant supervision and close observation.

The NCAA does not require drug testing programs at its institutional membership schools. Many colleges and universities along with professional sport teams, however, have implemented drug testing programs. In addition, the NCAA does perform drug testing at NCAA championship events and randomly selected regional events. The NCAA also visits all NCAA Division I schools twice per year to randomly drug test selected football and track-and-field athletes. Athletic trainers working with athletes should be familiar with the NCAA, USOC, and IOC banned substance lists. It must be noted that many OTC products and nutritional supplements may have substances that are banned by the NCAA and/or USOC; athletes should always make sure that the ingredients in these products are not banned before using them. Information concerning the NCAA drug testing program and the banned substance lists is available on the NCAA Web site (www.ncaa.org) and the USOC Web site (www.usoc.org).

 See **Drug Clearance Times**, found on the companion Web site at thePoint, for specific drugs and their approximate elimination time.

SUMMARY

1. Medications have chemical, generic, and brand names.

2. Pharmacokinetics is the process that explains a drug's entry into the body as well as its absorption, distribution, metabolization, and excretion.

3. The pharmacokinetic process determines the means by which a drug reaches a target site to either facilitate or inhibit an action.

4. The half-life of a drug, lipid solubility, therapeutic range, dosage, potency, and maximal efficacy all play a role in determining the drug's action and effect.

5. Common medications for the treatment of soft-tissue injuries include analgesics and antipyretics, NSAIDs, corticosteroids, muscle relaxants, topical antibiotics, antiseptics, and antifungal agents. Each of these drugs comes in both prescription and OTC forms.

6. Athletic trainers are not allowed to prescribe or dispense prescription medication.

7. Depending on state regulations, athletic trainers may be authorized by the team physician to administer a one-dose pack of an OTC medication when approved protocols warrant their use.

8. When providing OTC medications, a record log should be kept that indicates the individual's name, date, medication administered, reasons for administering the medication, and signature of the athletic trainer administering the medication.

9. OTC medications should be stored as directed on packaging labels and placed in a secure, locked cabinet.

10. Prescription medications should be kept in a secured and locked location under the direct supervision of a licensed physician or pharmacist.

11. Therapeutic medications, if not used as directed, can cause adverse reactions and, in some cases, toxicity and death.

12. Ergogenic aids are substances or devices that enhance energy production, energy use, or recovery to provide a competitive edge.

13. Current drug testing uses GC/MS.

APPLICATION QUESTIONS

1. An 18-year-old female gymnast sustained a second-degree lumbar strain. What two types of medications is the team physician likely to prescribe for this athlete? In filling the prescription, the generic brand of the medications will be supplied. What are possible generic names for each type of medication? What side effects may occur with each medication?

2. You are an intercollegiate athletic trainer. While in the weight training room, you overhear a member of the basketball team asking a teammate about the use of diuretics to help lose weight. How would you respond to this scenario? What suggestions can you make to help the athlete safely lose weight without the use of diuretics?

3. A 55-year-old male preparing for a tennis tournament complains of chronic pain associated with medial epicondylitis. What type of therapeutic medication might be used to relieve the pain and inflammation associated with this condition? Does the age of the individual present any additional concerns?

4. What are the responsibilities of an athletic trainer when using therapeutic medications for the treatment of sport-related injuries? When indications are used as part of the treatment protocol, how can athletic trainers protect themselves from possible litigation?

REFERENCES

1. National Collegiate Athletic Association. NCAA student-athlete substance use study: executive summary August 2014. http://www.ncaa.org/about/resources/research/ncaa-student-athlete-substance-use-study-executive-summary-august-2014. Accessed January 10, 2015.

2. Houglum J, Harrelson G. *Principles of Pharmacology for Athletic Trainers*. 2nd ed. Thorofare, NJ: Slack; 2011.

3. Roach S. *Pharmacology for Health Professionals*. Philadelphia, PA: Lippincott Williams & Wilkins; 2005.

4. Carl LL, Gallo JA, Johnson PR, eds. *Practical Pharmacology in Rehabilitation: Effects of Medication on Therapy*. Champaign, IL: Human Kinetics; 2014.

5. Epocrates. athenahealth, Inc. http://www.epocrates.com. Accessed January 10, 2015.

6. Green GA, Uryasz FD, Petr TA, et al. NCAA study of substance use and abuse habits of college student-athletes. *Clin J Sport Med*. 2001;11(1):51–56.

7. Warner DC, Schnepf G, Barrett MS, et al. Prevalence, attitudes, and behaviors related to the use of nonsteroidal anti-inflammatory drugs (NSAIDs) in student athletes. *J Adolesc Health*. 2002;30(3):150–153.

8. Gomez J; and the American Academy of Pediatrics Committee on Sports Medicine and Fitness.

Use of performance-enhancing substances. *Pediatrics*. 2005;115(4):1103–1106.

9. Parsons JT. Dispensing prescription medication. In: *2014-15 NCAA Sports Medicine Handbook*. Indianapolis, IN: National Collegiate Athletic Association; 2014:21–22. http://www.muhlenberg.edu/pdf/main/athletics/athletic_training/2014_15_Sports_Medicine_Handbook.pdf. Accessed January 15, 2015.

10. United States Olympic Committee. *Drug Free: U.S. Olympic Committee Drug Education Handbook*. Colorado Springs, CO: United States Olympic Committee; 1996.

11. Green GA, Puffer JC. Drugs and doping in athletes. In: Mellion MB, Walsh WM, Madden C, et al, eds. *Team Physician's Handbook*. Philadelphia, PA: Hanley & Belfus; 2002:180–197.

12. Graham TE. Caffeine and exercise: metabolism, endurance and performance. *Sports Med*. 2001;31(1):785–807.

13. Bahrke MS, Yesalis CE, eds. *Performance Enhancing Substances in Sport and Exercise*. Champaign, IL: Human Kinetics; 2002.

14. Ahrendt DM. Ergogenic aids: counseling the athlete. *Am Fam Physician*. 2001;63(5):913–922.

15. Higdon JV, Frei B. Coffee and health: a review of recent human research. *Crit Rev Food Sci Nutr*. 2006;46(2):101–123.

16. Nelson DE, Mowery P, Tomar S, et al. Trends in smokeless tobacco use among adults and adolescents in the United States. *Am J Public Health*. 2006;96(5):897–905.

17. Cassisi NJ. Smokeless tobacco: is it worth the risk? *NCAA Sports Sciences Education Newsletter*. 2000:A1.

18. Johnston LD, O'Malley PM, Bachman JG, et al. *Monitoring the Future National Survey Results on Adolescent Drug Use: Overview of Key Findings, 2003*. Bethesda, MD: National Institute on Drug Abuse; 2004.

19. Chen YC, Lu RB, Peng GS, et al. Alcohol metabolism and cardiovascular response in an alcoholic patient homozygous for the ALDH2*2 variant gene allele. *Alcohol Clin Exp Res*. 1999;23(12):1853–1860.

20. Diamond I, Jay CA. Alcoholism and alcohol abuse. In: Goldman L, Bennett JC, eds. *Cecil Textbook of Medicine*. Philadelphia, PA: WB Saunders; 2000:49–54.

21. Anish EJ. The senior athlete. In: Mellion MB, Walsh WM, Madden C, et al, eds. *Team Physician's Handbook*. Philadelphia, PA: Hanley & Belfus; 2002:95–107.

22. Dhar R, Stout CW, Link MS, et al. Cardiovascular toxicities of performance-enhancing substances in sports. *Mayo Clin Proc*. 2005;80(10):1307–1315.

23. Hartgens F, Kuipers H. Effects of androgenic-anabolic steroids in athletes. *Sports Med*. 2004;34(8):513–554.

24. Pope HG Jr, Kouri EM, Hudson JI. Effects of supraphysiologic doses of testosterone on mood and aggression in normal men: a randomized controlled trial. *Arch Gen Psychiatry*. 2000;57(2):133–140.

25. Thiblin I, Petersson A. Pharmacoepidemiology of anabolic androgenic steroids: a review. *Fundam Clin Pharmacol*. 2005;19(1):27–44.

26. Llewellyn W. *Anabolics 2000*. Aurora, CO: Williams Llewellyn; 2000.

27. Windisch PA, Papatheofanis FJ, Matuszewski KA. Recombinant human growth hormone for AIDS-associated wasting. *Ann Pharmacother*. 1998;32(4):437–445.

28. Dekhuijzen PH, Machiels HA, Heunks LM, et al. Athletes and doping: effects of drugs on the respiratory system. *Thorax*. 1999;54(11):1041–1046.

29. Mattay VS, Callicott JH, Bertolino A, et al. Effects of dextroamphetamine on cognitive performance and cortical activation. *Neuroimage*. 2000;12(3):268–275.

30. Munson BL. Myths and facts . . . about ephedrine use. *Nursing*. 2003;33(4):81.

31. Jacobs I, Pasternak H, Bell DG. Effects of ephedrine, caffeine, and their combination on muscular endurance. *Med Sci Sports Exerc*. 2003;35(6):987–994.

32. Sawka MN, Joyner MJ, Miles DS, et al. American College of Sports Medicine position stand. The use of blood doping as an ergogenic aid. *Med Sci Sports Exerc*. 1996;28(6):i–viii.

33. Metzl JD, Small E, Levine SR, et al. Creatine use among young athletes. *Pediatrics*. 2001;108(2):421–425.

34. Trojian T, Pengel B, Anderson JM. Sports supplements. In: Mellion MB, Walsh WM, Madden C, et al, eds. *Team Physician's Handbook*. Philadelphia, PA: Hanley & Belfus; 2002:198–210.

35. Greenwood M, Kreider RB, Melton C, et al. Creatine supplementation during college football training does not increase the incidence of cramping or injury. *Mol Cell Biochem*. 2003;244(1–2):83–88.

36. Bemben MG, Bemben DA, Loftiss DD, et al. Creatine supplementation during resistance training in college football athletes. *Med Sci Sports Exerc*. 2001;33(10):1667–1673.

37. Mayhew DL, Mayhew JL, Ware JS. Effects of long-term creatine supplementation on liver and kidney functions in American college football players. *Int J Sport Nutr Exerc Metab*. 2002;12(4):453–460.

38. Terjung RL, Clarkson P, Eichner ER, et al. American College of Sports Medicine roundtable. The physiological and health effects of oral creatine supplementation. *Med Sci Sports Exerc*. 2000;32(3):706–717.

39. Ventura R, Segura J. Detection of diuretic agents in doping control. *J Chromatogr B Biomed Appl*. 1996;687(1):127–144.

Therapeutic Modalities

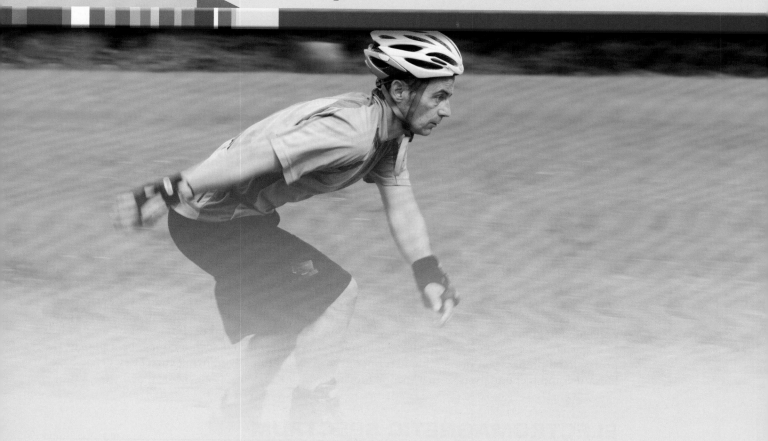

STUDENT OUTCOMES

1. Explain the principles associated with the electromagnetic spectrum and identify the types of energy found in the nonionizing range of the spectrum.

2. Explain the transfer of energy from one object to another and identify the factors that can affect this transfer.

3. Describe the physiological effects of cryotherapy and thermotherapy.

4. List the indications and contraindications for the various methods of cold and heat treatments, including ultrasound and diathermy.

5. Explain the principles that govern ultrasound, including the physiological effects and modes of application.

6. Explain the principles of electricity, and describe the different types of current.

7. Describe the various parameters that can be manipulated in electrotherapy to produce the desired effects.

8. Explain the various types of electrical-stimulating units and the use of each.

9. Describe the benefits attained in each of the five basic massage strokes and explain their application.

10. Explain the principles that govern traction and continuous passive motion.

INTRODUCTION

The ultimate goal of rehabilitation is to return the injured participant to activity in a pain-free and fully rehabilitated condition. The rehabilitation process must focus on controlling pain and inflammation and on regaining normal joint range of motion (ROM), flexibility, muscular strength, muscular endurance, coordination, and power. Therapeutic modalities and medications are used to create an optimal environment for injury repair by limiting the inflammatory process and breaking the pain–spasm cycle. Use of any modality depends on the supervising physician's exercise prescription as well as on the injury site and the type and severity of injury. An **indication** is a condition that could benefit from a specific modality, whereas a **contraindication** is a condition that could be adversely affected by a particular modality. In some cases, a modality may be indicated and contraindicated for the same condition. For example, thermotherapy may be contraindicated for tendinitis during the initial phase of the exercise program; however, once acute inflammation is controlled, heat therapy may be indicated. Frequent evaluation of the individual's progress (using patient outcomes) is necessary to ensure that the appropriate modality is being used.

This chapter initially addresses the basic principles associated with the electromagnetic spectrum and the factors affecting the transfer of energy. Then, the more common therapeutic modalities used in injury management are discussed. The material presented is a general overview of the various modalities. Because of the extensive information and clinical skills that are needed to adequately comprehend and apply therapeutic modalities in a clinical setting, this chapter should not be used in lieu of a specialized course on therapeutic techniques. It is essential that such a course be a part of the professional preparation of an athletic trainer as well as continually utilizing current evidence-based literature and meta-analysis of therapeutic modalities.

ELECTROMAGNETIC SPECTRUM

> **?** During practice, a lacrosse player sustains a contusion to the posterior aspect of the upper arm. A bag of crushed ice is applied to the injured area using a compression wrap. Should the ice bag be applied directly to the skin or over a layer of towel covering the skin? Explain the process of energy transmission between the ice bag and the underlying soft tissues.

On a daily basis, the environment is impacted by a variety of energy forms. Each form of energy falls under the category of **electromagnetic radiation** and can be located on an **electromagnetic spectrum** based on its wavelength or frequency (**Fig. 12.1**). Electrical therapeutic modalities are part of the electromagnetic spectrum, which is divided into two major zones: the ionizing range and the nonionizing range. Regardless of the range, electromagnetic energy has several common characteristics:

- Electromagnetic energy is composed of pure energy and does not have a mass.
- Energy travels at the speed of light (300 million meters per second).
- Energy waveforms travel in a straight line and can travel in a vacuum.
- Energy requires no transmission medium.

Ionizing Range

Energy in the ionizing range can readily alter the components of atoms (i.e., electrons, protons, and neutrons). This radiation can easily penetrate tissue to deposit energy within the cells. If the energy

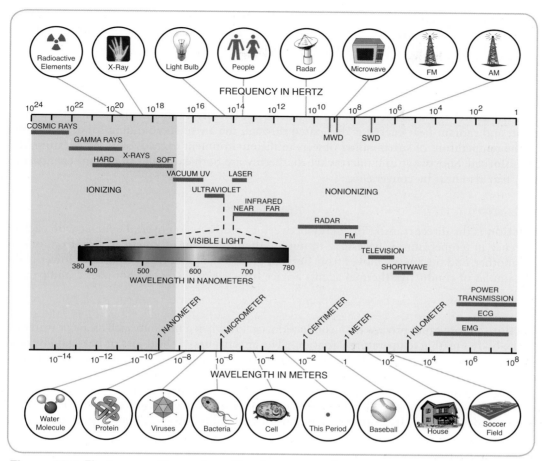

Figure 12.1. Electromagnetic spectrum. The electromagnetic spectrum covers a wide range of wavelengths and frequencies. UV, ultraviolet; ECG, electrocardiogram.

level is high enough, the cell loses its ability to regenerate, leading to cell death. Used diagnostically in radiography (i.e., in X-ray dosages below that required for cell death) and therapeutically to treat certain cancers (i.e., above the threshold), the level is strictly controlled and monitored to prevent injury to the patient. It is not used by athletic trainers or physical therapists.

Nonionizing Range

Energy in the nonionizing range commonly is used in the management of musculoskeletal injuries. This portion of the spectrum incorporates ultraviolet, visible, and infrared light. Electromagnetic waves are produced when the temperature rises and the electron activity increases. Ultraviolet light has a shorter wavelength than visible light; therefore, it is undetectable by the human eye. This energy source causes superficial chemical changes in the skin and is used to treat certain skin conditions; sunburns are an example of excessive exposure to ultraviolet rays. Wavelengths greater than visible light are called infrared light, or infrared energy. The infrared wavelengths closest to visible light are called near-infrared energy and can produce thermal effects 5 to 10 mm deep in tissue. The infrared wavelengths farthest from the visible are called far-infrared energy and result in more superficial heating of the skin (<2 mm deep). Energy forms with much longer wavelengths are collectively known as diathermy and can increase tissue temperature through a process called conversion. Microwave and shortwave diathermy are examples of this energy source.

Transfer of Energy

Electromagnetic energy can travel through a vacuum with no transfer medium. Energy moves from an area of high concentration to an area of lower concentration by energy carriers, such as mechanical waves, electrons, photons, and molecules. This energy flow in the form of heat involves the exchange of kinetic energy, or energy possessed by an object by virtue of its motion, and is transferred via radiation, conduction, convection, conversion, or evaporation.

Radiation

Radiation is the transfer of energy in the form of infrared waves (radiant energy) without physical contact. All matter radiates energy in the form of heat. Usually, body heat is warmer than the environment, and radiant heat energy is dissipated through the air to surrounding solid, cooler objects. When the temperature of surrounding objects in the environment exceeds skin temperature, radiant heat is absorbed. Shortwave and microwave diathermy are both examples of radiant energy transfer, but they can also heat by conversion.

Conduction

Conduction is the direct transfer of energy between two objects in physical contact with each other. A difference in temperature is necessary to initiate the movement of kinetic energy from one molecule to another, and the energy moves from an area of high temperature to an area of lower temperature. Examples of conductive thermal agents are ice bags, ice packs, moist hot packs, and paraffin.

Convection

Convection, a more rapid process than conduction, occurs when a medium such as air or water moves across the body, creating temperature variations. The effectiveness of heat loss or heat gain by conduction depends on the speed at which the air or water next to the body is moved away once it becomes warmed. For example, if air movement is slow, the air molecules next to the skin are warmed and act as insulation. In contrast, if warmer air molecules are continually replaced by cooler molecules (e.g., on a breezy day or in a room with a fan), heat loss increases as the air currents carry heat away. Fluidotherapy and whirlpools are examples of therapeutic modalities that exchange energy by convection.

Conversion

Conversion involves the changing of another energy form (e.g., sound, electricity, or a chemical agent) into heat. In ultrasound therapy, mechanical energy produced by high-frequency sound waves is converted to heat energy at tissue interfaces. In microwave diathermy, high electromagnetic energy is converted into heat, which can heat deep tissues. Chemical agents, such as liniments or balms, create heat by acting as counterirritants to superficial sensory nerve endings, thus reducing the transmission of pain from underlying nerves.

Evaporation

Heat loss can occur during evaporation as well. The body cools itself on a hot day when sweat forms as a liquid over the skin surface. The heat absorbed by the liquid cools the skin surface as the liquid changes into a gaseous state.

Factors Affecting Energy Transfer

When electromagnetic energy is transmitted in a vacuum, it travels in a straight line. When traveling through a physical medium, however, the path is influenced by the density of the medium, and the energy may be reflected, refracted, or absorbed by the material or may continue to pass through the material unaffected by its density (**Fig. 12.2**). **Reflection** occurs when the wave strikes an object and is bent

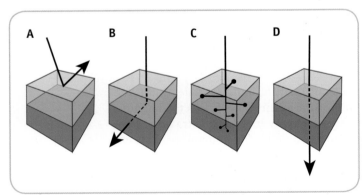

Figure 12.2. Factors affecting the transmission of energy. A, Reflection. The energy wave may be partially or fully reflected by the tissue layer. **B, Refraction.** The energy wave is bent as it strikes an interface between two different tissue layer densities. **C, Absorption.** Energy can be absorbed by one layer reducing the energy available to deeper tissues. **D, Transmission.** Any energy that is not reflected or absorbed by a tissue layer will continue to pass through the medium to the next layer, where it can again be reflected, refracted, absorbed, or transmitted through the tissue.

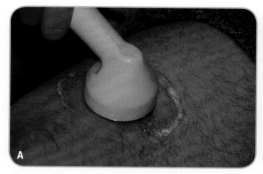
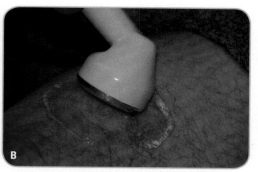

Figure 12.3. The cosine law. A, When energy is applied to a body part, the maximal effect occurs when energy rays strike the body at a right angle (90°). **B,** As the angle deviates from 90°, some of the energy is reflected away from the targeted site, thereby reducing the level of absorption. This concept is critical in the application of ultrasound.

back away from the material. An echo is an example of a reflected sound. The reflection itself may be complete or partial. **Refraction** is the deflection of waves because of a change in the speed of absorption as the wave passes between media of different densities. If energy passes through a high-density layer and enters a low-density layer, its speed increases. In contrast, if energy passes through a low-density layer and enters a high-density layer, its speed decreases. **Absorption** occurs when the wave passes through a medium, and its kinetic energy is either partially or totally assimilated by the tissue. Any energy that is not reflected or absorbed by a tissue layer passes through the layer until it strikes another layer with a different density, where it may again be reflected, refracted, absorbed, or transmitted through the medium. Each time the wave is partially reflected, refracted, or absorbed, the remaining energy available to the deeper tissues is reduced. This inverse relationship is called the **law of Grotthus-Draper:** The more energy the superficial tissues absorb, the less energy is available to be transmitted to the underlying tissues.

Effect of Energy on Tissue

To be effective, therapeutic modalities must be capable of producing the desired effects at the intended tissue depth. When energy is applied to the body, the maximal effect occurs when energy rays strike the body at a right angle (90°). As the angle deviates from 90°, some of the energy is reflected away from the target site, thereby reducing the level of absorption. The **cosine law (Fig. 12.3)** states that as the angle deviates from 90°, the energy varies with the cosine of the angle:

Effective energy = Energy × Cosine of the
angle of incidence

With radiant energy, a difference of ±10° from the right angle is considered to be within acceptable limits.[1] Another law that affects energy absorption is the **inverse square law (Fig. 12.4)**, which states that the intensity of radiant energy striking the tissues is directly proportional to the square of the distance between the source of the energy and the tissues:

$$E = \frac{E_S}{D^2}$$

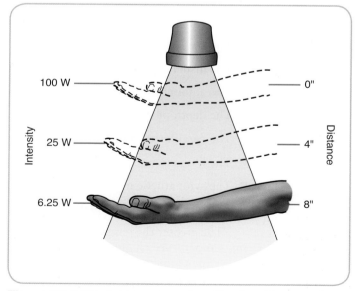

Figure 12.4. The inverse square law. Heating effect equals x(a). When the distance between the energy source and the skin is reduced by half, the heating effect is increased by fourfold (inverse of 1/2 = 2, and $2^2 = 4$).

Where

    E_S = amount of energy produced by the source,

    D^2 = square of the distance between the target and the source, and

    E = resulting energy absorbed by the tissue.

This means that each time the distance between the energy and the tissue is doubled, the intensity of the energy received by the tissue is reduced by a factor of four.

 The bag of crushed ice can be applied directly to the skin of the lacrosse player. Because the thermal energy is being transferred via conduction, application directly to the skin promotes a more efficient and effective transfer of cold to the injured area.

CRYOTHERAPY

 In treating the lacrosse player's contusion, for how long a period should the ice bag be applied? What contraindications may prohibit the use of cold in this case?

Cryotherapy describes multiple types of cold application that use the kind of electromagnetic energy classified as infrared radiation. When cold is applied to skin, which is a warmer object, heat is removed or lost; this is referred to as heat abstraction, or cooling. The most common modes of heat transfer with cold application are conduction and evaporation. Cold application causes vasoconstriction and decreased vascular permeability, which can lead to decreased cell metabolism, inflammation, circulation, pain perception, muscle spasm, muscle force production, and increased tissue stiffness.[2] The intent of cold application immediately following injury is to reduce the area of secondary injury, thus limiting the total amount of damaged tissue that needs repair. Depth of cold penetration can reach 4 to 5 cm and is dependent on the duration of treatment, the depth, and type of tissue. The longer the treatment, the greater the depth of cooling and the greater the decrease in temperature. The magnitude of temperature change depends on the following:

- The type of cooling modality (e.g., ice massage versus ice slush, where treatment temperature differs)
- The temperature difference between the cold object and soft tissue
- The use of a compression wrap to secure the cold agent
- The insulating medium between the skin and cold agent
- The amount of subcutaneous insulation (adipose tissue/fat)
- The depth of the target tissue
- The vascularity and thermal conductivity of the area being cooled
- The limb circumference
- The sympathetic nervous system
- The duration of the application

    The greater the temperature gradient between the skin and cooling source, the greater the resulting temperature change in the tissue. Likewise, the deeper the tissue, the more time is required to lower the temperature (e.g., treatment on a wrist versus a thigh). Adipose tissue acts as an insulator and resists heat transfer; both heat gain and heat loss. The amount of adipose tissue influences the degree and rate at which muscle is cooled and, conversely, the return to its precooled temperature.

    Cold therapy is used to lower the temperature in soft tissues (e.g., subcutaneous tissue, muscle, or joints), reduce pain, and control edema. Cold application leads to vasoconstriction at the cellular level and decreases tissue metabolism (i.e., decreases the need for oxygen), which reduces secondary hypoxia. Capillary permeability and pain are decreased, and the release of inflammatory mediators and prostaglandin synthesis is inhibited. As the temperature of peripheral nerves decreases, a corresponding decrease occurs in nerve conduction velocity across the nerve synapse, increasing the threshold required for nerves to fire. The gate theory of pain hypothesizes that cold inhibits pain transmission by stimulating large-diameter neurons in the spinal cord, acting as a counterirritant, which blocks pain perception. Because of the inhibition of nerves and muscle spindle activity, muscles in spasm are relaxed, breaking the pain–spasm cycle and leading to an **analgesic**, or pain-free, effect. During ice application, a decline in fast-twitch muscle fiber tension occurs, resulting in a more significant recruitment of slow-twitch muscle fibers, thereby increasing muscle endurance.[3]

Because vasoconstriction leads to a decrease in metabolic rate, inflammation, and pain, cryotherapy is the modality of choice during the acute phase of an injury. The therapeutic application of cold cools the surface skin temperature between 1° and 10°C (33° to 50°F)[4]; however, researchers have identified that maximal decreases in localized blood flow can occur at temperatures ranging from 12.83° to 15°C (55° to 59°F).[5,6] The desired therapeutic range of cooling can be obtained through the use of ice bags (e.g., crushed or cubed), commercial ice packs, ice cups (e.g., ice massage), and cold water baths (e.g., immersion or whirlpool). Recent technology also has provided new forms of cold application, such as the Cryo/Cuff or Game Ready or cold and compression therapy (CCT) units.

Cryotherapy is usually applied for 20 to 30 minutes several times a day for maximum cooling of both superficial and deep tissues. Treatment times may vary depending on the thickness of the adipose layer. When using ice packs, it was found that the time required to lower deep tissue temperature for selected skinfold thicknesses of 0 to 10 mm, 11 to 20 mm, 21 to 30 mm, and 31 to 40 mm were 12, 30, 40, and 60 minutes, respectively.[7] Barriers used between the ice application and skin also can affect heat abstraction. Research has shown that a dry towel or dry elastic wrap should not be used in treatment times of 30 minutes or less; rather, the cold agent should be applied directly to the skin for optimal therapeutic effects.[4,8] Using a compression wrap to secure the cold agent (e.g., ice pack) to the body part, however, produces a significant reduction in subcutaneous tissue temperatures as compared with simply placing the cold agent on the skin.[9] Ice application is continued during the first 24 to 72 hours after injury or until acute bleeding and capillary leakage have stopped, whichever is longer.

Another consideration is the length of time required to rewarm the injured area. Knight[4] has shown that except for the fingers, the rewarming time to approach normal body temperature is at least 90 minutes. This results in a treatment protocol of applying an ice pack for 20 to 30 minutes, followed by 90 minutes of rewarming. Fingers can rewarm more quickly, even following a 20- to 30-minute ice treatment, presumably because of their increased circulation. Fingers need only 20 to 30 minutes to rewarm.

One challenge, when working with athletes, is the practice of securing ice to an injury site in the athletic training room and having the individual walk to his or her residence. Intramuscular tissue temperature continually cools (34° to 28°C) at rest during the application of ice, which can be as great as 3.9° to 5.4°C cooler during a 20- to 30-minute treatment period. However, no change in intramuscular tissue temperature was shown during the same time period while walking.[10] The current trend of wrapping "to go" ice bags to the leg is not likely to achieve deep tissue cooling despite surface temperature decreases.

Certain methods of cryotherapy also may be used before ROM exercises and at the conclusion of an exercise bout (**Box 12.1**). Use of cold treatments before exercise is called **cryokinetics**. Cryokinetics alternates several bouts of cold using ice massage, ice packs, ice immersion, or iced towels with active exercise. The injured body part is numbed by applying cold for 10 to 20 minutes, and the individual is instructed to perform various progressive exercises. These exercises may begin with simple, non–weight-bearing ROM activities and progress to more complex, weight-bearing activities. All exercise bouts must be pain-free. As the mild anesthesia from the cold wears off, the body part is renumbed with a 3- to 5-minute cold treatment. The exercise bout is repeated three to four times each session. The session ends with exercise if the individual is able to participate in activity or with cold if the individual is not able to participate in activity.

Methods of cryotherapy include cold packs, ice massage, ice immersion, and cold and compression therapy units. Regardless of the methods of application, the individual feels four progressive sensations: cold, burning, aching, and **analgesia**.

BOX 12.1 Cryotherapy Application

Indications	Contraindications
Acute or chronic pain	Decreased cold sensitivity and/or hypersensitivity
Acute or chronic muscle spasm/guarding	Cold allergy/cold-induced urticaria
Acute inflammation or injury	Circulatory or sensory impairment
Postsurgical pain and edema	Raynaud phenomenon
Neuralgia	Advanced diabetes
Superficial first-degree burns	Hypertension
Used with exercises to:	Uncovered open wounds

Indications

Acute or chronic pain

Acute or chronic muscle spasm/guarding

Acute inflammation or injury

Postsurgical pain and edema

Neuralgia

Superficial first-degree burns

Used with exercises to:
- Facilitate mobilization
- Relieve pain
- Decrease muscle spasticity

Contraindications

Decreased cold sensitivity and/or hypersensitivity

Cold allergy/cold-induced urticaria

Circulatory or sensory impairment

Raynaud phenomenon

Advanced diabetes

Hypertension

Uncovered open wounds

Cardiac or respiratory disorders

Nerve palsy

Arthritis

Lupus

Cold Packs

Cold packs are administered in four common methods: plastic bags filled with crushed, flaked, or cubed ice; reusable cold gel packs; CCT units; and instant (chemical) cold packs. Most methods are inexpensive and maintain a constant temperature, making them very effective at cooling tissue.

Ice Bags

When filled with flaked ice or small cubes, ice bags can be safely applied to the skin for 30 to 40 minutes without danger of frostbite. Furthermore, ice packs can be molded to the body's contours, held in place by a compression wrap, and elevated above the heart to minimize swelling and pooling of fluids in the interstitial tissue spaces (**Fig. 12.5A**). During the initial treatments, the skin should be checked frequently for wheal or blister formation indicating an allergy to cold (**Fig. 12.5B**). A disadvantage of this application method is the cost of the ice machine, which can be expensive.

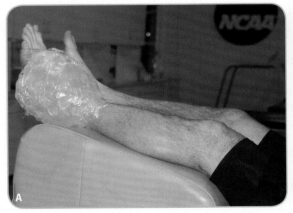
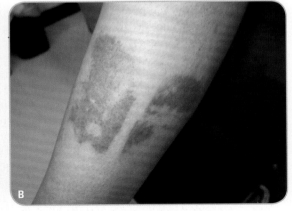

Figure 12.5. Ice treatments. A, Ice, compression, and elevation can reduce acute inflammation.
B, A slightly raised wheal formation may appear shortly after cold application in individuals who are sensitive to cold or who have cold allergies.

Reusable Cold Packs

Reusable commercial gel packs contain silica gel enclosed in a strong vinyl or plastic case, and they come in a variety of sizes to conform to the body's natural contours (**Fig. 12.6**). Used with compression and elevation, they are an effective method of cold application. The packs should be stored at a temperature of approximately −5°C (−23°F) for at least 2 hours before application.[2] Because the packs are stored at subzero temperatures, they may cause frostbite if used improperly. A wet towel or cloth should be placed between the pack and the skin to prevent frostbite and to maintain a hygienic surface for the reusable packs. Treatment time ranges from 15 to 20 minutes.

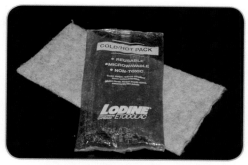

Figure 12.6. Commercial gel packs. Commercial gel packs come in a variety of sizes to conform to the body's natural contours.

Cold and Compression Therapy Units

CCT units use static, external compression and cold application to decrease blood flow to an extremity and to assist venous return, to decrease edema, and to increase the effective depth of cold penetration. In doing so, both pain and recovery time is decreased. Commercial circulating cold-water wraps, such as Cryo/Cuff (Aircast Inc, Summit, NJ), Polar Care (Breg Inc, Vista, CA), and **Game Ready** (CoolSystems Inc, Concord, CA), use ice water placed in an insulated thermos. When the thermos is raised above the body part, water flows into the pad wrapped around the injured extremity, maintaining cold compression for 5 to 7 hours (**Fig. 12.7A**). These often are applied after surgery over dressings and casts. Some CCT units provide a motorized, intermittent compression treatment when cooled water is circulated through a boot or sleeve around the injured body part, and the sleeve is inflated intermittently. This is done for 20 to 30 minutes several times a day to pump edematous fluid from the extremity (**Fig. 12.7B**). During deflation, the patient can perform active ROM exercises to enhance blood flow to the injured area. The unit can be used several times a day but never with a suspected compartment syndrome or fracture or in an individual with a peripheral vascular disease or impaired circulation.

Instant Cold Packs

Instant (chemical) cold packs are convenient to carry in an athletic training kit, can be disposed of after a single use, and can conform to a body part. Each bag contains two chemicals separated by a plastic barrier. When the barrier is ruptured, the chemicals mix, producing cold. Disadvantages of this type of application are the short duration of the cold application, the expense in using the pack only once, and the potential of the pack to tear or leak. The chemical substance that produces the cold has an alkaline pH, which can cause burns if the liquid substance comes in contact with the

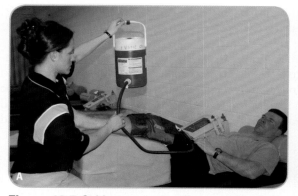
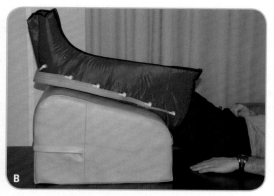

Figure 12.7. Cold compression therapy units. A, These devices provide circumferential cold compression around a specific body part. When the thermos is raised above the body part, water flows throughout the unit, maintaining cold compression for 5 to 7 hours. **B,** Some units have a motorized unit that can provide pressure or intermittent compression to an injured area to decrease edema.

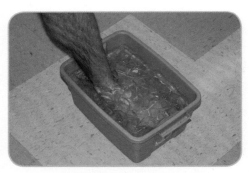

Figure 12.8. Ice immersion. This technique quickly reduces temperature over the entire surface area of a distal extremity. Toe caps may be used to prevent frostbite of the toes during the treatment.

skin. As such, the packs should never be squeezed or used in front of the face and, if possible, should be placed inside another plastic bag. Treatment ranges from 15 to 20 minutes. In longer treatments, the pack warms and becomes ineffective. Some commercial packs can be refrozen and reused.

Ice Massage

Ice massage is an inexpensive and effective method of cold application. Performed over a relatively small area, such as a muscle belly, a tendon, a bursa, or a trigger point, it produces significant cooling of the skin and a large, reactive **hyperemia**, or increase of blood flow into the region, once the treatment has ended. As such, it is not the treatment of choice in cases of acute injury. An ice massage is particularly useful for its analgesic effect in relieving pain that may inhibit stretching of a muscle, and it has been shown to decrease muscle soreness when combined with stretching.[2] It commonly is used before ROM exercises and deep friction massage when treating chronic tendinitis and muscle strains.

Treatment consists of water frozen in a cup, which is rubbed over an area 10 cm × 15 cm using small, overlapping, circular motions for 5 to 10 minutes. A continuous motion is used to prevent tissue damage. If this treatment is applied properly, skin temperature usually will not drop below 15°C (59°F); therefore, the risk of damaging tissue and producing frostbite is minimal.[2] A wooden tongue depressor frozen in the cup can provide a handle for easy application. During ice massage, the stages of cold, burning, and aching pass rapidly, within approximately 1 to 2 minutes. A prolonged aching or burning sensation may result if the area covered is too large or if a hypersensitive response occurs.

Ice Immersion

Ice immersion (ice slush bath) is used to reduce temperature quickly over the entire surface of a distal extremity (e.g., forearm, hand, ankle, or foot). A variety of containers or basins may be used. Because of the analgesic effect and the buoyancy of water, ice immersion and cold whirlpools often are used during the inflammatory phase to reduce an edema formation after a blunt injury. If the goal is to reduce an edema, placing the body part in a stationary position below the level of the heart keeps fluid in the body segment and is contraindicated. This can be avoided by placing a compression wrap over the body part before submersion and performing active muscle contractions. Neoprene toe caps may be used to reduce discomfort on the toes.

A bucket or cold whirlpool is filled with water and ice (**Fig. 12.8**). Bucket immersion in 4° to 10°C (40° to 50°F) water or a 10.0° to 15.6°C (50° to 60°F) whirlpool cools tissues as effectively as an ice pack. The lower the temperature, the shorter the duration of immersion. Treatment lasts from 10 to 15 minutes. When pain is relieved, the part is removed from the water, and functional movement patterns are performed. As pain returns, the area is reimmersed. The cycle continues three or four times.

Cold whirlpool baths also provide a hydromassaging effect. The intensity of the effect is controlled by the amount of air that is emitted through the electrical turbine. The turbine can be moved up and down or directed at a specific angle and locked in place. The whirlpool turbine should not be operated unless water totally covers the impeller. In addition to controlling acute inflammation, cold whirlpools can be used to decrease soft-tissue trauma and to increase active ROM after prolonged immobilization.

 The ice bag can be applied to the lacrosse player's injured upper arm for a period of 20 to 30 minutes. After a maximum of 90 minutes to allow for the rewarming of the area, another cold treatment should be initiated. This process should be followed throughout the remainder of the day. If the patient experiences any skin blanching, numbness, burning, or tingling sensations, the cold treatment should be stopped.

THERMOTHERAPY

? Following 5 days using cold treatments for the upper arm contusion, the lacrosse player shows significant improvement. The only significant finding is a slight decrease in strength as compared bilaterally with the uninvolved arm. Can the application of heat be advantageous during this stage in the healing process? What criteria would indicate that it is safe to use a heat modality at this time?

Thermotherapy, or heat application, typically is used during the second phase of rehabilitation to increase blood flow and to promote healing in the injured area (**Box 12.2**). If used during the acute inflammatory stage, heat application may overwhelm the injured blood and lymphatic vessels, leading to increased hemorrhage and edema. When applied at the appropriate time, however, heat can increase circulation and cellular metabolism; produce an analgesic, or sedative, effect; and assist in the resolution of pain and muscle-guarding spasms. Vasodilation and increased circulation result in an influx of oxygen and nutrients into the area to promote the healing of damaged tissues. Debris and waste products are removed from the injury site. Used before stretching exercises, joint mobilization, or active exercise, thermotherapy can increase the extensibility of connective tissue, leading to increased ROM. In the same manner as cold application, heat flow through tissue also varies with the type of tissue and is called thermal conductivity.

Superficial heating agents involve the transfer of heat through conduction, convection, and radiation. Common examples of superficial thermotherapy are warm whirlpools or immersion, moist heat packs, paraffin baths, fluidotherapy, and infrared lamps. Penetrating thermotherapy, including ultrasound, phonophoresis, and diathermy, is discussed in more detail later in this chapter.

To attain therapeutic effects from vigorous heating, tissue temperature must be elevated to between 40° and 45°C (104° to 113°F). Within these temperatures, hyperemia, which indicates increased blood flow, occurs. Potential tissue damage can occur with temperatures above this range; temperatures below this range are considered to be only mild heating and insufficient to stimulate cellular metabolism enough to cause therapeutic effects.[11,12] Changes in surface tissue temperature caused by superficial heating agents depend on the intensity of heat applied, the time of heat exposure, the volume of tissue exposed, and the thermal medium for surface heat.

The greatest degree of elevated temperature occurs in the skin and subcutaneous tissues within 0.5 cm of the skin surface. In areas with adequate circulation, temperature increases to its maximum within 6 to 8 minutes of exposure. Muscle temperature at depths of 1 to 2 cm increases to a lesser

---

BOX 12.2 Thermotherapy Application

Indications

Subacute or chronic injuries, to:

- Reduce swelling, edema, and ecchymosis
- Reduce muscle spasm/guarding

Subacute or chronic muscle spasm

Increase blood flow to:

- Increase ROM prior to activity
- Resolve hematoma
- Facilitate tissue healing
- Relieve joint contractures
- Fight infection

Contraindications

Acute inflammation or injuries

Impaired or poor circulation

Subacute or chronic pain

Advanced arthritis

Impaired or poor sensation

Impaired thermal regulation

Malignancy/neoplasms

Thrombophlebitis

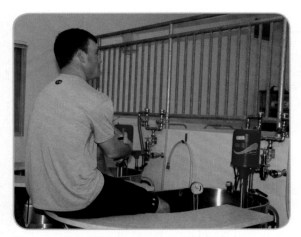

Figure 12.9. Whirlpools. Hot whirlpools increase superficial skin temperatures, leading to an analgesic effect that can reduce muscle spasm and pain, facilitate ROM exercises, and promote healing.

degree and requires a longer duration of exposure (i.e., 15 to 30 minutes) to reach peak values.[12] After peak temperatures are reached (i.e., approximately 7 to 9 minutes), a plateau effect or slight decrease in skin temperature is seen over the rest of the heat application. As mentioned, fat is an insulator and has a low thermal conductivity value. Therefore, tissues under a large amount of fat are minimally affected by superficial heating agents. To elevate deep tissues to the desired thermal levels without burning the skin and subcutaneous tissue, a deep-heating agent, such as continuous ultrasound or shortwave diathermy, should be selected.

Hydrotherapy Tanks

Whirlpool and hydrotherapy tanks combine warm or hot water with a hydromassaging effect to increase superficial skin temperature (**Fig. 12.9**). Tanks may be portable or fixed and include the more common extremity tanks and full-body therapeutic tubs, such as the Hubbard tank or walk tank.

Whirlpools are analgesic agents that relax muscle spasms, relieve joint pain and stiffness, provide mechanical debridement, and facilitate ROM exercises after prolonged immobilization. As with cold whirlpools and immersion baths, buoyancy facilitates increased ROM, and the hydromassaging effect is controlled by the amount of air that is emitted through the electrical turbine. The more agitation, the greater the water movement. The turbine can be moved up and down or directed at a specific angle and locked in place. Treatment time ranges from 20 to 30 minutes. Total body immersion exceeding 20 to 30 minutes can dehydrate the individual, leading to dizziness and a high body core temperature. Only the body parts being treated should be immersed. **Application Strategy 12.1** explains the use of this modality.

Many athletic training facilities also have large hydrotherapy tubs that can accommodate 4 to 16 athletes at a time. Because organic contaminants, high water temperature, and turbulence reduce the effectiveness of chlorine as a bacterial agent, infection with *Pseudomonas aeruginosa* causing folliculitis is an alarming and increasing problem associated with use of both hydrotherapy tanks and whirlpools. If an infection is to be prevented, these tubs must have an effective filtration and chlorination system. Chlorine and pH levels should be monitored hourly during periods of heavy use, and calcium hardness should be evaluated weekly.[13] The water temperature should not exceed 38.9°C (102°F). The water should be drained, superchlorinated, and refilled once a week. In an ideal setting, whirlpools should be drained, cleaned, and sanitized after each patient.

For safety reasons, ground-fault circuit interrupters (GFCIs) should be installed in all receptacles or in the circuit breaker box in the hydrotherapy area. They should be no more than 1.5 m away from the tanks. A sensor located within the GFCI monitors the current in the hot and neutral lines that feed the receptacle. Because the maximum safe transthoracic current (through intact skin) is deemed to be 5 mA, the GFCI activates at this level and immediately trips the circuit to disconnect all current to the receptacle. These receptacles should be inspected annually to ensure proper operation.

Moist Heat Packs

Heat packs provide superficial heat, transferring energy to the individual's skin by way of conduction. Each subsequent underlying tissue layer is heated through conduction from the overlying tissue, reaching a slightly deeper tissue level than occurs with a whirlpool. Like other forms of superficial heating, deeper tissues, including the musculature, are not significantly heated. The heat transfer is inhibited by subcutaneous fat, which acts as a thermal insulator, and by the increased blood flow through the area, which carries away externally applied heat. Hot packs most often are used to promote soft-tissue healing, to reduce pain and superficial muscle spasm while promoting general relaxation, and to improve tissue extensibility. The most efficient way to warm up the musculoskeletal tissue is with exercise (biking, elliptical trainer).

The pack consists of a canvas or nylon case filled with a hydrophilic silicate (or other hydrophilic substance) or with sand. The packs are stored in a hot water unit at a temperature ranging from

APPLICATION STRATEGY 12.1

Techniques for Using a Whirlpool Bath

1. Inspect the electrical system. To avoid electrical surges, make sure that ground-fault circuit breakers are used in the electrical outlet or in the circuit-breaker box.
2. Instruct the patient not to turn the turbine on or off or touch any electrical connections while in the whirlpool or while the body is wet.
3. Apply a whirlpool disinfectant according to the manufacturer's directions.
4. If an open wound is present on the body part being treated, add a disinfectant such as povidone, povidone-iodine, or sodium hypochlorite to the water.
5. Recommended temperature and treatment times include the following:

   Cold whirlpools   10°–16°C (55°–65°F) 5–15 minutes
   Hot whirlpools   32°–49°C (98°–110°F) 20–30 minutes
   Temperature and time is decreased as the body area being treated increases.

6. Assist the patient into the water and provide towels for padding and drying off.
7. Turn the turbine on and adjust the height to direct the water flow 6 to 8 in away from the injury site.
8. Instruct the patient to move the body part through the available ROM. This increases blood flow to the area, aids in the removal of debris, and improves balance and proprioception.
9. Turn the turbine off and remove the patient from the water. Dry the treated area and assist the patient from the whirlpool area.
10. Drain and cleanse the whirlpool tub after each use. Refill the tub with hot water (48.9°C [120.0°F]) to safely operate the turbine. Add a commercial disinfectant, antibacterial solution, or chlorine bleach to the water, following the manufacturer's directions. Run the turbine for at least 1 minute to allow the agent to cycle through the internal components. Drain the whirlpool.
11. Disinfect the interior hard-to-reach places with a brush and cleaner, paying attention to the external turbine, thermometer stem, drain, welds, and other areas that may harbor germs and organic material (blood, mucus). Thoroughly rinse the tub.
12. Clean the exterior of the tub with a stainless steel cleaner or other appropriate cleaner.
13. Cultures for bacterial and fungal agents should be conducted monthly from water samples in the whirlpool turbine and drain.
14. Have the whirlpool turbine inspected and the thermometer calibrated annually by a qualified service technician.

70° to 75°C (158° to 170°F) (**Fig. 12.10**). When removed from the water, a pack should be wrapped in a commercial padded cover or in six to eight layers of toweling and then placed directly over the injury site for 20 to 30 minutes. Commercial hot pack covers may need additional layers of toweling to ensure adequate insulation for the hot pack.

The pack should be secured and completely cover the area being treated. As with other forms of heat application, the patient should only feel a mild-to-moderate sensation of heat. The patient should never lie on top of the pack, because this may accelerate the rate of heat transfer, leading to burns on sensitive skin. Following 5 minutes of treatment, the area should be checked for any redness or signs of burning. At the conclusion of the treatment, the hot pack should be replaced in the heating unit for rewarming. It is strongly recommended that the hot pack temperature should be measured before use, because rewarming varies depending on the temperature of the hot pack before its return to the heating unit, on size of the heating unit, and on the number of used packs simultaneously returned for reheating.[14]

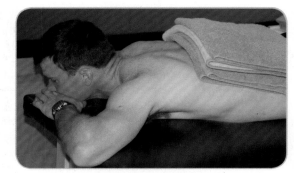

Figure 12.10. Moist hot packs. Moist heat treatments can burn sensitive skin. As such, the pack should be placed in a commercial padded towel or in six to eight layers of toweling, and the skin surface should be checked periodically for redness or signs of burning.

The hot packs should be checked regularly for leaks, and a hot pack should be discarded if any leaking occurs. This may become evident when cleaning the unit on a monthly basis. Hydrophilic silicate may accumulate on the bottom of the unit and should be removed so as not to interfere with the heating element.

Paraffin Baths

Paraffin baths provide heat to contoured bony areas of the body (e.g., feet, hands, or wrists). They are used to treat subacute or chronic rheumatoid arthritis associated with joint stiffness and decreased ROM as well as other common chronic injuries and diseases, such as systemic sclerosis.[15] A paraffin and mineral oil mixture (6:1 or 7:1 ratio) is heated in a unit at 45° to 54°C (113° to 129°F). The purpose of adding mineral oil is to lower the melting temperature of paraffin from 54°C (129°F) to between 45° and 50°C (113° to 122°F), thus making the mixture more comfortable for patients during the treatment.

Several methods of paraffin application may be employed; however, two principal methods of application are used: dip and wrap, and dip and reimmersed. For both methods, the body part should be thoroughly cleansed and dried, and all jewelry should be removed. The body part should be placed in a relaxed position and then dipped into the bath several times, each time allowing the previous coat to dry (**Fig. 12.11**). The patient should not move the fingers or toes so as not to break the seal of the glove being formed. In addition, outer layers of paraffin should not extend over new skin, because burning may occur. When completed, the body part should be wrapped in a plastic bag and towel to maintain heat and then elevated for 15 to 20 minutes (or until heat is no longer generated).

When using the dip and reimmersed method, after the formation of a wax glove, the body part covered by the glove is put back into the wax container for 10 to 20 minutes without moving it. This method results in a more vigorous response relative to temperature elevation and changes in blood flow. This technique should not be used in individuals predisposed to edema, however, or in those who cannot sit in the position required for treatment.

When the treatment is completed, the wax should be peeled off and returned to the bath, where it can be reused. The mineral oil in the wax helps to keep the skin soft and pliable during massage when treating a variety of hand and foot conditions. In comparison with other heat modalities, paraffin wax is not significantly better at decreasing pain or increasing joint ROM. It should not be used in patients with decreased sensation, open wounds, thin scars, skin rashes, or peripheral vascular disease.

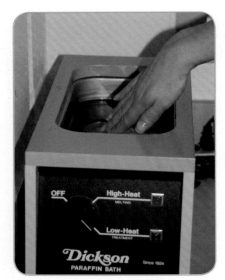

Figure 12.11. Paraffin bath. A thoroughly cleansed limb is dipped several times into the paraffin solution. The body part is then wrapped in plastic and a towel to maintain heat, or it can be reimmersed into the solution and held motionless for the duration of the treatment.

Fluidotherapy

Fluidotherapy is a dry thermal modality that transfers its energy (i.e., heat) to soft tissues by forced convection. Heat is transferred through the forced movements or agitation (blower action) in the unit chamber of heated air and Cellex particles, which are then circulated around the treated body part, making the fluidized bed behave with properties similar to those of liquids. Used to treat acute injuries and wounds, to decrease pain and swelling, and to increase ROM and inadequate blood flow, this modality is more effective than paraffin wax baths and warm whirlpool tubs at inducing absolute temperature increases in peripheral joint capsules and muscles.[16] Both the temperature and the amount of particle agitation can be varied. Treatment temperature ranges from 46° to 51°C (115° to 124°F).[11]

For optimal heating, the patient should remove all jewelry and wash the treated body parts before positioning the body area in the fluidotherapy chamber. A skin sensory heat discrimination test of the patient is mandatory before considering an application of this modality. This test consists of setting the amount of heat needed, the speed of particle agitation required, and the total treatment session duration.

Advantages of this superficial heating modality include that exercise can be performed during the treatment, higher treatment temperatures can be tolerated, and heat is distributed over the entire limb surface area with minimal to no pressure applied to the treated site. If a body part has an open wound, a plastic barrier or bag can be placed over the wound to prevent any fine cellulose particles from becoming embedded in the wound and to minimize the risk of cross-contamination. Treatment duration ranges from 15 to 20 minutes.

The lacrosse player's upper arm contusion showed significant improvement after 5 days of ice treatments. As long as the patient does not report point tenderness at the involved area, it probably is safe to move to a heat treatment. Heat can increase the local circulation and, in doing so, promote healing. It also can be used in conjunction with stretching and mild exercise to strengthen the injured muscle.

ULTRASOUND

 Two weeks after the injury, the lacrosse player is pain-free. There is a small, palpable, swollen area in the triceps at the spot where the force was sustained. What type of heat treatment would be most effective at this point in the healing process?

Superficial heating agents were discussed in the previous section. These agents produce temperature elevations in the skin and underlying subcutaneous tissues to a depth of 1 to 2 cm. Ultrasound uses high-frequency acoustic (sound) waves rather than electromagnetic energy to elicit thermal and non-thermal effects in deep tissue to depths of 3 cm or more. This transfer of energy takes place in the deep structures without causing excessive heating of the overlying superficial structures. The actual mechanism of ultrasound, produced via the **reverse piezoelectric effect**, converts electrical current to mechanical energy as it passes through a piezoelectric crystal (e.g., quartz, barium titanate, or lead zirconate titanate) housed in the transducer head. The vibration of the crystal results in organic molecules moving in longitudinal waves that move the energy into the deep tissues to produce temperature increases (i.e., thermal effects) as well as mechanical and chemical alterations (i.e., nonthermal effects). Thermal effects increase collagen tissue extensibility, blood flow, sensory and motor neuron velocity, and enzymatic activity and decrease muscle spasm, joint stiffness, inflammation, and pain. Nonthermal effects (i.e., mechanical effects) increase skin permeability, thus decreasing the inflammatory response, reducing pain, and facilitating the soft-tissue healing process. Both pulsed and continuous ultrasound reduces nerve conduction velocity of pain nerve fibers.

The Ultrasound Wave

Unlike electromagnetic energy, sound cannot travel in a vacuum. Sound waves, such as those produced by a human voice, diverge in all directions. This principle allows people to hear others talking while standing or being positioned behind them. As the frequency increases, the level of divergence decreases. Like sound waves, the frequencies used in therapeutic ultrasound produce collimated cylindrical beams, similar to a light beam leaving a flashlight, that have a width slightly smaller than the diameter of the transducer head. The **effective radiating area** is the portion of the transducer's surface area that actually produces the ultrasound wave.

Frequency and Attenuation

The frequency of ultrasound is measured in megahertz (MHz) and represents the number of waves (in millions) that occur in 1 second. Frequencies range between 0.75 and 3.0 MHz. For any given source of sound, the higher the frequency, the less the emerging sound beam diverges. For example, low-frequency ultrasound produces a more, widely diverging beam compared with high-frequency ultrasound, which produces a collimated beam. The more commonly used 1-MHz ultrasound heats tissue from 3 to 5 cm deep, whereas 3-MHz ultrasound heats tissue usually from 2 to 3 cm deep.[17,18]

Energy contained within a sound beam decreases as it travels through tissue. The level of absorption depends on the type of tissues to which it is applied. Tissues with high protein content (e.g., nerve and muscle tissue) absorb ultrasound readily. Deflection (i.e., reflection or refraction) is greater at heterogeneous (different or unrelated) tissue interfaces, especially at the bone–muscle interface. This deflection creates standing waves that increase heat. Ultrasound that is not absorbed or deflected is transmitted through the tissue.

The absorption of sound (and, therefore, attenuation) increases as the frequency increases. The higher the frequency, the more rapidly the molecules are forced to move against this friction. As the absorption increases, less sound energy is available to move through the tissue. The 1-MHz machine most often is used on individuals with a high percentage of subcutaneous body fat and whenever the desired effects are in the deeper structures. This ultrasound unit also has been used to stimulate collagen synthesis in tendon fibroblasts after an injury as well as cell division during periods of rapid cell proliferation.[19] In addition, it has been used on tendons on the second and fourth days after surgery to increase tensile strength. After the fifth day, however, application decreases tensile strength.[20]

The high-frequency, 3-MHz machine provides treatment to superficial tissues and tendons, with a depth of penetration between 1 and 2 cm (1/3 to 1/4 in). The low penetration depth is associated with limited transmission of energy, rapid absorption of energy, and higher heating rate in a relatively limited tissue depth.

Types of Waves

Sound waves can be produced as a continuous or pulsed wave. A continuous wave is one in which the sound intensity remains constant, whereas a pulsed wave is intermittently interrupted. Pulsed waves are further delineated by the fraction of time the sound is present over one pulse period or duty cycle. This is calculated with the following equation:

$$\text{Duty cycle} = \frac{\text{Duration of pulse (time on)} \times 100}{\text{Pulse period (time on + time off)}}$$

Typical duty cycles in the pulse mode range from 0.05 (5%) to 0.5 (50%), with the most commonly used duty cycle being 0.02 (20%).[21] Continuous ultrasound waves provide both thermal and nonthermal effects and are used when a deep, elevated tissue temperature is advisable. Pulsed ultrasound and low-intensity, continuous ultrasound produce primarily nonthermal effects and are used to facilitate repair and soft-tissue healing when a high increase in tissue temperature is not desired.

Intensity

Therapeutic intensities are expressed in Watts per square centimeter (W/cm^2) and range from 0.25 to 2.0 W/cm^2. The greater the intensity, the greater the resulting temperature elevation. Thermal temperature can increase 7° to 8°F up to 2.5 cm deep in the muscle after the application of ultrasound at 1.5 W/cm^2 for 10 minutes.[22] As mentioned, ultrasound waves are absorbed in those tissues that are highest in collagen content, and they are reflected at tissue interfaces, particularly between bone and muscle.

Clinical Uses

Ultrasound is used to manage several soft-tissue conditions, such as tendinitis, bursitis, and muscle spasm; to reabsorb calcium deposits in soft tissue; and to reduce joint contractures, pain, and scar tissue (**Box 12.3**). In other areas, musculoskeletal ultrasound frequently is used to determine the presence or absence of tendon tears or the extent of dermal injuries.[23,24] Wound healing is enhanced with low-intensity, pulsed ultrasound. It is recommended that ultrasound treatment should begin 2 weeks after an injury, during the proliferative phase of healing. An earlier treatment may increase inflammation and delay healing time. Tissue healing is thought to occur predominantly through nonthermal effects. An intensity of 0.5 to 1.0 W/cm^2 pulsed at 20% is recommended for superficial wounds. For skin lesions and ulcers, a frequency of 3 MHz or higher is recommended.[21]

Ultrasound often is used with other modalities. When used in conjunction with hot packs, muscle spasm and muscle guarding may be reduced. The hot pack produces superficial heating, and the ultrasound, using a 1-MHz ultrasound frequency, produces heating in the deeper tissues. Because ultrasound can increase the blood flow to deep tissues, this modality often is used with electrical stimulation units. The electrical current produces a muscle contraction or modulates pain; the ultrasound increases circulation and provides deep heating. This combination of treatment protocols can be effective in treating both trigger and acupuncture points.

Application

Because ultrasound waves cannot travel through air, a coupling agent is used between the transducer head and the skin to facilitate the passage of the waves. Coupling gels are applied liberally

BOX 12.3 Ultrasound Application

Indications	Contraindications
Deep tissue heating	Acute and postacute hemorrhage (continuous)
Acute inflammatory conditions (pulsed)	Infection
Chronic inflammatory conditions (pulsed or continuous)	Thrombophlebitis
Spasticity/muscle spasm	Areas of impaired circulation/sensation
Trigger areas	Over stress fracture sites or osteoporosis
Increase extensibility of collagen tissue	Over suspected malignancy/cancer
Joint adhesions/contractures	Over the pelvic or lumbar areas during menstruation or pregnancy
Neuroma	Over epiphyseal growth plates
Postacute myositis ossificans	Over the eyes, heart, skull, spine, or genitals
	Over active sites of infection or sepsis
	Over an implanted pacemaker
	Over exposed metal that penetrates the skin

over the area to be treated. The transducer head is then stroked slowly over the area (**Fig. 12.12**). Strokes are applied in small, continuous circles or longitudinal patterns to distribute the energy as evenly as possible at a rate of 4 cm per second to prevent **cavitation** (gas bubble formation) in deep tissues.[25] The total area covered usually is two- to threefold the size of the transducer head for every 5 minutes of exposure. If a larger area is covered, the effective dosage and elevated temperature changes that are delivered to any one region decrease. A firm, uniform amount of pressure exerted on the transducer head maximizes the transmission of acoustic energy between the sound head and the tissue interface.

A common alternate method for irregularly shaped areas (e.g., wrist, hand, ankle, or foot) is application under water. A rubber-type basin should be used for these treatments. For several reasons, metal containers and whirlpools should not be used for underwater treatments. If the treatment is given in a metal basin or whirlpool, some of the ultrasound energy is reflected off the metal, thus increasing the intensity in certain areas near the metal. In addition, water in a whirlpool often has a large number of air bubbles, which tend to reduce the transmission of ultrasound. This problem is even more pronounced if the turbine was used before the ultrasound treatment. Water treatments are indirect and generally have a 0.5- to 3-cm space between the patient and the sound head. Intensity is increased by 0.5 W/cm^2 to compensate for air and minerals in the water. Small air bubbles tend to accumulate on the face of the transducer head and the skin surface when this method is used. The clinician should quickly wipe off the accumulated bubbles during the treatment. No jewelry should be worn under the water surface. In addition, the clinician should hold the transducer head so that his or her hand is out of the water.

If for some reason the injured area cannot be immersed in water, a bladder technique may be used. A small balloon is filled with water or aqueous gel. To prevent blockage of the ultrasound energy, all air pockets must be eliminated. The ultrasound energy

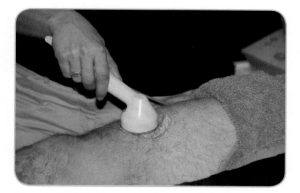

Figure 12.12. Ultrasound. A coupling agent is used between the transducer head and area being treated. The head is then moved in small circles or longitudinal strokes to distribute the energy as evenly as possible to prevent damage to the underlying tissues.

is transmitted from the transducer to the injured site through this bladder. Both sides of the balloon should be coated with gel to ensure good contact.

Research has shown that ultrasound treatments using gel in direct contact with the patient produce more heat than is produced with ultrasound administered indirectly underwater.[26–30] A reusable gel pad is another method of application over bony protuberances or irregular surfaces. These pads, when used with ultrasound gel, have been found to be more effective than using the traditional water bath immersion method.[30] Intensity for both gel and underwater treatment is determined by the stage of injury, the mode used (i.e., pulsed or continuous), the desired depth of penetration, and patient tolerance. The patient may feel a mild, warm sensation.

When the goal of treatment is to elevate tissue temperature over a large quantity of soft tissue (e.g., hip or back), a continuous-wave mode with intensities as high as 1.5 to 2.0 W/cm^2 typically is used. A lower intensity (0.5 to 1.0 W/cm^2) and a higher frequency are used over areas with less soft-tissue coverage and where bone is closer to the skin surface. At tissue–bone interfaces, approximately 35% of the ultrasound beam is reflected, resulting in an increased intensity in the soft tissue overlying the bone, particularly the periosteum.[26] Elevated temperatures should be maintained for at least 5 minutes after the patient reports the sensation of gentle heat to allow an increase in extensibility. If heat production in tissues greater than 3 cm deep is the desired effect, 10 minutes of treatment after the patient reports the sensation of heat is the minimum.[29]

Phonophoresis

Phonophoresis is a technique in which the mechanical effects of ultrasound are used to enhance percutaneous absorption of anti-inflammatory drugs (e.g., cortisol, dexamethasone, and **salicylates**) and local analgesics (e.g., lidocaine) through the skin to the underlying tissues. One advantage of this modality is that the drug is delivered directly to the site where the effect is sought. Phonophoresis is believed to accelerate functional recovery by decreasing pain and promoting healing. High ultrasound intensities have been used to deliver these medications to depths of 5 to 6 cm subcutaneously into skeletal muscle and peripheral nerves.[31] Pulsed-wave ultrasound appears to be more effective than continuous-wave ultrasound in decreasing inflammation.[32]

This technique is used during the postacute stage in conditions to treat painful trigger points, bursitis, contusions, or other chronic soft-tissue conditions, such as epicondylitis.[21,33] Phonophoresis also may be helpful in treating neuropathic pain, including phantom pain and central pain.[34] The standard coupling gel is replaced by a gel or cream containing the medication. Commercial chemp-ads impregnated with the medication also are readily available and may be used in lieu of the traditional medicated ointment applicators. Continuous ultrasound is used, because tissue permeability is increased by the thermal effects and, therefore, the medication is more easily absorbed. Treatment occurs at a lower intensity (i.e., 1.0 to 1.5 W/cm^2) for 5 to 15 minutes.

Ultrasound would be an accepted treatment for the small, palpable, swollen area in the triceps. Ultrasound can provide both thermal and nonthermal effects to increase circulation, blood flow, and tissue extensibility and to reduce hematoma formation and to optimize the healing process.

SHORTWAVE DIATHERMY

 In treating the lacrosse player's triceps contusion, would diathermy be an accepted treatment?

Diathermy, which literally means "to heat through," uses electromagnetic energy from the nonionizing radio frequency part of the spectrum. Because the duration of the impulses is so short, no ion movement occurs. The result is no stimulation of motor or sensory nerves.

Two types of generators are used for heating. One places two condenser plates (capacitive or condenser field) on either side of the injured area, thus placing the patient in the electrical circuit. The other method uses an induction coil (induction field) wrapped around the body part that places the patient in an electromagnetic field. Heating is uneven, because different tissues resist energy at different levels, an application of **Joule's law**, which states that the greater the resistance or impedance, the more heat is developed. Tissues with a high fluid content, such as skeletal muscle and areas surrounding joints, absorb more of the energy and are heated to a greater extent, whereas fat is not heated as much. Because the applicators are not in contact with the skin, this method can be used for heating skeletal muscle when the skin is abraded so long as an edema is not present.

Shortwave diathermy can be delivered as either a continuous or a pulsed form. The rapid vibration of the continuous shortwave diathermy (CSWD) waves is absorbed by the body and converted into heat by the resisting tissues. This elicits deep, penetrating thermal effects and is used primarily in chronic conditions. When these waves are interrupted at regular intervals, pulsed (or bursts of) radio frequency energy are delivered to the tissues and are referred to as pulsed radio frequency radiation (PRFR). PRFR may produce either thermal or nonthermal effects on tissues. Low power produces nonthermal effects, and high power produces thermal effects. Pulsed shortwave diathermy may be used in acute and subacute conditions, preventing tissue temperatures from rising too fast or too high.

Therapeutic devices that deliver CSWD and PRFR use high-frequency alternating currents to oscillate at specified radio frequencies between 10 and 50 MHz. The most commonly used radio frequency is 27.12 MHz. Microwave diathermy, another form of electromagnetic radiation, can be directed toward the body and reflected from the skin; it uses ultrahigh frequencies (UHF) at 2,450 MHz. Microwave diathermy is seldom used today, however, and is not discussed in this section.

Continuous Shortwave Diathermy

The goal of CSWD is to raise tissue temperature to within the physiologically effective range of 37.5° to 44.0°C (99.5° to 111.2°F) in deeper tissues (2.5 to 5.0 cm). This is done by introducing a high-frequency electrical current with a power output of 80 to 120 W. The depth of penetration and the extent of heat production depends on wave frequency, the electrical properties of the tissues receiving the electromagnetic energy, and the type of applicator used.

The physiological effects known to occur with other therapeutic heat treatments also are produced with CSWD. Mild heating usually is desired in acute musculoskeletal conditions, whereas vigorous heating may be needed in chronic conditions. Because the effects occur in deeper tissue, CSWD is used to increase the extensibility of deep collagen tissue, to decrease joint stiffness, to relieve deep pain and muscle spasm, to increase blood flow, to assist in the resolution of inflammation, and to facilitate the healing of soft-tissue injuries in the postacute stage (**Box 12.4**).

Pulsed Shortwave Diathermy

Pulsed shortwave diathermy (PSWD) is known by several names, including pulsed electromagnetic fields, pulsed electromagnetic energy, and PRFR. A relatively new type of diathermy, it uses a timing circuit to electrically interrupt the 27.12-MHz waves and produce bursts, or pulse trains, containing a series of high-frequency, sine wave oscillations. Each pulse train has a preset "time on" and is separated from successive pulse trains by a "time off," which is determined by the pulse repetition rate, or frequency. The pulse frequency can be varied from 1 to 700 pulses per second by turning the pulse-frequency control on the equipment operation panel.

The production of heat in tissues depends on the manipulation of peak pulse power, pulse frequency, and pulse duration. The measure of heat production is the mean power, which is lower than the power that is delivered (80 to 120 W) during most CSWD treatments. Nonthermal effects may be produced at mean power levels below 38 W; thermal effects are produced when mean power levels exceed 38 W. Mean power levels between 38 and 120 W are appropriate for the treatment of acute and subacute inflammatory conditions and have been shown to assist in the absorption of hematomas, the reduction of ankle swelling, and the stimulation of collagen formation. PSWD is applied to the patient in the same manner as CSWD. Most PSWD devices have the drum type of inductive applicator. Therefore, one could expect less heating of superficial fat and more heating of tissues such as the superficial muscle, which has a high electrolyte level. Indications and contradictions are the same for PSWD as for CSWD.

BOX 12.4 Diathermy Applications

Indications

Chronic inflammation (bursitis, tendinitis, myositis, osteoarthritis, etc.)

Joint capsule contractures

Degenerative joint disease

Sacroiliac strains

Acute or chronic pain

Subacute inflammation

Deep muscle spasms

Ankylosing spondylitis

Osteoarthritis

Chronic pelvic inflammatory disease

Epicondylitis

Contraindications

Over internally and externally worn metal objects

Over metal surgical implants

Metal objects within immediate area

Unshielded cardiac pacemaker

Peripheral vascular disease

Patients with hemophilia

Sensitive areas, including over:

- Lumbar, pelvic, or abdominal areas in women with metallic intrauterine devices
- Ischemic, hemorrhagic, malignant, and acutely inflamed tissues
- Eyes, face, skull, genitals, and swollen joints
- Moist wound dressings, clothing, or perspiration
- Pregnant abdomen
- Epiphyseal plates in children

 Shortwave diathermy can provide deep heating to tissues with a higher water content, such as muscle. It is important to recognize, however, that the extent of muscle heating can be inhibited by the thickness of the subcutaneous fat layer. As such, other modalities may be more effective in providing a deep heat treatment.

ELECTROTHERAPY

 In conjunction with a heat treatment for the lacrosse player's upper arm contusion, what type of electrotherapy could be used to elicit a muscle contraction and, in doing so, decrease muscle guarding and atrophy?

Electrical therapy is a popular therapeutic modality that can be applied to injured or immobilized muscles during the early stages of a therapeutic exercise program, when the muscle is at its weakest. The various forms of electrotherapy are used to decrease pain; increase blood flow, ROM, and muscle strength; reeducate muscle; facilitate the absorption of anti-inflammatory, analgesic, or anesthetic drugs to the injured area; and promote wound healing. An understanding of the clinical use of electrical stimulation requires an understanding of the basic principles of electricity.

Principles of Electricity

Electrical energy flows between two points. In an atom, protons are positively charged, electrons are negatively charged, and neutrons have no charge. Equal numbers of protons and electrons produce balanced neutrality in the atom. The transfer of energy from one atom to the next involves the movement of electrons only from the nucleus, thereby creating an electrical imbalance.

This subtraction and addition of electrons causes atoms to become electrically charged, and such atoms are then called ions. An ion that has more electrons is said to be negatively charged; an ion that has more protons is said to be positively charged. Ions of similar charge repel each another, whereas ions of dissimilar charge attract one another. The strength of the force and the distance between ions determine how quickly the transfer of energy occurs.

Types of Currents

Four types of electrical currents can be applied to tissues (**Fig. 12.13**). Two types fall under the category of continuous current: direct and alternating. Direct current (DC) is a continuous, one-directional flow of ions and is used to modulate pain, elicit a muscle contraction, or produce ion movement. Alternating current (AC) is a continuous, two-directional flow of ions used to modulate pain or elicit a muscle contraction. A third classification, pulsed current, represents a type of current that has been modulated to produce specific biophysical effects. With this type of current, a flow of ions in a DC or AC is briefly interrupted. The current may be one-directional (monophasic), two-directional (biphasic), or polyphasic (pertains to pulsed currents that usually contain three or more pulses grouped together). These groups of pulses are interrupted for short periods of time and repeat themselves at regular intervals. Pulsed currents are used in interferential and so-called Russian currents. In therapeutic use, each current can be manipulated by altering the frequency, intensity, and duration of the wave or pulse.

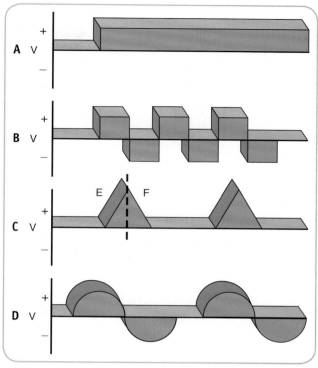

Figure 12.13. Four basic currents. The shape of the waveforms can be altered by changing the rate of rise and the rate of decay. **A,** DC with square wave. **B,** AC with square wave. **C,** Monophasic with triangular wave. *E,* rate of rise; *F,* rate of decay. **D,** Biphasic with sine wave.

Current Modifications

Once the basic current type is known, several parameters can be manipulated for the desired effects. The more common parameters include the amplitude, frequency, pulse duration, pulse charge, electrode setup, polarity, mode, duty cycle, and duration of treatment.[35] An electrical unit with the prescribed current type should be selected, and then the modifications indicated for the desired effect should be applied.

Amplitude

Amplitude is a measure of the force, or intensity, that drives the current. The maximum amplitude is the top, or highest, point of each phase. The term is synonymous with **voltage** and is measured in millivolts (mV), although some units use milliampere (mA) as a measure of amplitude. Voltage causes the ions to move, but the actual movement is called the **current**. If the current is presented graphically, the voltage is represented by the magnitude of the wave. If resistance remains the same, an increase in voltage will increase the amperage (i.e., the rate of current flow). An average current can be increased by increasing the pulse duration, increasing the pulse frequency, or some combination of the two.

Mediums that facilitate the movement of the ions are called **conductors** and include water, blood, and electrolyte solutions (e.g., sweat). Mediums that inhibit the movement of the ions are called **resistors** and include the skin, fat, and lotion. The combination of voltage, current, and resistance is measured in ohms (Ω). The **Ohm law** ($I = V / R$) states that current (I) in a conductor increases as the driving force (V) becomes larger or as resistance (R) is decreased. For example, 1 V is the amount of electrical force required to send a current of 1 A through a resistance of 1 Ω.

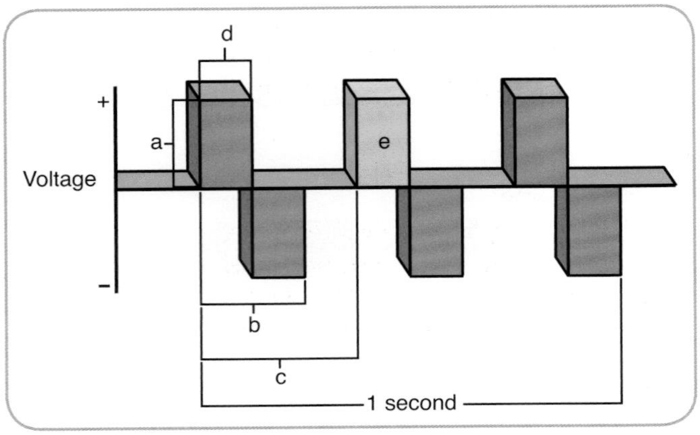

Figure 12.14. Graphic illustration of a biphasic current. *a*, amplitude (intensity); *b*, pulse duration; *c*, interpulse interval; *d*, phase duration; *e*, phase charge. Frequency, three pulses per second.

Frequency

Frequency refers to the number of waveform cycles per second (cps) or hertz (Hz) with AC, the number of pulses per second (pps) with monophasic or biphasic current, or the number of bursts per second (bps) with Russian stimulation. One purpose in altering frequency is to control the force of muscle contractions during neuromuscular stimulation. Low-frequency stimulation (<15 pps) causes the muscle to twitch with each pulse, cycle, or burst. As the frequency increases (15 to 40 pps), stimulation minimizes the relaxation phase of the muscle contraction. At higher frequencies (>40 pps), the stimulation is so fast that no relaxation occurs and a sustained, maximal contraction (tetany) is generated. Therefore, if the intent is to fatigue a muscle, the clinician can choose the appropriate frequency to bring about this effect.

Pulse Duration

Phase duration, or current duration as it is sometimes called, refers to the length of time that current is flowing. Pulse duration is the length of a single pulse of a monophasic or biphasic current. In a biphasic current, the sum of the two phases represents the pulse duration, whereas in a monophasic current, the phase and pulse duration are synonymous. The time between each subsequent pulse is called the interpulse interval. The combined time of the pulse duration and the interpulse interval is referred to as the pulse period. More powerful muscle contractions are generated with a pulse duration of 300 to 500 μs. A duration of less than 1 μs will not stimulate denervated muscle, regardless of the current's amplitude.

Pulse Charge

In a single phase, the pulse charge, or the quantity of an electrical current, is the product of the phase duration and amplitude and represents the total amount of electricity being delivered to the individual during each pulse. Amplitude, pulse duration, interpulse interval, phase duration, and phase charge are illustrated in **Figure 12.14**.

Electrode Setup

Electrical currents are introduced into the body through electrodes and a conducting medium. The smaller active pad has the greatest current density and brings the current into the body. The active electrode ranges from a very small pad to one that is 4-in square. Water or an electrolyte gel is used to obtain high conductivity. The arrangement of the pads depends on the polarity of the active pad, not on the number or size. If only one active electrode is used, or if the active electrodes are of the same charge, the arrangement is monopolar. This pattern requires the use of a large dispersal pad to take on the charge opposite that of the active pad and, in doing so, completes the circuit. The dispersal pad, from which the electrons leave the body, should be as large as possible to reduce current density. With the low current density, no sensation should be felt beneath the dispersal pad. When the active pads are of opposite charges, the arrangement is bipolar. Because this arrangement provides a complete circuit, no dispersal pad is necessary. Interferential stimulation requires a quadripolar electrode arrangement; this is nothing more than a bipolar arrangement from two channels where the currents cross at the treatment site. This electrode arrangement can be seen in **Figure 12.15**.

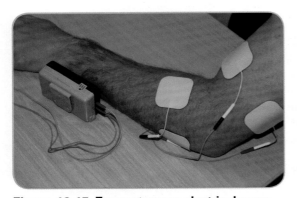

Figure 12.15. Transcutaneous electrical nerve stimulation. A transcutaneous electrical nerve stimulation unit is used to decrease acute and chronic pain to an injured area.

The pads should be placed at least one pad width apart. The closer the pads are, the shallower and more isolated the contraction; the farther apart the pads are, the deeper and more generalized the contraction. The physiological effects can occur anywhere between the pads but usually occur at the active electrode, because current density is greatest at this point.

Polarity

Polarity refers to the direction of current flow and can be toward either a positive or a negative pole. During DC and monophasic stimulation, the active electrode(s) can be either positive or negative, and current will flow in a predetermined direction (away from the negative electrode). During AC or biphasic stimulation, the polarity of the active pads alternates between positive and negative with each phase of the current.

Mode

In a monopolar arrangement, the term mode refers to the alternating (reciprocating) or continuous flow of current through the active electrodes. The term alternating means that the active electrodes receive current on an alternating basis, whereas with continuous flow, each electrode receives current throughout the treatment period. In neuromuscular stimulation, another popular mode is ramped, or surge, amplitude. The amplitude builds gradually to the desired level, which improves patient comfort and safety by preventing sudden, powerful muscle contractions.

Duty Cycle

Duty cycle refers to the ratio of the amount of time that current is flowing (i.e., on time) to the amount of time it is not flowing (i.e., off time). Used in neuromuscular stimulation, the duty cycle simulates repetitions and rest so as to delay the onset of fatigue. In edema formation, it creates a muscle pump. With neuromuscular stimulation, the recommended duty cycle should be 1:4 or 20% initially (i.e., 10 seconds on and 40 seconds off) and should gradually increase as fatigability decreases. Manual control of the duty cycle is necessary to prevent discomfort for the patient.

Duration of Treatment

The duration of treatment is the total time during which the patient is subjected to electrical stimulation. Many units have internal timers. Treatment duration typically is 15 to 30 minutes.

Electrical Stimulating Units

Several different types of electrical stimulating units are available (**Box 12.5**). Although it would be much easier to name the units based on the types of current that characterize the stimulation devices, this is not the case. Names often are used to show distinction between the characteristics, indications, and parameters of the various units. Unfortunately, many units could fall under the same general title. To complicate matters further, many common names, such as Galvanic, Faradic, and Russian stimulation, are still used.

Transcutaneous Electrical Nerve Stimulation

By varying the selection and setting of pulse duration, pulse/burst frequency, and current amplitude, clinicians can program transcutaneous electrical nerve stimulation (TENS) units to deliver one of the five basic therapeutic modes (**Table 12.1**)[11]:

1. Conventional TENS units typically are portable, biphasic generators with parameters that allow pain control via electrical pulses having short duration, high frequency, and low-to-comfortable current amplitude.

2. Acupuncture-like TENS has electrical pulses of long duration, low frequency, and comfortable-to-tolerable current amplitude. It is called acupuncture-like because the pulse frequency is low, resembling that used in acupuncture therapy.

BOX 12.5 Application of Neuromuscular Electrical Stimulation

TENS	Indications	Contraindications
	↓ Posttraumatic pain, acute and chronic	Patients with pacemakers
	↓ Postsurgical pain	Pregnancy (abdominal and/or pelvic area)
	↑ Analgesia	Pain of unknown origin
High-voltage pulsed	**Indications**	**Contraindications**
	↑ Circulation and joint mobility	Pacemakers
	↑ Muscle reeducation and strength	Pain of unknown origin
	↑ Wound and fracture healing	Pregnancy (abdominal and/or pelvic area)
	↑ Nonunion fracture healing	Thrombophlebitis
	↓ Muscle spasm/spasticity	Superficial skin lesions or infections
	↓ Pain and edema	Cancerous lesions over suspected fracture sites
	↓ Disuse atrophy	
	Denervation of peripheral nerve injuries	
Interferential	**Indications**	**Contraindications**
	↑ Circulation and wound healing	Pacemakers
	↓ Pain, acute and chronic	Pregnancy (abdominal and/or pelvic area)
	↓ Reduction of muscle spasm/guarding	Thrombophlebitis
	↓ Posttraumatic and chronic edema	Pain of unknown origin
	↓ Abdominal organ dysfunction	Prolonged use (may increase muscle soreness)
Low-intensity stimulation	**Indications**	**Contraindications**
	↑ Nonunion wound healing	Malignancy
	↑ Fracture healing	Hypersensitive skin
	Iontophoresis	Allergies to certain drugs

TENS, transcutaneous electrical nerve stimulation.

3. Brief-intense TENS has electrical pulses of long duration, high frequency, and comfortable-to-tolerable current amplitude. It gets its name because the duration of application is briefer and the current amplitude is higher than in the other modes, triggering a somewhat brief yet intense stimulation during treatment.

4. Burst TENS delivers bursts of pulses, not individual pulses, of low frequency at comfortable current amplitude.

5. Modulation TENS delivers random electronic modulation of pulse duration, pulse frequency, and current amplitude.

TABLE 12.1 The Five Classic Modes of TENS Therapy and Their Respective Biophysical and Physiological Characteristics

	CONVENTIONAL	ACUPUNCTURE-LIKE	BRIEF-INTENSE	BURST	MODULATION
Pulse duration	Short ($<$150 μs)	Long ($>$150 μs)	Long (150 μs)	N/A	Variable
Frequency	High ($>$120 Hz)	Low ($<$10 Hz)	High ($>$120 Hz)	Low ($<$10 Hz)	Variable
Current amplitude	Comfortable	Comfortable/tolerable	Comfortable/tolerable	Comfortable	Variable
Nerve fibers preferentially depolarized	S	S-M	S-M-N	S-M	Variable
Preferential mechanism of pain modulation	Nonopiate	Opiate	Opiate	Opiate	Variable
Onset of analgesia	Rapid (within minutes)	Slow (within hours)	Rapid (within minutes)	Slow (within hours)	Variable
Duration of analgesia	Short ($<$ few hours)	Long ($>$ hours)	Long ($>$ few hours)	Long ($>$ few hours)	Variable

N/A, not available; *S,* sensory; *S-M,* sensory-motor; *S-M-N,* sensory-motor-nociceptive.

Printed with permission from Bélanger AY. *Therapeutic Electrophysical Agents: Evidence Behind Practice.* Baltimore, MD: Lippincott Williams & Wilkins; 2009:31.

The units can produce analgesia and can decrease acute and chronic pain as well as pain associated with delayed-onset muscle soreness, although the duration of analgesia is unpredictable. TENS has also been shown to be effective in providing short-term pain relief in low back pain but is not as statistically effective as anterior–posterior joint mobilization or transdermal analgesic patches.[36] Often, TENS is used continuously after surgery in a 30- to 60-minute session, several times a day. It is thought that TENS works to override the body's internal signals of pain (gate theory of pain) or to stimulate the release of endorphins, a strong, opiate-like substance produced by the body. The unit uses small, carbonized silicone electrodes to transmit electrical pulses through the skin (**Fig. 12.16**). Most units are small enough to be worn on a belt and are battery-powered. The electrodes are taped on the skin over or around the painful site, but they also may be secured along the peripheral or spinal nerve pathways. For individuals who have allergic reactions to the tape adhesive or who develop skin abrasions from repeated applications, electrodes that are self-adhering are available.

High-Voltage Pulsed Stimulation

High-voltage pulsed stimulation uses a monophasic current with a twin-peak waveform, a relatively short pulse duration and a long interpulse interval, and an amplitude range above 150 mV. The short-phase duration activates sensory and type II motor nerves without stimulating pain fibers. High-voltage pulsed stimulation often is used to reeducate muscle; increase joint mobility; promote dermal wound healing; and decrease pain, edema, muscle spasm, and muscle atrophy, but it is ineffective in reducing the soreness, loss of ROM, and loss of strength associated with delayed-onset muscle soreness.[37]

Neuromuscular Electrical Stimulation

Neuromuscular electrical stimulation (NMES) units are designed to elicit a muscle contraction of moderately

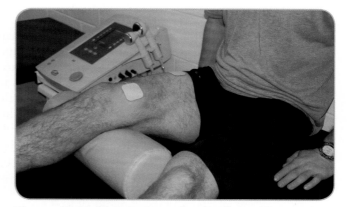

Figure 12.16. Electrical muscle stimulation. These units are used to stimulate muscle to maintain muscle size and strength during immobilization, to reeducate muscles, to prevent muscle atrophy, and to increase blood flow to tissues and to thereby decrease pain and spasm.

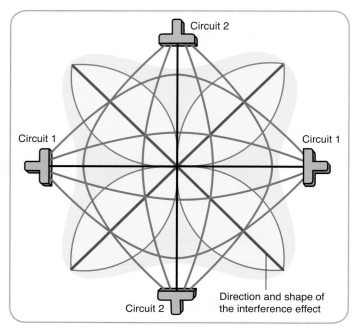

Figure 12.17. Interferential current. When arranged in a square alignment, the quadripolar electrode setup actually is a bipolar arrangement from two channels. An electric field is created where the currents cross between the lines of the electrical current flow. The maximum interference effect takes place near the center over the treatment site.

high intensity with relatively little patient discomfort, and they typically involve biphasic currents with a duty cycle. High-voltage electrical stimulation uses an output of 100 to 500 V to reduce edema, pain, and muscle spasm during the acute phase. It also is used to exercise muscle and delay atrophy, maintain muscle size and strength during periods of immobilization, reeducate muscles, and increase blood flow to tissues (**Fig. 12.16**). DC is used primarily to stimulate denervated muscle and to enhance wound healing as well as during iontophoresis.

Interferential Stimulation

An interferential current uses two separate generators and a quadripolar electrode arrangement to produce two simultaneous AC electrical currents acting on the tissues. The two paired pads are placed perpendicular to each other, and the current crosses at the midpoint (**Fig. 12.17**). A predictable pattern of interference occurs as the interference effects branch off at 45° angles from the center of the treatment in the shape of a four-leaf clover. Tissues within this area receive the maximal treatment effect. When the electrodes are placed properly, the stimulation should be felt only between the electrodes, not under the electrodes. Most medium-frequency, sinusoidal currents used to generate interferential current have a medium-frequency range of 3,000 to 5,000 Hz and are programmable to deliver beats (or envelopes) of interferential current at a low-frequency range of approximately 1 to 200 bps.[11] The higher frequencies lower skin resistance, thus eliciting a stronger response with less current intensity. Furthermore, sensory perception is decreased between the pads, allowing the use of a higher current, which increases stimulation. The amplitude and/or beat frequency can be modulated throughout the treatment by selecting the scan or sweep mode, respectively. Interferential stimulation is used to decrease pain, acute and chronic edema, and muscle spasm; to strengthen weakened muscles; to improve blood flow to an area; to heal chronic wounds; and to relieve abdominal organ dysfunction.

Low-Intensity Stimulation

Low-intensity stimulation (LIS) is the current term to replace the units originally called microcurrent electrical nerve stimulators (MENS) units. LIS units are available in a variety of waveforms, from modified monophasic to biphasic square waves. The units tend to be applied at a subsensory or very low sensory level, with a current operating at less than 1,000 μA. The devices deliver an electrical current to the body with approximately 1/1,000 the amperage of TENS but with a pulse duration that may be up to 2,500-fold longer. The stimulation pathway is not designed to stimulate peripheral nerves to elicit a muscle contraction but rather is used to reduce acute and chronic pain and inflammation, reduce edema, and facilitate healing in superficial wounds, sprains, strains, fractures, and neuropathies. The efficacy of microcurrent therapy and, subsequently, of LIS units is based primarily on anecdotal evidence rather than on valid research. It is posited that the current mimics the normal electrical current within the body, which is disrupted with injury, and, in doing so, reduces pain and spasms and improves healing.[38] Several studies have shown that microcurrent is ineffective at reducing pain and increasing muscle function associated with delayed-onset muscle soreness.[39,40]

Galvanic Stimulation

Galvanic stimulation is the common name for any stimulator using DC.

Russian Current

Russian current is a type of neuromuscular stimulation that uses AC, with frequencies ranging from 2,000 to 10,000 Hz. The current is generated in bursts, with interburst intervals. The number of bursts per second can be manipulated within the therapeutic range. For example, a high-frequency AC easily penetrates the skin and provides a high-amplitude, low-frequency current to the muscle. Russian electrical stimulation is designed to produce an isometric contraction and is useful in muscle reeducation. Because it induces an isometric rather than an isotonic contraction, strength gains do not transfer across the entire joint but instead are restricted to a narrow arc on either side of the joint angle at which the muscle is stimulated. Russian current, however, does permit the individual to contract actively along with the stimulation, provides an adequate work-to-rest interval, and usually is comfortable for the individual.

Faradic Current

Faradic current is a specialized, asymmetrical biphasic wave. Although popular in the past, it now is thought to have little benefit over symmetrical waves.[37]

Iontophoresis

Iontophoresis uses a DC monophasic waveform with a peak current amplitude of up to 5 mA. The current drives charged molecules from certain medications, such as anti-inflammatories (dexamethasone), anesthetics (lidocaine), or analgesics (aspirin or acetaminophen), into damaged tissue. It is used as a local anesthetic to treat inflammatory conditions, such as arthritis, myositis ossifans, and plantar fasciitis; myofascial pain syndrome; and skin conditions by reducing edema. Contraindications include an allergy to the ion being used, decreased sensation, and placement of electrodes directly over unhealed or partially healed skin wounds or new scar tissue. No contact should exist between metal or carbon–rubber electrode components and the skin, and electrodes should never be removed or rearranged until the unit has been turned off.

Iontophoresis is noninvasive and painless, uses a sterile application, and is excellent for those patients who fear injections. It yields tissue concentrations that are lower than those achieved with injections but greater than those with oral administration, because it avoids enzymatic breakdown in the gastrointestinal tract. A major disadvantage of this treatment is the electrolysis of NaCl in the body by DC. Electrolysis produces an increased pH (acidic) condition at the cathode (negative electrode) and a decreased pH (alkaline) condition at the anode (postive electrode). These pH changes can lead to tissue burns, especially with high intensities or prolonged application. Therefore, the negative electrode should be large, perhaps twice the size of the positive electrode, to reduce current density. With the newer controlled generators and buffered electrodes, clinicians can selectively decrease the current density under the anode to decrease the incidence of burns.

Before treatment, the skin must be thoroughly cleansed. Next, well-saturated electrodes are applied over the most focal point of tissue inflammation or pain unless skin irritation is visible. The polarity of the medication determines which electrode is used to drive the molecules into the skin. The medication is placed under the active (delivery) electrode with the same polarity. The return electrode is placed 4 to 6 in away. When the current is applied, the molecules are pushed away from the active electrode and into the skin toward the injured site. The medication can penetrate 6 to 20 mm below the skin surfaces and, in many instances, can reach the depth of tendinous structures, although the dose of the medication reaching this depth is not universally accepted. This localized treatment often is preferred over more disruptive systemic treatments.

 The use of ultrasound and a high-voltage pulsed stimulator or interferential stimulation will increase blood flow to the involved muscle. The electrical current can stimulate a muscle contraction to produce muscle pumping, can retard atrophy, and can strengthen the muscle.

LASER THERAPY

 Laser therapy uses specific wavelengths of laser light that, when absorbed, can lead to specific physiological responses in the body. What medical conditions might benefit from the use of laser therapy?

Low-level laser (LLL) therapy is a broad term for the application of light to provide therapeutic treatments for orthopedic injuries, skin conditions, and psychological problems such as depression and seasonal affective disorder. Devices include light-emitting diodes (LEDs), superluminous diodes (SLDs), fluorescent lamps, infrared lamps, ultraviolet (UV) lamps, diachronic lamps, and very bright incandescent light bulbs.[41] A laser, an acronym for *l*ight *a*mplification by *s*timulated *e*mission of *r*adiation, is a device that transforms electromagnetic energy of various frequencies in or near the range of visible light into an extremely intense, small, and nearly nondivergent beam of monochromatic radiation with all its waves in phase. The basic theoretical premise is that specific wavelengths of laser light, when absorbed, lead to specific physiological responses in the body. With recent advances in technology, the use of nonlaser devices, such as LEDs, SLDs, and polarized polychromic light, have been used to deliver light of a specific wavelength to the body.[41]

Although light therapy, also known as phototherapy, has been popular outside of the United States since the early 1970s, its use in the United States has recently gained in popularity since 2002 when the U.S. Food and Drug Administration (FDA) cleared specific models of LLLs, LEDs, and SLDs to treat musculoskeletal conditions, particularly for wound management, soft-tissue healing, and pain relief.[41]

To produce laser radiation, the device must have an energy source, a mechanical structure, and a lasing medium, either gas, liquid, chemical, crystal, or semiconductor. The more common LLLs use helium-neon (HeNe, a gas), gallium-aluminum-arsenide (GaAlAs, a diode or semiconductor), and gallium arsenide (GaAs, a semiconductor).[42] The effect of a laser is largely determined by the level of energy it emits. High-energy lasers (>500 mW), such as those used in surgery, are thermal in nature, meaning that they have a heating effect and may be used to destroy tissue. In contrast, LLLs, also called cold lasers or soft lasers, are athermic, meaning they do not directly heat tissues. They do, however, increase blood flow to the treatment site, thereby causing a slight measurable increase in tissue temperature with their use. Therapeutic modality lasers emit low levels of energy (<500 mW).

There is great discrepancy in the literature on the exact mechanisms by which laser light impacts tissues. It is thought that the application of a laser can increase mast cell release, promote interleukin-6 (an inflammatory regulatory substance) formation, and decrease dermal necrosis during the cellular phase of healing; increase collagen formation, degranulation, and myofibroblast conversion during the collagenization phase of healing; and promote wound contraction and tensile strength/stress during the remodeling phase of healing.[43] The literature is also split as to the effectiveness of pain relief. Overall, studies have found that laser therapy is effective at reducing pain and increasing function in acute musculoskeletal trauma,[44] carpal tunnel syndrome,[45] myofascial pain,[46,47] osteoarthritis,[48] trigger points,[46,47] neck pain,[49] and low back pain.[50]

Most lasers use a single laser probe to deliver light of a specific wavelength to tissues. More recently, cluster probes have been developed to apply multiple wavelengths to a larger area during treatment. Application involves two methods: a grid application or a scanning application. In the grid application, imagine a series of 1 cm² grid lines around the treatment site with the laser applied to each square for a predetermined time. In the scanning application, the probe is moved back and forth over the treatment area at a slow and steady rate, similar to an ultrasound treatment. Once the target area has been treated, a second treatment is applied with the probe moving at 90° to the first pass. The laser probe should have gentle contact with the skin surface to minimize divergence and reflection and should be perpendicular to the target area. With open wounds, the probe should be held close but not touching the wound. The use of a sterile, transparent film placed over the wound will allow the probe to be in near contact with the damaged tissue.

Lasers with shorter wavelengths have less depth of penetration than do lasers with longer wavelengths. Wavelengths in the near to middle infrared spectrum (1,000 to 1,350 nm) appear to penetrate deepest—3 to 5 mm—whereas shorter wavelengths may only penetrate <1 to 2 mm.[43]

Laser therapy has been found to be effective in reducing pain and increasing function in acute musculoskeletal trauma, carpal tunnel syndrome, myofascial pain, osteoarthritis, trigger points, neck and low back pain.

OTHER TREATMENT MODALITIES

 Electrical modalities are not always available for use by athletic trainers. What other treatment modalities might be used to promote healing of the lacrosse player's upper arm contusion?

Many of the electrotherapeutic modalities are costly and may not be readily available in all clinical settings. In addition, state licensure laws may prohibit an athletic trainer from using certain modalities in some settings. As such, it becomes necessary to use other treatment modalities to achieve the same results.

Massage

Massage involves the manipulation of soft tissues to increase cutaneous circulation, cell metabolism, and venous and lymphatic flow to assist in the removal of edema; to stretch superficial scar tissue; to alleviate soft-tissue adhesions; and to decrease neuromuscular excitability (**Box 12.6**). As a result, relaxation, pain relief, edema reduction, and increased ROM can be achieved. To reduce friction between the patient's skin and hand, particularly over hairy areas, lubricants (i.e., massage lotion, peanut oil, coconut oil, mineral oil) often are used. These lubricants should have a lanolin base or be alcohol-free. Massage involves five basic strokes (**Table 12.2**):

1. Effleurage (stroking)

2. Pétrissage (kneading)

3. Tapotement (percussion)

4. Vibration

5. Friction

Effleurage is a superficial, longitudinal stroke to relax the patient. When applied toward the heart, it reduces swelling and aids in venous return. It is the most commonly used stroke, and it

---

BOX 12.6 Application of Therapeutic Massage

Indications	Contraindications
Increase local circulation	Acute contusions, sprains, and strains
Increase venous and lymphatic flow	Over fracture sites
Reduce pain (analgesia)	Over open lesions or skin conditions
Reduce muscle spasm	Conditions such as acute phlebitis, thrombosis, severe varicose veins, cellulites, synovitis, arteriosclerosis, and cancerous regions
Stretch superficial scar tissue	
Improve systemic relaxation	
Chronic myositis, bursitis, tendinitis, tenosynovitis, fibrositis	

TABLE 12.2 Techniques of Massage

TECHNIQUE	USE	METHOD OF APPLICATION
Effleurage (stroking)	Relaxes patient Evenly distributes any lubricant Increases surface circulation	Gliding motion over the skin without any attempt to move deep muscles Apply pressure with the flat of the hand; fingers and thumbs spread; stroke toward the heart. Massage begins and ends with stroking.
Pétrissage (kneading)	Increases circulation Promotes venous and lymphatic return Breaks up adhesions in superficial connective tissue Increases elasticity of skin	Kneading manipulation that grasps and rolls the muscles under the fingers or hands
Tapotement (percussion)	Increases circulation Stimulates subcutaneous structures	Brisk hand blows in rapid succession: Hacking with ulnar border Slapping with flat hand Beating with half-closed fist Tapping with fingertips Cupping with arched hand
Vibration	Relaxes limb	Fine vibrations made with fingers pressed into a specific body part
Friction (rubbing)	Loosens fibrous scar tissue Aids in the absorption of edema Reduces inflammation Reduces muscular spasm	Small circular motions with the fingers, thumb, or heel of hand Transverse friction is done perpendicular to the fibers being massaged.

begins and ends each massage. Effleurage permits the clinician to evaluate the condition, distribute the lubricant, warm the skin and superficial tissue, and promote relaxation.

Pétrissage consists of pressing and rolling the muscles under the fingers and hands. This "milking" action over deep tissues and muscle increases venous and lymphatic return and removes metabolic waste products from the injured area. Furthermore, it breaks up adhesions within the underlying tissues, loosens fibrous tissue, and increases the elasticity of the skin.

Tapotement uses sharp, alternating, brisk hand movements, such as hacking, slapping, beating, cupping, and clapping, to increase blood flow and stimulate peripheral nerve endings. Because this technique is used for stimulation and not for relaxation, it is not used in most massage treatments.

Vibration consists of finite, gentle, and rhythmic movement of the fingers to vibrate the underlying tissues. It is used for relaxation or stimulation.

Friction is the deepest form of massage and consists of deep, circular motions performed by the thumb, knuckles, or ends of the fingers at right angles to the involved tissue. These deep circular movements can loosen adherent fibrous tissue (scars), aid in the absorption of an edema, and reduce localized muscular spasm. Transverse friction massage is a deep friction massage that is performed across the grain of the muscle, tendon sheath, or ligament. Cross-friction massage is the most effective technique and is used to break up adhesions and promote the healing of muscle and ligament tears.

One recent study found that blood flow did not significantly increase with effleurage, pétrissage, and tapotement on either a small or large muscle mass.[51] Another study found that manual massage did not have a significant impact on the recovery of muscle function following exercise or on any of the physiological factors associated with the recovery process.[52] In both studies, the researchers concluded that light exercise of the affected muscles probably is more effective than massage in improving muscle blood flow (thereby enhancing healing) and in temporarily reducing muscle soreness. Because the types and duration of massage typically are based on the preference of the individual and clinician, its use in athletic settings for these purposes should be questioned.

Traction

Traction is the process of drawing or pulling tension on a body segment. The most common forms involve lumbar and cervical traction. Spinal traction more commonly is used to treat small, herniated disk protrusions that may result in spinal nerve impingement, although it also may be used to treat a variety of other conditions (**Box 12.7**). The effects of spinal traction include distraction of the vertebral bodies, widening of the vertebral foramen, a combination of distraction and gliding of vertebral facets, and stretching and relaxing of the paraspinal muscles and ligamentous structures of the spinal segment.

A distractive force commonly is applied using a mechanical device or manually by a clinician. Traction may be applied continuously, through a low, distracting force for up to several hours; statically, with a sustained distracting force applied for the entire treatment time, usually 30 minutes; or intermittently, with a distracting force applied and released for several seconds repeatedly over the course of the treatment time. For example, in lumbar traction, a split table is used to eliminate friction. A special nonslip harness lined with vinyl is used to transfer the distractive force comfortably to the patient and stabilize the trunk and thoracic area while the lumbar spine is placed under traction. A distractive force, usually up to half the patient's body weight, is applied for 30 minutes daily for 2 to 4 weeks. Although intermittent traction tends to be more comfortable for the patient, sustained traction is more effective in treating lumbar disk problems. In cervical traction, the patient may be either supine or seated. Again, a nonslip cervical harness is secured under the chin and back of the head to transfer the distractive force comfortably to the patient. Recommended force ranges from 10 to 30 lb. Again, there are currently no clinically or statistically significant studies that support the use of traction as a therapeutic modality.

With manual traction, the clinician applies the distractive force for a few seconds or, sometimes, with a quick, sudden thrust. This method has been effective in reducing joint pain when the traction is applied within the normal range of joint movement. Because the clinician can feel the relaxation or resistance, it is possible to instantaneously change the patient's position, the direction of the force, the magnitude of the force, or the duration of the treatment, making manual traction more flexible and adaptable than mechanical traction.

Continuous Passive Motion

Continuous passive motion is a modality that applies an external force to move the joint through a preset arc of motion. It primarily is used postsurgically at the knee, after knee manipulation, or after stable fixation of intra-articular and extra-articular fractures of most joints, such as the hand, wrist, hip, shoulder, elbow, and ankle. It also may be used to improve wound healing, accelerate the clearance of a hemarthrosis, and prevent cartilage degeneration in septic arthritis (**Box 12.8**). The application is relatively pain-free and has been shown to stimulate the intrinsic healing process; maintain articular cartilage nutrition; reduce disuse effects, retard joint stiffness and the pain–spasm cycle; and benefit collagen remodeling, joint dynamics, and pain reduction.[1,53]

BOX 12.7 Application of Traction

Indications

Herniated disk protrusions

Spinal nerve impingement

Spinal nerve inflammation

Joint hypomobility

Narrowing of intervertebral foramen

Degenerative joint disease

Spondylolisthesis

Muscle spasm and guarding

Joint pain

Contraindications

Unstable vertebrae

Acute lumbago

Gross emphysema

S4 nerve root signs

Temporomandibular dysfunction

Patient discomfort

BOX 12.8 Application of Continuous Passive Motion

Indications

Postoperative rehabilitation to:

- Reduce pain
- Improve general circulation
- Enhance joint nutrition
- Prevent joint contractures
- Benefit collagen remodeling

Following knee manipulation

Following joint debridement

Following meniscal or osteochondral repair

Tendon lacerations

Contraindications

Noncompliant patient

If use would disrupt surgical repair, fracture fixation, or lead to hemorrhage in postoperative period

Malfunction of device

 Massage may be used after the acute phase has ended. Stroking and kneading toward the heart may provide some beneficial effects; however, mild exercise may be just as beneficial.

SUMMARY

1. Rehabilitation begins immediately after injury assessment with the use of therapeutic modalities to limit pain, inflammation, and a loss of ROM.

2. Therapeutic modalities, with the exception of ultrasound, fall within the electromagnetic spectrum based on their wavelength or frequency. All electromagnetic energy is pure energy that travels in a straight line at the speed of light (300 million meters per second) in a vacuum.

3. Depending on the medium, energy can be reflected, refracted, absorbed, or transmitted.

4. Common therapeutic modalities include cryotherapy, thermotherapy, ultrasound, diathermy, electrical stimulation, massage, traction, continuous passive motion, and medications to promote healing. Although many are used every day in treating musculoskeletal injuries, many others must be used under the direction of a physician or a licensed health care provider. Being a technician and merely applying a modality is not an acceptable athletic training practice.

5. Cryotherapy is used to decrease pain, inflammation, and muscle guarding and spasm as well as to facilitate mobilization.

6. Thermotherapy is used to treat subacute or chronic injuries to reduce swelling, edema, ecchymosis, and muscle spasm; to increase blood flow and ROM; to facilitate tissue healing; to relieve joint contractures; and to fight an infection.

7. Ultrasound produces both thermal and nonthermal effects. Thermal effects include increased blood flow, extensibility of collagen tissue, sensory and motor nerve conduction velocity, and enzymatic activity as well as decreased muscle spasm, joint stiffness, inflammation, and pain. Nonthermal effects include decreased edema; increased blood flow, cell membrane and vascular wall permeability, protein synthesis, and tissue regeneration; and the promotion of healing.

8. Diathermy is used to treat joint inflammation (e.g., bursitis, tendinitis, and synovitis), joint capsule contractures, subacute and chronic inflammatory conditions in deep-tissue layers, osteoarthritis, ankylosing spondylitis, and chronic pelvic inflammatory disease.

9. Electrotherapy is used to decrease pain, reeducate peripheral nerves, delay denervation and disuse atrophy by stimulating muscle contractions, reduce posttraumatic edema, and maintain ROM by reducing muscle spasm, inhibiting spasticity, reeducating partially denervated muscle, and facilitating voluntary motor function.

10. Iontophoresis is used to introduce ions into the body tissues by means of a direct electrical current. This treatment is beneficial in reducing inflammation, muscle spasm, ischemia, and edema.

11. Massage involves the manipulation of the soft tissues to increase cutaneous circulation, cell metabolism, and venous and lymphatic flow to assist in the removal of edema; to stretch superficial scar tissue; to alleviate soft-tissue adhesions; and to decrease neuromuscular excitability. Strokes include effleurage, pétrissage, tapotement, vibration, and friction massage.

12. Traction is the process of drawing or pulling tension on a body segment and commonly is used on the spine to treat herniated disk protrusion, spinal nerve inflammation or impingement, narrowing of intervertebral foramen, and muscle spasm and pain.

13. Continuous passive motion applies an external force to move the joint through a preset arc of motion and primarily is used postsurgically at the knee, after knee manipulation, or after the stable fixation of intra-articular and extra-articular fractures of most joints.

14. Because of the complexity of each of the therapeutic modalities, students should enroll in a separate therapeutic modalities class, permitting practice and demonstration of proper clinical skills associated with the application of therapeutic modalities.

15. While using any modality, if the individual begins to show signs of pain, swelling, discomfort, tingling, or loss of sensation, the treatment should be stopped and the individual should be reevaluated to determine if the selected modality is appropriate for the current phase of healing.

APPLICATION QUESTIONS

1. You are a newly hired high school athletic trainer. As you survey the space allocated for the athletic training room, you notice that there is only one electrical outlet. What factors should you consider prior to plugging any item into that outlet?

2. A field hockey player has chronic low back pain. What type of therapy (heat or cold) treatment would you use with this athlete prior to practice? Following practice? Why?

3. An athlete has sustained an acute ankle sprain. What type of modality might you use to manage this acute injury? How might your management differ after 48 hours postinjury? Why?

4. A shot putter sustained a strain to the triceps muscle. After applying the protect, rest, ice, compression, and elevation (PRICE) principle, what other modality can be combined with PRICE to decrease pain, muscle spasms, and edema? Why?

5. An athlete sustained a hamstring strain 3 days ago. There is no swelling. The athlete reports mild discomfort when flexing and extending the knee. What modalities could be used to decrease the athlete's discomfort and increase the ROM of the hamstring muscles? Of those selected, which ones are more effective at relieving pain and muscle soreness?

6. You are the only athletic trainer at a high school. The family physician of one of the athlete's suggests massage as a strategy for breaking up soft-tissue adhesions associated with a recent shoulder surgery. The parents of the athlete ask you to perform the massage treatments right before each practice. How would you respond to their request? Why?

REFERENCES

1. Starkey C. *Therapeutic Modalities for Athletic Trainers*. 3rd ed. Philadelphia, PA: FA Davis; 2013.

2. Nolan TP Jr. Technical aspects of therapeutic modalities. In: Michlovitz SL, Nolan TP Jr, eds. *Modalities for Therapeutic Intervention*. 4th ed. Philadelphia, PA: FA Davis; 2005:41–181.

3. Kimura IF, Thompson GT, Gulick DT. The effect of cryotherapy on eccentric plantar flexion peak torque and endurance. *J Athl Train*. 1997;32(2):124–126.

4. Knight KL. *Cryotherapy in Sport Injury Management*. Champaign, IL: Human Kinetics; 1995.

5. Knight KL, Bryan KS, Halvorsen JM. Circulatory changes in the forearm in 1, 5, 10, and 15°C water. *Int J Sports Med*. 1981;4:281.

6. Ho SS, Illgen RL, Meyer RW, et al. Comparison of various icing times in decreasing bone metabolism and blood flow in the knee. *Am J Sports Med*. 1995;23(1):74–76.

7. Otte JW, Merrick MA, Ingersoll CD, et al. Subcutaneous adipose tissue thickness alters cooling time during cryotherapy. *Arch Phys Med Rehabil*. 2002;83(11):1501–1505.

8. Tsang KK, Buxton BP, Guion WK, et al. The effects of cryotherapy applied through various barriers. *J Sports Rehabil*. 1997;(4):343–354.

9. Danielson R, Jaeger J, Rippetoe J, et al. Differences in skin surface temperature and pressure during the application of various cold and compression devices. *J Athl Train*. 1997;32(2):S34.

10. Bender AL, Kramer EE, Brucker JB, et al. Local ice-bag application and triceps surae muscle temperature during treadmill walking. *J Athl Train*. 2005;40(4):271–275.

11. Bélanger AY. *Therapeutic Electrophysical Agents: Evidence Behind Practice*. Baltimore, MD: Lippincott Williams & Wilkins; 2009.

12. Michlovitz SL, Rennie S. Heat therapy modalities: beyond fake and bake. In: Michlovitz SL, Nolan TP Jr, eds. *Modalities for Therapeutic Intervention*. Philadelphia, PA: FA Davis; 2005:61–78.

13. Walsh MT. Hydrotherapy: the use of water as a therapeutic agent. In: Michlovitz SL, ed. *Thermal Agents in Rehabilitation*. Philadelphia, PA: FA Davis; 1996:139–167.

14. Kaiser DA, Knight KL, Huff JM, et al. Hot-pack warming in 4- and 8-pack Hydrocollator® units. *J Sport Rehabil*. 2004;13(2):103–113.

15. Sandqvist G, Akesson A, Eklund M. Evaluation of paraffin bath treatment in patients with systemic sclerosis. *Disabil Rehabil*. 2004;26(16):981–987.

16. Borrell RM, Parker R, Henley EJ, et al. Comparison of in vivo temperatures produced by hydrotherapy, paraffin wax treatment, and fluidotherapy. *Phys Ther*. 1980;60(10):1273–1276.

17. Hayes BT, Sandrey MA, Merrick MA, et al. The differences between 1-MHz and 3-MHz ultrasound in the heating of subcutaneous tissues. *J Athl Train*. 2001;36(2):S92.

18. Schneider NC, Walsh CT, Lemley SF, et al. 3 MHz continuous ultrasound can elevate tissue temperature at 3-cm depth. *Phys Ther*. 2001;81:A8.

19. Ramirez A, Schwane JA, McFarland C, et al. The effect of ultrasound on collagen synthesis and fibroblast proliferation in vitro. *Med Sci Sports Exerc*. 1997;29(3):326–332.

20. Houglum PA. Soft tissue healing and its impact on rehabilitation. *J Sport Rehabil*. 1992;1(1):19–39.

21. Sparrow KJ. Therapeutic ultrasound. In: Michlovitz SL, Nolan TP Jr, eds. *Modalities for Therapeutic Intervention*. 4th ed. Philadelphia, PA: FA Davis; 2005:79–86.

22. Draper DO, Sunderland S. Examination of the law of Grotthus-Draper: does ultrasound penetrate subcutaneous fat in humans. *J Athl Train*. 1993;28(3):246–250.

23. Grant TH, Kelikian AS, Jereb SE, et al. Ultrasound diagnosis of peroneal tendon tears. A surgical correlation. *J Bone Joint Surg Am*. 2005;87(8):1788–1794.

24. Loudon JK, Cagle PE, Dyson M. High-frequency ultrasound: an overview of potential uses in physical therapy. *Phys Ther Rev*. 2005;10(4):209–215.

25. Klucinec B. The effectiveness of the aquaflex gel pad in transmission of acoustic energy. *J Athl Train*. 1996;31(4):313–317.

26. Draper DO, Castel JC, Castel D. Rate of temperature increase in human muscle during 1 MHz and 3 MHz continuous ultrasound. *J Orthop Sports Phys Ther*. 1995;22(4):142–150.

27. Forrest G, Rosen K. Ultrasound treatments in degassed water. *J Sport Rehabil*. 1992;1(4):284–289.

28. Merrick MA, Mihalyov MR, Roethemeier JL, et al. A comparison of intramuscular temperatures during ultrasound treatments with coupling gel or gel pads. *J Orthop Sports Phys Ther*. 2002;32(5):216–220.

29. Draper DO. Ten mistakes commonly made with ultrasound use: current research sheds light on myths. *Athl Train Sports Health Care Perspect*. 1996;2:95–107.

30. Klucinec B, Scheidler M, Denegar C, et al. Transmissivity of coupling agents used to deliver ultrasound through indirect methods. *J Orthop Sports Phys Ther*. 2000;30(5):263–269.

31. Ciccone CD, Leggin BG, Callamaro JJ. Effects of ultrasound and trolamine salicylate phonophoresis on delayed-onset muscle soreness. *Phys Ther*. 1991;71(9):666–675.

32. Cagnie B, Vinck E, Rimbaut S, et al. Phonophoresis versus topical application of ketoprofen: comparison between tissue and plasma levels. *Phys Ther*. 2003;83(8):707–712.

33. Başkurt F, Ozcan A, Algun C. Comparison of effects of phonophoresis and iontophoresis of

naproxen in the treatment of lateral epicondylitis. *Clin Rehabil.* 2003;17(1):96–100.

34. Hsieh YL. Effects of ultrasound and diclofenac phonophoresis on inflammatory pain relief: suppression of inducible nitric oxide synthase in arthritic rats. *Phys Ther.* 2006;86(1):39–49.

35. Johnston TE. Muscle weakness and loss of motor performance. In: Michlovitz SL, Nolan TP Jr, eds. *Modalities for Therapeutic Intervention.* 4th ed. Philadelphia, PA: FA Davis; 2005:41–181.

36. Jarzem PF, Harvey EJ, Arcaro N, et al. Transcutaneous electrical nerve stimulation [TENS] for short-term treatment of low back pain—randomized double blind crossover study of sham versus conventional TENS. *J Musculoskelet Pain.* 2005;13(2):11–17.

37. Butterfield DL, Draper DO, Ricard MD, et al. The effects of high-volt pulsed current electrical stimulation on delayed-onset muscle soreness. *J Athl Train.* 1997;32(1):15–20.

38. Holcomb WR. A practical guide to electrical therapy. *J Sport Rehabil.* 1997;6(3):272–282.

39. Bonacci JA, Higbie EJ. Effects of microcurrent treatment on perceived pain and muscle strength following eccentric exercise. *J Athl Train.* 1997; 32(2):119–123.

40. Denegar CR, Yoho AP, Borowicz AJ, et al. The effects of low-volt, microamperage stimulation on delayed onset muscle soreness. *J Sport Rehabil.* 1992;1(2):95–102.

41. Knight KL, Hopkins T. Laser and light therapy. In: Knight KL, Draper DO, eds. *Therapeutic Modalities: The Art and Science.* 2nd ed. Baltimore, MD: Lippincott Williams & Wilkins; 2013: 399–417.

42. Karu TI, Afanasyeva NI, Kolyakov SF, et al. Changes in absorbance of monolayer of living cells induced by laser radiation at 633, 670, and 820 nm. *IEEE J Select Top Quantum Electron.* 2001;7(6):982–988.

43. Baxter GD. *Therapeutic Lasers: Theory and Practice.* Edinburgh, United Kingdom: Churchill Livingstone; 1994.

44. Enwemeka CS, Parker JC, Dowdy DS, et al. The efficacy of low-power lasers in tissue repair and pain control: a meta-analysis. *Photomed Laser Surg.* 2004;22(4):323–329.

45. Naeser MA, Hahn KA, Lieberman BE, et al. Carpal tunnel syndrome pain treated with low-level laser and microamperes transcutaneous electric nerve stimulation: a controlled study. *Arch Phys Med Rehabil.* 2002;83(7):978–988.

46. Simunovic Z. Low level laser therapy with trigger points technique: a clinical study on 243 patients. *J Clin Laser Med Surg.* 1996;14(4):163–167.

47. Simunovic Z, Trobonjaca T, Trobonjaca Z. Treatment of medial and lateral epicondylitis—tennis and golfer's elbow—with low level laser therapy: a multicenter double blind, placebo-controlled clinical study on 324 patients. *J Clin Laser Med Surg.* 1998;16(3):145–151.

48. Brosseau L, Welch V, Wells G, et al. Low level laser therapy for osteoarthritis and rheumatoid arthritis: a metaanalysis. *J Rheumatol.* 2000; 27(8):1961–1969.

49. Chow RT, Barnsley L. Systematic review of the literature of low-level laser therapy (LLLT) in the management of neck pain. *Lasers Surg Med.* 2005;37(1):46–52.

50. Basford JR, Sheffield CG, Harmsen WS. Laser therapy: a randomized, controlled trial of the effects of low-intensity Nd:YAG laser irradiation on musculoskeletal back pain. *Arch Phys Med Rehabil.* 1999;80(6):647–652.

51. Shoemaker JK, Tiidus PM, Mader R. Failure of manual massage to alter limb blood flow: measures by Doppler ultrasound. *Med Sci Sports Exerc.* 1997;29(5):610–614.

52. Tiidus PM. Manual massage and recovery of muscle function following exercise: a literature review. *J Orthop Sports Phys Ther.* 1997; 25(2):107–112.

53. Chiarello CM, Gundersen L, O'Halloran T. The effect of continuous passive motion duration and increment on range of motion in total knee arthroplasty patients. *J Orthop Sports Phys Ther.* 1997; 25(2):119–127.

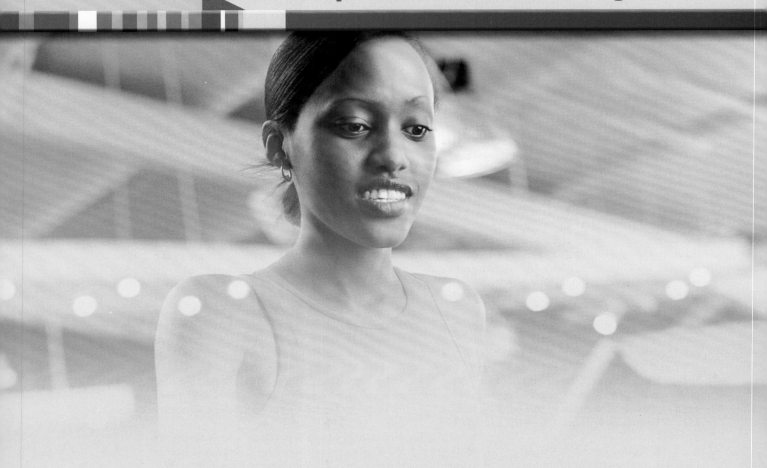

CHAPTER

13

Therapeutic Exercise Program

STUDENT OUTCOMES

1. Explain the principles of the cognitive model used to describe an individual's adjustment to injury.

2. Identify various psychological influences that can affect an injured individual, and describe strategies or intervention techniques used to overcome these influences.

3. Explain the importance of dealing with the psychological concerns that an individual may develop during a therapeutic exercise program.

4. Identify key factors in the development of a therapeutic exercise program.

5. Describe the four phases of a therapeutic exercise program, including the goals of these phases and the methodology of implementation.

6. Utilize limb symmetry measures and patient outcomes in return to play decisions.

7. List the criteria used to clear an individual to return to full participation in sports and physical activities.

INTRODUCTION

The ultimate goal of therapeutic exercise is to return the injured participant to pain-free and full return to activity. To accomplish this, attention must focus on modulating pain and restoring normal joint range of motion (ROM), kinematics, flexibility, muscular strength, endurance, coordination, and power. Furthermore, cardiovascular endurance and strength in the entire body must be maintained. An understanding of each component is necessary within a well-organized, individualized therapeutic exercise program.

In this chapter, a therapeutic exercise program will be explained following the SOAP (Subjective evaluation, Objective evaluation, Assessment, and Plan) note format. Phases of a therapeutic exercise program are presented, including criteria used to determine when an individual is ready to progress in the program and, ultimately, to participate in sports or physical activities. Practical application of the material for the various body segments is included in Chapters 14 through 22.

DEVELOPING A THERAPEUTIC EXERCISE PROGRAM

> **?** A female distance runner diagnosed with plantar fasciitis complains of pain with weight bearing that radiates up the medial side of the heel as well as across the lateral side of the foot. In addition, passive extension of the great toe and dorsiflexion of the ankle increase pain and discomfort. What short- and long-term goals could the athletic trainer and the athlete establish for a therapeutic exercise program? How should progress be measured?

In designing an individualized therapeutic exercise program, several sequential steps help to identify the needs of the patient:

1. Assess the present level of function and dysfunction from girth measurements, goniometric assessment, strength tests, neurological assessment, stress tests, functional tests, and patient outcomes.

2. Organize and interpret the assessment to identify compensatory factors that have contributed to the injury. Establish short- and long-term goals to return the individual safely to participation.

3. Develop and supervise the treatment plan, incorporating therapeutic exercise, therapeutic modalities, and medication as well as activity modification.

4. Reassess the progress of the plan and adjust as needed.

The process is dependent on the patient's progress and adaptation to the therapeutic exercise program.

Assess the Patient

The subjective evaluation (i.e., history of the injury) is recorded in the **subjective**, or S, portion of the SOAP note. This information should include the primary complaint, mechanism of injury, characteristics of the symptoms, functional impairments, previous injuries to the area, and family and medical history. The objective evaluation (i.e., observation and inspection, palpation, and physical examination tests) establishes a baseline of measurable information and is recorded in the **objective**, or O, portion of the SOAP note. This information documents the visual analysis of the injury site, symmetry, and appearance; determines the presence of a possible fracture; identifies abnormal clinical findings in the bony and soft-tissue structures; and measures ROM and strength (i.e., active, passive, and resisted ROM); stress tests for ligamentous and capsular integrity, neurological, and vascular testing; and sport-specific functional testing. In paired body segments, the dysfunction of the injured body part is always compared with the noninjured body part to establish standards for bilateral functional status.

Interpret the Assessment

When an assessment is completed, the data must be interpreted to identify factors outside the normal limits for an individual of the same age and fitness level. Specifically, primary deficits or weaknesses must be defined. These deficits, along with secondary problems resulting from prolonged immobilization, extended inactivity, or lack of intervention, are organized into a priority list of concerns. Examples of major concerns may include decreased ROM, muscle weakness or stiffness, joint contractures, sensory changes, inability to walk without a limp, or increased pain with activity. Physical limitations are then identified to determine the individual's present functional status. For example, normal gait and bilateral equal ROM should be documented. Specific problems are then recorded in a section called the problem list, which is a part of the **assessment**, or **A**, portion of the SOAP note.

Establish Goals

Next, long-term goals are established for the individual's expected level of performance at the conclusion of the exercise program. These goals typically focus on deficits in performing activities of daily living (ADLs) and might include bilateral equal ROM, flexibility, muscular strength, endurance, and power; relaxation training; and restoration of coordination and cardiovascular endurance. Then, short-term goals are developed to address the specific component skills needed to reach the long-term goals. The athletic trainer and patient should discuss and develop the goals. The individual must feel like a part of the process, because this may educate and motivate the individual to work harder to attain the stated goals. Many sport-specific factors, such as the demands of the sport; position played; time remaining in the season; regular season versus postseason or tournament play; game rules and regulations regarding prosthetic braces or safety equipment; location, nature, and severity of injury; and the mental state of the individual, may affect goal development.

The short-term goals are developed in a graduated sequence to address the list of problems identified during the assessment. For example, a high-priority short-term goal is the control of pain, inflammation, and spasms. Each short-term goal should be moderately difficult yet realistic. Specific subgoals should include an estimated timetable for attaining each one. These subgoals are time-dependent but are not fixed, because it is important to consider individual differences in preinjury fitness and participation status, severity of injury, motivation to complete the goals, and subsequent improvement. Constant reinforcement from the athletic trainer to achieve the subgoals can be an incentive to continually progress toward the long-term goals. Long- and short-term goals may be recorded in the **assessment**, or **A**, portion of the SOAP note; however, many athletic trainers choose to begin the **treatment plan**, or **P**, portion of the SOAP note with the objectives.

 An example of **short-term goals** can be seen on the companion Web site at thePoint.

Develop and Supervise the Treatment Plan

Any therapeutic exercise and modality used to achieve the goals is recorded in the plan section of the SOAP note along with any medications prescribed by the physician. To return the individual safely to participation, the therapeutic exercise program is divided into four phases. The termination of one phase and the initiation of the next may overlap; however, each phase has a specific role. In phase 1, the inflammatory response, pain, swelling, and ecchymosis are controlled. Phase 2 focuses on regaining any deficits in ROM at the affected joint and restoring proprioception. Phase 3 involves restoring muscle strength, endurance, and power in the affected limb. Phase 4 prepares the individual to return to activity and includes sport-specific skill training, regaining coordination, and improving cardiovascular conditioning. These phases and their expected outcomes are discussed in more detail later in this chapter, and **Box 13.1** lists the various phases of a therapeutic exercise program.

Each phase of the exercise program must be supervised and documented. In addition, progress notes should be completed on a weekly or biweekly basis or updated any time there is a change made to the rehabilitation plan. In many health care settings, these records also are used for third-party reimbursement of services rendered and, should litigation occur, provide documentation of services rendered.

BOX 13.1 Phases of the Therapeutic Exercise Program

Phase 1: Control Inflammation

- Control the inflammatory stage and minimize scar tissue with cryotherapy using **PRICE** principles (**p**rotect, **r**estrict activity, **i**ce, **c**ompression, and **e**levation).
- Instruct the patient on relaxation and coping techniques.
- Maintain ROM, joint flexibility, strength, endurance, and power in the unaffected body parts.
- Maintain cardiovascular endurance.

Phase 2: Restore Motion

- Restore ROM to within 80% of normal in the unaffected limb.
- Restore joint flexibility to that observed in the unaffected limb.
- Begin proprioceptive stimulation through closed isotonic chain exercises.
- Begin pain-free, isometric strengthening exercises on the affected limb.
- Begin unresisted, pain-free functional patterns of sport/activity-specific motion.
- Maintain muscular strength, endurance, and power in the unaffected muscles.
- Maintain cardiovascular endurance.

Phase 3: Develop Muscular Strength, Power, and Endurance

- Restore full ROM and proprioception in the affected limb.
- Restore muscular strength, endurance, and power using progressive resisted exercise.
- Maintain cardiovascular endurance.
- Initiate minimal-to-moderate resistance in sport/activity-specific functional patterns.

Phase 4: Return to Sport/Physical Activity

- Analyze skill performance and correct biomechanical inefficiencies in motion.
- Improve muscular strength, endurance, and power.
- Restore coordination and balance.
- Improve cardiovascular endurance.
- Increase sport/activity-specific functional patterns and return to protected activity as tolerated.

Reassess the Progress of the Program

Short-term goals should be flexible enough to accommodate the progress of the individual. For example, if therapeutic modalities or medications are used and the individual attains a short-term goal sooner than expected, a new short-term goal should be written. Some conditions, however, such as edema, hemorrhage, muscle spasm, atrophy, or infection, may impede the healing process and delay the attainment of a short-term goal. Periodic measurement of girth, ROM, muscle strength, endurance, power, and cardiovascular fitness determine whether progress occurs. If progress is not seen, the individual should be reevaluated. The athletic trainer must determine if the delay is caused by physical problems, noncompliance, or psychological influences, necessitating referral to the appropriate specialist (e.g., physician or clinical psychologist). The individual should continue to progress through the short-term goals until the long-term goals are attained and the individual is cleared for full activity.

Long-term goals for the distance runner might include pain-free ROM, flexibility, muscle strength, endurance, and power; maintenance of cardiovascular endurance; restoration of normal joint biomechanics; increased proprioception and coordination; restoration of bilateral function of ADLs; and pain-free, unlimited motion in sport-specific skills.

PHASE 1: CONTROLLING INFLAMMATION

Given the acute nature of the distance runner's plantar fasciitis, the acute care protocol was followed, including submersion of the foot in an ice bath. Would it be appropriate to begin any rehabilitation exercises during this initial phase of injury management?

Phase 1 of the exercise program begins immediately after injury assessment. The primary goal is to control inflammation by limiting hemorrhage, edema, effusion, muscle spasm, and pain. The individual can move into phase 2 when the following criteria have been attained:

- Control of inflammation with minimal edema, swelling, muscle spasm, and pain

- ROM, joint flexibility, muscular strength, endurance, and power are maintained in the unaffected/uninjured areas of the body.

- Cardiovascular fitness is maintained at the preinjury level.

Collagenous scar formation, a natural component of the repair and regeneration of injured soft tissue, is less efficient and tolerant of tensile forces compared with the original mature tissue. The length of the inflammatory response is a key factor influencing the ultimate stability and function of scar tissue: The longer the inflammatory process progresses, the more likely the resulting scar tissue will be less dense and weaker in yielding to applied stress. Furthermore, immobilization for more than 2 or 3 weeks may lead to joint adhesions that inhibit the regeneration of muscle fiber. Therefore, all inflammatory symptoms need to be controlled as soon as possible. **PRICE**, a well-known acronym for **p**rotect, **r**estrict activity, **i**ce, **c**ompression, and **e**levation, is used to reduce acute symptoms at an injury site.

Control of Inflammation

Following trauma, hemorrhage and edema at the site of injury lead to a pooling of tissue fluids and blood products that increases pain and muscle spasm. The increased pressure decreases the flow of blood to the injury site, leading to hypoxia (a deficiency of oxygen). As pain continues, the threshold for pain is lowered. These events lead to the cyclical pattern of pain-spasm-hypoxia-pain. For this reason, cryotherapy (i.e., ice, compression, and elevation) is preferred during the acute inflammation stage to decrease circulation, cellular metabolism, the need for oxygen, and conduction velocity of nerve impulses to break the pain–spasm cycle. An elastic compression wrap can decrease hemorrhage and hematoma formation yet still expand in cases of extreme swelling. Elevation and active ROM uses gravity to reduce the pooling of fluids and pressure inside the venous and lymphatic vessels and thereby prevent fluid from filtering into the surrounding tissue spaces. The result is less tissue necrosis and local waste, leading to a shorter inflammatory phase. **Application Strategy 13.1** explains acute care of soft-tissue injuries using the PRICE principle.

Cryotherapy, intermittent compression, and therapeutic exercise may be used to control hemorrhage and eliminate edema. Electrical muscle stimulation (EMS) is not currently recommended as a means to improve function, reduce edema, or decrease pain in the treatment of acute lateral ankle sprains.[1] Electrical therapy also has been shown to decrease pain and muscle spasm, strengthen weakened muscles, improve blood flow to an area, and enhance the healing rate of injured tendons.

APPLICATION STRATEGY 13.1

Acute Care of Soft-Tissue Injuries

Ice Application

- Apply crushed ice for 30 minutes directly to the skin (40 minutes for a large muscle mass, such as the quadriceps).
- Ice applications should be repeated every 2 hours when awake (every hour if the athlete is active) and may extend to more than 72 hours postinjury.
- Skin temperature can indicate when acute swelling has subsided. For example, if the area (compared bilaterally) feels warm to the touch, swelling continues. If in doubt, extend the time of a cold application.

Compression

- On an extremity, apply the wrap in a distal-to-proximal direction to avoid forcing extracellular fluid into the distal digits.
- Take a distal pulse after applying the wrap to ensure that the wrap is not overly tight.
- Felt horseshoe pads placed around the malleolus may be combined with an elastic wrap or tape to limit ankle swelling.
- Maintain compression continuously on the injury for the first 24 hours.

Elevation

- Elevate the body part 6–10 in above the level of the heart.
- While sleeping, place a hard suitcase between the mattress and box spring, or place the extremity on a series of pillows.

Restrict Activity and Protect the Area

- If the individual is unable to walk without a limp, fit the person for crutches and apply an appropriate protective device to limit unnecessary movement of the injured joint.
- If the individual has an upper extremity injury and is unable to move the limb without pain, fit the person with an appropriate sling or brace.

Transcutaneous electrical nerve stimulation (TENS) also may be used to limit pain (see Chapter 12). The modality of choice is determined by the size and location of the injured area, the availability of the modality, and the preference of the supervising health care provider. A decision to discontinue treatment and move to another modality should be based on the cessation of inflammation. Increased tissue temperature may indicate that inflammation is still present as well as swelling and redness in the involved body part.

Effects of Immobilization

The effects of immobilization on various tissues of the body have been extensively covered in the literature. It is well accepted that muscle tension, muscle and ligament atrophy, decreased circulation, and loss of motion prolong the repair and regeneration of damaged tissues. As determined by the physician, it is indicated to maintain partial to full weight bearing in the lower extremity in order to maintain strength.

Muscle

Immobilization can lead to a loss of muscle strength within 24 hours. This is manifested by decreases in muscle fiber size, total muscle weight, size and number of mitochondria (the energy source of the cell), muscle tension produced, and resting levels of glycogen and adenosine triphosphate, which reduces muscle endurance. Motor nerves become less efficient in recruiting and stimulating muscle fibers. Immobilization also increases muscle fatigability as a result of decreased oxidative capacity. The rate of loss appears to be more rapid during the initial days of immobilization; however, after 5 to 7 days, the loss of muscle mass diminishes.[2] Although both slow-twitch (type I) and fast-twitch (type II) muscle fibers atrophy, it generally is accepted that greater degeneration occurs in slow-twitch fibers with immobilization and that muscles immobilized in a lengthened or neutral position maintain muscle weight and the fiber cross-sectional area better than muscles immobilized in a shortened position. When shortened, the length of the fibers decreases, leading to increased connective tissue and reduced muscle extensibility. Muscles immobilized in a shortened position atrophy faster and have a greater loss of contractile function.

Articular Cartilage

The greatest impact of immobilization occurs in the articular cartilage, where adverse changes appear within 1 week of immobilization. The specific effects depend on the length of immobilization, the position of the joint, and joint loading. Intermittent loading and unloading of synovial joints is necessary to ensure the proper metabolic exchange necessary for normal function. Constant contact with opposing bone ends can lead to pressure necrosis and cartilage cell (chondrocyte) death. In contrast, noncontact between two surfaces promotes the growth of connective tissue into the joint. Diminished weight bearing, as well as loading and unloading, also can increase bone resorption. In general, articular cartilage softens and decreases in thickness. Immobilization for longer than 30 days can lead to progressive osteoarthritis.

Ligaments

Similar to bone, ligaments adapt to normal stress by remodeling in response to the mechanical demands that are placed on them. Stress leads to a stiffer, stronger ligament, whereas immobilization leads to a weaker, more compliant structure. This causes a decrease in the tensile strength, thus reducing the ability of ligaments to provide joint stability.

Bone

Mechanical strain on a bone affects the osteoblastic (bone cell formation) and osteoclastic (bone cell resorption) activity on the bone surface. Accordingly, the effects of immobilization on bone are similar to those on other connective tissues. Limited weight-bearing and muscle activity lead to bone loss, which can be detected as early as 2 weeks after immobilization.[2] As immobilization time increases, bone resorption occurs, resulting in the bones becoming more brittle and highly susceptible to fracture. Disuse atrophy appears to increase bone loss at a rate 5- to 20-fold greater than that resulting from metabolic disorders affecting bone.[3] Therefore, non–weight-bearing immobilization should be limited to as short a time as possible.

Effects of Remobilization

Early controlled mobilization can speed the healing process. Bone and soft tissue respond to the physical demands that are placed on them, causing the formation of collagen to remodel or realign along the lines of stress, and thereby promoting healthy joint biomechanics (**Wolff law**). Continuous passive motion can prevent joint adhesions and stiffness and can decrease joint hemarthrosis (blood in the joint) and pain. Early motion, as well as loading and unloading of joints, through partial weight-bearing exercise, maintain joint lubrication to nourish articular cartilage, menisci, and ligaments. This leads to an optimal environment for proper collagen fibril formation. Tissues recover at different rates with mobilization: Muscle recovers more quickly, and articular cartilage and bone respond least favorably.

Muscle

Muscle regeneration begins within 3 to 5 days after mobilization. Both fast-twitch and slow-twitch muscle fibers can completely recover after 6 weeks. Muscle contractile activity rapidly increases protein synthesis; however, maximal isometric tension may not return to normal until 4 months after mobilized activity. The use of electrotherapy (i.e., EMS) may be helpful in reeducating muscles, limiting pain and spasms, and decreasing effusion through the pumping action of the contracting muscle. Unfortunately, neither EMS nor isometric exercise has been shown to prevent disuse atrophy.

Articular Cartilage

The effects of immobilization, whether with contact or with a loss of contact between joint surfaces, can adversely interfere with cartilage nutrition. Articular cartilage generally responds favorably to mechanical stimuli, with structural modifications noted after exercise. Soft-tissue changes are reversible if immobilization does not exceed 30 days; these structural changes may not be reversible if immobilization exceeds 30 days.

Ligaments

The bone–ligament junction recovers more slowly than the mechanical properties in the midportion of the ligament. In addition, other nontraumatized ligaments weaken with disuse. Recovery depends on the duration of immobilization. Studies have shown that following 12 weeks of immobilization, a recovery of 50% of normal strength in a healing ligament is found after 6 months, 80% after 1 year, and 100% after 1 to 3 years, depending on the type of stresses placed on the ligament and on the prevention of repeated injury.[4] Although the properties of ligaments return to normal with remobilization, the bone–ligament junction takes longer to return to normal. This factor must be considered when planning a rehabilitation program.

Bone

Although bone lost during immobilization may be regained, the period of recovery can be several-fold greater than the period of immobilization. In disuse osteoporosis, a condition involving reduced quantity of bone tissue, bone loss may not be reversible on remobilization of the limb. Isotonic and isometric exercises during the immobilization period can decrease some bone loss and hasten recovery after returning to a normal loading environment.

Protection After Injury

The type of protection selected and the length of activity modification depend on the severity of the injury, the structures damaged, and the philosophy of the supervising health care provider. Several materials, including elastic wraps, tape, pads, slings, hinged braces, splints, walking boots, and crutches, can be used to protect the area; many of these items were discussed and illustrated in Chapter 4. If an individual cannot walk without pain or walks with a limp, crutches should be recommended (**Application Strategy 13.2**).

See **Daily Adjusted Progressive Resistance Exercise Program** on the companion Web site at thePoint.

Restricted activity does not imply cessation of activity but rather means relative rest—that is, decreasing activity to a level below that required in sport but tolerated by the recently injured tissue or joint. **Detraining**, or a loss of the benefits gained in physical training, can occur after only 1 to 2 weeks of nonactivity, with significant decreases measured in both metabolic and working capacities.[5] Strengthening exercises in a weight-lifting program can be alternated with cardiovascular exercises, such as jogging on an antigravity treadmill, swimming or water running, or use of a stationary bike or upper body ergometer. These exercises can prevent the individual from experiencing depression as a result of inactivity and can be done simultaneously with phase 1 exercises as long as the injured area is not irritated or inflamed.

 In addition to cold treatments for the control of inflammation, it would be appropriate to initiate gentle stretching exercises during this phase. The particular areas that should be stretched include the Achilles tendon and the toe flexor tendons. In addition, general body strength and cardiovascular endurance exercise can be performed as long as the injured area is not irritated.

APPLICATION STRATEGY 13.2

Fitting and Using Crutches and Canes

Fitting Crutches

1. Have the individual stand erect in flat shoes with the feet close together.
2. Place the crutch tip 2 in in front and 6 in from the outer sole of the shoe.
3. Adjust crutch height to allow a space of about two finger widths between the crutch pad and the axillary skinfold to avoid undue pressure on neurovascular structures.
4. Adjust the hand grip so the elbow is flexed 25°–30° and is at the level of the hip joint (greater trochanter).

Fitting for a Cane

1. Place the individual in the same position as previous. Adjust the hand grip so the elbow is flexed at 25°–30° and is at the level of the hip joint (greater trochanter).

Swing Through Gait (Non–Weight-Bearing)

1. Stand on the uninvolved leg. Lean forward and place both crutches and the involved leg approximately 12–24 in in front of the body.
2. Body weight should rest on the hands, not the axillary pads.
3. With the good leg, step through the crutches as if taking a normal step. Repeat the process.
4. If possible, the involved leg should be extended while swinging forward to prevent atrophy of the quadriceps muscles.

Three-Point Gait (Partial Weight Bearing)

1. This is indicated when one extremity can support the body weight, and the injured extremity is to be touched down or to bear weight partially.
2. As tolerated, place as much body weight as possible onto the involved leg, taking the rest of the weight on the hands.
3. Make sure a good heel-to-toe technique is used, whereby the heel strikes first, then the weight is shifted to the ball of the foot.
4. Increase the amount of weight bearing by decreasing the force transferred through the arms; mimic a normal gait.

Going Up and Down Stairs

1. Place both crutches under the arm opposite the handrail.
2. To go **up** the stairs, step **up with the uninvolved leg** while leaning on the rail.
3. To go **down** the stairs, place the crutches down on the next step and step **down with the involved leg**.

Using One Crutch or Cane

1. Place one crutch or cane on the uninvolved side and move it forward with the involved leg.
2. Do not lean heavily on the crutch or cane.

PHASE 2: RESTORATION OF MOTION

? The acute inflammatory symptoms associated with the plantar fasciitis have subsided. In the ongoing treatment of the plantar fasciitis, what type of exercises should be encouraged at this point during the rehabilitation process? Are there any modalities that could be used to supplement the exercise program?

Phase 2 begins immediately after the inflammation is controlled. This phase focuses on restoring ROM and flexibility at the injured site as well as on continuing to maintain general body strength and cardiovascular endurance. This phase may begin as early as 4 days after the injury, when swelling has stopped, or may have to wait until several weeks after the injury. The injured site may still be tender to the touch, but it is not as painful as in the earlier phase. Also, pain is much less evident on passive and active ROM (AROM). If the patient is in an immobilizer or splint, the splint should be removed for treatment and exercise. The splint then can be replaced to support and protect the injured site. The individual can move into phase 3 when the following criteria have been completed:

- Inflammation and pain are under control.

- ROM is within 80% of normal in the unaffected limb.

- Bilateral joint flexibility is restored, and proprioception is regained.

- Cardiovascular endurance and general body strength are maintained at the preinjury level.

An assessment of normal ROM should be done with a goniometer on the paired, uninjured joint (see Chapter 5). Cryotherapy or EMS may be used before exercise to decrease perceived pain, or thermotherapy may be used to warm the tissues and increase circulation to the region. When the tissue is warmed, friction massage, instrument-assisted soft-tissue mobilization, or joint mobilization may be helpful to break up scar tissue to regain normal motion.

Progression in this phase begins gradually, with the restoration of ROM, proprioception, and total joint flexibility. Factors that limit joint motion include bony block; joint adhesions; muscle tightness; tight skin or inelastic, dense scar tissue; swelling; pain; and fat or other soft tissues that block normal motion. Prolonged immobilization can lead to muscles losing their flexibility and assuming a shortened position, which is referred to as a **contracture**. Similar to muscle tissue, however, connective tissue adaptively shortens if immobilized. Connective tissue and muscles may be lengthened through passive and active stretching as well as proprioceptive neuromuscular facilitation exercises. However, fascial tissue forms a whole-body, continuous three-dimensional viscoelastic matrix of structural support that surrounds and penetrates skeletal muscle, joints, organs, nerves, and vascular beds. The classical concept of its mere passive role in force transmission has recently been disproven with evidence suggesting contractile elements enabling a modulating role in force generation and also mechanosensory fine-tuning.[6]

Passive Range of Motion

Two types of movement must be present for normal motion to occur around a joint. Physiological motion, measured by a goniometer, occurs in the cardinal movement planes of flexion–extension, abduction–adduction, and rotation. Accessory motion, also referred to as **arthrokinematics**, is an involuntary joint motion that occurs simultaneously with physiological motion, but it cannot be measured precisely. Accessory movements involve the spinning, rolling, or gliding of one articular surface relative to another. Normal accessory movement must be present for full physiological ROM to occur. If any accessory motion component is limited, normal physiological motion will not occur.

Limited passive ROM (PROM) is called **hypomobility**. These discrete limitations of motion prevent a pain-free return to competition and predispose an individual to microtraumatic injuries that reinflame the original injury or create compensations in other parts of the body. Restoring PROM prevents degenerative joint changes and promotes healing.

Joint Mobilization

Joint mobilization uses various oscillating forces, applied in the open-packed position, to "free up" stiff or "fixed" joints. The oscillations produce several key benefits in the healing process:

- Breaking up adhesions and relieving capsular restrictions

- Distracting impacted tissues

- Increasing lubrication for normal articular cartilage

- Reducing pain and muscle tension

- Restoring full ROM and facilitating healing

BOX 13.2 Contraindications to Joint Mobilization

- Acute inflammation
- Hypermobility
- Osteoporosis
- Advanced osteoarthritis
- Infections
- Premature stressing of surgical structures

- Congenital bone deformities
- Malignancy
- Rheumatoid arthritis
- Fractures
- Neurological signs
- Vascular disease

Joint mobilization is contraindicated in several instances (**Box 13.2**). Maitland[7] described five grades of mobilization:

- **Grade I:** a small-amplitude movement at the beginning of the available ROM; used when pain and spasms limit movement early in the ROM

- **Grade II:** a large-amplitude movement within the available ROM; used when spasms limit movement sooner with a quick oscillation than with a slow one or when slowly increasing pain restricts movement halfway into the range

- **Grade III:** a large-amplitude movement up to the pathological limit in the ROM; used when pain and resistance from spasms, inert tissue tension, or tissue compression limit movement near the end of the ROM

- **Grade IV:** a small-amplitude movement at the very end of the ROM used when resistance limits movement in the absence of pain and spasm.

- **Grade V:** a small-amplitude, quick thrust delivered at the end of the ROM, usually accompanied by a popping sound called a manipulation used when minimal resistance limits the end of the ROM. Manipulation is most effectively accomplished by the velocity rather than the force of the thrust.

Grading is based on the amplitude of the movement and where within the available ROM that the force is applied. Grades I and IV are small-amplitude movements performed at the beginning and end of the ROM, respectively. Grades II and III are large-amplitude movements. Grade II tends to be applied in the midrange of movement, whereas grade III is performed up to the pathological limit of the available ROM. Grade V is the manipulation grade and is a small-amplitude thrust beyond the end range of a joint's restricted motion. Grades I and II joint mobilizations are used primarily to decrease joint pain, and grades III and IV joint mobilizations are used to increase joint ROM and reduce joint stiffness. Proper training is necessary prior to performing grade V mobilizations.

In performing joint mobilization, the individual is placed in a comfortable position, with the joint placed in an open-packed position. This allows the surrounding tissues to be as lax as possible and the intracapsular space to be at its largest. The direction of force is dependent on the contour of the joint surface of the structure being mobilized. The concave–convex rule states that when the concave surface is stationary and the convex surface is mobilized, a glide of the convex segment should be in the direction opposite to the restriction of joint movement. If the convex articular surface is stationary and the concave surface is mobilized, however, gliding of the concave segment should be in the same direction as the restriction of joint movement (**Fig. 13.1**). Typical treatment involves a series of three to six mobilizations lasting from 30 to 60 seconds, with one to three oscillations per second.[7] **Figure 13.2** demonstrates joint mobilization techniques.

Flexibility

Flexibility is the total ROM at a joint that occurs pain-free in each of the planes of motion. Joint flexibility is a combination of normal joint mechanics, mobility of soft tissues, and muscle extensibility. For example, the hip joint may have full PROM, but when doing active hip flexion from a seated position, as in touching one's toes, resistance from tight hamstrings may limit full hip flexion. This type of resistance may be generated from tension in muscle fibers or connective tissue.

Muscles contain two primary proprioceptors that can be stimulated during stretching—namely, the muscle spindles and the Golgi tendon organs. Because muscle spindles lie parallel to muscle fibers, they stretch with the muscle. When stimulated, the spindle sensory fibers discharge and, through reflex action in the spinal cord, initiate impulses to cause the muscle to contract reflexively, thus inhibiting the stretch. Muscles that perform the desired movement are called **agonists**. Unlike muscle spindles, Golgi tendon organs are connected in a series of fibers located in tendons and joint ligaments, and they respond to muscle tension rather than to muscle length. If the stretch continues for an extended time (i.e., longer than 6 to 8 seconds), the Golgi tendons are stimulated. This stimulus, unlike the stimulus from muscle spindles, causes a reflex inhibition in the **antagonist** muscles, and this sensory mechanism protects the musculotendinous unit from excessive tensile forces that could damage muscle fibers.

Flexibility can be increased through active stretching, passive stretching, or a combination of the two. **Active stretching** includes flexibility exercises performed by the patient without outside assistance from another individual. For example, a **static stretch** produces movement that is slow and deliberate and has been found to increase hamstring flexibility.[8,9] Golgi tendon organs are able to override impulses from the muscle spindles, leading to a safer, more effective muscle stretch. When the muscle is stretched to the point at which a mild burn is felt, the joint position is maintained statically for approximately 15 seconds and then is repeated several times. **Box 13.3** outlines guidelines for static stretching to improve flexibility.

Passive stretching includes several short- and long-term stretches with the use of equipment or another person to assist in the stretch activity. An example of this occurs when the clinician stabilizes the proximal segment of a joint and then moves the patient's limb through the available ROM, applying a slight stretch at the end of the motion. The patient should feel a stretch or tension but no pain. In a long-term stretch, a static stretch is applied from 20 to 30 minutes; however, little research exists on a definitive time.

Proprioceptive neuromuscular facilitation uses both active and passive stretching to promote and hasten the response of the neuromuscular system through the stimulation of the proprioceptors (**Fig. 13.3**). The patient should be taught how to perform the exercise through cutaneous and auditory input. Often, the individual looks at the moving limb while the clinician moves the limb from the starting to terminal position. Verbal cues are used to coordinate voluntary effort with reflex responses. Words such as "push" or "pull" commonly are used to ask for an isotonic contraction. "Hold" may be used for an isometric or stabilizing contraction, followed by "relax." Manual (cutaneous contact) helps to influence the direction of motion and to facilitate a maximal response, because reflex responses are

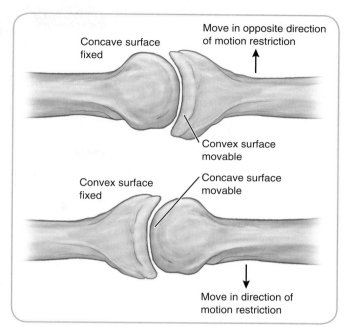

Figure 13.1. Concave–convex rule. If the joint surface to be moved is convex, it should be mobilized in the direction opposite that of the motion restriction. If the joint surface of the body segment being moved is concave, it should be moved in the direction of the motion restriction.

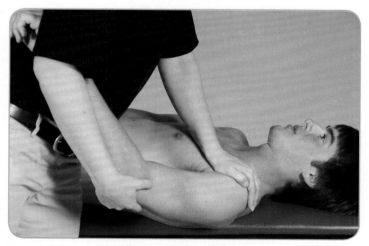

Figure 13.2. Joint mobilization technique. Posterior humeral glide uses one hand to stabilize the humerus at the elbow while the other hand glides the humeral head in a posterior direction to increase flexion and medial rotation at the joint.

BOX 13.3 Guidelines for Static Stretching to Improve Flexibility

1. Stretching is facilitated by warm body tissues; therefore, a brief warm-up is recommended. If unable to jog lightly, stretching may be performed after a superficial heat treatment.

2. In the designated stretch position, the individual should move to a position in which a sensation of tension is felt.

3. No bouncing should be associated with the stretch. The stretch position should be held for 10–30 seconds, until a sense of relaxation occurs. The individual should be aware of the feeling of relaxation or "letting go." Repeat the stretch six to eight times.

4. Breathing should be performed rhythmically and slowly. The individual should exhale during the actual stretch.

5. It is important to avoid being overly aggressive in stretching. Increased flexibility may not be noticed for 4–6 weeks.

6. If an area is particularly resistant to stretching, then partner stretching or proprioceptive neuromuscular facilitation may be used.

7. Vigorous stretching of tissues should be avoided in the following conditions:

   - After a recent fracture

   - After prolonged immobilization

   - With acute inflammation or infection in or around the joint

   - With a bony block that limits motion

   - With muscle contractures or when joint adhesions limit motion

   - With acute pain during stretching

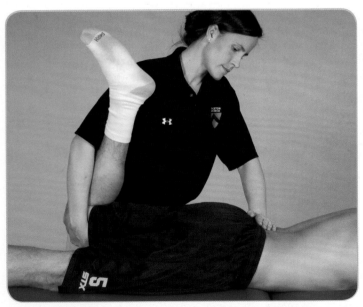

Figure 13.3. Proprioceptive neuromuscular facilitation. In performing proprioceptive neuromuscular facilitation stretching techniques, the athletic trainer passively stretches a muscle group. In this picture, the hip flexors are being stretched. When slight tension is felt, the individual isometrically contracts the muscle group against resistance for 3, 6, or 10 seconds. The muscle is then passively stretched. This process is repeated four or five times.

greatly affected by pressure receptors. Current research indicates that static stretching had a negative effect on explosive performances up to 24 hours poststretching on muscles in the lower extremity. Conversely, the dynamic stretching of the same muscle groups is highly recommended 24 hours before performing sprint and long jump performances. In conclusion, the positive effects of dynamic stretching on explosive performances seem to persist for 24 hours.[10] Once the injury has healed and the participant has return to activity, dynamic stretching is preferred prior to participation in activity.

These exercises increase flexibility in one muscle group (i.e., agonist) and simultaneously improve strength in another muscle group (i.e., antagonist). Furthermore, if instituted early in the exercise program, proprioceptive neuromuscular facilitation stretches can aid in elongating scar tissue. As scar tissue matures and increases in density, it becomes less receptive to short-term stretches and may require prolonged stretching to achieve deformational changes in the tissue.

The proprioceptive neuromuscular facilitation techniques recruit muscle contractions in a coordinated pattern as agonists and antagonists move through an ROM. One technique uses active **inhibition,** whereby the muscle group reflexively

> ### BOX 13.4 Active Inhibition Techniques
>
> To stretch the hamstring group on a single leg using the three separate proprioceptive neuromuscular facilitation techniques, the following guidelines should be followed:
>
> **Contract–Relax**
>
> 1. The thigh is stabilized and the hip passively flexed into the agonist pattern until limitation is felt in the hamstrings.
> 2. The individual performs an isotonic contraction with the hamstrings through the antagonist pattern.
> 3. A passive stretch is applied into the agonist pattern until limitation is felt, and the sequence is repeated.
>
> **Hold–Relax**
>
> 1. The leg is passively moved into the agonist pattern until resistance is felt in the hamstrings.
> 2. The individual performs an isometric contraction to "hold" the position for approximately 10 seconds.
> 3. The individual should relax for approximately 5 seconds.
> 4. A passive stretch is applied into the agonist pattern until limitation is felt, and the sequence is repeated.
>
> **Slow Reversal–Hold–Relax**
>
> 1. The individual consciously relaxes the hamstring muscles while doing a concentric contraction of the quadriceps muscles into the agonist pattern.
> 2. The individual performs an isometric contraction, against resistance, into the antagonist pattern for 10 seconds.
> 3. The individual should relax for approximately 10 seconds.
> 4. The individual actively moves the body part further into the agonist pattern, and the sequence is repeated.

relaxes before the stretching maneuver. Common methods include contract–relax, hold–relax, and slow reversal–hold–relax (**Box 13.4**). The clinician stabilizes the limb to be exercised. Alternating contractions and passive stretching of a group of muscles are then performed. Contractions may be held for 3, 6, or 10 seconds, with similar results obtained.[11]

A second technique, known as **reciprocal inhibition**, uses active agonist contractions to relax a tight antagonist muscle. In this technique, the individual contracts, against resistance, the muscle opposite the tight muscle. This causes a reciprocal inhibition of the tight muscle, leading to muscle lengthening. An advantage to proprioceptive neuromuscular facilitation exercise is the ability to stretch a tight muscle that may be painful or in the early stages of healing. In addition, movement can occur in a single plane or in a diagonal pattern that mimics actual skill performance.

Active Assisted Range of Motion

Frequently, PROM at the injured joint may be greater than active motion, perhaps because of muscle weakness. A person may be able to sit on top of a table and slide the leg across the tabletop away from the body to fully extend the knee. If, however, the individual sits at the edge of the table with the legs hanging over the edge and then attempts to straighten the knee, the individual may be unable to move the limb voluntarily into full extension. In this situation, normal joint mechanics exist and full PROM is present. To attain full AROM, however, the individual may require some assistance from an athletic trainer, a mechanical device, or the opposite limb (active assisted ROM). Working the limb through available pain-free motion with assistance restores normal AROM more quickly than working the limb within limited voluntary motion.

Active Range of Motion

AROM exercises performed by the individual enhance circulation through a pumping action during muscular contraction and relaxation. Full, pain-free AROM need not be achieved before strength exercises are initiated; however, performance of skills and drills, such as throwing or full squats, which require full pain-free ROM or certain agility drills, must be delayed until proper joint mechanics are restored. AROM exercises should be relatively painless and may be facilitated during certain stages of the program by completing the exercises in a whirlpool to provide an analgesic effect and to relieve the stress of gravity on sensitive structures. Examples of AROM exercises include spelling out the letters of the alphabet with the ankle and using a wand or cane with the upper extremity to improve active assisted ROM.

Resisted Range of Motion

Resisted ROM may be either static or dynamic. Static movement is measured with an isometric muscle contraction and can be used during phases 1 and 2 of the exercise program in a pain-free arc of motion. Dynamic resisted motion (dynamic strengthening) is discussed in the next section.

Isometric training measures a muscle's maximum potential to produce static force. The muscle is at a constant tension, whereas muscle length and the joint angle remain the same. For example, standing in a doorway and pushing outward against the door frame produces a maximal muscle contraction, but joints of the upper extremity do not appear to move. In performing an isometric contraction, a maximal force is generated against an object, such as the clinician's hand, for approximately 10 seconds and is repeated 10 times per set. Contractions, performed every 20° throughout the available ROM, are called multiangle isometric exercises.

Isometric exercise is useful when

1. Motion is contraindicated by pathology or bracing.

2. Motion is limited because of muscle weakness at a particular angle, called a sticking point.

3. A painful arc is present.

4. Prescribed postsurgical.

Isometric strength exercises are the least effective training method, because although circumference and strength increase, strength gains are limited to a range of 10° on either side of the joint angle. In addition, during isometric exercise, an adverse, rapid increase in blood pressure can occur when the breath is held against a closed glottis. This occurrence, referred to as the **Valsalva effect**, can be avoided with proper breathing.

Proprioception

Proprioception is a specialized variation of the sensory modality of touch that encompasses the sensation of joint movement (**kinesthesia**) and joint position. Sensory receptors located in the skin, muscles, tendons, ligaments, and joints provide input into the central nervous system relative to tissue deformation. Visual and vestibular centers also contribute afferent information to the central nervous system regarding body position and balance. The ability to sense body position is mediated by cutaneous, muscle, and joint mechanoreceptors.

Joint Mechanoreceptors

Joint mechanoreceptors are found in the joint capsule, ligaments, menisci, labra, and fat pads, and they include four types of nerve endings: Ruffini corpuscles, Golgi receptors, Pacinian corpuscles, and free nerve endings. Ruffini corpuscles are sensitive to intra-articular pressure and stretching of the joint capsule. Golgi receptors are intraligamentous and become active when the ligaments are stressed at the end ranges of joint movement. Pacinian corpuscles are sensitive to high-frequency vibration and pressure. Free nerve endings are sensitive to mechanical stress and the deformation and loading of soft tissues that comprise the joint.

Muscle Mechanoreceptors

As mentioned, the receptors found in muscle and tendons are the muscle spindles and the Golgi tendon organs. Muscle spindles are innervated by both afferent and efferent fibers and can detect not only muscle length but also, and more importantly, the rate of change in muscle length. Golgi tendon organs respond to both contraction and stretching of the musculotendinous junction. If the stretch continues for an extended time (i.e., longer than 6 to 8 seconds), the Golgi tendons are stimulated, causing a reflex inhibition in the antagonist muscles. This sensory mechanism protects the musculotendinous unit from excessive tensile forces that could damage muscle fibers.

Regaining Proprioception

Balance involves positioning the body's center of gravity over a base of support through the integration of information received from the various proprioceptors within the body. Even when the body appears motionless, a constant postural sway is caused by a series of muscle contractions that correct and maintain a dynamic equilibrium in an upright position. When balance is disrupted, as in falling forward or stumbling, the response is primarily automatic and reflexive. An injury or illness can interrupt the neuromuscular feedback mechanisms. Restoration of the proprioceptive feedback is necessary for promoting dynamic joints and functional stability to prevent reinjury.

Proprioceptive exercises must be specific to the type of activity that the individual will encounter during participation in a sport and physical activity. In general, the progression of activities to develop dynamic, reactive neuromuscular control is achieved through a progression that moves from slow speed to high speed, low force to high force, and controlled to uncontrolled activities. A single-leg stance test (e.g., stork stand) requires the individual to maintain balance while standing on one leg for a specified time with the eyes closed. The clinician looks for any tendency to sway or fall to one side. In the next stage, with the eyes open, the patient can progress to playing catch with a ball. This exercise can be made more difficult by having the patient balance on a trampoline while playing catch with a ball. Use of an Airex pad might begin with bilateral balancing and progress to one-legged balancing, dribbling a basketball, or playing catch with a ball. Many of these exercises can be adapted to the upper extremity. An individual can begin in a push-up position and shift his or her weight from one hand to another or perform isometric or isotonic press-ups, balance on one hand, balance on a BOSU ball or ball, or walk on the hands over material of different densities or heights.

Open Versus Closed Kinetic Chain Exercises

A common error in developing an exercise program is failure to assess the proximal and distal segments of the entire extremity, or kinetic chain. A **kinematic chain** is a series of interrelated joints that constitute a complex motor unit, constructed so that motion at one joint will produce motion at the other joints in a predictable manner. Whereas kinematics describe the appearance of motion, **kinetics** involves the forces, whether internal (e.g., muscle contractions or connective tissue restraints) or external (e.g., gravity, inertia, or segmental masses) that affect motion. Initially, a closed kinetic chain (CKC) was characterized as the distal segment of the extremity in an erect, weight-bearing position, such as the lower extremity when a person is weight bearing. Subsequently, when the distal segment of the extremity is free to move without causing motion at another joint, such as when non–weight-bearing, the system was referred to as an open kinetic chain (OKC). When force is applied, the distal segment may function independently or in unison with the other joints. Movements of the more proximal joints are affected by OKC and CKC positions. For example, the rotational components of the ankle, knee, and hip reverse direction when moving from an OKC to CKC position.

Because of incongruities between the lower and upper extremity, particularly in the shoulder region, several authors have challenged the traditional definition of OKC and CKC positions.[12–14] Stabilizing muscles in the scapulothoracic region produces a joint compression force that stabilizes the glenohumeral joint in much the same manner as a CKC in the lower extremity. Although debate continues on defining CKC and OKC relative to the upper extremity, there remains a general agreement that both CKC and OKC exercises should be incorporated into an upper and lower extremity rehabilitation program.

Injury and subsequent immobilization can affect the proprioceptors in the skeletal muscles, tendons, and joints. In rehabilitation, it is critical that CKC activities be used to retrain joints and muscle proprioceptors to respond to sensory input. CKC exercises are recommended because they

- Stimulate and reeducate the proprioceptors

- Increase joint stability and congruity

- Provide greater joint compressive forces

- Exercise multiple joints through weight bearing and muscular contractions

- Better control velocity and torque

- Reduce shear forces

- Increase muscle coactivation

- Allow better use of the specific adaptations to imposed demands (SAID) principle

- Permit more functional patterns of movement (including spiral and diagonal) and greater specificity for athletic activities

- Facilitate postural and dynamic stabilization mechanics

In contrast, OKC exercises can isolate a specific muscle group for intense strength and endurance exercises. In addition, they can develop strength in very weak muscles that may not function properly in a CKC system because of muscle substitution. Although OKC exercises may produce great gains in peak force production, these exercises usually are limited to one joint in a single plane (uniplanar) and have greater potential for joint shear, limited functional application, and limited eccentric and proprioceptive retraining. OKC exercises, however, can assist in developing a patient–athletic trainer rapport through uniplanar and multiplanar manual therapeutic techniques. **Figure 13.4** illustrates OKC and CKC chain exercises for the lower extremity.

When ROM has been achieved, repetition of motion through actual skill movements can improve coordination and joint mechanics as the individual progresses into phase 3 of the program. For example, a pitcher may begin throwing without resistance or force application in front of a mirror to visualize the action. This also can motivate the individual to continue to progress in the therapeutic exercise program.

 During phase 2, passive stretching and AROM exercises should be conducted. In particular, stretching and strengthening of both the intrinsic and extrinsic muscles of the foot and ankle should be major parts of the rehabilitation plan. Cryotherapy, thermotherapy, EMS, joint mobilization, or massage can complement the exercise program as needed.

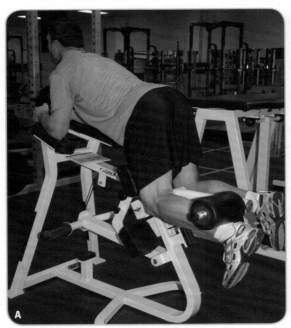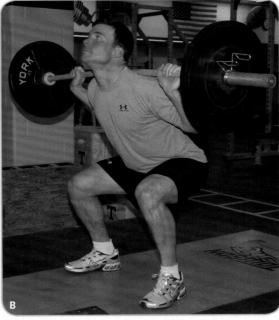

Figure 13.4. Open and closed kinetic chain exercises for the lower extremity. A, Open kinetic chain exercise for the hamstrings. **B,** Closed kinetic chain exercise for the hip and knee extensors.

PHASE 3: DEVELOPING MUSCULAR STRENGTH, ENDURANCE, AND POWER

 The distance runner has full, pain-free ROM. She wants to resume her running workouts. Is it advisable for her to do so at this time? What is the likelihood that reinjury will occur?

Phase 3 focuses on developing muscular strength, endurance, and power in the injured extremity as compared with the uninjured extremity. The individual can move into phase 4 when the following criteria have been completed:

■ Bilateral ROM and joint flexibility are restored.

■ Muscular strength, endurance, and power in the affected limb are equal or near equal to those in the unaffected limb.

■ Cardiovascular endurance and general body strength are equal to or better than the preinjury levels.

■ Score on Y balance test ≤4 cm and four hop testing scores at 80% to 90%.

■ Sport-specific functional patterns are completed using mild to moderate resistance.

■ The individual is psychologically ready to return to protected activity.

Muscular Strength

Strength is the ability of a muscle or a group of muscles to produce force in one maximal effort. Although static strength (isometric strengthening) is used during phases 1 and 2 in a pain-free arc of motion, dynamic strengthening is preferred during phase 3 of the program. Two types of contractions occur in dynamic strength: **concentric**, in which a shortening of muscle fibers decreases the angle of the associated joint, and **eccentric**, in which the muscle resists its own lengthening so that the joint angle increases during the contraction. Concentric and eccentric contractions also may be referred to as positive and negative work, respectively. Concentric contractions work to accelerate a limb; for example, the gluteus maximus and quadriceps muscles concentrically contract to accelerate the body upward from a crouched position. In contrast, eccentric contractions work to decelerate a limb and provide shock absorption, especially during high-velocity dynamic activities. For example, the shoulder external rotators decelerate the shoulder during the follow-through phase of the overhead throw, and hamstrings act to decelerate the body when running.

Eccentric contractions generate greater force than isometric contractions, and isometric contractions generate greater force than concentric contractions. In addition, less tension is required in an eccentric contraction. One major disadvantage of eccentric training, however, is delayed-onset muscle soreness, which is defined as muscular pain or discomfort 1 to 5 days following unusual muscular exertion. Delayed-onset muscle soreness is associated with joint swelling and weakness, which may last after the cessation of pain. This differs from acute-onset muscle soreness, in which pain during exercise ceases after the exercise bout is completed. To prevent the onset of delayed-onset muscle soreness, eccentric exercises should progress gradually. Remember to train specific muscles based on how they primarily function producing positive or negative work. Dynamic muscle strength is gained through isotonic or isokinetic exercise (**Fig. 13.5**).

Isotonic Training (Variable Speed/Fixed Resistance)

A more common method of strength training is isotonic exercise or, as it sometimes is called, **progressive resistive exercise**. In this technique, a maximal muscle contraction generates a force to move a constant load throughout the ROM at a variable speed. Both concentric and eccentric contractions are possible with free weights, elastic or rubber tubing, body weight exercises, and

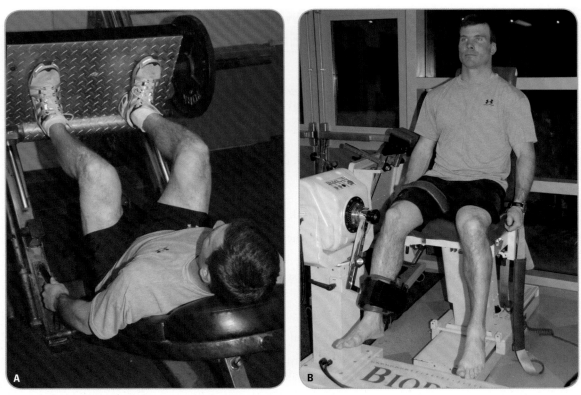

Figure 13.5. Dynamic muscle strengthening. Dynamic strength may be gained through **(A)** isotonic exercise or **(B)** isokinetic exercise.

weight machines. Free weights are inexpensive and can be used in diagonal patterns for sport- or activity-specific skills, but adding or removing weights from the bars can be troublesome. In addition, a spotter may be required for safety purposes to avoid heavy weights being dropped. Thera-Band, or surgical tubing, is inexpensive and easy to set up, can be used in diagonal patterns for sport- or activity-specific skills, and can be adjusted to the patient's level of strength using bands of different tension. Weights on commercial machines can be changed quickly and easily. Using several stations of free weights and commercial machines, an individual can perform circuit training to strengthen multiple muscle groups in a single exercise session. Typically, however, the machines are large and expensive, work in only a single plane of motion, and may not match the biomechanical makeup or body size of the individual.

Isotonic training permits the exercise of multiple joints simultaneously, both eccentric and concentric contractions, and weight-bearing CKC exercises. A disadvantage is that when a load is applied, the muscle can only move that load through the ROM with as much force as the muscle provides at its weakest point. Variable resistance machines provide minimal resistance where the ability to produce force is comparatively lower (i.e., early and late in the ROM) and greatest resistance where the muscle is at its optimal length tension and mechanical advantage (i.e., usually the midrange). The axis of rotation generates an isokinetic-like effect, but angular velocity cannot be controlled.

Isokinetic Training (Fixed Speed/Variable Resistance)

Isokinetic training, or accommodating resistance, allows an individual to provide muscular overload and angular movement to rotate a lever arm at a controlled velocity or fixed speed. Theoretically, isokinetic training should activate the maximum number of motor units, which consistently overloads muscles and achieves maximum tension-developing or force-output capacity at every point in the ROM, even at the relatively "weaker" joint angles. Cybex, Biodex, and Kin Com are examples of equipment that use this strength training method. Coupled with a computer and appropriate software, torque-motion curves, total work, average power, and measures of torque to body weight can be instantaneously calculated to provide immediate, objective measurements to the individual and clinician.

Two advantages of isokinetic training are that a muscle group can be exercised to its maximum potential throughout the full ROM and that the dynamometer's resistance mechanism essentially disengages if pain is experienced by the patient. As the muscles fatigue, however, isokinetic resistance decreases. In contrast, with an isotonic contraction, because the resistance is constant as the muscle fatigues, the muscle must either recruit additional motor units, thus increasing muscle force, or fail to perform the complete repetition. It is hypothesized that during rehabilitation, isotonic training is more effective than isokinetic training in achieving rapid gains in strength during training using the daily adjusted progressive resistance exercise (DAPRE) technique.[15] Two other disadvantages are the cost of the machine, computer, and software package (ranging from $25,000 to $60,000) and the fact that most available machines permit only OKC exercises. For this reason, isokinetic training should be used in conjunction with other modes of resistance training.

Muscular Endurance

Muscular endurance is the ability of muscle tissue to exert repetitive tension over an extended period of time. The rate of muscle fatigue is related to the endurance level of the muscle (i.e., the more rapidly the muscle fatigues, the lower the muscle endurance). A direct relationship exists between muscle strength and muscle endurance. As muscle endurance is developed, density in the capillary beds increases, providing a greater blood supply, and thus, a greater oxygen supply to the working muscle. Increases in muscle endurance may influence gains in strength; however, the development of strength has not been shown to increase muscle endurance. Muscular endurance is gained by lifting low weights at a faster contractile velocity with more repetitions in the exercise session or with the use of stationary bikes or aquatic therapy, an elliptical, a StairMaster, or a slide board.

Muscular Power

Muscular power is the ability of muscle to produce force in a given time. Power training is started after the injured limb has regained at least 80% of the muscle strength in the unaffected limb. Regaining power involves weight training at higher contractile velocities or using plyometric exercises.

Plyometric training employs the inherent stretch–recoil characteristics of skeletal muscle through an initial, rapid eccentric (loading) prestretching of a muscle, thereby activating the stretch reflex to produce tension before initiating an explosive concentric contraction of the muscle. This stretch produces a strong stimulus at the level of the spinal cord, which causes an explosive reflex concentric contraction. The greater the stretch from the muscle's resting length immediately before the concentric contraction, the greater the load the muscle can lift or overcome. Injury can result if the individual does not have full ROM, flexibility, and near normal strength before beginning these exercises. Many of the anterior cruciate ligament (ACL) injury prevention programs use plyometric exercises in order to develop explosive power and correct improper jumping mechanics. Examples of plyometric exercises include a standing jump, multiple jumps, box jumps or drop jumping from a height, single- or double-leg hops, bounding, leaps, and skips. In the upper extremity, a medicine ball, surgical tubing, plyoback, and boxes can be used. Performing jumping and skipping exercises on grass or mats reduces the impact on the lower extremity during landing by reducing ground reaction force. These exercises should be performed every 3 days to allow the muscles to recover from fatigue.

Functional Application of Exercise

Strength, endurance, and power can only be increased by using the **overload principle**, which states that physiological improvements occur only when an individual physically demands more than normally is required of the muscles. This philosophy is based on the SAID principle, which states that the body responds to a given demand with a specific and predictable adaptation. Overload is achieved by manipulating the intensity, duration, frequency, specificity, speed, and progression in the exercise program.

Intensity

Intensity reflects both the caloric cost of the work and the specific energy systems that are activated. Strength gains depend primarily on the intensity of the overload, not on the specific training method used to improve strength. The DAPRE of Knight[16] is an objective method of increasing resistance as the individual's strength increases or decreases. A fixed percentage of the maximum weight for a single repetition is lifted during the first and second sets. Maximum repetitions of the resistance maximum are lifted during the third set. Adaptations to the amount of weight lifted are then increased or decreased accordingly during the fourth set and during the first set of the next session. The DAPRE guidelines are based on the concept that if the working weight is ideal, the individual can perform six repetitions when told to perform as many as possible. If the individual can perform more than six repetitions, the weight is too light. Conversely, if the individual cannot lift six repetitions, the weight is too heavy.

For individuals with chronic injuries or early postoperative rehabilitation, the DAPRE method may not be appropriate. Instead, a high-repetition, low-weight exercise may be more productive, particularly during the early phases. High weights potentially can cause a breakdown of the supporting soft-tissue structures and exacerbate the condition. Use of smaller weights and submaximal intensities can stimulate blood flow and limit tissue damage. To gain strength and endurance, higher repetitions are required. The individual begins with two or three sets of 10 repetitions, progressing to five sets of 10 repetitions as tolerated. When the individual can perform 50 repetitions, 1 lb may be added and the repetitions can be reduced to three sets of 10 repetitions. All exercises should be performed slowly, concentrating on proper technique. As strength increases, the DAPRE method or other type of progressive resistance exercise schedule may be used.

Duration

Duration refers to the estimated time that it will take to return the individual to full (100%) activity; more commonly, however, duration refers to the length of a single exercise session. The time can shorten if pain, swelling, or muscle soreness occurs. In general, the individual must participate in at least 20 minutes of continuous activity, with the heart rate (HR) elevated to at least 70% of maximal. This is particularly important when increasing cardiovascular endurance, which will be explained later in this chapter.

Frequency

Frequency refers to the number of exercise sessions per day or week. Although exercise performed twice daily yields greater improvement than exercise performed once daily, in most cases, the exercise program should be conducted three to four times per week. It is critical not to work the same muscle groups on successive days to allow recovery from fatigue and muscle soreness. If daily bouts are planned, strength and power exercises may be alternated with cardiovascular conditioning, or exercises for the lower extremity may alternate with exercises for the upper extremity.

Specificity

An exercise program must address the specific needs of the patient. For example, exercises that mimic the throwing action will benefit a baseball pitcher but are not applicable to a football lineman. If exercises simulate actual skills used in the individual's sport or activity, the patient is more likely to be motivated and compliant with the exercise program. The type of exercise (e.g., isometric, isotonic, or isokinetic) also is important. Individuals who rely on eccentric loading also must include eccentric training in their rehabilitation program. Rhythm, or velocity, also has been shown to be specific to that required for the sport skill, with the greatest gains in strength consistently occurring at training speeds.[17]

Speed

Speed refers to the rate at which the exercise is performed. Initially, exercises should be performed in a slow, deliberate manner, at a rate of approximately 60° per second, with emphasis placed on concentric and eccentric contractions. The individual should exercise throughout the full ROM, pausing at the end of the exercise. Large muscle groups should be exercised first, followed by the smaller groups. In addition, the exercise speed should be varied. As strength, endurance, and power increase, functional movements should increase in speed. Surgical tubing can be used to develop a high-speed regimen to produce concentric and eccentric synergistic patterns, and isokinetic units also may be used at the highest speeds.

Progression

In an effort to maintain motivation and compliance, an objective improvement should occur each day, whether this is an increase in repetitions or intensity. Muscular strength is improved with a minimum of 3 days per week of training that includes 12 to 15 repetitions per bout of 8 to 10 exercises for the major muscle groups.[5] If the individual complains of pain, swelling, or residual muscle soreness, the program may need to be decreased or varied in intensity. An orderly progression should move from ROM exercises to isometric, isotonic, isokinetic, and functional activities however, progressing from low to high intensity with ever increasing demands on the patient as the healing process allows.

 Before permitting the distance runner to resume running workouts, her muscle strength, endurance, and power in the affected limb, in addition to full and pain-free ROM, must be at or near the levels of the unaffected limb to prevent reinjury.

PHASE 4: RETURN TO SPORT/PHYSICAL ACTIVITY

? The distance runner has full ROM and near normal strength in the affected limb. She has maintained cardiovascular endurance by swimming and using an upper body ergometer. What additional factors need to be considered to prepare this patient for a return to full activity?

The individual can return to the sport activity as soon as muscle strength, endurance, and power are restored. During phase 4, the individual also should correct any biomechanical inefficiency in motion and movement dysfunction; restore coordination and muscle strength, endurance, and power in sport-specific skills; and improve cardiovascular endurance. The individual may be returned to activity if the following goals are attained:

- Coordination and balance are normal.

- Sport-specific functional patterns are restored in the injured extremity.

- Muscle strength, endurance, and power in the affected limb are equal to those in the unaffected limb.

- Cardiovascular endurance is equal to or greater than the preinjury level.

- Quantitative testing should be completed: Examples include four hop test for the lower extremity, isometric strength tests measurements, Y balance test, and patient outcome scales specific to the injured body part.[18]

- The individual receives clearance to return to participation by the supervising physician.

Coordination

Coordination refers to the body's ability to execute smooth, fluid, accurate, and controlled movements. Simple movement, such as combing hair, involves a complex muscular interaction using the appropriate speed, distance, direction, rhythm, and muscle tension to execute the task. Coordination may be divided into two categories: gross motor movements involving large muscle groups and fine motor movements using small groups. Gross motor movements involve activities such as standing, walking, skipping, and running. Fine motor movements are seen in precise actions, particularly with the fingers, such as picking up a coin off a table, clutching an opponent's jersey, or picking up a ground ball with a glove. Coordination and proprioception are directly linked. When an injury occurs and the limb is immobilized, sensory input from proprioceptors and motor commands are disrupted, resulting in an alteration of coordination.

Performing CKC activities during phase 2 of the exercise program can help to restore proprioceptive input and improve coordination. Constant repetition of motor activities using sensory cues (i.e., tactile, visual, or proprioceptive) or increasing the speed of the activity over time can help a patient continue to develop coordination during phases 3 and 4. A wobble board, teeter board, Pro Fitter, or Biomechanical Ankle Platform System (BAPS) board often is used to improve sensory cues and balance in the lower extremity. Proprioceptive neuromuscular facilitation patterns and the Pro Fitter also may be used to improve sensory cues in the upper and lower extremities. Although the resistance-band protocol is common in rehabilitation, the proprioceptive neuromuscular facilitation strength protocol is also an effective treatment to improve strength in individuals with chronic ankle instability. Both protocols showed clinical benefits in strength and perceived instability. To improve functional outcomes, clinicians should consider using additional multiplanar and multijoint exercises.[18]

Sport/Activity-Specific Skill Conditioning

Because different sports require different skills, therapeutic exercise should progress to the load and speed that are expected for the individual's sport or physical activity. For example, a baseball player performs skills at different speeds and intensities than a football lineman. Therefore, exercises must be coupled with functional training or with specificity of training related to the physical demands of the sport.

As ROM, muscular strength, and coordination are restored, the individual should work the affected extremity through functional diagonal and sport-specific patterns. For example, during phase 3, a baseball pitcher may have been moving the injured arm through the throwing pattern with mild-to-moderate resistance. During phase 4, the individual should increase resistance and speed of motion. Working with a ball attached to surgical tubing, the individual can develop a kinesthetic awareness in a functional pattern. When controlled motion is done without pain, actual throwing can begin. Initially, short throws with low intensity can be used, progressing to longer throws with low intensity. As the player feels more comfortable and is pain-free with the action, the number of throws and their intensity are increased. Similar programs can be developed for other sports or physical activities. Other sport/activity-specific skills that can be performed at this level include sprint work, agility runs, figure eights, side stepping, shuttle runs, and interval training (i.e., alternating periods of intense work and active recovery).

Cardiovascular Endurance

Cardiovascular endurance, commonly called aerobic capacity, is the body's ability to sustain submaximal exercise over an extended period and depends on the efficiency of the pulmonary and cardiovascular systems. When an injured individual is unable to continue or chooses to stop aerobic training, detraining occurs within 1 to 2 weeks.[5] If the individual returns to activity without a high cardiovascular endurance level, fatigue sets in quickly, placing the individual at risk for reinjury.

Similar to strength training, maintaining and improving cardiovascular endurance is influenced by an interaction of frequency, duration, and intensity. The American College of Sports Medicine (ACSM) recommends that aerobic training be moderate-intensity aerobic physical activity for a minimum of 30 minutes per exercise session on 5 or more days per week or vigorous-intensity aerobic activity for a minimum of 20 minutes on 3 or more days.[5,19] If added consideration is needed to preserve bone health during adulthood, the ACSM recommends 30 to 60 minutes of weight-bearing cardiovascular exercises three to five times per week in addition to resistance exercises two or three times per week.[20] The targeted HR can be calculated in two manners:

1. An estimated HRmax for both men and women is approximately 220 bpm. HR is related to age, with HRmax decreasing as an individual ages. A relatively simple calculation is

$$HRmax = 220 - Age$$

With a 20-year-old individual working at 80% of maximum, the calculation is $0.8 \times (220 - 20)$, or 160 bpm.

2. Another commonly used formula (Karvonen formula) assumes that the targeted range of the HR is between 60% and 90% of HRmax. This calculation is

$$\text{Target HR range} = [(\text{HRmax} - \text{HRrest}) \times 0.60 \text{ and } 0.90] + \text{HRrest}$$

where HRrest is the individual's resting HR. If an individual's HRmax is 180 bpm and the HRrest is 60 bpm, this method yields a target HR range between 132 and 168 bpm.

Non–weight-bearing exercises, such as swimming, rowing, biking, or use of the upper body ergometer, can be helpful early during the therapeutic program, particularly if the individual has a lower extremity injury. Walking, cross-country skiing, jumping rope, or running can be performed as the condition improves.

> In preparing the distance runner for a return to her sport, modifications in running workouts must be addressed because it would not be appropriate for the athlete to continue at her previous level of training. Ongoing management of the condition should be addressed as well. In particular, the athlete should be informed about signs and symptoms that would warrant a decrease in activity and a return to more intensive rehabilitation. Finally, the documentation needed to clear the distance runner for return to activity, including a doctor's medical clearance, should be completed. It is important to remember that all written documentation of the exercise program and written medical clearance should be placed in the patient's file and stored in a safe, secure location for a minimum of 3 to 5 years. With changes in insurance reimbursement, proper documentation is critical for all athletic trainers.

SUMMARY

1. Rehabilitation begins immediately after the injury assessment and includes the following actions:

   - The level of function and dysfunction is assessed.

   - Results are organized and interpreted.

   - A list of patient problems is formulated.

   - Long- and short-term goals are established.

   - A treatment plan is developed, including therapeutic exercises, modalities, and medications.

   - The program is then supervised and periodically reassessed with appropriate changes made.

2. Phase 1 of the therapeutic exercise program should focus on patient education and control of inflammation, muscle spasm, and pain.

3. Phase 2 should regain any deficits in ROM and proprioception at the affected joint as compared with the unaffected joint.

4. Phase 3 should regain muscular strength, endurance, and power in the affected limb.

5. Phase 4 prepares the individual to return to activity and includes an analysis of motion, sport/activity-specific skill training, regaining coordination, and cardiovascular conditioning.

6. At the conclusion of the rehabilitation program, the supervising physician determines if the individual is ready to return to full activity. This decision should be based on a review of the individual's ROM and flexibility; muscular strength, endurance, and power; biomechanical skill; proprioception and coordination; and cardiovascular endurance.

7. If additional protective bracing, padding, or taping is necessary to enable the individual to return safely to activity, this should be documented in the individual's file. In addition, it should be stressed that use of any protective device should not replace a maintenance program of conditioning exercises.

8. The athletic trainer should keep a watchful eye on the individual as he or she returns to activity. If the individual begins to show signs of pain, swelling, or discomfort or if skill performance deteriorates, the individual should be reevaluated to determine whether activity should continue or the therapeutic exercise program needs to be reinstituted.

APPLICATION QUESTIONS

1. A football running back had knee surgery to repair a menisci injury. The supervising physician has suggested the inclusion of CKC exercises in the rehabilitation process. What are the advantages of CKC exercises?

2. A 21-year-old male hurdler has tight hamstrings. How can proprioceptive neuromuscular facilitation exercises be used to decrease the tightness of the hamstrings? What exercises might you consider using?

3. You are a high school athletic trainer with a limited budget. What type of rehabilitative equipment can you purchase to increase muscle strength, endurance, and power without overextending the budget?

4. An 18-year-old field hockey player has been diagnosed with Achilles tendinitis. Her current symptoms include increased pain with active plantar flexion and accompanying muscle weakness in plantar flexion. What short- and long-term goals might you suggest for her therapeutic exercise program?

5. A collegiate basketball player sustained a grade 2 inversion ankle sprain. What specific exercises would you suggest to improve the individual's proprioception?

6. A 32-year-old professional golfer sustained a lumbar strain, which resulted in an inability to practice or play competitively for 3 weeks. He has now completed phase 4 of the therapeutic exercise program for the injury. How will you determine his readiness to return to full activity and competition?

REFERENCES

1. Feger MA, Goetschius J, Love H, et al. Electrical stimulation as a treatment intervention to improve function, edema or pain following acute lateral ankle sprains: a systematic review. *Phys Ther Sport*. 2015;16(4):361–369.
2. Mangine B, Nuzzo G, Harrelson GL. Physiologic factors of rehabilitation. In: Andrews JR, Harrelson GL, Wilk KE, eds. *Physical Rehabilitation of the Injured Athlete*. 3rd ed. Philadelphia: WB Saunders; 2004:13–33.
3. Mazess RB, Whedon GD. Immobilization and bone. *Calcif Tissue Int*. 1983;35(3): 265–267.
4. Konin JG, Harrelson GL, Leaver-Dunn D. Range of motion and flexibility. In: Andrews JR, Harrelson GL, Wilk KE, eds. *Physical Rehabilitation*
of the Injured Athlete. 3rd ed. Philadelphia, PA: WB Saunders; 2004:136–156.
5. McArdle WD, Katch FI, Katch VL. *Exercise Physiology: Energy, Nutrition, and Human Performance*. 6th ed. Baltimore, MD: Lippincott Williams & Wilkins; 2007.
6. Klingler W, Velders M, Hoppe K, et al. Clinical relevance of fascial tissue and dysfunctions. *Curr Pain Headache Rep*. 2014;18(8):439.
7. Maitland GD. *Extremity Manipulation*. London, United Kingdom: Butterworth; 1977.
8. O'Sullivan K, Murray E, Sainsbury D. The effect of warm-up, static stretching and dynamic stretching on hamstring flexibility in previously injured subjects. *BMC Musculoskelet Disord*. 2009;10:37.

9. Davis DS, Ashby PE, McCale KL, et al. The effectiveness of 3 stretching techniques on hamstring flexibility using consistent stretching parameters. *J Strength Cond Res.* 2005;19(1):27–32.

10. Haddad M, Dridi A, Chtara M, et al. Static stretching can impair explosive performance for at least 24 hours. *J Strength Cond Res.* 2014;28(1):140–146.

11. Nelson KC, Cornelius WL. The relationship between isometric contraction durations and improvement in shoulder joint range of motion. *J Sports Med Phys Fitness.* 1991;31(3):385–388.

12. Wilk KE, Arrigo CA, Andrews JR. Closed and open kinetic chain exercise for the upper extremity. *J Sport Rehabil.* 1996;5(1):88–102.

13. Lephart SM, Henry TJ. Functional rehabilitation for the upper and lower extremity. *Orthop Clin North Am.* 1995;26(3):579–592.

14. Dillman CJ, Murray TA, Hintermeister RA. Biomechanical differences of open and closed chain exercises with respect to the shoulder. *J Sport Rehabil.* 1994;3(3):228–238.

15. Knight KL, Ingersoll CD, Bartholomew JB. Isotonic contractions might be more effective than isokinetic contractions in developing muscle strength. *J Sport Rehabil.* 2001;10(2):124–131.

16. Knight KL. Rehabilitating chondromalacia patellae. *Phys Sportsmed.* 1979;7(10):147–148.

17. Dale RB, Harrelson GL, Leaver-Dunn D. Principles of rehabilitation. In: Andrews JR, Harrelson GL, Wilk KE, eds. *Physical Rehabilitation of the Injured Athlete.* 3rd ed. Philadelphia: WB Saunders; 2004:157–188.

18. Hall EA, Docherty CL, Simon J, et al. Strength-training protocols to improve deficits in participants with chronic ankle instability: a randomized controlled trial. *J Athl Train.* 2015;50(1):36–44.

19. Haskell WL, Lee IM, Pate RR, et al. Physical activity and public health: updated recommendation for adults from the American College of Sports Medicine and the American Heart Association. *Circulation.* 2007;116(9):1081–1093.

20. Kohrt WM, Bloomfield SA, Little KD, et al. American College of Sports Medicine position stand: physical activity and bone health. *Med Sci Sports Exerc.* 2004;36(11):1985–1996.

Conditions of the Lower Extremity

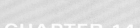
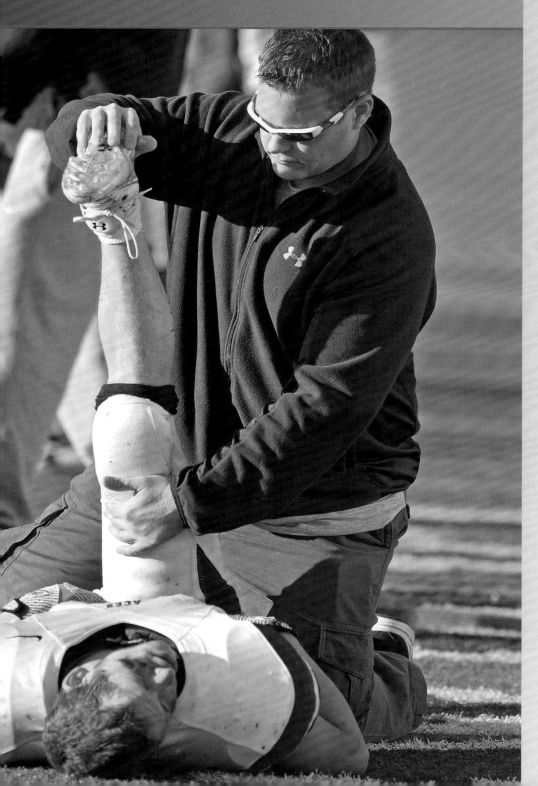

Lower Leg, Ankle, and Foot Conditions

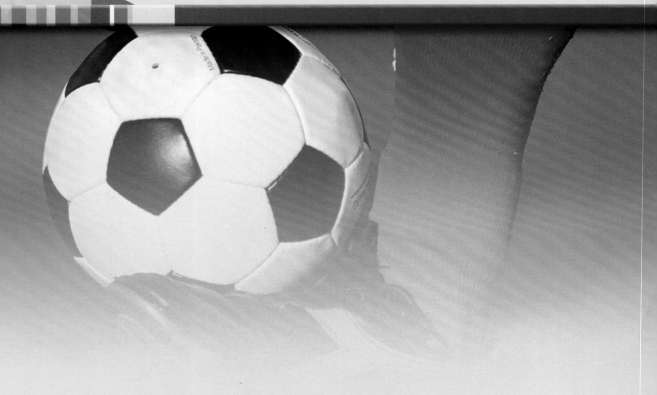

STUDENT OUTCOMES

1. Identify the major bony and soft-tissue structures of the lower leg, ankle, and foot.

2. Identify the various ligamentous structures that support the lower leg, ankle, and foot.

3. Identify the plantar arches and explain their function.

4. Describe the motions of the foot and ankle and identify the muscles that produce them.

5. Explain the general principles to prevent injuries to the lower leg, ankle, and foot.

6. Describe a thorough assessment of the lower leg, ankle, and foot.

7. Describe the common injuries to and conditions of the knee in physically active individuals (including sprains, dislocations, contusions, strains, bursitis, and vascular and neural disorders).

8. Explain the management strategies for common injuries and conditions of the lower leg, ankle, and foot.

9. List the various types of fractures that can occur at the lower leg, ankle, and foot and explain their management.

10. Explain the basic principles associated with rehabilitation of injuries to the lower leg, ankle, and foot.

INTRODUCTION

Because of the essential roles played by the lower leg, ankle, and foot during sport and physical activities, injuries to this region are common. Sport participation often places both acute and chronic overloads on the lower extremity, leading to sprains, strains, fractures, and overuse injuries. In particular, basketball, soccer, and football participants sustain a high incidence of injury to this region.[1-3] Lateral ankle sprains are the most common of all sports-related injuries, accounting for approximately 25% of injuries to the musculoskeletal system.[4] Increasingly, it is being recognized that repeated ankle sprains can result in functional instability of the ankle, which predisposes the individual to further injury.[5]

This chapter begins with an anatomical review and biomechanical overview of the lower leg, ankle, and foot. Next, prevention of injury is discussed, followed by a step-by-step injury assessment of the region. Finally, details on specific injuries and their management, including examples of rehabilitative exercises, are provided.

ANATOMY OF THE LOWER LEG, ANKLE, AND FOOT

The lower leg, ankle, and foot are composed of numerous bones and articulations (**Fig. 14.1**). They provide a foundation of support for the upright body, enabling propulsion through space, adaptation to uneven terrain, and absorption of shock.

Forefoot

The three major regions of the foot are the forefoot, midfoot, and hindfoot. The forefoot is composed of 5 metatarsals and 14 phalanges, along with numerous joints. In conjunction with the midfoot region, the forefoot forms interdependent longitudinal and transverse arches to support and distribute body weight throughout the foot.

Metatarsophalangeal and Interphalangeal Joints

The metatarsophalangeal (MTP) joint is a condyloid joint with a close-packed position in full extension. The proximal interphalangeal (PIP) and distal interphalangeal (DIP) joints are hinge joints that also have a close-packed position in full extension (**Fig. 14.1**). Numerous ligaments reinforce both sets of joints. Each MTP joint is surrounded by an articular and fibrous joint capsule, the plantar side of which is reinforced by the plantar fascia and thickened portions of the capsule (i.e., plantar ligament). The medial and lateral joint capsules are reinforced by collateral ligaments. The PIP and DIP joints are reinforced by the plantar and dorsal joint capsule and the collateral ligaments. The toes function to smooth the weight shift to the opposite foot during walking and help to maintain stability during weight bearing by pressing against the ground when necessary. The first digit is referred to as the hallux, or "great toe," and is the main body stabilizer during walking or running.

The first MTP joint has two sesamoid bones, which are located on the plantar surface of the joint to share in weight bearing. The sesamoid bones serve as anatomical pulleys for the flexor hallucis brevis muscle and protect the flexor hallucis longus muscle tendon from weight-bearing trauma as it passes between the two bones.

Tarsometatarsal and Intermetatarsal Joints

The deep transverse metatarsal ligament interconnects the five metatarsals. Both the tarsometatarsal and intermetatarsal joints are of the gliding type with the close-packed position in supination. These joints enable the foot to adapt to uneven surfaces during gait.

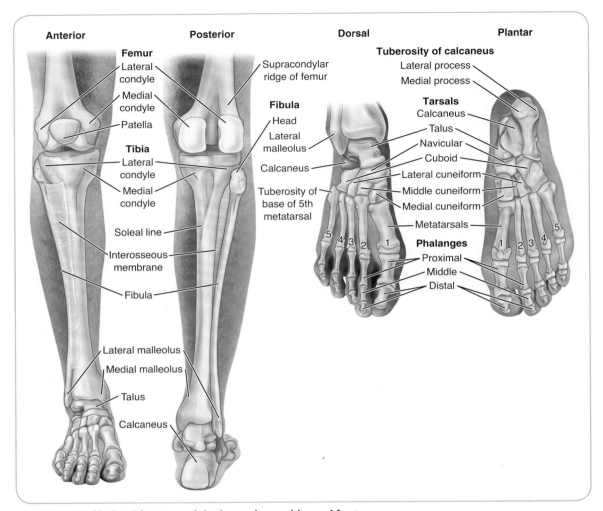

Figure 14.1. Skeletal features of the lower leg, ankle, and foot.

Midfoot

The midfoot region encompasses the navicular, cuboid, and three cuneiform bones as well as their articulations. The navicular, like its counterpart in the wrist, the scaphoid, helps to bridge movements between the hindfoot and forefoot.

Transverse Tarsal Joint

The transverse tarsal (or midtarsal) joint consists of two side-by-side articulations—namely, the calcaneocuboid joint on the lateral side and the talonavicular on the medial side. Collectively, these two joints are called the transverse tarsal joint, because they are adjacent and function as a unit.

The calcaneocuboid joint is a saddle-shaped joint with a close-packed position in supination. The joint is nonaxial and permits only limited gliding motion. It is supported by the bifurcate ligament, the plantar and dorsal calcaneocuboid ligaments, and the long plantar ligament. The most important of these, the long plantar ligament, extends inferiorly between the calcaneus and the cuboid and then continues distally to the base of the 2nd, 3rd, and 4th metatarsals, contributing significantly to transverse tarsal joint stability.

Because the talus moves simultaneously on the calcaneus and navicular, the term talocalcaneonavicular (TCN) joint often is used to describe the combined action of the talonavicular and subtalar joints. The TCN is a modified ball-and-socket joint with a close-packed position in supination. Movements at the joint include gliding and rotation. Three ligaments support the joint—namely, the plantar calcaneonavicular (spring) ligament inferiorly, the deltoid ligament medially, and the bifurcate ligament laterally (**Fig. 14.2**).

Because the subtalar joint is mechanically linked to the TCN and transverse tarsal joints, any motion at the subtalar joint produces similar motions at the transverse tarsal joints. For example, when the TCN is fully supinated and locked, the midfoot region is supinated and rigid. When the TCN is pronated and loose packed, the midfoot region is mobile and loose.

Other Midtarsal Joints

The remaining joints of the midfoot region include the cuneonavicular, cuboideonavicular, cuneocuboid, and intercuneiform. These joints provide gliding and rotation for the midfoot with a close-packed position in supination. They are bound together by several ligaments. When the midfoot (i.e., TCN) is locked in supination, these joints function in a compensatory manner to pronate the forefoot and increase stability. When the hindfoot is pronated, these joints supinate the forefoot to keep the foot flat on the surface.

Hindfoot

The hindfoot includes the calcaneus and talus. Rising off the anteromedial surface of the calcaneus is the sustentaculum tali, which largely supports the talus. Located on the inferior surface of the sustentaculum tali is a groove through which the flexor hallucis longus tendon passes. The peroneal tubercle projects out of the lateral side of the calcaneus and splits the two peroneal tendons as they course inferior to the lateral malleolus. The peroneus brevis tendon runs superior to the tubercle; the peroneus longus tendon runs inferior to the tubercle.

The talus is saddle-shaped and serves as the critical link between the foot and the ankle. It has several functional articulations, the two most important of which being the talocrural joint and the subtalar joint. Both serve a unique role in the integrated function of the lower leg, ankle, and foot.

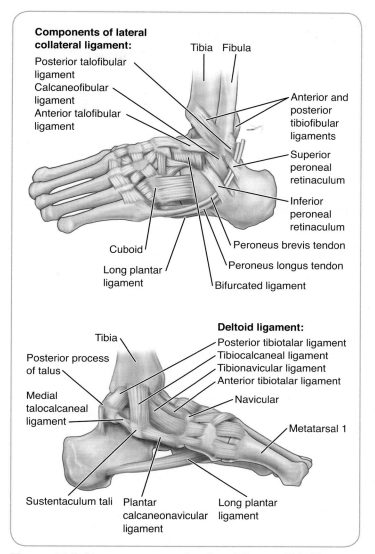

Figure 14.2. Ligaments supporting the midfoot and hindfoot region. Lateral view (top). Medial view (bottom).

Talocrural Joint

The talocrural (i.e., ankle) joint is a uniaxial, modified synovial hinge joint formed by the talus, tibia, and lateral malleolus of the fibula. The concave end of the weight-bearing tibia mates with the convex superior surface of the talus to form the roof and medial border of the ankle mortise. The fibula assists with weight bearing, supporting approximately 17% of the load on the leg[6]; serves as a site for muscle and ligamentous attachments; and forms the lateral border of the ankle mortise. The lateral malleolus extends farther distally than the medial malleolus; hence, eversion is more seriously limited than inversion. The dome of the talus is wider anteriorly than posteriorly. Therefore, the joint's close-packed position is maximum dorsiflexion.

Although the joint capsule is thin and especially weak anteriorly and posteriorly, a number of strong ligaments cross the ankle and enhance stability (**Table 14.1**). The four separate bands of the medial collateral ligament (more commonly called the deltoid ligament) cross the ankle medially. The anterior tibiotalar and tibionavicular ligaments are taut when the subtalar joint is plantar flexed, whereas the tibiocalcaneal and posterior tibiotalar ligaments are taut during dorsiflexion.

TABLE 14.1 Ligaments of the Talocrural Joint

	PROXIMAL ATTACHMENT	DISTAL ATTACHMENT
MEDIAL COLLATERAL LIGAMENTS		
Anterior tibiotalar	Anteromedial aspect of medial malleolus	Superior portion of medial talus
Tibiocalcaneal	Apex of medial malleolus	Calcaneus directly below medial malleolus
Posterior tibiotalar	Posterior aspect of medial malleolus	Posterior portion of the talus
Tibionavicular	Distal and slightly posterior to the anterior tibiotalar	Medial aspect of the navicular
LATERAL COLLATERAL LIGAMENTS		
Anterior talofibular	Anterolateral surface of lateral malleolus	Talus near the sinus tarsi
Calcaneofibular	Posterior apex of lateral malleolus	Courses 133° inferiorly and posteriorly to attach on calcaneus
Posterior talofibular	Posterolateral border of lateral malleolus	Posterior talus and calcaneus

Forces producing stress on the medial aspect of the ankle typically cause an avulsion fracture of the medial malleolus rather than tearing the deltoid ligament.

The lateral side of the ankle is supported by three ligaments. The anterior talofibular ligament (ATFL) is taut and resists inversion during plantar flexion and limits anterior translation of the talus on the tibia. The calcaneofibular ligament (CFL) is taut in the extreme range of dorsiflexion and is the primary restraint of talar inversion within the mid-range of motion (ROM). The posterior talofibular ligament (PTFL) is the strongest of the lateral ligaments and limits posterior displacement of the talus on the tibia. The relative weakness of these lateral ligaments as compared with the deltoid ligament, coupled with the fact of less bony stability laterally compared with medially, contributes to a higher frequency of lateral ankle sprains.

Subtalar Joint

As the name suggests, the subtalar joint lies beneath the talus, where facets of the talus articulate with the sustentaculum tali on the superior calcaneus. Obliquely crossing the talus and calcaneus is the tarsal canal, a sulcus that allows attachment of an intraarticular ligament. Because no muscles attach to the talus, the stability of the subtalar joint is derived from several small ligaments. The talocalcaneal interosseous ligament lies in the tarsal canal, divides the subtalar joint into two articular cavities, serves as an axis for talar tilt, and contributes substantially to joint stability, particularly during supination (**Fig. 14.3**). Four small talocalcaneal ligaments form interconnections between the talus and calcaneus, and the CFL and tibiocalcaneal fascicle of the deltoid ligament add support. The close-packed position for the joint occurs under vertical loading with internal rotation.

The subtalar joint behaves as a flexible structure, with motion occurring only through stretching of ligaments during weight bearing.[7] Motion at the subtalar joint involves "male" ovoid bone surfaces sliding over reciprocally shaped "female" ovoid bone surfaces. The subtalar joint functions essentially as a uniaxial joint with an orientation roughly in line with

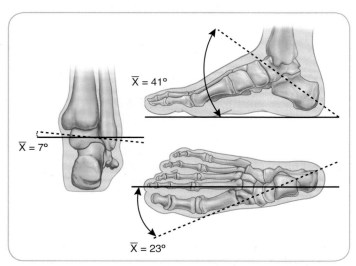

$\overline{X} = 41°$

$\overline{X} = 7°$

$\overline{X} = 23°$

Figure 14.3. Subtalar joint. The axis of rotation at the subtalar joint lies oblique to the sagittal and frontal planes.

the inversion/eversion axis of the foot, although the orientation of the subtalar joint axis varies appreciably across individuals.[8]

Tibiofibular Joints

The tibia and fibula articulate at both the proximal and distal ends (**Fig. 14.1**). The proximal, or superior, tibiofibular joint is a plantar synovial joint that is tightly reinforced with anterior and posterior ligaments. The inferior, or distal, tibiofibular joint is a syndesmosis, where dense fibrous tissue binds the bones together. No joint capsule exists, but the joint is supported by the anterior and posterior tibiofibular ligaments as well as by an extension of the interosseous membrane, the crural interosseous ligament. This structural arrangement allows some rotation and slight abduction (spreading) while still maintaining joint integrity. The strength of the crural interosseous ligament is such that strong lateral stresses often fracture the fibula rather than tear the membrane, although excessive eversion or dorsiflexion can result in sufficient widening of the ankle mortise to injure the ligaments supporting the syndesmosis.

Plantar Arches

The bones and supporting ligamentous structures in the tarsal and metatarsal regions of the foot form interdependent longitudinal and transverse arches (**Fig. 14.4**). They function to support and distribute body weight from the talus through the foot, through changing weight-bearing conditions, and over varying terrain. The longitudinal arch runs from the anteroinferior calcaneus to the metatarsal heads. Because the arch is higher medially than laterally, the medial side usually is the point of reference, with the navicular bone serving as the point of reference between the anterior and posterior ascending spans.

The transverse arch runs across the anterior tarsals and metatarsals. The foundation of the arch is the medial cuneiform, with the apex of the arch formed by the 2nd metatarsal. The arch is reduced at the level of the metatarsal heads, with all metatarsals aligned parallel to the weight-bearing surface for even distribution of body weight. Structural support is derived from the intermetatarsal ligaments and the transverse head of the adductor hallucis muscle.

The primary supporting structures of the plantar arches, in order of importance, are the calcaneonavicular (i.e., spring) ligament, long plantar ligament, plantar fascia (i.e., plantar aponeurosis), and short plantar (i.e., plantar calcaneocuboid) ligament (**Fig. 14.5**). When muscle tension is present, the muscles of the foot, particularly the tibialis posterior, contribute support to the arches and joints as they cross them.

The plantar fascia, or plantar aponeurosis, is a specialized, thick, interconnected band of fascia that covers the plantar surface of the foot, providing support for

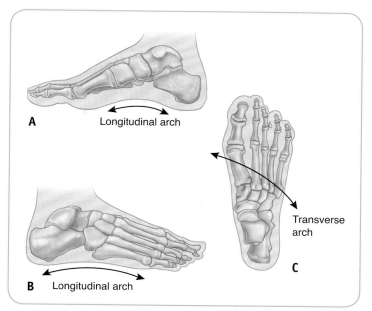

Figure 14.4. Arches of the foot. A, Medial view. **B,** Lateral view. **C,** Dorsal view.

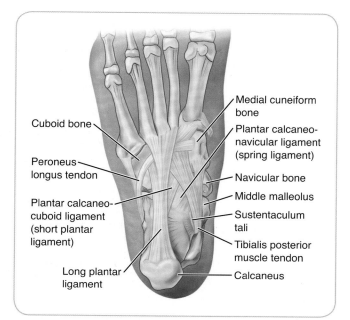

Figure 14.5. Medial longitudinal arch. The medial longitudinal arch is supported by the calcaneonavicular (spring) ligament, short plantar ligament, long plantar ligament, plantar aponeurosis, and tibialis posterior muscle tendon.

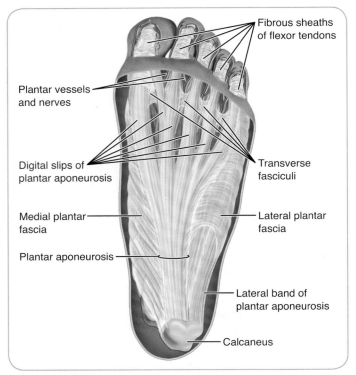

Figure 14.6. Plantar fascia. The plantar fascia stores mechanical energy each time the foot deforms during the weight-bearing phase of the gait cycle.

the longitudinal arch (**Fig. 14.6**). It has three distinct slips. The central slip extends from the posteromedial calcaneal tubercle and inserts into the distal plantar aspects of the proximal phalanges of each toe, where it attaches with deep transverse metatarsal ligaments. As the central slip courses down the length of the foot, it gives off two other slips, one deviating medially and the other laterally. The plantar fascia is the single greatest contributor to the stability of the arch of the foot, providing approximately 80% of arch stiffness.[9] During the weight-bearing phase of the gait cycle, the plantar fascia stretches on the order of 9% to 12% of resting length, functioning like a spring to store mechanical energy that is released to help the foot push off from the surface.[10] Stretching the Achilles tendon may elongate the plantar fascia, because both structures attach to the calcaneus.

Muscles of the Lower Leg and Foot

A large number of muscles cross the ankle (**Figs. 14.7** and **14.8**). Identifying the actions of these muscles is complicated by the fact that several muscles are two-joint muscles.

Thick sheaths of fascia divide the muscles of the leg into four compartments—namely, the anterior,

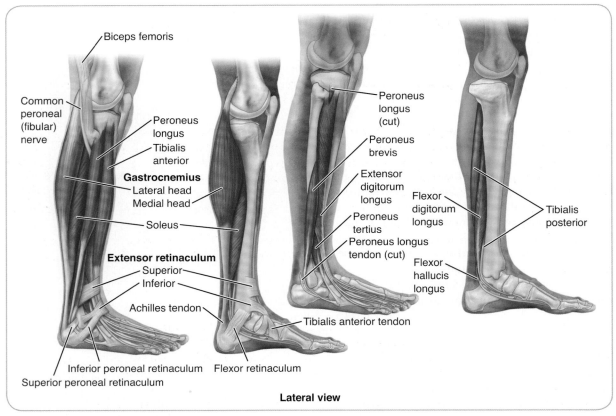

Lateral view

Figure 14.7. Muscles of the lower leg and foot. Lateral and medial views.

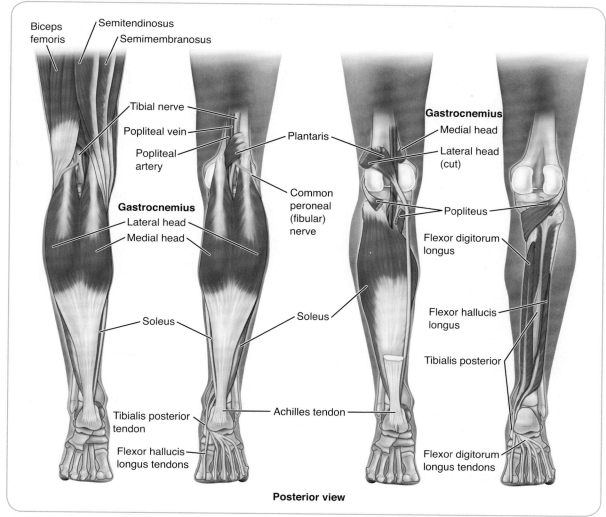

Posterior view

Figure 14.8. Muscles of the lower leg and foot. Posterior view.

deep posterior, superficial posterior, and lateral compartments. The anterior compartment contains the tibialis anterior, extensor digitorum longus, extensor hallucis longus, and peroneus tertius. Muscles in the deep posterior compartment include the tibialis posterior, flexor digitorum longus, tibialis posterior artery, tibial nerve, and flexor hallucis longus. The superficial posterior compartment contains the gastrocnemius, soleus, and plantaris, and the lateral compartment contains the peroneus longus and peroneus brevis.

The foot contains both intrinsic and extrinsic muscles. An intrinsic muscle has both attachments contained within the foot (**Figs. 14.9** and **14.10**), whereas an extrinsic muscle has one attachment outside the foot.

See **Major Muscles of the Foot and Leg**, available on the companion Web site at thePoint, for a summary of the attachments and primary actions of the major extrinsic muscles of the lower leg, ankle, and foot.

Nerves of the Lower Leg, Ankle, and Foot

The sciatic nerve and its branches provide primary innervation for the lower leg, ankle, and foot. Traveling down the posterior aspect of the leg from the lumbosacral spine, the sciatic nerve branches into smaller nerves just proximal to the popliteal fossa. The major branches are the tibial nerve, which innervates the posterior aspect of the leg, and the common peroneal nerve, which spawns the deep and superficial peroneal nerves.

The tibial nerve (L4 through S3) passes through the popliteal fossa and down the leg between the superficial and deep muscles in the posterior compartment of the leg (see **Fig. 15.4**). It continues

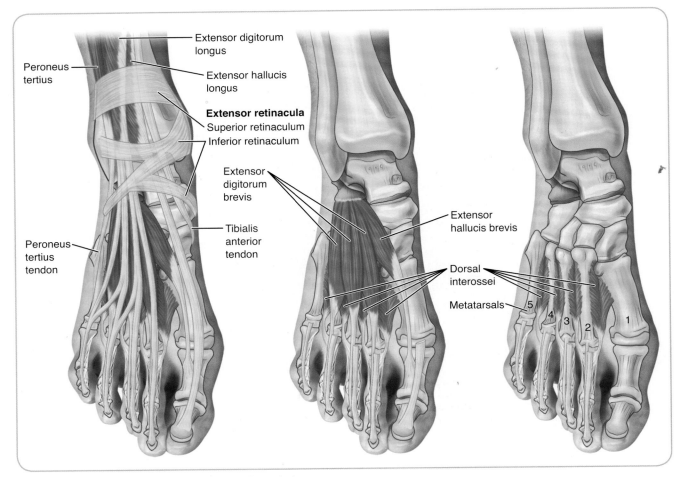

Figure 14.9. Intrinsic muscles of the foot. Dorsal view.

medially behind the medial malleolus with the posterior tibial artery to become the medial and lateral plantar nerves. The saphenous nerve (L2 through L4), which branches from the femoral nerve, supplies cutaneous innervation to the medial aspect of the ankle.

The common peroneal nerve passes laterally around the neck of the fibula to the anterolateral leg, where it splits into the deep and superficial peroneal nerves (see **Fig. 15.4**). The deep peroneal nerve (L4 through S1) innervates the anterior compartment, which contains the ankle dorsiflexors and toe extensors and then courses over the dorsum of the foot to innervate the skin between the first and second toes. The superficial peroneal nerve (L5 through S2) innervates the lateral compartment, which contains the primary evertor muscles, and provides cutaneous innervation to the second through fourth toes. The sural nerve (L4 through S2), a branch from both the common peroneal and tibial nerves, supplies cutaneous innervation to the lateral aspect of the ankle, heel, and foot. Given the extensiveness of the sciatic nerve supply to the lower extremity, it is no surprise that impingement of the sciatic nerve by a herniated disk in the lumbosacral region often results in pain, numbness, and/or impaired function in the foot and ankle region.

Blood Vessels of the Lower Leg, Ankle, and Foot

The blood supply to the lower leg, ankle, and foot enters the lower extremity as the femoral artery (**Fig. 14.11**). The femoral artery becomes the popliteal artery proximal and posterior to the knee and then branches into the anterior and posterior tibial arteries just distal to the knee. The anterior tibial artery becomes the dorsalis pedis artery to supply the dorsum of the foot. The posterior tibial artery gives off several branches that supply the posterior and lateral compartments and the plantar region of the foot.

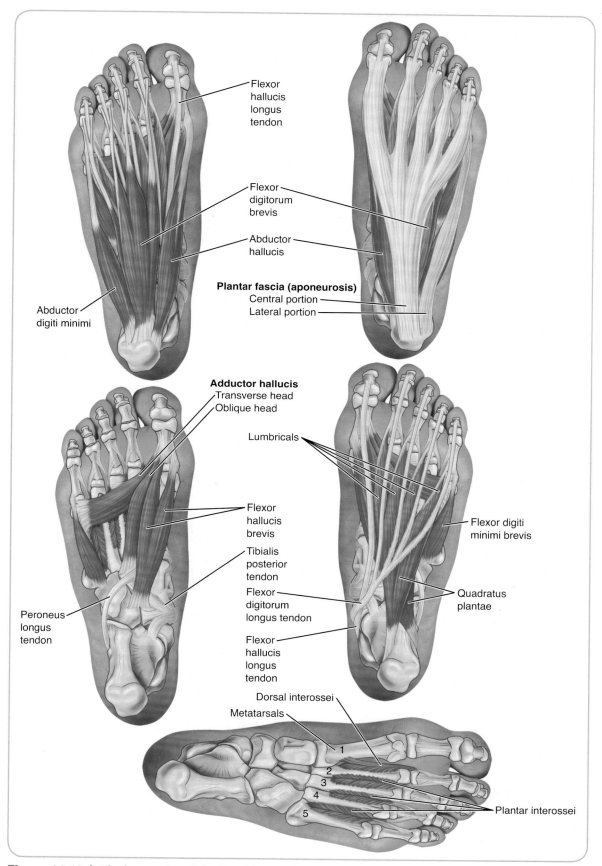

Figure 14.10. Intrinsic muscles of the foot. Plantar view.

KINEMATICS OF THE LOWER LEG, ANKLE, AND FOOT

As discussed in *Chapter 8: Assessment of Body Alignment, Posture, and Gait*, evaluation of the kinematics of gait during walking and running can provide important clues for the likelihood of injuries. Understanding the kinematics of the lower leg, ankle, and foot is imperative to accurately diagnose pathology and create appropriate prevention strategies and therapeutic exercise programs. If needed, please review the gait assessment information shared in Chapter 8.

PREVENTION OF LOWER LEG, ANKLE, AND FOOT CONDITIONS

Several steps can reduce the incidence or severity of injury. These include the use of appropriate protective equipment, footwear, and physical conditioning.

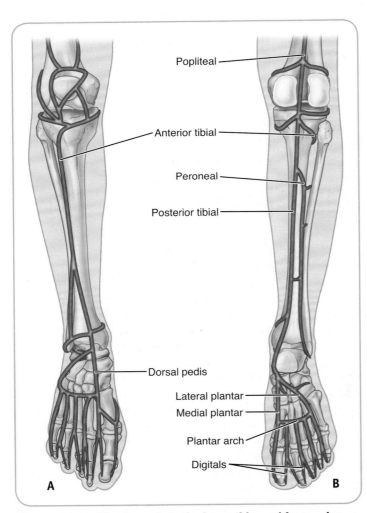

Figure 14.11. Blood supply to the leg, ankle, and foot region. A, The dorsalis pedis artery is easily palpated in the midfoot region between the second and third tendons of the extensor digitorum longus. **B,** The posterior tibial artery can be palpated just posterior to the medial malleolus.

Labels in figure:
Popliteal
Anterior tibial
Peroneal
Posterior tibial
Dorsal pedis
Lateral plantar
Medial plantar
Plantar arch
Digitals
A
B

Protective Equipment

The use of protective braces and equipment for the lower leg, ankle, and foot is discussed in Chapter 3. Shin pads can protect the anterior tibial area from a direct impact by a ball, bat, stick, or kick from a foot. Taping and commercial ankle braces are commonly used ankle injury prevention strategies; however, the literature supports that players with prior ankle injury derive the greatest benefit from taping or bracing over players with no existing ankle pathology.[11] Commercial ankle braces come in three categories: lace-up brace, semirigid orthosis, or air-bladder brace (see **Fig. 3.9**). A lace-up brace can limit all ankle motions, whereas semirigid orthoses and air-bladder braces limit only inversion and eversion. In general, ankle braces are more effective than taping the ankle to reduce injuries, are easier for the wearer to apply independently, do not produce some of the skin irritation associated with adhesive tape, provide better comfort and fit, and are more cost-effective and comfortable to wear. Specific foot conditions can be padded and supported with a variety of products, including inner soles, semirigid orthotics, rigid orthotics, antishock heel lifts, heel cups, or commercially available pads and devices. Adhesive felt (e.g., moleskin), felt, and foam also can be cut to construct similar pads to protect specific areas.

Physical Conditioning

Physical conditioning is one of the strongest defenses against injury. It is recommended that the injury prevention program be implemented 3 months prior to the start of the season and take a multi-intervention strategy approach focusing on balance, neuromuscular control, leg muscle strength, hip muscle strength, and ankle ROM. Examples of exercises for improving balance and neuromuscular control include incorporating aspects of the Balance Error Scoring System, the Star Excursion Balance Test, the Biodex Balance System, and other balance activities on hard and soft surfaces, stable and unstable surfaces, and in single, double, and tandem stance positions. The use of **functional** exercises to stimulate activation and strength of muscles controlling ankle eversion, inversion, plantar flexion, and dorsiflexion as well as muscles responsible for hip extensors and abductors should be incorporated into the injury prevention program. Exercises should target both concentric and eccentric activation. Before initiating strategies to target increasing ROM, it is important to assess if motion is limited. The motion of specific interest is dorsiflexion. If dorsiflexion is limited, joint mobilization techniques should be included as part of the injury prevention strategy to help improve ankle arthrokinematics and osteokinematics.[11]

Application Strategy 14.1 demonstrates several exercises that can be used to prevent injuries to the lower leg, ankle, and foot.

Footwear

The demands of a particular activity require adaptations in shoe design and selection. In field sports, shoes may have a flat-sole, long-cleat, short-cleat, or multicleated design. Cleats should be positioned under the major weight-bearing joints of the foot and should not be felt through the sole of the shoe. Shoe models with flat cleats or screw-in cleats, or pivot-disk models, have been shown to reduce the incidence of anterior cruciate ligament injuries when compared to shoes with the longer, irregular cleats. In individuals with arch problems, the shoe should include adequate forefoot, arch, and heel support. In all cases, individuals should select shoes based on the demands of the activity. Shoe selection and guidelines for fitting shoes are discussed in detail in Chapter 3.

ASSESSMENT OF THE LOWER LEG, ANKLE, AND FOOT CONDITIONS

> **?** A cross-country runner reports to the athletic training room complaining of pain along the plantar surface of the left foot. How should the assessment of this injury progress to determine the extent and severity of injury?

Initial assessment of the lower leg, ankle, and foot is usually conducted in three different situations. The first is the on-field (or sideline) evaluation of the acutely injured patient. In the acute setting, it is important to first assess for and treat any life-threatening conditions that may be present before focusing on the orthopedic injury. Next, assess for and treat obvious fractures, dislocations, and severe bleeding if present. Finally, assess for and treat other soft-tissue damage. When conducting an on-field evaluation of the acutely injured patient, the goals are to determine (1) the type and severity of damage the patient has sustained; (2) immediate first aid and care needed; (3) if referral is needed, the urgency of the referral, and to whom the patient should be referred; (4) the manner in which the patient will be removed from the playing field; and (5) the patient's participation status.

The second situation is the nonacute evaluation of the patient who has had ongoing pain or disability. When conducting an evaluation of a nonacutely injured patient, the goals are to determine (1) which structures have been injured, (2) the severity of the injury, (3) the cause of the injury, (4) strategies to address the patient's pain and dysfunction and restore normal function, and (5) participation status.

The third situation is with patients who will need longer and more complex therapeutic intervention due to the complexity, seriousness, or severity of injury. When conducting an evaluation of a patient in the clinic setting, the goals are to determine the patient's (1) baseline function, disability, and pain; (2) goals for recovery; (3) strategies to address function, disability, and pain that incorporate the patient's goals; and (4) return to participation.

The following information describes the assessment process for evaluating the lower leg, foot, and ankle. The exact content, sequence, and tools utilized will vary depending on the situation in which the evaluation is conducted.

See **Application Strategy: Lower Leg, Ankle, and Foot Evaluation**, available on the companion Web site at thePoint.

APPLICATION STRATEGY 14.1

Exercises to Prevent Injury to the Lower Leg

Intrinsic Muscle Exercises of the Foot

1. **Plantar fascia stretch.** Place a towel around the toes and slowly overextend the toes. Dorsiflex the ankle to stretch the Achilles tendon.
2. **Towel crunches.** Place a towel between the plantar surfaces of the toes and feet. Push the toes and feet together, crunching the towel between the toes.

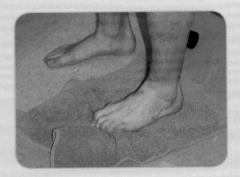

3. **Toe curls.** With the foot resting on a towel, slowly curl the toes under, bunching the towel beneath the foot. (Variation: Use two feet or a book or small weight on the towel for added resistance.)
4. **Picking up objects.** Pick up small objects, such as marbles or dice, with the toes and place them in a nearby container, or use therapeutic putty to work the toe flexors.
5. **Shin curls.** Slide the plantar surface of the foot up the opposite shin, moving distal to proximal.
6. **Unilateral balance activities.** Stand on uneven surfaces with the eyes first open and then closed.
7. **BAPS board.** In a seated position, roll the board slowly clockwise and then counterclockwise 20 times.

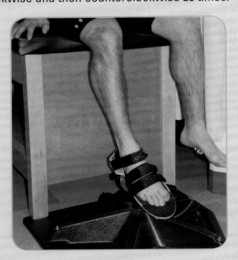

Ankle/Lower Leg Muscle Exercises

1. **Ankle alphabet.** Using only the ankle and foot, trace the letters of the alphabet from A to Z three times with capital letters and three times with lowercase letters.

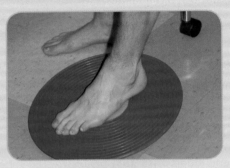

2. **Triceps surae stretch.** Keeping the leg straight and the heel on the floor, lean against a wall or stand on a slant board until tension is felt in the calf muscles. To isolate the soleus, bend both knees. Point the toes outward, straight ahead, and inward to stretch the various fibers of the Achilles tendon.

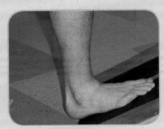

3. **Thera-Band or surgical tubing exercises.** Secure the Thera-Band or tubing around a table leg and do resisted dorsiflexion, plantar flexion, inversion, and eversion.

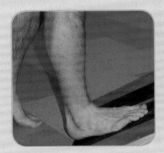
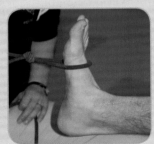

4. **Unilateral balance exercises.** Balance on the opposite leg while doing Thera-Band exercises.
5. **BAPS board.** In a standing position, balance on the involved foot; repeat several times. Additional challenges, such as using no support or dribbling with a basketball while balancing, can be added.

HISTORY

The injury assessment of the cross-country runner should begin with a history. What questions need to be asked to identify the cause and extent of this injury?

Many conditions in the lower leg, ankle, and foot are related to family history; congenital deformities; poor technique; and recent changes in the training program, surface, or foot attire. The assessment begins by asking questions related to the mechanism of injury, associated symptoms, progression of the symptoms, any disabilities that may have resulted from the injury, and related medical history. For example, an acute onset should lead one to suspect bony trauma or an acute ankle sprain until ruled out. A gradual onset of pain may signal inflammation from overuse of a muscle or the plantar fascia or the development of a stress fracture. Particular attention should be given to recent changes in the distance, duration, or intensity of training; each component can lead to overuse injuries. Medial heel pain may indicate plantar fasciitis or, if in the middle of the plantar heel area, a heel spur. Pain in the medial arch can be a sign of a fallen medial longitudinal arch or tarsal tunnel syndrome. Pain around either malleolus may indicate an ankle sprain. Pain posterior to the lateral malleolus can signify peroneal tendinitis, subluxation, or dislocation or even sural nerve entrapment. Pain posterior to the medial malleolus may reflect tendinitis or rupture of the tibialis posterior.

See **Application Strategy: Developing a History of the Injury**, available on the companion Web site at thePoint, for specific questions related to the lower leg, ankle, and foot.

The cross-country runner should be asked questions that address when, where, and how the injury occurred; intensity, location, and type of pain; when the pain begins (e.g., when getting out of bed, while sitting, while walking, during exercise, or at night); how long the condition has been present; how long the pain lasts; if the pain has changed or stayed the same; if the pain is worse before, during, or after activity; activities that aggravate or alleviate the symptoms; changes in training; changes in footwear; and previous injury, treatment, and medication. This is an example of a history that is appropriate for a patient with a nonacute injury.

OBSERVATION AND INSPECTION

The cross-country runner reports pain on the plantar, medial heel that has been present for the past 5 days. The pain is worse after rest but is particularly severe with the first few steps in the morning. The runner indicates that he has increased both the intensity and distance of his daily runs over the past 7 days. Explain the observation component in the ongoing assessment of the cross-country runner.

Both lower legs should be clearly visible to denote symmetry, any congenital deformity, swelling, discoloration, hypertrophy, muscular atrophy, or previous surgical incisions. The individual should wear running shorts to allow full view of the lower extremity. In addition, the individual should bring the shoes that normally are worn when pain is present so that they can be inspected for unusual wear, which could be indicative of a biomechanical abnormality that may be affecting the knee.

In an ambulatory patient, observation begins with the completion of a postural examination. Any bilateral gross deformity, swelling, or redness in the toes, foot, or ankle should be noted. The foot should be observed for the presence or absence of an arch on weight bearing and non–weight bearing. A supple, or flexible, flatfoot appears to be flattened when weight bearing but produces an obvious arch when non–weight bearing. In contrast, a rigid flatfoot appears to be flattened on weight bearing and non–weight bearing. It is important to note if the foot is in a pronated, neutral, or supinated position (**Box 14.1**).

See **Application Strategy: Postural Assessment of the Lower Leg, Ankle, and Foot**, found on the companion Web site at thePoint, for specific areas to focus on in the lower extremity.

BOX 14.1 Common Injuries Associated with Foot Deformities

Pes Cavus	Pes Planus
Plantar fasciitis	Tibialis posterior tendinitis
Metatarsalgia	Achilles tendinitis
Stress fractures of the tarsals and metatarsals	Plantar fasciitis
Peroneal tendinitis	Sesamoid disorders
Sesamoid disorders	Medial tibial stress syndrome
Iliotibial band friction syndrome	Patellofemoral pain

Next, the clinician should instruct the individual to lie prone on a table with the feet and ankles extended over the end of the table to determine the talar neutral position. In assessing the left foot, the clinician places the right thumb and index finger on the anterior aspect of the foot spanning the talar dome. Using the left hand, the clinician grasps the foot from the lateral side and then inverts and everts the ankle and foot until the neutral position of the foot is determined (**Fig. 14.12**). The neutral position is identified when the talus is aligned symmetrically between the thumb and index finger. When talar neutral is determined, the relationship of the forefoot and rearfoot alignment should be noted. This may be done in the non–weight-bearing position, the weight-bearing position, or both. The following conditions may be present with the calcaneus and talus in neutral position:

- **Forefoot varus.** The 1st metatarsal is elevated relative to the 5th metatarsal.
- **Forefoot valgus.** The 5th metatarsal is elevated relative to the 1st metatarsal.
- **Rearfoot varus.** The calcaneus is inverted relative to the long axis of the tibia, which may result from a varus tibial alignment.
- **Rearfoot valgus.** The calcaneus is everted relative to the long axis of the tibia, which may result from a valgus tibial alignment.

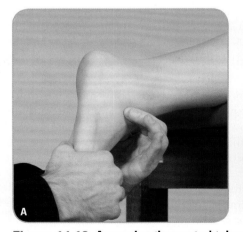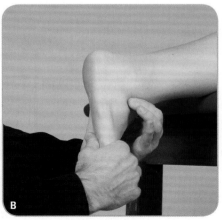

Figure 14.12. Assessing the neutral talar position. A and B, The clinician places the thumb and index fingers on the anterior aspect of the foot spanning the talar dome. Using the other hand, the clinician grasps the foot from the lateral side and then inverts and everts the ankle and foot until the neutral position of the foot is determined.

The mobility of the first ray (i.e., the first tarsometatarsal joint extending into the first MTP joint) should be assessed. If the first ray is slightly plantar flexed at the tarsometatarsal joint, this causes the ray to be situated inferior to the remaining four rays. This often is associated with a cavus foot, as is a rigid ray. In contrast, hypermobility of the first ray is associated with pes planus.

The clinician should then instruct the individual to walk barefoot and observe the individual from an anterior, posterior, and lateral view. It is important to note any abnormalities in gait, favoring of one limb, heel–toe floor contact, and heel alignment. The gait analysis should be repeated with the individual wearing shoes and any orthoses.

Finally, the injury site should be inspected for obvious deformities, discoloration, edema, scars that might indicate previous surgery, and general condition of the skin. A bilateral comparison should be performed. In contrast, the observation and inspection for a patient with an acute injury consists of inspecting for bleeding, deformity, swelling, discoloration, antalgic gait, and reaction to pain.

 Observation of the cross-country runner should include a full postural assessment and gait analysis. The specific injury site should be inspected for obvious deformities, discoloration, edema, scars that might indicate previous surgery, and general condition of the skin.

PALPATION

? The observation of the cross-country runner reveals no abnormal findings. Explain palpation specific to the injury sustained by the cross-country runner.

The individual should be seated on an examination table, with the foot and ankle extended beyond the table's edge. Bilateral palpation should be performed to determine temperature, swelling, point tenderness, crepitus, deformity, muscle spasm, and cutaneous sensation. Pulses can be taken at the posterior tibial artery behind the medial malleolus and at the dorsalis pedis artery on the dorsum of the foot.

Palpation should proceed proximal to distal, but the area anticipated to be most painful should be left to last. The following structures should be palpated:

Anterior and Medial Palpation

1. Shaft of the tibia

2. Medial malleolus

3. Posterior tibial artery

4. Tibialis posterior, flexor digitorum longus, and flexor hallucis longus muscles and tendons

5. Deltoid ligament

6. Sustentaculum tali (one finger width inferior to the medial malleolus)

7. Talar dome and neck (plantar flexion exposes this area)

8. Joint capsule

9. Tibialis anterior, extensor hallucis longus, extensor digitorum longus muscles and tendons, and dorsalis pedis artery

10. Navicular bone and tubercle of the navicular

11. Medial, middle, and lateral cuneiforms

12. Calcaneonavicular ligament (i.e., spring ligament)

13. Medial calcaneus

14. Plantar fascia

15. Head of 1st metatarsal, sesamoid bones, and great toe

16. Second metatarsal and second toe

Anterior and Lateral Palpation

1. Head of the fibula as well as peroneal longus and brevis

2. Distal tibiofibular joint and ligament

3. Lateral malleolus

4. ATFL, PTFL, CFL, peroneal tubercle, and peroneal tendons

5. Sinus tarsi (indentation over the talus next to the muscle belly of the extensor digitorum brevis)

6. Joint capsule and dome of the talus (plantar flex the foot)

7. Cuboid bone

8. Styloid process of the 5th metatarsal as well as shafts of the 3rd, 4th, and 5th metatarsals

9. Third through fifth toes

Posterior Palpation

1. Triceps surae and Achilles tendon

2. Calcaneus, calcaneal bursa, and retrocalcaneal bursa

3. Posterior aspect of the heel pad and calcaneus

When evaluating the acutely injured patient, only the structures in the painful area and those adjacent to the area are palpated. Findings such as extreme point tenderness, deformity, and crepitus suggest a more significant injury and warrant conducting specific special tests to confirm or rule out potential pathologies. For example, if a fracture is suspected, percussion and compression tests should be administered before moving the limb. Examples of these techniques are provided in **Application Strategy 14.2.**

APPLICATION STRATEGY 14.2

Determining a Fracture in the Lower Leg and Foot

- **Percussion.** Tapping on the head of the fibula or tibial shaft can be used to detect a fracture of the malleolus. Tapping on the ends of the toes along the long axis of the bone may detect a phalangeal fracture.
- **Bump test.** Strike the bottom of the heel with the palm to drive the talus into the mortise. Increased pain may indicate an osteochondral fracture, malleolar fracture, or increased mortise spread.
- **Squeeze test.** Compress the tibia and fibula together just distal to the knee. This causes the distal malleoli to distract. Increased pain distally may indicate a fracture.
- **Circumferential squeeze test.** Encircle the midfoot with the hand and slowly squeeze the metatarsal heads. Increased pain may indicate a tarsal or metatarsal fracture.
- **Vibration.** Place a vibrating tuning fork near the suspected fracture site. Increased localized pain is a positive sign.
- **Compression/distraction.** Compress the ends of the toes and metatarsals along the long axis of the bone. Follow this with distraction along the long axis. If a fracture is present, compression should increase pain, but distraction should decrease pain. If distraction increases pain, the injury may be a joint sprain.

The clinician should also make use of specific clinical prediction rules to help guide decision making regarding treatment options. The Ottawa ankle rules (OARs) have been found to be useful in the clinical setting.[11] The OARs are clinical prediction rules designed to assist the clinician in determining the need to refer the patient for radiographic imaging to detect potential fractures of the ankle and midfoot. The OARs are presented in **Figure 14.13**.

 In the continued assessment of the cross-country runner, the bony and soft-tissue structures on the plantar aspect of the foot should be palpated for point tenderness, swelling, deformity, sensation, or other signs of trauma.

PHYSICAL EXAMINATION TESTS

? The cross-country runner has point tenderness over the medial calcaneal tubercle. Explain the physical examination of the cross-country runner.

Physical examination testing should be performed in a comfortable position, with the individual lying on a table with feet hanging over the end or with the individual sitting. Bilateral comparison is used to assess normal level of function. When evaluating the acutely injured patient, the physical examination is usually conducted in the position the patient is found. It is important not to move an acutely injured patient until serious injury has been ruled out.

Functional Tests

The clinician should determine the available ROM in ankle dorsiflexion–plantar flexion, supination–pronation, toe flexion–extension, and toe abduction–adduction. Remember that in the acute setting, testing ROM may be contraindicated, based on findings obtained in the history, inspection, and palpation portions of the examination process.

Active Movements

Active movements, depicted in **Figure 8.8**, are best performed with the individual sitting on a table, with the leg flexed over the end of the table. The thigh and knee must be stabilized. Actions that

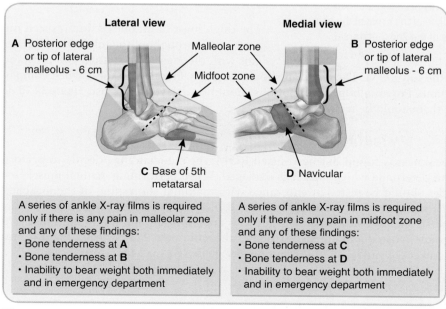

Figure 14.13. Clinical predictions rules: Ottawa ankle rules.

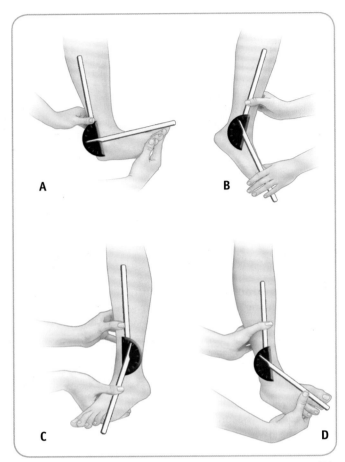

Figure 14.14. Goniometry measurement. Ankle dorsiflexion **(A)** and plantar flexion **(B)**. Center the fulcrum over the lateral malleolus. Align the proximal arm along the fibula using the head of the fibula for reference. Align the distal arm parallel to the midline of the 5th metatarsal. Pronation **(C)** and supination **(D)**. Center the fulcrum over the anterior ankle midway between the malleoli. Align the proximal arm with the midline of the crest of the tibia. Align the distal arm with the midline of the 2nd metatarsal.

may cause pain should be performed last to prevent any painful symptoms from overflowing into the next movement. The motions that should be assessed, and the normal ROM for each, are as follows:

- Dorsiflexion of the ankle (20°)
- Plantar flexion of the ankle (30° to 50°)
- Pronation (15° to 30°)
- Supination (45° to 60°)
- Toe extension
- Toe flexion
- Toe abduction and adduction

Passive Range of Motion

If the individual is able to perform full ROM during active movements, gentle pressure is applied at the extremes of motion to determine end feel. The end feel for dorsiflexion, plantar flexion, pronation, supination, and toe flexion and extension is tissue stretch. If the individual is unable to perform full active movements, passive movement should be performed to determine available ROM and end feel. ROM is measured most often when evaluating patients in nonacute situations. Obtaining baseline ROM measurements through the use of a goniometer provides a benchmark that the clinician can use to assess if the patient is improving. After the initial measurements are taken, measures taken throughout the rehabilitation process can be compared with the initial baseline numbers. **Figure 14.14** demonstrates proper positioning for goniometry measurement at the ankle.

Resisted Range of Motion

The thigh must be stabilized and resisted muscle testing performed throughout the full ROM. The assessment begins with the muscle on stretch, and resistance is applied throughout the full ROM. The clinician should note any muscle weakness when compared with the uninvolved limb. Potentially painful motions should be delayed until last. **Figure 14.15** demonstrates the motions that should be tested.

Manual Muscle Testing

If pain or weakness is found during resisted ROM, the clinician may decide to perform a manual muscle test to determine which muscle is damaged. When performing manual muscle testing, class I and II muscles should be tested at end range with maximal shortening of the muscle.[12] One-joint muscles that concentrically contract through the ROM are considered class I muscles. Class I muscles are short and strong. In contrast, class II muscles are two-joint and multijoint muscles that actively shorten all joints crossed and are also strong at the end range. Several class I and II muscles are involved with lower leg, ankle, and foot motion. See **Table 14.2** for MMT positioning.

Stress Tests for Ligament Laxity

From information gathered during the history, observation, inspection, and palpation, the clinician determines which tests will assess the condition most effectively. Special tests are used to confirm

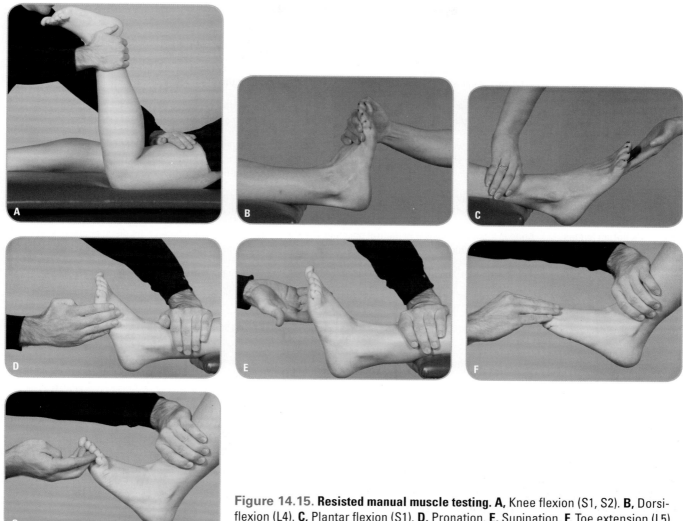

Figure 14.15. **Resisted manual muscle testing. A,** Knee flexion (S1, S2). **B,** Dorsiflexion (L4). **C,** Plantar flexion (S1). **D,** Pronation. **E,** Supination. **F,** Toe extension (L5). **G,** Toe flexion.

clinical impressions formulated during the history and early portion of the physical examination.[13] Although several tests are described in this text, only those tests that are deemed to be absolutely necessary should be performed. Important to note is that the clinical accuracy of joint stability tests increases when performed prior to onset of swelling.[11] Therefore, performing joint stability prior to onset of joint effusion is imperative to formulating an early accurate diagnosis.

Anterior Drawer Test

This test assesses collateral ligament integrity of the ankle. While the individual is supine and the foot is extended beyond the table, the clinician stabilizes the tibia and fibula in one hand and cups the individual's heel in the other hand. Testing of both the anterior talofibular and deltoid ligaments involves applying a straight anterior movement with slight dorsiflexion (**Fig. 14.16A**). If the entire dome of the talus shifts equally forward, it indicates both medial and lateral ligament damage. The ATFL and anterolateral capsule can be isolated by applying a straight anterior movement with slight plantar flexion and inversion. A positive test results in the lateral side of the talus shifting forward, indicating anterolateral rotary instability. The clinician should correlate mechanism of injury, pain, and areas of tenderness with the results of the anterior drawer test to determine involved structures. The diagnostic accuracy of the anterior drawer test increases when performed 5 days postinjury as compared to performing the test after 48 hours of injury.[11]

TABLE 14.2 Manual Muscle Testing of Lower Leg and Ankle Muscles

MUSCLE	JOINT POSITIONING	APPLY PRESSURE
Extensor hallucis longus	Ankle is in slight plantar flexion. MTP and IP joints of great toe are extended.	To dorsal aspect of the distal and proximal phalanges of the great toe in the direction of flexion
Extensor digitorum longus	Ankle is in slight plantar flexion, either everted or inverted, with the 2nd–5th digits in full extension.	To the dorsal aspect of the 2nd–5th digits in the direction of flexion
Tibialis anterior	Knee is flexed with ankle in dorsiflexion and inversion. Great toe should not be extended.	To the medial and dorsal aspect of the foot, along the 1st metatarsal, in the direction of eversion and plantar flexion
Flexor hallucis longus	Ankle is midway between dorsiflexion and plantar flexion with first IP joint flexed.	To the plantar surface of the distal phalanx of the 2nd–5th digits, in the direction of flexion
Flexor digitorum longus	Knee is flexed with ankle in neutral position. The distal IP joints of 2nd–5th digits are flexed.	To the plantar surface of the distal phalanges, in the direction of flexion
Tibialis posterior	Ankle is plantar flexed with foot inverted.	To the medial and plantar aspect of the foot in the direction of DF and EV

IP, interphalangeal; *DF*, dorsiflexion; *EV*, eversion.

From Kendall FP, McCreary EK, Provance PG, et al. *Muscles: Testing and Function with Posture and Pain.* 5th ed. Baltimore, MD: Lippincott Williams & Wilkins; 2005.

Talar Tilt

The calcaneofibular and deltoid ligaments are tested with the patient's foot and ankle in the same position described for the anterior drawer test. Maintaining the calcaneus in normal anatomical position (90° of flexion), the clinician slowly rocks the talus between inversion and eversion (**Fig. 14.16B**). Inversion tests the CFL, and eversion tests the deltoid ligament. The diagnostic accuracy of the talar tilt test increases when performed 5 days postinjury as compared to performing the test after 48 hours of injury.[11]

External Rotation (Kleiger) Test

A variation of the talar tilt test for deltoid ligament instability is the external rotation, or Kleiger, test. Being careful not to compress the joint, the lower leg is stabilized proximal to the distal tibiofibular syndesmosis.

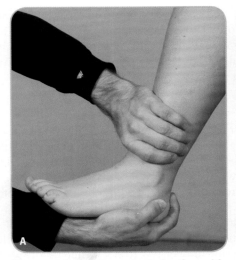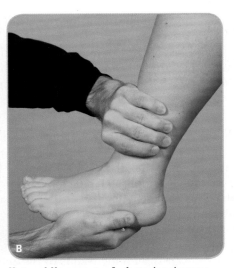

Figure 14.16. Stress tests for the ankle collateral ligaments. A, Anterior drawer test. **B,** Talar tilt test.

While the foot is in a neutral position, the clinician grasps the medial side of the foot and then rotates the foot laterally (i.e., external rotation) (**Fig. 14.17**). If this motion elicits pain over the medial joint line, it indicates damage to the deltoid ligament, whereas pain in the area above the talus over the anterior tibiofibular ligament indicates injury to the syndesmosis. Syndesmosis sprains are also referred to as a high ankle sprain.

Glide Tests

Ligaments in the metatarsal and tarsal region of the foot are assessed through the use of glide tests to determine the amount of "play" or motion within the joint. Joints that have excessive joint play as compared to the noninvolved joint are said to be hypermobile. Joints that have restricted joint play as compared to the noninvolved joint are said to be hypomobile. When assessing for the presence of a sprain in the acutely injured patient, increased joint play and pain are positive findings.

Intermetatarsal glide test assesses the integrity of the ligaments between the metatarsals. The test is performed by stabilizing one metatarsal while gliding the adjacent metatarsal from dorsal to ventral and ventral to dorsal.

Tarsometatarsal glide test is used to assess the integrity of the ligaments of the tarsometatarsal joints. The test is performed by stabilizing a tarsal bone while gliding the adjacent metatarsal from dorsal to ventral and ventral for dorsal. For example, the clinician stabilizes the medial or first cuneiform while gliding the 1st metatarsal.

Intertarsal glide test is used to assess the integrity of the ligaments between the tarsals. To perform the test, the clinician stabilizes one tarsal (e.g., the cuboid) while gliding the adjacent tarsal (the navicular).

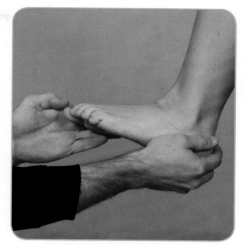

Figure 14.17. Kleiger test (external rotation test). The clinician passively dorsiflexes the ankle and rotates the foot laterally. Pain in the area of the lateral malleolus indicates injury to the syndesmosis.

Varus and Valgus Stress Test

Varus and valgus stress tests are used to examine the integrity of the lateral stabilizing structures of the MTP joints and the interphalangeal (IP) joints. The varus stress test stresses the lateral collateral ligament (or fibular collateral ligament), whereas the valgus stress test stresses the medial collateral ligament (or tibial collateral ligament). It is difficult to perform these tests on the second to fourth MTP joints and is more easily applied to all IP joints. To perform the test, the joint should first be in full extension, and the clinician should stabilize the bone just proximal and distal to the joint being assessed. Then, either a valgus (for the valgus stress test) or a varus (for the varus stress test) stress is placed on the joint. Degree of joint laxity is used to determine degree of sprain. If no pain or joint opening is noted in full extension, the joint should be flexed slightly and the test repeated.

Special Tests

A variety of special tests can be used for detecting injury or related pathology involving the lower leg, ankle, and foot.

Thompson Test for Achilles Tendon Rupture

While the individual is prone on a table, the clinician squeezes the calf muscles. A normal response is slight plantar flexion. A positive test, indicating a rupture of the gastrocnemius–soleus complex or Achilles tendon, is indicated by the absence of plantar flexion (**Fig. 14.18**). The amount of motion should always be compared with the uninjured side, because some plantar flexion may occur if the plantaris muscle is intact. The magnitude of contraction, however, is significantly reduced compared with that of the uninvolved leg.

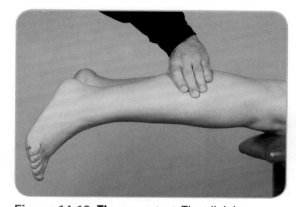

Figure 14.18. Thompson test. The clinician performs passive compression of the calf muscles. This should produce slight plantar flexion at the ankle. If no plantar flexion occurs, a possible rupture of the gastrocnemius–soleus complex or the Achilles tendon should be suspected.

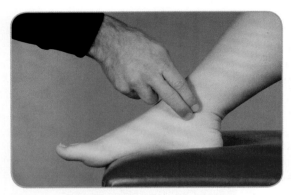

Figure 14.19. Tinel sign. The clinician taps the posterior tibial nerve, which may produce numbing, tingling, and paresthesia, indicating the presence of a possible tarsal tunnel syndrome.

Homans Sign

To test for deep venous thrombosis (DVT), the individual must be supine on a table. The clinician dorsiflexes the foot of the involved leg with the knee in extension. Pain in the calf indicates a positive Homans sign. Tenderness also may be elicited with palpation of the calf. In addition, pallor or swelling in the leg may be accompanied by an absence of the dorsalis pedis pulse.

Tinel Sign

To determine the presence of tarsal tunnel syndrome, the clinician should tap the posterior tibial nerve as it courses posterior to the medial malleolus (**Fig. 14.19**). The test is positive if numbness, tingling, and paresthesia occur.

Thumb Index Squeeze Test

With a sensitivity of 96% and 96% accuracy, the thumb index squeeze test is the most clinically useful test for detecting the presence of Morton neuroma.[14] To perform the test, locate the sensitive area on the foot and place your thumb on the plantar surface of the foot and the index finger on the dorsal aspect and squeeze. Pain is a positive finding for the presence of Morton neuroma.[14]

Neurological Tests

Neurological integrity is assessed with isometric muscle testing of the myotomes, reflex testing, and sensation in the segmental dermatomes and peripheral nerve cutaneous patterns.

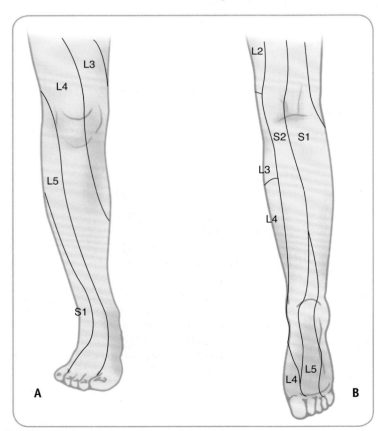

Figure 14.20. Dermatomes for the lower leg, ankle, and foot. A, Anterior. **B,** Posterior.

Myotomes

Isometric muscle testing should be performed in the following motions to test specific segmental myotomes:

- Knee extension (L3)
- Ankle dorsiflexion (L4)
- Toe extension (L5)
- Ankle plantar flexion, foot eversion, or hip extension (S1)

Reflexes

Reflexes in the lower leg region include the patella (L3, L4) and Achilles tendon reflex (S1). These are discussed in Chapter 15 and demonstrated in **Figure 15.22**.

Cutaneous Patterns

The segmental nerve dermatome patterns for the pelvis, hip, and thigh are demonstrated in **Figure 14.20**. The peripheral nerve cutaneous patterns are demonstrated in **Figure 14.21**.

Activity-Specific Functional Tests

Once the patient has achieved his or her rehabilitation goals, the patient should be assessed on his or her readiness to return to participation. Functional tests should be performed pain-free before clearing any individual for return to activity. Functional tests may sometimes be referred to as return to play guidelines. These may include any or all of the following:

- Squatting with both heels maintained on the floor
- Going up on the toes at least 20 times without pain
- Walking on the toes for 20 to 30 ft
- Balancing on one foot at a time
- Running straight ahead, stopping, and running backward
- Running figure eights with large circles that slowly decrease in size
- Running at an angle sideways and making V-cuts
- Jumping rope for at least 1 minute
- Jumping straight up and then going to a 90° squat

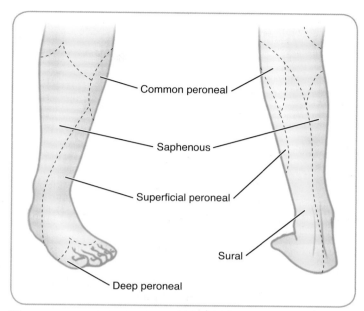

Figure 14.21. Peripheral nerve distribution in the lower leg, ankle, and foot.

 The physical examination of the cross-country runner should include active, passive, and restricted ROM of the foot and ankle; stretching the plantar aspect of the foot by having the athlete extend the toes while passively dorsiflexing the foot; fracture assessment; and performance of functional activities (e.g., walking and running).

TOE AND FOOT CONDITIONS

? A defensive back reports throbbing pain on the plantar side of the great toe of the right foot that has been present for the last 2 days. The athlete does not recall a specific mechanism or time of onset. The pain increases significantly when the athlete pushes off the right foot to block an opponent. For the past 3 days, the team was forced to practice indoors on a composite-type floor. What injury should be suspected, and why?

Many individuals are at risk for toe and foot problems because of a leg length discrepancy, postural deviation, muscle dysfunction (e.g., muscle imbalance), or malalignment syndrome (e.g., pes cavus, pes planus, pes equinus, and hammer or claw toes) (**Fig. 14.22**). In particular, pes cavus (e.g., high arch and rigid foot) and pes planus (e.g., flatfoot and mobile foot) are associated with several common injuries (**Box 14.1**). Typically, when compared to a man's foot, a woman's foot has a narrower hindfoot, a relatively increased forefoot-to-hindfoot width, and increased pronation, and, because of fashion trends and societal pressures, women tend to wear shoes that have narrow toe boxes and narrow midfoot design. High heels shift the forefoot forward into the toe box, causing crowding of the toes and a tight heel cord. Consequently, women tend to be more prone to hallux valgus deformities, bunionettes, hammer toes, and neuromas.[15] Other skin conditions commonly seen at the foot include calluses, corns, athlete's foot, and plantar warts, all of which are discussed in Chapter 32.

Toe Deformities

Most toe deformities are minor and can be treated conservatively. A few deformities require surgical intervention to correct serious structural malalignment.

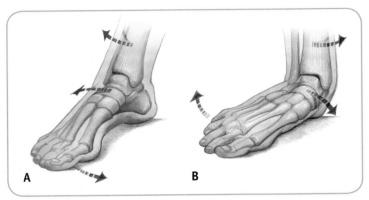

Figure 14.22. Common foot deformities. A, Pes cavus. **B,** Pes planus.

Hallux Rigidus

■ Etiology

Degenerative arthritis in the first MTP joint, associated with pain and limited motion, is known as hallux rigidus. Activities that involve running and jumping may predispose an individual to this condition as a result of degenerative changes resulting from direct injury, hyperextension injury, or varus/valgus stress.[16]

■ Signs and Symptoms

The individual presents with a tender and enlarged first MTP joint, loss of motion, and difficulty wearing shoes with an elevated heel. A hallmark sign is restricted toe extension (dorsiflexion), usually less than 60°, because of a ridge of osteophytes that can be palpated easily along the dorsal aspect of the metatarsal head.

■ Management

Conservative management includes ice, wearing low-heeled shoes with adequate width and depth to accommodate the increased bulk of the joint, nonsteroidal anti-inflammatory drugs (NSAIDs), and therapeutic mobilization. Individuals can add a Morton extension to their orthosis or use a rigid insole or shoe to reduce stress across the joint. Steroid injections may help if chronic inflammation is present. If conservative measures fail to resolve the symptoms within 6 months, surgery is indicated. Spurs may be removed through a cheilectomy, which can improve motion and reduce, but not eliminate, pain. An arthrodesis procedure may be suggested to fuse or resect the proximal portion of the proximal phalanx. Both techniques have a good or excellent outcome.[17]

Hallux Valgus

■ Etiology

Prolonged pressure against the medial aspect of the first MTP joint can lead to thickening of the medial capsule and bursa (i.e., bunion), resulting in a severe valgus deformity of the great toe (**Fig. 14.23**). The most common cause is wearing poorly fitted shoes with a narrow toe box, but it also can be caused by heredity, metatarsus primus varus, pes planus, rheumatoid arthritis, and neurological disorders.

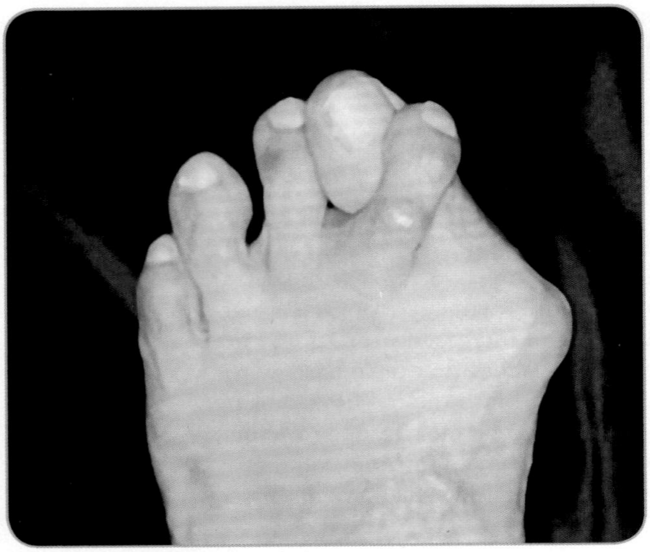

■ Signs and Symptoms

Many individuals with the deformity are asymptomatic. [*no symptoms*] Those with symptoms complain of pain over the MTP joint and have difficulty wearing shoes because of the medial prominence and associated overlapping toe deformity. The condition may also cause the 2nd metatarsal to bear more weight, leading to a callus under the second metatarsal head.

■ Management

Treatment varies depending on the degree of deformity and the severity of symptoms. Wide, soft shoes with a broad toe box and sufficient insole padding are critical for comfort. Orthoses that support the longitudinal arch and redistribute the pressure areas also may provide some relief. If conservative measures fail, surgery may correct the deformity, but this does not necessarily improve activity performance. Rehabilitation can take from 4 to 6 months.[17]

Figure 14.23. Hallux valgus. Hallux valgus is an abnormality in which the great toe is deviated laterally and may overlap the second toe. An enlarged, painful, inflamed bursa (bunion) may form on the medial side.

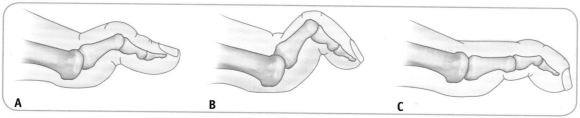

Figure 14.24. Toe deformities. A, Hammer toe. **B,** Claw toe. **C,** Mallet toe.

Claw, Hammer, and Mallet Toe

■ Etiology

Other lesser toe deformities may be congenital but more often develop because of improperly fitted shoes, neuromuscular disease, arthritis, or trauma. A **hammer toe** is extended at the MTP joint, flexed at the PIP joint, and hyperextended at the DIP joint (**Fig. 14.24**). **Claw toe** involves hyperextension of the MTP joint and flexion of the DIP and PIP joints. A **mallet toe** is in neutral position at the MTP and PIP joints but flexed at the DIP joint.

■ Signs and Symptoms

Each condition can lead to painful callus formation on the dorsum of the IP joints. Pressure against the shoe and under the metatarsal head, particularly the second toe, is caused by the retrograde pressure on the long toe.

■ Management

These conditions are difficult to treat conservatively. A metatarsal pad may help control symptoms, but surgery may be necessary to rectify tendon lengthening, capsulotomy, and/or ligament release. For more significant deformities, resection of the head of the proximal phalanx may be necessary to treat the condition.

Ingrown Toenail

■ Etiology

Although ingrown toenails are common, they are preventable with proper hygiene and nail care. Toenails should be long enough to extend beyond the underlying skin but short enough so as not to push into the toe box of the shoe. Toenails should be trimmed straight across to prevent the edges from growing under the skin on the side of the nail. In addition, properly fitted shoes and socks should be worn.

■ Signs and Symptoms

Improper cutting of the nail, improper shoe size, and constant sliding of the foot inside the shoe can traumatize the nail, causing its edge to grow into the lateral nail fold and surrounding skin. The nail margin reddens and becomes painful. If a fungal or bacterial infection is present, the condition is called **paronychia**.

■ Management

Two methods to treat this condition are discussed in **Application Strategy 14.3**.

Metatarsalgia

■ Etiology

General discomfort around the metatarsal heads is called **metatarsalgia**, or Morton metatarsalgia. Although often related to participation in sport and physical activity, other factors, such as age, arthritic disease, gout, and diabetes, can predispose an individual to metatarsal pain (**Box 14.2**).

APPLICATION STRATEGY 14.3

Management of an Ingrown Toenail

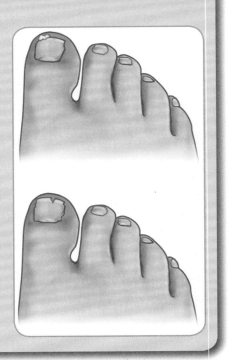

Method 1

- Soak the involved toe in hot water (108°–116°F) until the nail bed is soft (usually 10–15 minutes).
- Lift the edge of the nail and place a small piece of cotton or tissue under the nail to elevate the nail out of the skinfold.
- Apply antiseptic to the area and cover with a sterile dressing.
- Repeat the procedure daily, keeping the area clean and dry.
- *If a purulent infection is present, the individual should be referred to a physician for antibiotics and drainage of the infection.*

Method 2

- Soak the toe as in the preceding and cut a "V" in the center of the nail.
- As the nail grows, its edges pull toward the center, drawing the nail edges from under the skin.
- Apply an antiseptic, cover with a sterile dressing, and keep the area clean and dry.
- *If a purulent infection is present, the individual should be referred to a physician for antibiotics and drainage of the infection.*

BOX 14.2 Factors Leading to Metatarsalgia

Intrinsic Factors

- Excessive body weight
- Limited extensibility of the triceps surae complex
- Fallen metatarsal arch
- Valgus heel
- Hammer toes
- Pes planus or pes cavus

Extrinsic Factors

- Narrow toe box
- Improperly placed shoe cleats
- Improper technique (e.g., in a cyclist, poor foot position or rigid high gears at low cadence)
- Landing incorrectly from a height
- Repetitive jumping or excessive running
- Running style that puts undue pressure on the forefoot

■ **Signs and Symptoms**

Constant overloading of the transverse ligaments leads to flattening of the transverse arch, resulting in callus formation over the middle three metatarsal heads, particularly the second. The patient will complain of pain generalized in the metatarsal region and will have a gradual onset in intensity and duration.

■ **Management**

Treatment involves reducing the load on the metatarsal heads through activity modification, footwear examination, metatarsal pads or bars, and strengthening the intrinsic muscles of the foot.

Bunions

Etiology

Bunions generally are found on the medial aspect of the MTP joint of the great toe but also can occur on the lateral aspect of the fifth toe (i.e., a bunionette or tailor's bunion). Pronation of the foot, prolonged pronation during gait, contractures of the Achilles tendon, arthritis, and generalized ligamentous laxity between the first and second metatarsal heads can produce a thickening on the medial side of the first metatarsal head as it constantly rubs against the inside of the shoe.

Signs and Symptoms

As the condition worsens, the great toe may shift laterally and overlap the second toe, leading to a rigid, nonfunctional hallux valgus deformity (**Fig. 14.23**). This condition is exacerbated by high heels and pointed toe boxes in shoes, factors that account for a higher incidence of the condition in women compared to men.

Management

Once the deformity occurs, little can be done to correct the condition. Strapping the great toe as closely to proper anatomical position as possible and wearing wider shoes can provide some relief, but surgical correction is indicated in severe cases.

Retrocalcaneal Bursitis

Etiology

External pressure from a constrictive heel cup, coupled with excessive pronation or a varus hindfoot, can lead to swelling, erythema, and irritation of the retrocalcaneal bursa located between the Achilles tendon and calcaneus (**Fig. 14.25**). The posterior calcaneal bursa also can be irritated.

Signs and Symptoms

Pain is elicited on palpation of the soft tissue just anterior to the Achilles tendon, and the skin may be thickened, especially on the lateral side. Active plantar flexion during push-off compresses the bursa between the tendon and bone, leading to increased pain.

Management

Standard acute care, NSAIDs, stretching exercises for the Achilles tendon, shoe modification, or a heel lift may provide some relief. Radiographs may show calcification in the bursa. If so, excision of the bursa may be indicated if conservative treatment fails. Injection with steroids is not recommended.[16]

Occasionally, an inflamed bursa can lead to a dramatic, large mass referred to as a "pump bump," which is common among female figure skaters and

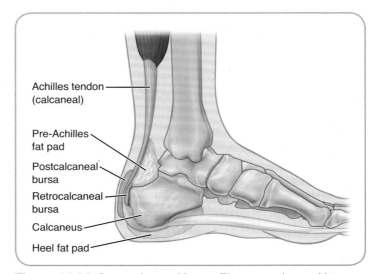

Figure 14.25. Retrocalcaneal bursa. The retrocalcaneal bursa commonly is inflamed when it is pinched between the Achilles tendon and calcaneus during plantar flexion.

runners (i.e., runner's bump). The condition also may be called **os calcis exostosis**. This bump may be related to an underlying bony spur caused by frequent microtrauma or microavulsions surrounding the distal attachment of the Achilles tendon. An additional Achilles tendinopathy above the insertion may be present when the symptoms have been present for more than 3 months. Conservative treatment is similar to that of retrocalcaneal bursitis. Open (preferably with tendinopathy) or endoscopic excision is recommended. Steroid injections should not be used because of the risk of Achilles tendon rupture.[16]

 The defensive back may have a turf toe. The injury could be the result of repeated hyperextension. The change in surface to a more rigid and less giving surface as well as use of inappropriate footwear could have contributed to this injury.

CONTUSIONS

? A soccer player was kicked in the anterolateral aspect of the lower leg. The athlete continued to play the remaining 10 minutes of the game. Twenty minutes after the game ended, however, the athlete reported severe pain to the area. Inspection revealed a firm mass and tight skin over the injured site. What condition should be suspected, and what further assessment should be performed?

Contusions of the foot and leg result from direct trauma, such as dropping a weight on the foot or being stepped on, kicked, or hit by a speeding ball or implement. Many of these injuries are minor and easily treated with standard acute care. A few injuries, however, can result in complications, such as excessive hemorrhage, periosteal irritation, nerve damage, or damage to tendon sheaths, leading to tenosynovitis.

Foot Contusions

Etiology

Compression on the midfoot can be painful and may damage the extensor tendons or lead to a fracture of the metatarsals or phalanges. During weight bearing, contusions of the plantar aspect of the forefoot may result from a cleat or spike irritating the ball of the foot. A contusion to the hindfoot, called a **heel bruise**, can be more serious. Elastic adipose tissue lies between the thick skin and the plantar aspect of the calcaneus to cushion and protect the inferior portion of the calcaneus from trauma. It is constantly subjected to extreme stress in running, jumping, and changing directions. Excessive body weight, age, poorly cushioned or worn-out running shoes, increases in training, and hard, uneven training surfaces can predispose an individual to this condition.

Signs and Symptoms

Pain, swelling, and ecchymosis may be present at the site of the contusion. Walking barefoot is particularly painful. Underlying skeletal structures should be assessed for presence of crepitus, which may suggest a fracture.

Management

Application of cold to minimize pain and inflammation, followed by regular use of a heel cup or doughnut pad, can minimize the condition. Despite excellent care, the condition may persist for months. Repairing or replacing the object, along with ice therapy to reduce immediate hemorrhage and discomfort, usually is sufficient to remedy the situation.

Lower Leg Contusions

Etiology

A contusion to the tibia, commonly called a **shin bruise**, may occur in soccer, field hockey, baseball, softball, football, or activities in which the lower leg is subjected to high-impact forces. The shin is particularly void of natural subcutaneous fat and is vulnerable to direct blows that irritate the periosteal tissue around the tibia. Participants should always wear appropriate shin guards to protect this highly vulnerable area.

Signs and Symptoms

Contusions of the anterior shin can be extremely painful. Localized swelling may be evident and dorsiflexion will be painful. Contusions to the gastrocnemius result in immediate pain, weakness, and partial loss of motion. Hemorrhage and muscle spasm quickly lead to a tender, firm, easily palpable mass.

Management

Although painful, the condition can be managed effectively with ice, compression, elevation, and rest. A doughnut pad or additional shin protection can allow the individual to participate within pain tolerance levels. For a gastrocnemius contusion, it is important when applying ice to keep the muscle on stretch to decrease muscle spasm. If the condition does not improve in 2 to 3 days, ultrasound may be used, to assist in breaking up the hematoma.

Acute Compartment Syndrome

Etiology

An acute compartment syndrome occurs when increased pressure within a limited or nonyielding space compromises the local venous pressure and obstructs the neurovascular network. In the lower leg, it tends to be caused by a direct blow to the anterolateral aspect of the tibia or by a tibial fracture. The anterior compartment is particularly at risk, because it is bounded by the tibia medially, the interosseous membrane posteriorly, the fibula laterally, and a tough fascial sheath anteriorly. Although an acute compartment syndrome occurs less frequently than the more common chronic exertional compartment syndrome, the acute syndrome is considered to be a medical and surgical emergency because of the compromised neurovascular functions. Compartment syndrome should be considered if there is a recent history of trauma, excessive exercise, vascular injury, or prolonged, externally applied pressure.

Signs and Symptoms

Signs and symptoms include increasing severe pain and swelling that appear to be out of proportion to the clinical situation. A firm mass, tight skin (because it has been stretched to its limits), loss of sensation on the dorsal aspect between the great and second toes, and diminished pulse at the dorsalis pedis are delayed and dangerous signs. A normal pulse, however, does not rule out the syndrome. Acute compartment syndrome can produce functional abnormalities within 30 minutes of the onset of hemorrhage. Immediate action is necessary, because irreversible damage can occur within 12 to 24 hours.

Management

Immediate care involves ice and total rest. Compression is not recommended, because the compartment already is unduly compressed and additional external compression only hastens the deterioration. In addition, the limb must not be elevated, because this decreases arterial pressure and further compromises capillary filling. Referral to a physician for immediate care is absolutely necessary.

If numbness in the foot is present, intercompartmental pressure is measured using either a slit catheter or a solid-state intracompartmental catheter. If the pressure ranges between 30 and 40 mm Hg (normal range, 0 to 10 mm Hg), the individual is watched carefully, and repeated measurements are taken until symptoms subside. If the pressure ranges from 40 to 60 mm Hg, a surgical release of the fascia (i.e., fasciotomy) is required to prevent permanent tissue damage.

 The soccer player may have an acute compartment syndrome. In the continued assessment of the athlete, the following should be examined: sensation between the first and second toes on the dorsum of the foot, circulation at the dorsalis pedis pulse, and active ROM, particularly the motions of dorsiflexion and eversion.

FOOT AND ANKLE SPRAINS

 A 30-year-old recreational basketball player has sustained a grade II lateral ankle sprain. What is the immediate management for this condition?

Sprains to the foot and ankle region are common in sports, particularly among those individuals who play on badly maintained fields. In many sports, cleated shoes become fixed to the ground while the limb continues to rotate around it. In addition, the very nature of changing directions places an inordinate amount of strain on the ankle region. Other methods of injury include stepping in a hole, stepping off a curb, stepping on an opponent's foot, or rolling the foot off the surface.

Toe Sprains and Dislocations

Turf Toe

■ Etiology

A sprain of the plantar capsular ligament of the first MTP joint, called turf toe, results from forced hyperextension or hyperflexion of the great toe (i.e., jamming the toe into the end of the shoe). Hyperextension causes the sesamoid bones to be drawn forward to bear weight under the first metatarsal head. Repetitive overload also can lead to injury, particularly when associated with a valgus stress. Because of forced hyperflexion of the MTP joint while kicking an instep ball strike, soccer players often irritate the dorsal capsular structures of the first MTP joint; the condition is then called reverse turf toe.

■ Signs and Symptoms

With regular turf toe, the individual has pain, tenderness, and swelling on the plantar aspect of the MTP joint of the great toe. Great toe extension is extremely painful. Because the sesamoid bones are located in the tendons of the flexor hallucis brevis, this condition sometimes is associated with tearing of the flexor tendons, fracture of the sesamoid bones, bone bruises, and osteochondral fractures in the metatarsal head. With reverse turf toe, symptoms are similar, except pain is noted dorsally over the joint and passive flexion of the toe is painful.

■ Management

Initial treatment for mild sprains involves standard acute care (i.e., ice, compression, elevation, and rest), NSAIDs, and protection from excessive motion. Taping to limit motion at the MTP joint, use of a metatarsal pad to lower stress on the 1st metatarsal, or use of a rigid shoe or forefoot plate may be helpful. In moderate-to-severe cases, the individual may need to be restricted from activity until symptoms disappear (i.e., usually 3 to 6 weeks).

Metatarsophalangeal and Interphalangeal Joint Injury

■ Etiology

Sprains and dislocations to the MTP and IP joints of the toes may occur by tripping or stubbing the toe. Varus and valgus forces more commonly affect the first and fifth toes rather than the middle three.

■ Signs and Symptoms

Pain, immediate swelling, dysfunction, and, if dislocated, gross deformity will be evident. Tenderness over the lateral aspects of the joint suggests damage to the collateral ligament, whereas tenderness on the volar or dorsal surfaces may be indicative of joint capsule, extensor hood mechanism, or volar plate damage.

■ Management

Depending on the location and severity of pain, adequate strapping, arch supports, and limited weight bearing are warranted during the acute stage. If the condition does not improve, the individual should be referred to a physician to rule out a possible avulsion fracture at the tarsal joints, but closed reduction and strapping to the next toe for 10 to 14 days usually are sufficient to remedy the problem. Reconditioning exercises should include ROM and strengthening for the intrinsic muscles of the foot.

Midfoot Sprains

■ Etiology
Midfoot sprains often result from severe dorsiflexion, plantar flexion, or pronation. Although the condition is seen in basketball and soccer players, it is more frequent among those who participate in activities where the foot is unsupported, such as in gymnastics or dance (in which slippers are typically worn) or in track athletes who wear running flats.

■ Signs and Symptoms
If the midfoot is sprained, pain and swelling will be deep on the medial aspect of the foot and weight bearing may be too painful.

Mechanisms of Injury for Ankle Sprains

Ankle sprains are the most common injury in recreational and competitive sports. They are classified as grade I (first degree), grade II (second degree), and grade III (third degree) based on the progression of the anatomical structures damaged and the subsequent disability (**Table 14.3**).[11] Ankle sprains generally are caused by severe medial (i.e., supination or inversion) and lateral (i.e., pronation or eversion) rotation motions. Excessive supination of the foot (i.e., adduction, inversion, and plantar flexion) results when the plantar aspect of the foot is turned inward, toward the midline of the body, which commonly is referred to as an inversion sprain. Excessive pronation (i.e., abduction, eversion, and dorsiflexion) results when the plantar aspect of the foot is turned laterally, which is referred to as an eversion sprain.

Inversion Ankle Sprains

Etiology

Acute inversion (i.e., lateral) sprains often occur while changing directions rapidly. Interestingly, injury typically involves the unloaded foot and ankle (or, more accurately, just at the moment of loading) with a plantar flexion and inversion force. In plantar flexion, the ATFL is taut and the CFL is relatively loose, whereas in dorsiflexion, the opposite is true. The medial and lateral malleoli project downward over the talus to form a mortise–tenon joint. The lateral malleolus projects farther downward than the medial, thus limiting lateral talar shifts. As stress is initially applied to the ankle during plantar flexion and inversion, the ATFL first stretches. If the strain continues, the ankle loses ligamentous stability in its neutral position. The medial malleolus acts as a fulcrum to further the inversion and stretches or ruptures the CFL (**Fig. 14.26**). The overlying inner wall of the peroneal tendon sheath lies adjacent to the CFL and can absorb some strain to prevent injury to this ligament. If the peroneal

TABLE 14.3 Mechanisms of Common Ankle Sprains and Resulting Ligament Damage

MECHANISM	FIRST (MILD)	SECOND (MODERATE)	THIRD (SEVERE)
Inversion and plantar flexion	Anterior talofibular stretched	Partial tear of anterior talofibular, with calcaneofibular stretched	Rupture of anterior talofibular and calcaneofibular, with posterior talofibular and tibiofibular torn
Inversion	Calcaneofibular stretched	Calcaneofibular torn, and anterior talofibular stretched	Rupture of calcaneofibular, and anterior talofibular with posterior talofibular stretched
Dorsiflexion eversion	Tibiofibular stretched, deltoid stretched, or an avulsion fracture of medial malleolus	Partial tear of tibiofibular, partial tear of deltoid and tibiofibular	Rupture of tibiofibular, rupture of deltoid, and interosseous membrane with possible fibular fracture above syndesmosis

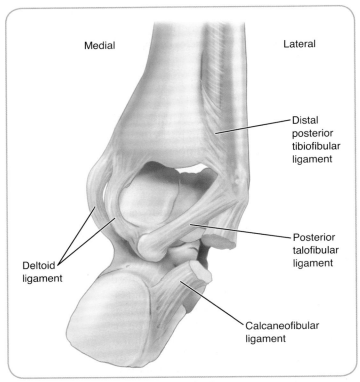

Figure 14.26. Inversion ankle sprain. During inversion, the medial malleolus acts as a fulcrum to further invert the talus, leading to stretching or tearing of the calcaneofibular ligament.

muscles are weak, however, they are unable to stabilize the joint, leading to tearing of the CFL. In severe injuries, the PTFL also is involved. As the ankle joint becomes unstable, the talus can pinch the deltoid ligament against the medial malleolus, which leads to injury on both sides of the ankle joint.

Signs and Symptoms

The individual usually describes experiencing a twisting, bending, or rolling action of the ankle. The individual may report hearing or feeling a cracking or tearing sound at the time of injury. In a grade I injury, the ligament has been stretched, resulting in slight or minimal tearing of fibers. An individual with a grade I ankle sprain may be able to bear weight immediately after injury and may even attempt to "walk it off" because the ankle feels stable. Initially, pain and swelling, if occurring at all, are mild. There is minimal point tenderness. In a grade II injury, the ligament has sustained greater damage with moderate tearing of the fibers. Swelling and tenderness are localized over the injured structure and may extend to surrounding tissue. Ecchymosis or bruising may occur, especially in the hours after the injury was sustained. The individual may be able to bear some weight and will definitely walk with an antalgic gait. The patient will be tender over the involved structures during palpation and the area may feel warm. A complete tear or rupture of a ligament is considered to be a grade III sprain. The ankle is unstable and swelling, and ecchymosis is rapid and diffuse. The individual demonstrates functional and clinical instability and will be unable to bear weight or walk with a normal gait. **Table 14.4** summarizes the signs and symptoms of the various grades of sprains of ligaments on the lateral aspect of the ankle.

Immediate assessment should distinguish the severity of injury, because swelling may soon obscure the level of instability. The same mechanisms that result in ligamentous damage may also result in damage to other musculoskeletal structures such as muscles, bones, and cartilage and should be considered when assessing the acutely injured ankle. A more focused discussion of these additional injuries is discussed later within this chapter.

TABLE 14.4 Signs and Symptoms of a Lateral Ankle Sprain	
DEGREE	**SIGNS AND SYMPTOMS**
First	Pain and swelling on anterolateral aspect of lateral malleolus Point tenderness over ATFL No laxity with stress tests
Second	Tearing or popping sensation felt on lateral aspect; pain and swelling on anterolateral and inferior aspect of lateral malleolus Painful palpation over ATFL and CFL; also may be tender over PTFL, deltoid ligament, and anterior capsule area Positive anterior drawer and talar tilt test
Third	Tearing or popping sensation felt on lateral aspect, with diffuse swelling over entire lateral aspect, with or without anterior swelling; can be very painful or absent pain Positive anterior drawer and talar tilt test

Management

Initial treatment should consist of standard acute care (i.e., cold, compression, elevation, and protected rest), nonsteroidal anti-inflammatory medication, and restricted activity. Crutches should be used if the individual is unable to bear weight. When treating grade I and II injuries, the use of functional exercise has been found to be more effective than prolonged immobilization.[11] Individuals with moderate-to-severe sprains should be referred immediately to a physician. Radiographs can determine damage to the syndesmosis or detect an osteochondral fracture to the dome of the talus. In individuals with a history of ankle sprains, the use of prophylactic taping or bracing in conjunction with a rehabilitation program that includes balance and coordination training for at least 6 weeks after injury can reduce the risk of recurrent sprains.[18] Mechanical stability may still be present for up to 1 year after injury.[19] The focus of rehabilitation should include strengthening the peroneals, stretching the heel cord, proprioceptive training, and establishing normal joint motion.[11] **Application Strategy 14.4** summarizes the management of lateral ankle sprains.

Eversion Ankle Sprains

Etiology

Eversion (i.e., medial) ankle sprains involve injury to the medial, deltoid-shaped talocrural ligaments (i.e., deltoid ligament) and may result from forced dorsiflexion and eversion, such as landing from a long jump with the foot abducted or landing on another player's foot. Most injuries to the deltoid ligament are associated with a fibula fracture, syndesmotic injury, or severe lateral ankle sprain. Individuals with pronated or hypermobile feet tend to be at a greater risk for eversion injuries.

The talar dome is wider anteriorly than posteriorly. During dorsiflexion, the talus fits more firmly in the mortise supported by the distal anterior tibiofibular ligament. During excessive dorsiflexion and eversion, the talus is thrust laterally against the longer fibula, resulting in either a mild sprain to the deltoid ligament or, if the force is great enough, a lateral malleolar fracture. If the force continues after the fracture occurs, the deltoid ligament may be ruptured or may remain intact, avulsing a small bony fragment from the medial malleolus and leading to a bimalleolar fracture. In either case, the distal anterior tibiofibular ligament and interosseous membrane may be torn, producing total instability of the ankle joint and eventual degeneration (**Fig. 14.27**).

APPLICATION STRATEGY 14.4

Management Algorithm for a Lateral Ankle Sprain

1. Use a compression wrap to secure crushed ice packs directly to the skin as quickly as possible following the injury; apply the ice for 30 minutes.
2. Do not place a towel or elastic wrap (dry or wet) between the crushed ice pack and skin (reduces effectiveness of treatment).
3. Elevate foot and ankle 6–10 in above the level of the heart.
4. After initial ice treatment,

   - Remove ice pack.
   - Replace compression wrap.
   - Continue elevation.

5. Apply a horseshoe pad and open basket weave with tape and/or elastic wrap to protect the area.
6. Instruct the individual to reapply a crushed ice pack regularly until going to bed:

   - Every 2 hours
   - Every hour if active between applications (crutch walking, showering)

7. If limping,

   - Fit with crutches.
   - Reassess in the morning.
   - Start rehabilitation.

If fracture is suspected, the individual should be referred to a physician.

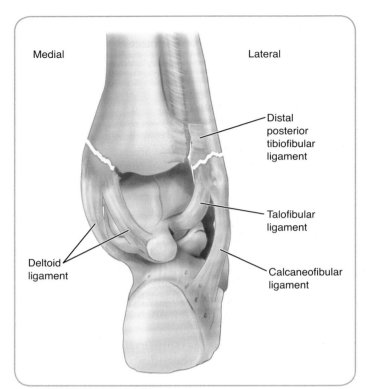

Figure 14.27. Eversion ankle sprain. During a severe eversion ankle sprain, the lateral malleolus can fracture, the deltoid ligament can avulse the medial malleolus, and the distal tibiofibular joint can be disrupted.

Signs and Symptoms

In mild to moderate injuries, the individual often is unable to recall the mechanism of injury. There may be some initial pain at the ankle when it was traumatized, but as the ankle returns to its normal anatomical position, pain often subsides and the individual continues to be active. In attempts to run or put pressure on the area, pain intensifies but the individual may not make the connection between the pain and the earlier injury. Swelling may not be as evident as a lateral sprain, because hemorrhage occurs deep in the leg and is not readily visible. Swelling may occur just posterior to the lateral malleolus, between it and the Achilles tendon. Point tenderness can be elicited over the deltoid ligament and distal anterior tibiofibular ligaments as well as the anterior and posterior joint lines. In severe injuries, passive motion may be pain-free in all motions except dorsiflexion. In a fracture of the malleoli, pain is evident over the fracture site and increases with any movement of the mortise. Percussion and heel strike produce increased pain.

Management

Initial management is the same as that of a lateral ankle sprain. Appropriate immobilization with a rigid posterior or vacuum splint is necessary. Referral to a physician is warranted. Surgical repair generally is indicated when a fracture or ligamentous disruption of the syndesmosis is involved.

Syndesmosis Sprain

Etiology

The most common mechanism involves an external rotation fracture mechanism. With this, the foot is planted fixed on the ground with internal rotation of the leg and body with respect to the foot, resulting in relative external rotation of the talus within the mortise and creating an external rotation force on the fibular with respect to the tibia.[20] As a result, the fibula separates from the tibia, disrupting the distal tibiofibular ligament, and potentially injuring the deltoid ligament. Injury to the distal tibiofibular syndesmosis (i.e., a "high" ankle sprain) often goes undetected, resulting in a longer recovery time and a greater disability than with the more frequent lateral ankle sprain.

Signs and Symptoms

The area of maximum point tenderness usually is over the anterolateral tibiofibular joint but may also be posteromedial at the level of the ankle joint. The degree of pain and swelling can be significant. The individual will have difficulty bearing weight and pushing off the ground on the injured ankle. The most commonly injured ligament (and a source of anterolateral ankle impingement) is the anterior inferior tibiofibular ligament, and the least injured ligament is the posterior inferior tibiofibular ligament, although the interosseous ligament may also be variably injured.[21] Assessment rests on six specific tests:

1. Syndesmosis ligament palpation

2. Passive dorsiflexion test

3. Anterior and posterior translation of the fibula (fibula translation test)

4. Medial and lateral translation of the talus (Cotton test)

5. Stabilizing the lower leg with one hand while applying an external rotation force to the ankle (external rotation test)

6. Compressing the proximal tibia and fibula while asking about pain at the ankle ("squeeze test")

Management

Treatment for syndesmotic sprains is more conservative than treatment provided for a lateral ankle sprain. In the acute stage, the patient should be non–weight-bearing and be fitted for an ankle boot in order to immobilize the joint to allow for healing and repair of tissues.[11] Referral to a physician is warranted for radiographic confirmation to assess for fractures, bony avulsions (10% to 50% occur off the tibia), and the mortise alignment of the tibia, talus, and fibula. A grade I high ankle sprain is treated with immobilization in a long, semirigid pneumatic stirrup brace that extends to just below the knee for up to 3 weeks. The individual may return to physical activity with protective taping and a heel lift.[21] A grade II injury involves 3 to 6 weeks of non–weight bearing, including stabilization with a fracture brace for 3 to 4 weeks, followed by a pneumatic stirrup brace for an additional 3 weeks. Application of cold should continue until swelling is reduced. Initially, weight bearing should be permitted with crutches, and weaning off of the crutches is done as tolerated. Participation in sports and physical activity may be delayed for up to 3 months after the initial treatment begins. If the injury involves no fracture but widening of the joint mortise is seen on stress radiographs, surgery is recommended.[22]

Subtalar Sprain

Etiology

The ligaments associated with the lateral subtalar joint are the CFL (spanning both the ankle and subtalar joints), the inferior extensor retinaculum, the lateral talocalcaneal ligament, the cervical ligament (just anterior to the tibiocalcaneal), and the interosseous ligament. The most common mechanism is believed to be dorsiflexion and supination. This position places the CFL in a position of maximal tightness. Further supination can lead to rupture of the CFL, followed by tearing of the cervical ligament and the interosseous tibiocalcaneal ligament.[22]

Signs and Symptoms

The individual often complains of a sensation of the ankle "turning inward" or "turning over." Individuals with this problem consistently watch the ground when they walk and are uncomfortable when running on uneven surfaces. Assessment of chronic subtalar instability varies only slightly from that of ankle instability; the conditions may coexist. The anterior drawer test should be negative in isolated subtalar instability but positive with ankle instability. A subtle finding with subtalar instability, however, is increased rotation of the calcaneus under the talus on the anterior drawer test. A definitive diagnosis can be established only with stress radiographs.

Management

Conservative treatment includes standard acute care, strengthening of the peroneals, stretching the heel cord, proprioceptive training, and use of a brace if needed. Functional exercises should be incorporated earlier into the rehabilitation process for grade I and II ankle sprains.[11] High-grade subtalar sprains (as determined by examination and imaging studies) are treated with 2 weeks of non–weight bearing in a below-knee cast, followed by 4 weeks in a commercial walker boot.[22] Chronic instability may necessitate surgical repair.

Subtalar Dislocation

Etiology

Another serious sprain that involves the subtalar joint results from a fall from a height (as in basketball or volleyball). The foot lands in inversion, disrupting the interosseous talocalcaneal and talonavicular ligaments. If the foot lands in dorsiflexion and

The clinician should activate the emergency action plan, including summoning emergency medical services (EMS). While waiting for EMS to arrive, the clinician should monitor the patient for shock and treat as necessary. Neurovascular function should be monitored as well.

inversion, the CFL also is ruptured. When the dislocation occurs, the injury is better known as "basketball foot."

Signs and Symptoms

Extreme pain and total loss of function are present. Gross deformity at the subtalar joint may not be clearly visible. The foot may appear to be pale and feel cold to the touch if neurovascular damage is present. The individual may show signs of shock.

Management

Because of the potential for peroneal tendon entrapment and neurovascular damage, leading to reduced blood supply to the foot, this dislocation is considered to be a medical emergency.

> The immediate management of the grade II ankle sprain sustained by the 30-year-old recreational basketball player should include standard acute care (i.e., ice, compression, elevation, and protected rest). Application of a horseshoe pad or open basket weave strapping and an elastic wrap can be used for compression. The patient should be fitted with crutches and referred to a physician.

TENDINOPATHIES OF THE FOOT AND LOWER LEG

> A 55-year-old woman preparing to compete in a recreational badminton tournament reports to a sports medicine clinic complaining of pain and swelling behind the medial malleolus and of pain in the arch when arising in the morning. Observation reveals pes planus. During resisted muscle testing, plantar flexion and inversion are weak. What muscle is involved in this injury, and how should this condition be managed?

Tendinopathies of the foot and lower leg are relatively common and encompass a wide spectrum of conditions ranging from tendinitis to tenosynovitis to partial and complete ruptures. The tendons most often involved in the foot and ankle include the Achilles, posterior tibialis, peroneal brevis, and peroneal longus tendons. In contrast to acute traumatic tendinous injury, these injuries most often involve repetitive submaximal loading of the tissues, resulting in repetitive microtraumas.

Strains and Tendinitis

Etiology

Muscle strains seldom occur in the lower extremity, except in the gastrocnemius–soleus complex. Instead, injury occurs to the musculotendinous junction or to the tendon itself. Most of the tendons in the lower leg have a synovial sheath surrounding the tendon; the Achilles tendon, which has a peritendon sheath that is not synovial, is an exception. Several factors can predispose an individual to tendinitis (**Box 14.3**). Common sites for tendon injuries include the following:

■ The Achilles tendon just proximal to its insertion into the calcaneus

■ The tibialis posterior just behind the medial malleolus

■ The tibialis anterior on the dorsum of the foot just under the extensor retinaculum

■ The peroneal tendons just behind the lateral malleolus and at the distal attachment on the base of the 5th metatarsal

Signs and Symptoms

Common signs and symptoms include a history of stiffness following a period of inactivity (e.g., morning stiffness), localized tenderness over the tendon, possible swelling or thickness in the tendon and peritendon tissues, pain with passive stretching, and pain with active and resisted motion.

BOX 14.3 Predisposing Factors for Tendinitis in the Lower Leg

- Training errors that include the following:
  - Lack of flexibility in the gastrocnemius–soleus muscles
  - Poor training surface or sudden change from soft to hard surface, or vice versa
  - Sudden changes in training intensity or program (e.g., adding hills, sprints, or distance)
  - Inadequate work-to-rest ratio that may lead to early muscle fatigue
  - Returning to participation too quickly following injury
- Direct trauma
- Infection from a penetrating wound into the tendon
- Abnormal foot mechanics producing friction among the shoe, tendon, and bony structure
- Poor footwear that is not properly fitted to foot

Management

In the majority of cases, treatment of muscle strains, tendinitis, or peritendinitis is conservative. If mechanical problems are present, they should be addressed first so that recovery can occur. Early exercises should be within the levels of pain tolerance and should not be too strenuous. Ice massage, active ROM exercises with elastic tubing for resistance, stretching of the Achilles tendon, and eccentric calf exercises are recommended during the early phase of rehabilitation.

Foot Strains

Etiology

Foot strains, caused by a direct blow or chronic overuse, often affect the intrinsic and extrinsic muscles of the foot. The tibialis anterior and the toe extensor tendons may be injured as a result of having the feet repeatedly stepped on or by having the shoelaces tied too tightly.

Signs and Symptoms

Pain, localized edema, inflammation, and adhesions may be present. During assessment, the involved tendons have pain on passive stretching and with active and resisted motion. Palpation over the tendon during active motion may reveal a sound similar to that heard when crunching a snowball together; hence, the sound is called "snowball" crepitation.

Management

Treatment involves standard acute care, NSAIDs, and strapping to limit active motion of the tendon. ROM and strengthening exercises should be started after acute pain has subsided.

Peroneal Tendinopathies

Etiology

Peroneal tendon injuries are less common than injury to the Achilles and posterior tibial tendons. Mechanisms of injury may include forceful passive dorsiflexion, as occurs when a skier catches the tip of the ski and falls forward; exploding off a slightly pronated foot, as when a football player is in a three-point stance and makes a forward surge; or being kicked from behind in the vicinity of the lateral malleolus. Tendinitis of the peroneus longus causes pain as the tendon passes beneath the cuboid toward its insertion on the plantar aspect of the metatarsal. Another problem that may exist involves the retinaculum that holds the tendons in place on the posterior aspect of the lateral malleolus. If this retinaculum gives way, the tendons slip forward over the lateral malleolus but usually return spontaneously. This condition can be overlooked or confused with an ankle sprain because it gives a feeling of instability and pain over the lateral malleolus. Partial tears of both the peroneus longus and brevis tendons have been linked to persistent lateral ankle pain and chronic lateral ankle instability.[23]

Signs and Symptoms

During an acute injury in which the reticulum ruptures, a cracking sensation, followed by intense pain and an inability to walk, is reported. Swelling and tenderness is localized over the posterosuperior aspect of the lateral malleolus rather than the anteroinferior aspect, as in an inversion ankle sprain. A hallmark symptom is extreme discomfort or apprehension during attempted eversion of the foot against resistance. If done immediately after injury, the dislocated tendons may be palpated during resisted dorsiflexion and eversion; however, swelling may soon obscure the dislocation. In a chronic injury, the individual complains primarily of instability; a "giving way"; or a slippage around the ankle, with little discomfort.

Management

Treatment is symptomatic with standard acute care. Acute injuries may respond to cast immobilization. External padding and strapping may help to stabilize the tendons, but because of the high rate of recurrence in the active population, surgery often is required.

Posterior Tibialis Tendon Dysfunction

Etiology

Posterior tibialis tendon dysfunction (PTTD) reflects the loss of support from the spring, deltoid, and talocalcaneal interosseous ligaments as well as from the talonavicular capsule and the plantar fascia.[24] PTTD is a common cause of painful acquired flatfoot deformity and is associated with substantial functional problems leading to significant morbidity. Individuals with a planovalgus foot, or flatfoot with pronation and loss of arch, are predisposed to this common injury. These individuals frequently have a loss of hindfoot inversion and difficulty in negotiating uneven ground and in climbing and descending stairs. Unfortunately, the problem frequently is missed, because progressive pronation is insidious and relatively painless. Overuse occasionally superimposes an acute injury by producing longitudinal tears or tethering, leading to dysfunction.

Signs and Symptoms

Three levels of dysfunction have been identified in the posterior tibialis muscle. In stage I, the individual has pain and swelling along the course of the tendon. Pain, tenderness, and swelling also may be present behind the medial malleolus, and there may be an accompanying aching discomfort in the medial longitudinal arch. Because the length of the tendon is normal, a single heel raise can be performed. The flatfoot deformity is minimal, alignment of the hindfoot and forefoot is normal, and the subtalar joint remains flexible.

In stage II, the individual is unable to perform a single heel raise because of attenuation or disruption of the posterior tibial tendon. Weakness is evident in plantar flexion and inversion. The tendon is enlarged, elongated, and functionally incompetent. The foot adopts a pes planovalgus position (flatfoot) with collapse of the medial longitudinal arch, hindfoot valgus and subtalar eversion, and forefoot abduction through the talonavicular joint. The subtalar joint remains flexible, and with the ankle in plantar flexion, the talonavicular joint can be reduced.

Stage III presents with the individual being unable to perform a single heel raise and a more severe flatfoot deformity. The pes planovalgus deformity is fixed, and the laterally subluxed navicular cannot be reduced. If the tendon is ruptured, a painful pop is felt, resulting in an immediate flatfoot deformity (acquired pes planus).

Management

Early treatment of PTTD depends on the severity of injury and may include standard acute care, NSAIDs, restricted activity, and a corrective orthosis, such as the University of California

Biomechanics Laboratory brace, molded ankle–foot orthosis, or articulated molded ankle–foot orthosis.[24] The goal of early treatment is to control the progressive valgus of the calcaneus. Modalities (e.g., phonophoresis and iontophoresis, icing, and heat), eccentric strengthening, and hands-on physical therapy also are necessary early in the rehabilitation process. If nonoperative or conservative treatment fails, surgery is indicated, because the progression of dysfunction may be rapid and disabling. In the early stages of dysfunction, soft-tissue surgical procedures, such as tendon debridement or tenosynovectomy, may halt the progression of deterioration. Surgical release with tenolysis and/or augmentation by another tendon may be necessary early on to prevent irreversible bony/joint changes. Surgical procedures involving osteotomies and arthrodesis are necessary once a flatfoot deformity develops.[24]

Gastrocnemius Muscle Strain

Etiology

Strains to the medial head of the gastrocnemius often are seen in tennis players older than 40 years, hence, the nickname "tennis leg." Common mechanisms are forced dorsiflexion while the knee is extended, forced knee extension while the foot is dorsiflexed, and muscular fatigue with fluid-electrolyte depletion and muscle cramping.

If related to muscle cramping, the strain commonly is attributed to dehydration (particularly in the heat), electrolyte imbalance, or prolonged muscle fatigue that stimulates cramping followed by an actual tear in the muscle fibers. Acute spasms may awaken an individual in the night following a day of strenuous exercise. Acute cramps are best treated with ice, pressure, and slow stretch of the muscle as it begins to relax. Prevention of this condition involves adequate water intake during strenuous activity and a regular stretching program for the gastrocnemius–soleus complex. When participation extends over 2 hours in hot weather, increased water intake with a weak electrolyte solution should be ensured during and after strenuous activity.

Signs and Symptoms

In an acute strain, the individual experiences a sudden, painful, tearing sensation in the calf muscles, primarily at the musculotendinous junction between the muscles and Achilles tendon or in the medial head of the gastrocnemius muscle (**Fig. 14.28**). Immediate pain, swelling, loss of function, and stiffness are common. Later, ecchymosis progresses down the leg into the foot and ankle.

Management

Acute management consists of standard acute care to control inflammation, restricted activity, gentle stretching of the gastrocnemius, heel lifts, and a progressive strengthening program. In more severe cases, immobilization and non–weight bearing may be necessary to allow the muscle to heal fully.

Achilles Tendon Disorders

Etiology

Achilles tendon disorders occur most often in athletes and, of those, most often in individuals who are involved in running sports. Inappropriately generalized as "Achilles tendinitis," posterior heel pain resulting from an overuse injury of the foot and ankle actually encompasses a myriad of distinct and often coexisting pathological disorders with both inflammatory and degenerative etiologies. Common intrinsic risk factors that can predispose an individual to disorders of the Achilles tendon include several foot malalignment and biomechanical faults, such as hyperpronation of the foot;

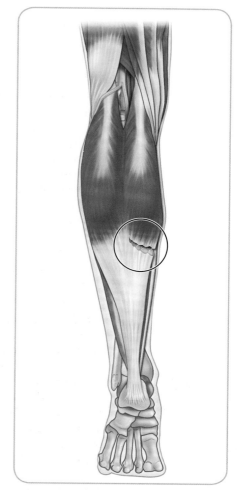

Figure 14.28. Gastrocnemius muscle strain. The medial head of the gastrocnemius muscle commonly is strained in individuals older than 40 years. A defect often can be palpated at the musculotendinous junction.

limited mobility of the subtalar joint and limited ROM of the ankle joint; leg length discrepancy; varus deformity of the forefoot and increased hindfoot inversion; decreased ankle dorsiflexion with the knee in extension; poor vascularity; genetic makeup; and gender, age, endocrine, or metabolic factors. Extrinsic factors that may lead to the disorder include changes in shoes or running surface; a sudden increase in workload (e.g., distance or intensity) or change in exercise environment (e.g., training on hard, slippery, or slanting surfaces); poor technique; and monotonous, asymmetric, and specialized training.[25]

When intrinsic and extrinsic factors are involved, microtraumatic changes occur in the Achilles tendon from different force contributions of the gastrocnemius and soleus, producing abnormal loading concentrations within the tendon and frictional forces between the fibrils leading to localized fiber damage. The tendon is relatively avascular at approximately 0.8 in (2 cm) above its distal insertion into the calcaneus, which is the site of the most torque on the tendon. This area is highly vulnerable to partial tears, with secondary nodule formation and degenerative cysts seen in **tendinosis**.

Signs and Symptoms

Acute signs and symptoms include an aching or burning pain in the posterior heel, which increases with passive dorsiflexion and resisted plantar flexion, such as going up onto the toes. Point tenderness and crepitus can be elicited at the bony insertion or 1 to 3 cm above the insertion. There also can be associated retrocalcaneal bursitis. Palpation may reveal local nodules either within the tendon, which moves during dorsiflexion and plantar flexion, or in the peritendon, which does not move during these motions.

Chronic signs and symptoms include pain that is worse after exercise within days of a change in activity levels or training techniques. The tendon often becomes thickened, and pain is localized on the posterolateral heel. The gastrocnemius–soleus complex is tight, which may result from tendon adhesions, muscle spasm, or inflexibility. Radiographs usually show a prominent posterosuperior calcaneus (Haglund deformity), and calcific spurring often occurs at the bone–tendon interface. Pathologically, the tendon demonstrates chronic degeneration rather than inflammation. Rest may relieve symptoms, but return to activity reactivates the pain, generally within a few training sessions.

A tendinopathy poses the risk of complete rupture of the tendon. Magnetic resonance imaging often is needed for accurate diagnosis.

Management

The goal of treatment is to minimize pain, prevent further degeneration, and allow the individual to return to baseline activity. Initial conservative treatment involves standard acute care, activity modification, and correcting factors that cause load imbalance and repetitive strain on the tendon and surrounding structures. Complete restriction of activity may be necessary for 3 weeks. Active stretching of the Achilles tendon before and after activity, along with a full strengthening program for the gastrocnemius–soleus complex, including eccentric loading, is initiated immediately after acute pain has subsided. Use of oral NSAIDs or steroidal pain relievers to control inflammation remains controversial. Recently, some success has been seen in ultrasound-guided injections of polidocanol, a sclerosing agent, to decrease the neovascularization and symptoms of chronic midportion Achilles tendinosis.[26] Operative treatment is recommended for individuals who do not respond to a 3- to 6-month trial of appropriate conservative treatment. Surgery usually involves excision of fibrotic adhesions and degenerated nodules or decompression of the tendon by longitudinal tenotomies.[27]

Achilles Tendon Rupture

Etiology

Acute rupture of the Achilles tendon probably is the most severe acute muscular problem in the lower leg. It more commonly is seen in individuals from 30 to 50 years of age.[28] The usual mechanism is a push-off of the forefoot while the knee is extending, which is a common move in many propulsive activities. Tendinous ruptures usually occur 1 to 2 in proximal to the distal attachment of the tendon on the calcaneus.

Signs and Symptoms

The individual hears and feels a characteristic "pop" in the posterior ankle and reports a feeling of being shot or kicked in the heel. Clinical signs and symptoms include a visible defect in the tendon, inability to stand on tiptoes or even balance on the affected leg, swelling and bruising around the malleoli, excessive passive dorsiflexion, and a positive Thompson test (**Fig. 14.18**). Because the peroneal longus, peroneal brevis, and muscles in the deep posterior compartment are still intact, the individual may limp or walk with the foot and leg externally rotated, because this does not require push-off with the superficial calf muscles.

Management

A compression wrap should be applied from the toes to the knee. The leg and foot can be immobilized in a posterior splint. The individual should be referred immediately to a physician. Nonoperative treatment offers excellent functional results for partial tears in older, noncompetitive individuals. With delayed diagnosis or in highly competitive individuals, surgical repair provides better push-off strength and prevents over elongation of the tendon and, in doing so, lowers the risk for reinjury. The course of action depends on the supervising physician, but in either case, full ROM and strength may not be achieved until 6 months after the injury.

The 55-year-old badminton player has tenosynovitis of the tibialis posterior. Pes planus, along with weakness in plantar flexion and inversion, provide evidence of the muscle involved. Management of the condition includes standard acute care. In addition, the patient should be advised to wear shoes with better arch support. If the condition does not improve, the patient should be referred to a physician.

OVERUSE CONDITIONS

? A slightly overweight, novice runner is in the third week of training for a 10K run. He reports the following symptoms: excruciating pain in the anteromedial hindfoot on arising in the morning, which disappears within 5 to 10 minutes; point tenderness just distal to the medial calcaneal tubercle; and pain that increases with weight bearing. What condition may be present, and how should this injury be managed?

Repetitive microscopic injury to tendinous structures can lead to chronic inflammation that overwhelms the tissue's ability to repair itself. Other factors, such as faulty biomechanics, poor cushioning or stiff-soled shoes, or excessive downhill running, also can inflame the tendons. Several overuse conditions are common in specific sports, such as plantar fasciitis in running; medial tibial stress syndrome in football, dance, or running; and exertional compartment syndrome in soccer or distance running. Many individuals complain of vague leg pain but have no history of a specific injury that caused the pain, differentiating these conditions from an acute muscle strain. A common complaint is pain caused by activity.

Plantar Fasciitis

Etiology

Plantar fasciitis is the most common hindfoot problem in runners and affects approximately 10% of the population during the course of a lifetime.[29] Extrinsic factors that increase the incidence of the condition include training errors, improper footwear, and participating on unyielding surfaces. Intrinsic factors include pes cavus or pes planus, decreased planar flexion strength, reduced flexibility of the plantar flexor muscles (e.g., Achilles tendon), excessive or prolonged pronation, and torsional malalignment. These factors can overload the plantar fascia's origin on the anteromedial aspect of the calcaneus during weight-bearing activities. In a chronic condition, entrapment of the first branch of the lateral plantar nerve can contribute to the pain syndrome. Entrapment of the posterior tibial or medial calcaneal nerve (i.e., tarsal tunnel syndrome) may mimic or complicate the condition.

Signs and Symptoms

The individual reports pain on the plantar, medial heel that is relieved with activity but that recurs after rest. Pain increases with weight bearing and may radiate up the medial side of the heel and, occasionally, across the lateral side of the foot. It is particularly severe with the first few steps in the morning, particularly in the proximal, plantar, medial heel, but diminishes within 5 to 10 minutes. Pain and stiffness are related to muscle spasm and splinting of the fascia secondary to inflammation. Point tenderness is elicited over or just distal to the medial tubercle of the calcaneus and increases with passive great toe extension and dorsiflexion of the ankle. If the lateral plantar nerve is involved, tenderness also is noted at the proximal, superior abductor hallucis muscle. A tight heel cord with decreased dorsiflexion of the ankle is seen in approximately 70% of patients who have unilateral symptoms.[30]

Management

Treatment involves standard acute care. Following completion of the inflammatory stage, therapeutic modalities used to alleviate symptoms may include ice, deep friction massage, ultrasound, and electrical muscle stimulation. Achilles tendon stretching exercises, stretching of the toe flexor tendons, strengthening of the peroneal and posterior tibial muscles, NSAIDs, and a soft heel lift may be helpful. A moleskin plantar fascia strap or figure eight arch strapping is an effective means of support. Circular strips of tape around the foot are contraindicated, however, because they may overstretch the fascia and prolong recovery. Use of a viscoelastic heel cushion and/or orthoses along with a corticosteroid injection may be needed. Night splinting to hold the heel cord under mild tension may be used as well. Surgery or noninvasive ultrasonic treatment should be considered after 6 to 12 months.[16] **Application Strategy 14.5** highlights the management of plantar fasciitis.

Medial Tibial Stress Syndrome

Etiology

Medial tibial stress syndrome (MTSS) is a **periostitis** along the posteromedial tibial border, usually in the distal third that is not associated with a stress fracture or compartment syndrome. MTSS is one of the most common causes of exercise-induced leg pain.[2] Although originally thought to be related to stress along the posterior tibialis muscle and tendon causing myositis, fasciitis, and periostitis, it is now believed to be related to periostitis of the soleus insertion along the posteromedial tibial border or the flexor digitorum longus. The soleus makes up the medial third of the heel cord as it inserts into the calcaneus. Excessive or prolonged pronation of the foot causes an eccentric contraction of the soleus, resulting in the periostitis that produces the pain. Other contributing factors include recent changes in running distance, speed, form, stretching, footwear, and running surface and being female.[31]

APPLICATION STRATEGY 14.5

Management of Plantar Fasciitis

- Use immediate ice therapy and NSAIDs.
- Use a shock-absorbing soft heel pad or soft plantar arch pad.
- Figure eight arch strapping or night splints may relieve acute symptoms.
- Use aggressive Achilles tendon stretching for 2–4 minutes, three to four times a day, with the toes straight ahead, the toes in, and the toes out.
- Use gentle isometric contractions initially for intrinsic muscles of the foot.
- Progress to active ROM exercise within pain-free ranges: toe curls, marble pick-up, towel crunches, and towel curls.
- Strengthen the intrinsic and extrinsic leg muscles.
- Maintain body fitness and strength, as well as aerobic fitness, with non–weight-bearing activities.
- The physician may administer cortisone injections into the plantar fascia aponeurosis.

Signs and Symptoms

Typically seen in runners or jumpers, the pain can occur at any point in the workout and typically is characterized as a dull ache, although it occasionally can be sharp and penetrating. As activity continues, pain diminishes only to recur hours after activity has ceased. During later stages, pain is present before, during, and after activity and may restrict performance. Point tenderness is elicited in a 3- to 6-cm area along the distal posteromedial tibial border. Pain is aggravated by resisted plantar flexion or by standing on tiptoe. An associated varus alignment of the lower extremity, including a greater Achilles tendon angle, often is present. In experienced runners, the condition usually is secondary to mechanical abnormalities, such as the following:

- Increased Achilles tendon angle (during stance phase and while running)
- Greater Achilles tendon angle between heel strike and maximal pronation
- Greater passive subtalar motion in inversion and eversion

Management

To relieve acute symptoms, 5 to 7 days of rest are essential. Other modalities (e.g., cryotherapy, NSAIDs, cortisone injections, heel pads, casting, crutches, and activity modification) have not been shown to be as effective as rest alone. Pain-free stretching of both the anterior and posterior musculature helps to improve joint mobility, increase muscle and tendon strength as well as coordination, and aid the musculoskeletal system in adapting to the physical demands of a specific sport. If the condition does not improve, possible stress fractures to the tibia should be ruled out through appropriate radiograph or scanning procedures. Analysis of the individual's running motion, foot alignment, running surface, and footwear may prevent recurrence. **Application Strategy 14.6** summarizes the management of MTSS.

Exertional Compartment Syndrome

Etiology

Exertional compartment syndrome (ECS) is characterized by exercise-induced pain and swelling that is relieved by rest. The two most frequently affected compartments are the anterior and deep posterior, but the lateral, superficial posterior, and "fifth" compartment around the tibialis posterior muscle may also be affected. Whereas acute ECS generally occurs in relatively sedentary people who undertake strenuous exercise, chronic ECS usually is seen in well-conditioned individuals younger than 40 years.

Signs and Symptoms

Chronic ECS is often described as a tight, cramp-like, or squeezing ache and sense of fullness, both of which are felt over the involved compartment. The condition often affects both legs. Symptoms are relieved with rest, usually within 20 minutes of exercise, only to recur if exercise is resumed.

APPLICATION STRATEGY 14.6

Management of Medial Tibial Stress Syndrome

- Five to 7 days of rest is essential.
- Ice, compression, elevation, and NSAIDs may help to relieve acute symptoms.
- Determine if a stress fracture is present.
- Evaluate and correct any foot malalignment or problems in technique.
- Change the running surface and, possibly, shoes.
- Increase muscle flexibility in the anterior and posterior compartments.
- Increase strength in all muscles of the lower leg and foot.

Activity-related pain begins at a predictable time after starting exercise or after reaching a certain level of intensity, and the pain increases if the training persists. Many individuals with anterior compartment involvement describe mild foot drop or paresthesia (or both) on the dorsum of the foot and demonstrate fascial defects or hernias, usually in the distal third of the leg over the intramuscular septum.

Evaluation should be performed after the individual has exercised strenuously enough to reproduce the symptoms. The exercise produces swelling and tenderness in the involved compartments and increased leg girth. Tenderness, if present, may be located in the middle third of the tibia, although many individuals have no focal pain. Vibration with a tuning fork produces no pain, as one typically sees in a stress fracture. Likewise, pain is not present in the distal leg, which corresponds with MTSS. To confirm the diagnosis, intracompartmental pressure must be measured (see "Acute Compartment Syndrome" section).

Management

Treatment involves assessing extrinsic factors (e.g., training patterns, technique, shoe design, and training surface) and intrinsic factors (e.g., foot alignment, especially hindfoot pronation, muscle imbalance, and flexibility). In minor conditions, ice massage, NSAIDs, and occasionally, diuretics may assist, along with stretching and strengthening of the involved compartment muscles, orthotics, and relative rest. If symptoms persist for 6 to 12 weeks of conservative care, or in cases with extreme pressure elevation, fasciotomy is recommended; unlike a fasciotomy for acute ECS, this may be limited to complete release of the involved compartments.

The runner may have plantar fasciitis. As part of the assessment, it is important to check foot alignment, gait, and shoes for problems that may have contributed to the condition. Stretching of the toe flexors and Achilles tendon should be a major part of the treatment plan.

VASCULAR AND NEURAL DISORDERS

? A figure skater is complaining of bilateral numbness in the posterolateral aspect of the leg along the Achilles tendon that has been present for the past 2 to 3 weeks. No history of trauma to the ankle is noted. The skater reveals that she routinely spirals her laces tightly around the proximal portion of each boot and then applies several circular bands of white tape to hold them in place. Could this technique impair the vascular or neural function of the lower leg, and how should this situation be managed?

Vascular and neural disorders of the lower leg are rare in sports but can occur. Vascular disorders typically involve occlusion of venous blood in the calf region; neural involvement typically affects the distal ankle and foot region. In either case, any change in circulation, sensation, or function should signal referral to a physician.

Venous Disorders
Etiology

By way of contraction of smooth and skeletal muscles, blood within the superficial venous system, as well as the deep venous system, is pushed, or "milked," back to the heart and lungs for elimination or metabolism. In some cases, particularly with inactivity following fracture or surgery, prolonged bed rest, and increasing age, this system becomes inefficient, leading to a reduced blood flow. The accumulated blood products may form a clot that can grow in size, depending on the vessel in which it is contained, causing partial or complete blockage. When symptoms are present for 14 days or fewer or when imaging studies confirm the condition, it is called acute DVT.[32] The deep calf veins are most frequently involved, but involvement of the popliteal, superficial femoral, and iliofemoral vein segments also is common. An **embolism** occurs when a loosened thrombus circulates from a larger vessel to a smaller one, subsequently obstructing circulation. When the obstruction occurs in the veins of the lungs, it is called a pulmonary embolism. Because the risk factors for DVT include a sedentary lifestyle, smoking, obesity, and prolonged periods of inactivity, DVT rarely is seen in an active population.[33]

Signs and Symptoms

DVT typically is asymptomatic and may not become apparent until a pulmonary embolism occurs. The most reliable signs are paresthesia in the area, chronic swelling and edema in the involved extremity, engorged veins, ecchymosis formation with a blue hue, and a positive Homans sign.

Management

Immediate referral to a physician is warranted. Treatment involves anticoagulant therapy, leg elevation, compression stockings, and ambulation in individuals who are clinically stable and for whom it is medically indicated. Functional neuromuscular stimulation of the gastrocnemius and tibialis anterior may help to activate the physiologic muscle pump while moving venous blood back to the central circulation to prevent DVT.

Neurological Conditions

Impingement of nerves in the lower leg and foot is rare but does happen. Three such conditions involve the compression of the interdigital nerves as they bifurcate at the metatarsal heads (i.e., plantar interdigital neuroma), the posterior tibial nerve beneath the flexor retinaculum and behind the medial malleolus (i.e., tarsal tunnel syndrome), and the sural nerve as it courses behind the lateral malleolus and into the lateral aspect of the foot.

Plantar Interdigital Neuroma

■ Etiology

A plantar interdigital neuroma (i.e., Morton neuroma) is a common source of forefoot pain and is 10 times more common in women than in men; women in their 30s and 40s who wear high-fashion shoes are particularly vulnerable.[34] Trauma or repetitive stress caused by tight-fitting shoes or a pronated foot can lead to abnormal pressure on the plantar digital nerves as they are compressed between the metatarsal heads and transverse intermetatarsal ligament. It typically occurs at the web space between the 3rd and 4th metatarsals (i.e., second and third intermetatarsal spaces) and, to a lesser extent, between the 2nd and 3rd metatarsals (**Fig. 14.29**).

■ Signs and Symptoms

The individual may initially describe a sensation of having a stone or hot coal in the shoe that worsens when standing. Tingling or burning, radiating to the toes, along with intermittent symptoms of a sharp, shock-like sensation into the involved toes is commonly reported. Pain subsides when activity is stopped or when the shoe is removed. In fact, the desire to remove the shoe and massage the foot is a classic indicator of

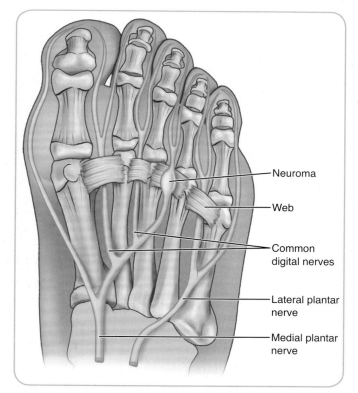

Figure 14.29. Plantar's neuroma. Plantar's neuroma (Morton neuroma) is caused by pinching of the interdigital nerve between the metatarsal heads. While weight bearing in shoes, the individual has an agonizing pain on the lateral side of the foot that is relieved when barefoot.

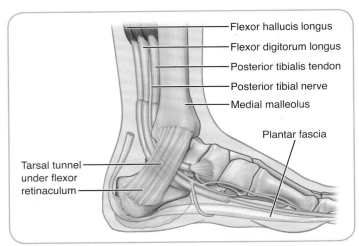

Figure 14.30. Tarsal tunnel syndrome. The posterior tibial nerve can become constricted beneath the tarsal tunnel roof formed by the flexor retinaculum.

a neuroma. The clinician may be able to palpate a painful mass, elicit increased pain by squeezing the mass between the index finger and thumb.[14]

■ Management

Conservative management involves a metatarsal pad placed just proximal to the metatarsal heads and wearing a broad, soft-soled shoe with a low heel. The focus is to preserve and maximize flexion at the lesser toe MTP joints to prevent and treat the condition. NSAIDs and massage over the affected area once or twice a day may also help. Local corticosteroid injections or surgical excision of the nerve may be necessary to remedy persistent pain.[34]

Tarsal Tunnel Syndrome

■ Etiology

Tarsal tunnel syndrome occurs when the posterior tibial nerve, or one of its branches, becomes constricted beneath the fibrous roof of the flexor retinaculum of the foot (**Fig. 14.30**). Entrapment most often occurs at the anteroinferior aspect of the canal, where the nerve winds around the medial malleolus. Space-occupying lesions that have been identified as causes for tarsal tunnel syndrome include ganglions, varicosities, lipomas, tenosynovitis, fibrosis, and synovial hypertrophy.[35] The lateral plantar nerve branch tends to be affected more frequently than the medial branch. The condition often is linked to hyperpronation or an excessive heel varus or valgus deformity that leads to stress or traction on the nerve with impingement.

■ Signs and Symptoms

Clinically, the individual complains of tingling and/or numbness around the medial malleolus radiating into the sole and heel (particularly with entrapment of the lateral plantar nerve) and hyperesthesia in the distribution of the posterior tibial nerve. The pain is often worse with activity, certain shoes that the patient may find aggravating, or standing, and the pain can be relieved by rest.[35] Hyperdorsiflexion, external rotation, and eversion may reproduce symptoms similar to those during provocative tests for carpal tunnel syndrome. One of the most reliable signs is a positive Tinel sign—namely, tingling elicited by tapping along the course of the nerve (**Fig. 14.19**).

■ Management

Conservative management involves rest, NSAIDs, orthoses (especially in individuals with hyperpronation), and gradual return to activity. A one-time injection of cortisone and lidocaine without epinephrine may be given into the tarsal tunnel, but if symptoms persist and other causes of heel pain are eliminated, surgical release may be necessary to relieve symptoms. Rehabilitation takes longer than with carpal tunnel syndrome because of the dependent weight-bearing requirements.[16]

Sural Nerve Entrapment

Etiology

The sural nerve, which is formed from branches of the tibial and peroneal nerves, provides cutaneous innervation to the lateral lower leg and foot. It passes distally along the lateral margin of the Achilles tendon to emerge from the fascia of the leg proximal to the lateral malleolus. After providing lateral calcaneal branches to the ankle and heel, the nerve passes behind the lateral malleolus and continues along the lateral border of the foot to extend to the fifth toe as the lateral dorsal cutaneous nerve. In addition to being vulnerable to compression from tight-fitting skates, boots, and shoes, the nerve can be irritated by fibrous adhesions that result from repetitive inversion ankle injuries or by ganglia that may form in the peroneal tendon sheath. Peripheral sural nerve neuropathy related to diabetes also may be a cause of paresthesia in this area.

Signs and Symptoms

Symptoms of sural nerve involvement include numbness in the affected area with decreased temperature sensation along the dorsolateral aspect of the foot, a burning sensation, local tenderness over the sural nerve, and reproduction of the symptoms by compression over the nerve (i.e., positive Tinel sign).

Management

Conservative treatment may be as simple as changing the lacing of the skates, boots, or shoes; however, surgical intervention may be necessary to correct the problem.

 The figure skater may have compressed the sural nerve with the tight laces and tape. The individual should be referred to a physician to determine the extent of injury to the nerve. The skater should be advised to change the way that she laces her boots.

FRACTURES

 In addition to Sever disease, what conditions could lead to heel pain in young athletes?

Fractures in the foot and lower leg region seldom result from a single traumatic episode. Often, repetitive microtraumas lead to apophyseal or stress fractures. Tensile forces associated with severe ankle sprains can lead to avulsion fractures of the 5th metatarsal, or severe twisting can lead to displaced and undisplaced fractures in the foot, ankle, or lower leg. A combination of forces can lead to a traumatic fracture dislocation.

Freiberg Disease

Etiology

Freiberg disease is a painful avascular necrosis of the second or, rarely, third metatarsal head that often is seen in active adolescents aged 14 to 18 years before closure of the epiphysis.

Signs and Symptoms

The condition can lead to diffuse pain in the forefoot region.

Management

Early detection is best treated by a metatarsal pad or bar to unload the involved metatarsal head and activity modification to eliminate excessive running and jumping. If pain persists and deformity develops with degenerative osteophytes, surgical resection of the distal metatarsal head may be necessary.

Sever Disease

Etiology

Sever disease, or calcaneal apophysitis, frequently is seen in 7- to 10-year-old children. It is associated with growth spurts, decreased heel cord and hamstring flexibility, and other biomechanical abnormalities contributing to poor shock absorption (e.g., forefoot varus, hallux valgus, pes cavus, pes planus, and more commonly, forefoot pronation). Because the apophyseal plate is vertically oriented, it is particularly susceptible to shearing stresses from the gastrocnemius. Hard surfaces, poor-quality or worn-out athletic shoes, being kicked in the region, or landing off-balance also may precipitate the condition.

Signs and Symptoms

The individual complains of unilateral or bilateral, intermittent or continuous, posterior heel pain that occurs shortly after beginning a new sport or season. Pain tends to be worse during and after activity but improves with rest. Although gait may be normal, the child may walk with a limp or exhibit a forceful heel strike. Point tenderness can be elicited at or just anterior to the insertion of the Achilles tendon along the posterior border of the calcaneus. Mediolateral compression (i.e., squeeze test) of the calcaneus over the lower third of the posterior calcaneus elicits pain, as does standing on the tiptoes (i.e., positive Sever sign). Heel cord flexibility is tested by passive dorsiflexion of the foot with the knee extended. Other conditions that may lead to heel pain should be ruled out before determining the treatment plan (**Box 14.4**).

Management

Following standard acute care, the individual should be referred to a physician for further care. The condition usually resolves itself with closure of the apophysis. Until that time, rest, ice, NSAIDs, heel lifts, heel cups, strapping the foot in slight plantar flexion to relieve some strain on the Achilles tendon, and activity modification usually relieve symptoms. Heel cord flexibility and strengthening exercises of the dorsiflexors are recommended. Resistant cases may benefit from a nighttime dorsiflexion splint.

Stress Fractures

Stress fractures often are seen in running and jumping activities, particularly after a significant increase in training mileage or a change in surface, intensity, or shoe type. Women with **amenorrhea** of longer than 6 months' duration and **oligomenorrhea** have a higher incidence of stress fractures of the foot and leg; however, women who use oral contraceptives tend to have significantly fewer stress fractures compared with nonusers.[16]

Stress fractures can be generally classified as noncritical and critical. Noncritical stress fractures of the lower leg, foot, and ankle include the medial tibia; fibula; and the 2nd, 3rd, and 4th metatarsals. The neck of the 2nd metatarsal is the most common location for a stress fracture, although it also is seen on the 4th and 5th metatarsals. Critical stress fractures require special attention because of a higher rate of nonunion. Common sites include the anterior tibia, medial malleolus, talus, navicular, 5th metatarsal, and sesamoids.

Etiology

Stress fractures of the lower leg, ankle, and foot are commonly caused by repetitive stress that leads to a summation point in the bone accompanying muscle fatigue, a change in ground surfaces (moving from grass to pavement), or an overload caused by muscle contraction. The resulting loss in shock absorption increases stress on the bone and periosteum. In the tibia, most stress fractures occur at the junction of the middle and distal thirds (most common site), the posteromedial tibial plateau, or just distal to the tibial tuberosity. Fibular stress fractures usually occur in the distal metadiaphyseal region. Because the fibula has a minimal role in weight bearing, it is believed that fibular stress fractures result from muscle traction and torsional forces.[25]

Signs and Symptoms

Pain from a stress fracture begins insidiously, increasing with activity and decreasing with rest; pain usually is limited to the fracture site. A stress fracture of the talus, for example, commonly involves the lateral body near the junction of the body with the lateral process of the talus. The patient may present with prolonged pain (i.e., several months in duration) following an ankle sprain despite full rehabilitation. Excessive subtalar pronation is felt to predispose an individual to talar stress fractures by allowing impingement of the lateral process of the calcaneus on the concave posterolateral corner of the talus.[25] Stress fractures of the calcaneus produce significant pain on heel strike. The individual often has a history of a substantial increase in the individual's activity level, particularly in distance runners. Palpation reveals maximum pain on the medial and lateral aspects of the plantar-calcaneal tuberosity. The most common site is the upper posterior margin, just anterior to the apophyseal plate and at a right angle to the normal trabecular pattern.[25] Squeezing the calcaneus produces pain.

Stress fractures of the navicular are seen in jumpers, ballet dancers, and equestrians because of the nature of foot positions as well as the motions and inevitable stresses that are produced in the midfoot. Often seen in young men, this fracture is difficult to assess. A high degree of suspicion is required when an individual complains of generalized foot pain on the dorsomedial aspect of the midfoot brought on by activity and relieved with rest. During the advanced stages, overlying swelling and pain on walking become evident.

The two sesamoid bones of the great toe can carry threefold the body's weight with leg-based activity. These bones often are fractured as a result of constant weight bearing on a hyperextended great toe or because of prolonged pronation during running. Individuals with pes cavus or tight plantar fascia are predisposed to this injury because of the large tensile forces placed on the bones. Pain and swelling are present on the ball of the foot, and the individual is unable to roll through the foot to stand on the toes. Radiographs may be inconclusive, because it is common in the general population for sesamoid bones to be bipartite.

Management

Pain can be elicited with percussion, a tuning fork, or ultrasound over the fracture site. Encircling the forefoot or calcaneus with the hand and squeezing the fingers together produce added discomfort. Following standard acute care, the individual should be referred to a physician. Frequently, early radiographs are negative, but periosteal reaction or cortical thickening can be seen 2 to 4 weeks later (**Fig. 14.31**). Bone scans and magnetic resonance images are more sensitive and usually reveal the presence of a fracture long before it becomes evident on radiographs.

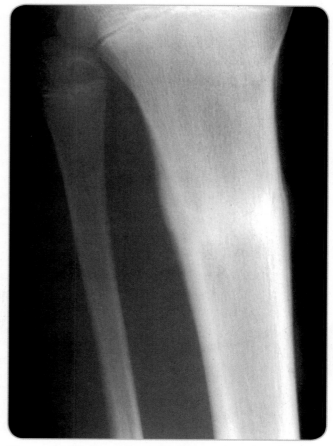

Figure 14.31. Stress fractures. Notice the sclerosis and widened cortices associated with bone healing.

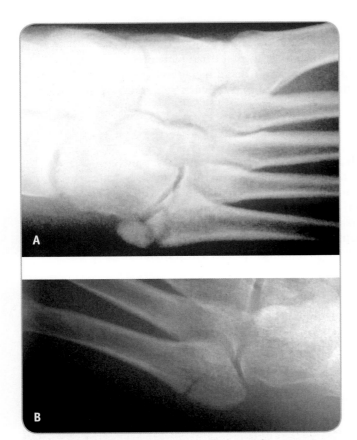

Figure 14.32. Avulsion fractures. A, A type I transverse fracture into the proximal shaft of the 5th metatarsal often is overlooked in cases of an inversion ankle sprain, resulting in a nonunion fracture. **B,** A type II fracture involves the styloid process of the 5th metatarsal.

Treatment usually requires relative rest, ice therapy, NSAIDs, stretching and strengthening exercises, and correcting any mechanical abnormalities that may have contributed to the condition. Protected weight bearing, a stiff shoe, a rigid orthosis, or a walking cast may be indicated in fractures of the metatarsals, calcaneus, or tibia. Wearing stiff-soled shoes or a heel cup may be helpful in cases with stress fractures of the sesamoid bones and calcaneus, respectively. The individual should be completely asymptomatic before returning to participation, which generally is seen in 6 to 8 weeks.

Avulsion Fractures

Etiology

Avulsion fractures may occur at the site of any ligamentous or tendinous attachment and as a result of a sudden, powerful twist or stretch of the body part. Severe eversion ankle sprains may cause the deltoid ligament to avulse a portion of the distal medial malleolus rather than tearing of the ligament. Inversion ankle sprains can provide sufficient overload to cause the plantar aponeurosis or peroneus brevis tendon to be pulled from the bone, avulsing the base of the 5th metatarsal (i.e., the so-called dancer's fracture). If the styloid process is avulsed, it is called a type II fracture and has an excellent prognosis, with healing occurring within 4 to 6 weeks.

Signs and Symptoms

Avulsion fractures are painful directly over the fracture site. Pain increases with a traction force applied to the joint or bony attachment. A much more complicated avulsion fracture that is seen in sprinters and jumpers involves a type I transverse fracture into the proximal shaft of the 5th metatarsal at the junction of the diaphysis and metaphysis, called a **Jones fracture** (**Fig. 14.32**). It often is overlooked in conjunction with a severe ankle sprain that involves plantar flexion and a strong adduction force to the forefoot. Because of low vascularization and high stresses at this site, Jones fractures are associated with a poor outcome; nonunions and delayed unions are common.

Management

Following standard acute care, the individual should be referred to a physician. Treatment involves non–weight-bearing immobilization for 6 to 10 weeks, followed by use of a walking cast or orthosis for an additional 4 weeks. Physical activity should be avoided until clinical and radiographic evidence of union appears, typically by 8 to 12 weeks. Displaced fractures may require open reduction and internal fixation. After screw fixation, progressive weight bearing is initiated at 2 weeks, with return to running in 7 weeks. When bone grafting is used, running activities are delayed for 12 weeks to allow bony healing.[25]

Osteochondral Fracture of the Talus

Etiology

Severe ankle sprains can impinge the dome of the talus against the malleoli, leading to a fracture of the cartilaginous cover. Anterolateral fractures account for 43% of osteochondral lesions, are wafer-shaped, and result from forceful inversion and dorsiflexion. Posteromedial fractures account for 57% of osteochondral fractures and are cup-shaped. They result from forceful inversion and plantar flexion (**Fig. 14.33**). The fragment may remain nondisplaced or float freely in the joint. Osteochondritis dissecans of the talus can develop if the fragment, particularly one of the corners, floats freely in the ankle joint, thus losing its blood supply.

Signs and Symptoms

Symptoms may be nonspecific and include a deep, aching pain that is aggravated by activity, recurrent ankle swelling, ankle instability and stiffness, occasional crepitus, clicking, and locking (if displaced). Passive plantar flexion and palpation of the anterolateral and posteromedial corner of the talus elicit point tenderness. A palpable lesion or crepitus may be felt on the corners.

Management

If pain and joint effusion persist after an inversion ankle sprain or ankle fracture, or if symptoms return after an asymptomatic period, a more serious underlying condition should be suspected, and referral to a physician is warranted. Limited weight bearing (and/or immobilization) and NSAIDs are used to treat undisplaced fractures. Arthroscopic excision or repair usually is necessary in cases with displaced fractures.

Displaced Fractures and Fracture Dislocations

Severe fractures result from direct compression in acute trauma (e.g., falling from a height or being stepped on) or from combined compression and shearing forces (e.g., as occurs during a severe twisting action). Because of the proximity of major blood vessels and nerves, many displaced and undisplaced fractures necessitate immediate immobilization and referral to the nearest trauma center.

Forefoot Fractures

Etiology

Phalangeal fractures are caused by an axial load (e.g., jamming the toe into an immovable object) or direct trauma (e.g., crushing injury). Most are minor injuries, with the exception of a fracture to the great toe.

Signs and Symptoms

Metatarsal fractures are classified according to their anatomical location (i.e., neck, shaft, or base). A single fracture tends to be minimally displaced because of the restraining forces of the intermetatarsal ligaments.

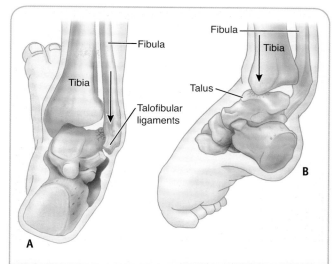

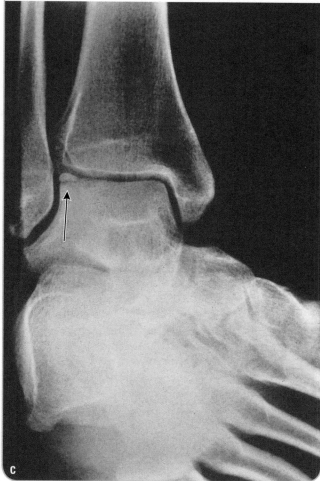

Figure 14.33. Osteochondral fractures. A, Forceful inversion of a dorsiflexed ankle can produce damage to the anterolateral talar dome. **B,** Forceful inversion of a plantar-flexed ankle can produce damage to the posteromedial aspect of the dome. **C,** Radiograph of an osteochondral lesion on the lateral aspect of the talus.

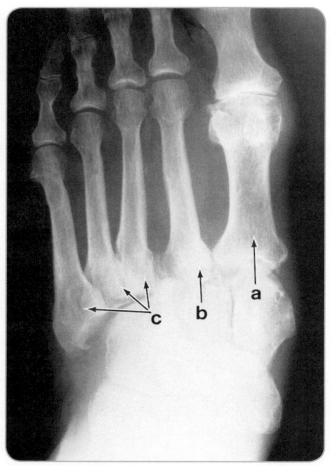

Figure 14.34. Lisfranc injury. Radiograph of a Lisfranc injury: *(a)* 1st metatarsal; *(b)* 2nd metatarsal; and *(c)* 3rd, 4th, and 5th metatarsals, which have been dislocated laterally.

Swelling and pain are localized over the fracture site, and pain increases with weight bearing. Swelling, ecchymosis, and pain are present; the individual is able to walk but may have problems with footwear. Most tenderness resolves in 3 to 4 weeks.

Management

If the bony fragment is nondisplaced, buddy padding, splinting, and wearing a wooden shoe or a shoe with a wide toe box may help. If the great toe is fractured, a walking cast with a toe plate, or a wooden shoe and crutches, is helpful; if displaced, surgery may be necessary to prevent osteoarthritis. Metatarsal fractures are treated with a short slipper cast or wooden shoe for 6 weeks, with weight bearing as tolerated.

Tarsal Fractures

Lisfranc Injury

■ Etiology

A **Lisfranc injury** involves disruption of the tarsometatarsal joint, with or without an associated fracture, and is notorious for delayed diagnosis (**Fig. 14.34**). The typical mechanism is a severe twisting injury (e.g., a football player falls onto the heel of another player's plantar-flexed foot) that causes an axial load along the metatarsals.

■ Signs and Symptoms

The 1st metatarsal typically is dislocated from the first cuneiform, whereas the other four metatarsals are laterally displaced, usually in combination with a fracture at the base of the 2nd metatarsal. Because the supply of blood to the forefoot can be compromised by the dislocation and subsequent swelling, a compartment syndrome may develop and create a serious injury. If assessed soon after the injury, the fracture may appear to be unremarkable until massive swelling sets in. A history of severe midfoot pain, paresthesia, or swelling along the midfoot region with variable flattening of the arch or abduction of the forefoot should signal a serious condition.

■ Management

A nondisplaced Lisfranc injury can be treated in a short-leg, nonwalking cast for 6 weeks, followed by 6 weeks in a short-leg, walking cast. Most injuries require open reduction and internal fixation.

Talus Fracture

■ Etiology

A fracture of the lateral process of the talus and neck of the talus, which is rare, is caused by acute hyperdorsiflexion with inversion. Posterior fractures of the talus are seen in individuals aged 15 to 30 years, particularly in those activities requiring forced plantar flexion of the foot, such as ballet or soccer, and may be either acute or stress-related.

■ Signs and Symptoms

Severe posterior pain is present when jumping, running, or kicking with the instep of the foot, and this pain is increased on forced plantar flexion and resisted great toe flexion, stemming from the close proximity of the flexor hallucis longus tendon to the fractured process. Moderate to severe edema, tenderness, and ecchymosis may be present.

■ Management
Because of the potential devastating complication of avascular necrosis of the talus, talar neck fractures need immediate immobilization and referral to a physician.

Calcaneus Fractures

■ Etiology
Traumatic fractures of the calcaneus are rare, but when they do occur, such fractures commonly are caused by high-energy axial loads. Occasionally, fractures occur at the anterior process either by forceful plantar flexion and adduction or by compression. Nearly 75% of calcaneus fractures extend into the subtalar joint.

■ Signs and Symptoms
Symptoms include severe heel pain, an inability to walk, and palpable, intense pain directly over the process, located just distal to the sinus tarsi.

■ Management
Initial treatment of intra-articular fractures includes immobilization in a bulky dressing and splint, with ice and elevation to control edema. Nondisplaced extra-articular calcaneal fractures can be treated with a short-leg cast or walking boot for approximately 6 weeks. Most displaced fractures must be repaired surgically, but patients typically experience residual stiffness of their subtalar joint that can adversely affect future athletic performance.

Tibia–Fibula Fractures

Etiology

In an inversion sprain, the medial malleolus typically is fractured at the level of the talar dome, or the injury may occur as a spiral fracture at the distal tibial metaphysis. Eversion and dorsiflexion injuries lead to spiral or comminuted fractures of the lateral malleolus. In lateral malleolar fractures, the risks for a bimalleolar fracture are high when the deltoid ligament avulses the medial malleolus.

A **Maisonneuve fracture** is an eversion-type injury of the ankle, with an associated fracture of the proximal third of the fibula, commonly at the junction of the proximal and middle thirds of the shaft (**Fig. 14.35**). The tibiofibular syndesmosis is disrupted, and either a tear of the tibiofibular ligament or a fracture of the medial malleolus also is present. The more proximal the location of the fibular fracture, the more damage to the interosseous membrane between the tibia and fibula, because the membrane is always disrupted up to the fracture site. The typical mechanism is external rotation of the foot.

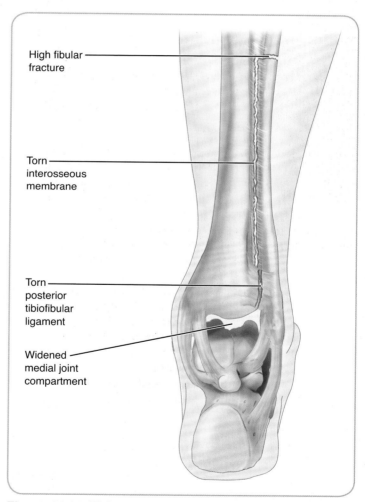

Figure 14.35. Maisonneuve fracture. The classic fracture occurs at the junction of the proximal and middle thirds of the fibula. The tibiofibular syndesmosis is disrupted, and the interosseous membrane is torn up the level of the fracture. The tibiotalar (medial) joint compartment is widened because of lateral subluxation of the talus.

(Figure labels:) High fibular fracture; Torn interosseous membrane; Torn posterior tibiofibular ligament; Widened medial joint compartment

Nearly 60% of tibial fractures involve the middle and lower thirds of the tibia. Whether open or closed, this fracture is associated with complications such as delayed union, nonunion, or malunion. The most common cause of an isolated tibial fracture is torsional force, resulting in a spiral or oblique fracture of the lower third of the tibia.

Fracture dislocations usually are caused by landing from a height with the foot in excessive eversion or inversion or by being kicked from behind while the foot is firmly planted on the ground. Typically, the foot is displaced laterally at a gross angle to the lower leg, and extreme pain is present. This position can compromise the posterior tibial artery and nerve.

Signs and Symptoms

In a simple tibial or fibular fracture, often a crack is heard, and the individual is unable to bear weight on the injured extremity because of intense pain. Gross deformity, gross bone motion at the suspected fracture site, crepitus, immediate swelling, extreme pain, or pain with motion should signal immediate action.

With a Maisonneuve fracture, deformity may or may not be present. The individual presents with tenderness over the deltoid ligament and the fracture site on the proximal fibula. Any proximal fibular tenderness after a twisting injury calls for radiographs of the ankle, the tibia, and the fibula. A high fibular fracture often requires open reduction and internal fixation between the distal fibula and tibia to maintain the normal relationship of the bones while ligament healing occurs. The screws generally are removed 8 to 12 weeks after surgery.

Because shock is possible in serious traumatic fractures, the emergency action plan should be activated. In some settings, this will include summoning EMS to immobilize and transport the individual to the nearest medical facility. Suspected disruption of the tarsometatarsal joint (i.e., Lisfranc fracture) and fractures with suspected neurovascular compromise should be immobilized in a noncircumferential bulky splint to prevent complications from further compression.

Management

Management of lower leg, ankle, and foot fractures involves removing the shoe and sock to expose the injured area. If a fracture is suspected, the clinician should perform percussion, compression, and distraction before any movement of the limb. Depending on the site, the techniques listed in **Application Strategy 14.2** may be helpful. The clinician also should assess the neurovascular integrity of the limb before and after immobilization by taking a distal pulse at the posterior tibial artery and/or dorsalis pedis artery or by blanching the toenails to determine capillary refill. The clinician should note the skin color of the foot and toes and should feel the toes for warmth. Sensation can be assessed by using the pulp of the fingers to stroke the top of the distal metatarsal heads and by asking the individual if the stroke was felt. The action is then repeated using the fingernail.

Nondisplaced malleoli fractures are treated conservatively, with cast immobilization for 4 to 6 weeks, followed by a functional brace until the fracture is completely healed. Displaced fractures involving joint stability require surgical intervention with open reduction and internal fixation. Healing after surgery usually takes 2 to 3 months or longer, followed by extensive rehabilitation. Internal fixation with plates and screws often is necessary to stabilize tibial fractures; however, some individuals may experience a high rate of infection as a complication of internal fixation.

In addition to Sever disease, the following conditions could lead to heel pain in young athletes: plantar fasciitis, heel fat pad syndrome, Achilles tendinitis/strain, retrocalcaneal bursitis, calcaneal stress fracture, calcaneal exostosis, contusion infection, tarsal coalition, and tarsal tunnel syndrome.

REHABILITATION

The cross-country runner has plantar fasciitis. What exercises should now be included in the rehabilitation program?

Rehabilitation exercises for the lower leg, ankle, and foot can be initiated during the acute inflammatory phase as long as the condition is not further irritated. For example, while icing an ankle, the gastrocnemius and soleus can be passively stretched, or strengthening exercises for the foot intrinsic muscles can be started. Pain and swelling dictate the amount of exercise that can be tolerated and may necessitate restricted weight bearing. The rehabilitation program should restore motion and proprioception, maintain cardiovascular fitness, and improve muscular strength, endurance, and power, predominantly through closed chain exercises.

Restoration of Motion

Application Strategy 14.1 provided several ROM exercises that can be performed non–weight bearing. For example, towel pulls stretching the Achilles tendon, writing the alphabet in large circles, picking up objects with the toes and combining the action with shin curls, and use of a biomechanical ankle platform system (BAPS) board can each be done in a seated position. As pain subsides and weight bearing is initiated, Achilles tendon stretches, toe raises, balance exercises, and use of a BAPS board can be completed in a standing position.

Restoration of Proprioception and Balance

Proprioception and balance must be regained to allow safe return to sport participation. Early exercises may include shifting one's weight while on crutches, performing bilateral minisquats, or using a BAPS board in a seated position. As balance improves, BAPS board exercises can progress to partial weight bearing while supported by a table and then to full weight-bearing exercises. Running in place on a minitramp and use of a slide board are closed chain exercises that also improve proprioception and balance.

Muscular Strength, Endurance, and Power

Early emphasis is placed on strengthening the foot's intrinsic muscles. Towel crunches are demonstrated in **Application Strategy 14.1**. As the condition allows, toe raises and Thera-Band or surgical tubing exercises are added. Use of a multiaxial ankle machine, toe raises with weights, squats and lunges, and isokinetic exercises continue to strengthen the lower leg musculature. During later stages, jogging, running side to side, and multiangle plyometrics can assist the individual in a gradual return to sport participation.

Cardiovascular Fitness

Maintenance of cardiovascular fitness can begin immediately after injury with use of an upper body ergometer or hydrotherapeutic exercise. Running in deep water and performing sport-specific exercises can provide mild resistance in a non–weight-bearing medium. When ROM is adequate, a stationary bicycle may be used. Light jogging, running backward, and running side to side should increase in both intensity and duration to facilitate return to activity. **Application Strategy 14.7** lists several rehabilitation exercises that may be incorporated in a complete program for the lower leg.

In addition to exercises, the individual should be assessed for biomechanical anomalies, and appropriate orthotics should be fabricated to correct any malalignment. Following an ankle injury, it may be necessary to provide external support to the ankle region. Following completion of the rehabilitation program and clearance for full participation, a proper maintenance program of stretching and strengthening exercises should be provided.

 The rehabilitation program for the cross-country runner with plantar fasciitis should include aggressive Achilles tendon stretching for 2 to 4 minutes, three to four times a day, with toes straight ahead, toes in, and toes out; gentle isometric contractions for intrinsic muscles of the foot, progressing to active ROM exercises within pain-free ranges (e.g., toe curls, marble pick-up, towel crunches, and towel curls) to strengthen the intrinsic and extrinsic muscles of the leg; and general fitness (i.e., strength and aerobic conditioning) with non–weight-bearing activities.

APPLICATION STRATEGY 14.7

Rehabilitation Exercises for the Lower Leg

1. **Phase 1.** Control inflammation. Minimize inversion and eversion exercises to allow healing. Dorsiflexion and plantar flexion should be performed within the limits of pain. Exercises should be combined with ice therapy or electrical stimulation with elevation. Use those exercises listed in Application Strategy 14.1 as tolerated.
   - Plantar fascia stretch
   - Towel crunches
   - Toe curls
   - Picking up objects
   - BAPS board in seated position
   - Triceps surae stretch, non–weight bearing
   - Pool therapy or upper body ergometer (UBE) exercises for cardiovascular fitness

2. **Phase 2.** As pain and tenderness subside, initiate inversion and eversion ROM. Initiate strengthening exercises as tolerated. Include the following:
   - Shin curls
   - Ankle alphabet
   - Triceps surae stretch, standing position
   - Toe raises
   - Elastic tubing exercises in dorsiflexion, plantar flexion, inversion, and eversion
   - Unilateral balance BAPS board activities with support
   - Pool therapy, UBE, and stationary bike (if tolerated) for cardiovascular fitness

3. **Phase 3**
   - Toe raises with weights
   - Multiaxial ankle machine
   - Squats and lunges
   - Balance exercises with challenges, such as dribbling while balancing on one leg, performing elastic band exercises while balancing on one leg, or balancing on an uneven surface
   - Straight-ahead jogging, if able to walk without a limp

4. **Phase 4.** (Use external support for the ankle as needed.)
   - Isokinetic exercises to work functional speeds
   - Multiangle plyometrics, including single- and double-limb jumping, front to front, side to side, and diagonals
   - Side-to-side running
   - Running backward
   - Jumping for height and distance (long jump)
   - Slide board
   - Gradual return to activity with protection

SUMMARY

1. The true ankle (talocrural) joint is the mortise–tenon joint between the tibia, fibula, and talus. Plantar flexion and dorsiflexion occur at this joint. Motion at the subtalar joint occurs in an oblique direction. The combination of calcaneal inversion, foot adduction, and plantar flexion is known as supination; the combination of calcaneal eversion, foot abduction, and dorsiflexion is known as pronation.

2. The primary supporting structures of the plantar arches are the calcaneonavicular (i.e., spring) ligament, long plantar ligament, plantar fascia (plantar aponeurosis), and short plantar (plantar calcaneocuboid) ligament. In addition, the tibialis posterior provides some support.

3. Congenital abnormalities, leg length discrepancy, muscle dysfunction (e.g., muscle imbalance), or a malalignment syndrome (e.g., pes cavus, pes planus, pes equinus, and hammer or claw toes) can predispose an individual to several chronic injuries.

4. Generalized forefoot pain may result from intrinsic factors (e.g., excessive body weight, limited flexibility of the Achilles tendon, pronation, valgus heel, hammer toes, fallen metatarsal arch, pes planus, or pes cavus) or from extrinsic factors (e.g., narrow toe box, improperly placed shoe cleats, repetitive jumping or running, or landing poorly from a height).

5. An acute anterior compartment syndrome is a medical emergency. Signs and symptoms include a recent history of trauma; a palpable, firm mass in the anterior compartment; tight skin; and a diminished dorsalis pedis pulse.

6. Ankle sprains are classified as grade I, II, or III based on the progression of the anatomical structures that are damaged and the subsequent disability. In lateral ankle sprains involving plantar flexion and inversion, the ATFL is torn first, followed by the calcaneal fibular ligament. In eversion ankle sprains, the deltoid ligament is injured, and an associated avulsion fracture of one or both malleoli also may be present.

7. Common sites for tendon injuries include the Achilles tendon just proximal to its insertion into the calcaneus, the tibialis posterior just behind the medial malleolus, the tibialis anterior just under the extensor retinaculum, and the peroneal tendons behind the lateral malleolus or at the distal attachment on the styloid process of the 5th metatarsal.

8. Injury to the tibialis posterior results in weakness in plantar flexion and inversion and may lead to acquired pes planus.

9. Risk factors for Achilles tendinitis include a tight heel cord, foot malalignment deformities, recent change in shoes or running surface, sudden increase in workload (e.g., distance or intensity), or changes in the exercise environment (e.g., changing footwear, or excessive hill climbing or impact-loading activities [e.g., jumping]).

10. MTSS is a periostitis along the posteromedial tibial border, usually in the distal third that is not associated with a stress fracture or compartment syndrome. Signs and symptoms include point tenderness in a 3- to 6-cm area along the distal posteromedial tibial border as well as pain and weakness with resisted plantar flexion or standing on tiptoe.

11. ECS is characterized by exercise-induced pain and swelling that are relieved by rest. The anterior compartment most frequently is affected, and in such cases, mild foot drop or paresthesia (or both) may be present. Fascial defects or hernias also may be present in the distal third of the leg over the anterior intramuscular septum.

12. Nerve impingement may involve the interdigital nerves as they bifurcate at the metatarsal heads (i.e., plantar interdigital neuroma), posterior tibial nerve beneath the flexor retinaculum and behind the medial malleolus, or sural nerve as it courses behind the lateral malleolus into the lateral foot.

13. Fractures of the lower leg, ankle, and foot may involve the following:

   ■ Freiberg disease (i.e., avascular necrosis of the second metatarsal head)

   ■ Sever disease (i.e., calcaneal apophysis)

   ■ Stress fractures (most commonly the neck of the 2nd metatarsal)

   ■ Avulsion fractures (e.g., styloid process of the 5th metatarsal and the medial and lateral malleoli)

   ■ Osteochondral fractures (e.g., talar dome)

   ■ Displaced fractures or fracture dislocations

14. Pain may be referred to the lower leg, ankle, and foot from the lumbar spine, hip, or knee.

15. Conditions that warrant special attention include the following:

   - Obvious deformity suggesting a dislocation, fracture, or ruptured Achilles tendon

   - Significant loss of motion or weakness in a myotome

   - Excessive joint swelling

   - Possible epiphyseal or apophyseal injuries

   - Abnormal reflexes or sensation or an absent or weak pulse

   - Gross joint instability

   - Any unexplained pain

16. Functional tests should be performed pain-free without limp or antalgic gait before clearing any individual for return to activity. In addition, the individual should have bilaterally equal ROM, strength, and proprioception as well as an appropriate cardiovascular fitness level before being allowed to return to activity. When necessary, protective equipment or braces should be used to prevent reinjury.

APPLICATION QUESTIONS

1. An 18-year-old cross-country runner comes to the athletic training room complaining of pain along the plantar surface of his left foot. Following the history and observation components of the exam, you learn that the runner has been increasing his distance and running more frequently on street-like surfaces. He has pain when he wakes in the morning, but the pain diminishes as he completes his morning routine (i.e., getting ready for classes). After he runs, the pain returns. His shoes are somewhat old and worn. He has some pes planus on the left foot when compared with the right foot. There is minor swelling along the longitudinal medial border but no discoloration. How should the testing components and palpations proceed with this history?

2. A 16-year-old soccer player has an aching pain on the posterior calcaneus just above the attachment of the Achilles tendon. When the tendon is palpated, it does not hurt, but when you reach around the tendon and squeeze into the soft-tissue area just anterior to the tendon, it is very painful. What condition might you suspect? What may have contributed to this condition? How should the injury be managed?

3. A middle-aged tennis player reports pain and swelling behind the medial malleolus and pain in the arch when arising in the morning. Observation reveals that the individual has pes planus. During resisted muscle testing, plantar flexion and inversion are weak. What muscles are involved in this injury? What exercises would you recommend to address this injury?

4. A 22-year-old ice hockey player is complaining of bilateral numbness in the posterolateral aspect of the leg along the Achilles tendon for the past 2 to 3 weeks. There is no history of trauma to the ankle, but he admits that, in order to provide better support for the ankles, he routinely spiraled his laces tightly around the proximal portion of each ice hockey boot and then applied several circular bands of white tape to hold them in place. Could this technique impair the vascular or neural function of the lower leg? What structures may be impacted by his actions? What recommendations could be made to manage the injury?

5. A soccer athlete "rolled" her foot during the game and is now complaining of lateral ankle pain during the timeout. What special tests could you do to determine whether this ankle injury is a grade I or grade II sprain?

6. A high school lacrosse player accidentally stepped in a hole, inverting the ankle. Although she stayed off the ankle and iced it during the night, the ankle appeared swollen and discolored the next morning and continued to hurt on weight bearing. How would you manage this injury?

7. A softball player sprained the right ankle a week ago. Following standard acute care and partial weight bearing, the swelling and pain have significantly decreased around the lateral malleolus, but pain is still present on the styloid process of the 5th metatarsal. What additional injury may be present? What would you recommend for further management of the injury?

8. Prevention and rehabilitation for injuries to the foot, ankle, and lower leg typically include strengthening exercises. What exercises can be used to strengthen both the intrinsic and extrinsic muscles of the foot?

9. What factors that contribute to the development of metatarsalgia can be addressed in the prevention or management of this condition to alleviate pain?

REFERENCES

1. Borowski LA, Yard EE, Fields SK, et al. The epidemiology of US high school basketball injuries, 2005-2007. *Am J Sports Med.* 2008;36(12):2328–2335.
2. Koutures CG, Gregory AJ. Injuries in youth soccer. *Pediatrics.* 2010;125(2):410–414.
3. Meyers MC. Incidence, mechanisms, and severity of game-related college football injuries on Field-Turf versus natural grass: a 3-year prospective study. *Am J Sports Med.* 2010;38(4):687–697.
4. Khan W, Oragui E, Akagha E. Common fractures and injuries of the ankle and foot: functional anatomy, imaging, classification and management. *J Perioper Pract.* 2010;20(7):249–258.
5. Munn J, Sullivan SJ, Schneiders AG. Evidence of sensorimotor deficits in functional ankle instability: a systematic review with meta-analysis. *J Sci Med Sport.* 2010;13(1):2–12.
6. Wang Q, Whittle M, Cunningham J, et al. Fibula and its ligaments in load transmission and ankle joint stability. *Clin Orthop Relat Res.* 1996;(330):261–270.
7. Leardini A, Stagni R, O'Connor JJ. Mobility of the subtalar joint in the intact ankle complex. *J Biomech.* 2001;34(6):805–809.
8. Goto A, Moritomo H, Itohara T, et al. Three-dimensional in vivo kinematics of the subtalar joint during dorsi-plantarflexion and inversion-eversion. *Foot Ankle Int.* 2009;30(5):432–438.
9. Iaquinto JM, Wayne JS. Computational model of the lower leg and foot/ankle complex: application to arch stability. *J Biomech Eng.* 2010;132(2):021009.
10. Gefen A. The in vivo elastic properties of the plantar fascia during the contact phase of walking. *Foot Ankle Int.* 2003;24(3):238–244.
11. Kaminski TW, Hertel J, Amendola N, et al. National Athletic Trainers' Association position statement: conservative management and prevention of ankle sprains in athletes. *J Athl Train.* 2013;48(4):528–545.

12. Kendall FP, McCreary EK, Provance PG, et al. *Muscles: Testing and Function with Posture and Pain.* 5th ed. Baltimore, MD: Lippincott Williams & Wilkins; 2005.
13. Schwieterman B, Haas D, Columber K, et al. Diagnostic accuracy of physical examination tests of the ankle/foot complex: a systematic review. *Int J Sports Phys Ther.* 2013;8(4):416–426.
14. Mahadevan D, Venkatesan M, Bhatt R, et al. Diagnostic accuracy of clinical tests for Morton's neuroma compared with ultrasonography. *J Foot Ankle Surg.* 2015;54(4):549–553.
15. McClure SK, Adams JE, Dahm DL. Common musculoskeletal disorders in women. *Mayo Clin Proc.* 2005;80(6):796–802.
16. McBryde AM Jr, Hoffman JL. Injuries to the foot and ankle in athletes. *South Med J.* 2004;97(8):738–741.
17. Coughlin MJ, Shurnas PS. Hallux rigidus. *J Bone Joint Surg Am.* 2004;86(1 suppl 2):119–130.
18. Olmsted-Kramer LC, Hertel J. Preventing recurrent lateral ankle sprains: an evidence-based approach. *Athl Ther Today.* 2004;9(6):19–22.
19. Hubbard TJ, Hicks-Little CA. Ankle ligament healing after an acute ankle sprain: an evidence-based approach. *J Athl Train.* 2008;43(5):523–529.
20. Williams GN, Jones MH, Amendola A. Syndesmotic ankle sprains in athletes. *Am J Sports Med.* 2007;35(7):1197–1207.
21. Smith AH, Bach BR Jr. High ankle sprains: minimizing the frustration of a prolonged recovery. *Phys Sportsmed.* 2004;32(12):39–43.
22. Mullen JE, O'Malley MJ. Sprains—residual instability of subtalar, Lisfranc joints, and turf toe. *Clin Sports Med.* 2004;23(1):97–121.
23. Molloy R, Tisdel C. Failed treatment of peroneal tendon injuries. *Foot Ankle Clin.* 2003;8(1):115–129.
24. Gluck GS, Heckman DS, Parekh SG. Tendon disorders of the foot and ankle, part 3: the posterior tibial tendon. *Am J Sports Med.* 2010;38(10):2133–2144.

25. Wilder RP, Sethi S. Overuse injuries: tendinopathies, stress fractures, compartment syndrome, and shin splints. *Clin Sports Med.* 2004;23(1):55–81.

26. Ohberg L, Alfredson H. Ultrasound guided sclerosis of neovessels in painful chronic Achilles tendinosis: pilot study of a new treatment. *Br J Sports Med.* 2002;36(3):173–175.

27. Glaser T, Poddar S, Tweed B, et al. Clinical inquiries. What's the best way to treat Achilles tendonopathy? *J Fam Pract.* 2008;57(4):261–263.

28. Brown DE. Ankle and leg injuries. In: Mellion MB, Walsh WM, Madden C, et al, eds. *The Team Physician's Handbook.* 3rd ed. Philadelphia, PA: Hanley & Belfus; 2002:509–519.

29. Riddle DL, Pulisic M, Pidcoe P, et al. Risk factors for plantar fasciitis: a matched case-control study. *J Bone Joint Surg Am.* 2003;85-A(5):872–877.

30. Shea M, Fields KB. Plantar fasciitis: prescribing effective treatments. *Phys Sportsmed.* 2002;30(7):21–25.

31. Moen MH, Tol JL, Weir A, et al. Medial tibial stress syndrome: a critical review. *Sports Med.* 2009;39(7):523–546.

32. Lookstein RA, Giordano CF. Deep vein thrombosis: endovascular management. *Mt Sinai J Med.* 2010;77(3):286–295.

33. Fleming A, Frey D. Extensive venous thrombosis in a runner: progression of symptoms key to diagnosis. *Phys Sportsmed.* 2005;33(1):34–36.

34. Recognizing and treating Morton's neuroma. *Harv Womens Health Watch.* 2009;16(6):5–6.

35. Hudes K. Conservative management of a case of tarsal tunnel syndrome. *J Can Chiropr Assoc.* 2010;54(2):100–106.

Knee Conditions

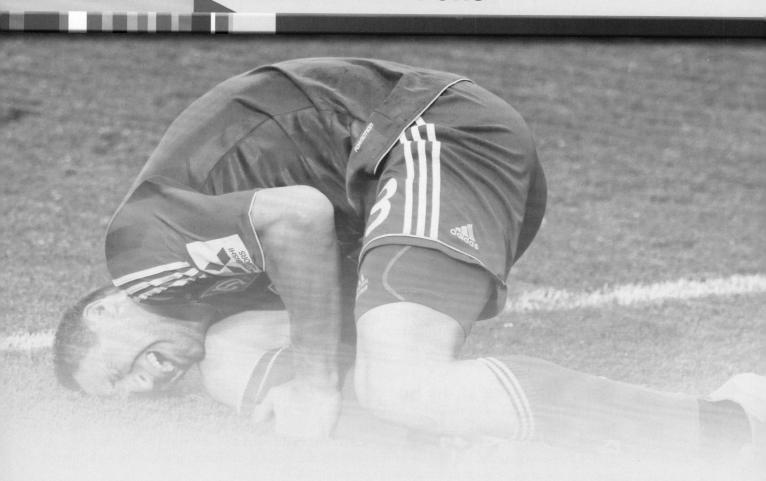

katatonia82 / Shutterstock.com

STUDENT OUTCOMES

1. Identify the major bony and soft-tissue structures of the knee region.

2. Identify the primary and secondary ligamentous restraints of the knee.

3. Describe the motions of the knee and identify the muscles that produce them.

4. Describe the forces that produce the loading patterns responsible for common injuries at the knee.

5. Explain the general principles used to prevent injuries to the knee.

6. Describe a thorough assessment of the knee and patellofemoral joint.

7. Describe the common injuries to and conditions of the knee in physically active patients (including sprains, dislocations, contusions, strains, bursitis, meniscal tears, and by patellofemoral pain).

8. Explain the management strategies for common injuries and conditions of the knee.

9. List the various types of fractures that can occur at the knee and explain their management.

10. Explain the basic principles associated with rehabilitation of the knee.

INTRODUCTION

The knee is a complex joint that frequently is injured in physical activity. When walking and running, the knee moves through a considerable range of motion (ROM) while bearing loads equivalent to 3 to 4 times body weight. Because the knee is positioned between the two longest bones in the body (i.e., the femur and the tibia), the potential exists for creating large, injurious torques at the joint. These factors, coupled with minimal bony stability, make the knee susceptible to injury. Knee injuries comprise approximately 60% of all sport injuries, being the predominant site of injury among runners and one of the most frequently injured joints for all sport participants.[1–3]

This chapter begins with a review of the anatomy of the knee and a discussion of the associated kinematics and kinetics. General principles to prevent injuries are presented followed by a step-by-step injury assessment of the region. Discussion regarding common injuries to the knee complex and examples of rehabilitative exercises are then included.

ANATOMY OF THE KNEE

The knee is a large, synovial joint that includes three articulations within the joint capsule. The weight-bearing joints are the two condylar articulations of the tibiofemoral joint; the third articulation is the patellofemoral joint. The soft-tissue connections of the proximal tibiofibular joint also exert a minor influence on knee motion.

Bony Structure of the Knee

The proximal bone of the knee joint is the femur. The prominent posterior ridge of the femur, the linea aspera, serves as an attachment for many of the muscles that move the hip and knee. The distal portion of the femur broadens to form the medial and lateral epicondyles. The area between the epicondyles on the anterior surface of the femur is the femoral trochlea, through which the patella glides as the knee moves into flexion and extension (**Fig. 15.1**).

The lateral epicondyle is wider than the medial epicondyle. Arising from the most superior crest of the medial epicondyle is the palpable adductor tubercle. Inferior to each epicondyle are the medial and lateral condyles, with the medial condyle being the longer. Sharing a common anterior surface, these condyles bifurcate posteriorly and are separated by the deep intercondylar notch.

Corresponding to the femoral condyles are the medial and lateral tibial plateaus with conformations that are complex and asymmetric.[4] To accommodate for the longer medial femoral condyle, the medial tibial plateau is 50% larger than the lateral tibial plateau. Separating the two tibial plateaus are the intercondylar eminences, which are raised areas that match the femur's intercondylar notch. The anterior aspect of the tibia includes the prominent tibial tubercle, which serves as the distal attachment of the infrapatellar ligament.

The patella is a sesamoid bone located in the quadriceps (patellar) tendon. It improves the biomechanical function of the extensor mechanism and protects the anterior portion of the knee. The fibula is not a direct part of the knee joint. The head of the fibula, however, does serve as a site for several soft-tissue attachments that support and stabilize the knee.

Tibiofemoral Joint

The distal femur and proximal tibia articulate to form two side-by-side condyloid joints that collectively are known as the tibiofemoral joint (see **Fig. 15.1**). These joints function together primarily as a modified hinge joint. Because of the restricting ligaments, some lateral and rotational motions are allowed at the knee. The medial and lateral condyles of the femur differ somewhat in size, shape, and orientation. As a result, the tibia rotates laterally on the femur during the last few degrees of extension to produce a "locking" of the knee. This phenomenon, known as the "screwing-home" mechanism, brings the knee into the close-packed position of full extension.

Menisci

The menisci, which also are known as semilunar cartilages because of their half-moon shapes, are disks of fibrocartilage firmly attached to the superior plateaus of the tibia by the coronary ligaments and joint capsule. They provide several functional advantages, including absorption and dissipation of force and significantly improved congruency of the joint surfaces to even the distribution of stress across

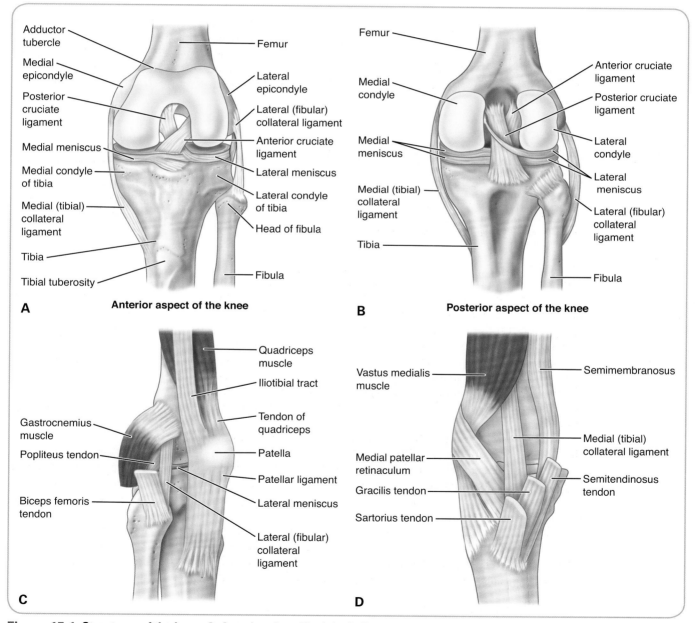

Figure 15.1. Structures of the knee. A, Anterior view. The joint is flexed, and the patella is removed. **B, Posterior view.** The knee is in extension. **C, Lateral view. D, Medial view.** *(continued)*

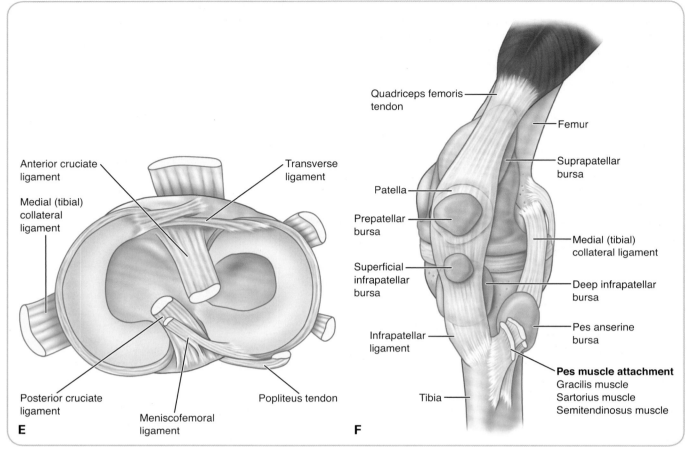

Figure 15.1. *(continued)* **E, Superior surface of the tibia. F, Bursae of the knee.**

the joint (**Box 15.1**).[5] In addition, because 74% of the total weight of the menisci is water, much of the fluid is squeezed out into the joint space when the knee undergoes compression during weight bearing, which provides lubrication to promote gliding of the joint structures.[6] The menisci also increase knee stability by serving as soft-tissue restraints that resist anterior tibial displacement.

When viewed in cross-section, the menisci are thicker along the lateral margin and thinner on the medial margin, serving to deepen the concavities of the tibial plateaus. When viewed from above, the medial meniscus is semicircular, whereas the lateral meniscus is somewhat more circular (see **Fig. 15.1**). The inner edges of both menisci are unattached to the bone, but the two ends of

---

BOX 15.1 Functions of the Menisci

- Deepen the articulation and fill the gaps that occur during knee motion.
- Aid in lubrication and nutrition of the joint.
- Reduce friction during movement.
- Increase area of contact between the condyles, thus improving weight distribution.
- Provide shock absorption by dissipating stress over the articular cartilage, thus decreasing cartilage deterioration.
- Assist the ligaments and capsule in preventing hyperextension.
- Prevent the joint capsule from entering the joint during the locking mechanism by directing the movement of the femoral articular condyles.

the menisci, known as the anterior and posterior horns, are attached to the intercondylar tubercles. The anterior horns of each meniscus are joined to each other by the transverse ligament and are connected to the infrapatellar tendon via the patellomeniscal ligaments.

The medial meniscus has an attachment to the deep medial collateral ligament (MCL) and fibers from the semimembranosus muscle. It is injured much more frequently than the lateral meniscus, in part because the medial meniscus is more securely attached to the tibia and, therefore, is less mobile.

In comparison, the lateral meniscus is a smaller and more freely movable structure. In addition to its attachments to the joint capsule, intercondylar tubercles, and transverse ligament, the lateral meniscus is attached to the posterior cruciate ligament through the meniscofemoral ligament (ligament of Wrisberg) and to the popliteus muscle via the joint capsule and coronary ligament. Contraction of the popliteus serves to retract the lateral meniscus. During flexion and extension of the knee, the medial and lateral menisci move posteriorly and anteriorly, respectively. The outer third of each meniscus is innervated and contains nociceptors that, when a meniscus is injured, send signals of pain to the brain.[7] The outer most portion of each meniscus is also the most vascularized portion of the structure, whereas the inner most portion of the structure is the least vascularized portion.[8] Injuries occurring to the vascularized portions of the menisci have a greater chance of healing than injuries occurring in the avascular region.

Joint Capsule and Bursae

The thin articular capsule at the knee is large and lax, encompassing both the tibiofemoral and patellofemoral joints. Anteriorly, it extends approximately 2.5 cm above the patella to attach along the edges of the superior patellar surface. The deep bursa formed by this capsule above the patella, known as the suprapatellar bursa, is the largest in the body (**Fig. 15.1F**). The suprapatellar bursa lies between the femur and quadriceps femoris tendon, and it functions to reduce friction between the two structures.

Posteriorly, two other bursae communicate with the joint capsule—namely, the subpopliteal and semimembranosus bursae. The subpopliteal bursa lies between the lateral condyle of the femur and the popliteal muscle. The semimembranosus bursa lies between the medial head of the gastrocnemius and the semimembranosus tendon.

During flexion and extension, synovial fluid moves throughout the bursal recesses to lubricate the articular surfaces. In extension, the gastrocnemius and subpopliteal bursae are compressed, driving the synovial fluid anteriorly. In flexion, the suprapatellar bursa is compressed, forcing the fluid posteriorly. When the knee is in a semiflexed or open-packed position, the synovial fluid is under the least amount of pressure; this position provides relief of pain caused by swelling in the joint capsule and surrounding bursae.

Four other key bursae are associated with the knee but not contained in the joint capsule—namely, the prepatellar, superficial infrapatellar, deep infrapatellar bursae, and pes anserine bursa. The prepatellar bursa is located between the skin and anterior surface of the patella, allowing free movement of the skin over the patella during flexion and extension. The superficial infrapatellar bursa is located between the skin and patellar tendon. Inflammation of this bursa caused by excessive kneeling sometimes is referred to as "housemaid's knee." The deep infrapatellar bursa is located between the tibial tubercle and the infrapatellar tendon, and it is separated from the joint cavity by the infrapatellar fat pad. This bursa reduces friction between the ligament and the bony tubercle. The pes anserine bursa is located between the MCL and the sartorius, gracilis, and semitendinosus tendons and distal to the joint line, in close proximity and posterior to the MCL. Images of knee bursa can be seen in **Figure 15.1F**.

Ligaments of the Knee

Because the shallow articular surfaces of the tibiofemoral joint contribute minimally to knee stability, the stabilizing role of the ligaments crossing the knee is of great significance. Two major ligaments of the knee are the anterior and posterior cruciate ligaments (see **Fig. 15.1**). The name cruciate is derived from the fact that the two ligaments cross each other, with anterior and posterior referring to their respective tibial attachments. These ligaments are termed intracapsular ligaments, because they are located within the articular capsule and extrasynovial ligaments because they lie outside the synovial cavity.

The anterior cruciate ligament (ACL) stretches from the anterior aspect of the intercondyloid fossa of the tibia just medial and posterior to the anterior tibial spine in a superoposterior direction to the posteromedial surface of the lateral condyle of the femur. The ACL is a critical stabilizer that prevents the following:

■ Anterior translation (movement) of the tibia on a fixed femur

■ Posterior translation of the femur on a fixed tibia

■ Internal and external rotation of the tibia on the femur

■ Hyperextension of the tibia

The ACL has two discrete bands—namely, an anteromedial and a posterolateral bundle. Occasionally, a third, intermediate band also is present. When the knee is fully extended, the femoral attachment of the anteromedial bundle is anterior to the attachment of the posterolateral bundle. When the knee is flexed, the positions are reversed, causing the ACL to wind on itself. The result of this action is that varying portions of the ACL are taut as the knee moves through a normal ROM. When the knee is fully extended, the posterolateral bundle is taut; when the knee is fully flexed, the anteromedial bundle is taut.[9] Generally, loads on the ACL correspond to anteriorly directed shear force at the knee.[10] During gait, this force is maximum in early stance and small in late stance. The ACL frequently is subject to deceleration injuries; internal tibial torque is the most dangerous loading mechanism, particularly when combined with an anterior tibial force.[11]

The shorter and stronger posterior cruciate ligament (PCL) runs from the posterior aspect of the tibial intercondyloid fossa in an anterosuperior direction to the lateral anteromedial condyle of the femur. It consists of a large anterolateral and a smaller posteromedial bundle. The PCL is considered the primary stabilizer of the knee, and it resists posterior displacement of the tibia on a fixed femur. The posterior fibers of the PCL are taut when the knee is fully extended, and the anterior fibers are taut when it is fully flexed.

The medial and lateral collateral ligaments also are referred to as the tibial and fibular collateral ligaments, respectively, after their distal attachments (see **Fig. 15.1**). Formed by two layers, the deep fibers of the MCL merge with the joint capsule and medial meniscus to connect the medial epicondyle of the femur to the medial tibia. The superficial layer originates from a broad band just below the adductor tubercle and is separated from the deep layer by a bursa. The two layers insert just below the pes anserinus, the common attachment of the semitendinosus, sartorius, and gracilis, thereby positioning the ligament to resist medially directed shear (i.e., valgus) and rotational forces acting on the knee. As a unit, the MCL is taut in complete extension. In midrange, its posterior fibers are the tautest; in complete flexion, the anterior fibers are the most taut.

The lateral collateral ligament (LCL) connects the lateral epicondyle of the femur to the head of the fibula, contributing to lateral stability of the knee. The ligament is separated from the lateral meniscus by a small fat pad. The LCL is the primary restraint against varus forces when the knee is between full extension and 30° of flexion, and it provides secondary restraint against external rotation of the tibia on the femur. The LCL is highly innervated and includes Ruffini endings, Golgi tendon organs, and free nerve endings, all of which can contribute to an indistinct pain when the knee is injured.[12]

Other Structures Stabilizing the Knee

Several other structures contribute to knee integrity. Posteriorly, the oblique popliteal ligament forms an extension of the semimembranosus tendon, and the arcuate popliteal ligament connects the lateral condyle of the femur to the head of the fibula. These two ligaments, which are called the arcuate–popliteal complex, provide support to the posterior joint capsule. The complex limits anterior displacement of the tibia relative to the femur as well as hyperextension and hyperflexion of the knee. It becomes taut during internal and external tibial rotation and during valgus and varus loading of the knee.

Although the knee is only partially surrounded by a joint capsule, the capsule is reinforced by several tendons, including the expanded tendons of the quadriceps, the tendon of the semimembranosus, and the iliotibial (IT) band. Laterally, the IT band is a broad, thickened band of fascia that

TABLE 15.1 Structures Contributing to the Stability of the Knee

TIBIAL MOTION	PRIMARY RESTRAINTS	SECONDARY RESTRAINTS
Anterior translation	ACL	MCL, LCL, middle third of the mediolateral capsule, IT band
Posterior translation	PCL	MCL, LCL, posterior third of the mediolateral capsule, popliteus tendon, anterior and posterior meniscofemoral ligaments
Valgus rotation	MCL	ACL, PCL, posterior capsule when the knee is fully extended
Varus rotation	LCL	ACL, PCL, posterior capsule when the knee is fully extended
Lateral rotation	MCL, LCL	Popliteus corner, ACL, PCL
Medial rotation	ACL, PCL	Anteroposterior meniscofemoral ligaments

extends from the tensor fasciae latae over the lateral epicondyle of the femur to the Gerdy tubercle on the lateral tibial plateau. The IT band is well supplied with free nerve endings that transmit signals for pain and proprioception to the brain, enhancing the structure's ability to promote lateral knee stability. The tissue under the IT band is a lateral extension and invagination of the knee joint capsule. **Table 15.1** lists the structures providing stability to the knee, including primary and secondary restraints.

Patellofemoral Joint

The patella (i.e., the kneecap) is a triangular bone that rests between the femoral condyles to form the patellofemoral joint (**Fig. 15.2**). The posterior surface of the patella is composed of three distinct facets, although the number, size, and shape of these facets vary from person to person.[13] A central, vertical ridge separates the medial and lateral regions, each having a superior, middle, and inferior articular surface. The odd facet, lying medial to the medial facet, has no articular subdivisions. The thickest articular cartilage in the body covers these facets, with the cartilage ranging up to 5 mm in thickness.[13]

In the sagittal plane, the patella serves to increase the angle of pull of the patellar tendon on the tibia, thereby improving the mechanical advantage of the quadriceps muscles to produce knee extension. Patellar positioning is both maintained and restrained by the patellar retinaculum. The lateral retinaculum originates from the vastus lateralis and the IT band and inserts on the patella's lateral border. The medial retinaculum originates from the distal portion of the vastus medialis and adductor magnus, and it inserts on the medial border of the patella. The superior portion of the knee's joint capsule thickens and inserts on the patella's superior border, forming the medial and lateral patellofemoral ligaments.

The Q-angle is defined as the angle between the line of resultant force produced by the quadriceps

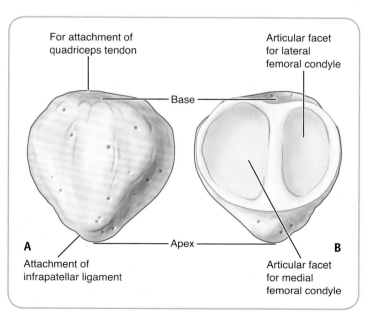

Figure 15.2. Patella. A, Anterior view. **B,** Posterior view.

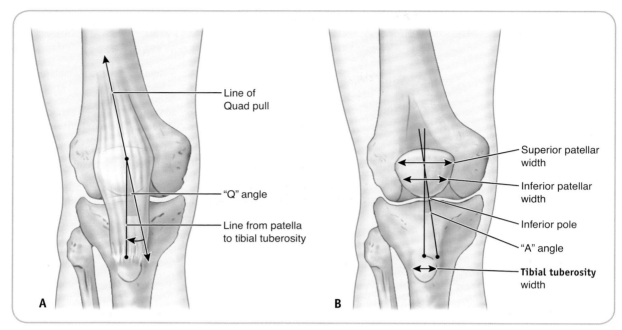

Figure 15.3. Angles at the knee. A, The Q-angle is formed between the line of quadriceps pull and the imaginary line connecting the center of the patella to the center of the tibial tubercle. **B,** The A-angle measures the relationship of the patella to the tibial tubercle.

muscles and the line of the patellar tendon (**Fig. 15.3A**). One line is drawn from the middle of the patella to the anterior superior iliac spine of the ilium, and a second line is drawn from the tibial tubercle through the center of the patella. When the knee is fully extended during weight bearing, the normal Q-angle ranges from approximately 12° in males to approximately 22° in females.[14] A Q-angle of less than 12° or greater than 22° is considered to be abnormal and can predispose patients to patellar injuries or degeneration. Cadaver studies show that increasing the Q-angle increases lateral patellofemoral contact pressures and could promote lateral patellar dislocation, whereas decreasing the Q-angle could increase the medial tibiofemoral contact pressure.[15] Factors that contribute to an increased angle in women include a wider pelvis, increased femoral anteversion, increased knee valgus, external tibial torsion, increased ligamentous laxity, and hyperpronation of the foot.

Another measurement, similar to the Q-angle, is the A-angle, which measures the relationship of the patella to the tibial tubercle (**Fig. 15.3B**). This measurement consists of a vertical line that divides the patella in half. A second line is drawn from the tibial tubercle to the apex of the inferior pole of the patella. An A-angle of greater than 35° has been linked to increased patellofemoral pain, although some have questioned the reliability of this measurement because of the difficulty in consistently finding appropriate landmarks.

Muscles Crossing the Knee

See **Muscles Acting on the Knee**, available on the companion Web site at thePoint, for a summary of these muscles, including their attachments, primary actions, and innervation.

The muscles of the knee develop tension to produce motion at the knee and contribute to the knee's stability.

Nerves of the Knee

The tibial nerve (L4, L5, S1 to S3) is the largest and most medial continuation of the sciatic nerve. It innervates all the muscles in the hamstring group except for the short head of the biceps femoris, and it also supplies all muscles in the calf of the leg (**Fig. 15.4**).

The common peroneal nerve (L4, L5, S1, S2) is the lateral branch of the sciatic nerve (see **Fig. 15.4**). It innervates the short head of the biceps femoris in the thigh and then circles around the Gerdy tubercle, or the lateral tubercle of the proximal tibia, with a radius of approximately 45 mm.[16] Proceeding inferiorly, it passes through the popliteal fossa to wind laterally along the subcutaneous

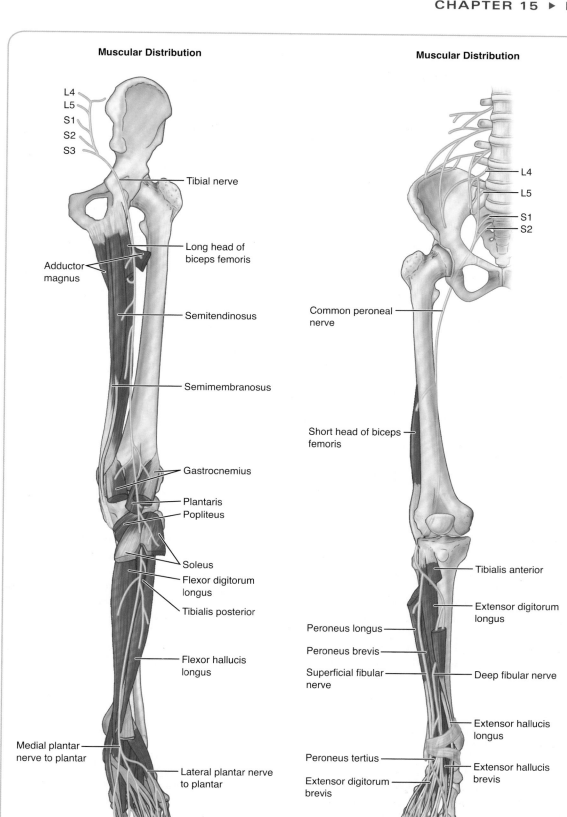

Muscular Distribution

L4
L5
S1
S2
S3

Tibial nerve

Adductor magnus

Long head of biceps femoris

Semitendinosus

Semimembranosus

Gastrocnemius

Plantaris
Popliteus

Soleus
Flexor digitorum longus
Tibialis posterior

Flexor hallucis longus

Medial plantar nerve to plantar

Lateral plantar nerve to plantar

A

Muscular Distribution

L4
L5
S1
S2

Common peroneal nerve

Short head of biceps femoris

Tibialis anterior

Extensor digitorum longus

Peroneus longus

Peroneus brevis

Superficial fibular nerve

Deep fibular nerve

Extensor hallucis longus

Peroneus tertius

Extensor hallucis brevis

Extensor digitorum brevis

B

Figure 15.4. Innervation of the knee. A, Anterior view. **B,** Posterior view.

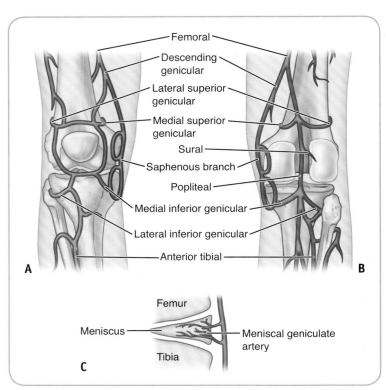

Figure 15.5. Collateral circulation around the knee. A, Anterior view. **B,** Posterior view. **C,** Circulation to meniscus.

surface to just below the proximal head of the fibula, where it can be easily damaged. As it passes between the fibula and the peroneus longus muscle, it subdivides into the superficial and deep peroneal nerves. An articular branch to the knee may arise either from the deep peroneal nerve or from both the deep and superficial peroneal nerves as a terminal branch of the common peroneal nerve.

The femoral nerve (L2 to L4) courses down the anterior aspect of the thigh adjacent to the femoral artery to supply the quadriceps group. The L2 and L3 branches of the femoral nerve also innervate the sartorius.

The Blood Vessels of the Knee

Just proximal to the knee, the main branch of the femoral artery becomes the popliteal artery. The popliteal artery courses through the popliteal fossa and then branches, forming the medial and lateral superior genicular, the middle genicular, and the medial and lateral inferior genicular arteries that supply the knee (Fig. 15.5). The superior and inferior genicular arteries intertwine with each other about the knee.

KINEMATICS AND MAJOR MUSCLE ACTIONS OF THE KNEE

The knee functions primarily as a hinge joint. The different shapes of the femoral condyles, however, serve to complicate joint function.

Flexion and Extension

The primary motions permitted at the tibiofemoral joint are flexion and extension. Knee flexion is performed primarily by the hamstrings and is assisted by the popliteus, gastrocnemius, gracilis, and sartorius. In addition, the flexor musculature has a secondary responsibility of rotating the tibia. The flexors attaching on the tibia's medial side (i.e., semitendinosus, semimembranosus, gracilis, and sartorius) internally rotate the tibia, whereas those attaching on the lateral side (i.e., biceps femoris) externally rotate the tibia. Knee extension is carried out by the quadriceps femoris muscle group. Although the name implies four muscles, most clinicians describe five—namely, the vastus lateralis, vastus intermedius, vastus medialis, vastus medialis oblique (VMO), and rectus femoris. The VMO is a discrete group of fibers arising from the medial femoral condyle and the fascia of the adductor magnus. Each muscle has a common attachment on the tibial tubercle via the patella and infrapatellar ligament.

In the terminal 20° of knee extension, the tibia externally rotates approximately 15° in what is called the "screw-home" mechanism. In full extension, the joint's close-packed position, maximal bony contact occurs between the femur and tibia, resulting in the joint being anatomically "locked." This rotation occurs because the articulating surface of the medial condyle of the femur is longer than that of the lateral condyle in this locked position, rendering motion almost completely impossible. Initiation of flexion from a position of full extension requires that the knee first be "unlocked." The role of "locksmith" in the closed kinetic chain is provided by the popliteus, which acts to externally rotate the femur with respect to the tibia and, in doing so, frees the joint for motion.

Once the knee is unlocked from full extension, bony contact is diminished, and motion in the transverse and frontal planes becomes freer. In an open kinetic chain, contraction of the popliteus causes internal rotation of the tibia on the femur. As the knee moves into flexion, the medial femoral condyle moves very little anteroposteriorly, but the lateral femoral condyle rolls back and the point of femorotibial contact shifts posteriorly, producing internal rotation of the tibia, with 120° of flexion accompanied by 20° of internal tibial rotation.[17] This motion is facilitated by the inferior sloping of the lateral compartment of the tibial plateau. The reverse occurs during extension as the lateral femoral condyle of the femur slides anteriorly on the tibia.

Rotation and Passive Abduction and Adduction

The rotational capability of the tibia with respect to the femur is maximal at approximately 90° of knee flexion. A few degrees of passive abduction and adduction are permitted when the joint is positioned in the vicinity of 30° of flexion.

Knee Motion During the Gait

During midstance of normal gait, the knee is flexed to approximately 20°, internally rotated approximately 5°, and slightly abducted. Knee motion during the swing phase includes approximately 70° of flexion, 15° of external rotation, and 5° of adduction. Gait is explained in more detail in Chapter 8.

Patellofemoral Joint Motion

During movements of knee flexion and extension, the patella glides in the trochlear groove, primarily in a vertical direction, with an excursion of as much as 8 cm. When the knee is fully extended, the inferior pole of the patella rests on the distal portion of the femoral shaft, just proximal to the femoral groove. During flexion, the patella makes initial contact with the groove at 10° to 20° of flexion, and it becomes seated within the groove as the knee approaches 20° to 30°. In this position, the lateral border of the trochlea is prominent, forming a barrier against lateral displacement of the patella. The inferior border of the patella tilts upward and medially during knee flexion, with the contact area increasingly shifted superiorly on the medial and lateral facets of the posterior patella.[18,19] The patella also undergoes medial and lateral displacement as the tibia is rotated laterally and medially, respectively, with the center of the patella following a circular path during knee flexion/extension.[20]

Tracking of the patella against the femur is dependent on the direction of the net force produced by the attached quadriceps. The vastus lateralis tends to pull the patella laterally in the direction of the muscle's action line, parallel to the femoral shaft. The IT band and lateral extensor retinaculum also exert a lateral force on the patella, and IT band tightness can cause maltracking of the patella.[21] Although considerable debate exists regarding its role, the VMO seems to oppose the lateral pull of the vastus lateralis and, in doing so, keeps the patella centered in the patellofemoral groove. If the magnitude of the force produced by the vastus lateralis exceeds that produced by the VMO, the patella is pulled laterally out of its groove during tracking. Mistracking of the patella during knee flexion–extension can be extremely painful and lead to several chronic patellofemoral conditions.

KINETICS OF THE KNEE

Because the knee is positioned between the body's two longest bony levers (i.e., the femur and the tibia), the potential for torque and force development at the knee is significant. The key role played by the knee during weight bearing makes the knee subject to large forces during the gait cycle.

Forces at the Tibiofemoral Joints

Weight bearing and tension development in muscles crossing the knee are the predominant forces acting at the tibiofemoral joints, with both contributing to joint compression. The medial compartment sustains the majority of the load during stance, with compressive force at the joint reaching an estimated threefold body weight during the stance phase of gait, increasing to around three- to sixfold body weight during stair climbing.[22,23] Comparison of front and back squat exercises shows significantly higher knee compressive forces during the back squat as compared to the front squat, with shear forces at the knee during squat exercises being small and posteriorly directed.[24] During sport participation, knee forces undoubtedly are large, although quantitative estimates are lacking. Tension in the knee extensors also increases lateral stability of the knee, with tension in the knee flexors contributing to medial stability.

The menisci assist with force absorption at the knee, behaving as a rubberlike elastic material at high loading frequencies and as a more viscous force dissipator at lower loading frequencies.[25] The medial two-thirds of each meniscus have an internal structure that is particularly well suited to resisting compression. The menisci also serve to distribute force from the femur over a broader area and, in doing so, reduce the magnitude of joint stress. Tibiofemoral joint stress is an estimated threefold higher during weight bearing when the menisci have been removed. Because the menisci also serve to protect the articulating bone surfaces from wear, knees that have undergone complete or partial meniscectomies still may function adequately, but such knees are more likely to develop degenerative conditions.

Forces at the Patellofemoral Joint

Compressive force at the patellofemoral joint has been found to be half the body weight during normal walking gait, increasing up to eightfold body weight during stair climbing.[23] During stair climbing, there is an increase in patellofemoral pressure, lateral force distribution, and lateral patellar tilt.[26]

PREVENTION OF KNEE CONDITIONS

Because many of the muscles that move the knee also move the hip, prevention of knee injuries must focus on a well-rounded physical conditioning program. Although much debate continues as to the effectiveness of prophylactic knee braces (see Chapter 3), recent rule changes and improved shoe design have contributed significantly to a reduction of injuries at the knee.

Physical Conditioning

The development of a well-rounded physical conditioning program is the key to injury prevention. Exercises should include flexibility and muscular strength, endurance, and power as well as speed, agility, balance, and cardiovascular fitness. Lack of flexibility can predispose a patient to muscular strains. Exercises should focus on general flexibility and may be performed either alone or with a partner using proprioceptive neuromuscular facilitation stretching techniques. In particular, stretching exercises should focus on the quadriceps, hamstrings, gastrocnemius, IT band, and adductors. Because many of these muscles contribute to knee stability, strengthening programs also should focus on these muscle groups. Warm-up exercises (e.g., jogging, high-knee skipping, muscle activation, balance training with different jumping exercises, strength and core stability such as sit-ups) may reduce the incidence of knee injuries. When designing ACL injury prevention programs for females, specific attention needs to be focused on "core-based programs" that emphasize increasing hip abduction strength and muscle recruitment and overall neuromuscular training of the trunk muscles.[27] Specific exercises to prevent injury to the musculature that moves the knee are provided in **Application Strategy 15.1**. Additional exercises for muscles that cross the hip region are demonstrated in **Application Strategy 16.1**. Many of these exercises can be supplemented with tubing to add resistance to the exercise.

Rule Changes

Rule changes in contact sports, particularly football, have significantly reduced injuries to the knee region. Specifically, modifications in acceptable techniques that prohibit blocking at or below the knee and blocking from behind have reduced traumatic injuries. Proper training methods on correct technique should continue throughout the season to ensure compliance with specific rules designed to prevent injury.

APPLICATION STRATEGY 15.1

Exercises to Prevent Injury at the Knee

Closed chain exercises involve all the joints in the lower extremity and engage both agonist and antagonist muscle groups.

1. **Body weight squats.** Starting position is with feet slightly wider than shoulder width apart, with toes pointed forward. Motion is initiated at the hips, and the body is lowered as if to sit on a chair. Knees should not extend beyond toes. In the ending position, body should be equally centered between hips, knees and hips flex to 90°, with torso upright. Hands may be held in front of body for balance. To return standing, extend hips and knees while keeping the chest upright.

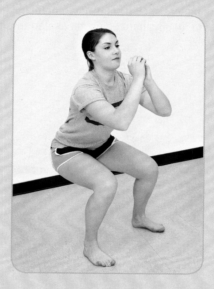

2. **Body weight squat progression.** As the patient shows gains in strength and endurance and demonstrates improved proprioception, the patient can progress to performing squats on an unstable platform, with or without weights.

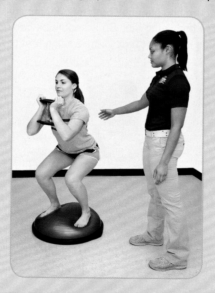

(continued)

3. **Body weight lunge.** Patients will feel this exercise in their gluteal muscles, hamstrings, and quadriceps. Starting position is in standing with feet shoulder width apart. Hands may rest on hips or be held in front of body. One foot is kept stationary while the opposing limb is moved forward, as if stepping or lunging forward. Weight is transferred from back limb to front limb as patient begins to bend knee of back limb. The front knee should be directly over the ankle and should not extend beyond the foot. The back knee should not touch the ground, and weight is on the toes, not the foot. Attempt to maintain a 90° angle at the ankle, knee, and hip of both limbs. Torso should be balanced over hips and chest upright. To regain standing position, push off with front limb to step back into starting position. A basic lunge is performed on stationary platform. As the patient shows gains in strength and endurance and demonstrates improved proprioception, the patient can progress to lunging onto an unstable platform.

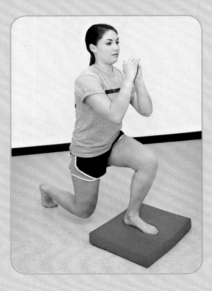

4. **Step-ups.** Make sure bench or box is secure and stand on both feet, facing step up box. Keeping torso upright, lift one limb onto box and extend hip and knee to raise body onto box. Body should be balanced over hips and lead knee should point in same direction as the lead foot, keeping knee over foot. Bring trailing foot to rest beside lead foot on the top of the box.

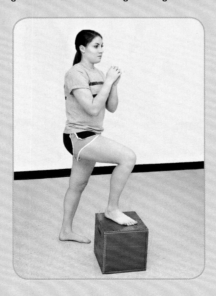

(continued)

5. **Step-up progression.** To increase difficulty and recruit additional muscle groups and movements, do not drop trailing leg to box but rather continue the motion and bring the trailing leg into 90° of flexion before returning to the floor.

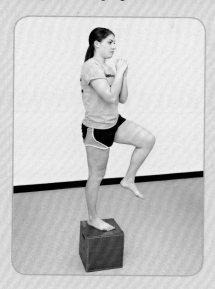

6. **Roman deadlifts (RDLs).** RDLs are considered one of the best closed chain exercises for posterior chain muscles of the lower extremity. RDLs can be performed as a double-leg or single-leg exercise and standing on a flat or raised surface. Back should remain straight, shoulders should remain "down and back" (retracted position), core stable, hips and shoulders squared forward. Knee of standing leg should remain forward in line with toes, but knee should not be totally locked out (soft knee position).

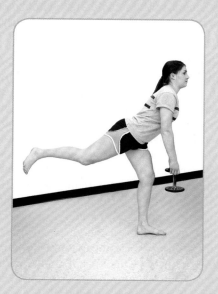

Shoe Design

Shoe design is discussed in Chapter 3. In field sports, shoes may have a flat-sole, long-cleat, short-cleat, or multicleated design. The cleats should be properly positioned under the major weight-bearing joints of the foot and should not be felt through the sole of the shoe. Although cleat pattern and type had previously been thought to predispose football athletes to knee injury, new research suggests that it is the interface between the turf and the stiffness of the upper portion of the shoe that is the greater risk factor to consider. Artificial turf and stiff uppers appear to have the greatest impact on rotational function.[28]

ASSESSING KNEE CONDITIONS

 A female high school basketball player is complaining of a deep, aching pain in the knee during activity. How should the assessment of this injury progress to determine the extent and severity of injury?

The lower extremity works as a unit to provide motion, and the knee plays a major role in supporting the body during dynamic and static activities. Biomechanical problems at the foot and hip can directly affect strain on the knee. As such, assessment of the knee complex must encompass an overview of the entire lower extremity. Refer to **Table 15.3** for a summary of the various knee instabilities, the tests used, and the injured structures as indicated by the various positive tests.

 See **Special Tests for the Knee and Application Strategy: Knee Evaluation**, both available on the companion Web site at thePoint.

HISTORY

 The injury assessment of the female high school basketball player should begin with a history. What questions need to be asked to identify the cause and extent of this injury?

Conditions at the knee can be related to family history, age, congenital deformities, mechanical dysfunction, and recent changes in training programs, surfaces, or foot attire. Assessment should begin by gathering information on the mechanism of injury, associated symptoms, progression of the symptoms, any disabilities that may have resulted from the injury, and related medical history. Injuries seldom occur in an absolute frontal or sagittal plane; instead, most injuries involve a fixed, weight-bearing foot, with the patient trying to change directions or pivot. These acute, noncontact injuries most likely involve a rotational stress on the knee, which may injure several structures.

 See **Application Strategy: Developing a History of the Injury**, available on the companion Web site at thePoint, for specific questions related to the knee.

Sprains of the collateral ligaments usually result in pain directly over the injury site, and the patient may describe medial/lateral instability. Injury to the ACL may be described as "deep in the knee" or "under the kneecap," whereas pain associated with a PCL tear is located in the posterior knee near the proximal attachment of the gastrocnemius. Unlike ACL injuries, PCL injuries usually do not cause incapacitating pain but, rather, produce vague symptoms, such as unsteadiness or insecurity of the knee. Patients with meniscal injuries frequently report knee pain after twisting their leg while the foot is bearing their full weight.

The patient also may describe an associated pop or snap or other unusual sensation at the time of injury. Hearing a "pop" is a classic sign of an ACL tear. Patients with an ACL tear may also describe a feeling of instability as if the lower leg is sliding out from under the thigh. Symptoms such as locking of the knee may indicate a meniscal tear; "giving way" may indicate a patellar subluxation or internal derangement of the knee. Pain following extended periods of sitting, the "moviegoer's" or "theater" sign, usually indicates prolonged pressure being placed on one of the patellar facets. Patients who have symptoms of patellar instability may have had a dislocation or recurrent subluxation.

The high school basketball player should be asked questions that address when, where, and how the injury occurred; intensity, location, and type of pain; when the pain begins (e.g., when you get out of bed, while sitting, while walking, during exercise, or at night); how long the condition been has present; how long the pain lasts; if the pain has changed or stayed the same; if the pain is worse before, during, or after activity; activities that aggravate or alleviate the symptoms; changes in training; changes in footwear; and previous injury, treatment, and medication. It is also important to allow the patient to describe sensations other than pain that she may be experiencing, such as catching, locking, snapping, or creaking. Check for episodes of instability and clarify what motions cause the instability, if any, to occur. Even though you will be assessing for presence of swelling, discoloration, fever, and areas of tenderness during the physical examination, check with the patient to see if these were present previously and, if so, when they resolved.

OBSERVATION AND INSPECTION

? The female high school basketball player indicates a deep, aching pain in the knee during activity that began 7 to 10 days ago. The patient cannot identify a specific mechanism of injury. She reports no episodes of instability; denies experiencing any popping, catching, or locking; and has not noticed any swelling in the area. She reports that practice has been taking place in two facilities. One gym has hardwood floors, and the other gym has composite flooring. She reports that there has been increased focus on cardiovascular conditioning during the past 2 weeks of practice. Explain the observation component in the ongoing assessment of the basketball player.

Both legs should be clearly visible to check symmetry, any congenital deformity, swelling, discoloration, hypertrophy, muscle atrophy, or previous surgical incisions. The patient should wear running shorts to allow a full view of the entire lower extremity. In addition, the patient should bring the shoes normally worn when pain is present so that they can be inspected for unusual wear, which could be indicative of a biomechanical abnormality.

The injured knee should be placed on a folded towel or pillow at 30° of flexion to relieve any strain on the joint structures. The injury site should be inspected for obvious deformities, discoloration, swelling, or scars that might indicate previous surgery. Swelling proximal to the patella may indicate suprapatellar bursitis or quadriceps involvement. Swelling distal to the patella may indicate patellar tendinitis, fat pad contusion, or internal derangement. Posterior swelling may indicate a Baker cyst, gastrocnemius strain, or venous thrombosis. Medial swelling over the pes anserine may indicate bursitis or tendinitis. Girth measurements should be taken to determine the presence of swelling. One measurement should be at the joint line; subsequent measurements should be taken at 2-in increments (1-in for smaller patients) above the superior pole of the patella.

For patients seeking assistance with nonacute injuries, identifying the presence of faulty posture, malalignments, and other structural differences may assist the clinicians in discovering not only the injury but also factors they may predispose the patient to specific conditions as well as factors that may be the cause of the patient's pain. Faulty posture or congenital abnormalities can increase stress on any joint. In an ambulatory patient, observation should include a thorough postural examination. It is important to observe the alignment of the femur on the tibia. Normally, the angle between the femoral and tibial shafts ranges from 180° to 195°. An angle of less than 180° is called **genu valgum** (i.e., "knock knee"); an angle of greater than 195° is called **genu varum** (i.e., "bowlegs"). Hyperextension, or posterior bowing of the knee, is called **genu recurvatum**.

When evaluating a patient with a chronic condition, the clinician should observe patella alignment for any abnormalities (**Box 15.2**). A high-riding patella exposes the infrapatellar fat pad, leading to a double hump when viewed from the lateral side (i.e., "camel sign"). Although some misalignments may be observed during a postural examination, radiographs often are required to establish a definitive diagnosis.

Patella alta	High-riding patella caused by a long patellar tendon
Patella baja	Low-riding patella caused by a short patellar tendon
Squinting patella	Medial-riding patella caused by hip anteversion (internal rotation of the femur) or internal tibial rotation
"Frog-eyed" patella	Lateral-riding patella caused by hip retroversion (external rotation of the femur) or external tibial rotation

Tibial torsion should be evaluated. Normally, the patella faces straight ahead while the foot faces slightly lateral (i.e., Fick angle). Medial torsion is associated with genu varum, in which the feet point toward each other, resulting in a "pigeon-toed" foot deformity. Genu valgum is associated with lateral tibial torsion, in which the feet point outward. When standing, most people exhibit a lateral tibial torsion. Femoral torsion, or anteversion (see Chapter 16), can impact the position of the patella relative to the femur and tibia.

While the patient is seated, the clinician should observe whether the tibial tubercles are directly below the patella or are displaced laterally by more than 10°, indicating an increased tubercle sulcus angle. Lateral displacement of the tubercle suggests bony patellofemoral malalignment and predisposition to lateral patellar tracking. The clinician should ask the patient to actively extend and flex the knee and should observe the dynamic tracking of the patella. The patella should be palpated for crepitus during the movement and compared with the contralateral knee. Although asymptomatic crepitus is common in certain patients, symptomatic crepitus in the injured knee may indicate articular cartilage damage on the patella or trochlea.

 See **Application Strategy: Postural Assessment of the Knee Region**, found on the companion Web site at thePoint.

Following completion of a static examination, the clinician should observe the patient walking. This observation should include an anterior, posterior, and lateral view, with the clinician noting any abnormalities in gait, favoring of one limb, tibial torsion, increased Q-angle, or inability to perform a fluid motion.

 Observation of the basketball player should include a full postural assessment and gait analysis. In particular, it is important to note the presence of pes planus, pes cavus, foot pronation, foot supination, genu varum, genu valgum, tibial torsion, patella alta, Q-angle, and leg length discrepancies. The specific injury site should be inspected for obvious deformities, discoloration, edema, scars that might indicate previous surgery, and the general condition of the skin.

PALPATION

 Observation of the female basketball player reveals an increased Q-angle, genu valgum, and excessive foot pronation. Explain palpation specific to the injury sustained by the basketball player.

Bilateral palpation can determine temperature, swelling, point tenderness, crepitus, deformity, muscle spasm, and cutaneous sensation. Vascular pulses can be taken at the popliteal artery in the posterior knee, posterior tibial artery behind the medial malleolus, and dorsalis pedis artery in the dorsum of the foot.

Palpation should move proximal to distal, leaving the most painful area until last. The patient should be non–weight bearing, with a pillow placed under the knee to relax the limb. It may be necessary to change knee position to palpate certain structures more effectively. For example, meniscal lesions are best palpated at 45°; the joint line is more prominent at 90°. Externally rotating the knee exposes the anteromedial border of the medial meniscus; internally rotating the knee exposes the lateral meniscus.

Extreme pain or point tenderness during palpation of bony structures may indicate a fracture. Compression, distraction, and percussion also may be used to detect fracture. For example, compression at the distal tibia and fibula causes distraction at the proximal tibiofibular joint. Percussion or tapping on the malleoli, or use of a tuning fork, may produce positive signs at the fracture site as well.

Palpation should proceed proximal to distal, but the area anticipated to be the most painful should be left to last. The following structures should be palpated:

Anterior Palpation

1. Quadriceps muscles, adductor muscles, and sartorius

2. Patellar surface, edges, and retinaculum

3. Patellar tendon, fat pad, tibial tubercle, medial and lateral tibial plateaus, and bursa. When the knee is extended, the infrapatellar fat pad can be palpated on the medial and lateral sides of the patellar tendon.

4. Patella plica (medial to the patella, with the knee flexed at 45°)

5. Medial femoral condyle and epicondyle and MCL

6. Pes anserinus

7. IT band, lateral femoral condyle and epicondyle, LCL, and head of fibula. The LCL can be palpated further by having the patient place the foot of the affected limb on the knee of the unaffected leg while palpating the lateral joint line.

8. While the knee is flexed at 90°, the tibiofemoral joint line, medial and lateral tibial plateaus, medial and lateral femoral condyles, and adductor muscles should be palpated.

Posterior Palpation with Knee Slightly Flexed

1. Popliteal fossa for Baker cyst and popliteal artery

2. Popliteus muscle in posterolateral corner

3. Hamstring muscles and gastrocnemius

Palpation for Swelling

Two special tests are used to determine if the swelling is intra-articular or extra-articular. Intra-articular swelling feels heavy and mushy, because blood often is mixed with the synovial fluid. Extra-articular swelling is light and fluid and can easily be moved between the fingers from one side to the other.

Brush or Stroke Test (Milking) for Joint Swelling

This test differentiates between synovial thickening and joint effusion. With effusion, the knee assumes a resting position of 15° to 25° of flexion, which allows the synovial cavity maximum capacity for holding fluid. Beginning below the medial joint line, the clinician strokes two or three times toward the patient's hip, moving proximal to the suprapatellar pouch (**Fig. 15.6A**). Next, using the opposite hand,

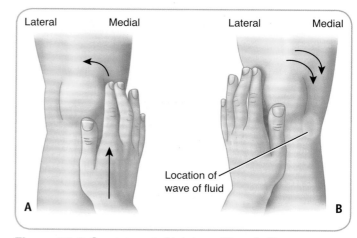

Figure 15.6. Assessment of joint swelling. A, To assess joint swelling, the clinician strokes the medial side of the knee several times, toward the hip. **B,** Using the opposite hand, the clinician strokes down the lateral side of the patella and notes any wave of fluid as it moves to the medial side of the joint.

the clinician strokes down the lateral side of the patella (**Fig. 15.6B**). An effusion is present if a wave of fluid passes to the medial side of the joint and bulges just below the medial, distal portion of the patella.

Ballotable Patella Test

While the knee is relaxed, the clinician pushes the patella downward, into the patellofemoral groove (**Fig. 15.7**). If swelling is intra-articular, the fluid under the patella causes it to rebound, exhibiting the outlines of the floating patella. If the swelling is extra-articular, a click or definite stopping point is felt when the patella strikes the patellofemoral groove. The outline of the patella usually is obscured by extra-articular swelling, typically seen with a ruptured bursa.

> Bilateral palpation of the basketball player's knee, with a particular focus on the patella, should include examining for presence of swelling, point tenderness, deformity, crepitus, temperature, other signs of trauma, and patellofemoral joint pain.

PHYSICAL EXAMINATION TESTS

> **?** In palpating the basketball player's patella, point tenderness is elicited over the lateral facet. In addition, pain and crepitus are elicited when the patella is manually compressed into the patellofemoral groove. Explain the physical examination of the basketball player.

Physical examination tests are performed with the patient in a comfortable position, preferably supine. Pain and muscle spasm can restrict motion and cause an inaccurate result. The limb should not be forced through any sudden motions. It may be necessary to place a rolled towel under the knee to relieve strain on the joint structures.

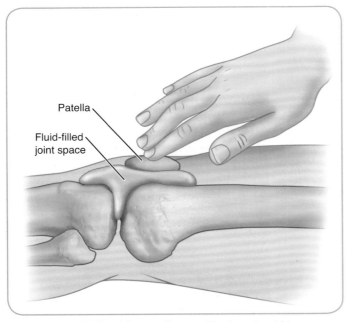

Figure 15.7. Ballotable patella test. The leg should be relaxed. The clinician gently pushes the patella downward into the groove. If joint effusion is present, the patella rebounds and floats back up.

Patella

Fluid-filled joint space

Functional Tests

The clinician should determine the available ROM in knee flexion–extension and medial-lateral rotation of the tibia on the femur. Bilateral comparison with the noninjured knee is critical to determine normal or abnormal movement.

Active Movements

Active movements can first be performed while the patient is sitting, with the leg flexed over the end of the table, and then repeated in a prone or supine position. The thigh must be stabilized, and the most painful movements performed last to prevent painful symptoms from overflowing into the next movement. If assessing an acutely injured patient while still at the site where the injury occurred, the clinician may have to assess active ROM in the position in which the patient is most comfortable. The motions that should be assessed and the normal ROM for each are as follows:

- Knee flexion (0° to 135°)
- Knee extension (0° to 15°)

- Medial rotation of the tibia on the femur (20° to 30°) with the knee flexed at 90°

- Lateral rotation of the tibia on the femur (30° to 40°) with the knee flexed at 90°

Measuring ROM at the knee with a goniometer is not usually done during on-field or sideline assessment of injury but rather during follow-up evaluations and throughout the rehabilitation process. Measuring joint ROM with a goniometer is demonstrated in **Figure 15.8**.

Passive Range of Motion

If the patient is able to perform full ROM during active movements, the clinician should apply gentle pressure at the extremes of motion to determine end feel. The end feel for flexion is tissue approximation. The end feel for extension is medial rotation, and that for lateral rotation is tissue stretch. Patellar motion should be performed passively, before palpation for point tenderness.

Resisted Muscle Testing

To assess resisted ROM testing, the clinician must stabilize the hip during testing to prevent muscle substitution. The assessment begins with the muscles

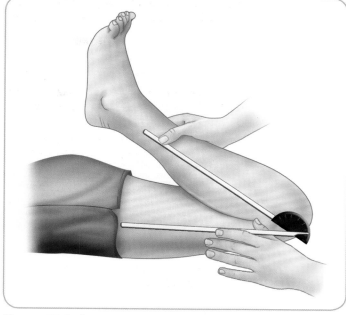

Figure 15.8. Goniometry measurement for knee flexion and extension. Center the fulcrum over the lateral epicondyle of the femur. Using the greater trochanter for reference, align the proximal arm along the femur. Align the distal arm in line with the lateral malleolus.

on stretch, and resistance is applied throughout the full ROM. The clinician should note any muscle weakness when compared with the uninvolved limb. Potentially painful motions should be delayed until last.

The patient is in a seated position during testing of extension, internal, and external rotation of the tibiofemoral joint. During knee extension, any abnormal tibial movement or excessive pain from patellar compression should be noted. When assessing tibiofemoral flexion, the patient is a prone position. **Figure 15.9** demonstrates motions that should be tested.

Manual Muscle Testing

If pain or weakness is found during resisted ROM, the clinician may decide to perform a manual muscle test to determine which muscle is damaged. When performing manual muscle testing, class I and II muscles should be tested at end range with maximal shortening of the muscle.[29] One-joint muscles that concentrically contract through the ROM are considered class I muscles. Class I muscles are short and strong. In contrast, class II muscles are two-joint and multijoint muscles that actively shorten all joints crossed and are also strong at the end range. Several class I and II muscles are involved with lower leg, ankle, and foot motion. See **Table 15.2** for manual muscle testing positioning.

Stress Tests

From information gathered during the history, observation, inspection, and palpation, the clinician determines which tests will assess the condition most effectively. Only those tests deemed to be absolutely necessary should be performed. If ACL damage is suspected, tests for anterior cruciate instability should be performed as soon as possible, before swelling, joint effusion, and muscle spasm occludes the extent of instability. Possible structures injured with the various positive tests for unidirectional and multidirectional instability are listed in **Table 15.3** and are not repeated in this section, except when necessary to explain the test.

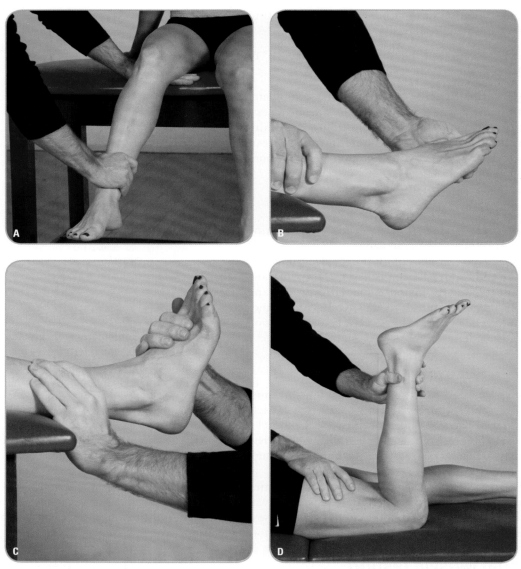

Figure 15.9. Resisted range of motion testing. A, Knee extension (L3). **B,** Ankle plantar flexion (S1). **C,** Ankle dorsiflexion (L4). **D,** Knee flexion (S1, S2). Myotomes are listed in parentheses.

TABLE 15.2 Manual Muscle Testing of Knee

MUSCLE	JOINT POSITIONING	APPLY PRESSURE
Semitendinosus/ semimembranosus	The knee should be flexed between 50° and 70° with the thigh in medial rotation and toes pointed toward the midline. Patient is in a prone position.	To the distal aspect of the leg in the direction of knee extension. With opposite hand, stabilize thigh.
Biceps femoris	With the patient prone, the knee should be placed in about 50° to 70° of flexion with the thigh in slight lateral flexion and the toes pointed away from the midline.	To the distal aspect of the leg in the direction of knee extension. With opposite hand, stabilize thigh.
Rectus femoris	Patient should be seated with knees lower legs handing off the table. Ask patient to fully extend testing limb.	To the anterior aspect of the distal leg, in the direction of flexion

Wong M. *Pocket Orthopaedics: Evidence-Based Survival Guide*. Sudbury, MA: Jones and Bartlett; 2010:318.

TABLE 15.3 Classification of Knee Instability and Structures Injured

INSTABILITY	STRESS TEST	POSSIBLE STRUCTURES INJURED IF TEST IS POSITIVE
Straight valgus (medial)	Abduction (valgus) stress with knee in full extension	1. MCL 2. Oblique popliteal ligament 3. Posteromedial capsule 4. ACL 5. PCL 6. Medial quadriceps expansion 7. Semimembranosus muscle
	Abduction (valgus) stress with knee slightly flexed (20°–30°)	1. MCL 2. Oblique popliteal ligament 3. PCL
Straight varus (lateral)	Adduction (varus) stress with knee in full extension	1. LCL 2. Posterolateral capsule 3. Arcuate–popliteus complex 4. Biceps femoris tendon 5. ACL 6. PCL 7. Lateral gastrocnemius muscle
	Adduction (varus) stress with knee slightly flexed (20°–30°) and tibia laterally rotated	1. LCL 2. Posterolateral capsule 3. Arcuate–popliteus complex 4. IT band 5. Biceps femoris tendon
Straight anterior	Anterior drawer test (90° knee flexion)	1. ACL (anteromedial bundle) 2. Posterolateral and posteromedial capsule 3. Deep MCL 4. IT band 5. Oblique popliteal ligament 6. Arcuate–popliteus complex
	Lachman test Modified Lachman test	1. ACL (anteromedial bundle) 2. Oblique popliteal ligament 3. Arcuate–popliteus complex
Straight posterior	Posterior sag (gravity) test Posterior drawer sign Reverse Lachman test	1. PCL (anterolateral bundle) 2. Arcuate–popliteus complex 3. Oblique popliteal ligament 4. ACL
Anteromedial rotary	Slocum drawer test (tibia externally rotated)	1. MCL 2. Oblique popliteal ligament 3. Anteromedial and posteromedial capsule 4. ACL
Anterolateral rotary	Slocum drawer test (tibia internally rotated) Lateral pivot shift test Jerk test Slocum ALRI Cross-over test Flexion-rotation drawer test	1. ACL 2. Anterolateral and posterolateral capsule 3. Arcuate–popliteus complex 4. LCL 5. IT band 6. Lateral meniscus

(continued)

TABLE 15.3 Classification of Knee Instability and Structures Injured *(continued)*

Posteromedial rotary	Posteromedial drawer test Posteromedial pivot shift test	1. PCL 2. Oblique popliteal ligament 3. MCL 4. Semimembranosus muscle 5. Posteromedial capsule 6. ACL
Posterolateral rotary	Posterolateral drawer test External rotation recurvatum test	1. PCL 2. Arcuate–popliteus complex 3. LCL 4. Biceps femoris tendon 5. Posterolateral capsule 6. ACL

Straight Anterior Instability

■ Anterior Drawer Test

The patient is supine, with the hip flexed at 45° and the knee flexed at 90°. The clinician stabilizes the foot by placing it under the thigh to prevent any tibial rotation. In this position, the ACL is nearly parallel to the tibial plateau. The clinician places both thumbs on either side of the patellar tendon to palpate the anteromedial and anterolateral joint line and to determine anterior translation as the tibia is drawn forward on the femur. The fingers are placed in the popliteal fossa to ensure that the hamstrings are relaxed. A step-off at the medial tibial plateau should first be palpated to ensure the proper starting position (see "Posterior Drawer Test" section). While palpating the joint line, apply an alternating anterior (i.e., anterior drawer) and posterior (i.e., posterior drawer) displacement force on the proximal tibia (**Fig. 15.10A**). Stability can be visualized from a lateral view or palpated with the thumb at the joint line. The knee is tested with the foot in neutral rotation, external rotation, and finally, internal rotation. The amount of translation and the end point are compared with those for the contralateral knee. The sensitivity of the anterior drawer test has not been found to be consistently strong, with scores reported from .25 to .60.[30,31] However, the test appears to have higher specificity, with scores reported from .85 to .96.[30,31] The clinician should be aware that the anterior drawer test is not as effective as Lachman test for a variety of reasons (**Box 15.3**).

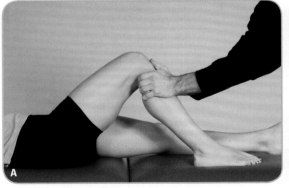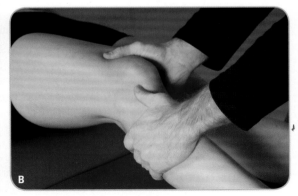

Figure 15.10. Anterior cruciate ligament tests. A, Drawer test. The knee is flexed, and the clinician applies an anterior and posterior displacement force on the proximal tibia. **B, Lachman test.** Using one hand to stabilize the femur, the clinician applies firm pressure on the posterior proximal tibia in an attempt to move the tibia anteriorly.

BOX 15.3 Limitations of the Anterior Drawer Test

- Gravity also has an effect.

- Guarding by the hamstrings group can mask anterior displacement of the tibia on the femur.

- The triangular shape of the meniscus can form a block against anterior movement of the tibia.

- A displaced "bucket-handle" meniscal tear can block anterior movement.

- Knee flexion at 90° may lead to anterior displacement of tibia, masking further displacement during the test.

- Increased pain is elicited in an acute injury at 90° of flexion, masking the true extent of injury.

- If the PCL is absent, anterior movement to the neutral position can be misread as abnormal anterior displacement.

- Because the knee is flexed at 90°, only the anteromedial bundle is tested.

■ Lachman Test

Lachman test isolates the posterolateral bundle of the ACL. The patient is supine, with the knee joint at 20° to 30° of flexion. When the knee is in slight flexion, the ACL is the primary restraining force that prevents anterior translation, because the secondary restraints are relaxed. The clinician stabilizes the femur with one hand while placing the other hand over the proximal tibia to displace the tibia anteriorly (**Fig. 15.10B**). If the patient has heavy, muscular legs, or the clinician is unable to appropriately manually support the patient's leg, a small support, such as a pillow or tightly rolled towel, can be placed under the femur. A positive sign results in a "mushy" or soft end feel when the tibia is moved anterior in relation to the femur. When the tibia is in slight internal rotation, anterior displacement indicates additional damage to the IT band and to the anterior and middle lateral capsule. When the tibia is in slight external rotation, anterior displacement indicates damage to the ACL, MCL, and medial meniscus. The Lachman test has a sensitivity of .87 and a specificity of .96, indicating that the Lachman test is a strong clinical tool to use for assessing the presence of ACL tears.[31]

■ Modified (Prone) Lachman Test

This test is used to differentiate abnormal tibiofemoral glide caused by tears of the ACL from glide caused by PCL deficiencies. It often is favored over the traditional Lachman position when the patient has large thighs or the clinician has small hands, because the weight of the femur is supported by the examination table and the tibia may be supported by the clinician's thigh or forearm.[32] The patient is in a prone position, and the knee is flexed at 30°. The clinician supports the tibia with one hand while palpating either side of the joint line. The other hand applies a downward pressure on the proximal portion of the posterior tibia (**Fig. 15.11**). The clinician notes any anterior tibial displacement. Positive anterior translation found with an anterior drawer, Lachman test, or modified Lachman test indicates a tear of the ACL. Positive anterior translation with the anterior drawer test or Lachman test and a negative modified Lachman test indicate a tear in the PCL.

Straight Posterior Instability

■ Posterior Sag (Gravity) Test

The true posterior sag test is performed in a supine position, feet resting on the table with the hips flexed at 45° and the knees at 90°. When viewed laterally, a loss of tibial tubercle prominence in a PCL-deficient knee is evident when the tibia falls back or sags on the femur because of gravitational forces. A variation of the posterior sag test is **Godfrey test**. To perform the Godfrey test, the patient is placed in 90° of hip and

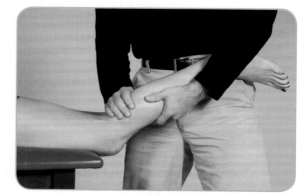

Figure 15.11. Modified Lachman test. The clinician applies downward pressure on the proximal posterior tibia and notes any anterior translation.

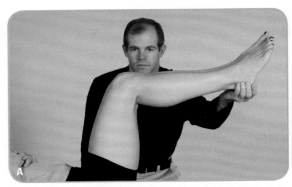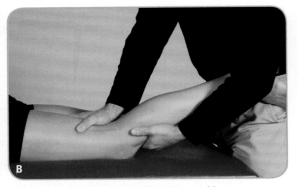

Figure 15.12. Posterior cruciate ligament tests. A, Posterior sag (gravity) test. The hips and knees are flexed, and the clinician looks from the side and compares the anterior contours of both legs. If one leg sags back and the prominence of the tibial tubercle is lost, the posterior cruciate may be damaged (Godfrey sign). **B, Reverse Lachman test.** The clinician stabilizes the femur with one hand while the other lifts the tibia up (superiorly). Any posterior translation and the quality of the end feel is noted.

knee flexion. The clinician holds both relaxed legs distally to prevent manual reduction of the tibia and moves to the side of the patient, looking for the position of the tibia as it sags back on the femur (**Fig. 15.12A**) This maneuver is called Godfrey sign. Godfrey test is a very useful clinical tool, with strong sensitivity (.79 to 1.00) and strong specificity (1.00).[31] It is important to note the sag, because if the sag goes unnoticed, it may produce a false-positive Lachman test.

■ Posterior Drawer Test

The evidence supports that the posterior drawer test is a clinical relevant test for assessing for the presence of PCL injury. Both the sensitivity and specificity scores are in the 90th percentile.[30] To perform the test, place the patient in the same pose as described for the anterior drawer test. The clinician initially observes the resting position of the tibial plateau in relation to the femoral condyles. When the knee is flexed to 90°, the medial tibial plateau normally lies approximately 1 cm anterior to the medial femoral condyle. This can be felt by running the thumb or index finger down the medial femoral condyle toward the tibia. In a PCL-deficient knee, this relationship is not present. The clinician then applies a posteriorly directed force to the tibia (see **Fig. 15.10A**). The knee is tested with the foot in neutral position, external rotation, and finally, internal rotation. Isolated PCL tears often produce only minimal posterior translation when the secondary restraints of the knee, particularly the posterior capsule and the posteromedial and posterolateral structures, are intact.

False-negative results can occur with a displaced bucket-handle meniscal tear, hamstring or quadriceps spasm, or hemarthrosis.

■ Reverse Lachman Test

Positioning of the patient is identical to that in the modified Lachman test. While the patient is prone and the knee flexed to between 20° and 30°, the clinician holds the distal femur to the table and grasps the proximal tibia (**Fig. 15.12B**). Using the hand on the femur to stabilize the thigh and ensure that the hamstrings are relaxed, the clinician lifts the proximal tibia posteriorly (up), noting the amount of translation and the quality of end point. A false-positive test may occur if the ACL is torn, allowing gravity to cause an anterior shift of the tibia. The test is not as sensitive for detecting a torn PCL, because the PCL functions more at 90° of knee flexion.

Straight Valgus Instability

■ Abduction (Valgus Stress) Test

Although the valgus stress test has been found to have poor specificity (.17), the test is highly sensitive, with scores ranging from .86 to 1.00.[29,30] To perform the test, the patient is placed supine, with the leg in full extension. The clinician places the heel of one hand on the lateral joint line, and the other hand stabilizes the distal lower leg. Next, a lateral or valgus force is applied at the joint line with the

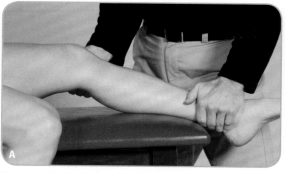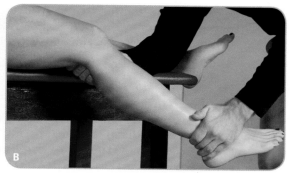

Figure 15.13. Valgus and varus stress tests. A, Valgus stress test. The knee is flexed at 30° to isolate the MCL. The clinician applies a gentle valgus stress at the knee joint while moving the lower leg laterally. The test is repeated with the knee fully extended. **B, Varus stress test.** The knee is flexed at 30° to isolate the LCL. The clinician applies a varus stress at the knee joint while moving the lower leg medially. The test is repeated with the knee fully extended.

lower leg stabilized in slight lateral rotation (**Fig. 15.13A**). If positive, joint opening will occur (i.e., the tibia abducts) and indicates primary damage involving the structures of the medial joint capsule. The tibial collateral ligament or MCL is isolated by flexing the knee at 30° and repeating the valgus stress.

Straight Varus Instability

▪ Adduction (Varus Stress) Test

The knee is placed in the same position as for the abduction test, but a medial force (i.e., varus stress) is applied at the knee joint (**Fig. 15.13B**). Laxity in full extension indicates major instability and damage to the fibular collateral ligament, popliteus, and posterolateral capsule. When testing at 20° to 30° of flexion, which is the true test for one-plane lateral instability, a positive test indicates damage to the fibular collateral ligament. The varus stress test has been found to range in sensitivity from .25 to .75 yet has been found to be highly specific of .98.[30]

Anteromedial Rotary Instability

▪ Slocum Drawer Test

Think of the Slocum drawer test as a spin-off of the anterior drawer test, with the focus being on assessing for anteromedial rotary instability (AMRI), instead of just liner anterior instability. The clinician should consider performing the Slocum drawer test when the history, inspection, and palpation point toward an ACL injury but the anterior drawer and Lachman tests are negative. This test is performed in the same position as the anterior drawer test, but with the tibia externally rotated (toes pointed outward) 15° (**Fig. 15.14A**). In this position, when an anterior drawer force is applied,

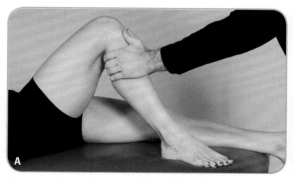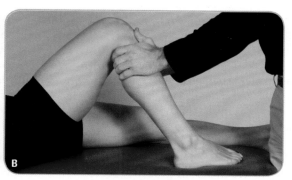

Figure 15.14. Slocum drawer test. A, An anterior drawer force is applied for AMRI with the tibia externally rotated 15°. **B,** Anterolateral rotary instability is tested with the tibia internally rotated 25° to 30°.

the majority of anterior translation occurs on the medial side of the knee. If the amount of anterior translation is the same or increases, AMRI is present, indicating injury to the MCL, oblique popliteal ligament, posteromedial capsule, and ACL (posteromedial corner).

Anterolateral Rotary Instability

■ Slocum Drawer Test
This test also is performed in the same position as the anterior drawer test; with the tibia internally (toes pointing toward midline) rotated 25° to 30° (**Fig. 15.14B**). In this position, the majority of anterior translation occurs on the lateral side of the knee. If the anterior translation increases or does not decrease, anterolateral rotary instability (ALRI) is present.

■ Lateral Pivot Shift Test
This test duplicates the anterior subluxation/reduction phenomenon that occurs during functional activities in ACL-deficient knees. During the test, the tibia moves away from the femur on the lateral side (but rotates medially) and moves anteriorly in relation to the femur. While supine, the hip is flexed at 30° with no abduction. The clinician places one hand behind the head of the fibula, and the other hand holds the foot while internally rotating the lower leg approximately 20°. A valgus force is applied to the knee while maintaining the internal rotation; the knee is moved from extension into flexion (**Fig. 15.15**). If the ACL is torn, the femur displaces posteriorly when the knee is placed in 10° to 20° of flexion. As the knee continues to flex, the IT band changes its angle of pull from that of an extensor to that of a flexor. When the knee reaches 30° to 40° of flexion, the IT band causes the tibia to reduce or slide backward, resulting in a noticeable "clunk." The pivot shift test has been found to have little clinical relevance in patients with osteoarthritis present within the knee[33] or when used on conscious patients.[34] The pivot shift test seems to be most appropriate to be used within nonarthritic patients under anesthesia.[33,34]

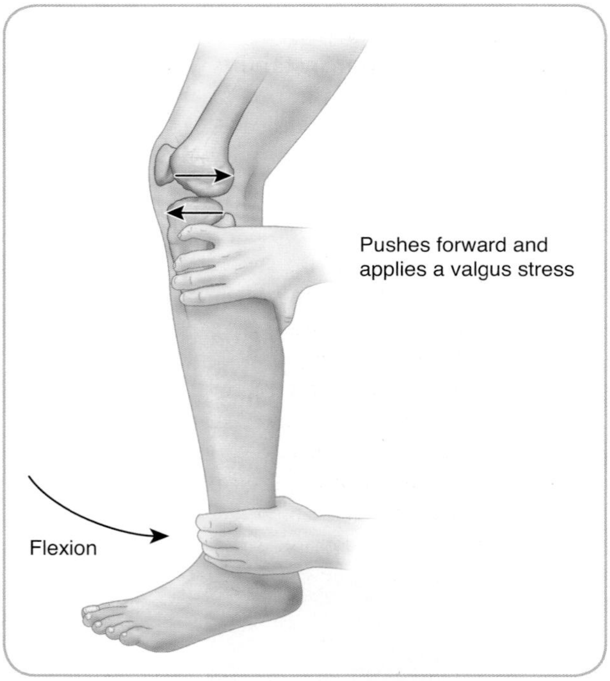

■ Cross-Over Test
The patient is weight bearing on the involved limb and asked to step across and in front of the involved leg with the uninvolved leg, in essence rotating on the involved limb (**Fig. 15.16**). Because the foot of the weight-bearing leg remains fixed, the lateral femoral condyle is allowed to displace posteriorly relative to the tibia in the presence of laxity in the lateral capsular restraints. This motion will assess for presence of ALRI. Next, the patient is instructed to return to the starting position and then step behind and in back of the involved limb with the uninvolved leg. The foot of the involved limb should always remain in contact with the floor. Stepping behind assesses for the presence of AMRI. Pain, instability, or apprehension is a positive finding for this test.

Posteromedial Rotary Instability

■ Hughston Posteromedial Drawer Test
This test combines what you already know about the *posterior drawer test* and *Slocum test*. The patient is supine with the knee flexed to 80° to 90° and the hip at 45°, which is similar to the position the patient is in for the posterior drawer test. The clinician medially rotates the patient's foot (toes pointed toward midline) and sits on the foot to stabilize it, which is similar to the Slocum test. Next, the clinician pushes the tibia posteriorly. If the tibia displaces or

Pushes forward and applies a valgus stress

Flexion

Figure 15.15. Lateral pivot shift test. While the hip is flexed and abducted 30° and is relaxed in slight medial rotation, the clinician places the heel of one hand behind the head of the fibula while the other hand grasps the distal tibia and 20° of internal tibial rotation is maintained. Next, the clinician applies a valgus force while the knee is slowly flexed. When the knee reaches 30° to 40° of flexion, the IT band causes the tibia to reduce or slide backward, giving a noticeable "clunk."

rotates posteriorly on the medial aspect by an excessive amount relative to the normal knee, the test is positive, indicating posteromedial rotary instability.

Posterolateral Rotary Instability

■ Hughston Posterolateral Drawer Test

The patient is in the same position as the Hughston posteromedial drawer test but with the foot laterally rotated or toes pointed away from the midline. The tibia is pushed posteriorly. If the tibia displaces or rotates posteriorly on the lateral aspect by an excessive amount relative to the normal knee, this indicates posterolateral rotary instability but only if the PCL is torn.

■ External Rotation Recurvatum Test

With the patient supine and the lower limbs relaxed, the clinician gently grasps the big toes of each foot and lifts both feet off the table (**Fig. 15.17**). The patient is told to keep the quadriceps relaxed. While elevating the legs, the clinician watches the tibial tubercles. If the test is positive, the affected knee goes into relative hyperextension on the lateral aspect, with the tibia and tibial tubercle rotating laterally. The affected knee appears to have genu varum, with damage to the PCL and LCL, arcuate ligament complex, posterolateral joint capsule, and biceps femoris.

Special Tests

A variety of special tests can be used for detecting injury or related pathology involving the knee.

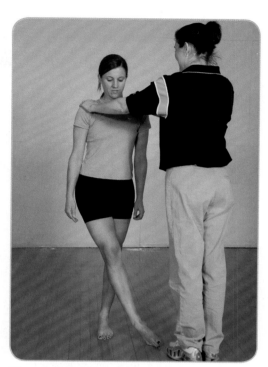

Figure 15.16. Cross-over test. Stepping across the injured leg determines ALRI. Stepping behind the injured leg can determine AMRI.

Tests for Meniscal Lesions

■ McMurray Test

While the patient is supine, the clinician flexes the knee and hip to about 90°. The clinician should place the fingers of one hand along the medial and lateral joint line of the knee under examination, the opposite hand is used to grasp the distal aspect of the leg. The clinician then slowly moves the patient's knee and hip into increased flexion while externally rotating the tibia. Next, slowly extend the knee and hip while keeping hand contact with the joint line (**Fig. 15.18**). This action attempts to trap the displaced posterior horn of the medial meniscus in the joint and produce an audible and palpable click or thud. Next, the clinician returns the leg to the starting position while internally rotating and extending the knee and hip. This motion places stress on the posterior horn of the lateral meniscus. Each test is repeated several times. Sharp pain along the joint line and/or a palpable click in conjunction with pain is a positive finding. The McMurray test has moderate sensitivity (.49) and moderate to good specificity (.79).[31]

■ Thessaly Test

To perform the Thessaly test, the patient is asked to stand flat-footed on the noninvolved leg and then flex the involved knee 5°. The clinician should grasp the outstretched hands of the patient in order to provide support and balance. The patient is then instructed to internally and externally rotate his or her torso three times while the knee remains flexed. The procedure is then again repeated with the knee flexed at 20°. Once that the patient is familiar with how to perform the test, the test is then repeated on the involved limb. A positive finding occurs when the patient complains of joint line pain or experiencing a locking or catching sensation. At 20° of flexion, the Thessaly test is reported to have a diagnostic accuracy of 94% in detecting medial meniscus injury and a 96% diagnostic accuracy of detecting lateral meniscal tears. The Thessaly test was also found to produce limited false-positive and false-negative findings.[35]

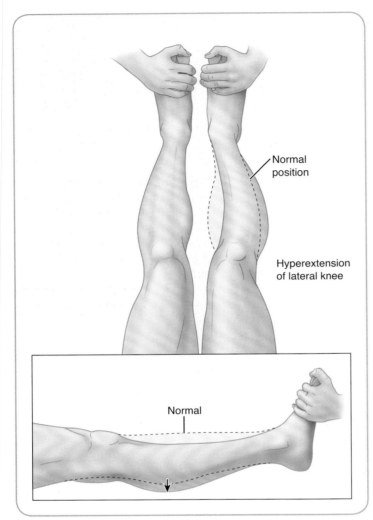

Figure 15.17. External rotation recurvatum test. The clinician grasps the big toes of each foot and then lifts both feet off the table. It is important that the patient keeps the quadriceps relaxed. In a positive test, the affected knee becomes hyperextended on the lateral aspect, with the tibia and tibial tubercle rotating laterally.

Tests for Tibiofibular Instability

■ Proximal Tibiofibular Syndesmosis Test

While the patient is supine and the knees are flexed at approximately 90° and feet resting on the table, the clinician stabilizes the tibia with one hand while the other hand grasps the proximal fibular head. In this position, the clinician attempts to displace the fibular head anteriorly and posteriorly. A positive test is indicated by any perceived movement of the fibula on the tibia. An anterior shift indicates damage to the proximal posterior tibiofibular ligament; posterior displacement indicates damage to the proximal anterior tibiofibular ligament.

Plica Tests

■ Mediopatellar Plica Test

While the patient is supine, the clinician flexes the affected knee to 30°. Next, the clinician moves the patella medially in an effort to cause pain, which would indicate a positive test. The pain is caused by pinching the edge of the plica between the medial femoral condyle and patella.

■ Plica "Stutter" Test

This is done with the patient seated on the edge of the examination table, with both knees flexed to 90°. The clinician places a finger over the patella and instructs the patient to extend the knee slowly. If the test is positive, the patella stutters or jumps between 45° and 60° of flexion (0° being full extension). The test is only effective if the patient has no joint swelling.

Tests for Patellofemoral Dysfunction

Because the cause of patellofemoral pain syndrome is so complex, multiple tests exist to examine this condition. However, no clear evidence has been found to establish the diagnostic accuracy of the majority of these tests due to the complex nature of patellofemoral dysfunction.[36] The tests included within this text are the ones most commonly used to assess patellofemoral dysfunction.

■ Patellar Mobility

When assessing a patient complaining of knee pain, patella mobility should be evaluated. While holding the patella in neutral position, the clinician should attempt to displace the patella first medially and then laterally. Medial glide of the patella stresses the lateral patellar retinaculum and the other soft-tissue restraints. Lateral glide stresses the medial patellar retinaculum, the VMO, and the knee's medial joint capsule. The patella should move half its width (one to two quadrants of the size of the patella) in both directions, with an end feel of tissue stretch (**Fig. 15.19**). Movement of one quadrant or less is called a hypomobile patella; movement of three quadrants or more is a hypermobile patella, indicating laxity of the restraints. The medial and lateral patellar glide test is moderately sensitive (.53).[31]

A hypermobile lateral glide may predispose the patient to a laterally subluxating or dislocating patella. If lateral displacement produces apprehension or reproduces symptoms of a subluxation (apprehension test), the test is considered to be positive, indicating patellar instability. The apprehension test for patellar instability has strong specificity (.86) but poor sensitivity (.35).[31] Comparing superior and inferior patellar glide sometimes can reveal side-to-side differences, especially in patients who have undergone surgery.

While the patient is supine, the patellar tilt test should be performed. The clinician grasps the patella, pushing down on the medial edge, and attempts to rotate the patella in the coronal plane to determine if the lateral patellar tilt can be corrected to "neutral" (i.e., when the patella's anterior surface comes parallel to the surface of the examination table). Normal tilt is between 0° and 15°. This test has poor to moderate reliability (.21 to .47) and may not be a clinically useful test.[31]

Patella Compression (Grind Test)

To assess articular pain resulting from irritation of subchondral bone, the clinician compresses the patella in the trochlea at various degrees of flexion. Normally, the patella enters the trochlea at 10° to 15° of knee flexion, so pressure applied in full extension does not directly produce articular compression between the patella and trochlea. As such, it is necessary to place a rolled towel under the knee, flexing the knee at approximately 20°. In this position, the clinician compresses the patella into the patellofemoral groove (**Fig. 15.20A**). The distal portion of the patella is articulating. Pain with compression in this range suggests a lesion in the distal patellar or proximal trochlear area. Conversely, as knee flexion increases, the patella is drawn distally in the trochlea, causing the area of articulation to be more proximal on the patella. Pain with compression in flexion suggests a more proximal patellar lesion. The test is considered to be positive if pain is felt or a grinding sound is heard, indicating pathology of the patellar articular cartilage.

Clarke Sign

Using the web of the hand, the clinician places the hand just proximal to the superior pole of the patella (**Fig. 15.20B**). The patient is instructed to contract the quadriceps while the clinician gently pushes downward. If the patient can hold the contraction without pain, the test is considered to be negative; if the patient has pain and is unable to hold the contraction, the test is considered to be positive for chondromalacia patellae. This test can elicit pain in any patient if the pressure is significant. Therefore, it is imperative to repeat the procedure several times with increasing pressure in full knee extension and at 30°, 60°, and 90° of knee flexion. However, the Clarke sign has been found to have very limited clinical usefulness due to the great variation in how the test is described and performed, resulting in poor reliability, sensitivity, and specificity.[37]

Waldron Test

The clinician palpates the patella while the patient does several slow, deep knee bends. Any crepitus, pain, "catching," or improper tracking of the patella should be noted. If any of these signs or symptoms occurs

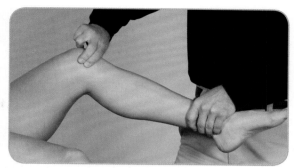

Figure 15.18. McMurray test. The hip and knee are flexed, and the clinician stabilizes the lower leg with one hand and laterally rotates the tibia. The other hand is placed over the anterior knee with the fingers on the joint line. The clinician slowly extends the leg. If a loose body is in the medial meniscus, this action causes a snap or click. Internally rotating the leg and repeating the test with the thumb over the lateral joint line tests for lateral meniscus damage.

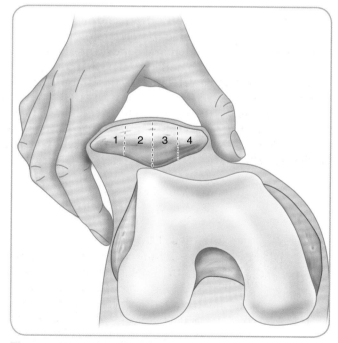

Figure 15.19. Patellar glide. Passive lateral glide of the patella demonstrating subluxation to its second quadrant. Hypomobility is manifested by less than one quadrant of displacement; hypermobility is manifested by three or more quadrants (greater than half of patellar width).

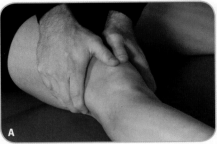
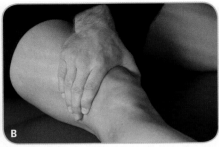
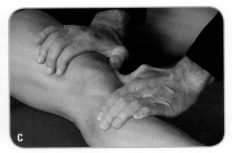

Figure 15.20. Patellofemoral dysfunction. A, Patella compression or grind test. Pain on compression of the patella indicates pathology of the patella articular cartilage. **B, Clarke sign.** Slight compression is applied just proximal to the superior pole of the patella while the patient contracts the quadriceps. The test is positive for chondromalacia patella if the patient has pain or is unable to hold the contraction. **C, Patellar apprehension test.** The clinician gently displaces the patella laterally. The test is positive for a subluxating patella if the patient shows apprehension.

simultaneously, the test is considered to be positive for chondromalacia patellae. The Waldron test has been found to have both low positive and negative likelihood ratios, suggesting the test may provide little relevant clinical information regarding the presence or absence of conditions relating to patellofemoral syndrome.[38]

■ Patellar Apprehension Test

While the knee is in a relaxed position, the clinician pushes the patella laterally (**Fig. 15.20C**). If the patient voluntarily or involuntarily shows apprehension, the test is considered to be positive for a subluxating patella.

Tests for Iliotibial Band Friction Syndrome

■ Noble Compression Test

The Noble compression test is used to assess for inflammation of the IT band fibers that cross the lateral femoral condyle or of the underlying bursa (**Fig. 15.21A**). The patient is supine on a table, with the hip and knee flexed at 45°. The clinician applies pressure with the thumb directly over, or 1 to 2 cm proximal to, the lateral epicondyle of the femur and passively lowers the leg and extends the

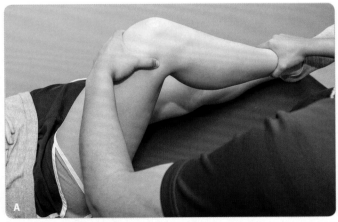
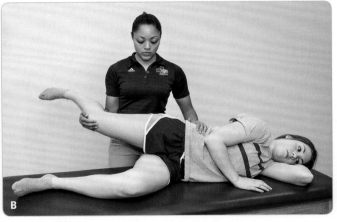

Figure 15.21. Tests for iliotibial band friction syndrome. A, Noble compression test. The hip and knee are flexed at 90°. The clinician applies thumb pressure over the lateral epicondyle of the femur as the leg is extended. Pain at or near 30° of flexion indicates iliotibial band (ITB) syndrome. **B, Ober test.** The clinician passively abducts and slightly extends the hip. Then, the clinician slowly lowers the extended leg. If the ITB is tight, the leg remains in the abducted position.

knee. As the knee moves to 30° of knee flexion, a positive response is severe pain similar to that caused during activity.

■ Ober Test

Although the Ober test does not assess specifically for iliotibial band syndrome (ITBS), the test is used to assess for the presences of a tight or contracted IT band, which is thought to contribute to ITBS.[39] The patient lies on the side with the lower leg slightly flexed at the hip and knee for stability. The knee of the upper or affected limb is flexed to 90°. The clinician stabilizes the pelvis with one hand to prevent the pelvis from shifting posteriorly during the test. Next, the clinician passively abducts and slightly extends the hip of the upper or affected limb so that the IT band passes over the greater trochanter (**Fig. 15.21B**). Although the original Ober test called for the knee to be flexed at 90°, the IT band has a greater stretch if the knee is extended.[39] The clinician slowly lowers the upper leg. If the IT band is tight, the leg will remain in the abducted position.

Neurological Tests

Neurological integrity is assessed with isometric muscle testing of the myotomes, reflex testing, and sensation in the segmental dermatomes and peripheral nerve cutaneous patterns.

Myotomes

Isometric muscle testing should be performed in the following motions to test specific segmental myotomes:

- Hip flexion (L1, L2)
- Knee extension (L3)
- Ankle dorsiflexion (L4)
- Toe extension (L5)
- Ankle plantar flexion, foot eversion, or hip extension (S1)
- Knee flexion (S2)

Reflexes

Reflexes in the lower leg region include the patella (L3, L4) and Achilles tendon reflex (S1) (**Fig. 15.22**). The patellar reflex is tested with the patient seated on the end of a table so that the knee is flexed at 90°. The clinician strikes the tendon with the flat end of the reflex hammer using a crisp, wrist-flexion action. A normal reflex exhibits a slight, jerking motion in extension. In testing the Achilles tendon reflex, the clinician slightly dorsiflexes the ankle to place the tendon on stretch and taps the tendon with the flat end of the reflex hammer. An alternate position is to have the patient lie prone

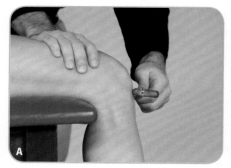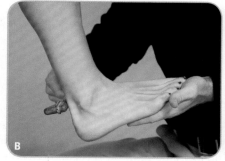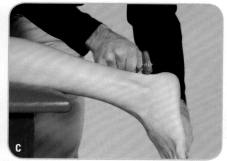

Figure 15.22. Reflex testing. A, The patellar reflex. **B,** The Achilles reflex. **C,** Alternate position for the Achilles reflex.

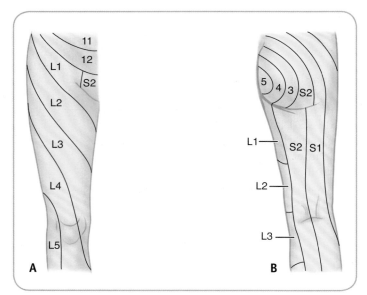

Figure 15.23. Segmental nerve dermatome patterns. A, Anterior view. **B,** Posterior view.

on a table or place the knee on a chair, with the foot extended beyond the edge. A normal reflex should elicit a slight plantar flexion jerk.

Cutaneous Patterns

The segmental nerve dermatome patterns for the pelvis, hip, and thigh are demonstrated in **Figure 15.23.** The peripheral nerve cutaneous patterns are demonstrated in **Figure 15.24.**

Activity-Specific Functional Tests

Functional tests should be performed before clearing the patient for return to participation. These tests should be performed pain-free, without a limp or antalgic gait. Examples of functional tests include forward running, cross-over stepping, running figure eights or V-cuts, side-step running, and carioca running. When appropriate, functional braces or protective supportive devices should be used to prevent reinjury.

The physical examination of the basketball player should include active ROM, passive ROM, and restricted ROM for knee flexion and extension and for internal and external tibial rotation. In addition, a battery of tests assessing for possible causes and presence of patellofemoral pain syndrome should be performed.

CONTUSIONS

? A volleyball player fell on the knee and felt an intense pain on the anterior of the joint. Pain is palpable on either side of the patellar tendon but not directly on the tendon. The patient reports a "catching" sensation. Extreme pain is felt with forced knee extension. What condition should be suspected, and how should the injury be managed?

Etiology

Contusions at the knee result from compressive forces (i.e., a kick or falling on the knee). The infrapatellar fat pad may become entrapped between the femur and tibia or inflamed during arthroscopy, leading to a tender, puffy, fat pad contusion. The common peroneal nerve leaves the popliteal space and winds around the fibular neck to supply motor and sensory function to the anterior and lateral compartments of the lower leg (see **Fig. 15.4**). A kick or blow to the posterolateral aspect of the knee can compress this nerve, leading to temporary or permanent paralysis. The nerve also may be injured by prolonged compression from a knee brace or elastic wrap, prolonged squatting (e.g., baseball or softball catcher), or traction caused by a varus stress or hyperextension at the knee.

Signs and Symptoms

General signs and symptoms of any contusion are localized tenderness, pain, swelling, and ecchymosis. With a fat pad contusion, locking, catching, giving way, palpable pain on either side of the patellar tendon, and extreme pain on forced extension may be present. In a mild acute injury to the peroneal nerve, an immediate "shocking" feeling of pain may radiate down the lateral aspect of the leg and foot. If the actual nerve is not damaged, tingling and numbness may persist for several minutes. In severe cases (i.e., when the nerve is crushed), initial pain is not immediately followed by tingling or numbness. Rather, as swelling increases within the nerve sheath, muscle weakness in dorsiflexion or eversion as well as loss of sensation on the dorsum of the foot, particularly between the great and second toes, may progressively occur days or weeks later.

Management

Following a full assessment to rule out fracture and major ligament damage, initial treatment includes ice, compression, elevation, rest, and nonsteroidal anti-inflammatory drugs (NSAIDs). Participation in sport and physical activity usually is not limited; however, the area should be protected to prevent further insult. If any signs of sensory changes or motor weakness become evident, the patient should be referred to a physician.

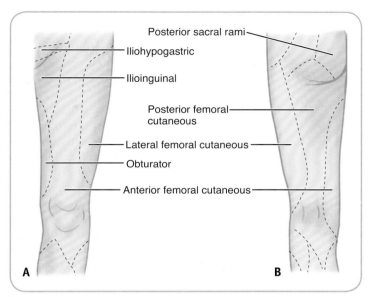

Figure 15.24. Peripheral nerve sensory distribution patterns. A, Anterior view. **B,** Posterior view.

 The volleyball player probably contused the infrapatellar fat pad during the fall onto the knee. Standard acute care (i.e., ice, compression, elevation, and protected rest) should be sufficient to address the injury.

BURSITIS

? As part of rehabilitation for a shoulder injury, a 30-year-old man is maintaining cardio-vascular fitness by using a stationary bike. Following 1 week on the bike, the patient complains of pain on the proximal, medial tibia just distal to the knee joint. The pain is particularly evident after his workout. What structure may be inflamed, and are there any factors that may contribute to this condition?

Etiology

Bursitis can be caused by direct trauma, overuse, infections, metabolic abnormalities, rheumatic afflictions, and **neoplasms** (tumors). Compressive forces from a direct blow can be associated with a grossly distended, warm bursal sac filled with bloody effusion, called a hemabursa. Repeated insult can lead to the more common chronic bursitis, in which the bursal wall thickens and, when filled with fluid, appears to be distended. Inflammation of the pes anserine bursa typically develops from friction, but it also may occur in direct trauma. It often is seen in runners, cyclists, and swimmers who are subjected to excessive valgus stress at the knee or in patients who have tight hamstrings.

Signs and Symptoms

Common symptoms of bursitis include swelling and pain in the prepatellar region (i.e., **prepatellar bursitis**), in the distal patellar tendon region (i.e., deep **infrapatellar bursitis**), in the proximal medial tibia (i.e., **pes anserine bursitis**), or over the medial joint line (i.e., **tibial collateral ligament bursitis**).

Inflammation of the deep infrapatellar bursa due to overuse and subsequent friction between the patellar tendon and the structures behind it (i.e., fat pad and tibia) is often confused with

Osgood-Schlatter disease in adolescents and with patellar tendinitis in older patients. In extension, the fat pad is squeezed between the patellar tendon and tibia and often extends beyond the sides of the tendon. Careful palpation over the distal patellar tendon and noting the specific area of tenderness will determine which condition is present. In flexion, bursitis is indicated by pain deep to the patellar tendon. In extension, pain palpated on either side of the patellar tendon indicates a fat pad contusion.

If the pes anserine bursa is inflamed, point tenderness, localized swelling, and crepitation may be palpated beneath the pes tendons (usually 2 cm below the medial joint line). When inflamed, contraction of the hamstring muscles, rotational movements of the tibia, and direct pressure over the bursa produce pain. Inflammation of this bursa is commonly seen in middle-aged or older, overweight women, many of whom also have osteoarthritis of the knee.[40] To avoid recurrence, the patient should begin an extensive flexibility program for the hamstrings and gastrocnemius–soleus complex.

The term **Baker cyst** identifies almost any synovial herniation of the posterior joint capsule or bursitis on the posterior aspect of the knee. With no posterior obstruction, internal derangement injuries (i.e., meniscal problems, cruciate ligament tears, or arthritis) commonly lead to joint effusion that expands into the bursal sac. The semimembranosus bursa most commonly is involved, because it often communicates with the joint capsule. A soft, tumorous mass can be palpated in the medial popliteal space and may or may not be painful. A Baker cyst does not pose a serious problem, although it may be bothersome during full flexion or extension of the knee.

Abrasions or penetrating injuries can lead to infected bursitis caused by bacteria entering broken skin. This condition differs from acute bursitis because of the localized and intense redness, increased pain, enlarged regional lymph nodes, spreading cellulitis, and subsequent fever and malaise. If infection is suspected, immediate referral to a physician is warranted for proper cleansing, irrigation, and closure (often with a drain). The infection can enter the lymph system, causing pyarthrosis, or suppurative arthritis, at the knee.

Management

Treatment consists of ice therapy, a compressive wrap, NSAIDs, avoiding activities that irritate the condition, or total rest until acute symptoms subside. A protective foam, or doughnut, pad may protect the area from further insult. A risk of infection exists if the skin is broken during the initial injury, in which case the patient should be referred to a physician immediately. The physician may culture any aspirated fluid to detect bacteria and subsequently prescribe medication.

Corticosteroid injections may be administered by the physician in cases of chronic or persistent bursitis when other means of treatment have been ineffective in decreasing inflammation.[40] Because these injections can weaken surrounding tendons or ligaments, they should not be injected close to these structures.

The 30-year-old man using the stationary bike to maintain cardiovascular fitness could have pes anserine bursitis. Tight hamstrings and excessive valgus stress placed on the knee during the pedaling motion can predispose a patient to this injury. In addition to standard acute care, this patient should begin an extensive flexibility program for the hamstrings and gastrocnemius–soleus complex.

LIGAMENTOUS CONDITIONS

? A basketball player decelerated, set the left foot, and then forcefully pushed off the left leg to perform a right-handed layup shot. The player felt a sudden popping sensation and intense pain, and then the knee collapsed. Initial evaluation revealed point tenderness on the anteromedial joint line. The basketball player has swelling but no signs of deformity. What structures might be involved with this injury?

BOX 15.4 Signs and Symptoms of Ligament Failure

Minimal Ligament Failure (Distraction, <5 mm)

- Less than one-third of the fibers are torn.
- Mild swelling and pain are localized over the injury site (with the MCL, pain is in the proximal 1–2 in).
- Active and passive ROM are normal, and muscular strength is normal or slightly decreased.
- No joint laxity is apparent during the stress test.
- Definite end feel is present.

Partial Ligament Failure (Distraction, 5–10 mm)

- One- to two-thirds of the ligament is damaged, with microtears present.
- Localized swelling and joint effusion may result from deep capsular tears, meniscal damage, or cruciate ligament damage.
- Pain is sharp and may be either transient or lasting.
- Patient may complain of instability and an inability to walk with the heel on the ground.
- ROM is decreased initially by pain and hamstring muscle spasm and later by soft-tissue swelling or effusion.
- Inability to fully extend the knee actively
- Visible translation of the tibia during stress tests

Complete Ligament Failure (Distraction, >10 mm)

- More than two-thirds of the ligament is ruptured.
- Swelling is diffuse, indicating severe capsular tear and damage to intracapsular structures.
- Pain is initially sharp and often disappears within a minute.
- Patient is aware of the feeling of instability or the knee giving way.
- Significant loss of ROM
- Visible distraction of greater than 10 mm during stress testing may appear as a subluxation.

Knee joint stability depends on a static, passive system of support from its ligaments and capsular structures. The American Academy of Orthopaedic Surgeons (AAOS) classifies ligamentous injuries at the knee according to the functional disruption of a specific ligament, or amount of laxity (**Box 15.4**), and the direction of laxity. Clinicians often refer to minimal ligament failure as a grade I injury, partial ligament failure as a grade II injury, and complete disruption as grade III. The AAOS identifies four straight instabilities and four rotary instabilities (see **Table 15.3**). Knowing the knee position at impact and the direction the tibia displaces or rotates is beneficial in determining the damaged structures.

Unidirectional Instabilities

A straight plane (i.e., unidirectional) instability implies instability in one of the cardinal planes. Injury to the ACL or PCL produces instability in the sagittal plane, allowing equal anterior or posterior **translation** (i.e., shifting) of the medial and lateral tibial plateaus on the femur. Injury to the MCL and LCL leads to valgus or varus instability in the frontal plane. Although several structures may be damaged, the resulting instability involves a single plane.

Straight Medial Instability

■ Etiology

In straight medial instability, the MCL is damaged. This is known as a **valgus instability**. Lateral or valgus forces cause tension on the medial aspect of the knee, potentially damaging the MCL and posteromedial capsular ligaments as well as the PCL (**Fig. 15.25A**). Damage occurs more often when the valgus force is applied with the limb in a weight-bearing position or closed kinetic chain.

■ Signs and Symptoms

A grade I sprain is characterized by mild point tenderness on the medial joint line and/or MCL, little or no joint effusion, full ROM that may include some discomfort, and a stable joint when doing the

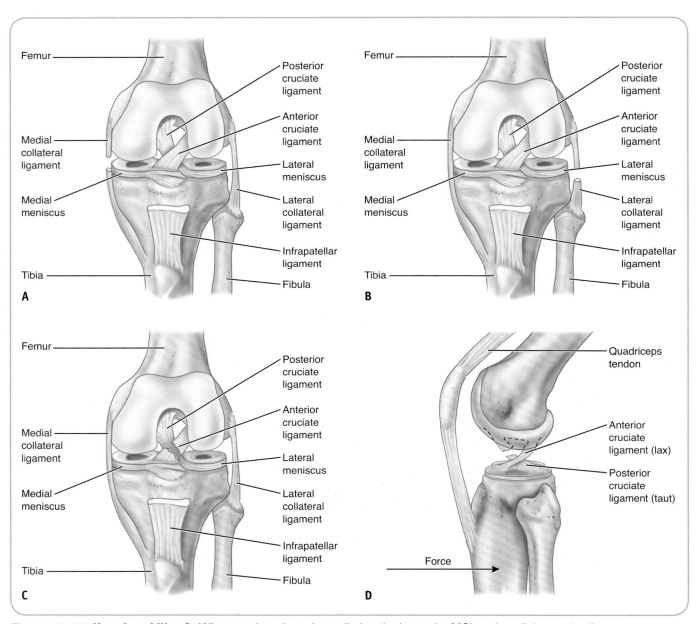

Figure 15.25. Knee instability. A, When a valgus force is applied to the knee, the MCL and medial capsular ligaments are damaged, leading to valgus laxity. **B,** An isolated varus force damages the LCL, leading to varus laxity. **C,** When changing directions during deceleration, the ACL can be damaged. **D,** During hyperextension of the knee or when the knee is flexed and the tibia is driven posterior, the PCL can be damaged.

valgus stress test. A **positive valgus test in 30°** of flexion with a soft end feel indicates at least a grade II injury to the middle third of the capsular ligament and MCL. The patient may be unable to fully extend the leg and often walks on the ball of the foot, unable to keep the heel flat on the ground and will complain of tenderness over the MCL and joint line when palpated. A grade III MCL injury often has no significant intra-articular effusion, but if such effusion is found, injuries to the cruciate ligaments, patella, or meniscus should be assessed. A grade III injury has a positive valgus test with significant joint laxity, a soft or even absent end point because of a complete tear of the MCL, usually at the femoral attachment. **A positive valgus stress test in full extension** suggests MCL and medial joint capsule involvement.

Straight Lateral Instability

■ Etiology

Straight lateral instability, or **varus instability**, results from medial forces that produce tension on the lateral compartment, damaging the LCL, lateral capsular ligaments, PCL, and joint structures (**Fig. 15.25B**). This isolated injury is rare, because the biceps femoris, IT band, and popliteus provide a strong stabilizing effect. A potential mechanism for this injury can be seen in the sport of wrestling, in which an opponent often is between the patient's legs and is able to deliver an excessive varus force that can lead to injury.

■ Signs and Symptoms

Damage to the LCL has the same general signs and symptoms that are associated with an MCL sprain. The patient may experience lateral knee pain that is described as sharp. Swelling is minimal, because the ligament is not attached to the joint capsule. Instability is subtle, because other structures are intact. A positive varus test in 30° of flexion, however, should confirm damage to the ligament. A positive varus stress test in full extension may indicate damage to the lateral joint capsule and LCL. If tenderness is detected on the head of the fibula, an avulsion fracture or peroneal nerve injury may be present, although these injuries usually are associated with more severe knee injuries.

Straight Anterior Instability

■ Etiology

In a straight anterior instability, both tibial plateaus sublux anteriorly by an equal amount when an anterior drawer test is performed. This translation is resisted by the ACL. Isolated anterior instability is rare; instead, an anteromedial or anterolateral laxity usually occurs. Damage to the ACL commonly occurs during a cutting or turning maneuver, landing, or sudden deceleration (**Fig. 15.25C**).

The rate of ACL injuries is higher in women than in men, particularly for those women who are involved with jumping and pivoting sports.[41] Several theories have been put forth to explain this phenomenon, and recent research has begun to look at muscle strength imbalance between the hamstrings and quadriceps in both men and women. During a landing/deceleration maneuver, flexion movements are occurring at the hip and knee. Simultaneous eccentric contractions of the quadriceps to stabilize the knee and of the hamstrings to stabilize the hip decelerate the horizontal velocity of the body. The hamstrings also act to neutralize the tendency of the quadriceps to cause anterior tibial translation. If the muscles are unable to meet the demand of stabilization, inert internal tissues, such as ligaments, cartilage, and bone, are at risk for injury. Therefore, a deficit in eccentric hamstrings strength relative to eccentric quadriceps strength could predispose a patient to an ACL injury. Prophylactic bracing has not been shown to prevent ACL injuries.[40–42]

See **Possible Factors Influencing Increased Rate of Anterior Cruciate Ligament Injuries in Women**, available on the companion Web site at thePoint.

■ Signs and Symptoms

In approximately 80% of ACL injuries, patients experience a popping, snapping, or tearing sensation, and in a similar percentage of cases, patients note a rapid onset (i.e., usually within 3 hours) of swelling (hemarthrosis). Pain can range from minimal and transient to severe and lasting. It may be described as being deep in the knee but more often is felt anterior, on either side of the patellar tendon, or laterally, on the joint line. Weight bearing leads to a feeling of the knee giving way or as "the leg slipping out from under the knee." The high incidence of damage to other internal structures necessitates immediate referral to a physician. Positive Lachman and/or anterior drawer tests suggest ACL damage.

Straight Posterior Instability

■ Etiology
In straight posterior instability, the medial and lateral tibial plateaus have equal translation posteriorly in a neutral position without rotation. The PCL, along with the arcuate complex and oblique popliteal ligament, provides nearly all resistance to prevent this motion. Hyperextension is the most common mechanism for injury. The PCL, however, also can be damaged during a fall on a flexed knee with the foot plantar flexed, resulting in a blow to the tibial tubercle that drives the tibia posteriorly (**Fig. 15.25D**).

■ Signs and Symptoms
In milder cases, intense pain and a sense of stretching are felt in the posterior aspect of the knee. In a total rupture, a characteristic pop or snap is felt and heard, and this may be followed by autonomic symptoms of dizziness, sweating, faintness, or slight nausea.[43] A large effusion and hemarthrosis usually occur within the first 2 hours after the acute injury. Knee extension is limited because of the effusion and stretching of the posterior capsule and gastrocnemius. A positive posterior sag (gravity) test or reverse Lachman test confirms damage to the PCL. When the PCL is torn, the extensor mechanism, including the patella and the patellar tendon, forcefully holds the tibia in a reduced position, which results in increased patellofemoral pressure. Increased patellofemoral loading also is caused by a vector change resulting from posterior tibial displacement. This concept may explain complaints of patellofemoral pain in patients with PCL-deficient knees.

Multidirectional Instabilities

Although unidirectional instability involves damage that results in instability to a single plane, multidirectional instability involves instability in more than one plane. This injury also is called a multiplane or rotary instability.

Anteromedial Rotary Instability

■ Etiology
AMRI results from anterior external rotation of the medial tibia condyle on the femur, leading to damage of the medial compartment ligaments and oblique popliteal ligament (**Fig. 15.26**). This instability can be accentuated by a tear of the medial meniscus and ACL. Although referred to as the "unhappy triad," the MCL is the primary ligamentous restraint to this motion. In AMRI, valgus stress testing at 0° and 30° of flexion is positive. In addition, increased anterior translation of the medial tibial plateau is noted when a Slocum drawer test or Lachman test is performed with the tibia externally rotated. A more functional test for assessing rotary instability is the cross-over test.

Anterolateral Rotary Instability

■ Etiology
ALRI is a characteristic of an anterior internal subluxation of the lateral tibial condyle on the femur. The ACL is the primary structure damaged by this instability, but the IT band and lateral capsule ligaments also can be damaged. The injury typically is caused by a sudden deceleration and cutting maneuver, and it is the most frequent rotary instability at the knee. In anterolateral instability, the Slocum drawer test with the tibia internally rotated, Slocum ALRI test, and cross-over test show increased anterior translation of the lateral tibial plateau.

Posteromedial Rotary Instability

■ Etiology
In posteromedial rotary instability, the medial tibial plateau shifts posteriorly on the femur and opens medially. This is a severe injury and is indicative of damage to the superficial MCL, posteromedial

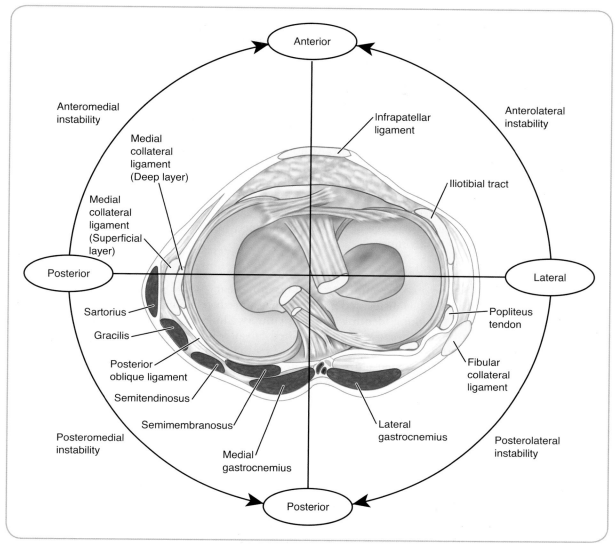

Figure 15.26. Instabilities at the knee.

capsule, oblique popliteal ligament, and both cruciate ligaments. Injury of the posteromedial capsule is suspected if joint space opening and a soft end point are apparent on valgus stress at 0°. The posteromedial drawer test and posteromedial pivot shift test are positive.

Posterolateral Rotary Instability

■ Etiology

In posterolateral rotary instability, a greater posterior translation of the lateral tibial plateau is noted, as compared to the medial tibial plateau, when a posterior drawer force is applied. This injury often is caused by a sudden anteromedial force that brings the knee joint from near-full extension into hyperextension. This mechanism, when combined with a varus moment, disrupts the posterolateral structures, which include the PCL, arcuate–popliteal complex, posterolateral capsule, and LCL. Other mechanisms may include a combined hyperextension and external rotation force, contact and noncontact hyperextension, severe varus bending moment, and severe tibial external rotation torque.[43] Injury of the posterolateral capsule is suspected if joint space opening and a soft end point are apparent on varus stress at 0° and 30°. In addition, the posterolateral drawer and external rotation recurvatum tests are positive.

Knee Dislocations

■ Etiology

Knee dislocations and less severe multiligament injuries make up approximately 20% of all grade III knee ligament injuries. Frequent two-ligament injuries include the ACL-MCL (most common), PCL-MCL, ACL-LCL, and ACL-PCL. Damage to only two ligaments does not result in enough translation of the joint to cause neurovascular injury. The exception, however, is injury to the LCL and a cruciate ligament that results in enough lateral opening to damage the peroneal nerve.

A minimum of three ligaments must be torn for the knee to dislocate. Most often, this involves the ACL, PCL, and one collateral ligament. Although dislocations may occur in any direction, the most common is in an anterior or posterior direction. As with any dislocation, additional damage can occur to other joint structures, including the ligaments, capsular structures, menisci, articular surfaces, tendons, and neurovascular structures. Associated injuries include vascular damage in 20% to 40% of knee dislocations and nerve damage in 20% to 30%. Posterior knee dislocations are associated with the highest incidence of damage to the popliteal artery; posterolateral rotary dislocations have the highest incidence of nerve injury.

■ Signs and Symptoms

The patient may describe a severe injury to the knee and hear a loud pop. Deformity of the knee may be present if the knee has dislocated and remained unreduced. Knee dislocations often reduce spontaneously, however, making identification difficult. Swelling occurs within the first few hours, but swelling may not be large because of an associated capsular injury and extravasation of the hemarthrosis. It is critical to identify the dislocated knee by the ligamentous structures that have been disrupted. If a vascular injury is left untreated or not repaired within 8 hours after injury, the amputation rate is 86%. If surgery is completed within 6 to 8 hours, however, the amputation rate drops to 11%. Associated nerve injury has a poor prognosis regardless of the treatment.

Management of Ligament Conditions

Injuries involving minimal ligament failure are managed conservatively, with ice application, compression, elevation, and protected rest until acute symptoms subside. A compression wrap, consisting of an inverted horseshoe around the patella secured by an elastic wrap, can be used with a knee immobilizer to reduce swelling. Cryotherapy and NSAIDs are used to reduce pain and inflammation. In suspected ACL injuries, radiographs should be obtained to rule out an associated intraarticular fracture. Avulsion fractures of the tibial eminence may occur, particularly in adults older than 35 years who have some associated osteopenia. Magnetic resonance imaging can clarify the diagnosis.

In consultation with a physician, a moderate injury with partial ligament failure is managed with ice, compression, elevation, and protected rest for 24 to 72 hours. Crutches are used until the patient walks without a limp. Progression to partial weight bearing with heel-to-toe gait can begin as tolerated. Rehabilitation should be initiated as soon as acute symptoms subside. ROM exercises should include assisted knee flexion and knee extension. Isometric exercises of the quadriceps and straight leg raises in all directions should progress to resisted exercises throughout the full ROM. Closed chain strengthening exercises and maintenance of ROM can be supplemented with cardiovascular exercises as tolerated.

The physician may determine that surgical repair is necessary for injuries in which isolated complete ligament failure has occurred or in which more than one major ligament is involved. Surgical reconstruction is based on the degree of laxity, activity-specific demands, hours per week of activity, intensity of activity, frequency of instability, and associated repairable meniscal tear. Reconstruction usually is delayed at least 3 weeks postinjury to allow swelling to decrease and ROM to increase. **Application Strategy 15.2** describes the management and rehabilitation of a mild ACL injury.

 The basketball player may have sustained an injury to the medial meniscus, the ACL, or the MCL. Additional assessment is necessary to confirm the involved structure.

APPLICATION STRATEGY 15.2

Management of an Anterior Cruciate Ligament Injury

Phase 1

1. Protect, restrict activity, ice, compression, elevation, and rest with a knee immobilizer to reduce swelling.
2. Use crutches if the patient cannot bear weight without pain.
3. ROM exercises within pain-free limits
   - Heel slides
   - Prone knee flexion, assisted with the opposite leg
   - Passive knee extension in a supine or seated position
4. Strengthening exercises
   - Bent leg raises in all directions
   - Multiangle isometric exercises for the quadriceps, hamstrings, and hip adductors
5. Cardiovascular fitness: upper body ergometer and unilateral leg cycling

Phase 2

1. ROM. Continue exercises to regain full ROM.
2. Unilateral balance activities. See Application Strategy 15.1 and progress as tolerated.
3. Strengthening exercises
   - Perform slow, controlled, eccentric closed chain exercises, such as two-legged squats to 60°, step-ups, step-downs, and lateral step-ups.
   - Calf raises (seated position) can progress to standing position when pain-free.
   - Perform straight leg raises in all directions, with tubing added as tolerated.

Phase 3

1. ROM. Maintain full ROM and flexibility in the lower extremity.
2. Strengthening
   - Hip leg press and squats
   - Toe raises with weights
   - Lunges
   - Isokinetic open and closed chain exercises
3. Cardiovascular fitness
   - Bilateral, minimal tension cycling if 110°–115° of knee flexion is present. Avoid full knee extension.
   - Pool running, swimming with a flutter kick, jogging in place on a trampoline, and power walking

Phase 4

1. Balance and proprioception. Continue exercises from the preceding.
2. Functional activities
   - Running drills, such as circles, figure eights, cross-over steps (cariocas), and jumping with double limb/single limb progressing from standing in place, front to back, to diagonals
   - Multidirectional, high-speed balance drills are added after the patient can run 2–3 miles.
   - Jumping, bounding, and skipping (plyometrics)
   - Slide board

MENISCAL CONDITIONS

 A 40-year-old golfer complains of mild swelling and tenderness on the medial joint line. Slight joint effusion is present, and pain can be elicited with rotation of the tibia on the femur and during extreme knee flexion. What injury may be present, and what is the management for this injury?

Etiology

Menisci, which become stiffer and less resilient with age, are injured in manners similar to the ligamentous structures. In addition to compression and tensile forces, shearing forces caused when the femur rotates on a fixed tibia trap the posterior horns of both menisci, leading to some tearing. Tears are classified according to age, location, or axis of orientation. Medial meniscus damage is more common than lateral meniscus damage because of the lower mobility of the structure.

Longitudinal tears result from a twisting motion when the foot is fixed and the knee is flexed (**Fig. 15.27A**). This action produces compression and torsion on the posterior peripheral attachment. The tear can be partial, affecting only the peripheral segment of the meniscus, or a complete tearing of the inner substance of the meniscus. A **"bucket-handle"** tear occurs when an entire longitudinal segment is displaced medially toward the center of the tibia (**Fig. 15.27B**). This tear can lead to locking of the knee at approximately 10° flexion; however, this only occurs in approximately 40% of complete meniscal tears.

Horizontal cleavage tears result from degeneration and often affect the posteromedial portion of the meniscus (**Fig. 15.27C**). With age, shearing forces from rotational motions tear the inner substance of the meniscus. If detached, momentary locking, associated pain, and instability may occur. A parrot-beak tear is actually two tears that commonly occur in the middle segment of the lateral menisci, leading to the characteristic shape of a parrot's beak. It is seen more frequently in patients with a history of previous trauma or some cystic pathology that makes the meniscus more fixed at its periphery (**Fig. 15.27D**).

Signs and Symptoms

Meniscal injuries are difficult to assess, both because they are not innervated by nociceptors and because only 10% to 30% of the peripheral medial meniscus border and 10% to 25% of the lateral meniscus border receive direct blood supply. The patient may describe performing a cutting or rotational maneuver and experiencing sharp, stab-like pain in the joint line at the time of injury. Localized pain and joint-line tenderness near the collateral ligament probably are the most common findings. Anterior joint-line pain rarely reflects meniscal pathology unless a bucket-handle or ruptured bucket-handle tear is present. Because the meniscal periphery is attached to the synovial lining, tensile forces may cause synovial inflammation and slight joint effusion more than 12 hours after the initial injury. Pain occurs on rotation and extreme flexion of the knee. The patient may also describing episodes of instability, such as the knee "giving out" or locking. In the initial assessment, it is important to determine whether the knee lacked full extension from the time of injury (i.e., locked knee from displaced fragment) or lacked full extension the next day (i.e., pseudolocking from a hamstring spasm).

A chronic degenerative meniscal tear often results from multiple episodes of minimal trauma leading to almost no pain, disability, or swelling, although atrophy of the quadriceps may be present. Recurrent locking is typical. Chronic tears in the absence of degeneration have point tenderness only over the site of the lesion. The patient may experience a popping, grinding, or clicking sensation that can lead to the knee buckling or giving way. Special tests used to identify meniscal injuries that

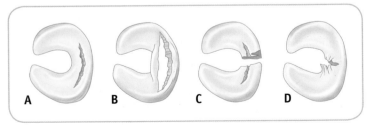

Figure 15.27. Meniscal tears. A, Longitudinal. **B,** Bucket-handle. **C,** Horizontal. **D,** Parrot-beak.

APPLICATION STRATEGY 15.3

Management of a Partial Meniscectomy

Phase 1

1. Protect, restrict activity, ice, compression, elevation, and bracing to reduce swelling. Use crutches if needed.
2. ROM exercises within pain-free limits
   - Heel slides
   - Supine wall slides
   - Prone knee flexion, assisted with the opposite leg
   - Passive knee extension in a supine or seated position

Phase 2

1. ROM. Continue exercises as tolerated.
2. Unilateral balance activities. See Application Strategy 15.1.
3. Strengthening exercises. Include the following:
   - Multiangle isometric exercises for the quadriceps, hamstrings, and hip adductors
   - Straight leg raises in all directions. Add tubing or ankle weights during later stages.
   - Short-arc quadriceps extension exercises. Place a pillow or bolster under the knee to support the knee at 45° of flexion. Extend the knee, and hold for 10 seconds. Add ankle weights to increase resistance.
   - Toe raises from a seated position can progress to standing position when pain-free.
   - Straight leg raises in all directions, with tubing added as tolerated
4. Cardiovascular fitness
   - Use upper body ergometer and a stationary cycle with bilateral minimal tension if 115°–120° of knee flexion is present. Avoid full knee extension.

Phase 3

1. ROM. Maintain full ROM and flexibility in the lower extremity.
2. Strengthening
   - Hip leg press and squats
   - Toe raises with weights
   - Lunges
   - Isokinetic open and closed chain exercises
3. Cardiovascular fitness
   - Pool running, swimming with a flutter kick, jogging on a trampoline, and power walking

Phase 4 (Return to Activity)

1. Maintain ROM, flexibility, strength, and balance.
2. Functional activities. See Application Strategy 15.2.

have been found to be clinically useful include Thessaly and McMurray tests.[44] However, if the patient has also sustained a concurrent ACL injury, diagnostic accuracy of the Thessaly test is diminished.[31]

Management

Initial treatment depends on the extent of damage. Mild cases with no ligamentous instability are managed with standard acute care, including ice, compression, elevation, protected rest, NSAIDs, and use of crutches as needed. Isometric strengthening exercises can be initiated when swelling has subsided. Application Strategy 15.3 summarizes the initial management and suggested rehabilitation exercises for a mild meniscal injury.

If joint effusion is extensive, immediate referral to a physician is warranted. Immediate referral also is necessary if the knee is locked and cannot be spontaneously reduced.

Bucket-handle tear segments can be excised surgically without removing the total meniscus, although regeneration of the centrally displaced portion will not occur. Arthroscopic meniscectomy is performed as an outpatient procedure under local anesthesia, with return to function following partial meniscectomy within 2 to 6 weeks. Total meniscectomy increases rotary instability and can lead to arthritis.

 The golfer has mild joint effusion and pain on the medial joint line that increases with rotation and extreme flexion of the knee. This suggests a possible chronic meniscal tear. This patient should be referred to a physician.

PATELLAR AND RELATED CONDITIONS

? A high school wrestler complains of an aching pain on the lateral side of the patella that increases during the workout. Slight effusion is present in the patellofemoral joint, and pain is elicited over the lateral patellar border. Intense pain is felt when the patella is pushed downward into the patellofemoral groove. What factors may contribute to this condition, and what long-term management should be considered after acute symptoms have subsided?

The patellofemoral joint is the region most commonly associated with anterior knee pain. Patellar tracking disorders and instability within the joint, along with obesity, direct trauma, and repetitive motions, all contribute to a variety of injuries. Patellofemoral pain may be classified into mechanical causes (e.g., patellar subluxation or dislocation), inflammatory causes (e.g., prepatellar bursitis or patellar tendinitis), and other causes (e.g., reflex sympathetic dystrophy or tumors). Other terms in the literature to describe anterior knee pain include patellofemoral arthralgia, patellar pain, patellar pain syndrome, and patellofemoral stress syndrome.

The main dynamic stabilizer is the quadriceps mechanism. More accurately called the **extensor mechanism**, it is made up of the vastus lateralis, vastus intermedius, vastus medialis, and rectus femoris, each of which is innervated by the femoral nerve. The vastus medialis has two heads, the superior longus head (vastus medialis longus) and the VMO. The VMO fibers approach the patella at a 55° angle. Although the VMO is incapable of producing knee extension, it provides a dynamic restraint to forces that would laterally displace the patella. Atrophy of this muscle nearly always is evident in patellofemoral dysfunction. The pes anserinus muscle group and the biceps femur influence patellar stability, because they control tibial internal and external rotation, which can significantly influence patellar tracking.

The static stabilizers include the anteriorly projected, lateral aspect of the femoral sulcus, the extensor retinaculum, IT band, quadriceps tendon, and patellar tendon. Oblique condensations of the retinacula produce the patellofemoral ligament and the medial and lateral patellotibial ligaments (**Fig. 15.28**). The structures that resist medial displacement of the patella (i.e., lateral retinaculum and IT band) are thicker and stronger than the soft-tissue structures that resist lateral displacement forces (i.e., medial

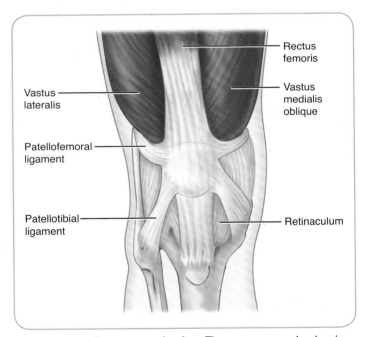

Rectus femoris

Vastus medialis oblique

Vastus lateralis

Patellofemoral ligament

Patellotibial ligament

Retinaculum

Figure 15.28. Extensor mechanism. The extensor mechanism is composed of dynamic and static stabilizers. Working together, they combine rolling and gliding motions to place the femur and patella in specific positions to effect the deceleration mechanism of the patellofemoral articulation and provide stability and function at the knee.

BOX 15.5 Causes of Patellofemoral Pain

- Patellar instability caused by
  - Abnormally shaped medial patellar facet
  - Shallow patellofemoral (trochlear) groove
  - Variable length and width of the patellar tendon
  - Patella alta (high-riding patella)
- Weak VMO or VMO dysplasia
- Hypermobility of the patella caused by
  - Muscle atrophy after an injury
  - Tightness of the lateral retinaculum, IT band, and hamstrings
- Anatomical malalignment caused by
  - Shallow patellofemoral groove
  - Excessive femoral anteversion or external tibial rotation
  - Genu valgum or genu recurvatum
  - Increased Q-angle
  - Excessive foot pronation
- Plica syndromes and repetitive minor trauma

---

retinaculum and lateral aspect of femoral sulcus). The patellar tendon resists superior displacement forces on the patella, whereas the quadriceps tendon resists inferior displacement of the patella. Both medial and lateral retinacula assist in knee extension even though the patellar tendon may be ruptured.

Deficiencies in stabilization of the extensor mechanism can be caused by several abnormalities of the patellofemoral region (**Box 15.5**), which can lead to anterior knee pain. Each condition can be counterbalanced in a healthy knee by the triangular shape of the patella, depth of the patellofemoral groove, and limiting action of the static ligamentous structures. Failure of medial structures to restrain the patella in a balanced position, or the presence of bony anomalies, can result in lateral tilting or lateral excursion of the patella, which in turn leads to patellofemoral **arthralgia**, or severe joint pain.

Patellofemoral Pain Syndrome

Etiology

Patellofemoral pain syndrome, also called lateral patellar compression syndrome, is pain in the patellofemoral joint without documented instability. The condition often occurs when either the VMO is weak or the lateral retinaculum that holds the patella firmly to the femoral condyle is excessively tight. Pain results when a tense lateral retinaculum passes over the trochlear groove or when increased patellofemoral stresses are transferred from the articular cartilage to pain fibers in the subchondral bone.

Signs and Symptoms

The patient may report a dull, aching pain in the anterior knee that is made worse by squatting, sitting in a tight space with the knee flexed, and descending stairs or slopes. Point tenderness can be located over the lateral facet of the patella, with intense pain and crepitus elicited when the patella is manually compressed into the patellofemoral groove. Synovial inflammation also may be present.

Management

Treatment involves standard acute care and NSAIDs. The entire lower extremity should be assessed for gait characteristics, flexibility, and strength of the proximal and distal portions. It is important to determine the presence of decreased rotation or strength in the lateral rotators of the hip as well as tightness in the hamstrings, quadriceps, and Achilles tendon. The McConnell taping technique uses passive taping of the patella to correct patellar position and tracking. The technique should be used in conjunction with corrective exercises to address the cause of the condition and is not intended to be used indefinitely. Patellofemoral support devices may be used to prevent lateral displacement of the patella, or orthotics may be employed to correct foot malalignment conditions.

Rehabilitation should focus on recruiting the VMO, normalizing patella mobility, and increasing flexibility and muscle control of the lower extremity. Closed chain exercises often are preferred because of the decrease in patellofemoral compression forces. Examples of closed kinetic chain exercises include knee flexion of 30° to 70° and lateral steps up of from 1 to 8 in to allow eccentric and concentric movements. Eccentric quadriceps strengthening is emphasized, because the quadriceps muscle is an important decelerator. Strengthening of the hip muscles to prevent adduction and internal rotation is critical to allow the progression of closed chain exercises. Restoring proprioception also is critical in re-establishing neuromuscular control. Weight-training programs that load the patellofemoral joint, such as bent-knee exercises, should be avoided. Resisted terminal knee extension exercises, straight leg raises in hip flexion and adduction, and quadriceps isometric, isotonic, and high-speed isokinetic exercises in a 60° to 90° arc may be performed. If the VMO is not monitored using biofeedback devices, proper recruitment is difficult to determine.

Chondromalacia Patellae

Etiology

Chondromalacia patellae is a true degeneration in the articular cartilage of the patella that results when compressive forces exceed the normal physical range or when alterations in patellar excursion produce abnormal shear forces that damage the articular surface. Because articular cartilage does not contain nerve endings, chondromalacia should not be considered as the true source of anterior knee pain. Chondromalacia is a surgical finding that represents areas of hyaline cartilage trauma or aberrant loading; it is not the cause of pain. The medial and lateral patellar facets are most commonly involved. The condition is confirmed when pain results from Clarke sign and Waldron test. Chondromalacia has four stages, which are detailed in **Figure 15.29**.

Management

Asymptomatic chondromalacia does not require treatment; if the condition becomes symptomatic, standard acute care is the appropriate protocol. Most patients respond well to mild anti-inflammatory medication, quadriceps strengthening, and a hamstring flexibility program. All resisted exercises with knee extension from a fully flexed position, crouches, and deep knee bends should be avoided, because these positions may aggravate the condition. A knee sleeve with a patellar cutout may be helpful. If this does not reduce the symptoms, the condition may require surgical intervention, such as arthroscopic patellar debridement, lateral retinacular release, extensor mechanism realignment, or elevation of the tibial tubercle to relieve patellar compression forces.

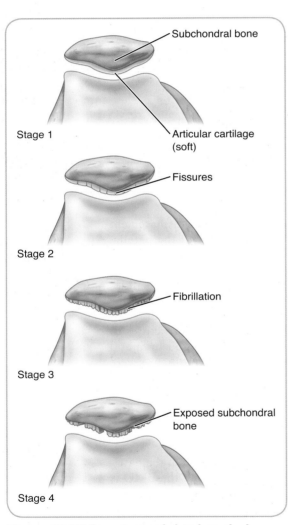

Figure 15.29. Four stages of chondromalacia patellae. Stage 1 involves softening or blistering of the cartilage. Stage 2 reveals fissures in the cartilage. Stage 3 is reached when fibrillation of the cartilage occurs, causing a "crabmeat" appearance. Stage 4 reveals cartilage defects with subchondral bone exposed.

Patellar Instability and Dislocations

Etiology

Patellar instability occurs when the patella has normal or abnormal alignment in the trochlear groove but is displaced by internal or external forces. Displacement can range from microinstability to subluxation or gross dislocation. Factors that may lead to congenital malalignment of the extensor mechanism include VMO dysplasia, vastus lateralis hypertrophy, high and lateral patellar posture, increased Q-angle, and bony deformity.

Signs and Symptoms

In a subluxation, transient partial displacement of the patella from the femoral trochlea may occur acutely, as in a patellar dislocation, or be intermittent, with spontaneous reduction of the displacement. The patient may or may not have a history of complete dislocation or patellofemoral pain but reports a feeling of the patella slipping when cutting, twisting, or pivoting. Joint effusion may develop, but it improves rapidly when the patient resumes activity.

Chronic subluxations produce less swelling, pain, and disability. The condition is verified by observing patellar position during active knee flexion and extension and by a positive patellar apprehension test. The patellar apprehension test should only be performed in the absence of obvious deformity. A patient with patellofemoral stress syndrome is not apprehensive with this test, whereas one with patellar pain resulting from subluxation resists any attempt to displace the patella laterally.

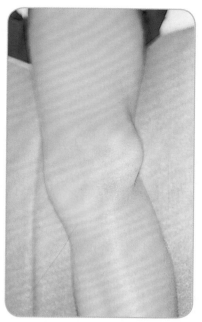

Figure 15.30. Dislocated patella. A dislocated patella often displaces laterally and is accompanied by an audible pop and violent collapse of the knee following deceleration involving a cutting maneuver.

Acute patellar subluxations and dislocations appear the same and generally occur during deceleration with a cutting maneuver (**Fig. 15.30**). Distinguishing one from the other depends on patient history. In a dislocation, the patient reports that the patella moved and had to be pushed back into place; with a subluxation, the patient reports that the patella slipped out and then went back into place spontaneously. The majority of the medial muscular and retinacular attachments are torn from the medial aspect of the patella, leading to an audible pop and violent collapse of the knee. Localized tenderness also may occur along the medial extensor retinaculum or at the adductor tubercle, which is the origin of the medial patellofemoral ligament. In addition, there may be localized tenderness along the peripheral edge of the lateral femoral condyle, where impaction from the patella occurs with flexion of the knee.

Typically, a traumatic displacement has acute effusion associated with a hemarthrosis occurring within the first 2 hours. A dislocation without acute effusion should signal chronic laxity; the tissues are so lax that the patella moves in and out of the groove without traumatizing surrounding tissues. The clinician should palpate the area to assess any defects in the medial retinaculum and VMO before they are obscured by swelling. Occasionally, a fracture of the patella or lateral femoral condyle occurs, resulting in a loose, bony fragment in the joint.

Management

Treatment includes ice, elevation, immobilization, and immediate referral to a physician. Following reduction of the dislocation by the physician, aspiration of the hemarthrosis may be indicated for comfort or to determine the presence of fat in the blood secondary to an osteochondral fracture. Immobilization of a first-time dislocation is only needed to control acute symptoms and is followed by an extensive rehabilitation program and functional patellar bracing. During immobilization, isometric quadriceps exercises and straight leg raises can be performed. When immobilization is removed, a full rehabilitative program to strengthen the dynamic stabilizers of the patellofemoral joint, particularly the VMO, and a flexibility program for the hamstrings and IT band should be initiated. A knee sleeve with a lateral pad to restrict lateral excursion and activity modification may be helpful. Most patients with patellofemoral tracking disorders and instability can improve and return to activity without surgical intervention. An obvious disruption of the VMO insertion into the medial patellar edge, however, or a rupture of the medial patellofemoral ligament from the adductor tubercles responds best with early surgical repair.[45]

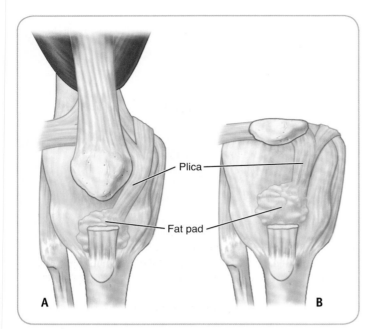

Figure 15.31. Patella plica. The patella plica is a fold in the synovial lining of the knee joint that can become inflamed and thickened by trauma where it extends over the femoral condyle or by microtrauma from overuse. **A,** Fully extended. **B,** Flexion of 90°.

Patella Plica Syndrome
Etiology

The patella plica shelf is a fold in the synovial lining that projects into the joint cavity. This congenital abnormality is a remnant of the embryological walls that divide the knee into medial, lateral, and suprapatellar pouches. Typically, it is crescent-shaped and extends from the infrapatellar fat pad medially (medial plica), loops around the femoral condyle, crosses under the quadriceps tendon in the suprapatellar region (suprapatellar plica), and then passes laterally over the lateral femoral condyle to the lateral retinaculum (**Fig. 15.31**). Normally, a synovial plica remains asymptomatic until traumatized by a direct blow to the capsule or it becomes inflamed and thickened from overuse, resulting from friction caused as the plica bowstrings across the medial femoral condyle. This bowstringing results in two reservoirs for synovial fluid—namely, a suprapatellar reservoir and the cavity of the knee joint itself.

Signs and Symptoms

Anterior knee pain comes on gradually and is aggravated by quadriceps exercises. Approximately 25% of cases have a positive "moviegoer sign" (i.e., pain with prolonged sitting). As the patient stands and begins to walk, a sharp pain is felt for 8 to 10 steps and then disappears. The pain is caused by the plica being maximally stretched and impinged within the patellofemoral joint. As the articularis genus muscle contracts several times, it elevates the plica enough to prevent further impingement. Occasionally, adhesions in the plica lead to a distinctive pop or snap as the patient extends the knee, or pseudolocking may occur over the medial patellofemoral joint, mimicking a torn meniscus. Assessment reveals slight joint effusion, palpable pain, and crepitus in the medial and lateral retinacular regions, particularly along the edge of the medial femoral condyle with the knee flexed at 45°. The test for medial synovial plica and the stutter test are positive.

Management

Treatment is symptomatic, with ice therapy, NSAIDs, activity modification, phonophoresis, and use of an external patellar support device. The condition may improve with hamstring stretching, heel cord stretching, and VMO strengthening exercises, especially if the VMO is dysplastic (abnormally developed). If the condition warrants, the plica shelf can be removed arthroscopically.

Patellar Tendinitis (Jumper's Knee)
Etiology

The patellar tendon frequently becomes inflamed and tender from repetitive or eccentric knee extension activities; these occur in running and in sports, such as volleyball and basketball, in which jumping is a critical action, hence, the name "jumper's knee." Patellar subluxation, patellofemoral stress syndrome, and other conditions also can overload the patellar tendon, predisposing a patient to this condition. Extrinsic factors that can lead to the condition include frequency of training, years of play, playing surface, type of training, stretching and warm-up practices, and type of shoe that is worn. Some intrinsic factors that may have a role in contributing to the condition include lower extremity malalignment, leg length discrepancies, muscle imbalance, anthropometric variables, muscle length, and muscle strength.[46]

Signs and Symptoms

Most patients will complain of chronic anterior knee pain of insidious onset, which might be described as a sharp or aching pain. Initially, pain after activity is concentrated on the inferior pole

APPLICATION STRATEGY 15.4

Management of Patellar Tendinitis

- Rest for 2–3 weeks to allow symptoms to subside.
- Modalities that may be used during the early stages of healing include heat therapy, electrical stimulation, phonophoresis, iontophoresis, and ultrasound.
- Transverse friction massage for 6–8 minutes.
- Initiate early flexibility exercises for the gastrocnemius–soleus complex, quadriceps, and hamstrings.
- Aquatic therapy during the early stages can reduce gravitational forces.
- Progressive resistance strengthening exercises may include the following:
  - Straight leg raises in all directions
  - Short-arc knee extension exercises
  - One-quarter knee squats
- Eccentric strengthening exercises for the quadriceps and dorsiflexors, such as drop squats (i.e., landing from a jump). Focus on the deceleration between the upward and downward phase. Increase deceleration as tolerated by the patient.
- Cardiovascular fitness should be maintained with exercises that do not involve powerful knee extension (i.e., upper body ergometer, swimming, and stationary bike with minimal tension).
- During the later stages, plyometrics may be incorporated (i.e., single-leg hop, double-leg hop, single-leg vertical jump, and bounding).
- A patellofemoral knee sleeve may reduce mobility of the patellar tendon during activity.

of the patella or the distal attachment of the patellar tendon on the tibial tubercle. As the condition progresses, pain is present at the beginning of activity, subsides during warm-up, and then reappears after activity. Increased pain often is reported while ascending and descending stairs or after prolonged sitting. Eventually, pain is present both during and after activity and can become too severe for the patient to participate. Pain can be elicited during passive knee flexion beyond 120° and during resisted knee extension. It also is common to find tightness in the hamstrings, quadriceps, and heel cord, with weakness in the ankle dorsiflexors. Chronic tendinitis occasionally may lead to cystic changes at the distal pole of the patella or ectopic calcification and nodule formation in the tendon.

Management

Immediate treatment involves standard acute care and NSAIDs. **Application Strategy 15.4** summarizes the management of patellar tendinitis.

Osgood-Schlatter Disease

Etiology

Osgood-Schlatter disease is a traction-type injury to the tibial apophysis where the patellar tendon attaches onto the tibial tubercle (**Fig. 15.32**). Osgood-Schlatter disease typically develops in girls between the ages of 8 and 13 years and in boys between the ages of 10 and 15 years at the beginning of their growth spurt. It is estimated that the condition occurs in 21% of adolescent athletes, compared with 4.5% of age-matched nonathletes.[47] The condition has been more common in boys, but with girls' increased participation in sports, the ratio may be equalizing.

Signs and Symptoms

Assessment of the condition usually is straightforward. Patients point to the tibial tubercle as the source of pain, and the tubercle appears to be enlarged and prominent. Patients report that pain generally occurs during activity and is relieved with rest. Point tenderness can be elicited directly over the tubercle, but ROM is unaffected. Pain is present at the extremes of knee extension and forced flexion. Severity is rated in three grades, depending on the duration of pain:

- **Grade I**—pain after activity that resolves within 24 hours
- **Grade II**—pain during and after activity that does not hinder performance and resolves within 24 hours

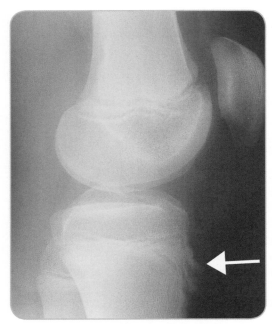

Figure 15.32. Patellar tendon traction-type injuries. Patellar tendon traction-type injuries may involve Sinding-Larsen-Johansson disease or Osgood-Schlatter disease. The location of pain typically defines which problem is present.

■ **Grade III**—continuous pain that limits sport performance and daily activities

Management

Treatment is symptomatic and self-limiting, but it may take 12 to 24 months for the condition to run its course. In most cases, activity is unrestricted unless pain is disabling. Shock-absorbent insoles in shoes may decrease peak stress on the tendon and tubercle. Application of cold for 20 minutes after activity should be beneficial, as should hamstrings and quadriceps stretching. Knee pads may protect the tibial tubercle when kneeling, or a knee strap (e.g., Cho-Pat straps) may decrease the traction forces on the tibial tubercle. The condition rectifies with closure of the apophysis, but a small percentage of patients develop a painful ossicle, which can necessitate surgical excision. Others may develop painful kneeling as adults.

Sinding-Larsen-Johansson Disease

Etiology

A condition similar to Osgood-Schlatter disease is **Sinding-Larsen-Johansson disease**, but the excessive strain occurs on the inferior patellar pole at the origin of the patellar tendon (see **Fig. 15.32**). The condition usually is seen in children 8 to 13 years of age.

Signs and Symptoms

The onset of pain over the inferior patellar pole is gradual and seen in children who are involved in running and jumping sports. The condition often is missed unless the clinician palpates the inferior patellar pole with the patient's knee extended and the patellar tendon relaxed. Repeating the examination with the knee flexed at 90° should reveal diminished tenderness as the patellar tendon becomes taut.

Management

Treatment is symptomatic and similar to that for Osgood-Schlatter disease. Symptoms generally resolve quickly with standard acute care, NSAIDs, and activity modification.

Extensor Tendon Rupture

Etiology

Extensor tendon ruptures can occur at the superior or inferior pole of the patella, the tibial tubercle, or within the patellar tendon itself. Ruptures result from powerful eccentric muscle contractions or in conjunction with severe ligamentous disruption at the knee. The rupture may be partial or total.

Signs and Symptoms

A partial rupture produces pain and muscle weakness in knee extension. If a total rupture occurs distal to the patella, assessment reveals a high-riding patella, a palpable defect over the tendon, and an inability to perform knee extension or perform a straight leg raise. If the quadriceps tendon is ruptured from the superior pole of the patella and the extensor retinaculum is still intact, knee extension is still possible, although it is weak and painful. Patients with a history of previous corticosteroid injections, anabolic steroid abuse, or use of systemic steroids are at a greater risk for tendon ruptures. Steroid use can cause softening or weakening of collagen fibers in the muscle tendon, predisposing the tendon to premature rupture.

Management

Treatment involves standard acute care, use of a knee immobilizer, fitting the patient for crutches, and immediate referral to a physician. Treatment depends on the location and displacement of any bony fragment. In partial ruptures involving a shredded tendon, wiring through the patella may be necessary to relieve tension on the healing tendon. Surgical repair is necessary in total ruptures.

Overall, the results of a delayed repair are less satisfactory than the results with an acute repair, but a delayed repair still provides an extensor mechanism and adequate function.[48]

 The high school wrestler complains of lateral patellofemoral pain that increases with certain maneuvers during practice. Precipitating factors that increase stress on the patellofemoral region include patellar instability, a weak VMO, hypermobility of the patella, and anatomical malalignment conditions. Following standard acute care, a total assessment of the lower extremity should be conducted to address deficiencies in muscle strength or biomechanical problems that contributed to the condition.

ILIOTIBIAL BAND FRICTION SYNDROME

? Following an evening practice session on the third day of preseason, a field hockey player complains of a sharp ache over the lateral epicondyle of the femur that has gotten progressively worse since the start of the week. A history reveals that the daily double sessions have concentrated on technique drills and conditioning exercises. Observation reveals excessive foot pronation and genu varum. What actions might be taken to reduce the pain and correct the injury?

A common condition in runners, cyclists, weight lifters, and volleyball players is IT band friction syndrome. The band originates on the lateral iliac crest and continues the line of pull from the tensor fasciae latae and gluteus maximus muscle; the deep fibers are associated with the lateral intermuscular septum. The distal fibers become thicker at their attachment on the Gerdy tubercle adjacent to the tibial tubercle on the lateral proximal tibia. The band drops posteriorly, behind the lateral femoral epicondyle, with knee flexion and then snaps forward over the epicondyle during extension (**Fig. 15.33**).

Etiology

Weight bearing increases compression and friction forces over the greater trochanter and lateral femoral condyle. Friction between the posterior edge of the IT band and underlying lateral femoral epicondyle is particularly intense near foot strike through foot contact (midstance). Patients with a malalignment problem are predisposed to this condition; see **Box 15.6** for a listing of predisposing factors.

Signs and Symptoms

Initially, pain is present over the lateral aspect of the knee after running a certain mileage, typically late in the run, but does not restrict distance or speed. As the condition progresses, the pain begins to occur earlier and earlier with distance and speed affected. Pain may be present while running uphill, downhill, and climbing stairs. With continued activity, the initial ache progresses into a more painful, sharp, stinging discomfort over the lateral femoral condyle approximately 2 to 3 cm above the lateral joint line and, occasionally, radiates distally to the tibial attachment or proximally up

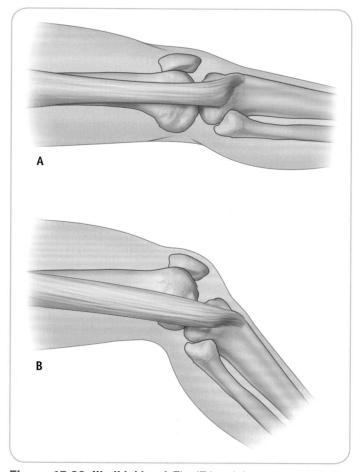

Figure 15.33. Iliotibial band. The IT band drops posteriorly behind the lateral femoral epicondyle during knee flexion and then snaps forward over the epicondyle during extension. Malalignment problems or constant irritation can inflame the IT band or lead to bursitis. **A,** Extension. **B,** Flexion.

> **BOX 15.6 Predisposing Factors for Iliotibial Band Friction Syndrome**
>
> - Genu varum
> - Excessive pronation in feet
> - Leg length discrepancy
> - Prominent greater trochanter of femur
> - Preexisting IT band tightness
> - Muscle weakness in knee extensors, knee flexors, and hip abductors
> - Training errors, such as excessive distance in a single run, increasing mileage too quickly, inadequate warm-up, and running on the same side of a crowned road

the thigh. Swelling may be noted at the distal IT band, and palpation of the affected limb may reveal multiple trigger points in the vastus lateralis, gluteus medius, and biceps femoris.[49] Palpation of these trigger points may cause referred pain to the lateral aspect of the affected knee. Flexion and extension of the knee may produce a creaking sound. Positive Noble and Ober compression tests confirm the condition. Magnetic resonance images have shown that the distal band becomes thickened and that the potential space deep to the IT band over the femoral epicondyle becomes inflamed and filled with fluid.[49] Eventually, pain restricts all running and becomes continuous during activities of daily living.

Management

The immediate treatment should be focused on alleviating inflammation with standard acute care and NSAIDs. Any activity that requires repeated knee flexion and extension should be limited. Functional exercises focusing on strengthening the posterior and lateral muscles of the hip and pelvis should be a core component of the corrective exercise program. **Application Strategy 15.5** describes the management of IT band friction syndrome.

> **APPLICATION STRATEGY 15.5**
>
> **Management of Iliotibial Band Friction Syndrome**
>
> - Ice, compression, elevation, NSAIDs, and rest until acute symptoms subside.
> - Roll out iliotibial band, hamstrings, and quadriceps using a foam roller.
> - Use dynamic warm-up exercises that function on hip and pelvis as well as lower leg muscle groups.
> - Use active release techniques for hip and thigh muscles.
> - Hill running should be avoided until asymptomatic.
> - Foot orthotics may correct some structural problems.
> - Non–weight-bearing strengthening exercises, such as leg lifts and isometric exercises for knee flexion, extension, hip abduction, and adduction, can be initiated when pain-free, followed by concentric and eccentric strengthening of the hip and thigh muscles.
> - Work on strengthening posterior chain muscles of the hip and pelvis through exercises such as claim shells, hip thrusts, side steps/shuffles, double- and single-leg squats and hip hikes.
> - Running or training should be modified to the point of little or minimal pain during activity. Initially, this may necessitate an easy pace on level ground, progressing to increased mileage while maintaining pain-free activity.
> - Cardiovascular fitness can be maintained with swimming; biking should be avoided.
> - Ice massage before and after running may be helpful.
> - Steroid injections may be used in resistant cases.
> - Full return to participation should be gauged on pain-free completion of all functional tests.

The field hockey player has IT band friction syndrome. The double sessions, coupled with the preexisting genu varum and pronated feet, have added strain to the IT band. Following standard acute care to control inflammation, an extensive flexibility program for the IT band should be initiated.

FRACTURES AND ASSOCIATED CONDITIONS

 A 14-year-old soccer player complains of an aching, diffuse pain in his right knee. The pain increases with strenuous activity and twisting motions. Because of the pain, he tends to walk with the leg externally rotated. What condition should be suspected, and what is the immediate management for this condition?

Traumatic fractures about the knee area are rare in sports competition, except for high-velocity sports, such as motorcycling and auto racing. These fractures usually are associated with multiple traumas. Other, more common fractures and associated bony conditions can occur with regular participation in sport and physical activity. Displaced and undisplaced fractures of the femoral shaft are discussed in Chapter 16.

Avulsion Fractures

Etiology

Direct trauma, excessive tensile forces from an explosive muscular contraction, repetitive overuse, or a tensile force can pull a ligament from its bony attachment. For example, getting kicked on the lateral aspect of the knee may avulse a portion of the lateral epicondyle, or the tibial tubercle may be avulsed when the extensor mechanism pulls a fragment away.

Signs and Symptoms

Localized pain and tenderness will occur over the bony site, and if displaced, a fragment may be palpated. If a musculotendinous unit is involved, muscle function is limited. When the anterior cruciate is involved, the bony fragment may lodge in the joint, causing the knee to lock.

Management

Treatment involves standard acute care and application of a knee immobilizer. The patient should be referred immediately to a physician for further care. If necessary, the patient should be fitted for crutches and instructed to use a non–weight-bearing gait en route to the physician.

Epiphyseal and Apophyseal Fractures

Adolescents in contact sports are particularly susceptible to epiphyseal fractures in the knee region. A shearing force across the cartilaginous growth plate may lead to disruption of growth and a shortened limb.

Tibial Tubercle Fractures

■ Etiology

The tibial tubercle, a common site for apophyseal fractures in boys, may occur as a result of Osgood-Schlatter disease. The typical patient is a muscular, well-developed patient who has almost reached skeletal maturity and who almost always is involved in a jumping sport, most commonly basketball. These fractures usually result from forced flexion of the knee against a straining quadriceps contraction or a violent quadriceps contraction against a fixed foot.

■ Signs and Symptoms

The patient has pain, ecchymosis, swelling, and tenderness directly over the tubercle. Difficulty going up and down stairs also is reported. When the fracture extends from the tubercle to the tibial epiphysis (type II) or through the secondary epiphysis and into the joint (type III), quadriceps insufficiency makes knee extension both painful and weak. In larger fractures involving extensive retinacular damage, the patella rides high, and knee extension is impossible.

■ Management

Treatment involves standard acute care and application of a knee immobilizer. The patient should be referred immediately to a physician for further care. If necessary, the patient should be fitted for crutches and instructed to use a non–weight-bearing gait en route to the physician. Displaced fractures need open reduction and internal fixation.

Distal Femoral Epiphyseal Fractures

■ Etiology

Fractures to the distal femoral epiphysis are 10-fold more common than proximal tibial fractures and are more serious because of possible arterial damage to the growth plate. They may occur at any age but often are seen in boys between 10 and 14 years of age. These fractures occur when a varus or valgus stress is applied on a fixed, weight-bearing foot, as when someone falls on the outer aspect of the knee while the foot is planted.

■ Signs and Symptoms

The patient complains of pain around the knee and is unable to bear weight on the injured leg.

■ Management

Treatment involves standard acute care and application of a knee immobilizer or vacuum splint. The patient should be referred immediately to a physician for further care. Undisplaced type I fractures usually are treated with closed reduction and casting and with use of crutches and protective weight bearing for 4 weeks, followed by rehabilitation to restore motion and strength. This fracture has a history of fairly good resolution, although such resolution may take weeks to occur. More serious fractures require internal fixation and may result in angular or leg length discrepancy.

Stress Fractures

■ Etiology

The femoral supracondylar region, medial tibial plateau, and tibia tubercle are common regions for stress fractures. These fractures occur when

■ Load on the bone is increased (e.g., jumping or high-impact activity).

■ The number of stresses on the bone increase (e.g., changes in training intensity, duration, frequency, or running surface, or unevenly worn shoes).

■ The surface area of the bone that receives the load is decreased (i.e., during the normal process of bone repair, certain portions of the bone remain immature and less able to tolerate stress for a period of time).

■ Signs and Symptoms

Localized pain before and after activity is relieved with rest and non–weight bearing. In a stress fracture of the medial tibial plateau, pain runs along the anteromedial aspect of the proximal tibia just below the joint line. Localized tenderness and edema are present, but initial radiographs of the stress fracture may be negative. As the condition progresses, pain becomes more persistent. Follow-up radiographs 3 weeks postinjury may show periosteal new bone development. Early bone scans are highly recommended.

■ Management

Once a stress fracture is identified, treatment involves rest, crutches, and/or casting.

Chondral and Osteochondral Fractures

Etiology

A chondral fracture is a fracture involving the articular cartilage at a joint. An osteochondral fracture involves the articular cartilage and the underlying bone (**Fig. 15.34**). These fractures result from compression with a direct blow to the knee, causing shearing or forceful rotation. A substantial amount of articular surface on the involved bone can be damaged.

Signs and Symptoms

The patient usually feels a painful "snap" and reports considerable pain and swelling within the first few hours after injury. Displaced fractures can cause locking of the joint and produce crepitation during ROM.

Management

Following standard acute care and immobilization in a vacuum splint, the patient should be referred immediately to a physician for further care. Aspiration of the joint often yields bloody fluid containing fat. Magnetic resonance images may be indicated, because some fractures may not appear on standard radiographs. Small fragments can be removed during arthroscopic surgery; internal fixation is necessary with larger fragments. Following surgery, ROM exercises are performed to improve articular cartilage nutrition, limit joint adhesions, and prevent muscular atrophy.

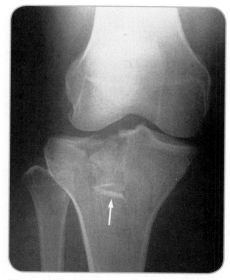

Figure 15.34. Osteochondral fracture. This traumatic osteochondral fracture involves the articular cartilage and sub-chondral bone on the medial epicondyle of the tibia.

Osteochondritis Dissecans

Etiology

Osteochondritis dissecans (OCD) occurs when a fragment of bone adjacent to the articular surface of a joint is deprived of its blood supply, leading to avascular necrosis (**Fig. 15.35**). The bone fragment may be in its normal anatomical location with a smooth articular surface (i.e., stable), or the lesion may displace and form a loose body within the joint space, leaving a defect in the articular cartilage (i.e., unstable). The cartilage remains healthy even if the fragment is loose, because cartilage is nourished by synovial fluid rather than a direct blood supply. Repetitive trauma and loss of mechanical support, however, may cause the cartilage to undergo softening and degenerative changes. Although found in other joints, it more commonly affects the knee joint, particularly in males from 10 to 20 years of age, with the femoral condyles accounting for 75% of all lesions. Of these, the medial femoral condyle accounts for 75% to 85% of all femoral lesions.[50] Causes include direct and indirect trauma, skeletal abnormalities associated with endocrine dysfunction, a prominent tibial spine that impacts the medial femoral condyle, and generalized ligamentous laxity.

See **Classification and Prognosis of Osteochondritis Dissecans**, available on the companion Web site at thePoint.

Signs and Symptoms

The most common symptom is an aching, diffuse pain, or swelling, with activity. Locking or giving way of the knee may develop as the disease progresses. Pain increases with strenuous activity and twisting motions, especially internal rotation of the tibia, which causes the medial tibial spine to strike the lateral aspect of the medial femoral condyle (the site of most OCD lesions). As a result, the patient walks with the affected leg externally rotated. Lesions of the lateral femoral condyle may produce a painful "clunk" with knee flexion and extension. Patients with OCD of the patella usually present with retropatellar pain and crepitus. Thigh circumference may be diminished because of muscle disuse atrophy.

Management

Following standard acute care and immobilization with a knee immobilizer or vacuum splint, the patient should be referred immediately to a physician for further care. Treatment depends on the age of the patient, the size and location of the lesion, and the radiographic appearance of the fragment and articular cartilage.

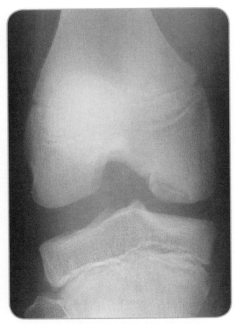

Figure 15.35. Osteochondritis dissecans. Osteochondritis dissecans occurs when a fragment of bone adjacent to the articular surface of a joint is deprived of its blood supply, leading to avascular necrosis. In this patient, a portion of the medial epicondyle of the femur is damaged.

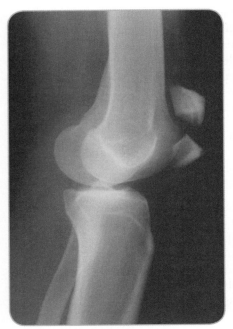

Figure 15.36. Traumatic patellar fracture. This radiograph provides a lateral view of a transverse fracture of the patella.

Patients in categories 1 and 2 (those younger than 20 years of age) are treated nonsurgically if the fragment has not separated. A soft knee immobilizer is worn, and activity is restricted for 1 to 2 weeks, with minimal weight bearing to control pain and initiate healing. Activities are then modified for 6 to 12 weeks; younger patients generally require a shorter period of activity modification compared with older patients. Rapid or strenuous movement of the lower extremities should be avoided, especially high-impact activities, such as running, cutting, and jumping. Plain radiographs usually reveal evidence of healing between 3 and 6 months after treatment. Full activity may be permitted once the following criteria are met:

- The patient is pain-free.

- Physical examination is normal, including full ROM, and no joint effusion or tenderness is present.

- Radiographic evidence of healing is present, as noted by disappearance of the radiolucent line that outlined the fragment.

If the patient is older than 20 years, the fragment is unstable (regardless of the patient's age), or a chronic lesion does not respond to conservative measures, internal fixation or removal of the fragment is indicated. Older patients do not heal as well, because degenerative joint changes may have already developed within the joint. For OCD lesions of the patella, conservative management often is unsuccessful, necessitating early surgical intervention to excise the fragment. For these patients, brief postsurgical immobilization followed by activity limitations usually brings about gradual healing.

Patellar Fractures

Etiology

Stress fractures of the patella are rare and typically involve the inferior pole of the patella. Traumatic fractures can be transverse, stellate or comminuted, or longitudinal (**Fig. 15.36**). Displaced patellar fractures, which generally are associated with disruption of the quadriceps retinaculum, require open reduction and internal fixation. These fractures occur as a result of a fall onto the knee, a direct blow to the knee, or an eccentric contraction of the quadriceps that overloads the intrinsic tensile strength of the bone, as occurs in jumping activities. Patellar fracture also is a rare complication of ACL reconstruction using a bone–patellar tendon–bone **autogenous** (i.e., from within the body) graft. These fractures occur an average of 7 weeks postsurgery and result from external trauma, rapid flexion movement while preventing a fall backward, or a twisting maneuver. A **bipartite** (i.e., having two parts) patella, although not a fracture, is present in 1% to 4% of patients and is more common in males than in females. It typically is seen on the superolateral corner of the patella and has rounded rather than sharp edges. The patient lacks point tenderness over the area and can maintain knee extension, which differentiates the condition from a true fracture.

Signs and Symptoms

Generally, 2 mm of articular incongruity signifies a displaced fracture, which produces diffuse extra-articular swelling on and about the knee. A portion of the patella is retracted proximally. A visible and palpable defect lies between the fragments, which are mobile. A straight leg raise is impossible to perform.

Management

Initial treatment involves ice, elevation, immobilization in a knee immobilizer, and immediate referral to a physician. Radiographs are needed for verification. Nondisplaced patellar fractures are treated nonoperatively, with either a long-leg cylinder cast or a knee immobilizer for 4 to 6 weeks. Partial weight bearing is then allowed, and a full rehabilitation program is initiated. Surgery is indicated in a displaced fracture with major disruption to the extensor mechanism.

 The 14-year-old soccer player may have OCD. Following standard acute care and immobilization with a knee immobilizer or vacuum splint, the patient should be referred immediately to a physician for further care.

REHABILITATION OF KNEE INJURIES

 The basketball player is diagnosed with patellofemoral syndrome. Explain the focus of a rehabilitation program for this condition.

A rehabilitation program attempts to minimize inflammation and the effects of immobilization by initiating early mobilization and controlled movement to allow healing tissues to be stressed gradually and progressively until normal joint function is restored. The rehabilitation program should restore motion and proprioception, maintain cardiovascular fitness, and improve muscular strength, endurance, and power, predominantly through closed chain exercises. Sample exercise programs for specific injuries are listed in **Application Strategies 15.1** to **15.5**.

Restoration of Motion

Some loss of motion occurs following most knee injuries. Passive ROM exercises normally can begin on the first day after injury. Because of potential damage to the graft, however, some concern has been raised about the use of continuous passive motion (CPM) machines following autogenous patellar tendon reconstruction of the ACL. The literature does support the early use of the CPM in this population.[51] The unit moves the knee through a protected ROM to stimulate the intrinsic healing process. The benefits of CPM following ACL surgery include the following:

- Maintaining articular cartilage nutrition and preventing articular cartilage degradation

- Preventing adhesions, joint stiffness, and muscle spasm

- Improving collagen remodeling and joint dynamics

- Reducing pain, thereby reducing amount of pain medication

- Decreasing joint swelling and effusion

- Producing no significant deleterious effects on the stability of the ligament

- Increasing knee ROM sooner

When a CPM machine is not needed, ROM exercises, such as the supine wall slide, heel slide, assisted knee flexion and extension, half squats, or proprioceptive neuromuscular facilitation stretching exercises, can be performed (**Fig. 15.37**). Extension usually is the most difficult motion to restore, and it is critical in achieving normal gait. The patient is placed prone, with the thigh resting on the table. The lower leg is extended off the end of the table. A weight can be added on the distal tibia so that a gradual stretch is achieved. Following the exercise bout, the knee should be iced in the supine position, with the heel elevated to assist with extension.

In addition to active and passive ROM exercises at the tibiofemoral joint, stretching exercises to improve passive glide of the patellofemoral joint, particularly medial glide, can stretch tight lateral structures to correct patellar positioning and tracking (**Fig. 15.38**). Normal passive glide of the patellofemoral joint should be restored before full flexion exercises, resisted exercises, or bicycling is initiated.

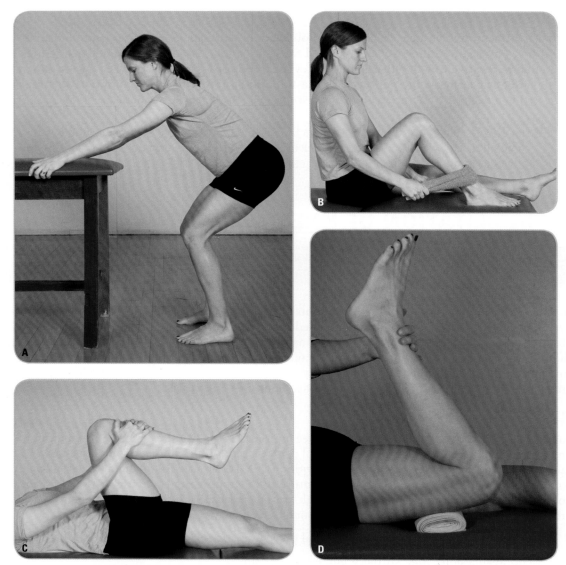

Figure 15.37. Range of motion exercises. A, Half squat. **B,** Assisted heel slide. **C,** Assisted knee flexion and hip flexion. **D,** Assisted knee flexion.

Restoration of Proprioception and Balance

Proprioception and balance must be regained to return safely to activity. During the early stages following injury, when weight bearing is allowed, closed chain exercises, such as shifting one's weight while on crutches, straight leg raises, bilateral minisquats, or use of a biomechanical ankle platform system (BAPS) board with support, may be helpful. As balance improves, unassisted use of the BAPS board, closed chain exercises, running in place on a minitramp, or use of a slide board may be incorporated along with other closed chain exercises that are used to develop strength.

Muscular Strength, Endurance, and Power

Early emphasis should be placed on strengthening the quadriceps femoris musculature, particularly the vastus medialis and VMO. These muscles aid in the stabilization of the patella both superiorly and medially. Isometric contractions, called quad sets, are performed at or near 0°, 45°, 60°, and 90° of flexion. Isometric hip adduction exercises also are used to recruit the VMO and can be performed by squeezing a rolled towel between the knees in a seated position. Open chain exercises may include straight leg raises in all directions, supplemented by ankle weights or tubing to increase resistance.

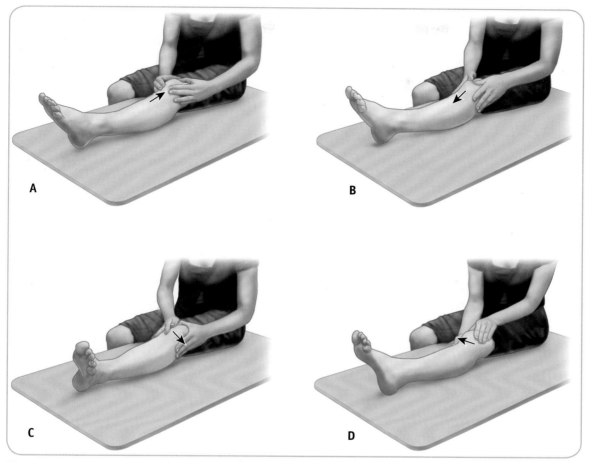

Figure 15.38. Patellar self-mobilization. A, Proximal. **B,** Distal. **C,** Medial. **D,** Lateral.

Knee extension and flexion exercises may be done with free weights or on several commercially available isotonic or isokinetic machines.

Closed chain exercises performed during weight bearing may include terminal knee extension (**Fig. 15.39**), step-ups, step-downs, lateral step-ups, minisquats from 0° to 40°, leg presses on a machine from 0° to 60°, or use of a stepping machine or stationary bicycle. Several of these exercises are detailed in **Application Strategy 15.1**. Closed chain exercises can be made progressively more difficult by increasing the resistance or speed of movement or by changing the patient's visual feedback (e.g., looking at the ceiling, looking at the floor, or closing the eyes). Ensuring proper performance of closed chain exercises is critical. For example, when doing a minisquat or leg press, if the hip is not strong enough to control adduction and internal rotation, the knee assumes a valgus alignment, with the foot pronated. This leads to an increased Q-angle, predisposing the patient to patellofemoral pain.

Plyometric jumping during the later stages of rehabilitation can be performed using small boxes and directional changes to improve power and proprioceptive function. Because of the increased eccentric contraction and the associated muscle microtrauma that results from the power maneuvers, these exercises should only be performed two or three times weekly.

Cardiovascular Fitness

Cardiovascular fitness exercises can begin immediately after injury with use of an upper body ergometer or hydrotherapeutic exercise. Running in water and performing sport-specific exercises in deep water can allow the patient to maintain activity-specific functional skills in a non–weight-bearing position. When ROM is adequate, a stationary bicycle may be used. The seat should be adjusted so that the knee is flexed by 15° to 30°. The patient should be instructed to pedal with the ball of the

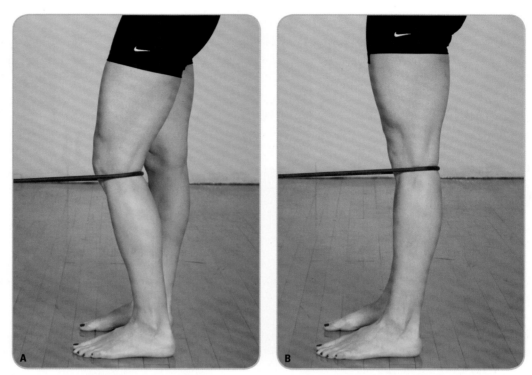

Figure 15.39. **Closed chain terminal extension. A,** Starting position. **B,** Ending position.

foot, using toe clips, and to pull through the bottom of the stroke. A low to moderate workload is recommended to reduce patellofemoral compressive forces. Other exercises, such as walking, light jogging, and functional activities, can progress as tolerated.

Rehabilitation for the basketball player with patellofemoral syndrome should focus on recruiting the VMO, normalizing patella mobility, and increasing flexibility and muscle control of the lower extremity. Resisted terminal knee extension exercises, straight leg raises in hip flexion and adduction, as well as quadriceps isometric, isotonic, and high-speed isokinetic exercises in a 60° to 90° arc may be performed. Closed chain exercises often are preferred because of the decrease in patellofemoral compression forces. Strengthening of the hip muscles to prevent adduction and internal rotation is critical to allow the progression of closed chain exercises. Restoring proprioception also is critical in reestablishing neuromuscular control. Weight training programs that load the patellofemoral joint, such as bent-knee exercises, should be avoided.

SUMMARY

1. The knee (tibiofemoral joint) functions primarily as a modified hinge joint, with some lateral and rotational motions allowed.

2. The cruciate ligaments are intracapsular and extrasynovial. They prevent anterior and posterior translation of the tibia on the femur. The ACL frequently is subject to deceleration injuries, with internal tibial torque being the most dangerous loading mechanism, particularly when combined with an anterior tibial force. The shorter and stronger PCL is considered to be the primary stabilizer of the knee.

3. The collateral ligaments prevent valgus (medial) and varus (lateral) stress at the knee.

4. The menisci aid in lubrication and nutrition of the joint, reduce friction during movement, provide shock absorption by dissipating stress over the articular cartilage, improve weight distribution, and help the capsule and ligaments to prevent hyperextension.

5. Tracking of the patella against the femur is dependent on the direction of the net force that is produced by the attached quadriceps. Factors such as patellar instability, a weak VMO, hypermobility of the patella, anatomical malalignment conditions, plica syndromes, or repetitive minor trauma can lead to chronic patellofemoral pain.

6. Because of its location, the prepatellar bursa is the bursa most commonly injured by compressive forces. The deep infrapatellar bursa often is inflamed by overuse and subsequent friction between the infrapatellar tendon and structures behind it (fat pad and tibia).

7. A straight plane instability implies instability in one of the cardinal planes. A multidirectional instability involves instability in more than one plane.

8. Isolated anterior instability is rare. Instead, an anteromedial or anterolateral laxity usually occurs. The rate of ACL injuries is higher in women, in part because of an imbalance of muscle strength as well as both intrinsic and extrinsic factors.

9. Menisci become stiffer and less resilient with age. Tears are classified according to age, location, or axis of orientation, and they include longitudinal, bucket-handle, horizontal, and parrot-beak. Because the menisci are not innervated by nociceptors, synovial inflammation and joint effusion may not develop for more than 12 hours after the initial injury.

10. Patellofemoral stress syndrome often occurs when either the VMO is weak or the lateral retinaculum that holds the patella firmly to the femoral condyle is excessively tight. This condition is much more common than chondromalacia patellae, which is a true degeneration in the articular cartilage of the patella.

11. Adolescents are particularly prone to Osgood-Schlatter disease, Sinding-Larsen-Johansson disease, and fractures to the distal femoral epiphysis.

12. Pain in the knee region can be referred from the lumbar spine, hip, or ankle.

13. A rehabilitation program should minimize inflammation and the effects of immobilization by initiating early mobilization and controlled movement to allow healing tissues to be stressed, gradually and progressively, until normal joint function is restored.

14. A patient should be referred to a physician if any of the following conditions are suspected:

   ■ Obvious deformity suggesting a dislocation or fracture

   ■ Significant loss of motion or locking of the knee

   ■ Excessive joint swelling

   ■ Gross joint instability

   ■ Reported sounds, such as popping, snapping, or clicking, or giving way of the knee

   ■ Possible epiphyseal injuries

   ■ Abnormal or absent reflexes

   ■ Abnormal sensations in either segmental dermatomes or peripheral cutaneous patterns

   ■ Absent or weak pulse

   ■ Weakness in a myotome

   ■ Any unexplained or chronic pain that disrupts a patient's play or performance

APPLICATION QUESTIONS

1. Shoe design, specifically cleat length and placement, has been associated with increased risk of ACL injury. What type of cleat length and placement would you recommend to athletes playing on a sod field if the goal is to reduce the risk of injury?

2. A 17-year-old female basketball player is complaining of a deep, aching pain in the knee during activity. What open-ended questions could be asked to determine the medical history of this injury? What factors would the athletic trainer be looking for during the inspection/observation of this injury?

3. A 37-year-old tennis player complains of mild swelling and tenderness on the medial joint line. Slight joint effusion is present, and pain can be elicited with external rotation of the tibia on a fixed femur, and during extreme knee flexion. In assessing this condition, what stress and special tests could be performed to determine the possible injury?

4. A 20-year-old basketball player fell on the court directly on the knee and felt an intense pain on the anterior aspect of the knee. There is palpable pain on either side of the patellar tendon but not directly on the tendon. When the knee is moved into full extension, pain significantly increases. What condition may be present? What is the immediate management for this injury?

5. A 27-year-old female reported to the athletic training room complaining of anteromedial knee pain. She does not remember when her knee began hurting, but it has gotten more painful over the past 2 weeks. She describes a locking sensation and increased deep pain going up and down stairs. How would you differentiate between patellofemoral pain with patellar maltracking and a medial meniscus tear?

6. A 30-year-old cyclist is complaining of pain on the proximal, medial tibia just distal to the knee joint. It has been bothersome for nearly 2 weeks, especially after the completion of the workout. What structure(s) may be inflamed? Are there any factors which may contribute to this condition?

7. A 13-year-old male participates on his school swimming and diving team. He is complaining of anterior (patellar) knee pain in his takeoff and landing leg used for diving. The pain has developed over the past month. How would you differentiate between Sinding-Larsen-Johansson disease and Osgood-Schlatter disease?

8. A cross-country runner complains of an aching pain on the lateral side of the patella that increases during the workout, particularly when running downhill. Slight effusion is present in the patellofemoral joint, and palpable pain is elicited over the lateral patellar border. Intense pain is felt when the patella is pushed downward into the patellofemoral groove. What factors may contribute to this condition? What long-term management might be considered after acute symptoms have subsided?

9. A patient has been diagnosed with patellofemoral stress syndrome. Your evaluation findings include an atrophied VMO and laterally displaced patella. One of the rehabilitation goals is to recruit the VMO. What type of exercises would be appropriate to implement?

REFERENCES

1. Rishiraj N, Taunton JE, Lloyd-Smith R, et al. The potential role of prophylactic/functional knee bracing in preventing knee ligament injury. *Sports Med*. 2009;39(11):937–960.
2. Bradley J, Honkamp NJ, Jost P, et al. Incidence and variance of knee injuries in elite college football players. *Am J Orthop (Belle Mead NJ)*. 2008;37(6):310–314.
3. Messier SP, Legault C, Schoenlank CR, et al. Risk factors and mechanisms of knee injury in runners. *Med Sci Sports Exerc*. 2008;40(11): 1873–1879.
4. Hashemi J, Chandrashekar N, Gill B, et al. The geometry of the tibial plateau and its influence on the biomechanics of the tibiofemoral joint. *J Bone Joint Surg Am*. 2008;90(12):2724–2734.

5. Englund M, Guermazi A, Lohmander LS. The meniscus in knee osteoarthritis. *Rheum Dis Clin North Am.* 2009;35(3):579–590.

6. Rath E, Richmond JC. The menisci: basic science and advances in treatment. *Br J Sports Med.* 2000;34(4):252–257.

7. Mine T, Kimura M, Sakka A, et al. Innervation of nociceptors in the menisci of the knee joint: an immunohistochemical study. *Arch Orthop Trauma Surg.* 2000;120(3–4):201–204.

8. Starkey C, Brown SD, eds. Knee pathologies. In: *Examination of Orthopedic & Athletic Injuries.* 4th ed. Philadelphia, PA: FA Davis; 2015:306.

9. Hosseini A, Gill TJ, Li G. In vivo anterior cruciate ligament elongation in response to axial tibial loads. *J Orthop Sci.* 2009;14(3):298–306.

10. Sell TC, Ferris CM, Abt JP, et al. Predictors of proximal tibia anterior shear force during a vertical stop-jump. *J Orthop Res.* 2007;25(12): 1589–1597.

11. Markolf KL, Burchfield DM, Shapiro MM, et al. Combined knee loading states that generate high anterior cruciate ligament forces. *J Orthop Res.* 1995;13(6):930–935.

12. Yan J, Sasaki W, Hitomi J. Anatomical study of the lateral collateral ligament and its circumference structures in the human knee joint. *Surg Radiol Anat.* 2010;32(2):99–106.

13. Yang B, Tan H, Yang L, et al. Correlating anatomy and congruence of the patellofemoral joint with cartilage lesions. *Orthopedics.* 2009;32(1):20.

14. Omololu BB, Ogunlade OS, Gopaldasani VK. Normal Q-angle in an adult Nigerian population. *Clin Orthop Relat Res.* 2009;467(8): 2073–2076.

15. Mizuno Y, Kumagai M, Mattessich SM, et al. Q-angle influences tibiofemoral and patellofemoral kinematics. *J Orthop Res.* 2001;19(5):834–840.

16. Rubel IF, Schwarzbard I, Leonard A, et al. Anatomic location of the peroneal nerve at the level of the proximal aspect of the tibia: Gerdy's safe zone. *J Bone Joint Surg Am.* 2004;86(8):1625–1628.

17. Johal P, Williams A, Wragg P, et al. Tibio-femoral movement in the living knee. A study of weight bearing and non-weight bearing knee kinematics using "interventional" MRI. *J Biomech.* 2005; 38(2):269–276.

18. Nakagawa S, Kadoya Y, Kobayashi A, et al. Kinematics of the patella in deep flexion. Analysis with magnetic resonance imaging. *J Bone Joint Surg Am.* 2003;85(7):1238–1242.

19. Moro-oka T, Matsuda S, Miura H, et al. Patellar tracking and patellofemoral geometry in deep knee flexion. *Clin Orthop Relat Res.* 2002;(394):161–168.

20. Iranpour F, Merican AM, Baena FR, et al. Patellofemoral joint kinematics: the circular path of the patella around the trochlear axis. *J Orthop Res.* 2010;28(5):589–594.

21. Merican AM, Amis AA. Iliotibial band tension affects patellofemoral and tibiofemoral kinematics. *J Biomech.* 2009;42(10):1539–1546.

22. Winby CR, Lloyd DG, Besier TF, et al. Muscle and external load contribution to knee joint contact loads during normal gait. *J Biomech.* 2009;42(14):2294–2300.

23. Costigan PA, Deluzio KJ, Wyss UP. Knee and hip kinetics during normal stair climbing. *Gait Posture.* 2002;16(1):31–37.

24. Gullett JC, Tillman MD, Gutierrez GM, et al. A biomechanical comparison of back and front squats in healthy trained individuals. *J Strength Cond Res.* 2009;23(1):284–292.

25. Bursac P, Arnoczky S, York A. Dynamic compressive behavior of human meniscus correlates with its extra-cellular matrix composition. *Biorheology.* 2009;46(3):227–237.

26. Goudakos IG, König C, Schöttle PB, et al. Stair climbing results in more challenging patellofemoral contact mechanics and kinematics than walking at early knee flexion under physiological-like quadriceps loading. *J Biomech.* 2009;42(15): 2590–2596.

27. Hewitt TE, Myer GD. The mechanistic connection between trunk, hip, knee, and anterior cruciate ligament injury. *Exerc Sport Sci Rev.* 2011; 39(4):161–166.

28. Villwock MR, Meyer EG, Powell JW, et al. Football playing surface and shoe design affect rotational traction. *Am J Sports Med.* 2009;37(3):518–525.

29. Kendall FP, McCreary EK, Provance PG, et al, eds. *Muscles: Testing and Function with Posture and Pain.* 5th ed. Baltimore, MD: Lippincott Williams & Wilkins; 2005.

30. Wong M. *Pocket Orthopaedics: Evidence-Based Survival Guide.* Sudbury, MA: Jones and Bartlett; 2010.

31. Starkey C, Brown SD. *Orthopedic & Athletic Injury Examination Handbook.* 3rd ed. Philadelphia, PA: FA Davis; 2015.

32. Norkus SA, Swartz EE, Floyd RT. Advantages of the prone Lachman test. *Athl Ther Today.* 2002;7(2):52–56.

33. Dodd M, Trompeter A, Harrison T, et al. The pivot shift test is of limited clinical relevance in the arthritic anterior cruciate ligament-deficient knee. *J Knee Surg.* 2010;23(3):131–135.

34. Matsushita T, Oka S, Nagamune K, et al. Differences in knee kinematics between awake and anesthetized patients during the Lachman and pivot-shift tests for anterior cruciate ligament deficiency. *Orthop J Sports Med.* 2013;1(1):1–6. http:// ojs.sagepub.com/content/1/1/2325967113487855 .full.pdf+html. Accessed July 1, 2015.

35. Karachalios T, Hantes M, Zibis AH, et al. Diagnostic accuracy of a new clinical test (the Thessaly test) for early detection of meniscal tears. *J Bone Joint Surg Am.* 2005;87(5):955–962.

36. Nunes GS, Stapait EL, Kirsten MH, et al. Clinical test for diagnosis of patellofemoral pain syndrome: systematic review with meta-analysis. *Phys Ther Sport*. 2013;14:54–59

37. Doberstein ST, Romeyn RL, Reineke DM. The diagnostic value of the Clarke sign in assessing chondromalacia patella. *J Athl Train*. 2008;43(2):190–196.

38. Nijs J, Van Geel C, Van der auwera C, et al. Diagnostic value of five clinical tests in patellofemoral pain syndrome. *Man Ther*. 2006;11(1):69–77.

39. Rosenthal MD. Clinical testing for extra-articular lateral knee pain. A modification and combination of tests. *N Am J Sports Phys Ther*. 2008;3(2):107–109.

40. Cardone DA, Tallia AF. Diagnostic and therapeutic injection of the hip and knee. *Am Fam Physician*. 2003;67(10):2147–2152.

41. Tyler TF, McHugh MP. Neuromuscular rehabilitation of a female Olympic ice hockey player following anterior cruciate ligament reconstruction. *J Orthop Sports Phys Ther*. 2001;31(10):577–587.

42. Marx RG. Functional bracing was no better than nonbracing after anterior cruciate ligament repair. *J Bone Joint Surg Am*. 2005;87(8):1890.

43. Walsh WM, Vanicek JJ. Knee injuries. In: Mellion MB, Walsh WM, Madden C, et al, eds. *The Team Physician's Handbook*. 3rd ed. Philadelphia, PA: Hanley & Belfus; 2002:490–508.

44. Horn A. Diagnostic accuracy of orthopedic special tests for meniscal injury. http://commons.pacificu.edu/ptcats/3. Published January 1, 2011. Accessed July 9, 2015.

45. Covey DC. Injuries of the posterolateral corner of the knee. *J Bone Joint Surg Am*. 2001;83(1):106–118.

46. Hale SA. Etiology of patellar tendinopathy in athletes. *J Sport Rehab*. 2005;14(3):259–276.

47. Wall EJ. Osgood-Schlatter disease: practical treatment for a self-limiting condition. *Phys Sportsmed*. 1998;26(3):29–34.

48. Greis PE, Lahav A, Holmstrom MC. Surgical treatment options for patella tendon rupture, part II: chronic. *Orthopedics*. 2005;28(8):765–769.

49. Khaund R, Flynn SH. Iliotibial band syndrome: a common source of knee pain. *Am Fam Physician*. 2005;71(8):1545–1550.

50. Johnson MP. Physical therapist management of an adult with osteochondritis dissecans of the knee. *Phys Ther*. 2005;85(7):665–675.

51. Weber MD, Woodall WB. Knee rehabilitation. In: Andrews JR, Wilk KE, Harrelson GL, eds. *Physical Rehabilitation of the Injured Athlete*. 3rd ed. Philadelphia, PA: WB Saunders; 2004:377–428.

16

Pelvic, Hip, and Thigh Conditions

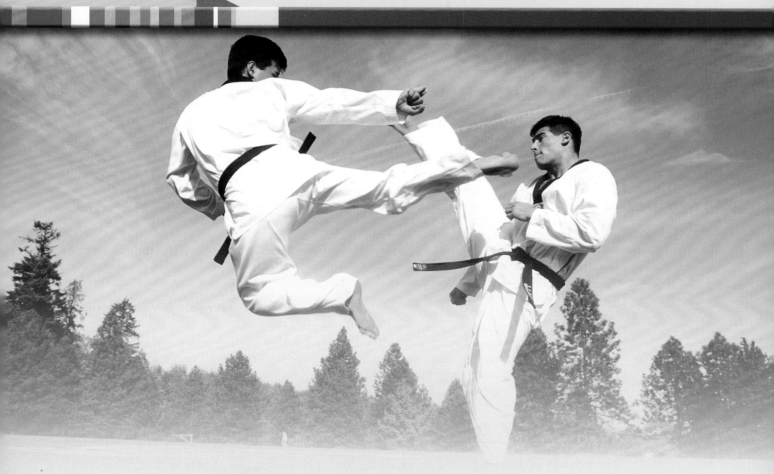

STUDENT OUTCOMES

1. Identify the major bony and soft-tissue structures of the pelvis, hip, and thigh.

2. Describe the functions of the various soft-tissue structures that support the sacroiliac joint, sacrococcygeal joint, and hip joint.

3. Describe the motions of the hip and identify the muscles that produce them.

4. List the major nerves and blood vessels that course through the pelvic and proximal femoral region.

5. Describe the forces that produce loading patterns responsible for common injuries of the pelvis, hip, and thigh.

6. Explain general principles used to prevent injuries to the pelvis, hip, and thigh.

7. Describe a thorough assessment of the pelvis, hip, and thigh.

8. Identify the common injuries and conditions sustained in the pelvis, hip, and thigh by physically active patients (including sprains, dislocations, contusions, strains, bursitis, and vascular and neural disorders).

9. Explain the management strategies for common injuries and conditions of the hip, pelvis, and thigh.

10. Describe the various types of fractures that can occur in the wrist and hand and explain their management.

11. Explain the general principles and techniques used in developing a rehabilitation exercise program for the pelvis, hip, and thigh.

INTRODUCTION

Although the pelvis, hip, and thigh have a sturdy anatomical composition, this region can be subjected to large, potentially injurious forces when patients engage in sports or exercise. For example, the soft tissues of the anterior thigh often sustain compressive forces, particularly during contact sports. Although the resulting contusions are not usually serious, mismanagement of these injuries can lead to more serious problems. Daily activities, such as sitting, walking, and climbing stairs, rarely involve stretching of the hamstrings. A lack of hamstring flexibility combined with an imbalance of strength between the hamstrings and the quadriceps place the physically active patient at higher risk for sustaining a hamstring strain.

Because of their strong bony stability, the hip and pelvis are seldom injured. Because the hip sustains repetitive forces of four- to sevenfold the body weight during walking and running, however, the joint is subject to stress-related injuries. Overuse injuries of the hip among athletes include stress fracture, avulsive injuries, snapping-hip syndrome, iliopsoas bursitis, femoroacetabular impingement syndrome, tendinosis, and tears of the gluteal musculature.[1,2]

This chapter begins with a review of the anatomy, kinematics, and kinetics of the pelvis, hip, and thigh. Next, preventative measures are discussed. A step-by-step process of injury assessment is followed by information regarding basic injuries to the region. Finally, examples of rehabilitation exercises for the region are presented.

ANATOMY OF THE PELVIS, HIP, AND THIGH

The pelvis, hip, and thigh have an extremely stable bony structure that is further reinforced by a number of large, strong ligaments and muscles. This region is well-suited anatomically for withstanding the large forces to which it is subjected during daily activities.

The Pelvis

The pelvis, or pelvic girdle, consists of a protective bony ring formed by four fused bones—namely, the two innominate bones, the sacrum and the coccyx (**Fig. 16.1**). The innominate bones articulate with each other anteriorly at the pubic symphysis and with the sacrum posteriorly at the sacroiliac (SI) joints. Each innominate bone consists of three fused bones—namely, the ilium, the ischium, and the pubis. Among these, the ilium forms the major portion of the innominate bone, including the prominent iliac crests. The anterior superior iliac spine (ASIS) is a readily palpable landmark on the iliac crest; the posterior superior iliac spine (PSIS) typically is marked by an indentation in the soft tissues just lateral to the sacrum. The pelvis protects the enclosed inner organs, transmits loads between the trunk and lower extremity, and provides a site for a number of major muscle attachments.

Sacroiliac Joints

The SI joints form the critical link between the two pelvic bones. Working with the pubic symphysis, they help to transfer the weight of the torso and skull to the lower limbs, provide elasticity to the pelvic ring, and conversely, act as a buffer to decrease impact forces from the foot as they are transmitted to the spine and upper body.

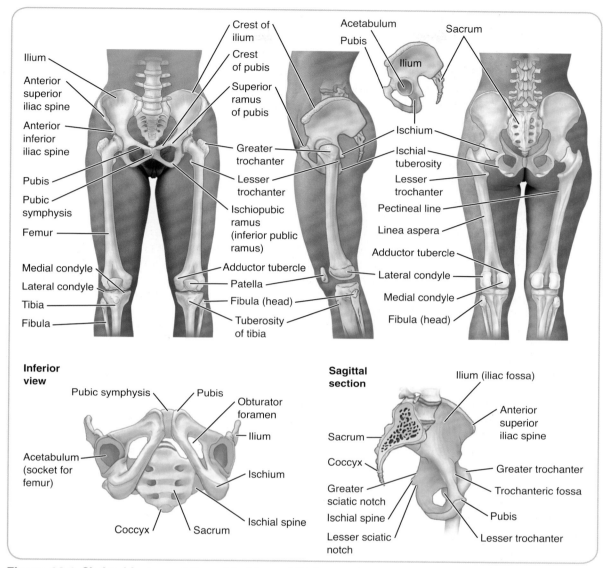

Figure 16.1. Skeletal features of the pelvis, hip, and thigh.

The SI joints are synovial as well as syndesmosis joints. The synovial portion of the joint is C-shaped, with the convex iliac surface of the "C" facing an anterior and inferior direction. The articular surface of the ilium is covered with fibrocartilage; the articular surface of the sacrum is covered with hyaline cartilage and is threefold thicker than that of the ilium. The size, shape, and texture of the articular surfaces vary across the lifespan. In children, the surfaces are smooth. In adults, irregular depressions and elevations are formed that fit into one another. As a result, the articulation is very strong and has a limited range of motion (ROM). In older patients, portions of the joint surfaces may be obliterated by adhesions.

The strong fibers of the interosseous SI ligaments bind the anterior portion of the ilium and the posterior portion of the sacrum, filling the void behind the articular surfaces of these bones (**Fig. 16.2**). The joint also is strengthened anteriorly and posteriorly by the dorsal and ventral SI ligaments. The dorsal SI ligament runs transversely to bind the posterior ilium to the upper portion of the sacrum, and vertical fibers connect the lower sacrum to the PSIS. The ventral SI ligament lines the anterior portion of the pelvic cavity, attaching onto the anterior portion of the sacrum. These SI ligaments, particularly the ventral bond, play a significant role in restricting movement at the SI joints and are stronger in males than in females.[3] Two accessory ligaments also assist in maintaining the stability of the SI joint. The sacrotuberous ligament arises from the ischium to merge with the inferior fibers of

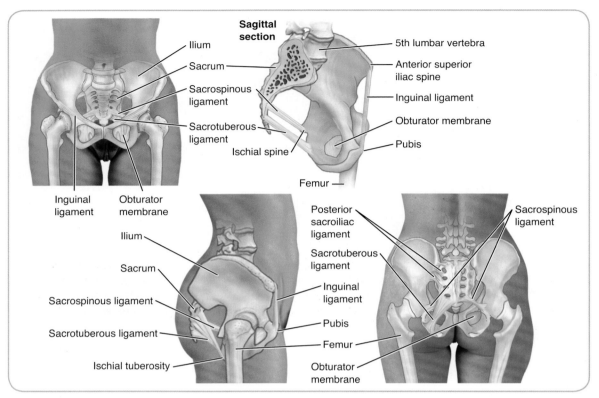

Figure 16.2. Ligaments of the pelvis and hip.

the dorsal SI ligaments. The sacrospinous ligament, indirectly supporting the sacrum, runs from the ischial spine and attaches to the coccyx.

Sacrococcygeal Joint

The sacrococcygeal joint usually is a fused line (i.e., symphysis) that is united by a fibrocartilaginous disk. Occasionally, the joint is freely movable and synovial, but with advanced age, the joint may fuse and be obliterated.

Pubic Symphysis

The pubic symphysis is a cartilaginous joint with a disk of fibrocartilage, called the interpubic disk, which is located between the two joint surfaces. A small degree of spreading, compression, and rotation occurs between the two halves of the pelvic girdle at this joint.

Bony Structure of the Thigh

The femur, a major weight-bearing bone, is the longest, largest, and strongest bone in the body (**Fig. 16.1**). The weakest component is the femoral neck, which is smaller in diameter than the rest of the bone and is weak internally, because it is composed primarily of cancellous bone. The head of the femur is angled at approximately 125° in the frontal plane, although it can vary from 90° to 135°. This relationship, known as the angle of inclination (**Fig. 16.3**), allows the femur to angle medially downward from the hip during the support phase of walking and running, producing single-leg support beneath the body's center of gravity. Because women have a wider pelvis, this angulation tends to be more pronounced than the angulation in men. Angles of inclination greater than 125° are termed coxa valga, and angles less than 125° are referred to as coxa vara.

In the transverse plane, the relationship between the femoral head and the femoral shaft is called the angle of torsion, which is approximately 12° (**Fig. 16.4**). A decreased angle between the femoral condyles and femoral head is called retroversion; an increased angle is called anteversion.

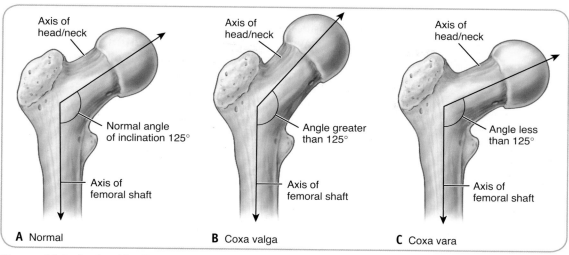

Figure 16.3. Angle of inclination. In the frontal plane, the femoral head normally assumes a 125° angle with the long axis of the femur **(A)**. This angle allows the femur to angle medially downward from the hip during the support phase of walking and running, producing single-leg support beneath the body's center of gravity. Because women have a wider pelvis, this angulation tends to be slightly increased, which is called coxa valga **(B)**; a decrease is called coxa vara **(C)**.

Retroversion causes a tendency for external rotation of the leg during the swing phase of gait, and anteversion causes the opposite tendency (i.e., toward internal rotation). Both are relatively common in children but tend to normalize with maturity.

The Hip Joint

The coxofemoral joint or hip is the articulation between the concave acetabulum of the pelvis and the head of the femur. It functions as a classic ball-and-socket joint (**Fig. 16.5**). The acetabulum angles obliquely in an inferior, anterior, and lateral direction. Because the socket is deep, it provides considerable bony stability to the joint. Both articulating surfaces are covered with friction-reducing joint cartilage. The cartilage on the acetabulum is thickened around the periphery, where it merges with the U-shaped fibrocartilaginous acetabular labrum, which further contributes to stability of the joint.

Hip Joint Capsule

The joint capsule of the hip is large and loose. It completely surrounds the joint, attaching to the labrum of the acetabular socket. The labrum forms a seal around the joint, with increased fluid pressure within the labrum contributing to lubrication of the joint.[4] The joint capsule also passes over a fat pad internally to join to the distal aspect of the femoral neck. Because the capsular fibers attaching to the femoral neck are arranged in a circular fashion, they are known as the zona orbicularis and are an important contributor to hip stability.

Ligaments of the Hip Joint

Several large, strong ligaments support the hip (**Fig. 16.2**). The anterior aspect of the hip includes the extremely strong, Y-shaped iliofemoral ligament, sometimes referred to as the **Y-ligament of Bigelow**. It extends from the anterior inferior iliac spine (AIIS) to the intertrochanteric line on the femur, enabling it to limit hip hyperextension. The pubofemoral ligament, which also is located anteriorly, connects the pubic ramus to the intertrochanteric line, limiting abduction and hyperextension of the hip. The ischiofemoral ligament reinforces the hip posteriorly, extending from the posterior acetabular rim of the ischium in a superior, lateral direction and attaching to the inner surface of the greater trochanter of the femur. The spiraling nature of this ligament causes it to limit extension of the hip. Tension in these major ligaments twists the head of the femur into the acetabulum on

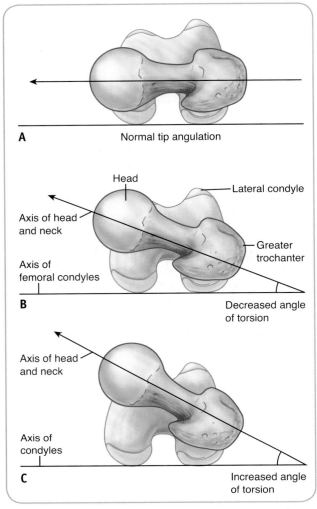

A   Normal tip angulation

Head

Lateral condyle

Axis of head and neck

Axis of femoral condyles

Greater trochanter

B   Decreased angle of torsion

Axis of head and neck

Axis of condyles

C   Increased angle of torsion

Figure 16.4. Angle of torsion. A, In the transverse plane, deviations may occur from the norm. **B,** A decreased angle between the femoral condyles and femoral head is called retroversion. **C,** An increased angle is called anteversion.

hip extension, as occurs when a person rises from a seated position.

Within the joint, the **ligamentum teres** serves as a conduit for the medial and lateral **circumflex arteries** but provides little support to the hip joint. The inguinal ligament, which runs from the ASIS and inserts at the pubic symphysis, contains the soft tissues as they course anteriorly from the trunk to the lower extremity. The structure demarcates the superior border of the femoral triangle.

Femoral Triangle

The femoral triangle is formed by the inguinal ligament superiorly, the sartorius laterally, and the adductor longus medially (**Fig. 16.6**). This region is significant in that the femoral nerve, artery, and vein are located within the area. The femoral pulse can be palpated as it crosses the crease between the thigh and the abdomen. In addition, with an infection of or active inflammation in the lower extremity, enlarged lymph nodes may be palpated in this region. Therefore, knowing where the borders of the femoral triangle are and the structures that are contacted within the triangle is important for conducting a skilled assessment of the area.

Bursae

Four primary bursae in the hip and pelvic region are frequently irritated during physical activity (**Fig. 16.7**). The **iliopectineal (iliopsoas) bursa** is positioned between the iliopsoas and articular capsule, serving to reduce the friction between these structures. The **deep trochanteric bursa** provides a cushion between the greater trochanter of the femur and the gluteus maximus at its attachment to the iliotibial tract. The **gluteofemoral bursa** separates the gluteus maximus from the origin of the vastus lateralis. Finally, the **ischial bursa** serves as a weight-bearing structure when a patient is seated, cushioning the ischial tuberosity where it passes over the gluteus maximus.

Q-Angle

The Q-angle is defined as the angle between the line of resultant force produced by the quadriceps muscles and the line of the patellar tendon (see **Fig. 15.3A**). One line is drawn from the middle of the patella to the ASIS of the ilium, and a second line is drawn from the tibial tubercle through the center of the patella. When the knee is fully extended during weight bearing, the normal Q-angle ranges from approximately 12° in males to approximately 22° in females.[5] There is evidence that an excessive Q-angle may predispose women to greater lateral displacement of the patella when the quadriceps is vigorously activated during physical activity.[6] The Q-angle is discussed in more detail in Chapter 15.

See **Muscles of the Hip**, available on the companion Web site at thePoint, for a summary of these muscles, including their attachments, primary actions, and innervation.

Muscles of the Hip Joint

A large number of muscles cross the hip (**Figs. 16.8** to **16.10**). Identifying the actions of these muscles is complicated by the fact that several muscles are two-joint muscles. These muscles, crossing both the hip and knee joints, are biomechanically efficient in their ability to simultaneously produce positive

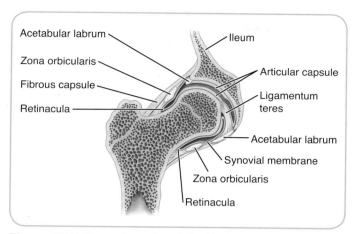

Figure 16.5. **Coronal section of the hip joint.** The epiphysis of the head of the femur is entirely within the joint capsule. The ligamentum teres is a synovial tube that is fixed superiorly at the fovea on the head of the femur and opens inferiorly at the acetabular foramen, where it is continuous with the synovial membrane covering the fat in the acetabular fossa. The ligament is taut during adduction of the hip joint, as occurs when crossing the legs.

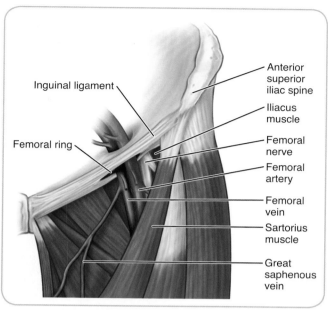

Figure 16.6. **Femoral triangle.** The triangle is bounded by the inguinal ligament superiorly, the adductor longus medially, and the sartorius laterally. The femoral artery, vein, and nerve pass through this area to enter the thigh.

work at one joint and negative work at the other, transferring energy between body segments and thus decreasing the metabolic cost of movement.[7] Excessive tightness in the hip muscles has been associated with development of chronic groin injury.[8] Weak external hip rotators are believed to contribute to the development of iliotibial band syndrome.[9]

Nerves of the Pelvis, Hip, and Thigh

The major nerve supply to the pelvis, hip, and thigh arises from the lumbar and sacral plexus. The lumbar plexus is formed from the first four lumbar spinal nerves (see **Fig. 22.4**). This plexus is typically found within the psoas major muscle but occasionally lies posterior to it.[10] The plexus innervates portions of the abdominal wall and psoas major, with branches into the thigh region. The largest branch is the femoral nerve (L2 through L4), which supplies the muscles and skin of the anterior thigh. Another branch, the obturator nerve (L2 through L4), provides innervation to the hip adductor muscles.

The sacral plexus is positioned just anterior to the lumbar plexus and has some intermingling of fibers with the lumbar plexus. The lower spinal nerves, including L4 through S4, spawn the sacral plexus (see **Fig. 22.5**). Twelve nerve branches arise from the sacral plexus. The major nerve is the sciatic nerve (L4, L5, and S1 through S3), which is the largest and longest single nerve in the body. The sciatic nerve passes through the greater sciatic notch of the pelvis, courses through the gluteus maximus muscle, and then innervates the hamstrings and adductor magnus. The tibial and common peroneal nerves that branch from the sciatic nerve in the posterior thigh region are discussed in Chapters 14 and 15.

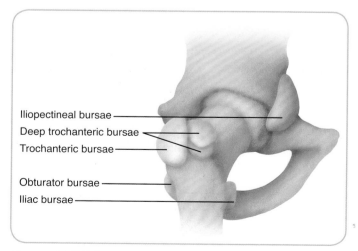

Figure 16.7. **Primary bursae of the hip and pelvis.**

text continues on page 497

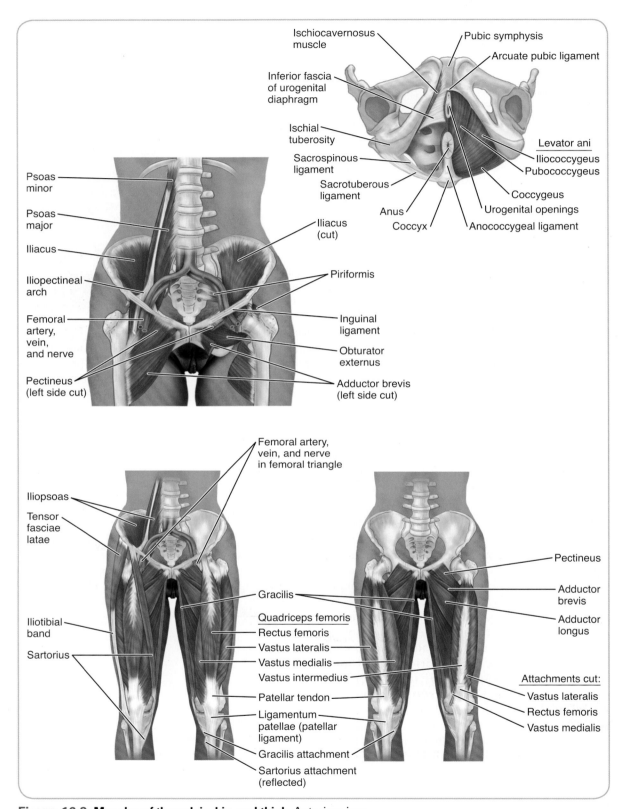

Figure 16.8. Muscles of the pelvis, hip, and thigh. Anterior view.

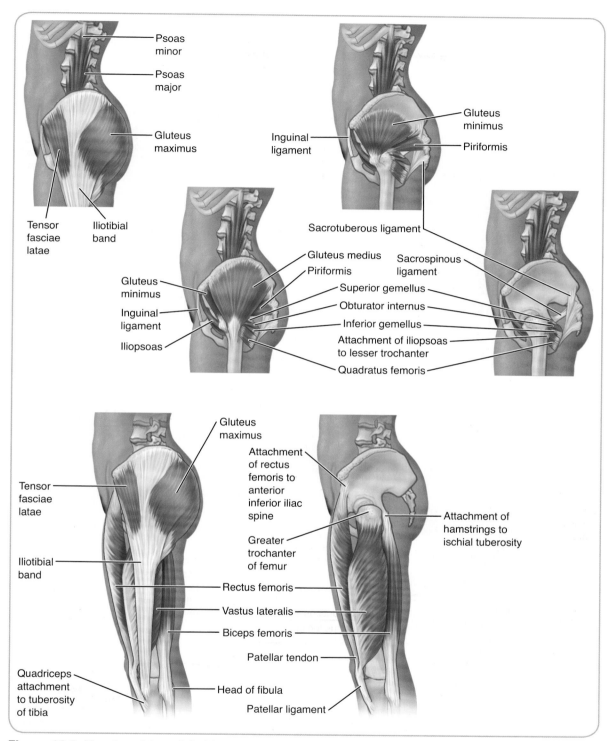

Figure 16.9. Muscles of the pelvis, hip, and thigh. Lateral view.

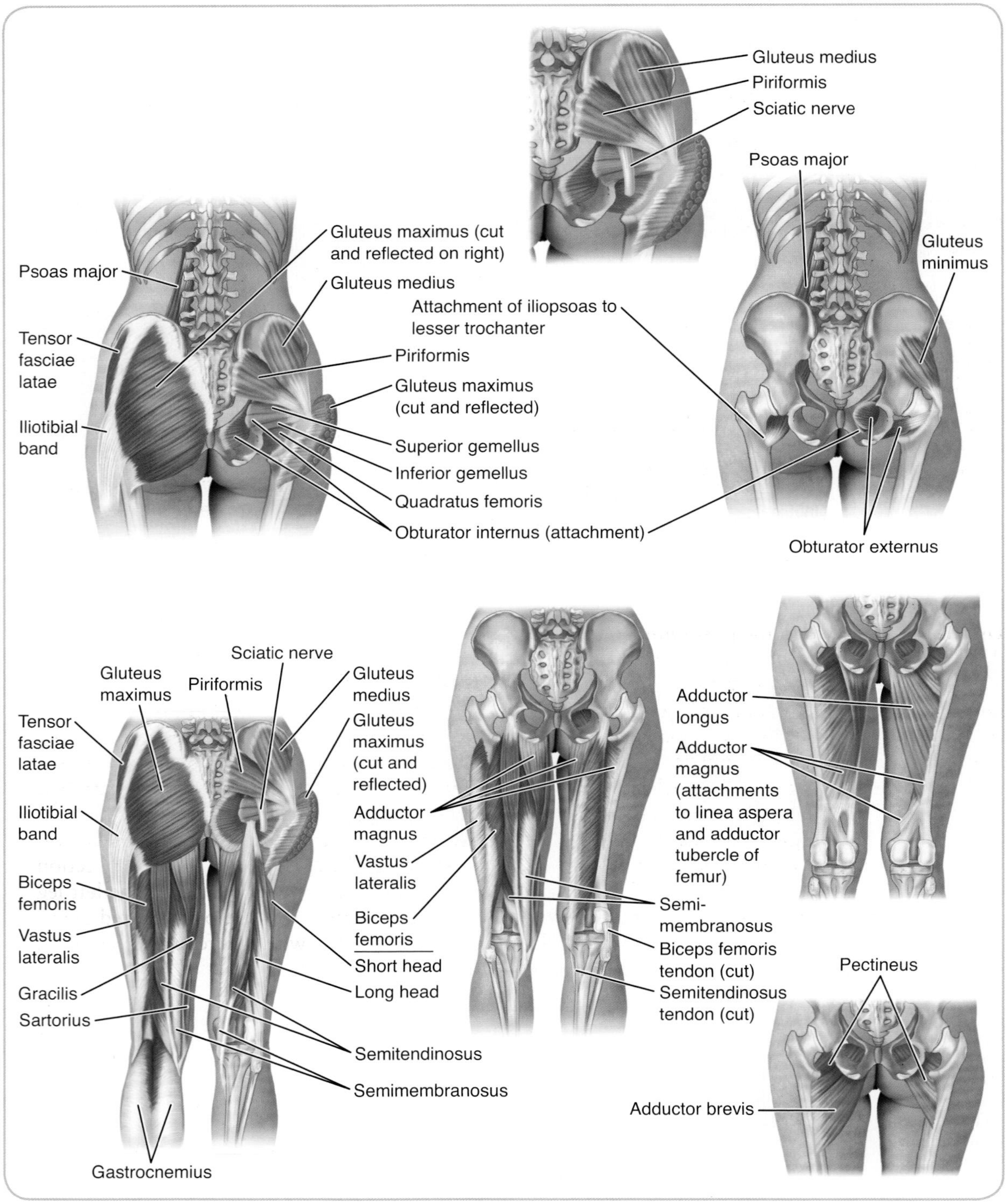

Figure 16.10. Muscles of the pelvis, hip, and thigh. Posterior view.

Blood Vessels of the Pelvis, Hip, and Thigh

The external iliac arteries become the femoral arteries at the level of the thighs (**Fig. 16.11**). The femoral artery gives off several branches in the thigh region, including the deep femoral artery, which serves the posterior and lateral thigh muscles, and the lateral and medial femoral circumflex arteries, which supply the region of the femoral head.

KINEMATICS AND MAJOR MUSCLE ACTIONS OF THE HIP

Because the hip is a ball-and-socket joint, the femur can move in all planes of motion. The massive muscles crossing the hip tend to limit ROM, however, particularly in the posterior direction.

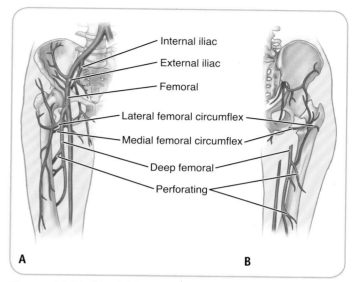

Figure 16.11. Arterial supply to the hip and thigh region. A, Anterior view. **B,** Posterior view.

Pelvic Positioning

During many activities, the positioning of the pelvic girdle facilitates motion of the femur at the hip. Also, treatment programs for patients with low back pain often include pelvic positioning exercises. The reference point for describing pelvic positioning is **pelvic neutral**, which occurs when the ASIS and the PSIS are in the same transverse plane (**Fig. 16.12**). **Anterior pelvic tilt** occurs with trunk or thigh extension, resulting in a bilateral shift of the ASIS downward (**Fig. 16.13A**), thus increasing lumbar lordosis. **Posterior pelvic tilt** (**Fig. 16.13B**) results in decreasing lumbar lordosis and occurs with trunk or thigh flexion. The pelvis can also tilt as well as rotate around the sacrum. **Lateral tilt** tends to occur naturally, as when shifting the body weight from one leg to the other during normal gait patterns and results with unilateral downward motion of one innominate with unilateral upward motion of opposing innominate (**Fig. 16.13C and D**). **Pelvic rotation** is defined by the direction in which the anterior aspect of the pelvis moves and occurs naturally when walking. As the left leg moves forward, the pelvis rotates to the right (see **Fig. 8.9**). Abnormally excessive or restricted pelvic position usually results in injury to the associated joints and muscles as well as affecting other areas in the kinetic chain.

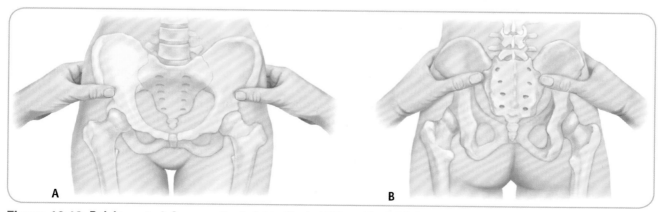

Figure 16.12. Pelvic neutral. Compare the height of both ASIS and both PSIS along with the iliac crests to determine pelvic neutral. If one side of the pelvis is higher than the other, lateral pelvic tilt is present. **A,** Anterior view. **B,** Posterior view.

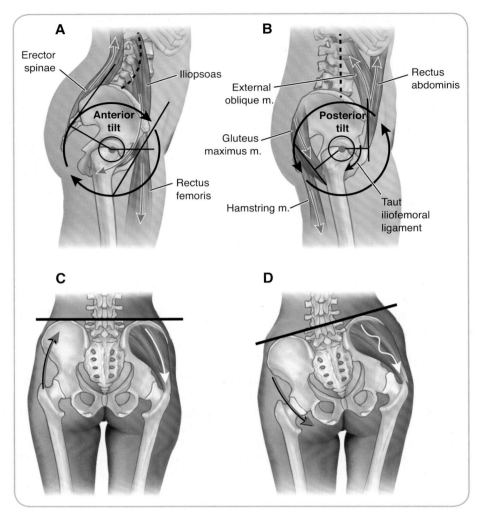

Figure 16.13. Pelvic positioning. A, Anterior pelvic tilt, the reverse action of trunk extension, causing a bilateral shift of the ASIS downward, thus increasing lumbar lordosis. **B,** Posterior pelvic tilt, the reverse action of trunk flexion, decreases lumbar lordosis and can lead to flat back. **C,** Pelvic left side elevation is the reverse action of trunk left lateral flexion (pelvic right side elevation is the reverse action of trunk right lateral flexion). In normal lateral pelvic positioning, the gluteus medius engages to stabilize the pelvis during gait **(C).** With a weak gluteus medius, an abnormal pelvic tilt and lateral spine flexion occurs **(D).**

Flexion

The major hip flexors are the iliacus and psoas major, which because of their common attachment at the femur are referred to jointly as the iliopsoas. Four other muscles cross the anterior aspect of the hip to contribute to hip flexion—namely, the pectineus, the rectus femoris, the sartorius, and the tensor fasciae latae. Because the rectus femoris is a two-joint muscle that is active during both hip flexion and knee extension, it functions more effectively as a hip flexor when the knee is in flexion, as occurs when a person kicks a ball. The sartorius also is a two-joint muscle. Crossing from the ASIS to the medial surface of the proximal tibia just below the tuberosity, the sartorius is the longest muscle in the body.

Extension

The hip extensors are the gluteus maximus and the three hamstrings—namely, the biceps femoris, the semitendinosus, and the semimembranosus. The gluteus maximus usually is active only when the hip is in flexion, as occurs during stair climbing or cycling, or when extension at the hip is resisted. The nickname "hamstrings" derives from the prominent tendons of the three muscles, which are readily palpable on the posterior aspect of the knee. The hamstrings cross both the hip and the knee, contributing to hip extension and knee flexion.

Abduction

The gluteus medius is the major abductor at the hip, with assistance from the gluteus minimus. The hip abductors are active in stabilizing the pelvis during single-leg support of the body and during the support phase of walking and running (see Chapter 8). For example, when body weight is supported by the right foot during walking, the right hip abductors contract isometrically and eccentrically to prevent the left side of the pelvis from being pulled downward by the weight of the swinging left leg. This allows the left leg to move freely through the swing phase without scuffing the toes. If the hip abductors are too weak to perform this function, lateral pelvic tilt occurs with every step.

Adduction

The hip adductors include the adductor longus, adductor brevis, and adductor magnus. These muscles are active during the swing phase of gait, bringing the foot beneath the body's center of gravity for placement during the support phase. The relatively weak gracilis assists with hip adduction. The hip adductors also contribute to flexion and internal rotation at the hip, especially when the femur is externally rotated. Strength and flexibility deficits in the hip adductors have been linked to increased risk of injury among ice hockey and soccer players.[11]

Medial and Lateral Rotation of the Femur

Although several muscles contribute to lateral rotation of the femur, six function solely as lateral rotators. These six muscles are the piriformis, gemellus superior, gemellus inferior, obturator internus, obturator externus, and quadratus femoris. The femur of the swinging leg rotates laterally to accommodate the lateral rotation of the pelvis during the stride.

The major medial rotator of the femur is the gluteus minimus, with assistance from the tensor fasciae latae, semitendinosus, semimembranosus, gluteus medius, and the four adductor muscles. The medial rotators are relatively weak; their estimated strength is approximately one-third that of the lateral rotators. **Table 16.1** summarizes the muscles responsible for the various motions at the hip joint.

KINETICS OF THE HIP

Forces at the Hip During Standing

The hip is a major weight-bearing joint that is subject to extremely high loads during sport participation. During upright standing, with weight evenly distributed on both legs, the weight supported

TABLE 16.1 Hip Movements and Involved Muscles

FLEXION	EXTENSION	ABDUCTION	ADDUCTION	MEDIAL ROTATION	LATERAL ROTATION
Iliopsoas	Gluteus maximus	Gluteus medius	Pectineus	Gluteus medius	Piriformis
Rectus femoris	Biceps femoris	Gluteus minimus	Adductor brevis	Gluteus minimus	Obturator internus
Pectineus	Biceps femoris	Gluteus minimus	Adductor magnus	Tensor fasciae latae	Obturator externus
Sartorius	Semitendinosus	Tensor fasciae latae	Adductor longus		Superior gemelli
Tensor fasciae latae	Semimembranosus	Sartorius	Adductor magnus		Inferior gemelli
	Adductor magnus	Piriformis	Gracilis		Quadratus femoris
					Gluteus maximus

at each hip is half the weight of the body segments above the hip. The total load on each hip in this situation is greater than the weight that is being supported, however, because tension in the large, strong hip muscles further adds to compression at the joint.

Forces at the Hip During Gait

Compression on the hip is approximately the same as body weight during the swing phase of normal walking gait but increases up to three- to sixfold the body weight during the stance phase.[3] Body weight, impact forces translated upward through the skeleton from the foot, and muscle tension contribute to this compressive load. Walking or running increases the forces on the hip. Use of a crutch or a cane on the side opposite an injured lower limb serves to more evenly distribute the load between the legs throughout the gait cycle. It is better to use no assistive device than to use a crutch or a cane on the same side as the lower extremity injury, because this actually increases joint forces on the injured side.[12]

PREVENTION OF PELVIC, HIP, AND THIGH CONDITIONS

The hip joint is well protected within the pelvic girdle and seldom is injured. Several factors, however, such as wearing protective equipment, wearing shoes with adequate cushioning and support, and participating in an extensive physical conditioning program, can further reduce the incidence of acute and chronic injuries to the region.

Protective Equipment

Several collision and contact sports require special pads composed of hard polyethylene covered with layers of specialized foam rubber to protect vulnerable areas, such as the iliac crests, sacrum and coccyx, and genital region. A girdle with special pockets can hold the pads in place. The male genital region is best protected by a protective cup placed in an athletic supporter. Special commercial thigh pads also may be used to prevent contusions to the anterior thigh, and neoprene sleeves can provide uniform compression, therapeutic warmth, and support for a quadriceps or hamstring strain. Many of these items can be seen in Chapter 3.

Physical Conditioning

Because several of the muscles in the pelvis, hip, and thigh are two-joint muscles, physical conditioning should include ROM and strengthening exercises for both the hip and the knee. **Application Strategy 16.1** demonstrates specific exercises for the hip flexors, extensors, adductors, abductors, and medial and lateral rotators. Exercises for the muscles that govern the knee are presented in Chapter 15.

Shoe Selection

Sport and physical activities take place on a variety of terrains and floor surfaces. Shoes should adequately cushion impact forces as well as support and guide the foot during the stance and final push-off phases of running, regardless of the terrain or surface. Inadequate cushioning in the heel region can transmit forces up the leg, leading to inflammation of the hip joint or stress fractures of the femoral neck or pubis. Therefore, it is important to purchase shoes that provide an adequate heel cushion and a thermoplastic heel counter, which can maintain its shape and firmness even during adverse weather conditions. The soles should be designed for the specific type of playing surface to avoid slipping or sliding.

ASSESSMENT OF PELVIC, HIP, AND THIGH CONDITIONS

 A high school basketball player reports to the athletic training room complaining of discomfort in the anterior thigh for the past 2 weeks. How should the assessment of this player progress to determine the extent and severity of injury?

APPLICATION STRATEGY `16.1`

Exercises to Prevent Injury at the Thigh, Hip, and Pelvis

The following exercises can be performed for motions at the hip. Exercises for the hamstrings, quadriceps, and iliotibial band, which also cross the knee joint, can be seen in Chapter 15.

1. **Hip flexor stretch (lunge).** Place the leg to be stretched in front. Bend the contralateral knee as the hips are moved forward. Keep the back straight. Alternate method: Place the foot on a chair or table and lean forward until a stretch is felt.

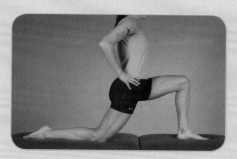

2. **Lateral rotator stretch, seated position.** Cross one leg over the thigh and place the elbow on the outside of the knee. Gently stretch the buttock muscles by pushing the bent knee across the body while keeping the pelvis on the floor.

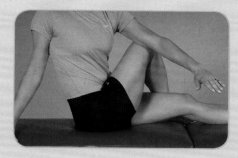

3. **Adductor stretch, standing position.** Place the leg to be stretched out to the side. Slowly bend the contralateral knee. Keep the hips in a neutral or extended position.

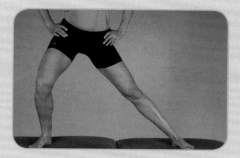

4. **Elastic tubing exercises.** Secure elastic tubing to a table. Perform hip flexion, extension, abduction, adduction, and medial and lateral rotation in a single plane or in multidirectional patterns.

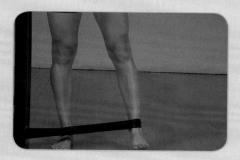

5. **Full squats.** A weight belt should be worn during this exercise. Place the feet at shoulder width or wider. Keep the back straight by keeping the chest out and the head up at all times. Flex the knees and hips to no greater than 90°. Begin the upward motion by extending the hips first.

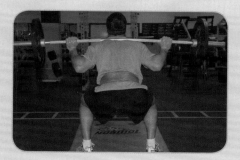

6. **Hip extension.** With the trunk stabilized and the back flat, extend the hip while keeping the knee flexed. Alternate legs.

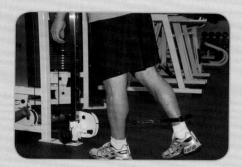

The lower extremity works as a unit to transmit load from the upper body to the ground through a closed kinetic chain. In the closed chain, the foot, ankle, leg, and hip also absorb force from the ground and dissipate the stress throughout the various structures. When excessive loads and stress exceed the yield points of a tissue, an injury occurs. Furthermore, the hip is a common site for referred pain from visceral, low back, and knee conditions. Evaluations therefore must be inclusive, particularly with adolescents who are complaining of groin pain. In the absence of direct trauma to the hip, or findings do not support the presence of an overuse injury and no improvement is seen in 2 to 5 days, always refer the patient to a physician to rule out serious underlying conditions.

See **Application Strategy: Hip Evaluation**, available on the companion Web site at thePoint.

HISTORY

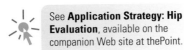

? The injury assessment of the basketball player should begin with a history. What questions need to be asked to identify the cause and extent of this injury?

Many conditions at the hip may be related to family history, age, congenital deformity, improper biomechanical execution of skills, and recent changes in training programs, surfaces, or foot attire. The clinician should gather information regarding the mechanism of injury; onset, duration, severity, and progression of symptoms; any disabilities that may have resulted from the injury; and related medical history. Because hip and back pain often coexists, take note of the relative severity of each type of pain. In addition, weakness, numbness, or paresthesia in the lower extremity suggests neural compression, which often occurs in the lumbar spine. For example, deep groin pain may originate in the hip joint itself or be referred from the lumbar spine or SI joint. **Box 16.1** lists other conditions that can cause groin pain. SI pathology almost always manifests itself with pain over the PSIS of the affected side. Mechanical symptoms such as locking, catching, popping, or sharp stabbing pain are indicators of a correctable problem, whereas pain in the absence of mechanical symptoms is a poorer predictor.[13] Examples suggesting a mechanical hip problem include symptoms present during the following:

- Nighttime
- Twisting, turning, or changing directions
- Seated position, especially with hip flexion
- Rising from a seated position (catching)
- Difficulty ascending and descending stairs

BOX 16.1 Conditions That Can Cause Groin Pain

- Referred pain from the bowel, bladder, testicle, kidney, abdomen, rectum, hip joint, SI joint, pubic symphysis, lymph nodes, or rectus abdominis muscle
- Pelvic inflammatory disease
- Urinary tract infections
- Apophysitis, stress fracture, or avulsion fracture
- Avascular necrosis of the femoral head, or slipped capital femoral epiphysis
- Osteitis pubis

- Toxic synovitis of the hip
- Lymphadenopathy
- Testicular torsion or rupture
- Hernia
- Testicular cancer and other neoplasms
- Osteoarthritis
- Ovarian cysts

- Entering and exiting an automobile
- Putting on shoes, socks, hose, etc.
- Dyspareunia (painful sexual intercourse)[13]

Critical to any history taking, the clinician should note any "red flags" such as fever, malaise, night sweats, weight loss, night pain, intravenous drug use, cancer history, or known immunocompromised state, which may indicate systemic problems that necessitate referral to a physician for further diagnostic testing.

> The high school basketball player should be asked questions that address when, where, and how the injury occurred; intensity, location, and type of pain; when the pain begins (e.g., when getting out of bed, while sitting, while walking, during exercise, or at night); how long the condition has been present; how long the pain lasts; if the pain has changed or stayed the same; if the pain is worse before, during, or after activity; activities that aggravate or alleviate the symptoms; as well as previous injury, treatment, and medication.

OBSERVATION AND INSPECTION

> **?** The basketball player reports having sustained a severe blow to the right anterior thigh 2 weeks earlier. He did not report the injury when it occurred. During today's practice, he received a mild blow to the same area. He complains of discomfort after the initial injury that became progressively worse. In particular, he reports pain and weakness during activity. Explain the observation component in the ongoing assessment of the basketball player.

In the examination room, the patient should wear shorts to allow full view of the lower extremity. This may not be possible during an on-field or on-site examination, however, because protective equipment or the uniform may obstruct the view. In these cases, determination of the condition may rest more heavily on palpation and stress tests. If the patient is nonambulatory, it is important to complete all observations, inspection, and palpation for possible fractures and dislocations before moving the patient.

In general, for non-acute, non–on-field/sideline evaluations, observation should include a full postural assessment and gait analysis. The patient should be viewed from anterior, lateral, and posterior positions. Although not necessary for the evaluation of our basketball player and his specific complaint, the position of the ilium relative to the SI joint should be noted in patients complaining

See **Application Strategy: Postural Assessment of the Hip Region**, found on the companion Web site at thePoint, for specific areas on which to focus in this region.

of back, hip, or groin pain with no known mechanism (**Fig. 16.14**). If contranutation occurs at the SI joint, it indicates anterior torsion of the joint or posterior rotation of the sacrum on the ilium on one side; the limb on that side probably is medially rotated. **Contranutation** occurs when, on one side, the ASIS is lower and the PSIS is higher. As a result, the iliac bones move apart, and the ischial tuberosities approximate. Contranutation is limited by the posterior SI ligaments; nutation is the backward rotation of the ilium on the sacrum. **Nutation** occurs when a person assumes a pelvic tilt position; contranutation occurs

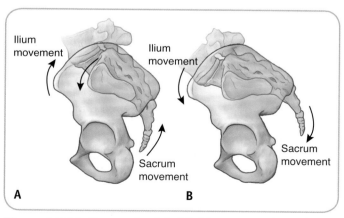

Figure 16.14. Abnormal pelvic tilt. Movements of nutation **(A)** and contranutation **(B)** occurring at the SI joint.

when a person assumes a lordotic or anterior pelvic tilt position. If nutation occurs on only one side, the ASIS is higher and the PSIS is lower on that side. The iliac innominate bones move together, and the ischial tuberosities move apart, resulting in an apparent or functional short leg on the same side. Nutation is limited by the anterior SI ligaments, the sacrospinous ligament, and the sacrotuberous ligament.

The symmetry in the region should be observed, noting any visible congenital deformity, such as excessive femoral torsion, abnormal positioning of the patella, toeing in, or toeing out. An increase in the angle of torsion greater than 15° (i.e., **anteversion**) is evidence of external femoral rotation characterized by a toe-out gait. When the angle is decreased (i.e., **retroversion**), the femur internally rotates, causing a toe-in position of the feet. An increase in the angle of inclination (i.e., coxa valga) may be visible through either **genu varum** or laterally positioned patellae. Decreases in this angle (i.e., coxa vara) may be visible with **genu valgum** or medially positioned, "squinting" patellae.

Following the completion of a static examination, the clinician should observe the patient walking. Gait should be observed, when possible, for six to eight full strides from an anterior, posterior, and lateral view, noting any abnormalities in stride length, internal or external rotation of the foot, pelvic rotation, and stance phase to determine if any actions cause pain or discomfort. With an abnormal gait, it is important to determine the onset of the limp, if the limp is constant or intermittent, and the activities that make the condition better or worse. For example, varying degrees of abductor lurch (also known as **Trendelenburg gait**) may be present as the patient attempts to place the center of gravity over the hip, reducing the forces on the joint. A short-leg limp may imply either iliotibial-band pathology or true or false leg length discrepancies.

 See **Application Strategy: Developing a History of the Injury**, available on the companion Web site at thePoint, for specific questions related to the pelvis, hip, and thigh region.

The specific site of injury should be inspected for obvious deformities, discoloration, edema, scars that might indicate previous surgery, and general condition of the skin. Snapping of the iliotibial band may be visually apparent as the tensor fasciae latae flips back and forth across the greater trochanter.

 Observation of the basketball player should include a full postural assessment and gait analysis. The specific site of injury should be inspected for obvious deformities, discoloration, edema, scars that might indicate previous surgery, and general condition of the skin.

PALPATION

 Observation of the basketball player reveals a swollen thigh (i.e., 3 cm larger than the uninvolved thigh). Explain palpation specific to the injury sustained by the basketball player.

Palpation of the hip and pelvis should begin with a systematic palpation of the lumbar spine prior to moving to the pelvic region. Bilateral palpation can determine temperature, swelling, point tenderness, crepitus, deformity, muscle spasm, and cutaneous sensation. Vascular pulses can be taken at the femoral artery in the groin, popliteal artery in the posterior knee, and posterior tibial artery and dorsalis pedis artery in the foot.

Pain during palpation of bony structures may indicate a displaced avulsion fracture or a femoral shaft fracture. Compression, distraction, percussion, or use of a tuning fork on specific bony landmarks also may be used to determine a possible fracture.

During palpation, the patient should be non–weight-bearing, preferably on a table. When the patient is prone on the table, a pillow should be placed under the hip and abdominal area to reduce strain on the low back region. Palpation should proceed proximal to distal, but the area anticipated to be the most painful should be palpated last. The following structures should be palpated.

Anterior Palpation

1. ASIS, AIIS, rectus femoris, and sartorius

2. Inguinal ligament, lymph nodes, pubic symphysis

3. Femoral triangle, femoral artery, iliopsoas bursa, and flexor and adductor muscles (i.e., pectineus, adductor brevis, adductor longus, adductor magnus, and gracilis)

4. Quadriceps muscles (i.e., vastus lateralis, rectus femoris, vastus medialis, and vastus intermedius)

Medial Palpation

1. Gracilis

2. Adductor longus, magnus, and brevis

Lateral Palpations

1. Iliac crest

2. Greater trochanter, trochanteric bursa (bursitis usually presents with pain in the posterior aspect of the greater trochanter)

3. Gluteus medius and gluteus minimus

4. Iliotibial band

5. Tensor fasciae latae

Posterior Palpation

1. Iliac crest and PSIS

2. Ischial tuberosity, ischial bursa, hamstring muscles (i.e., biceps femoris is lateral, and semitendinosus and semimembranosus are medial)

3. SI, lumbosacral, and sacrococcygeal joints

4. Median sacral crests

 Bilateral palpation should include point tenderness, swelling, muscle spasms, deformity, hardness or a firm mass, and skin temperature.

PHYSICAL EXAMINATION TESTS

? Palpation of the basketball player revealed a warm, firm, swollen thigh. A palpable mass was not detected. What physical examination findings would suggest that the patient has myositis ossificans?

The patient should be placed in a comfortable position for the physical examination. Depending on the history, some tests are compulsory, whereas others may be used to confirm or exclude suspected injury or pathology. Information collected during the history, inspection, and palpation phase of the examination process should always drive the decision regarding which clinical tests are needed. Caution should be used while moving through the assessment; bilateral comparison should always be performed.

Functional Tests

The clinician should determine the available ROM in hip flexion–extension, hip abduction–adduction, hip internal-external rotation, and knee flexion–extension. Bilateral comparison is critical to determine normal or abnormal movement.

Active Movements

Active movements can be performed in a seated or prone position. Active movements that are anticipated to be painful should be performed last to prevent painful symptoms from overflowing into the next movement.

The motions that should be assessed, and the normal ROM for each, are as follows:

- Knee extension (0° to 15°)

- Lateral rotation (40° to 60°)

- Medial rotation (30° to 40°)

- Hip flexion (110° to 120°) with knee flexed

- Abduction (30° to 50°)

- Adduction (30°)

- Knee flexion (0° to 135°)

- Hip extension (10° to 15°)

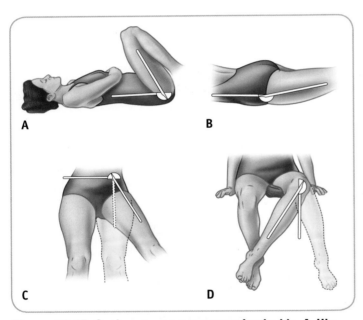

Figure 16.15. Goniometry measurements for the hip. A, Hip flexion. Center the fulcrum over the greater trochanter of the femur. Align the proximal arm with the lateral margin of the pelvis and then align the distal arm along the lateral midline of the femur, using the lateral epicondyle as reference. **B, Hip extension.** Alignment is the same as for measuring hip flexion, except that the patient is prone. **C, Hip abduction and adduction.** Center the fulcrum over the ASIS of the extremity being measured. Align the proximal arm along an imaginary horizontal line extending to the other ASIS and then align the distal arm along the middle of the femur, using the midline of the patella for reference. **D, Hip medial and lateral rotation.** Center the fulcrum over the anterior aspect of the patella. Align the proximal arm perpendicular to the floor and then align the distal arm, using the crest of the tibia and a point midway between the two malleoli for reference.

Loss of internal rotation suggests arthritis, effusion, a slipped capital femoral epiphysis, or muscle contractures. Excessive internal rotation with decreased external rotation suggests increased femoral anteversion. Significant side-to-side differences in rotational measurements, whether or not in the normal range, can suggest hip pathology.[13] Measuring ROM at the hip with a goniometer is demonstrated in **Figure 16.15**.

Passive Range of Motion

If the patient is able to perform full ROM during active movements, gentle pressure is applied at the extremes of motion to determine end feel. The end feel for hip flexion and adduction is tissue approximation; the end feel for hip extension, abduction, and medial and lateral rotation is tissue stretch. When testing passive movement, the aim is to reproduce the patient's symptoms, not just pain or discomfort.

Resisted Range of Motion

The hip must be stabilized and resisted muscle testing performed throughout the full ROM to eliminate recruitment of additional muscles other than the group being assessed. The assessment begins with the muscle on stretch, and resistance is applied throughout the full ROM. The clinician should note any muscle weakness when compared with the uninvolved limb. Potentially painful motions should be delayed until last. **Figure 16.16** demonstrates the motions that should be tested.

Manual Muscle Testing

If pain or weakness is found during resisted ROM, the clinician may decide to perform a manual muscle test to determine which muscle is damaged. When performing manual muscle testing, class I and II muscles should be tested at end range with maximal shortening of the

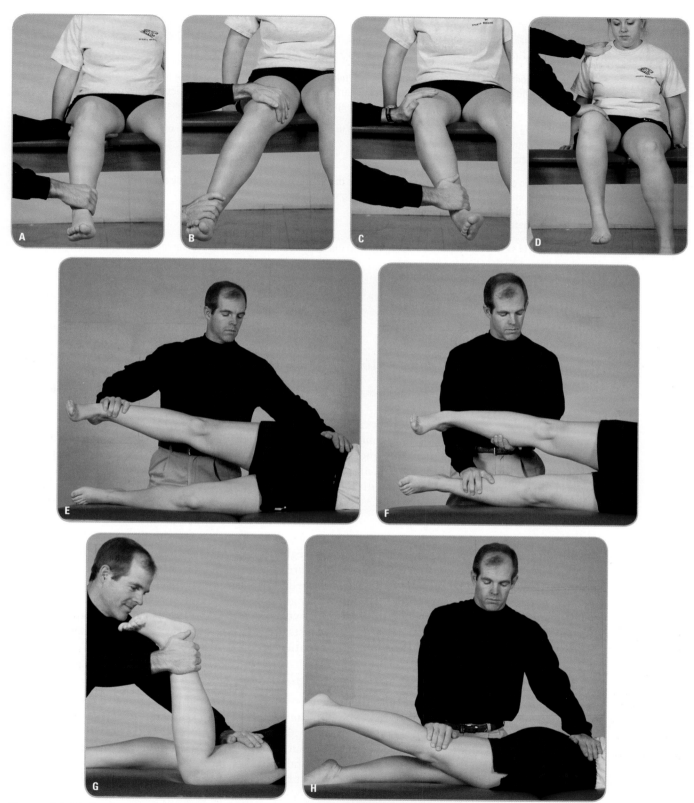

Figure 16.16. Resisted range of motion testing. A, Knee extension (L3). **B,** Internal hip rotation. **C,** External hip rotation. **D,** Hip flexion (L2). **E,** Hip abduction. **F,** Hip adduction. **G,** Knee flexion (S2). **H,** Hip extension (S1).

TABLE 16.2 Manual Muscle Testing of Lower Leg and Ankle Muscles

MUSCLE	JOINT POSITIONING	APPLY PRESSURE
Sartorius	Patient is supine with hip in lateral rotation, abducted, and flexed. Knee is also flexed.	While the patient attempts to move the foot of the affected leg from the starting position into a figure-four position, the clinician should attempt to apply resistance in opposition of this movement.
Tensor fasciae latae	The patient is supine, knee fully extended with hip slightly abducted, slightly flexed, and slightly medially rotated.	To the distal lateral leg in the direction of hip extension and adduction
Gluteus minimus	The patient is side lying on uninvolved leg. Involved hip should be abducted midway between neutral and fully abducted with no hip flexion, extension, or rotation occurring.	To the lateral aspect of the leg in the direction of adduction and very slight extension
Gluteus medius	The patient is side lying on uninvolved leg which should be flexed at the knee and hip. The pelvis should be rotated forward slightly with involved hip abducted in slight extension and slight external rotation.	To the distal lateral aspect of the lower leg, in the direction of adduction and slight flexion
Gluteus maximus	The patient is prone with knee flexed to at least 90° with hip extended.	To the posterior aspect of the thigh in the direction of thigh flexion

Adapted from Kendall FP, McCreary EK, Provance PG, et al. *Muscles: Testing and Function with Posture and Pain.* 5th ed. Baltimore, MD: Lippincott Williams & Wilkins; 2005.

muscle.[14] One-joint muscles that concentrically contract through the ROM are considered class I muscles. Class I muscles are short and strong. In contrast, class II muscles are two-joint and multijoint muscles that actively shorten all joints crossed and are also strong at the end range. Several class I and II muscles are involved with hip motion. See **Table 16.2** for MMT positioning.

Stress Tests

When using stress tests, only those tests that are absolutely necessary should be performed. While moving through the tests, the clinician should begin by applying gentle stress. The force should be applied several times with increasing overpressure. The presence of pain or joint laxity should be noted. The purposes of the first five tests described are to assess the patient for possible SI dysfunction. The tests are SI distraction (also known as gapping test), SI compression (also known as approximation test), thigh thrust, Patrick (also known as FABER), and Gaenslen (also known as pelvic torsion test).[15–17] If three or more of these five tests are found to be positive, there is strong evidence to indicate that the SI joint is the source of the patient's pain.[15–17]

Sacroiliac Distraction and Compression Test

To perform the **SI distraction test**, the patient is supine and the clinician applies a cross-arm pressure downward and outward to the ASIS with the thumbs (**Fig. 16.17**). Pain indicates a positive test. The SI distraction test has moderate sensitivity (.60) and strong specificity (.81).[18] To perform the *SI compression test, the patient is side lying.* Pressure is applied down through the anterior portion of the ilium, spreading the SI joint (**Fig. 16.18**). Unilateral gluteal or posterior leg pain may indicate a sprain to the anterior SI ligaments. The SI compression test has moderate sensitivity (.69) and specificity (.69).[18]

Patrick (FABER) Test

In a supine position, the foot and ankle of the involved leg are rested on the contralateral knee. Then, the flexed leg is slowly lowered into abduction (**Fig. 16.19**). The final position of **F**lexion, **AB**duction, and External **R**otation (FABER) at the hip should place the involved leg on the table, or at least near

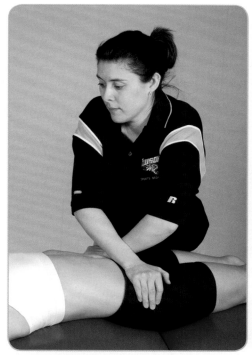

Figure 16.17. Sacroiliac distraction test. With the patient supine, the clinician uses a cross-arm maneuver and places the heel of each hand on the medial aspect of the patient's iliac crest bilaterally. Pressure is applied outward and downward, causing the anterior aspect of the SI joint to gap. Unilateral pain or posterior leg pain may indicate sprain to the anterior SI ligament.

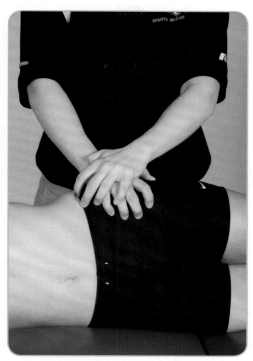

Figure 16.18. Sacroiliac compression test. With the patient side lying, the clinician applies a downward pressure over the iliac crest. Increased pain or feeling of pressure over the SI joints indicates possible sprain of the SI ligaments.

a horizontal position with the opposite leg. Overpressure on the knee of the involved leg and the contralateral iliac crest may produce pain in the SI joint on the side of the involved leg, denoting possible pathology. The Patrick test has moderate sensitivity (60) and poor specificity (29).[19]

Gaenslen Test

Gaenslen test is used to place a rotary stress on the SI joint by forcing one hip into hyperextension.[15-17] Several different ways to perform the Gaenslen test are described within the literature. The description provided within this test appears most frequently.[15-17] The patient is supine with the sacrum on the edge of the table. Next, the far leg (or one supported on table) is drawn onto the chest, while the near leg is allowed to hang off the side of the table. The clinician stabilizes the patient with one hand on the far ASIS and the one hand gently pushes the near leg into further extension (**Fig. 16.20**). The other leg is tested in a similar fashion for comparison. A positive test is indicated when the patient experiences pain in the SI joints. Gaenslen test is reported to have moderate (53) sensitivity and moderate to strong (71) specificity.[18]

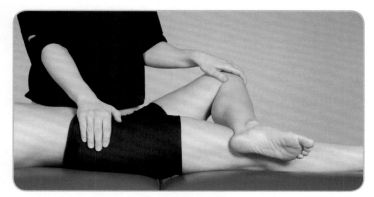

Figure 16.19. Patrick (FABER) test. Also called the figure-four test, the foot and ankle of the involved leg are rested on the contralateral knee. Overpressure on the knee of the involved leg and the contralateral iliac crest may produce pain in the SI joint on the side of the involved leg, indicating pathology.

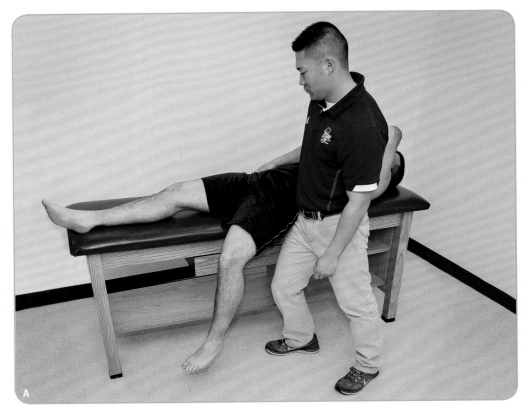

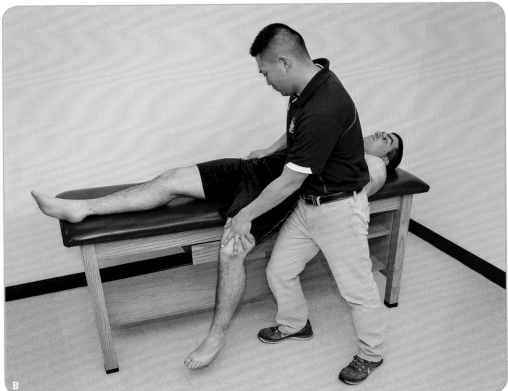

Figure 16.20. Gaenslen test. A, The patient is positioned so that the involved hip extends beyond the edge of the table. **B,** The clinician applies a downward force to the lower leg (symptomatic side) putting it into hyperextension at the hip while the other hand stabilizes the opposite iliac crest.

Thigh Thrust

The patient is supine with the knee and hip of the involved side both flexed to 90°, taking care not to adduct the hip (**Fig. 16.21**).[15,17] The clinician stabilizes the SI joint by placing one hand along the sacrum. With the opposing hand, the clinician applies a downward force through the femur of the affected limp and to the SI joint. The test is positive if pain is elicited within the SI joint. The thigh thrust has the highest (88) reported sensitivity of all SI joint dysfunction test with moderate (69) specificity.[17]

Leg Length Measurement

Nutation of the ilium on the sacrum results in decreased leg length, as does contranutation on the opposite side. If the iliac bone on one side is lower, the leg on that side usually is longer. Anatomical discrepancy, or true leg length, is measured in a supine position with the ASIS square, level, and balanced. The legs should be parallel to each other, with the heels approximately 6 to 8 in apart.

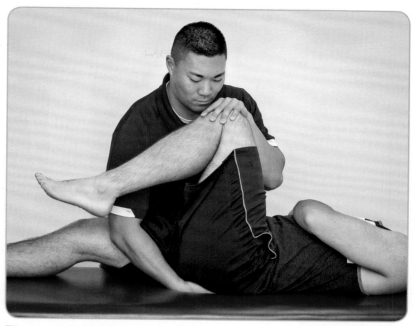

Figure 16.21. Thigh thrust test. This test is positive for SI joint dysfunction if pain is produced.

Using a flexible tape measure, the distance from the distal edge of the ASIS to the distal aspect of the medial malleolus of each ankle is measured (**Fig. 16.22A**). The measurement is repeated on the other side, and the results are then compared. A difference of 1.0 to 1.3 cm (0.5 to 1.0 in) is considered to be normal.

Apparent leg length discrepancies as a result of lateral pelvic tilt or flexion or adduction contractures are measured from the umbilicus to the medial malleolus of each ankle (**Fig. 16.22B**). The test is meaningful only if the result for true leg length discrepancy is negative.

Supine to Long Sit (Long Sitting Test)

Leg length discrepancies may also be associated with unilateral innominate rotations. The patient begins in a fully supine position (**Fig. 16.23A**) and is then instructed to perform two to three bridges (**Fig. 16.23B**) to release any muscle contractures that may influence the test. The clinician grasps the patient's ankles and passively moves the knees into full extension. Next, the clinician assesses leg length by examining alignment of the malleoli to one another (**Fig. 16.23C**). The patient is then instructed to sit up,

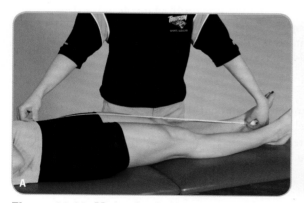
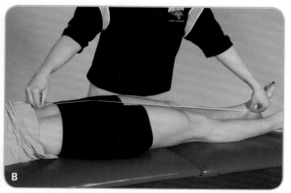

Figure 16.22. Measuring leg length. A, In measuring leg length, the pelvis should be square, level, and balanced. For anatomical discrepancy, or true leg length, the measure is from the ASIS to the distal aspect of the medial malleolus of each ankle. **B,** For apparent leg length discrepancies, the measure is from the umbilicus to the medial malleolus of each ankle.

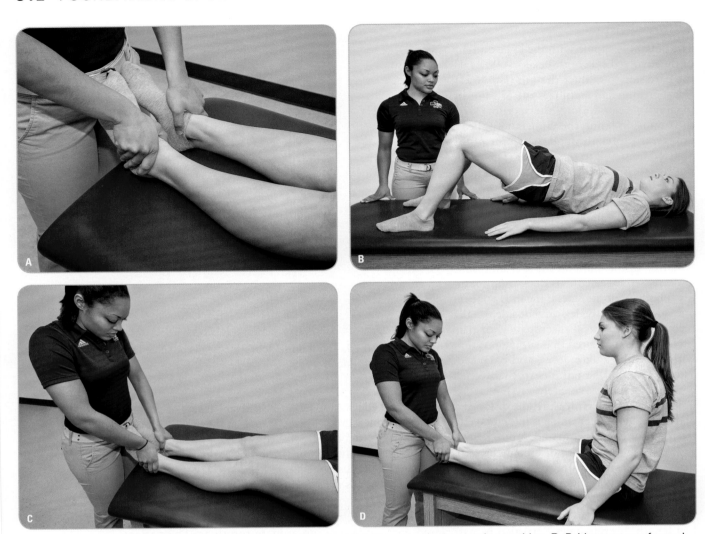

Figure 16.23. Supine to long sit (long sitting test). A, Patient is fully supine in the starting position. **B,** Bridges are performed to loosen muscle restrictions. **C,** The clinician passively extends the legs and measures leg length using malleoli alignment. **D,** Lengthening or shortening of a leg when compared to the nonmoving leg suggests innominate rotation.

if possible, without pushing on the table with hands for assistance. While the patient is moving from a supine to long sit position, the clinician is focused on watching how both malleoli move (**Fig. 16.23D**). If one leg appears to shorten in comparison to the opposite leg, the innominate on the side that moved is anteriorly rotated. If the leg appears to lengthen in comparison to the opposite leg, the innominate is posteriorly rotated. The supine to sit test has low (44) sensitivity with moderate (64) specificity.[18]

Ely Test

This test assesses the presence of a tight rectus femoris. The patient is prone. The clinician stabilizes the patient by placing one hand on the lower back. Grasping the ankle, the clinician slowly moves the knee into flexion. If the hip of the limb being tested moves into flexion and lifts off the table, the test is positive and implies tight rectus femoris (**Fig. 16.24**).

Thomas Test for Flexion Contractures

The Thomas test and Kendall test have long been confused. The Thomas test looks specifically for flexion contractions, whereas the Kendall test is utilized to identify which specific muscle is shortened. In essence, Kendall is a modification of the Thomas test, and thus, both are often referred to as the Thomas test or the Thomas-Kendall test.[14,19]

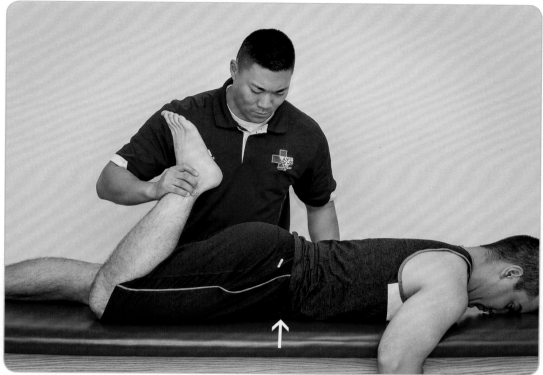

Figure 16.24. Ely test. The test is positive if the hip of the limb being tested moves into flexion and lifts off the table.

To perform the Thomas test, the patient is lying supine on a table. The clinician should note the presence of lumbar lordosis. If contractures are present, the clinician may be able to slip one's hand under the low back. Next, the patient is instructed to flex the uninvolved leg to the chest until the lordosis flattens. Moving the hip into further flexion will cause the pelvis to rotate and result in a false positive.[14] Once in position, the patient is instructed to hold that position while the clinician examines the opposite leg. If the test is negative, the straight leg (i.e., the involved leg) remains in contact with the table; if the test is positive, the straight leg rises off the table (**Fig. 16.25**). The Thomas test has yet to be validated.[18]

Kendall Test for Rectus Femoris Contracture

The patient lies supine on the table, with both knees flexed at 90° over the edge of the end of table. The patient flexes the unaffected knee to the chest to the point that the lordosis flattens and holds the leg in that position. Similar to the Thomas test, pulling the knee all the way to the chest will cause a posterior rotation of the pelvis, resulting in a false positive.[14] The other knee should remain flexed at 90°. If the knee slightly extends, a contracture in the rectus femoris may be present in that leg (**Fig. 16.26**). If the results are positive, the muscle is palpated for tightness to confirm the contracture. With no palpable tightness, the condition may be caused by tight joint structures (i.e., capsular or ligamentous). If the hip abducts during the test, it may result from iliotibial band tightness. Then, Ober test should be performed bilaterally.

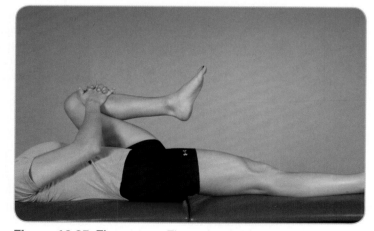

Figure 16.25. Thomas test. The patient is instructed to flex the uninvolved leg to the chest and hold it. A positive test occurs when the extended leg moves up off the table, indicating hip flexion contractures.

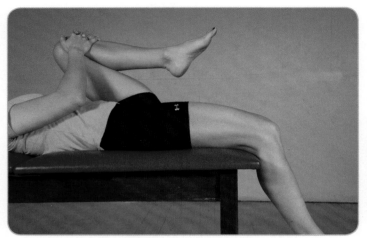

Figure 16.26. Kendall test. The Kendall test is similar to the Thomas test and can be considered a modification of the Thomas test. In the Kendall test, the patient lies supine, with both knees flexed over the edge end of the table. The uninvolved leg is flexed to the chest and held. A positive test occurs when the leg flexed over the end of the table extends beyond 90° and suggests rectus femoris shortening. If the extended leg is able to flex to 90° or more but the thigh remains off the table, the test is positive for iliopsoas tightness.

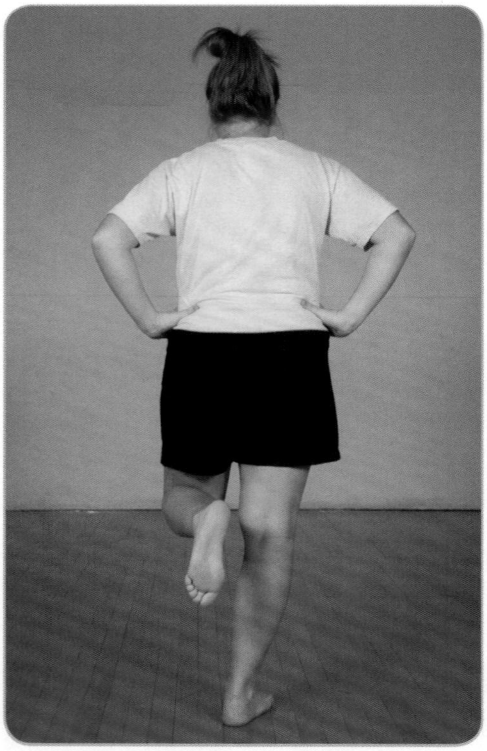

Figure 16.27. Trendelenburg test. This patient is demonstrating a negative test. A positive test is indicated by an inability to maintain equal PSIS levels due to a weak gluteus medius.

Ober Test

The patient is side lying, with the lower leg flexed at 90° at the hip and knee for stability. The patient may feel more secure if allowed to place one hand under his or her head and grasp the edge of the table with the opposite hand. The clinician stabilizes the pelvis with one hand to prevent the pelvis from shifting posteriorly during the test. Preventing the pelvis from rotating during the test is the key to successfully performing the test. Next, the clinician grasps the upper leg on the medial aspect of the flexed knee and abducts and slightly extends the hip so that the iliotibial tract passes over the greater trochanter (see **Fig. 15.21B**). Next, the clinician slowly lowers the upper leg. If the tensor fasciae latae, or iliotibial band, is tight, the leg remains in the abducted position. Although the original Ober test called for the knee to be flexed at 90°, the iliotibial tract has a greater stretch if the knee is extended. If the knee is flexed during the test, greater stress is placed on the femoral nerve, which may result in neurological signs (i.e., pain, tingling, or paresthesia). Therefore, having the knee in slight flexion appears to work best. No information regarding the diagnostic accuracy of this test has been reported.[20]

Hamstring Contracture Test

The **straight-leg raising test for hamstring shortness** is performed with the patient supine, legs extended and back and sacrum flat on table if possible. The clinician then passively flexes the hip with the leg in full extension and ankle relaxed.[14] If the patient can flex the hip to at least 90° and extend the knee to within 20° of full extension, the patient is said to have normal flexibility and does not indicate presence of hamstring shortening.[14,19]

Trendelenburg Test

The Trendelenburg test is used to assess for gluteus medius weakness. The patient is asked to balance on one leg while flexing the knee of the non–weight-bearing leg (**Fig. 16.27**). While the patient is balancing, the level of the pelvis is noted. If the pelvis on the side of the non–weight-bearing leg falls, the test is considered to be positive, indicating weakness or instability of the gluteus medius on the stance side. The Trendelenburg sign is both somewhat sensitive (73) and specific (77).[18]

Piriformis Test

The piriformis test is used to assess the piriformis muscle for tightness. Although many descriptions for performing this test are found, the description provided here appears most frequently in the literature.[18,21] The patient is in a side-lying position resting on the uninvolved leg. The involved hip is flexed at 60° with the knee flexed. The clinician stabilizes the involved hip with one hand and applies a downward pressure to the knee (**Fig. 16.28**). If the piriformis muscle is tight, pain will be elicited in the muscle. If the sciatic nerve is compressed by the piriformis muscle, the patient may experience sciatic-like symptoms. Resisted lateral rotation with the muscle on stretch (i.e., with the hip medially rotated) also may cause the same sciatica. This test is highly specific (83) and sensitive (88).[18]

Hip Scour Test

The hip scour test is used to identify the possible presence of osteoarthritis or damage to the articular cartilage within the hip. Sensitivity for this test has been reported as ranging from 50 to 91 with specificity scores of 29 to 75.[18,19] The patient is placed in a supine position. The clinician then fully flexes the patient's knee while simultaneously applying an axial load through the knee, into the hip joint. Combining axial loading with internal and external hip rotation and moving the hip into various degrees of flexion, the clinician attempts to "scour" the joint with the femoral head. The test is positive if the patient experiences pain, apprehension, or reproduction of symptoms.

Neurological Tests

Neurological integrity is assessed with the use of myotomes, reflexes, and cutaneous patterns, including segmental dermatomes and peripheral nerve patterns.

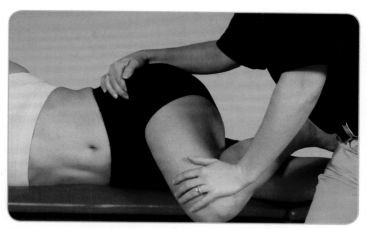

Figure 16.28. Piriformis test. The patient lies on the uninvolved side. The involved hip is flexed at 60°, and the knee is flexed. The clinician stabilizes the hip with one hand and applies a downward pressure to the knee. Pain over the piriformis muscle indicates a positive test.

Myotomes

Isometric muscle testing in the loose-packed position should be performed in the following motions to test specific segmental myotomes:

- Hip flexion (L1, L2)

- Knee extension (L3)

- Ankle dorsiflexion (L4)

- Toe extension (L5)

- Ankle plantar flexion, foot eversion, or hip extension (S1)

- Knee flexion (S2)

Reflexes

The pelvic or hip area has no specific reflexes to test. Other reflexes in the lower extremity include the patella (L3, L4) and Achilles tendon reflexes (S1).

Cutaneous Patterns

The segmental nerve dermatome patterns for the pelvis, hip, and thigh are demonstrated in **Figure 16.29**. The peripheral nerve cutaneous patterns are demonstrated in **Figure 16.30**.

Activity-Specific Functional Tests

Functional tests should be performed before clearing any patient to return to activity. The patient should be able to perform activities pain-free, with no limp or antalgic gait. Examples of functional activities include walking, going up and down stairs, jogging, squatting, jumping, running straight ahead, running sideways, and changing directions while running.

 Physical examination findings that would suggest that the basketball player has myositis ossificans include passive knee flexion limited to 20° to 30° and inability to perform active quadriceps contractions and straight leg raises.

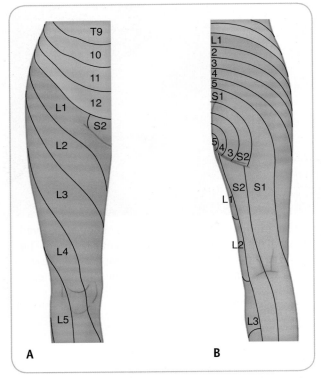

Figure 16.29. **Segmental nerve dermatome patterns for the pelvis, hip, and thigh. A**, Anterior view. **B**, Posterior view.

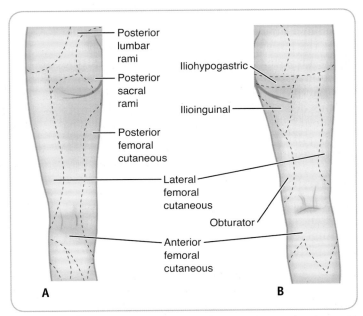

Figure 16.30. **Peripheral nerve cutaneous patterns for the pelvis, hip, and thigh. A**, Anterior view. **B**, Posterior view.

CONTUSIONS

 A volleyball athlete was digging for a ball and fell directly on her left hip. She experienced immediate severe pain and extreme tenderness over the iliac crest. What painful movements would confirm a suspected hip pointer?

Direct impact to soft tissue, such as a blow to the thigh or a fall onto a hard surface, causes a compressive force to crush soft tissue. Many factors affect the type and severity of injury sustained. The condition may be mild and resolve on its own in a matter of days, or the bleeding and swelling may be more extensive, resulting in a large, deep hematoma that takes months to resolve. Contusions may occur anywhere in the hip region but typically are seen on the crest of the ilium or in the quadriceps muscle group as was the case with the patient in the previous scenario who eventually developed myositis ossificans.

Hip Pointer

Etiology

A **hip pointer** generally refers to a contusion of the iliac crest over the tensor fasciae latae muscle belly with an associated hematoma, but the term also may be used to identify tearing of the external oblique muscle from the iliac crest, periostitis of the crest, and trochanteric contusions. Most injuries are sustained when a direct blow impacts the iliac crest.

Signs and Symptoms

Deep, rapid bleeding and swelling can be subperiosteal, intramuscular, or subcutaneous. Because so many trunk and abdominal muscles attach to the iliac crest, any movement of the trunk, including

TABLE 16.3 Signs and Symptoms of Hip Pointers	
INJURY	**SIGNS AND SYMPTOMS**
Grade I	Normal gait and normal posture Slight pain on palpation Little or no swelling present Full trunk range of motion Return to activity may take 3–7 days
Grade II	Abnormal gait pattern Posture may be slightly flexed toward the side of injury. Noticeable pain on palpation of iliac crest, with visible swelling Active trunk ROM is painful and limited, especially lateral flexion to the opposite side and trunk rotation. Return to activity may take 5–14 days.
Grade III	Severe pain, swelling, and ecchymosis Gait is slow, with short stride length and swing through. Posture may have severe tilt to injured side. Trunk range of motion is painful and limited in all directions. Return to activity may take 14–21 days.

coughing, laughing, and even breathing, is painful. Immediate pain, discoloration, spasm, and loss of function prevent the patient from rotating the trunk or laterally flexing the trunk toward the injured side. Extreme tenderness is present over the iliac crest, and abdominal muscle spasm may be present. Within 24 to 48 hours, the swelling is more diffuse, and ecchymosis is evident. In severe injury, the patient may be unable to walk or bear weight, even with crutches, because of the intense pain caused by muscular tension at the injury site. **Table 16.3** lists the signs and symptoms of the various grades of hip pointers.

Management

Treatment involves ice, compression, and total rest during the first 2 to 3 days following injury. Mild stretching and electrical stimulation to the muscles during icing may reduce secondary muscle spasm. If intense pain is palpated directly over the iliac crest, the patient should be referred to a physician to rule out a fracture of the iliac crest, because the same mechanism of injury may cause both injuries.

In an uncomplicated hip pointer, the patient can return to activity in 3 to 7 days. To prevent reinjury, however, the area should be protected with a pad.

In a grade II or III injury, crutches should be used for ambulation. Analgesic medications for pain and nonsteroidal anti-inflammatory drugs (NSAIDs) are indicated after 48 hours. Later treatment may include heat therapy, ultrasound, transcutaneous electrical nerve stimulation (TENS), and pain-free ROM exercises as tolerated. As soon as pain-free active ROM exercise can be accomplished, the patient should progress to resistive exercise, including lower extremity and trunk strengthening. Return to activity should be gradual, with the patient possibly wearing a dense foam donut pad fitted into a custom-formed plastic shell or a compression garment to protect the area from further injury.

Quadriceps Contusion
Etiology

The most common site for a quadriceps contusion is the anterolateral thigh. If the contusion is located adjacent to the intermuscular septum, pain and hemorrhage tend to resolve more rapidly. Contusions within the muscle itself often are associated with greater tearing, hemorrhage, and pain and with a greater tendency toward abnormal pathology. Severity of the injury is almost always underestimated, leading to undertreatment.

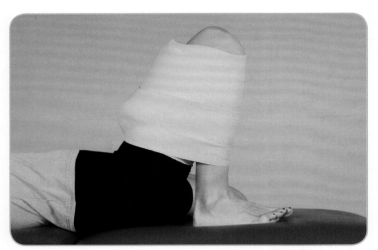

Figure 16.31. Management of a quadriceps contusion. Ice should be applied, with the knee in maximal flexion to place the muscles on stretch.

Signs and Symptoms

Pain and swelling may be extensive immediately after impact. In a mild (grade I) contusion, the patient has mild pain and swelling and is able to walk without a limp. Passive flexion beyond 90° may be painful, but resisted knee extension may cause less discomfort. In a moderate (grade II) contusion, the patient can flex the knee between 45° and 90° and walks with a noticeable limp. Swelling prevents the knee from being fully flexed. In a severe (grade III) contusion, little evidence of bruising is seen initially, but within 24 hours, progressive bleeding and swelling occur, preventing knee flexion beyond 45°. There may be a palpable, firm hematoma, resulting in an inability to contract the quadriceps or do a straight leg raise. The patient will require crutches for ambulation.

Management

For the first 24 to 48 hours, treatment involves application of ice and a compressive wrap applied with the knee in maximal flexion (**Fig. 16.31**). This position preserves the needed flexion and limits intramuscular bleeding and spasm. After 48 hours, reevaluation may necessitate continuation of the ice, compression, and flexion for another 12 to 24 hours. Continued swelling despite proper acute care protocol indicates continued hemorrhage. In these cases, immediate referral to a physician is necessary to assess the level of bleeding.

The patient should begin gentle passive and active, pain-free stretching with daily ice treatments and use of NSAIDs. If unable to perform a pain-free gait, the patient should be placed on crutches (non–weight-bearing) for 48 hours; as motion capability improves, partial weight bearing should be initiated. Proprioceptive neuromuscular facilitation exercise patterns may be used to strengthen, relax, or gain ROM. Isometric quadriceps strengthening and hamstrings resistive exercises can progress to an active stretching and progressive resistance strengthening program. Pulsed ultrasound or high-voltage galvanic stimulation may be helpful in the early stages to reduce edema. Continuous ultrasound, hydrotherapy, and massage should be avoided during the early stages, because they may irritate the inflammatory process but may be used during later stages to aid recovery.

When full ROM has been restored, full weight-bearing gait should be resumed; the progressive strengthening program can be expanded; and cycling, jogging, running, and functional activities specific to the sport can be incorporated. **Application Strategy 16.2** explains the care of a quadriceps contusion.

Myositis Ossificans

Etiology

Myositis ossificans is an abnormal ossification involving bone deposition within muscle tissue. It may stem from a single traumatic blow, or from repeated blows, to the quadriceps. Several risk factors following a quadriceps contusion can predispose a patient to this condition, including the following:

■ Innate predisposition to ectopic bone formation

■ Continuing to play after injury

■ Early massage, hydrotherapy, or thermotherapy during the acute stage

■ Passive, forceful stretching

APPLICATION STRATEGY 16.2

Management Algorithm for a Quadriceps Contusion

Acute Phase (First 24–48 Hours)

- Ice and compression with knee flexed at 120°
- Crutches with partial or no weight bearing
- Pain-free passive and active ROM
- NSAIDs after 24 hours

Subacute Phase (2–5 Days)

- Cryotherapy and passive stretching exercises
- NSAIDs
- Active ROM and pain-free resisted proprioceptive neuromuscular facilitation relaxation and strengthening exercises
- Continue partial weight bearing until 90° of flexion is attained
- High-voltage galvanic stimulation, hot packs, or hydromassage (when no swelling is present)
- Swimming with gentle kicking exercises

Final Phase

- Discontinue crutches (when no limp is present)
- Cycling, light jogging, or running as tolerated
- High-voltage galvanic stimulation
- Radiography at 3 weeks to rule out myositis ossificans

Return to Play

- ROM within 10° of that for the unaffected leg
- Bilaterally equal strength and endurance
- Work on jumping, starts, stops, changing directions, sprinting
- Must pass all functional tests
- Consider protective padding to prevent reinjury

- Too rapid a progression in the rehabilitation program

- Premature return to play

- Reinjury of same area

Common sites are the anterior and lateral thigh. Although the precise mechanism that triggers the bone formation has yet to be established, it is thought that during resolution of the hematoma, within a week after injury, the existing fibroblasts involved in the repair process begin to differentiate into osteoblasts. The evidence of calcification on a radiograph becomes visible after 2 to 4 weeks. As the calcification continues to progress, a palpable, firm mass can be felt in the deep tissues. After 6 to 7 weeks, the mass generally stops growing, and resorption occurs. Total resorption may not occur, however, leaving a visible, cortical-type bony lesion (**Fig. 16.32**).

Signs and Symptoms

Examination reveals a warm, firm, swollen thigh nearly 2 to 4 cm larger than the unaffected side. A palpable, painful mass may limit passive knee flexion to 20° to 30°. Active quadriceps contractions and straight leg raises may be impossible.

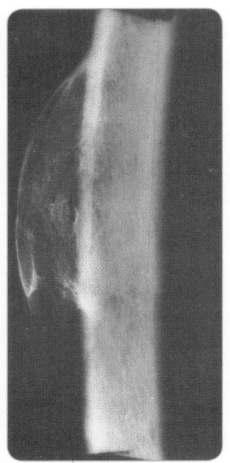

Figure 16.32. Myositis ossificans. In myositis ossificans, full resorption of the calcification may not occur, leaving a visible, cortical-type bony lesion.

Management

Immediate treatment includes ice, compression, elevation, crutches, and protected rest. The patient should be referred to a physician. NSAIDs are indicated only after 48 hours because they inhibit platelet function and promote hemorrhage. Once out of the acute phase and the area is no longer warm, ultrasound and light stretching may be implemented. If the condition does not respond to treatment, the patient should be referred back to the physician. Periodic radiographs generally are taken until the abnormal ossification matures, which typically occurs within 6 to 12 months. For cases in which the mass fails to reabsorb completely, many patients return safely to participation, using adequate protection to prevent injury from subsequent blows. Surgery is indicated only in cases where activity is limited by pain, weakness, and decreased ROM. Excision before the mass matures may result in reformation, with the new mass sometimes being larger than the original mass.

Acute Compartment Syndrome

Etiology

Compartment syndrome is defined as increased tissue pressure in a closed fascial compartment that compromises circulation to the nerves and muscles within that compartment. In the thigh, this condition can impact the anterior, posterior, or medial compartments. The condition often follows severe blunt trauma to the thigh but may also result from a crushing injury or fracture of the femur. Considered to be a true surgical emergency, it requires prompt clinical diagnosis and treatment.

Signs and Symptoms

The patient complains of a progressive, severe thigh pain that is often out of proportion to the injury. There will be severe swelling and induration of the involved compartment, increased thigh circumference, pain with passive stretch, weakness of the involved thigh muscles, or sensory or motor deficits in the distribution of the nerves contained in the involved compartment.[22]

- Anterior compartment
  - Pain increases during passive knee flexion with the hip extended.
  - Knee extension will be weak.
  - Sensory deficits occur in the lateral, intermediate, and medial thigh (femoral nerve cutaneous branches) and medial calf (saphenous nerve).
- Posterior compartment
  - Pain increases during passive knee extension with the hip in flexion.
  - Knee flexion, plantar flexion, and great toe extension will be weak.
  - Sensory deficits occur in the plantar foot (tibial branch), dorsal foot, and first web space (peroneal branch).
- Medial compartment
  - Pain increases during passive hip abduction with the knee extended.
  - Hip adduction will be weak.
  - Sensory deficits will occur in the proximal medial thigh (obturator nerve cutaneous branch).

Management

Ice should be applied to reduce swelling, and the patient should be immediately referred to a physician. Because motor function is difficult to assess in the presence of a large hematoma, diagnosis is based on measurements of compartment pressure as taken by a physician. Pressure readings of greater than 40 mm Hg usually indicate surgical intervention consisting of an incision, fasciotomy, and evacuation of the hematoma. Untreated compartment syndrome can lead to muscle necrosis, fibrosis, scarring, and limb contractures, whereas nerve injury can result from either a direct blow or compartment compression.[22,23]

> In the assessment of the volleyball player, the painful movements that would confirm a suspected hip pointer include active trunk motion, especially lateral flexion to the opposite side and trunk rotation. In addition, because so many trunk and abdominal muscles attach to the iliac crest, pain can be elicited from coughing, laughing, and even breathing.

BURSITIS

> A 36-year-old woman is complaining of pain while running. Pain is located on the posterolateral aspect of her hip near the greater trochanter and, occasionally, is accompanied by a snapping sensation. Further assessment suggests that the patient has snapping hip syndrome. Describe a rehabilitation program for this condition.

Bursitis is common in runners and joggers and typically affects the greater trochanteric bursa, iliopectineal (iliopsoas) bursa, and ischial bursa (**Fig. 16.7**). The most common mechanism is inflammation secondary to excessive friction or shear forces caused by overuse, but it may also be caused by direct trauma, such as falling on the lateral hip, arthritis, or regional muscle dysfunction.[24]

Greater Trochanteric Bursitis

Etiology

The greater trochanteric bursa lies between the greater trochanter and the gluteus maximus and tensor fasciae latae (iliotibial tract). Inflammation of this bursa is 4 times more common in women because of their wider pelvis and larger Q-angle.[25] It also is seen in runners who cross their feet over the midline as they run, thereby functionally increasing the Q-angle. Because streets are crowned to allow for runoff, patients who typically run on streets are at increased susceptibility for irritating the greater trochanteric bursa. The down leg (i.e., the leg closest to the gutter) usually is affected. Other factors that may increase the onset of greater trochanter pain syndrome include gluteus medius insertional dysfunction, hip osteoarthritis, lumbar spondylosis, excessive or rapidly increased mileage, frequent training on hard surfaces, poorly cushioned shoes, excessive pronation, leg length discrepancies, and iliotibial band syndrome.[25]

Signs and Symptoms

Trochanteric bursitis, or more recently called greater trochanter pain syndrome, is characterized by a burning or aching pain over or just posterior to the tip of the greater trochanter that intensifies with walking or exercises. The condition is aggravated by contraction of the hip abductors against resistance or during hip flexion and extension on weight bearing. Referred pain also may move distally into the lateral aspect of the thigh. If accompanied by a sudden, sharp pain that occurs during certain movements, it can be secondary to a snapping hip problem.

Iliopectineal Bursitis

Etiology

The iliopectineal (iliopsoas) bursa, which is the largest bursa in the body, lies under the iliopsoas muscle where it passes over the iliopectineal eminence in the pubis and inserts onto the lesser femoral trochanter. Repeated compression of the bursa against either the joint capsule of the hip or the lesser trochanter of the femur during sprinting or hill climbing may lead to several hip diseases, such as osteoarthritis, rheumatoid arthritis, and symptomatic iliopsoas syndrome.[26]

Signs and Symptoms

Pain is felt more medial and anterior to the joint and cannot be easily palpated. When the knee is supported to relax the muscles, point tenderness may be elicited with the hip and knee flexed and the leg externally rotated. Passive rotary motions at the hip and resisted hip flexion, abduction, and external rotation also may produce increased pain. Iliopectineal bursitis may be associated with symptoms of a **snapping hip syndrome** as well.

Ischial Bursitis

Etiology

Direct bruising from a fall can lead to compression of the ischial bursa. Often, however, the patient has a history of prolonged sitting, especially with the legs crossed or on a hard surface—commonly seen in rowing and crew. Although uncommon, it must be differentiated from a hamstring tear at the tendinous attachment or an epiphyseal fracture.

Signs and Symptoms

Pain is aggravated by prolonged sitting, uphill running, and even carrying a wallet in the back pocket. When the hip is flexed, point tenderness can be palpated directly over the ischial tuberosity. Pain increases with passive and resisted hip extension.

Management of Bursitis

Treatment for bursitis includes cryotherapy, deep friction massage, protected rest, NSAIDs, and a stretching program for the involved muscles. The use of ultrasound or interferential current also may be helpful. A postural examination and biomechanical analysis of the running motion performed by trained professionals can be used to determine if certain factors contributed to the patient's condition. Different shoes, orthotics, or alteration of the running technique may correct the problem and avoid recurrence. If the condition does not improve rapidly, a bone scan should be performed to rule out possible femoral neck stress fractures. Patients who do not respond to conservative treatment may require local injections with anesthetics and cortisone, or surgery may be necessary for a bursectomy, bony prominence resection, or tendon release.[25]

Snapping Hip Syndrome

Etiology

Chronic bursitis can lead to snapping hip syndrome, a benign condition very prevalent in dancers, runners, and cheerleaders that may develop secondary to a variety of both intra-articular and extra-articular causes (**Box 16.2**). The three types of the condition are as follows:

- **External.** The most prevalent and common cause is the movement of a thickened iliotibial band, tensor fasciae latae, or gluteus maximus tendon snapping over the greater trochanter during hip flexion, leading to trochanteric bursitis.

- **Internal.** The less common but more pronounced condition is caused by the iliopsoas tendon snapping over the anterior hip capsule, lesser trochanter, femoral head, or iliopectineal eminence.

- **Intra-articular.** Lesions of the joint, such as a labral tear, recurrent hip subluxation, osteochondral fractures, or intra-articular loose bodies, can lead to the condition.

Signs and Symptoms

Snapping hip syndrome is characterized by a snapping sensation, rather than pain, that is either heard or felt during certain motions at the hip. It usually occurs when a patient laterally rotates and flexes the hip joint while balancing on one leg. If the iliopsoas bursa is affected, the patient may complain of snapping, chronic pain, or both in the femoral triangle of the medial groin.

BOX 16.2 Causes of Snapping Hip Syndrome

Intra-articular Causes

- Osteocartilaginous nodules occurring in the synovial membrane of the joint (synovial chondromatosis)
- Loose bodies
- Osteocartilaginous exostosis
- Subluxation of the hip
- Negative pressure in the joint capsule

Extra-articular Causes

- Iliotibial band friction syndrome
- Snapping of the iliopsoas over the iliopectineal eminence on the medial aspect of the inferior ilium
- Snapping of the iliofemoral ligaments over the femoral head
- Snapping of the long head of the biceps femoris over the ischial tuberosity

---

Management

The condition usually is handled with limitation of hip motion, particularly limitation of extension by use of an elastic wrap. Ice and NSAIDs are used to relieve inflammation and pain. If associated with pain or a sense of hip joint instability, the patient should be referred to a physician. A rehabilitation program should address specific deficits, including stretching exercises for hip abduction and external rotation, muscle imbalance, poor training techniques, or poor biomechanics of movement.

> A rehabilitation program for the 36-year-old female diagnosed with snapping hip syndrome should address specific deficits: muscle tightness, muscle imbalance, poor training techniques, or poor biomechanics of movement.

SPRAINS AND DISLOCATIONS

> **?** A van transporting a collegiate swim team to a meet was involved in a multivehicle accident. The van was struck in the rear and forced into the vehicle in front of it. The assistant coach, sitting in the front seat on the passenger's side, was thrown into the dashboard of the vehicle. He is experiencing severe pain, and the hip is slightly flexed and internally rotated. Explain management for this condition.

Hip joint sprains are rare, both because of the multitude of movements allowed at the ball-and-socket joint and because of the level of protection provided by layers of muscles that add to its stability. Traumatic hip dislocations are rare with 85% to 90% of these in a posterior dislocation. This may largely result from the pliable cartilage composition of the acetabulum during the early- to mid-teen years. Associated injuries with a hip dislocation may include fractures of the femoral head, femoral neck, acetabulum, or a combination of these.[26]

Etiology

Injury can occur in violent, twisting actions or in catastrophic trauma when the knee strikes a stationary object (axial loading), such as during an automobile accident when the knee is driven into the dashboard. The impact of the knee with the hip in an adducted position leads to a posteriorly direct force, causing a posterior dislocation. In contrast, an anterior dislocation occurs when the hip is abducted and externally rotated.[26]

Signs and Symptoms

Symptoms of a mild or moderate hip joint sprain mimic those of synovitis, or stress fractures about the hip, and involve pain on hip rotation. Severe hip sprains and dislocations result in immediate intense pain and an inability to walk or even move the hip. The hip remains in a characteristic flexed and internally rotated position, indicating a posterosuperior dislocation (**Fig. 16.33**).

Management

Treatment for a mild to moderate sprain is symptomatic and may include cryotherapy, NSAIDs, rest, and protected weight bearing on crutches until walking is pain-free. Radiographs or bone scans usually are obtained to rule out degenerative joint disease, slipped femoral capital epiphysis, and femoral stress fractures.

 A hip dislocation is considered to be a medical emergency. As such, it requires activation of the emergency action plan, including summoning EMS.

In a hip dislocation, the patient should not be moved until emergency medical services (EMS) arrives. With a fracture to the posterior rim of the acetabulum or head of the femur, movement could damage the blood supply to the head of the femur and cause avascular necrosis or further damage to surrounding soft-tissue structures. The vital signs should be monitored frequently and the patient treated for shock. Because the sciatic nerve may be damaged, nerve function should be assessed by determining if the patient has full or partial sensation.

Management of the hip injury sustained by the assistant coach requires activation of the emergency action plan, including summoning EMS. While waiting for EMS to arrive, the clinician should maintain the airway, assess vital signs, check for nerve and circulatory impairment at the lower leg and ankle, and treat for shock as necessary. The patient should not be moved until EMS arrives.

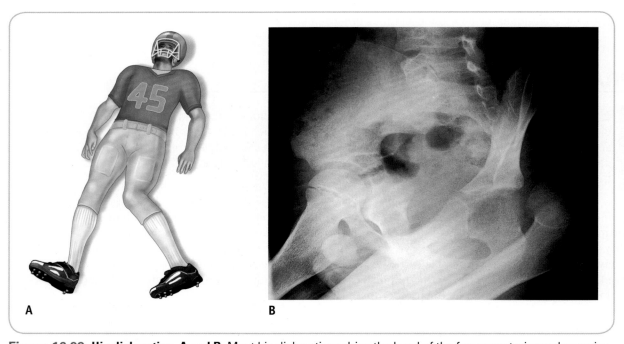

A

B

Figure 16.33. Hip dislocation. A and B, Most hip dislocations drive the head of the femur posterior and superior, leaving the leg in a characteristically flexed and internally rotated position.

STRAINS

 A first-base softball player stretches for an overthrown ball. During the stretch, the athlete feels a twinge in her left inner groin region. What painful movements would suggest an adductor strain?

Muscular strains of the hip and thigh muscles frequently are seen not only in sport but also in many occupations involving repetitive motions. Strains may range from mild to severe, with the severity of symptoms paralleling the amount of disruption to the fibers.

Quadriceps Strain

Etiology

Quadriceps strains are less common than hamstring strains. An explosive muscular contraction of the rectus femoris can lead to an avulsion fracture at the proximal attachment on the AIIS, but tears more commonly occur in the midsubstance of the muscle belly. Because the rectus femoris is the most superficial muscle of the quadriceps, any disruption in its continuity is easily visible. The vastus lateralis and vastus medialis are more rarely injured, but when an injury does occur, it usually involves the mid to upper third of the muscle belly.

Signs and Symptoms

In a grade I injury, the patient complains of tightness in the anterior thigh, but gait is normal. No swelling or pain can be palpated, although passive knee flexion beyond 90° may be painful. In a grade II injury, the patient reports a snapping or tearing sensation during an explosive jumping, kicking, or running motion, followed by immediate pain and loss of function. The knee may be held in extension as a means for protecting the injured area. Assessment reveals tenderness, swelling, a palpable defect if continuity is disrupted, discoloration, pain on passive knee flexion between 45° and 90°, and pain and weakness during resisted knee extension. Grade III strains are extremely painful, and ambulation is not possible. Palpation reveals an obvious defect in the muscle. Resisted knee extension is not possible, and ROM is severely limited. An isometric contraction may reveal a muscle bulge or defect in the quadriceps muscles, especially the rectus femoris of the thigh. **Box 16.3** lists the signs and symptoms of a quadriceps strain.

BOX 16.3 Signs and Symptoms of a Quadriceps Strain

- Snapping or tearing sensation at the AIIS or at midthigh during an explosive movement
- Increased pain or weakness elicited during the following:
  - Passive knee flexion
    - Grade I: 90° is painful
    - Grade II: Limited to 45°–90°
    - Grade III: Limited to <45°
  - Active knee extension with a flexed hip
  - Resisted knee extension
- Isolated rectus femoris strain produces increased pain and weakness during the following:
  - Passive knee flexion and hip extension
  - Active knee extension and hip flexion
  - Resisted hip flexion with the knee flexed at 45°

Hamstring Strains

Etiology

During the initial swing phase of gait, the hamstrings act to flex the knee. In the late swing, the hamstrings contract eccentrically to decelerate knee extension and reextend the hip in preparation for the stance phase. The hamstrings are the most frequently strained muscles in the body, and these strains typically are caused by either a rapid contraction of the muscle during a ballistic action or a violent stretch. Several factors can increase the risk of injury, including the following:

- Poor flexibility
- Poor posture
- Muscle imbalance
- Improper warm-up
- Muscle fatigue
- Lack of neuromuscular control
- Previous injury
- Overuse
- Improper technique

Signs and Symptoms

In mild strains, the patient complains of tightness and tension in the muscle. Passive stretching of the hamstrings may be painful. In second- and third-degree strains, the patient may report a tearing sensation or feeling a "pop," leading to immediate pain and weakness in knee flexion. In more severe cases, a sharp pain in the posterior thigh may occur during midstride. The patient limps and is unable to do a heel-strike or to fully extend the knee. Pain and muscle weakness are elicited during active knee flexion. If assessed early enough, a noticeable defect in the muscle belly may be palpated. Frequently, profuse swelling and ecchymosis become visible in the popliteal fossa 1 to 2 days after injury. Although rare, total rupture of the ischial origin can result from a sudden, forceful flexion of the hip joint when the knee is extended and the hamstring muscles contract powerfully. **Box 16.4** lists the signs and symptoms of a hamstring strain.

BOX 16.4 Signs and Symptoms of a Hamstring Strain

- History of poor posture, inflexibility, and muscle imbalance
- Injury often occurs when muscle function suddenly changes from a stabilizing knee flexor to an active hip extensor, as occurs in sprinting, and may occur midstride.
- Sharp pain in the posterior thigh
- Increased pain or weakness during the following:
  - Passive knee extension
  - Passive hip flexion
  - Active knee flexion
  - Active hip extension with an extended knee
  - Resisted knee flexion
    - Medial hamstrings—tibia internally rotated
    - Lateral hamstrings—tibia externally rotated
  - Resisted hip extension with an extended knee

A hamstring strain has a reputation of being both chronic and recurring. With such a high reoccurrence rate, great care and attention should be focused on both prevention and rehabilitation of this condition.[27] **Application Strategy 16.3** provides an outline of a comprehensive program for returning patients to activity who have sustained grade I and grade II hamstring strains.

Adductor (Groin) Strain

Etiology

Adductor strains are common in activities that require quick changes of direction as well as explosive propulsion and acceleration. A strength imbalance between the hip abductors and adductors may be a predisposing factor in many of these injuries. The more severe strains typically occur at the proximal attachment of the muscle on the hip, particularly the adductor longus. Milder strains tend to occur more distally, at the musculotendinous junction.

Signs and Symptoms

The patient often experiences an initial "twinge" or "pull" of the groin muscles and is unable to walk because of the intense, sharp pain. As the condition worsens, increased pain, stiffness, and weakness in hip adduction and flexion become apparent. Running straight ahead or backward may be tolerable, but any side-to-side movement leads to more discomfort and pain. Localized tenderness can be palpated on the ischiopubic ramus, lesser trochanter, or musculotendinous junction. Increased pain is felt during passive stretching with the hip extended, abducted, and externally rotated and with resisted hip adduction. Occasionally, a palpable defect may be found, indicating a more serious injury.

Gluteal Muscles

Etiology

Because of their size and strength, the gluteal muscles rarely are injured except in activities that require muscle overload, such as power weight lifting and rowing. Signs and symptoms are similar to those of other muscular strains and include the following:

- History of muscle overload or repetitive muscular contractions, as occurs in weight lifting or rowing
- Increased pain or weakness during the following:
  - Passive hip flexion with the knee flexed
  - Active hip extension with the knee flexed
  - Resisted hip extension with the knee flexed

Piriformis Syndrome

Etiology

The sciatic nerve passes through the sciatic notch beneath the piriformis muscle to travel into the posterior thigh (**Fig. 16.10**). In approximately 10% to 15% of the population, the nerve passes through or above the muscle, subjecting the nerve to compression from trauma, hemorrhage, or spasm of the piriformis muscle. More commonly, the peroneal portion of the nerve is compressed. The incidence of piriformis syndrome has been reported to be sixfold more prevalent in women than in men.[26] A history of prolonged sitting, stair climbing, and repetitive squatting and rising; recent increase in activity; or buttock trauma may be reported. Resulting symptoms may mimic those of a herniated lumbar disk with nerve root impingement. With a herniated disk, pain usually is increased on coughing, sneezing, or straining during defecation, indicating epidural involvement; such pain is not noted in a piriformis syndrome.

Signs and Symptoms

Low back pain is not usual, although the patient may complain of a dull ache in the midbuttock region; pain that worsens at night, particularly when turning from one side to the other in bed;

APPLICATION STRATEGY 16.3

Recommendations for Hamstring Strain Rehabilitation Program

The following protocols are recommended for use in treating grade I and grade II hamstring strains. The protocol is divided into three phases. Within each phase, recurring themes appear: protection, ice, NSAIDs, and therapeutic exercise.

Phase 1 (1–5 Days Postinjury)

Goal: Decrease intensity of pain and protect formation of scar tissue

- **Protection**
  - ROM should be limited by pain; do not exceed ranges that cause pain.
  - Shorten strides and use crutches if needed.
  - Allow leg for fully extend; do not keep knee flexed.
  - Assume normal gait as pain disappears.
- **Ice**
  - Ice two to three times per day for 20 minutes per session.
- **NSAIDs**
  - Attempt to manage pain with rest and ice.
  - NSAIDs may be used initially, but analgesics such as acetaminophen are a recommended alternative.
- **Therapeutic exercise**
  - Work on promoting neuromuscular control within the protected range.
  - Focus is on isometric exercise for the lumbopelvic muscle groups.
  - Single-leg balance exercises and frontal plane stepping drills
  - All exercise should be performed pain-free.
- **Criteria to progress to phase 2**
  - Normal walking stride without pain
  - Low-speed jogging without pain
  - Pain-free isometric contractions against submaximal resistance during prone knee flexion

Phase 2 (Varies)

Goal: Exercising within pain-free ROM and allowing healing to occur

- **Protection**
  - Avoid reaching end-range lengthening of hamstrings to avoid elongation and possible damage to the weakened musculotendon unit.
- **Ice**
  - Postexercise for pain control and inflammation
- **NSAIDs**
  - Should not be used during phase 2 as use may mask pain
  - Important to be able to detect pain in order to stress weakened tissue
- **Therapeutic exercise**
  - Work on promoting gradual controlled lengthening of musculature.
  - Emphasis is on neuromuscular control, agility drills, and trunk stabilization exercises.
  - Progressively increase speed and intensity, respectively.
  - Movements are in the transverse and frontal planes, gradually transitioning to sagittal plane.
  - Submaximal eccentric strengthening exercises near midlength of the muscle are initiated as part of functional movement patterns and not as isolated hamstring exercises.
  - Anaerobic training and sport skills are initiated, taking care to avoid end-range lengthening of the hamstrings or substantial eccentric work.
- **Criteria to progress to phase 3**
  - Full strength (5/5) without pain during a 1-repetition maximum effort isometric manual muscle test in prone with the knee flexed at 90°
  - Forward and backward jogging at 50% maximum speed without pain

APPLICATION STRATEGY 16.3 *(continued)*

Phase 3 (Varies)

A. Goal: Symptom-free, normal pain-free ROM, and improved neuromuscular control

- **Protection**
  - ROM is no longer limited; however, sprinting and explosive drills are prohibited at this stage.
- **Ice**
  - Postexercise for control of pain and inflammation as needed
- **Therapeutic exercise**
  - Agility and sport-specific drills should be emphasized that involve quick direction changes and technique training, respectively.
  - Trunk stabilization exercises should become more challenging by incorporating transverse plane motions and asymmetrical postures.
  - Emphasize functional movement patterns; eccentric hamstring strengthening should be progressed toward end ROM, with appropriate increases in resistance.
  - Incorporating sport-specific movements that involve a variety of head and trunk postures, as well as quick changes in those postures, is encouraged.
- **Criteria to progress to return to sport**
  - Return to unrestricted sporting activities once full ROM, strength, and functional abilities can be performed without complaints of pain or stiffness.
  - Patient should be able to complete four consecutive pain-free repetitions of maximum effort manual strength test in each prone knee flexion position (90° and 15°).

Adapted from Heiderscheit BC, Sherry MA, Silder A, et al. Hamstring strain injuries: recommendations for diagnosis, rehabilitation, and injury prevention. *J Orthop Sports Phys Ther.* 2010;40(2):67–81.

difficulty walking up stairs or on an incline; and weakness or numbness extending down the back of the leg. Assessment reveals point tenderness in the midbuttock region over the greater sciatic notch. Increased pain and weakness on active hip external rotation, passive hip flexion, adduction, and internal rotation, and resisted hip external rotation are present. The patient may stand with the leg in slight external rotation. Pain can be elicited with the patient supine and the hip flexed, adducted, and internally rotated (i.e., reverse Patrick test), because this stretches the piriformis muscle. Straight leg raising may be limited.

Management of Strains

Treatment for muscular strains involves immediate ice, compression, elevation, and protected rest. Whenever possible, the injured muscles should be iced in a stretched position. If the patient cannot walk with a normal gait, crutches should be used. With severe strains, a compression wrap may be indicated from the toe to the groin to prevent venous thrombosis and distal edema. NSAIDs typically are used for the first 7 to 10 days.

If the condition does not improve within 2 to 5 days, referral to a physician is necessary to rule out other underlying conditions. Nontraumatic diagnostic possibilities can include an avulsion fracture, osteitis pubis, myositis ossificans, hip joint disease, nerve entrapment, hernia-related conditions, urological disorders, and gynecological problems.

When the acute inflammatory phase has progressed to resolution of the hematoma, pain-free gentle stretching and isometric contractions can be initiated in conjunction with cryotherapy and electrical modalities. Compression shorts can provide symptomatic relief and expedite return to activity. If compression shorts are not available, a hip spica wrap or compressive wrap can provide both warmth and support. Active stretching, progressive resistance exercises, soft-tissue mobilization, as well as swimming, cycling, mild jogging, and stair climbing can begin when the region is pain-free and ROM is within 10° of the uninvolved limb. Several stretching and strengthening exercises are discussed in **Application Strategy 16.1**; other exercises for muscles crossing the knee joint can be seen in **Application Strategy 15.1**. When jogging is comfortable, skipping and rope jumping may be initiated. Rapid stops, starts, and changes in direction are not allowed until the patient can achieve full, pain-free motion. The patient should not return to activity until normal muscular strength and power are achieved.

 The softball player suspected of having an adductor strain would experience pain with the following movements: sliding sideways (no pain with running straight ahead or backward), passive hip abduction, active hip adduction, and resisted hip adduction.

VASCULAR AND NEURAL DISORDERS

? A 12-year-old soccer player is seen limping after a game. When asked about a possible injury, he reports that his groin and knee have hurt since the start of the season, nearly 10 weeks ago. When the parents are questioned about the pain, they report that the pain comes and goes. They have been having the child ice the hip and stretch the groin muscles but have not thought that the situation was serious enough to see a physician. What recommendations are appropriate?

Vascular disorders should be suspected in any lower extremity injury caused by a high-velocity, low-mass projectile and in an injury for which no physical findings support the continued discomfort. If an acute circulatory problem exists, the lower leg and foot may appear to be pale or cyanotic, be cool to the touch, or have diminished or totally absent pulse. In these cases, immobilization of the limb and transportation to the nearest medical center are warranted. Other vascular problems are more insidious but can be just as serious. Neural entrapment is very rare in the hip region, particularly as a result of sport participation.

Legg-Calvé-Perthes Disease

Etiology

Legg-Calvé-Perthes disease, or avascular necrosis of the capital femoral epiphysis, is a noninflammatory, self-limiting disorder of the hip seen more commonly in boys than girls and that typically occurs between the ages of 4 and 8 years but can occur up to 12 years of age.[28] It is considered to be an osteochondrosis condition of the femoral head caused by diminished blood supply to the capital region of the femur. This leads to a progressive necrosis of the bone and marrow of the epiphysis of the femoral head (**Fig. 16.34**). The natural history of the condition occurs in the following stages:

1. Edema develops at the synovial membrane and capsule over 1 to 6 weeks.

2. Necrosis of the femoral epiphysis occurs, lasting from several months to 1 year.

3. Regeneration/resorption lasts 1 to 3 years. Granulation tissue invades necrotic bone, leaving isolated areas of bone sequestered. Connective tissues invade the area, leading to resorption and replacement by new immature bone, which results in a weakened subchondral support system.

4. Repair occurs when new, normal bone replaces dead bone. Outcome is related to the percentage of epiphysis involved, age of the patient, and promptness of diagnosis.

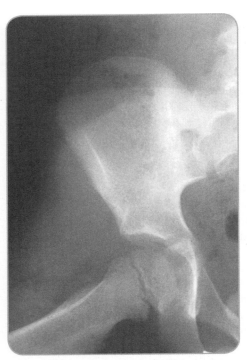

Figure 16.34. Osteochondrosis of the left femoral head (Legg-Calvé-Perthes disease). This picture demonstrates the destruction of articular cartilage.

Signs and Symptoms

The most common complaint is a gradual onset of a limp and mild hip or knee pain of several months' duration. The pain most often is referred to the groin region, but up to 15% of patients report knee pain as the primary symptom.[28] Pain generally is related to activity, which often contributes to delayed recognition. Examination reveals a decreased ROM in hip abduction, extension, and external rotation caused by muscle spasm in the hip flexors and adductors.

Management

Unexplained pain and a limp after activity that persists for more than 1 week after initial acute care necessitates immediate referral to a physician to rule out nontraumatic causes of the pain, such as a slipped capital femoral epiphysis, septic arthritis, transient synovitis, juvenile rheumatoid arthritis, or a bone tumor. Confirmation of the condition is made through radiographs, bone scans, or magnetic resonance images.

Treatment depends on the age of the patient, extent of femoral head damage, and the philosophy of the supervising physician. Nonoperative treatment may involve several different progressive protocols, including the following:

■ Therapy to improve hip ROM with NSAIDs

■ Non–weight bearing in a brace

■ Weight bearing in a brace that limits hip motion

■ Weight bearing in a brace that allows free movement

Treatment can be quite extensive, sometimes taking 1 to 2 years. It may involve immobilization, non–weight bearing, and possible surgery to prevent any further deformity of the femoral head caused by the avascular necrosis.

Venous Disorders

Etiology

A direct blow from a baseball, softball, puck, or helmet may damage a vein, causing thrombophlebitis or phlebothrombosis. **Thrombophlebitis** is an acute inflammation of a vein; **phlebothrombosis** is a thrombosis, or clotting, in a vein without overt inflammatory signs and symptoms. Phlebothrombosis is discussed in more detail in Chapter 15. Superficial thrombophlebitis is more painful and is often associated with varicose veins that are visible just under the skin. Deep venous thrombosis (DVT) is more dangerous and often cannot be seen or felt by the patient. Predisposing factors include obesity, smoking, surgery, hospitalization, cancer, and trauma. An increased incidence of complications from the condition is seen among patients who are older than 60 years, are male, have a history of DVT or prolonged bed rest, have bilateral superficial thrombophlebitis, and have infection in the involved leg.[29]

Signs and Symptoms

Superficial thrombophlebitis may present itself as an acute, red, hot, palpable, tender cord in the course of a superficial vein. Extension of superficial thrombophlebitis to the deep venous system occurs through the proximal long and short saphenous veins to the common femoral and popliteal veins, respectively, and through the perforating veins. The most reliable signs are chronic swelling and edema in the involved extremity and a positive Homans sign (**Fig. 16.35**).

Management

Treatment may involve a variety of actions. Superficial thrombophlebitis may include elevation of the leg, warm compresses, and medication to decrease pain and inflammation. External support with compression stockings or elastic bandages may help to reduce swelling. Treatment for

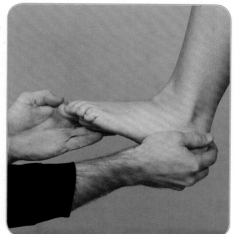

Figure 16.35. Homans sign.

DVT may involve anticoagulant (blood thinning) therapy with heparin (by injection) or warfarin (by mouth for longer term treatment).[30] Ambulation and lower extremity exercises, particularly with hydrotherapy, and avoidance of long-term sitting or standing in one position may also be helpful.

Toxic Synovitis

Etiology

An infrequent condition that occurs largely in children is **toxic synovitis** of the hip. It is the most common cause of acute hip pain in children ages 3 to 10 years and is not considered a disease in adults.

Signs and Symptoms

The transient inflammatory condition is characterized by a painful hip joint accompanied with an antalgic gait and limp. The condition usually affects only one hip.

Management

Early referral to a physician is necessary to rule out septic arthritis of the hip and other more serious conditions that may require surgery to drain the septic joint, relieve pressure, and preserve blood supply to the femoral head. Symptoms usually improve in 4 to 5 days. Rest is the key to treatment, along with appropriate medication and traction for prompt resolution.

Obturator Nerve Entrapment

Etiology

The obturator nerve is derived from the anterior portion of the lumbar plexus (L2 through L4). It innervates the adductor brevis, longus, and magnus; the obturator externus; and the gracilis as well as provides sensory innervation for the hip joint and the distal, medial thigh. A fascial entrapment of the obturator nerve may occur where it enters the thigh as a result of pelvic tumors, obturator hernias, or pelvic and proximal femoral fractures.

Signs and Symptoms

A characteristic clinical pattern of exercise-induced, medial thigh pain presents from the adductor muscle origin distally along the medial thigh. This pain may be described as vague groin or medial knee pain.

Management

With no abnormal findings during special stress tests for the hip and knee region, a patient who reports vague groin or medial knee pain should be referred to a physician. If the obturator nerve is entrapped, surgical intervention is necessary. Return to activity usually occurs within several weeks of treatment.

The soccer player's symptoms have been present for more than 10 weeks, and icing and stretching of the groin muscles have not improved the injury. Because of the age of the athlete, the vague groin and knee pain, and the length of time for the disability, which has now resulted in a noticeable limp, you should recommend that the child see a physician immediately. He may have Legg-Calvé-Perthes disease or another degenerative condition involving the hip joint.

HIP FRACTURES

? A rugby player is down on the field after receiving a severe blow to the anterior right thigh. The thigh is externally rotated and severely angulated, and the involved limb appears to be shorter than the uninvolved limb. The athlete is in severe pain. What injury should be expected? Explain and demonstrate management for this injury.

Major fractures of the pelvic girdle and hip often result from severe direct trauma. In some sports (e.g., football and ice hockey), the pelvic region usually is adequately protected by padding to prevent such injuries. Fractures that may be sustained in this region include avulsion and apophyseal fractures, epiphyseal fractures, and stress fractures.

Apophysitis and Avulsion Fractures
Etiology

Apophysitis and avulsion fractures will often occur during the adolescent growth period between 11 and 15 years of age, but many of the apophyseal sites do not unite with the bone until 18 to 25 years of age and, as such, continue to be prone to fracture. Repetitive apophyseal microtrauma and stress may produce traction cartilage abnormalities, whereas avulsion fractures usually result from a forceful, rapid eccentric muscle contraction that disrupts apophyseal bony integrity. Common sites for avulsion fractures include the following:

- The ASIS with the displacement of the sartorius
- The AIIS with displacement of the rectus femoris
- The ischial tuberosity with displacement of the hamstrings
- The lesser trochanter with displacement of the iliopsoas

Signs and Symptoms

With apophysitis, the patient usually presents with gradually increasing, localized, dull pain that is exacerbated by running. In contrast to an avulsion fracture, the patient complains of sudden, acute, localized pain that may radiate down the muscle. Examination reveals severe pain, swelling, and discoloration directly over the tendinous attachment on the bony landmark. In a completely displaced avulsion fracture, the patient may hear or feel a pop, and a gap may be palpated between the tendon's attachment and the bone. Pain increases with passive stretching of the involved muscle, active ROM, and resisted ROM.

Management

Depending on the injured site, immobilization from an elastic compression spica wrap may limit motion and decrease pain. Neoprene shorts may be helpful to provide warmth and compression. Ice, rest, modified activity, and protected weight bearing with crutches for 4 to 6 weeks if necessary should provide adequate healing for an undisplaced fracture. ROM exercises should be discouraged until the fracture has healed, but isometric exercises can be performed if pain-free. Most patients return to sport activity within 4 to 8 weeks if strength and motion have been restored.[25]

Slipped Capital Femoral Epiphysis
Etiology

The capital femoral epiphysis is the growth plate at the femoral head. A fracture to this area, sometimes referred to as adolescent coxa vara, is seen in adolescent boys from 12 to 15 years of age. In particular, the condition commonly is seen in obese adolescents with underdeveloped sexual characteristics and, occasionally, in rapidly growing, slender boys. In a slipped capital femoral epiphysis, the femoral head slips at the epiphyseal plate and displaces inferiorly and posteriorly relative to the femoral neck (**Fig. 16.36**). As the proximal femoral growth plate deteriorates, the patient begins to develop a painful limp with groin pain. Pain also may be referred to the anterior thigh or knee region. The condition may lead to synovitis of the hip and an accompanying psoas major spasm.

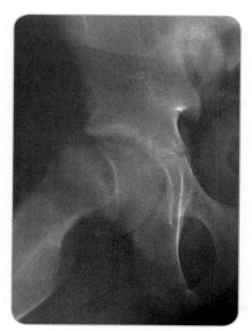

Figure 16.36. Slipped capital femoral epiphysis. An epiphyseal fracture, seen in adolescents from 12 to 15 years of age, occurs through the growth plate at the femoral head. A patient who sustains this fracture will not be able to rotate the femur internally.

Signs and Symptoms

Early signs and symptoms may go undetected. Frequently, the only complaint is diffuse knee pain. During later stages, the patient feels more comfortable holding the leg in slight flexion. The patient is unable to touch the abdomen with the thigh, because the hip externally rotates with flexion. The patient also is unable to rotate the femur internally or to stand on one leg. If the obturator nerve is damaged during the fracture, an aching pain may be referred to the groin, medial thigh, or knee.

Management

The patient should be fitted with crutches and referred to a physician for further assessment. Radiographs of the hip are necessary to confirm the condition and to rule out other possible conditions, such as tumors, bone cysts, and underlying osteochondromas. Prognosis is good with early detection, although those with more severe slips likely have residual deformity and progressive disability. Surgery is indicated in nearly all cases.

Stress Fractures

Etiology

Stress fractures of the pubic ramus, femoral neck, and proximal third of the femur are seen in patients who engage in extensive jogging or aerobic dance activities to the point of muscle fatigue. Several factors can increase the risk of sustaining a stress fracture, including the following:

- Sudden increase in training (mileage, intensity, or frequency)
- Change in running surface or terrain
- Improper footwear
- Biomechanical abnormalities (coxa vara)
- Nutritional and hormonal factors (anorexia, amenorrhea, osteopenia, malabsorption syndromes, and calcium deficiencies)
- Chronic glucocorticoid use, smoking, hyperparathyroidism, hyperthyroidism

Women are 3 to 10 times more likely to sustain a stress fracture than men. Rather than occurring from a sudden traumatic impact, stress fractures occur from either abnormal forces on normal bones (fatigue fractures) or normal forces on abnormal bones (insufficiency fractures).[25]

Signs and Symptoms

Signs and symptoms usually involve a diffuse or localized, aching pain in the anterior groin or thigh region during weight-bearing activity that is relieved with rest. Night pain is a frequent complaint. An antalgic gait may be present. A delay of at least 6 weeks between symptom onset and clinical diagnosis is not uncommon because the signs and symptoms may be subtle. Deep palpation in the inguinal area will produce discomfort, and diffuse or localized swelling may be present. Positive signs include increased pain on the extremes of hip motion, particularly internal rotation, adduction, and flexion; an abduction lurch; an inability to stand on the involved leg (i.e., positive Trendelenburg sign or "one-legged hop" test); and a positive fulcrum test (putting one arm under the affected leg and pushing downward on the distal thigh).

Management

Referral to a physician is necessary. Bone scans or magnetic resonance images frequently are used for early diagnosis. If the diagnosis is established early enough, rest is indicated for at least 1 to 4 weeks, with no weight-bearing activity until the fracture is completely healed. Stress fractures of the ischium and pubis may require 2 to 3 months of rest. Biking and swimming can help the patient to maintain cardiovascular fitness; however, during swimming, the whip kick and scissors kick should be avoided. Displaced stress fractures of the femoral neck require surgical pin fixation to prevent a complete fracture and avascular necrosis of the femoral head.

Osteitis Pubis

Etiology

Osteitis pubis is an inflammatory process involving continued stress on the pubic symphysis from repeated overload of the adductor muscles or repetitive running activities.

Signs and Symptoms

The most common complaint is a gradual onset of pain in the adductor musculature, which is aggravated by kicking, running, and pivoting on one leg. Sit-ups and abdominal muscular strengthening exercises will increase pain in the lower abdominal muscles and over the pubic symphysis. Pain also may radiate distally into the groin or medial thigh.

Management

Treatment is symptomatic with ice, protected rest, and NSAIDs until the condition is resolved. Prolonged rest extending over 2 to 3 months, however, may be necessary to alleviate symptoms. Hydrotherapy exercises may help in rehabilitation. Use of a stationary bike and light jogging may be added as tolerated.

Displaced and Nondisplaced Pelvic Fractures

Etiology

Major fractures of the pelvis seldom occur in sport participation except in activities such as equestrian sports, ice hockey, rugby, skiing, and football. Three distinct mechanisms are involved in traumatic pelvic fractures:

1. Avulsion or traction injury of the bony origin or attachment of muscle

2. Direct compression, with disruption of the pelvic osseous ring

3. Direct blow to the pelvis

Because the pelvis is a closed ring, an injury to one location in the pelvis can cause a contrecoup fracture or sprain on the other side of the pelvic ring. For example, if the superior and inferior pubic rami are fractured on the right side, the left side often has an SI disruption.

Signs and Symptoms

This crushing injury produces severe pain, total loss of function, and, in many cases, severe loss of blood, leading to hypovolemic shock. The extent of blood loss is unknown, because hemorrhage within the pelvic cavity is not visible. In addition, possible internal injuries to the genitourinary system, such as rupture of the bladder or laceration of the urethra, also may occur. In dramatic, severe fractures, this internal damage and subsequent shock can lead to death. A fracture to the pelvis can be assessed by applying slight compression to the sides of the ilium and the ASIS. Fractures of the acetabulum can be detected by placing gentle, upward pressure on the femur against the acetabulum.

Management

Fractures of the pelvis should be regarded as serious injuries with immediate referral to the nearest medical facility a priority. With the possibility of internal hemorrhaging, the patient should be stabilized, vital signs should be measured, and the patient treated for shock.

If a fracture is suspected, the emergency action plan, including summoning EMS, should be activated. While waiting for EMS to arrive, the clinician should assess vital signs and treat for shock as necessary.

Sacral and Coccygeal Fractures

Etiology

Fractures of the sacrum and coccyx rarely occur in sports. They typically are caused by a direct blow onto the sacrococcygeal area subsequent to a fall on the buttock region.

Signs and Symptoms

Direct impact leads to an extremely painful injury. Subsequent to pain, the patient is unable to sit.

Management

The patient should be referred immediately to a physician. These fractures usually heal within 6 weeks and without any functional impairment, but clinically healed fractures often show evidence of fibrous union. In rare cases, coccygodynia, or persistent severe pain, can occur. This condition is very difficult to treat because of the rich complex of pain nociceptors in the area. Return to activity should be restricted only if pain interferes with the activity.

Femoral Fractures

Etiology

Fractures of the femoral shaft can be very serious because of potential damage to the neurovascular structures from bony fragments. Femoral shaft fractures are caused by tremendous impact forces, such as shearing or torsion forces when an alpine skier falls, or from direct compressive forces, such as tackles in football, ice hockey, or rugby.

Signs and Symptoms

Fractures may be open or closed, but in either case, significant bleeding occurs at the fracture site. Signs and symptoms indicating a femoral fracture are listed in **Box 16.5**.

If a fracture is suspected, the emergency action plan, including summoning EMS, should be activated. This type of fracture is best immobilized in a traction splint, which should be applied only by trained personnel. While waiting for EMS to arrive, the clinician should assess vital signs and treat for shock as necessary. Any external bleeding should be covered with a dry, sterile dressing to protect the area from further contamination.

Management

It is not unusual for significant bleeding in the thigh to lead to hypovolemic shock, similar to that seen in pelvic fractures. Vascular damage may lead to impaired circulation distal to the injury, causing a pale, cold, pulseless foot. Distal neurovascular function should be assessed immediately and monitored frequently; this can be performed by palpating a pulse at the posterior tibial artery and dorsalis pedis artery, looking for pale skin at the foot, and feeling for cool skin temperature. Sensation testing can be performed by stroking the dorsum and plantar aspect of both feet.

Table 16.4 summarizes signs and symptoms of the various fractures seen in the pelvis and thigh region.

 The rugby player has signs and symptoms that suggest a fracture of the femoral shaft. The emergency action plan, including summoning EMS, should be activated. This fracture is best immobilized in a traction splint, which should be applied by trained personnel. While waiting for EMS to arrive, the clinician should maintain the airway, assess vital signs, check for nerve and circulatory impairment at the lower leg and ankle, and treat for shock as necessary.

BOX 16.5 Signs and Symptoms of Femoral Fractures

Displaced Fracture

- Shortened limb deformity
- Severe angulation with the thigh externally rotated
- Swelling into the soft tissues
- Severe pain
- Total loss of function
- Loss of, or change in, distal neurovascular functions

Nondisplaced Fractures

- Extreme pain on palpation
- Crepitation
- Muscle weakness
- Muscle spasm
- Swelling into the soft tissues

TABLE 16.4 Fractures and Associated Signs and Symptoms

FRACTURE	COMMON SITES	SIGNS AND SYMPTOMS
Avulsion and pain with apophyseal	ASIS AIIS Ischial tuberosity Lesser trochanter	Severe pain and tenderness over bony landmark Increased active motion of involved muscle
Epiphyseal	Capital femoral epiphysis	Unable to internally rotate the thigh Possible pain in groin, medial thigh, or knee
Stress	Pubis Femoral neck Proximal third of femur	May have point tenderness over fracture site Pain is worse before and after activity and is relieved with rest. Possible limp as the fracture progresses
Pelvic girdle	Wing of ilium or acetabulum	Severe pain over fracture site Total loss of function Positive fracture tests Show signs of shock
Femoral	Shaft of femur or femoral neck	Severe angulation with thigh externally rotated Shortened limb; swelling into soft tissue Severe pain and crepitation at fracture site Total loss of function and signs of shock Positive fracture tests Vascular damage may lead to pale, cold, pulseless foot.

REHABILITATION

> **?** In the first scenario, the basketball player sustained a blow to the anterior thigh 2 weeks ago followed by another blow during today's practice. The condition developed into myositis ossificans. The patient was referred to the team physician who recommended treatment including ice, compression, elevation, crutches, and protected rest. Is it advantageous to treat this condition using NSAIDs?

Rehabilitation of the hip area should restore motion and proprioception; improve muscular strength, endurance, and power; and maintain cardiovascular fitness. In addition to focusing on muscles that move the hip, exercises also should involve the muscles that govern the knee.

Restoration of Motion

ROM exercises for the hip region should focus on the hip flexors, extensors, abductors, adductors, medial and lateral rotators, and quadriceps and hamstrings. Several of the stretching exercises were demonstrated in **Application Strategy 16.1**; other ROM exercises for muscles crossing the knee joint appear in **Application Strategy 15.1**. These exercises can be active or passive, and they should include proprioceptive neuromuscular facilitation stretching techniques.

Restoration of Proprioception and Balance

Proprioception and balance are regained in the early stages of exercise, with activities such as shifting one's weight while on crutches, performing straight leg raises while weight bearing on one leg, performing bilateral minisquats, and using a biomechanical ankle platform system (BAPS) board, slide board, or minitramp. Straight leg raises can be further supplemented with ankle weights and elastic tubing. Attaching the tubing to the opposite limb from the one being worked can develop balance in one limb while strengthening the other. Movement patterns can work in a single plane or in multidirectional patterns.

Muscular Strength, Endurance, and Power

Isometric exercises may be used early to strengthen the muscle groups. Open chain exercises, such as straight leg raises, can be completed in a single plane or in multidirectional patterns and can be supplemented with ankle weights or tubing. Closed chain exercises may include minisquats and modified lunges and should progress to full squats and lunges. Resistance may be added with hand-held weights, a weighted bar, or use of a leg-press machine. A variety of commercial isotonic and isokinetic machines are available to strengthen the patient muscle groups using both open and closed chain techniques.

Cardiovascular Fitness

Cardiovascular fitness exercises can include early use of an upper body ergometer or hydrotherapeutic exercise. Running in water and performing sport-specific exercises in deeper water can allow the patient to maintain sport-specific functional skills in a non–weight-bearing position. When ROM is adequate, a stationary bike can be used, beginning with a light to moderate load and increasing the load as tolerated. A slide board also may be used. Light jogging can begin with one-quarter speed and progress to half-speed, three-quarter speed, and full sprints. Plyometric exercises, including jumping, skipping, and bounding, can be combined with running, side-to-side running, or cutting and changing directions. Timed sprints, shuttle runs, carioca runs, and hops or vertical jump tests may be used to measure return to full activity. Patients should not be cleared for participation until they have bilaterally equal ROM, balance, muscular strength, endurance, and power as well as an appropriate level of cardiovascular fitness for the specific sport.

 Use of NSAIDs is dependent on the stage of healing. Because the basketball player experienced repeated trauma to the same area, NSAIDs are not indicated for 48 hours postinjury because they inhibit platelet function and promote more hemorrhage.

SUMMARY

1. The SI joints help to transfer the weight of the torso and skull to the lower limbs, provide elasticity to the pelvic ring, and conversely, act as a buffer to decrease impact forces from the foot as they are transmitted to the spine and upper body.

2. The hip joint is the most stable joint in the body. It is protected by a deep, bony socket called the acetabulum and is stabilized by several strong ligaments, including the iliofemoral, pubofemoral, and ischiofemoral ligaments.

3. Compression on the hip is approximately the same as body weight during the swing phase of normal walking, but compression increases to at least sixfold body weight during the stance phase.

4. Muscle imbalance and dysfunction, congenital abnormalities, and postural deviations can predispose a patient to injury.

5. Contusions typically are seen on the crest of the ilium or in the quadriceps muscle group. Severe quadriceps contusions can lead to myositis ossificans or an acute compartment syndrome.

6. Bursitis can result from inflammation secondary to excessive friction or shear forces or can stem from a direct blow that causes bleeding in the bursa. The greater trochanteric bursa is the most commonly injured bursa.

7. The hamstrings are the most frequently strained muscle group in the body. Injuries typically are caused by a rapid contraction of the muscle during a ballistic action or by a violent stretch.

8. Adductor strains are common in activities that require quick changes of direction and explosive propulsion and acceleration.

9. Piriformis syndrome is sixfold more prevalent in women than in men, and it can mimic the signs and symptoms of a herniated lumbar disk problem with nerve root impingement.

10. In adolescents, any unexplained groin pain associated with a gradual onset of a limp should be referred to a physician to rule out Legg-Calvé-Perthes disease or a slipped capital femoral epiphysis.

11. Avulsion fractures may occur in patients who perform rapid moves involving sudden acceleration and deceleration, with the following sites being most affected:

   - **ASIS**—proximal sartorius muscle or tensor fasciae latae
   - **AIIS**—proximal rectus femoris muscles
   - **Ischial tuberosity**—proximal hamstrings attachment
   - **Lesser trochanter**—distal iliopsoas attachment

12. Physician referral is warranted if any of the following conditions are suspected:

   - Obvious deformity suggesting a dislocation or fracture
   - Significant loss of motion or palpable defect in a muscle
   - Severe joint disability that may be evident by a noticeable limp
   - Excessive soft-tissue swelling, particularly in the quadriceps
   - Any adolescent with groin pain that does not improve within 5 to 7 days or is associated with a gradual onset of a limp
   - Any abnormal or absent reflexes or weakness in a myotome
   - Abnormal sensations in either the segmental dermatomes or peripheral cutaneous patterns
   - Absent or weak pulse

13. Radiographs, bone scans, or magnetic resonance images can be used to rule out underlying bone cysts, tumors, osteochondromas, or congenital defects that could lead to permanent disability.

APPLICATION QUESTIONS

1. A 36-year-old woman is complaining of hip pain while running. Pain is located on the posterolateral aspect of her hip near the greater trochanter and is occasionally accompanied by a snapping sensation. What open-ended questions could be asked to develop a medical history of this injury?

2. An athlete has sustained a quadriceps strain. What signs and symptoms would one expect to see during the functional testing of this injury? If the injury were an isolated rectus femoris strain, what specific signs and symptoms would be evident during functional testing?

3. A football running back sustains an acute thigh contusion. How would this injury be immediately managed on the field?

4. During a track meet, a triple jumper sustains a left hamstring injury. In assessing the injury, how would one differentiate between a mild and moderate hamstring strain?

5. An aerobic dancer complains of pain over the right anterior groin that increases after weight-bearing activities but decreases with rest. The dancer also reports night pain in the same region. The dancer does not recall a specific injury but reports that the condition has been getting worse the last week. Deep palpation in the inguinal area produces moderate discomfort. What functional and special tests can be used to assess this injury? What injury(ies) may be present?

6. A tall, thin high school sophomore basketball player is complaining of diffuse knee and groin pain on the left side. It is uncomfortable to run and do shooting drills, and he notes that he cannot balance on his left leg or walk without a limp. What injury(ies) might be present with these symptoms? What would you suggest for the immediate management of these injuries? At what point would the athletic trainer refer this patient to a physician?

7. As the athletic trainer at a recreational soccer tournament, you notice a 12-year-old soccer player limping after a game. When asked about a possible injury, he reports that his groin and knee have hurt ever since the start of the season, nearly 10 weeks ago. In questioning the athlete's parents about the condition, they report that the pain comes and goes. They have been having the child ice the hip and stretch the groin muscles but did not think it was serious enough to see a physician. What recommendation might you make to the parents about this possible condition?

8. A first base softball player stretches for an overthrown ball. During the stretch, the athlete feels a twinge in her left inner groin region. After treatment, what sport-specific tests should this athlete perform to determine return to play?

9. As part of the rehabilitation of a moderate hamstring strain, what type of exercises should be initiated first: closed chain or open chain exercises? Why?

REFERENCES

1. Feeley BT, Powell JW, Muller MS, et al. Hip injuries and labral tears in the National Football League. *Am J Sports Med*. 2008;36(11):2187–2195.
2. Hodnett PA, Shelly MJ, MacMahon PJ, et al. MR imaging of overuse injuries of the hip. *Magn Reson Imaging Clin N Am*. 2009;17(4):667–679.
3. Steinke H, Hammer N, Slowik V, et al. Novel insights into the sacroiliac joint ligaments. *Spine (Phila Pa 1976)*. 2010;35(3):257–263.
4. Ito H, Song Y, Lindsey DP, et al. The proximal hip joint capsule and the zona orbicularis contribute to hip joint stability in distraction. *J Orthop Res*. 2009;27(8):989–995.
5. Omololu BB, Ogunlade OS, Gopaldasani VK. Normal Q-angle in an adult Nigerian population. *Clin Orthop Relat Res*. 2009;467(8):2073–2076.
6. Sarkar A, Razdan S, Yadav J, et al. Effect of isometric quadricep activation on "Q" angle in young females. *Indian J Physiol Pharmacol*. 2009;53(3):275–278.
7. Fraysse F, Dumas R, Cheze L, et al. Comparison of global and joint-to-joint methods for estimating the hip joint load and the muscle forces during walking. *J Biomech*. 2009;42(14):2357–2362.
8. Verrall GM, Slavotinek JP, Barnes PG, et al. Hip joint range of motion restriction precedes athletic chronic groin injury. *J Sci Med Sport*. 2007;10(6):463–466.
9. Noehren B, Schmitz A, Hempel R, et al. Assessment of strength, flexibility, and running mechanics in men with iliotibial band syndrome. *J Orthop Sports Phys Ther*. 2014;44(3):217–222.
10. Kirchmair L, Lirk P, Colvin J, et al. Lumbar plexus and psoas major muscle: not always as expected. *Reg Anesth Pain Med*. 2008;33(2):109–114.
11. Hrysomallis C. Hip adductors' strength, flexibility, and injury risk. *J Strength Cond Res*. 2009;23(5):1514–1517.
12. Chan GNY, Smith AW, Kirtley C, et al. Changes in knee moments with contralateral versus ipsilateral cane usage in females with knee osteoarthritis. *Clin Biomech (Bristol, Avon)*. 2005;20(4):396–404.
13. Domb BG, Brooks AG, Byrd JW. Clinical examination of the hip joint in athletes. *J Sport Rehabil*. 2009;18(1):3–23.
14. Kendall FP, McCreary EK, Provance PG, et al. *Muscles: Testing and Function with Posture and Pain*. 5th ed. Baltimore, MD: Lippincott Williams & Wilkins; 2005.
15. Laslett M. Evidence-based diagnosis and treatment of the painful sacroiliac joint. *J Man Manip Ther*. 2008;16(3):142–152.
16. Vanelderen P, Szadek K, Cohen SP, et al. Sacroiliac joint pain. *Pain Pract*. 2010;10(5):470–478.
17. Wong CK, Johnson EK. A narrative review of evidence-based recommendations for the physical examination of the lumbar spine, sacroiliac and hip complex. *Musculoskeletal Care*. 2012;10(3):149–161.
18. Wong M. *Pocket Orthopaedics: Evidence-Based Survival Guide*. Sudbury, MA: Jones & Bartlett; 2010.
19. Starkey C. Brown SD. *Orthopedic and Athletic Injury Handbook*. Philadelphia, PA: FA Davis; 2015.

20. Norkin CC, White DJ. *Measurement of Joint Motion: A Guide to Goniometry*. 4th ed. Philadelphia, PA: FA Davis; 2009.

21. MaGee DJ. *Orthopedic Physical Assessment*. St. Louis, MO: Elsevier Health Sciences; 2014.

22. Mithoefer K, Lhowe DW, Vrahas MS, et al. Functional outcome after acute compartment syndrome of the thigh. *J Bone Joint Surg Am*. 2006;88(4):729–737.

23. Newton M, Walker J. Acute quadriceps injury: a case study. *Emerg Nurse*. 2004;12(8):24–29.

24. Paluska SA. An overview of hip injuries in running. *Sports Med*. 2005;35(11):991–1014.

25. Sanders S, Tejwani N, Egol KA. Traumatic hip dislocation—a review. *Bull NYU Hosp Jt Dis*. 2010;68(2):91–96.

26. Esposito PW. Pelvis, hip, and thigh injuries. In: Mellion MB, Walsh WM, Madden C, et al, eds. *Team Physician's Handbook*. 3rd ed. Philadelphia, PA: Hanley & Belfus; 2002:480–489.

27. Heiderscheit BC, Sherry MA, Silder A, et al. Hamstring strain injuries: recommendations for diagnosis, rehabilitation, and injury prevention. *J Orthop Sports Phys Ther*. 2010;40(2):67–81.

28. Wise S. Current management and rehabilitation in Legg-Calvé Perthes disease. *Athl Ther Today*. 2010;15(4):30–35.

29. Kalodiki E, Nicolaides AN. Superficial thrombophlebitis and low-molecular-weight heparins. *Angiology*. 2002;53(6):659–663.

30. Torpy JM, Burke AE, Glass RM. JAMA patient page. Thrombophlebitis. *JAMA*. 2008;300(14):1718.

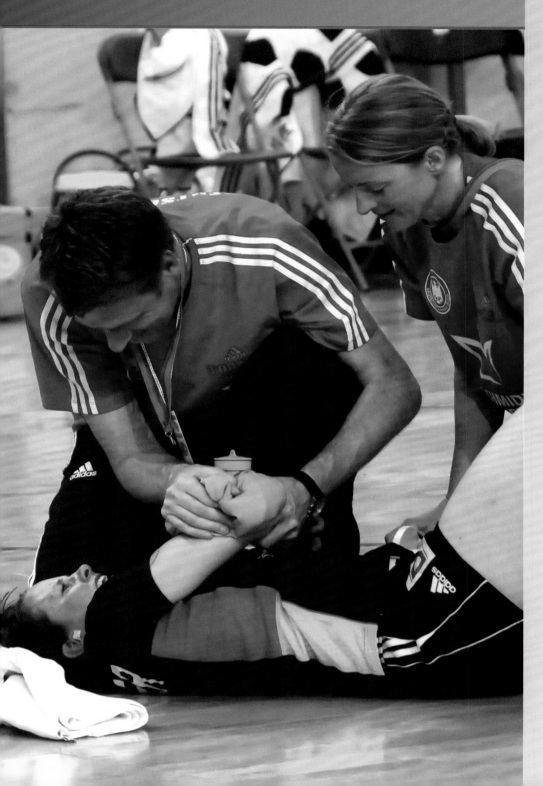

Conditions of the Upper Extremity

Shoulder Conditions

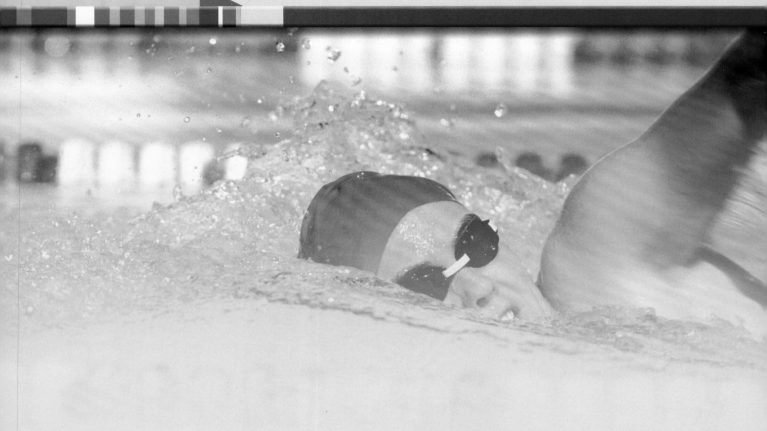

STUDENT OUTCOMES

1. Identify the major bony and soft-tissue structures of the shoulder.

2. List the major motions at the shoulder and the muscles that produce them.

3. Describe the phases of the throwing motion and list the common injuries sustained during each phase.

4. Explain the general principles used to prevent injuries to the shoulder.

5. Describe a thorough assessment of the shoulder region.

6. List the common mechanisms of injury that can lead to instability in the sternoclavicular, acromioclavicular, and glenohumeral joints.

7. Describe the common acute injuries and conditions sustained in the shoulder region by physically active patients.

8. Describe the soft-tissue pathology in the shoulder region that results from overuse.

9. Explain the management strategies for common injuries and conditions of the shoulder.

10. Explain general principles and techniques used in developing a rehabilitation exercise program for the shoulder complex.

INTRODUCTION

The loose structure of the shoulder complex enables extreme mobility but provides little stability. As a result, the shoulder is much more prone to injury compared to the hip. Common shoulder injuries include dislocations, clavicular fractures, muscle and tendon strains, rotator cuff tears, acromioclavicular (AC) sprains, bursitis, bicipital tendonitis, and impingement syndrome. Shoulder injuries commonly occur during activities involving an overhead motion, such as baseball, swimming, tennis, volleyball, and weight lifting.[1] In fact, shoulder pain is the most common musculoskeletal complaint among competitive swimmers and volleyball players, affecting 40% to 70% of swimmers and approximately 60% of volleyball players.[2,3] Dislocations of the shoulder articulations are not uncommon in contact sports, such as wrestling and football.[4,5]

This chapter begins with a review of the anatomy of the shoulder region, followed by a synopsis of the kinematics and kinetics of the shoulder joints. A discussion regarding prevention of injuries is followed by the assessment process. An overview of common injuries to the shoulder complex is presented as well as management of specific injuries. Examples of rehabilitation exercises then conclude the chapter.

ANATOMY OF THE SHOULDER

The arm articulates with the trunk at the shoulder, or pectoral girdle, which comprises the scapula and clavicle (**Figs. 17.1** and **17.2**). The shoulder region has five separate articulations:

1. The sternoclavicular (SC) joint

2. The AC joint

3. The coracoclavicular joint

4. The glenohumeral (GH) joint

5. The scapulothoracic joint

The articulation referred to specifically as the shoulder joint is the GH joint; the remaining articulations are collectively referred to as the shoulder girdle. The SC and AC joints enhance motion of the clavicle and scapula, enabling the GH joint to provide a greater range of motion (ROM).

Sternoclavicular Joint

As the name suggests, the SC joint consists of the articulation of the superior sternum, or manubrium, with the proximal clavicle. The SC joint is surrounded by a joint capsule that is thickened anteriorly and posteriorly by four ligaments, including the interclavicular, costoclavicular, and anterior and posterior SC ligaments (**Fig. 17.3**). The anterior SC ligament is a broad band supporting the anterior capsule, whereas the posterior SC ligament is smaller and weaker, providing support to the posterior capsule. The costoclavicular ligament runs from the clavicle to the 1st rib and its adjacent cartilage. The interclavicular ligament provides minimal support to the joint, runs between the two SC joints, and attaches to the manubrium. A substantial fibrocartilaginous disk is found between the manubrium and clavicle, which divides the joint almost completely in half. Because of its attachments, the disk adds significant strength to the joint and, in doing so, prevents medial displacement of the clavicle.

The SC joint enables rotation of the clavicle with respect to the sternum. The joint allows motion of the distal clavicle in superior, inferior, anterior, and posterior directions, along with some forward and backward rotation of the clavicle. As such, rotation occurs at the SC joint during motions such as shrugging the shoulders, reaching above the head, and most throwing-type activities. Because the 1st rib is joined by its cartilage to the manubrium just inferior to the joint, motion of the clavicle in the inferior direction is restricted.

The close-packed position for the SC joint occurs with maximal shoulder elevation. Although SC joint dislocations are uncommon, rapid diagnosis and treatment of posterior SC joint dislocations are important because of the proximity of the displaced medial clavicle to the great vessels.[6]

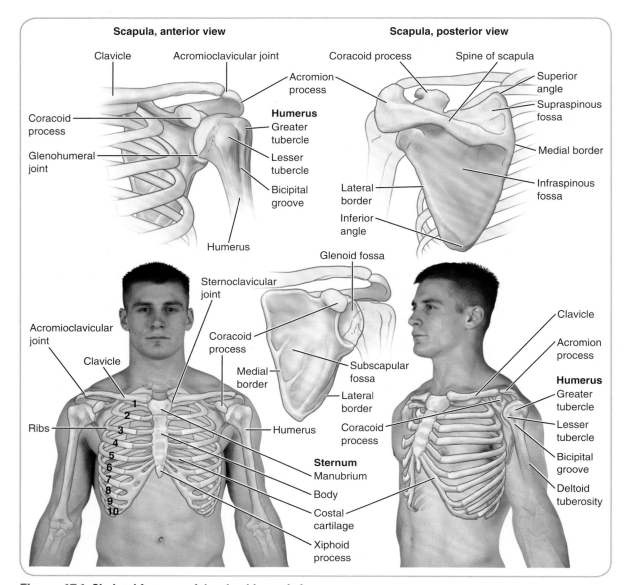

Figure 17.1. Skeletal features of the shoulder and chest.

Acromioclavicular Joint

The AC joint consists of the articulation of the medial facet of the acromion process of the scapula with the distal clavicle (**Fig. 17.3**). As an irregular, diarthrodial joint, limited motion is permitted in all three planes. Highly variable in structure, as many as three different morphological types of AC joint have been identified.[7] The joint is enclosed by a capsule, although the capsule is thinner than that of the SC joint. The strong superior and inferior AC ligaments cross the joint, providing stability. The coracoacromial ligament also attaches to the inferior lip of the AC joint to serve as a buffer between the rotator cuff muscles and the bony acromion process. This ligament is sometimes referred to as the "arch" ligament.

The close-packed position of the AC joint occurs when the humerus is abducted at 90°. Injuries to the AC joint account for nearly half of all athletic shoulder injuries, typically resulting from the force of a fall being absorbed by the shoulder when the arm is in adduction.[8]

Coracoclavicular Joint

The coracoclavicular joint is a syndesmosis in which the coracoid process of the scapula and the inferior surface of the clavicle are joined by the coracoclavicular ligament (**Fig. 17.3**). The coracoclavicular

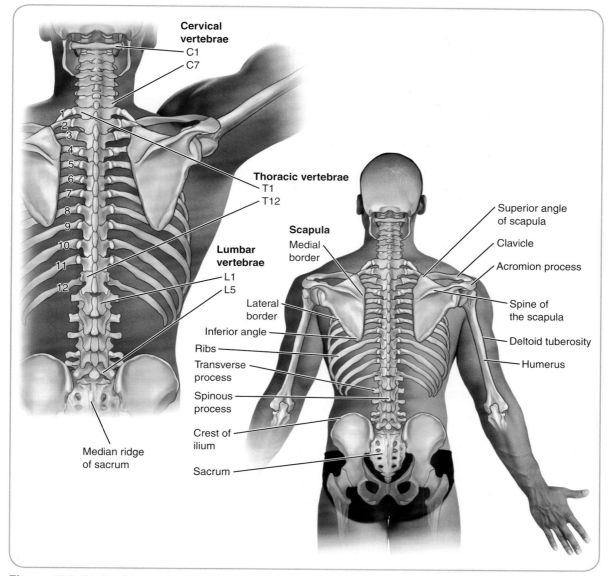

Figure 17.2. Skeletal features of the shoulder and upper back.

ligament, with its conoid and trapezoid branches, resists independent upward movement of the clavicle, downward movement of the scapula, and anteroposterior movement of the clavicle or scapula. Minimal movement is permitted at this joint. The coracoclavicular ligaments frequently are ruptured during contact sports, such as football, hockey, and rugby.[9]

Glenohumeral Joint

The GH joint is the articulation between the glenoid fossa of the scapula and the head of the humerus. Although the joint enables a greater total ROM than any other joint in the human body, it lacks bony stability. This partially results from the hemispheric head of the humerus, which has three- to fourfold the surface area as compared to the shallow glenoid fossa. Because the glenoid fossa also is less curved than the humeral head, the humerus not only rotates but also moves linearly across the surface of the glenoid fossa when humeral motion occurs. Humeral head translation is limited by muscle tension, which also limits rotation, during active positioning of the arm. The largest translations take place during passive movement of the arm at the extremes of the ROM.

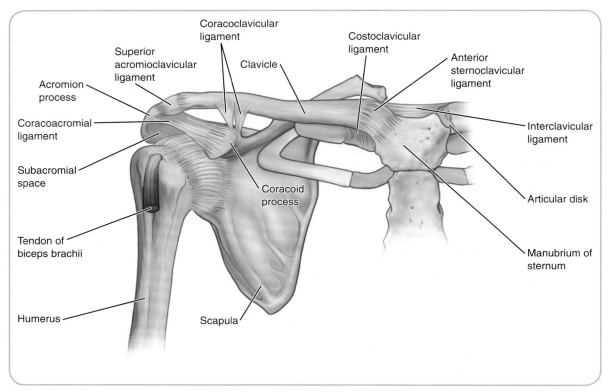

Figure 17.3. Ligaments of the shoulder girdle.

The glenoid fossa is somewhat deepened around its perimeter by the glenoid labrum, a narrow rim of fibrocartilage around the edge of the fossa. The GH joint capsule is joined by the superior, middle, and inferior GH ligaments on the anterior side and by the coracohumeral ligament on the superior side (**Fig. 17.4**). Although joint displacements can occur in anterior, posterior, and inferior directions, the strong coracohumeral ligament protects against superior dislocations. The inferior GH ligament is the thickest of the ligaments and reinforces the inferior capsule. It is the main static stabilizer in the abducted arm.

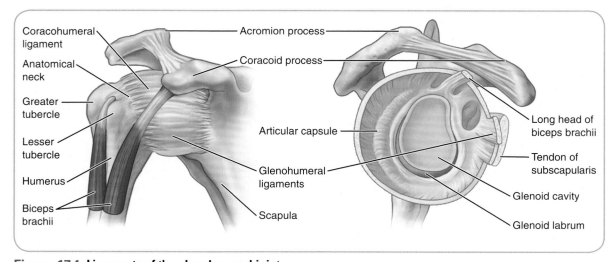

Figure 17.4. Ligaments of the glenohumeral joint.

The tendons of four muscles, including the supraspinatus, infraspinatus, teres minor, and subscapularis, also join the joint capsule. These muscles, which are referred to as the SITS muscles, after the first letter of each muscle's name, also are known as the rotator cuff muscles, both because they act to rotate the humerus and because their tendons merge to form a collagenous cuff around the joint. Tension in the rotator cuff muscles helps to hold the head of the humerus against the glenoid fossa, further contributing to joint stability. The joint is most stable in its close-packed position when the humerus is abducted and laterally rotated.

Scapulothoracic Joint

Because a muscle attaching to the scapula permits its motion with respect to the trunk or thorax, this region sometimes is described as the scapulothoracic joint. Muscles attaching to the scapula include the levator scapula, rhomboids, serratus anterior, pectoralis minor, subclavius, deltoid, subscapularis, supraspinatus, infraspinatus, teres major, teres minor, coracobrachialis, short head of the biceps brachii, long head of the triceps brachii, and the trapezius.

The scapular muscles perform two functions. The first is stabilization of the shoulder region. For example, when a barbell is lifted from the floor, the levator scapula, trapezius, and rhomboids develop tension to support the scapula and, in turn, the entire shoulder through the AC joint. The second is to facilitate movement of the upper extremity through appropriate positioning of the GH joint. For example, during an overhand throw, the rhomboids contract to move the entire shoulder posteriorly as the arm and hand move backward during the preparatory phase. As the arm and hand then move forward to execute the throw, tension in the rhomboids is released to permit forward movement of the shoulder, enabling medial rotation of the humerus. Abduction of the arm at the GH joint is facilitated by rotation of the scapula.

A detailed table providing the **muscles of the shoulder, including each muscle's proximal attachment, distal attachment, primary actions, and nerve innervation**, is available on the companion Web site at thePoint.

Muscles of the Shoulder

A large number of muscles cross the GH joint (**Figs. 17.5** and **17.6**). Because of the large ROM at the shoulder, however, the action produced by contraction of a given muscle can change with the orientation of the humerus, which complicates the process of identifying the actions of these muscles.

Bursae

The shoulder is surrounded by several bursae, including the subcoracoid, the subscapularis, and the most important, the subacromial. The subacromial bursa lies in the subacromial space, where it is surrounded by the acromion process of the scapula and the coracoacromial ligament above and the GH joint below (**Fig. 17.5**). The bursa cushions the rotator cuff muscles, particularly the supraspinatus, from the overlying bony acromion, and it provides the major component of the subacromial gliding mechanism. This bursa is supplied with free nerve endings, Ruffini endings, and Pacinian corpuscles and can become irritated when repeatedly compressed during overhead arm action.

Nerves of the Shoulder

Innervation of the upper extremity arises from the brachial plexus, branching primarily from the lower four cervical (C5–C8) and first thoracic (T1) spinal nerves (see **Fig. 21.9**). The brachial plexus is positioned between the anterior scalene and middle scalene muscles in approximately 60% of patients, with the C5 and/or C6 nerves coursing through or lying anterior to the anterior scalene in others. The ventral rami of these nerves divide into upper, middle, and lower trunks, which in turn separate into anterior and posterior divisions and then divide into lateral, medial, and posterior cords (see Chapter 21). This network of nerves passes between the clavicle and 1st rib at a distance approximately one-third of the length of the clavicle proximal to the GH joint. Injuries to the clavicle in this region can damage the brachial plexus. Major nerves arising from the brachial plexus that supply the shoulder region are the axillary (C5, C6), musculocutaneous (C5 through C7), dorsal scapular (C5), subscapular (C5, C6), suprascapular (C5, C6), and pectoral nerves (C5 through T1).

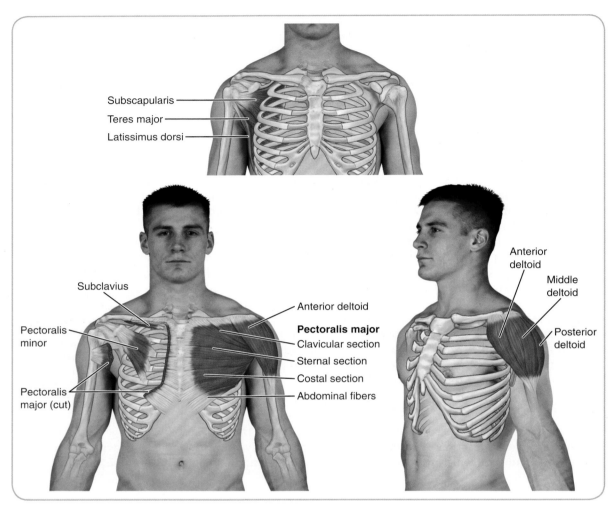

Figure 17.5. Muscles of the shoulder and chest.

Blood Vessels of the Shoulder

The subclavian artery passes beneath the clavicle to become the axillary artery, which provides the major blood supply to the shoulder (**Fig. 17.7**). Branches of the axillary artery include the thoracoacromial trunk, lateral thoracic artery, subscapular artery, and thoracodorsal artery as well as the anterior and posterior humeral circumflex arteries that supply the head of the humerus.

KINEMATICS AND MAJOR MUSCLE ACTIONS OF THE SHOULDER COMPLEX

The shoulder is the most freely movable joint in the body, with motion capability in all three planes (**Fig. 17.8**). Sagittal plane movements at the shoulder include flexion (i.e., elevation of the arm in an anterior direction), extension (i.e., return of the arm from a position of flexion to the side of the body), and hyperextension (i.e., elevation of the arm in a posterior direction). Frontal plane movements include abduction (i.e., elevation of the arm in a lateral direction) and adduction (i.e., return of the arm from a position of abduction to the side of the body). Transverse plane movements include horizontal adduction (i.e., a horizontally extended arm is moved medially) and horizontal abduction (i.e., a horizontally extended arm is moved laterally). The humerus also can rotate medially

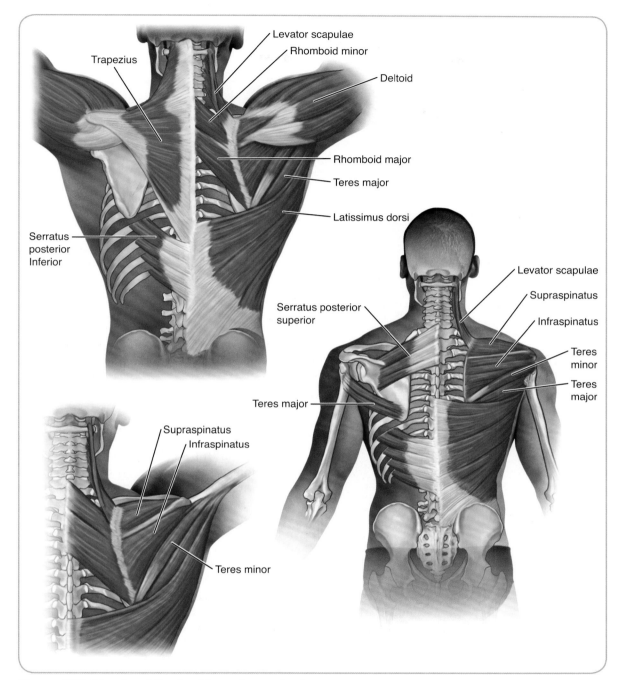

Figure 17.6. Muscles of the shoulder and upper back.

(i.e., the anterior face of the humerus is moved medially) and laterally (i.e., the anterior face of the humerus is moved laterally). Elevation of the humerus in all planes is facilitated by a coordinated and consistent scapular rotation.[10]

Throwing

Throwing and related motions can produce a variety of both acute and chronic injuries to the shoulder. Throwing styles vary from patient to patient, even across overarm, sidearm, and underarm styles of the throw. Further complicating matters, some sport skills—casually referred to as throwing—actually involve more of a pushing motion than a throwing motion. An example is

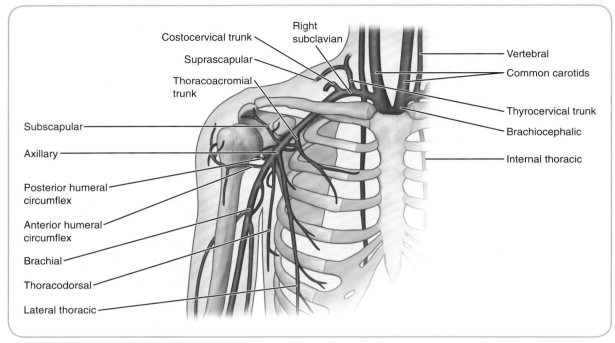

Figure 17.7. Blood supply to the shoulder.

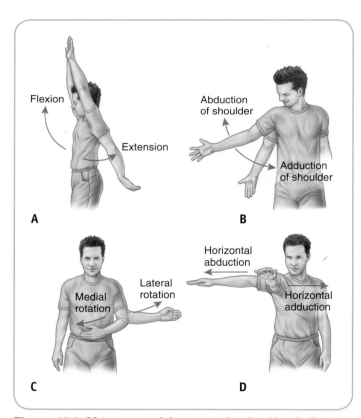

Figure 17.8. Movements of the arm at the shoulder. A, Flexion and extension. **B,** Abduction and adduction. **C,** Internal and external rotation. **D,** Horizontal abduction and adduction.

putting the shot. Nevertheless, overarm throwing can be described in distinct phases (**Table 17.1**).

Although skillful throwing involves the coordinated action of the entire body, this description focuses on the phases in which potential injury to the shoulder girdle and GH joint may occur. In the preparatory or cocking phase, the arm and hand are drawn behind the body through approximately 90° of abduction and 15° of horizontal abduction at the shoulder, accompanied by maximal external rotation of the humerus (170° to 180°), and shoulder distractive forces of 80% to 120% body weight are generated.[11] The combined motion causes heavy eccentric loading of the horizontal adductors and internal rotators of the shoulder. In particular, the subscapularis has its peak eccentric activity during the late cocking phase and serves to protect the anterior joint, which is under extreme tension. The pectoralis major and latissimus dorsi work eccentrically with the subscapularis to further protect the joint. This arm motion is facilitated by the action of the rhomboids contracting concentrically to pull the scapula and GH joint posteriorly, whereas the serratus anterior provides additional scapular stabilization. As the shoulder proceeds into horizontal abduction and external rotation, the humeral head tends to sublux, first posteriorly and then anteriorly, against the anterior capsule; consequently, tendinitis of the anterior muscle tendons is quite common.[12,13] Elbow extension

TABLE 17.1 Phases and Injuries of the Throwing Motion

PHASE	DESCRIPTION	COMMON INJURIES
Windup phase	From the first movement until the hands separate. The arms begin with a downward swing and then are raised overhead (gathered position). The shoulders and hips rotate as the arms go overhead; the body shifts from facing the target to being perpendicular to the line of throw. Balance is maintained on the "stance leg" as the lead leg or "stride leg" lifts up; the hip and knee flex at about the chest-high level.	—
Stride phase	From hand separation until the lead foot contacts the ground	—
Cocking phase	From foot contact until maximum shoulder external rotation	Anterior GH instability or subluxation Anteroinferior glenoid labral tears AC joint pathology Subacromial bursitis Strain to the medial rotators (i.e., pectoralis major and latissimus dorsi), biceps brachii, and triceps brachii Thoracic outlet syndrome
Acceleration phase	From maximum shoulder external rotation until ball release	Anterior subluxation Rotator cuff tendinitis or partial tears Subacromial bursitis Proximal humeral apophysitis Glenoid labral pathology Strain to the anterior deltoid, pectoralis major, subscapularis, or latissimus dorsi Bicipital tendinitis or biceps tendon subluxation
Deceleration and follow-through phase	From ball release until maximum shoulder internal rotation and balanced position is achieved	Rotator cuff tendinitis or partial tears Triceps tendinitis Biceps tendinitis or rupture Teres minor strain Posterior GH subluxation Posterior capsulitis Glenoid labral pathology AC joint pathology

begins just before maximal shoulder external rotation. This is immediately followed by the onset of humeral internal rotation.

During the acceleration or delivery phase, the ball is brought forward and released. Humeral horizontal adduction, elbow extension, and rapid internal rotation of the humerus at velocities that can exceed 7,000 deg/sec are produced by the pectoralis major, latissimus dorsi, and subscapularis and are coupled with relaxation of the rhomboids to enable anterior movement of the GH joint.[13] If the internal rotators are weak, however, the reduced ability to provide forceful arm depression can lead to increased external rotation, superior humeral migration, and impaired scapular rotation, which can cause or aggravate an impingement syndrome. During ball release, the elbow is almost fully extended and positioned slightly anterior to the trunk. Because throwing can involve a whip-like action of the arm, large stresses can be placed on the tendons, ligaments, and epiphyses of the throwing arm during delivery.[12]

Arm deceleration occurs after ball release and continues until maximal shoulder internal rotation occurs, and it consists primarily of a snap-like flexion of the wrist and pronation of the forearm. Large eccentric loads at the elbow and shoulder decelerate the arm. The infraspinatus, supraspinatus, teres major and minor, latissimus dorsi, and posterior deltoid play major roles in resisting shoulder distraction and anterior subluxation forces. If the rotator cuff muscles are weak, fatigued, or injured,

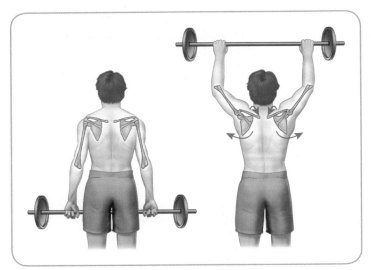

Figure 17.9. Scapulohumeral rhythm. The coordinated movement of the scapula needed to facilitate motion of the humerus is known as scapulohumeral rhythm. The arrows indicate the direction in which the scapulae must rotate to raise the arms.

the humeral head distracts and translates in an anterior direction, leading to stress on the posterior capsule. The serratus anterior contracts either concentrically or isometrically to decelerate scapular protraction and it is assisted by the middle trapezius and rhomboids. Injuries common to the specific phases of throwing are listed in **Table 17.1.**

Coordination of Shoulder Movements

The extensive ROM afforded by the shoulder results in part from the loose structure of the GH joint and in part from the proximity of the other shoulder articulations and the movement capabilities they provide. Movement at the shoulder typically involves some rotation at the SC, AC, and GH joints. For example, as the arm is elevated past 30° of abduction, or the first 45° to 60° of flexion, the scapula also rotates, contributing approximately one-third of the total rotational movement of the humerus. This important coordination of scapular and humeral movements, known as scapulohumeral rhythm, enables a much greater ROM at the shoulder than would occur if the scapula were fixed (**Fig. 17.9**). Also contributing to the first 90° of humeral elevation is the elevation of the clavicle through approximately 35° to 45° of motion at the SC joint. The AC joint contributes to overall movement capability as well, with rotation occurring during the first 30° of humeral elevation and then again as the arm is moved past 135°.[14]

Glenohumeral Flexion

The muscles that cross the GH joint anteriorly are positioned to contribute to flexion (**Figs. 17.5** and **17.6**). The anterior deltoid and clavicular pectoralis major are the primary shoulder flexors; the coracobrachialis and short head of the biceps brachii provide assistance. Because the biceps brachii also crosses the elbow joint, it is capable of exerting more force at the shoulder when the elbow is in full extension.

Glenohumeral Extension

When extension is not resisted, the action is caused by gravity. Eccentric contraction of the flexor muscles serves as a controlling or braking mechanism. When resistance to extension is offered, the posterior GH muscles, including the sternocostal pectoralis, latissimus dorsi, and teres major, act with assistance from the posterior deltoid and long head of the triceps brachii (**Figs. 17.5** and **17.6**).

Glenohumeral Abduction

The muscles superior to the GH joint produce abduction and include the middle deltoid and supraspinatus (**Fig. 17.5**). During the contribution of the middle deltoid, from approximately 90° through 180° of abduction, the infraspinatus, subscapularis, and teres minor produce inferiorly directed force to neutralize the superiorly directed, dislocating force produced by the middle deltoid. This action serves an important function in preventing impingement of the supraspinatus and subacromial bursa. The long head of the biceps brachii provides GH stability during abduction.

Glenohumeral Adduction

As with extension, adduction in the absence of resistance results from gravitational force, with the abductors controlling the speed of motion. When resistance is present, adduction is accomplished through the action of the muscles positioned on the inferior side of the GH joint, including the latissimus dorsi, teres major, and sternocostal pectoralis (**Fig. 17.5**). The short head of the biceps and long head of the triceps contribute minor assistance. When the arm is elevated above 90°, the coracobrachialis and subscapularis also assist.

TABLE 17.2 Primary Muscles Producing Movement at the Glenohumeral Joint

FLEXION	EXTENSION	ABDUCTION	ADDUCTION	MEDIAL ROTATION	LATERAL ROTATION
Anterior deltoid	Latissimus dorsi	Middle deltoid	Latissimus dorsi	Subscapularis	Infraspinatus
Pectoralis major (clavicular)	Pectoralis major (sternal)	Supraspinatus	Pectoralis major (sternal)	Teres major	Teres major
	Teres major		Teres major		

Lateral and Medial Rotation of the Humerus

Lateral rotators of the humerus lie on the posterior aspect of the humerus, including the infraspinatus and teres minor; the posterior deltoid provides assistance. Muscles on the anterior side of the humerus contribute to medial rotation; these include the subscapularis and teres major, with assistance from the pectoralis major, anterior deltoid, latissimus dorsi, and short head of the biceps (**Fig. 17.5**). **Table 17.2** summarizes the primary muscles that act on the arm.

KINETICS OF THE SHOULDER

Although the articulations of the shoulder girdle are interconnected, the GH joint sustains much greater loads compared to the other shoulder joints, primarily because the GH joint provides mechanical support for the entire arm. Although the weight of the arm is only approximately 9% of body weight, the length of the horizontally extended arm creates large torques that must be countered by the shoulder muscles. When these muscles contract to support the extended arm, large compression forces are generated inside the joint. The compression force acting on the articulating surfaces of the GH joint when the arm is abducted to 90° has been estimated to reach 50% of body weight.[14] This load is reduced by approximately half when the elbow is maximally flexed, but because of the shortened moment arm, the shoulder is considered to be a major load-bearing joint.

During the throwing motion, two critical instances increase the potential for shoulder injury. The first is during the cocking phase, when the arm has not quite reached maximum lateral rotation and a large internal rotation torque develops at the shoulder, heightening the possibility of a glenoid labral tear. The second occurs just after ball release, when both a large compression force and a large horizontal abduction torque are generated at the shoulder, creating the potential for rotator cuff tension failure and subacromial impingement.[12]

Muscles that attach to the humerus at small angles with respect to the glenoid fossa contribute more to shear than to compression at the joint. These muscles stabilize the humerus in the fossa when the contractions of the powerful muscles that move the humerus might otherwise dislocate the joint. Maximum shear force has been found to be present at the GH joint when the arm is elevated approximately 60°.[14]

PREVENTION OF SHOULDER CONDITIONS

Acute and chronic injuries to the shoulder complex are common in sport participation. Many contact and collision sports require some protective equipment, but in most cases, flexibility, physical conditioning, and proper technique are the primary factors that can reduce the risk of injury to this vulnerable area.

Protective Equipment

Contact and collision sports, such as football, lacrosse, and ice hockey, require shoulder pads to protect exposed bony protuberances from impact (see Chapter 3). Although shoulder pads do prevent some soft-tissue injuries in this region, they do not protect the GH joint from excessive motion. Several other commercial pads and braces that are used to protect the region are illustrated in Chapter 3.

Physical Conditioning

Lack of flexibility can predispose a patient to joint sprains and muscular strains. Warm-up exercises should focus on general joint flexibility and may be performed either alone or with a partner using proprioceptive neuromuscular facilitation (PNF) stretching techniques. Patients using the throwing motion in their sport should increase ROM in external rotation, because this has been shown to increase the velocity of the throwing arm and to decrease shearing forces on the GH joint. Several flexibility exercises for the shoulder complex are demonstrated in **Application Strategy 17.1**.

Strengthening programs should focus on muscles acting on both the GH and scapulothoracic regions. Strength in the infraspinatus, teres minor, and posterior shoulder musculature is necessary to

- Begin the cocking phase of throwing
- Fix the shoulder girdle during the acceleration phase
- Provide adequate muscle tension, with eccentric contractions, for smooth deceleration through the follow-through phase

A weakened supraspinatus is present in many chronic shoulder problems, particularly among throwers. Concentric and eccentric contractions with light resistance during the first 30° of abduction can strengthen this muscle. Strengthening the scapular stabilizers can be accomplished by doing push-ups or moving the arm through a resisted, diagonal pattern of external rotation and horizontal abduction. Other strengthening exercises are demonstrated in **Application Strategy 17.2**.

Proper Skill Technique

Coordinated muscle contractions are necessary for the smooth execution of the throwing motion. Any disruption in the sequencing of integrated movements can lead to additional stress on the GH joint and surrounding soft-tissue structures. High-speed photography, often used to record the mechanics of the throwing motion, can lead to early detection of improper technique. In addition to proper throwing technique, participants in contact and collision sports should be taught the shoulder-roll method of falling rather than falling on an outstretched arm. This technique reduces direct compression of the articular joints and disperses the force over a wider area.

ASSESSMENT OF SHOULDER CONDITIONS

> **?** A collegiate swimmer reports to the athletic training room with anterior pain in the right shoulder. How should the assessment of this injury progress to determine the extent and severity of injury?

The shoulder complex is a complicated region to assess because of the number of important structures that are located in such a small area. Furthermore, the biomechanical demands on each structure during overhead motion are not fully understood, so identification of all injured structures is difficult. As a result, each joint must be methodically assessed to determine any limitation of function. Improper biomechanical skill techniques are a leading cause of many acute and overuse injuries at the shoulder. Assessment of the patient's activity-specific techniques may determine if improper technique contributed to the injury. By correcting minor mechanical flaws in technique and identifying deficits in flexibility and strength, many shoulder injuries can be prevented. It also is important to remember that pain may be referred to the shoulder from the cervical region, heart, spleen, lungs, and other internal organs.

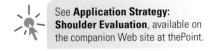

See **Application Strategy: Shoulder Evaluation**, available on the companion Web site at thePoint.

APPLICATION STRATEGY 17.1

Flexibility Exercises for the Shoulder Region

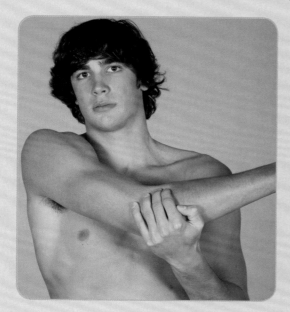

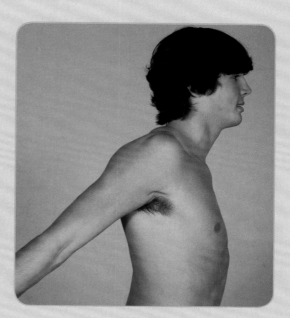

1. **Posterior capsular stretch.** Horizontally adduct the arm across the chest while the opposite hand assists the stretch.

3. **Anterior and posterior capsular stretch.** Hold on to both sides of a doorway with the hands behind the back. Straighten the arms while leaning forward. Repeat with the hands in front while leaning backward.

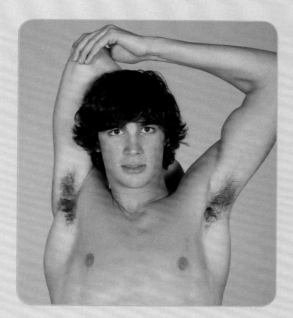

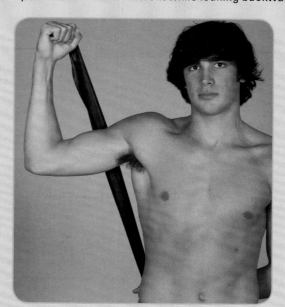

2. **Inferior capsular stretch.** Hold the involved arm over the head with the elbow flexed. Use the opposite hand to assist in the stretching. Add a side stretch.

4. **Medial and lateral rotators.** Using a towel, bat, or racquet, pull the arm to stretch it into lateral rotation. Repeat in medial rotation.

APPLICATION STRATEGY 17.2

Strengthening Exercises for the Shoulder Complex

1. Shoulder shrugs. Elevate the shoulders toward the ears and hold. Pull the shoulders back, pinch the shoulder blades together, and hold. Relax and repeat.
2. Scapular abduction (protraction). Lift the weight directly upward while also lifting the posterior shoulder from the table. Relax and repeat.
3. Scapular adduction (retraction). Perform bent-over rowing while flexing the elbows. When the end of the motion is reached, pinch the shoulder blades together and hold.
4. Bench press or incline press. Place the hands shoulder-width apart and push the barbell directly above the shoulder joint. This exercise should be performed with a spotter.
5. Bent arm lateral flies, supine position. Keeping the elbows slightly flexed, lift the dumbbells directly over the shoulders. Lower the dumbbells until they are parallel to the floor and then repeat. An alternate method is to move the dumbbells in a diagonal pattern. In the prone position, the exercise strengthens the trapezius.
6. Lateral pull-downs. In a seated position, grasp the handle and pull the bar behind the head. An alternate method is to pull the bar in front of the body.
7. Surgical tubing. Secure the tubing and then work in diagonal functional patterns similar to those skills experienced in a specific sport/activity.

HISTORY

 The injury assessment of the swimmer should begin with a history. What questions need to be asked to identify the cause and extent of this injury?

Questions about a shoulder injury should focus on the current primary complaint, past injuries to the region, and other factors that may have contributed to the current problem (e.g., referred pain, alterations in posture, change in technique, or overuse). Many conditions may be related to family history, age, improper biomechanical execution of skills, and recent changes in training programs. Because the shoulder and upper arm are common sites for referred pain from orthopedic or visceral origins, a complete examination of the cervical spine, thorax, and abdomen may be indicated, particularly when the patient presents a vague history of injury to the shoulder girdle.

 See **Application Strategy: Developing a History of the Injury**, available on the companion Web site at thePoint, for specific questions related to the shoulder region.

 The swimmer should be asked questions that address type of pain, changes in training regimen, strokes that are most painful, previous injuries and their treatment, and any medications being taken for the current injury.

OBSERVATION AND INSPECTION

 The history reveals a chronic injury. The swimmer reports a feeling of subluxation during the power phase of the crawl and butterfly strokes. The swimmer also complains of an inability to sleep on the right side of the body. Explain the observation component in the ongoing assessment of the swimmer.

On-site (e.g., field or court) assessment may be somewhat limited, because uniforms and protective equipment may obscure the region from observation and assessment. The clinician may need to reach under the protective pads to palpate the region and determine the presence of a possible fracture or major ligament damage. If necessary, the pads could be cut and gently removed to expose the area more fully. When conducting an assessment of an acute injury, the involved area should be inspected for presence of deformity, muscle guarding, bleeding, swelling, bruising, and dysfunction. The patient should be observed for signs of shock and reaction to pain. Following the initial examination, the patient may need to be removed from the on-site location to complete a more comprehensive assessment in the examination room.

When performing an evaluation of chronic or long-term injury, the patient should also be inspected for symmetry, hypertrophy, muscle atrophy, or previous surgical incisions. The affected limb should always be compared to the unaffected limb. The postural examination is an important component of the overall shoulder examination for patients presenting with long-term pain or dysfunction. The postural examination involves looking for faulty posture or congenital abnormalities that could place additional strain on the anatomical structures should be completed. The patient should be viewed from the anterior, lateral, and posterior views. The entire shoulder and arm should be as exposed as possible during the examination. Postural assessment is presented in Chapter 8 and should be reviewed if needed.

See **Application Strategy: Postural Assessment of the Shoulder Region**, available on the companion Web site at thePoint, for specific areas in which to focus for this region.

 Observation of the swimmer should include a postural assessment of the upper body. In addition, the injury site should be inspected for swelling, discoloration, deformity, muscle hypertrophy or atrophy, and other signs of existing or previous trauma.

PALPATION

? Observation of the swimmer reveals slight kyphosis. Otherwise, the patient has no abnormal findings. Explain the palpation for this injury.

Bilateral palpation can determine temperature, swelling, point tenderness, crepitus, deformity, muscle spasm, and cutaneous sensation. Increased skin temperature could indicate inflammation or infection; decreased skin temperature could indicate a reduction in circulation. Swelling should be differentiated between localized, extra-articular swelling and joint effusion. In the shoulder, intra-articular swelling prevents full adduction of the arm against the body. Crepitus may indicate an inflamed subacromial bursa, bicipital tenosynovitis, or irregular articular surface. Vascular pulses can be taken at the radial and ulnar arteries in the wrist, the brachial artery on the medial arm, or the axillary artery in the armpit.

Fractures can be assessed through palpation of pain at the fracture site, compression of the humeral head against the glenoid fossa, compression along the long axis of the humerus, percussion on a specific bony landmark, or use of a tuning fork. If a fracture or dislocation is suspected, circulatory and neural integrity distal to the site should be assessed immediately.

In general, when palpating the shoulder region, the clinician should stand behind the patient to begin bilateral palpation, which should move from proximal to distal. The areas that are anticipated to be most painful should be palpated last. The following structures should be palpated:

Anterior

1. Sternocleidomastoid muscle

2. SC joint, interclavicular ligament, SC ligament, and sternal end of the clavicle

3. Clavicle and costoclavicular ligament

4. AC joint, acromion process, and AC ligament

5. Coracoid process, pectoralis minor, short head of the biceps brachii, and coracoacromial ligament

6. Pectoralis major and anterior deltoid muscle

7. Greater tuberosity and the distal attachments of the supraspinatus, infraspinatus, and teres minor

8. Biceps brachii muscle and tendon. The bicipital groove should be palpated with the arm in external rotation. The lesser tubercle is medial to the groove where the subscapularis is attached.

9. Subacromial bursa and supraspinatus tendon. The arm should be in a position of extension.

Lateral

1. Middle deltoid muscle and greater tubercle

2. GH capsule

Posterior

1. Posterior deltoid and trapezius muscles

2. Spine of the scapula, medial and lateral borders, and inferior angle

3. Rhomboid muscles, latissimus dorsi, serratus anterior, levator scapulae, and scaleni

 Bilateral palpation includes bony and soft-tissue structures of the shoulder for point tenderness, swelling deformity, crepitus, sensation, and other signs of trauma.

PHYSICAL EXAMINATION TESTS

 Palpation reveals tenderness along the anterior and posterior GH joint. A click is felt during active shoulder abduction and external rotation. What anatomical structures could be involved with this injury, and what injury should be suspected?

The patient should be placed in a comfortable position for the physical examination. Depending on the history, some tests are compulsory, whereas others may be used to confirm or exclude suspected injury or pathology. Caution should be used while moving through the assessment, and bilateral comparison should always be performed.

Functional Tests

The arm and shoulder may act as an open kinetic chain when the hand is free to move or as a closed kinetic chain when the hand is fixed to a relatively immovable object. Depending on the activity-specific skills performed by the patient and when the pain occurs, the components of the kinetic chain can have different effects on the shoulder. The first movements to be performed are active movements.

Active Movements

Active movements may be performed in a seated or prone position. The movements that are expected to be most painful should be performed last. Because pain frequently is referred from the cervical region into the shoulder, active ROM should be performed initially at the neck. However, cervical spine involvement should be cleared or ruled out through history, inspection, and palpation prior to initiating active ROM. See Chapter 21 for discussion of cervical spine ROM testing. If pain is elicited on active motion at the neck, a full neck evaluation should be completed.

If no problems are noted during neck movement, the shoulder evaluation should continue. The patient should perform gross movement patterns at the shoulder, and the arms should be viewed from an anterior and a

 If findings are significant, and there is a high degree of suspicion of cervical spine involvement, the neck should be immobilized in a cervical collar, and the emergency action plan, including summoning emergency medical services, should be activated.

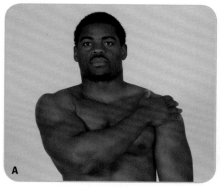 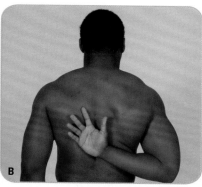 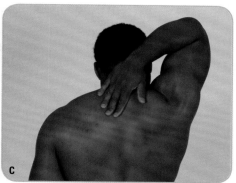

Figure 17.10. Apley scratch test. A, Medial rotation and adduction. The patient reaches in front of the head to touch the opposite shoulder. **B, Medial rotation, extension, and adduction.** The patient reaches behind the back to touch the inferior angle of the opposite scapula. **C, Abduction, flexion, and lateral rotation.** The patient reaches behind the head to touch the superior angle of the opposite scapula.

posterior view. When the clinician is standing behind the patient, it is important to note if the scapula and humerus move together in a freely coordinated motion. The scapula should not move until the humerus is elevated to at least 30°.

To facilitate active movement, Apley scratch test can be used to measure gross movement patterns at the shoulder and arm (**Fig. 17.10**). The advantage of these simple tests is that they quickly assess bilateral symmetry in gross motor movements. Any deficit can be easily seen and investigated in further detail.

The motions that should be assessed and the normal ROM for each are as follows:

- Shoulder abduction (170° to 180°)
- Shoulder flexion (160° to 180°)
- Shoulder extension (50° to 60°)
- Lateral or external rotation (80° to 90°)
- Medial or internal rotation (60° to 100°)
- Adduction (50° to 70°)
- Horizontal abduction/adduction (130°)
- Upward/downward rotation of the scapula

Goniometry measurements for the GH joint are illustrated in **Figure 17.11**.

Passive Range of Motion

If the patient is able to perform full ROM during active movements, gentle pressure should be applied at the extremes of motion to determine end feel. The normal end feels are as follows:

- **Tissue stretch**—shoulder flexion, extension, lateral rotation, medial rotation, abduction, and horizontal abduction

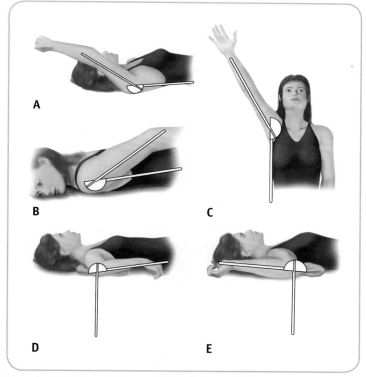

Figure 17.11. Goniometry measurements. A, Shoulder flexion. Align the proximal arm with the midaxillary line of the thorax with the fulcrum close to the acromion process. Align the distal arm along the humerus in line with the lateral epicondyle of the humerus. **B, Shoulder extension.** Use the same landmarks as for shoulder flexion. **C, Shoulder abduction.** The proximal arm is parallel to the midline of the sternum with the fulcrum close to the acromion process. Align the distal arm with the humerus using the medial epicondyle for reference. **D, Lateral rotation.** Flex the elbow at 90° with the fulcrum centered over the olecranon process. The proximal arm is placed perpendicular to the floor, with the distal arm aligned with the olecranon process and ulnar styloid process. **E, Medial rotation.** Use the same landmarks as for lateral rotation.

- Tissue **approximation**—shoulder adduction

- Tissue **stretch or approximation**—horizontal adduction of the shoulder

- **Bone-to-bone or tissue stretch**—abduction of the shoulder

Resisted Range of Motion

The hip and trunk should be stabilized during ROM testing to prevent any muscle substitution. This can be achieved through testing the patient in seated, supine, or prone position. The testing begins with the clinician placing the muscle on a stretch. In moving through the various motions, the clinician should apply gentle resistance throughout the full ROM. Motion should be assessed several times to note any weakness or fatigue. A painful arc is a common finding at the shoulder. As such, it is important to assess full ROM and to note if movement through an isolated ROM is particularly painful. Any sudden or jarring motions should be avoided, because this may lead to undue pain. Any lag or muscle weakness should be noted. Muscle actions that may cause extreme pain should be delayed until the final phase of resisted ROM testing. **Figure 17.12** demonstrates resisted scapular motions to be tested, and **Figure 17.13** demonstrates GH and elbow motions to be tested.

Manual Muscle Testing

If pain or weakness is found during resisted ROM, the clinician may decide to perform a manual muscle test to determine which muscle is damaged. To correctly apply the manual muscle testing techniques to the shoulder complex, the torso must be properly stabilized.[15] See **Table 17.3** for manual muscle testing procedures for the shoulder.

Stress Tests

By this point in the assessment, the history, observation, palpation, and functional testing should have established a strong suspicion regarding the structures that may be damaged. In using stress

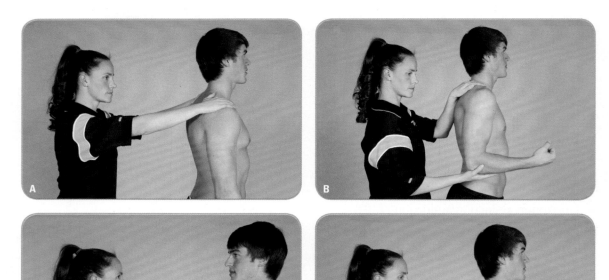

Figure 17.12. Resisted range of motion testing for the scapula. Myotomes are listed in parentheses. **A,** Elevation (C4). **B,** Depression. **C,** Protraction. **D,** Retraction.

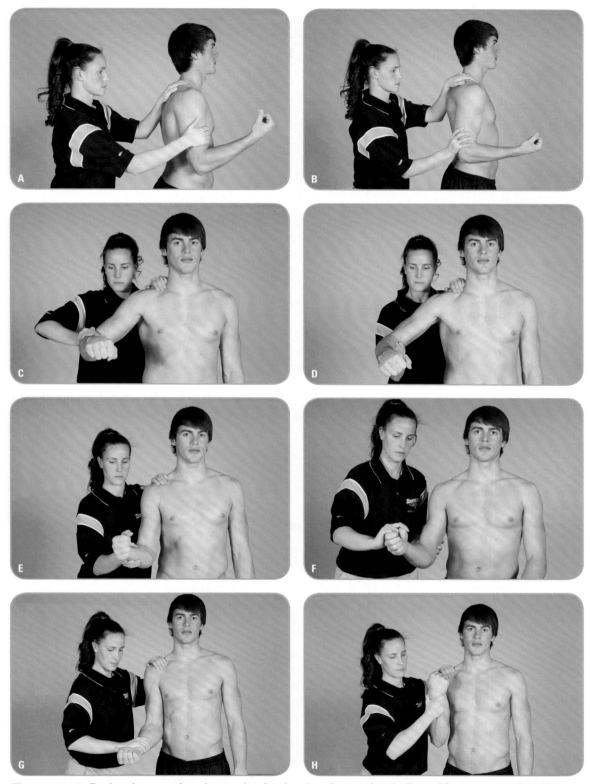

Figure 17.13. Resisted range of motion testing for the glenohumeral and elbow. Myotomes are listed in parentheses. **A,** Flexion. **B,** Extension. **C,** Abduction (C5). **D,** Adduction. **E,** External or lateral rotation. **F,** Internal or medial rotation. **G,** Elbow flexion (C6). **H,** Elbow extension (C7).

TABLE 17.3 Manual Muscle Testing of Selected Muscles of the Shoulder Complex

MUSCLE	JOINT POSITIONING	APPLY PRESSURE
Coracobrachialis	Patient is seated with forearm supinated, elbow completely flexed, and GH joint laterally rotated.	To the anteromedial surface of the lower one-third of the humerus in the direction of GH extension
Deltoid	Patient is seated with GH abducted to 90° without rotation. Elbow is flexed to 90°.	To the distal end of the humerus on the dorsal surface in the direction of adduction
Anterior deltoid	Patient is seated with GH abducted and slightly flexed with humerus in slight lateral rotation. Elbow is flexed to 90°.	To the anteromedial aspect of humerus in the direction of adduction and slight extension
Posterior deltoid	Patient is seated with GH abducted, in slight extension and slight medial rotation. Elbow is flexed to 90°.	To the posterolateral aspect of the humerus in the direction of adduction and flexion
Upper pectoralis major	Patient is supine, with GH joint in 90° of flexion and slight medial rotation and some adduction. Elbow is fully extended.	To the palmer surface of the forearm in the direction of horizontal abduction
Pectoralis minor	Patient is supine with shoulder protracted.	To the anterior aspect of the humeral head in the direction of retraction or toward the table
Latissimus dorsi	The patient is prone with GH extended and internally rotated so that forearm is in fully pronated. Patient looks away from testing side.	To the forearm in the direction of abduction and flexion
Rhomboid	Patient is prone with GH at 90° of horizontal abduction, elbow fully extended and thumb pointing down. Scapula should be adducted and elevated.	To the ulnar side of the forearm in a downward direction toward the floor
Upper trapezius	Patient is sitting with shoulder elevated and head laterally flexed *toward* testing side but rotated *away* from side being tested.	To the AC joint/top of shoulder in the opposite direction
Supraspinatus	Patient is standing with arm at side and facing away for side being tested.	To the forearm in the direction of adduction as the patient attempts to initiate abduction

For more in depth descriptions and illustrations, see Kendall FP, McCreary EK, Provance PG, et al. *Muscles: Testing and Function with Posture and Pain.* 5th ed. Baltimore, MD: Lippincott Williams & Wilkins; 2005.

tests, only those tests that are absolutely necessary should be performed (**Table 17.4**). In moving through the various tests, the clinician should begin with gentle stress and apply it several times to note any weakness or instability.

Test for Sternoclavicular Instability

SC instability can be determined by assessing the amount of joint play at SC. To assess **SC joint play**, the patient should be supine. The clinician gently grasps the midpoint of the clavicle and attempts to move the clavicle downward, upward, anteriorly, and posteriorly to determine any instability or increased pain.[16] Pain that is present in all movements may stem from an SC sprain, damage to the SC joint disk, or complete disruption of the joint capsule, which would indicate a possible dislocation or subluxation of the joint.

Tests for Acromioclavicular Joint Instability

■ Paxinos Sign
The patient sits with the affected arm by the side of the chest wall. The clinician's hand is placed over the affected shoulder so that the thumb rests under the posterolateral aspect of the acromion and the index and other fingers of the same or contralateral hand are placed superior to the midpart of the ipsilateral clavicle. The clinician then applies pressure to the acromion with the thumb in an

TABLE 17.4 Common Stress and Special Tests Performed at the Shoulder

JOINT	TEST
SC joint	SC instability test (SC joint play)
Acromioclavicular joint	AC instability test (AC joint play) AC distraction test (AC traction test) AC compression test (AC shear test)
GH instability, anterior	Apprehension test ("crank test") Relocation test Anterior load and shift test
GH instability, posterior	Posterior load and shift test Posterior apprehension test
GH instability, inferior	Sulcus sign
Labral lesions	Clunk test Compression rotation test
Impingement tests	Neer shoulder impingement test Anterior impingement test (Hawkins-Kennedy test)
Muscle tendon pathology	Serratus anterior weakness test Pectoralis major contracture test Lift-off test for subscapularis Drop arm test Empty can (Centinela) supraspinatus test Transverse humeral ligament test Yergason test Speed's test Ludington test
Thoracic outlet syndrome	Adson test Allen test Costoclavicular syndrome (military brace) test

anterosuperior direction and inferiorly to the midpart of the clavicular shaft with the index and long fingers. The test is positive if pain is felt or increased in the region of the AC joint. The Paxinos sign has high sensitivity (79).[17]

■ Acromioclavicular Instability Test

AC instability can be determined by assessing the amount joint play present at the AC. To assess **AC joint play**, the patient should be supine. The clinician gently grasps the midpoint of the clavicle and attempts to move the clavicle downward, upward, anteriorly, and posteriorly to determine any instability or increased pain. An inferior glide will stress the AC ligament while a superior glide stresses the conoid, trapezoid, and AC ligaments. The coracoclavicular ligament and AC ligament are stressed by an anterior glide and a posterior glide stresses the posterior aspect of the AC ligament. The clinician grasps the distal clavicle and applies pressure in all four directions to determine stability and any increase in pain.[16]

■ Acromioclavicular Distraction

This test is also referred to as the AC traction test and, as the name implies, involves applying a downward (or traction) force to the AC joint. Assessment involves grasping the arm of the involved shoulder in one hand and applying steady downward traction while palpating the joint with the other hand (**Fig. 17.14A**). A positive test produces pain and/or joint movement. If the AC joint is unstable, downward traction on the upper extremity leads to downward movement of the acromion process away from the clavicle.

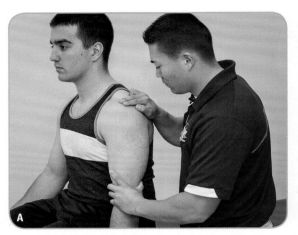
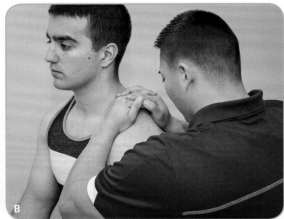

Figure 17.14. **Acromioclavicular testing. A,** AC traction. **B,** AC compression.

Acromioclavicular Compression Test

The AC compression test is also known as the AC shear test[18] and has reported sensitivity ranging from 41 to 100 and specificity ranging from 92 to 97.[19,20] To perform the test, the patient should be seated and in a relaxed position. The clinician places the heel of one hand over the clavicle and the heel of the opposite hand over the spine of the scapula and applies a gentle compression (**Fig. 17.14B**). Pain or abnormal motion at the AC joint is positive and implies AC joint instability.[18]

Tests for Glenohumeral Joint Instability

■ Apprehension Test ("Crank Test") for Anterior Instability

This test involves positioning the patient in a supine position and then slowly abducting and externally rotating the patient's humerus (**Fig. 17.15A**). If the patient does not allow passive movement to the extremes of motion or shows apprehension in his or her facial expression, the test is considered to be positive for chronic anterior subluxation or dislocation of the GH joint. This motion should always be done slowly to prevent recurrence of a dislocation. The apprehension test has moderate sensitivity (58) and strong specificity (78).[16]

■ Relocation Test for Anterior Instability

Position for this test is identical to the apprehension test. If the patient demonstrates a positive apprehension test, the clinician slowly applies a posterior stress to the arm (**Fig. 17.15B**). The patient's

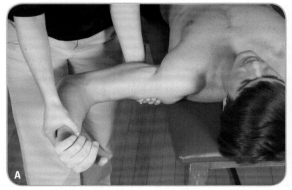
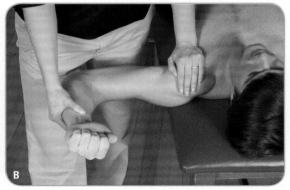

Figure 17.15. **Glenohumeral anterior instability. A, Apprehension or "crank" test.** The clinician should apply gentle pressure in an abducted and laterally rotated position. **B, Relocation test.** The clinician applies abduction and lateral rotation combined with posterior translation of the humerus.

apprehension and pain should diminish. In addition, further lateral rotation of the GH joint may be possible before the apprehension returns. This test is considered to be positive if pain decreases during the maneuver, even if the patient showed no apprehension. If the arm is released in the newly acquired range, any pain and forward translation of the humeral head indicates a positive sign. The resulting pain from this release procedure may be caused by anterior shoulder instability, labral lesion (i.e., Bankart or superior labrum anteroposterior [SLAP] lesion), or bicipital tendinitis.[16,18] The release should be performed slowly, because it may dislocate the joint, leading to distrust on the part of the patient. Lateral rotation should be released before the posterior stress is released.

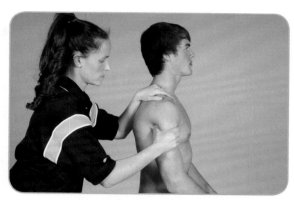

Figure 17.16. Load and shift test. The humerus is compressed into the glenoid to load the humeral head. Subsequently, the clinician pushes the humeral head anteriorly or posteriorly, noting the amount of shift or translation.

▪ Anterior Load and Shift Test

The load and shift test has a strong sensitivity (90) and specificity (85).[21] While the patient is seated and the test arm is resting on the thigh, the clinician stands or sits slightly behind the patient and stabilizes the shoulder with one hand over the clavicle and scapula. The head of the humerus is grasped with the clinician's other hand, placing the thumb over the posterior humeral head and the fingers over the anterior humeral head (**Fig. 17.16**). The clinician then gently pushes the humerus into the glenoid to "seat" it properly in the glenoid fossa. This is the "load" portion of the test, and it is necessary for true translation to occur. If the load is not applied, movement is greater, and the "feel" is altered. While pushing the humeral head anteriorly (i.e., assessing anterior instability) or posteriorly (i.e., assessing posterior instability), the amount of translation should be noted. This is the "shift" portion of the test. Normally, the head translates 0% to 25% of the diameter of the humeral head. The test is considered to be positive if translation is between 25% and 50% and the head feels as if it is riding over the glenoid rim but spontaneously reduces.[18]

▪ Posterior Load and Shift Test

In a posterior load and shift test, posterior translation of 50% of the humeral head is considered to be normal. Differences between the normal and injured sides should be bilaterally compared for the amount of translation and the ease with which that translation occurs. This comparison, along with the patient's symptoms, is considered to be more important than the amount of movement that occurs. If multidirectional instability is present, both anterior and posterior translation may be excessive on the affected side as compared to the normal side. The test also may be done in a supine position.[18]

▪ Posterior Apprehension Test

While the patient is supine, the arm is moved into forward flexion and internal rotation as a steady downward force is applied on the elbow to drive the humeral head posteriorly on the glenoid fossa (**Fig. 17.17**). While applying the axial load, the clinician horizontally adducts and medially rotates the arm. A positive test is indicated by apprehension, resistance to further motion, or reproduction of symptoms. Reproducing pain is more likely to occur than apprehension. A positive sign indicates a possible posterior dislocation.

▪ Sulcus Sign

The clinician applies traction to the humerus to determine the integrity of the supportive structures. If the space widens between the acromion process and humeral head, producing an indentation or "sulcus," the test is considered to be positive for

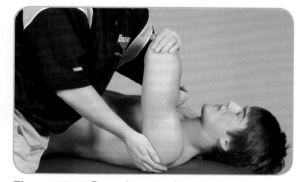

Figure 17.17. Posterior apprehension test. The clinician applies a steady downward force on the elbow to displace the humeral head posteriorly on the glenoid fossa.

inferior instability. In the sulcus test, only the humerus is distracted away from both the clavicle and scapula. In comparison, the AC distraction test involves distraction of both the humerus and scapula away from the clavicle. The sulcus sign has very low sensitivity (17) but strong specificity (93).[22]

Special Tests

A variety of special tests can be used for detecting shoulder injury or related pathology (e.g., labral lesions, impingement, muscle-tendon trauma, or thoracic outlet syndrome) (**Table 17.4**). In general, special tests occur across planes and are not graded.

Tests for Labral Lesions

■ Clunk Test

The clunk test is also referred to as the jerk test. Although the test has strong specificity (94), it is only moderately sensitive (52).[16] While the patient is supine, the clinician places one hand on the posterior aspect of the shoulder under the humeral head. Next, the humerus is grasped above the elbow, and the arm is fully abducted over the patient's head. The hand over the humeral head applies a slow push in an anterior direction while the other hand moves the humerus into lateral rotation (**Fig. 17.18A**). A positive test results in a clunk or grinding sound, indicating a tear of the labrum. This test also may cause apprehension if anterior instability is present.

■ Compression Rotation Test (Grind Test)

The patient is supine, with the arm positioned at approximately 20° of abduction and the elbow flexed. The humerus is slowly compressed into the glenoid fossa by pushing on the elbow with one hand while the other hand rotates the humerus medially and laterally (**Fig. 17.18B**). If a snapping or catching sensation is present as the humeral head is felt, the test is considered to be positive for a labral tear (i.e., Bankart or SLAP lesion). The grind test has poor to moderate sensitivity (38) and moderate to strong specificity (78).[16]

Tests for Shoulder Impingement

■ Neer Shoulder Impingement Test

The patient is seated and the arm is placed in anatomical position. First, the clinician stabilizes the posterior shoulder. Next, the clinician grasps the patient's arm at the elbow joint and passively moves the arm through forward flexion (**Fig. 17.19A**). An easy way to remember the name and action of the test is to passively move the patient's arm *NEAR* the *EAR*. The test is considered to be positive if pain occurs with motion, particularly near the end of the ROM. A positive test indicates impingement of the supraspinatus or the long head of the biceps tendon between the greater tuberosity of the

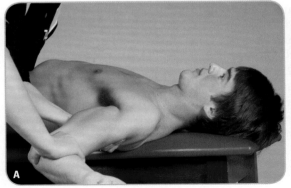
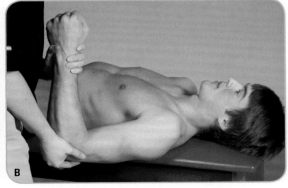

Figure 17.18. Glenoid labral pathology. A, Clunk test. Using the hand placed under the humeral head, the clinician applies an anterior force while the other hand rotates the humerus into lateral rotation. **B, Compression rotation test.** With the arm slightly abducted and the elbow flexed, the clinician applies a compression force along the long axis of the humerus while the other hand rotates the humerus medially and laterally.

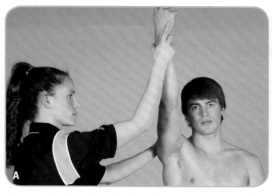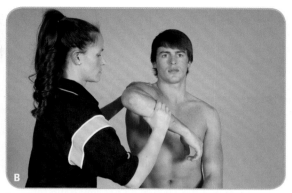

Figure 17.19. Anterior impingement tests. A, Neer shoulder impingement test. The arm is internally rotated and forcibly flexed forward to jam the greater tuberosity against the anteroinferior surface of the acromion. **B, Anterior impingement test.** An alternate method is to forcibly, medially rotate the proximal humerus when the arm is forward flexed to 90°. (This also is known as the Hawkins-Kennedy impingement test.)

humerus and acromion process or coracoacromial arch. The Neer impingement test has almost equal sensitivity (68) and specificity (68.7) with a positive likelihood ratio of 80.4%.[23]

■ Anterior Impingement Test (Hawkins-Kennedy Test)

This test involves internally rotating and abducting the humerus through shoulder flexion while depressing the scapula. This action forces the greater tubercle underneath the anteroinferior border of the acromion process. The arm is returned to 90° of abduction (with the elbow flexed at 90°) and then is horizontally adducted across the chest while maintaining internal rotation of the humerus (**Fig. 17.19B**). Pain or apprehension may indicate an overuse injury to the supraspinatus or biceps brachii tendon. This test also is called the Hawkins-Kennedy impingement test. This test has higher sensitivity (71.5) than specificity (66.3) with relative strong positive predictive value (79.7%).[23]

■ Painful Arc Sign

The patient is asked to actively abduct the arm through a full ROM if possible and is then asked to indicate if and when pain was experienced while performing the motion. The test is positive if pain was experienced between 60° and 120° of motion (**Fig. 17.20**). This test has a strong positive prediction value (88.2), with strong sensitivity (73.5) and specificity (81.1), indicating that it is a clinically useful test for detecting shoulder impingement.[23]

Tests for Muscle Tendon Pathology

■ Serratus Anterior Weakness

Weakness of the serratus anterior, often called winging of the scapula, is determined by having the patient perform a push-up against the wall. If the muscle is weak or the long thoracic nerve is injured, the medial border of the scapula pulls away from the chest wall.

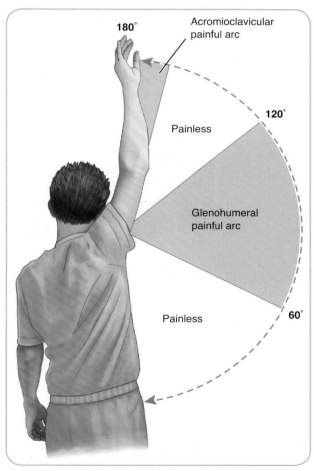

Figure 17.20. Painful arc sign. As the patient actively abducts the shoulder through full ROM, pain occurring between 60° and 120° is positive for impingement syndrome.

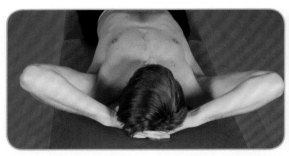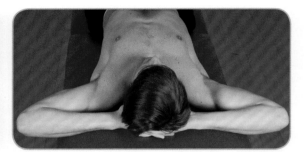

Figure 17.21. **Pectoralis major contracture test.** The patient begins by clasping both hands behind the head. The elbows are then slowly lowered to the table. A positive test, indicating a tight pectoralis major muscle, occurs if the elbows do not reach the table.

■ Pectoralis Major Contracture Test

The patient lies supine, with the hands clasped together behind the head. The patient is instructed to lower the arms until the elbows touch the examination table (**Fig. 17.21**). A positive test occurs if the elbows do not reach the table, indicating a tight pectoralis major muscle.

■ Lift-Off Test for Subscapularis

The patient stands with the dorsum of the hand on the lumbar region of the back. The patient is instructed to lift the hand away from the back (**Fig. 17.22**). An inability to perform this action indicates a lesion of the subscapularis muscle. Abnormal motion of the scapula during the test indicates scapular instability. If the medial border of the scapula wings during the test, the rhomboids also may be affected.

■ Drop Arm Test

This test assesses the integrity of the supraspinatus muscle and tendon. The patient is positioned with the shoulder abducted to 90° with no humeral rotation. The patient is instructed to slowly lower the arm to the side. The test is positive if the arm does not lower smoothly or increased pain is felt during the motion.

An alternate test is to abduct the arm to 90° with no rotation. The patient is instructed to hold that position while the clinician applies downward resistance to the distal end of the humerus (**Fig. 17.23A**). A positive test is indicated if the patient is unable to maintain the arm in the abducted position. The drop arm test has poor sensitivity (26.9) and strong specificity (88.4).[23]

■ Empty Can (Centinela) Test and Full Can Test for Supraspinatus Pathology

Both arms are positioned at 90° of abduction. The arms are then horizontally adducted approximately 30° to 60°, and the humerus is internally rotated, with the thumbs pointing downward ("empty can position") (**Fig. 17.23B**). The clinician applies a downward pressure proximal to the elbow. Pain and/or weakness should be assessed. The arms should rebound to the 90° abducted position. A positive test indicates a tear to the supraspinatus muscle or tendon. However, because the testing the supraspinatus in the "empty can" position also engages the middle deltoid and subscapularis, the specificity of the test is called into question.[24]

The **full can test**, which is identical to the empty can test except the humerus is externally rotated, as if holding a full can, is recommended (**Fig. 17.23C**). The subscapularis and middle deltoid are less active in this position[24] and is thought to be less pain provoking.[16]

■ Transverse Humeral Ligament Test

The patient is positioned with the shoulder in 90° of abduction and external rotation and the elbow flexed at 90°. The clinician places the fingers

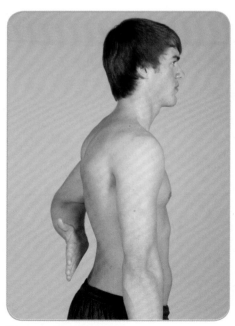

Figure 17.22. **Lift-off test.** Failure to lift the hand away from the small of the back indicates a weakened subscapularis muscle, scapular instability, or weak rhomboids.

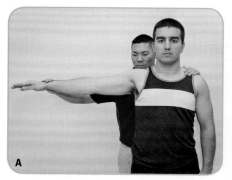
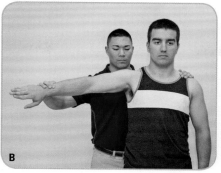
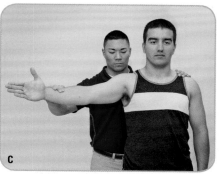

Figure 17.23. Supraspinatus testing. A, Drop arm test. The clinician instructs the patient to abduct the humerus to 90° and subsequently applies mild, downward pressure on the distal humerus. **B, Empty can test.** The patient horizontally adducts the arm approximately 30° to 60° with the humerus internally rotated. The clinician applies mild, downward pressure on the distal humerus. **C, Full can test.** The patient horizontally adducts the arm approximately 30° to 60° with the humerus in anatomical or neutral position. The clinician applies mild, downward pressure on the distal humerus.

over the bicipital groove. A torn transverse humeral ligament is indicated by an audible and/or palpable snap, which may be accompanied by pain, as the arm is moved into internal rotation (**Fig. 17.24**).

Yergason Test for Bicipital Tendinitis
The patient should be positioned with the arm stabilized against the body, the elbow flexed at 90°, and the forearm pronated. The clinician instructs the patient to supinate the forearm, flex the elbow, and externally rotate the humerus. Simultaneously, the clinician resists the motion with one hand while applying downward traction on the elbow with the other hand (**Fig. 17.25A**). The test is considered to be positive for biceps tendinopathy without the presence of popping.[16,22] If pain and popping or just popping/snapping present over the bicipital groove, the test is positive for tear of the transverse humeral ligament.[16]

Speed's Test for Bicipital Tendinitis
In this test, the tendon moves over the bone during movement rather than simply having tension applied to it. As such, it provides a more effective, accurate result than Yergason test.[18] The arm is supinated, with the elbow fully extended. The clinician places one hand over the bicipital groove and resists forward flexion of the arm with the other hand. A positive test results in tenderness over the groove (**Fig. 17.25B**). However, due to this test's low specificity (14) and high sensitivity (90), false positives may be found.[22]

Ludington Test for Biceps Brachii Pathology
The patient may sit or stand during this test. The patient's hands are placed on top of the head with the fingers interlocked. The clinician should stand behind the patient while palpating the long head of the biceps brachii tendon in the bicipital groove. The patient alternately contracts and relaxes the biceps brachii muscles (**Fig. 17.26**). If no contraction or tension is palpated on one side, a rupture of the long head of the biceps brachii likely is present.

Tests for Thoracic Outlet Syndrome

Adson Test
This test begins by having the clinician palpate the radial pulse. Next, the patient is instructed to turn the head toward the affected shoulder and extend the head. The clinician then slowly

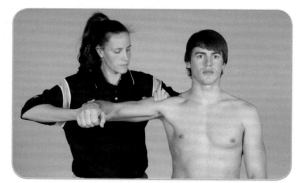

Figure 17.24. Transverse humeral ligament test. The patient is instructed to place the extended arm in 90° of abduction and external rotation. The clinician places one's fingers over the bicipital groove and moves the arm into internal rotation. In a positive test, an audible or palpable snap, which may be accompanied by pain, occurs during internal rotation.

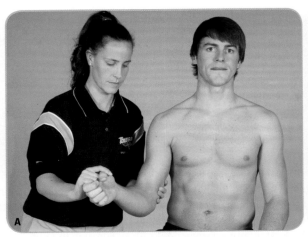
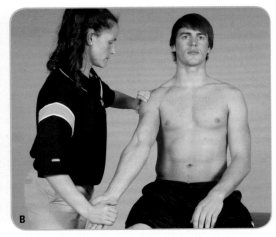

Figure 17.25. Bicipital tendinitis. A, Yergason test. The clinician stabilizes the flexed arm against the body, with the forearm pronated. The patient is asked to supinate the forearm, flex the elbow, and externally rotate the humerus. The clinician applies resistance throughout the ROM and, with the other hand, simultaneously applies downward traction on the elbow. **B, Speed's test.** The patient is instructed to supinate the hand, with the elbow fully extended. The clinician places one hand over the bicipital groove and resists forward flexion of the arm.

extends and laterally rotates the humerus (**Fig. 17.27A**). The patient is instructed to take a deep breath and hold it. A diminished or absent pulse indicates a positive test, verifying occlusion of the subclavian artery between the anterior and middle scalene muscles. This test sometimes is referred to as the anterior scalene syndrome test. Differing values for the diagnostic accuracy have been reported for the Adson test. One source reported Adson as having strong sensitivity (79) but poor specificity (7%),[16] whereas a second source reported strong specificity (89 to 100) for the Adson test without posting sensitivity values.[22] It appears that the results of the Adson test should be considered within the context of findings gathered throughout the examination process.

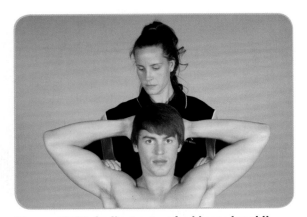

Figure 17.26. Ludington test for biceps brachii pathology. The clinician stands behind the patient and palpates the long head of the biceps brachii while the patient contracts the biceps by applying force to the top of the head. The test is positive for rupture of the long head of the biceps brachii tendon if decreased or no tension is felt under the involved tendon.

■ Allen Test

Similar to Adson test, the clinician palpates the radial pulse while the patient abducts the shoulder, flexes the elbow to 90°, and looks toward the opposite shoulder (**Fig. 17.27B**). Next, the clinician instructs the patient to take a deep breath and hold it. A diminished or absent pulse indicates a positive test, suggesting that the pectoralis minor muscle is compressing the neurovascular bundle. It is important to note, however, that this test often produces false positive results.

An alternate position, called the Halstead maneuver, is performed with the arm extended and the neck hyperextended and rotated to the opposite side. While palpating the radial pulse, the clinician applies a downward traction to the arm. An absent or diminished pulse indicates a positive test for thoracic outlet syndrome.

■ Costoclavicular Syndrome (Military Brace) Test

The patient stands in a relaxed position. The clinician stands behind the patient and palpates the radial pulse. Next, the patient retracts the shoulders as if coming to military attention. The clinician then extends and abducts the arm to 30° while the patient hyperextends the neck (**Fig. 17.28**). If the radial pulse diminishes or disappears, it indicates that the subclavian artery is being blocked by the costoclavicular structures of the shoulder.

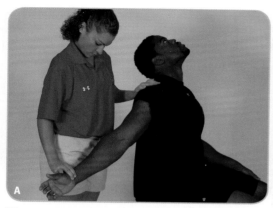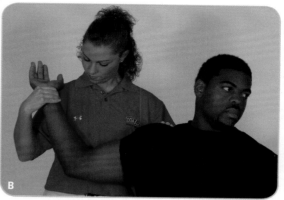

Figure 17.27. Thoracic outlet compression syndrome. A, Adson maneuver. The clinician extends and externally rotates the humerus while the patient extends the head. **B, Allen test.** The clinician abducts the shoulder and flexes the elbow while the patient looks toward the opposite shoulder. An alternate position is to extend the elbow and apply downward traction while the patient hyperextends the neck and rotates the head to the opposite side (Halstead maneuver).

Neurological Tests

Neurological integrity can be assessed with the use of myotomes, reflexes, and cutaneous patterns that include both the segmental dermatomes and peripheral nerve patterns.

Myotomes

Isometric muscle testing should be performed in the following motions to test specific myotomes in the upper extremity:

- Scapular elevation (C4) (**Fig. 17.12A**)

- Shoulder abduction (C5) (**Fig. 17.13C**)

- Elbow flexion and/or wrist extension (C6) (**Fig. 17.13G**)

- Elbow extension and/or wrist flexion (C7) (**Fig. 17.13H**)

- Thumb extension and/or ulnar deviation (C8)

- Abduction and/or adduction of the hand intrinsics (T1)

Reflexes

Reflexes in the upper extremity include the biceps (C5), brachioradialis (C6), and triceps (C7). The biceps reflex is tested with the patient's arm flexed and supported by the clinician's forearm. The clinician's thumb is placed over the biceps tendon, and the thumb is struck with the reflex hammer using a quick, downward thrust (**Fig. 17.29A**). A normal response is slight elbow flexion. The brachioradialis reflex is tested with the patient's arm flexed, forearm in a neutral position and resting on a support (**Fig. 17.29B**). Strike the tendon of the brachioradialis slightly proximal to the insertion at the base of the styloid process of the radius. A normal response is slight supination. To test the triceps reflex, passively extend the GH joint to 90° and support the limb at the distal humerus, just above the joint. The triceps reflex is tested with the patient's arm abducted and extended with the elbow flexed. The triceps tendon is placed on a slight stretch, and the triceps tendon is then tapped with the reflex hammer (**Fig. 17.29C**). A normal response is slight elbow extension.

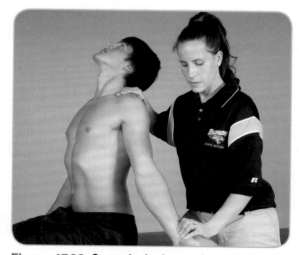

Figure 17.28. Costoclavicular syndrome test. The patient retracts the shoulders as if coming to military attention. The arm is extended and abducted approximately 30° while the head and neck are hyperextended. If the radial pulse disappears, it indicates that the subclavian artery is blocked by the costoclavicular structures in the shoulder.

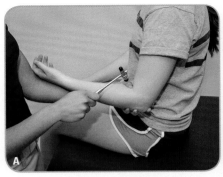
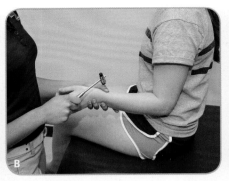
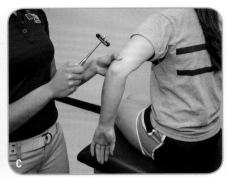

Figure 17.29. Reflex testing. A, Biceps reflex (C5). **B,** Brachioradialis reflect (C6). **C,** Triceps reflex (C7).

Cutaneous Patterns

The segmental nerve dermatome patterns for the shoulder region are illustrated in **Figure 17.30**. The peripheral nerve cutaneous patterns are illustrated in **Figure 17.31**. Bilateral testing should be performed for altered sensation with sharp and dull touch by running the open hand and fingernails over the neck, shoulder, anterior and posterior chest walls, and both sides of the arms.

Activity-Specific Functional Tests

Occasionally, activity-specific functional movements are the only activities that reproduce signs and symptoms. Throwing a ball, performing a swimming stroke, doing the arm part of jumping jacks, or performing an overhead serve or spike may replicate the painful pattern. The clinician should look for smooth, coupled motion of the scapulothoracic and GH joints. Disharmony constitutes scapulothoracic dyskinesia, which is an inability to perform fluid, voluntary movements. Based on knowledge of the mechanics of the motion, it may be possible to narrow down the few definitive results of the assessment to determine the actual injury. These movements also commonly are used to determine when the patient can return to participation in activity. All functional patterns should be fluid and pain-free.

 The assessment of the swimmer suggests that the humerus, glenoid fossa, glenoid labrum, rotator cuff muscles, and anterior GH ligament could be involved with this injury. The swimmer should be suspected of having recurrent GH dislocations or subluxations.

SPRAINS TO THE SHOULDER COMPLEX

? A soccer player fell on an outstretched arm. A physician diagnosed a type II AC sprain. What are the signs and symptoms of a type II AC sprain?

Ligamentous injuries to the SC, AC, and GH joints can result from compression, tension, and shearing forces occurring in a single episode or from repetitive overload. A common method of injury is a fall or direct hit on the lateral aspect of the acromion as well as a fall on an outstretched hand (FOSH). The force is transmitted first to the site of impact, then to the AC joint and the clavicle, and finally, to the SC joint. Failure can occur at any one of these sites. Acute sprains are common in hockey, rugby, football, soccer, equestrian sports, and the martial arts.

Sternoclavicular Joint Sprain

Etiology

The SC joint is the main axis of rotation for movements of the clavicle and scapula. The majority of injuries result from compression related to a direct blow, as when another participant lands on a supine patient or, more commonly, by indirect forces transmitted from a blow to the shoulder or a fall on an outstretched arm. The disruption typically drives the proximal clavicle superior, medial, and anterior, disrupting the costoclavicular and SC ligaments and leading to anterior displacement.

Signs and Symptoms

Grade I (first-degree) injuries are characterized by point tenderness and mild pain over the SC joint, with no visible deformity. The SC joint play test will elicit pain and or motion. Grade II (second-degree) injuries involve a joint subluxation that leads to bruising, swelling, and pain. The patient is unable to horizontally adduct the arm without considerable pain and may hold the arm forward and close to the body, supporting it across the chest, which indicates disruption of the stabilizing ligaments. In addition, scapular protraction and retraction can reproduce pain associated with ligamentous or disk damage. Grade III (third-degree) sprains involve a prominent displacement of the sternal end of the clavicle and may involve a fracture. The patient has a complete rupture of the SC and costoclavicular ligaments. Pain is severe when the shoulders are brought together by a lateral force.

Although rare, posterior, or retrosternal displacement is more serious because of the potential injury to the esophagus, trachea, internal thoracic artery and vein, and brachiocephalic and subclavian artery and vein. The most common mechanism of injury is a blow to the posterolateral aspect of the shoulder with the arm adducted and flexed, such as a fall on the shoulder that displaces the distal clavicle anteriorly.[25] This action may occur during a piling-on injury in football; less commonly, the injury may be caused by a direct blow to the anteromedial end of the clavicle. The patient has a palpable depression between the sternal end of the clavicle and manubrium, is unable to perform shoulder protraction, and may have difficulty swallowing and breathing. The patient also may complain of numbness and weakness of the upper extremity secondary to the compression of structures in the thoracic inlet. If the venous vascular vessels are impinged, the patient may have venous congestion or engorgement in the ipsilateral arm and a diminished radial pulse.[25]

Management

Grade I sprains of the SC joint are treated with rest, ice, and anti-inflammatory drugs. The arm may be immobilized with a sling for 1 to 2 weeks, followed by early ROM exercises. Grade II sprains may require longer immobilization (3 to 6 weeks) in a sling or a soft figure eight brace, followed by ROM exercises.

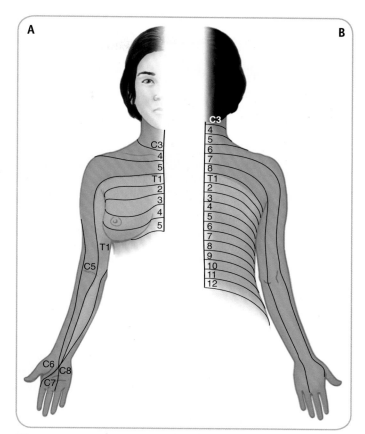

Figure 17.30. Dermatome patterns for the shoulder region. A, Anterior view. **B,** Posterior view.

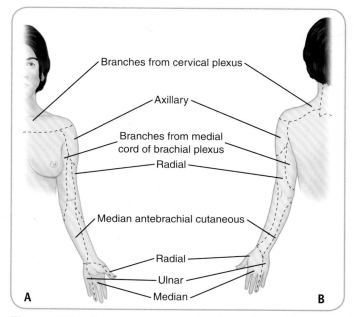

Figure 17.31. Cutaneous patterns for the peripheral nerves. A, Anterior view. **B,** Posterior view.

TABLE 17.5 Management of a Sternoclavicular Sprain

SIGNS AND SYMPTOMS	FIRST DEGREE	SECOND DEGREE	THIRD DEGREE
Deformity	None	Slight prominence of medial end of the clavicle	Gross prominence of medial end of the clavicle
Swelling	Slight	Moderate	Severe
Palpable pain	Mild	Moderate	Severe
Movement	Usually unlimited but may have discomfort with movement	Unable to abduct the arm or horizontally adduct the arm across the chest without noticeable pain	Limited as in second degree but pain is more severe
Treatment	Ice, rest, and immobilization with sling/swathe	Ice, rest, immobilization with figure eight or clavicular strap with a sling for 3–4 weeks. Initiate strengthening program after 3–4 weeks.	Apply a figure eight immobilizer with scapulas retracted. Immediately refer to a physician. Check radial pulse, respiration, and ability to swallow. If significant findings are present, activate the emergency action plan.

Grade III sprains require immediate reduction of the dislocation by a physician. Immobilization usually is maintained by a Velpeau bandage, soft figure eight brace, clavicle strap harness, or bulky pressure pad over the medial clavicle for 4 to 6 weeks. Scar tissue may form, but typically, no function is lost. There remains, however, a high incidence of recurrent SC sprains. When immobilization is discontinued, the arm motion should still be protected for an additional 2 weeks. Elbow exercises and shoulder ROM can be started at 3 weeks.[26] Surgical intervention may be necessary in the treatment of recurrent anterior SC joint or trauma that results in significant cosmetic issues. **Table 17.5** summarizes the signs and symptoms as well as the management of anterior SC sprains.

 Posterior displacement can become life-threatening, and the emergency plan, including summoning emergency medical services, should be activated.

Acromioclavicular Joint Sprain

Etiology

The AC joint is weak and easily injured by a direct blow, fall on the point of the shoulder (called a shoulder pointer), or force transmitted up the long axis of the humerus during a fall with the humerus in an adducted position. In these cases, the acromion is driven away from the clavicle, or vice versa. Although often referred to as a "separated shoulder," ruptures of the AC and/or coracoclavicular ligaments can result in an AC dislocation; therefore, they are more correctly referred to as "sprains."

Classification of Injury

Like other joint injuries, AC sprains may be classified as first degree (i.e., mild), second degree (i.e., moderate), or third degree (i.e., severe). Because of the complexity of the joint, however, AC sprains often are classified as types I to VI based on the extent of ligamentous damage, degree of instability, and direction in which the clavicle displaces relative to the acromion and coracoid process (**Table 17.6**).

Signs and Symptoms

All special tests used to assess AC joint injury will be positive; however, the amount of pain and/or motion elicited will help to determine degree of damage. Type I injuries have no disruption of the AC or coracoclavicular ligaments. Minimal swelling and pain are present over the joint line and increase with abduction past 90°. The injury is inherently stable, and pain is self-limiting.

Type II injuries result from a more severe blow to the shoulder. The AC ligaments are torn, but the coracoclavicular ligament, only minimally sprained, is intact. Vertical stability is maintained, but

TABLE 17.6 Classification of Acromioclavicular Joint Sprains

GRADE	DEGREE	INJURED STRUCTURES
Type I	First	Stretch or partial damage of the AC ligament and capsule
Type II	Second	Rupture of AC ligament and partial strain of coracoclavicular ligament
Type III	Second	Rupture of AC ligament and coracoclavicular ligament
Type IV–VI	Third	Rupture of AC ligament and coracoclavicular ligament and tearing of deltoid and trapezius fascia

sagittal plane stability is compromised. The clavicle rides above the level of the acromion, and a minor step or gap is present at the joint line. Pain increases when the distal clavicle is depressed or moved in an anterior-posterior direction and during passive horizontal adduction.

Type III injuries have complete disruption of the AC and coracoclavicular ligaments, resulting in visible prominence of the distal clavicle. The patient will have obvious swelling and bruising and, more significantly, depression or drooping of the shoulder girdle.

Higher grade injuries (types IV to VI) (**Fig. 17.32**) are caused by more violent forces. Extensive mobility and pain in the area may signify tearing of the deltoid and trapezius muscle attachments at the distal clavicle. These rare injuries must be carefully evaluated for associated neurological injuries.

Management

Type I and II injuries are treated with rest, ice, and nonsteroidal anti-inflammatory drugs (NSAIDs), followed by ROM exercises as tolerated. Immobilization in a sling for 1 to 3 weeks is necessary only if pain is present. The patient may return to activity when pain and strength permit normal use of the extremity, but the area should be padded to protect it from further insult. The majority of type I and II injuries heal without complications. Occasionally, however, persistent limiting pain may necessitate a cortisone injection to diminish inflammation. Rehabilitation involves regaining ROM and, once ROM is bilaterally equal, beginning a progressive resistance exercise program.

The management of type III injuries is controversial, because they are managed both operatively and nonoperatively. Most type III injuries are treated conservatively, with 90% to 100% having satisfactory results. Nonsurgical treatment involves immobilization in a sling for 2 to 4 weeks, followed by pendulum exercises, elbow ROM exercises, isometrics in all planes, and rope-and-pulley exercises for shoulder flexion and abduction as tolerated. If treatment includes surgery, pendulum and isometric exercises in all planes are encouraged during the initial stages of rehabilitation, although abduction and flexion to 90° are limited for approximately 3 to 4 weeks. Rehabilitation should focus on strengthening the rotator cuff and scapula stabilizers and on restoring neuromuscular control and arthrokinematics. Return to activity may take as

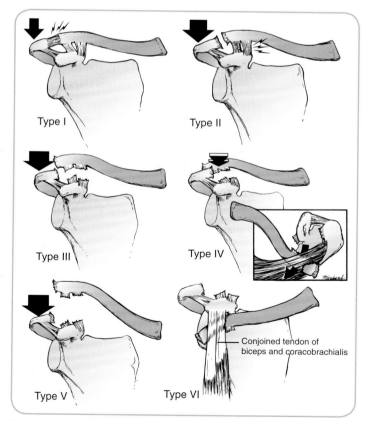

Figure 17.32. Rockwood classification for acromioclavicular joint injury. (From Tornetta P, Court-Brown C, Heckman J, et al. *Rockwood and Green's Fractures in Adults*. 8th ed. Philadelphia, PA: Wolters Kluwer; 2014.)

TABLE 17.7 Management of an Acromioclavicular Sprain

SIGNS AND SYMPTOMS	TYPE I	TYPE II	TYPE III
Deformity	None; ligaments are still intact.	Slight elevation of lateral clavicle; AC ligaments are disrupted, but coracoclavicular is still intact.	Prominent elevation of clavicle AC ligaments and coracoclavicular ligaments are disrupted.
Swelling	Slight	Moderate	Severe
Palpable pain	Mild over joint line	Moderate with downward pressure on distal clavicle; palpable gap or minor step present; snapping may be felt on horizontal adduction.	Severe on palpation and depression of acromion process; definite palpable step deformity present.
Movement	Usually unlimited but may have some discomfort on abduction greater than 90°	Unable to abduct the arm or horizontally adduct the arm across the chest without noticeable pain	Limited as in type II but pain is more severe
Stability	No instability	Some instability	Demonstrable instability
Treatment	Ice, NSAIDs, regain full ROM and strength; return to activity as tolerated, with protection	Ice, NSAIDs, immobilize with sling; TENS, interferential EMS for pain relief; ultrasound; strengthening and stability exercises; return to activity with protection	Ice, immobilize, and immediately refer to physician; if treated conservatively, deformity remains, but function should be within normal limits.

EMS, electrical muscle stimulation; *TENS*, transcutaneous electrical nerve stimulation.

long as 10 to 12 weeks, depending on the restoration of full, pain-free ROM and the stability of the joint. Participation in contact sports usually is permitted 3 to 5 months after the injury, depending on functional recovery.

In severe cases (types IV to VI) involving total disruption of the supporting ligaments, intra-articular disk damage, or an intra-articular fracture, open or arthroscopic intervention may be necessary. Immobilization may be necessary for as long as 4 to 6 weeks. The patient is permitted to use the arm for most activities of daily living but is restricted from active forward elevation or abduction. Pushing, pulling, or carrying more than 5 lb also is prohibited. In approximately 6 weeks, a progressive ROM and strengthening regimen begins. Complete sport and physical activity participation usually is not permitted until isokinetic testing shows results equal to those of the contralateral side, which occurs approximately 6 months after surgery. **Table 17.7** summarizes the signs and symptoms as well as the management of AC sprains.

Glenohumeral Joint Sprain

Etiology

Damage to the GH joint can occur when the arm is forcefully abducted (e.g., when making an arm tackle in football), but such damage more commonly is caused by excessive shoulder external rotation and extension (i.e., arm in the overhead position). When the arm rotates externally, the anterior capsule and GH ligaments are stretched or torn, causing the humeral head to slip out of the glenoid fossa in an anterior-inferior direction (**Fig. 17.33**). A direct blow or forceful movement that pushes the humerus posteriorly also can result in damage to the joint capsule.

Signs and Symptoms

In a first-degree injury, the anterior shoulder is particularly painful to palpation and movement, especially when the mechanism of injury is reproduced. Active ROM may be slightly limited, but pain does not occur on adduction or internal rotation, in contrast to a muscular strain. A second-degree sprain produces some joint laxity. In addition, pain, swelling, and bruising usually are significant, and ROM, particularly abduction, is limited.

Management

Treatment includes cryotherapy, rest, and immobilization with a sling during the initial 12 to 24 hours. NSAIDs can be administered after the first 48 hours so as to inhibit the early stages of the healing process. Early emphasis is placed on pain-free ROM exercises, elastic-band strengthening, and PNF exercises. Exercises to regain full external rotation and abduction should be delayed for at least 3 weeks to allow capsular healing. A more extensive resistance program can be started as tolerated.

Glenohumeral Instability

GH instability is based on joint play movements, or the relative displacement of the humeral head in the glenoid fossa, and may be classified as anterior, posterior, inferior, or multidirectional instability. Instability may result from poorly developed musculature; a decrease in the proprioceptive properties of the dynamic stabilizes of the GH joint as well as scapular dyskinesia or prior injury.[27] Instability can range from a vague sense of shoulder dysfunction (atraumatic instability) to noticeable hypermobility with activities of daily living. Although GH instability can occur in any direction, most acute dislocations are anterior, with posterior dislocations being the second most frequent.

Anterior Instability

■ Etiology

Anterior instability may result from a blow to the posterolateral aspect of the shoulder, but it is more commonly caused by excessive indirect forces that push the arm into abduction, external rotation, and extension.

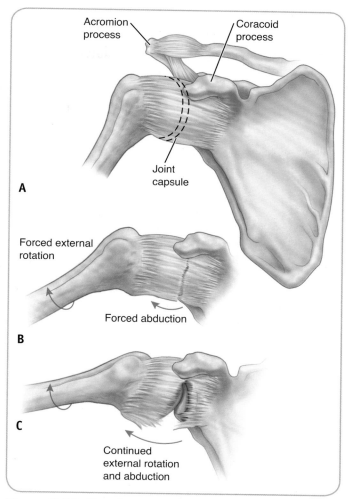

Figure 17.33. Glenohumeral sprains. A, Normal abduction with some stretching of the fibers. **B,** Forced external rotation and abduction with minimal tears to the joint capsule, leading to a moderate or second-degree sprain. **C,** Continuation of the forced movement causes a third-degree sprain or shoulder dislocation.

■ Signs and Symptoms

Failure of the capsule ligamentous complex, particularly the middle and inferior GH ligaments, allows the head of humerus to slide forward. If excessive, the head of the humerus may dislocate and lodge under the anteroinferior portion of the glenoid fossa adjacent to the coracoid process. As the humerus slides forward, either during a dislocation or due to chronic instability, the inferior GH ligament may be avulsed from the anterior lip of the labrum or in combination with a portion of the labrum. This condition is referred to as a **Bankart lesion**.

A patient with anterior shoulder instability may complain of vague pain within the shoulder, an inability to sleep resting on the shoulder at night, and a sense of abnormal motion within the joint. Tenderness may be elicited when palpating the anterior GH structures. Active ROM may reveal abnormal movement, and the patient may report feeling clicking within the joint if additional structures have been injured.[27] Because deformity is associated with dislocations and not instability, it is appropriate to use clinical test to assess for the presence of instability. In the presence of anterior instability, the shoulder apprehension test, the shoulder relocation test, and the anterior load and shift test may be positive.[27]

Posterior Instability

■ Etiology

The prevalence of posterior GH instability is becoming more common among young athletes making up about 10% of the instability events.[28] Acutely, the instability will arise when a posterior force is directed along the long axis of the humerus with the humerus flexed and internally rotated. This action often is associated with blocking in football. Although a single traumatic episode may lead to posterior instability, the condition more commonly results from a series of accumulated microtraumatic episodes. Excessive glenoid retroversion and increased internal and external rotation strength are thought to be factors that place a patient at risk for developing posterior instability.[28]

Inferior Instability

■ Etiology

Inferior instability is rare. The primary restraint against inferior translation is the superior GH ligament. When the arm is abducted 45° in neutral rotation, the anterior portion of the inferior GH ligament is the primary restraint; when the arm is at 90° of abduction, the entire GH ligament, particularly the posterior band, is responsible for restricting inferior displacement. Superior translation is limited by the coracoacromial arch and acromion process.

Multidirectional Instability

■ Etiology

Multidirectional instability (MDI) of the shoulder occurs when damage takes place in more than one plane. Acutely, most, if not all, anterior and posterior dislocations are associated with some preexisting, inferior laxity or laxity in the opposite direction. If the damage caused by the initial injury is not properly treated with a comprehensive rehabilitation program, the condition may become chronic, leading to further injury and complications.

■ Signs and Symptoms

Pain and/or instability can occur during simple tasks, such as picking up a box or backpack. The pain may be described as a chronic aching that increases with increased use of the shoulder. It is essential that a shoulder evaluation differentiate between unidirectional and MDI. To assess for the presence of MDI, multiple clinical tests should be used to stress the joint in multiple planes such as anterior and posterior load and shift, posterior drawer, and sulcus sign tests. Failure to identify MDI and, subsequently, provision of treatment only for a unidirectional instability can significantly alter joint mechanics and predispose the patient to continued instability in one or more planes. If the patient presents with or describe clicking within the joint, a labral tear should also be suspected.

■ Management

Treatment is initially conservative, with 50% to 70% of patients responding favorably to rehabilitation and activity modification. Rehabilitation should focus on restoring muscle function and balance; increasing the proprioceptive properties of the dynamic stabilizes of the GH joint as well as assessing for and treating scapular dyskinesia if present.[27] Surgical repair is indicated for patients who do not respond to conservative measures.

Glenohumeral Dislocation and Subluxation

The GH joint is the most frequently dislocated major joint in the body. A GH dislocation occurs when the humeral head moves out of the glenoid fossa, causing complete disruption to the joint. Ninety percent of shoulder dislocations are anterior; posterior dislocations rank second in occurrence. Inferior dislocations are rare and often are accompanied by neurovascular injury and fracture.[28] A subluxation occurs when the humeral head slides out of the joint, but a portion remains within the joint and can also be described as a partial dislocation. Both dislocations and subluxations can be acute or chronic.

Acute Dislocations

■ Etiology

The same forces that may cause a sprain of the GH joint capsule may also result in a dislocation. Acute dislocations may have an associated fracture or nerve damage. Therefore, this injury is considered to be serious, and it necessitates immediate transportation to the nearest medical facility for reduction.

■ Signs and Symptoms

An initial dislocation presents with intense pain. Recurrent dislocations may be less painful. Tingling and numbness may extend down the arm into the hand. In a first-time anterior dislocation, the injured arm often is held in slight abduction (20° to 30°) and external rotation and is stabilized against the body by the opposite hand. Visually, a sharp contour on the affected shoulder, with a prominent acromion process and flattened deltoid can be seen when compared with the smooth deltoid outline on the unaffected shoulder. The humeral head may be palpated in the axilla anterior to the acromion and resting adjacent to the coracoid process. The patient will not allow the arm to be brought across the chest and may assume a guarding posture where the patient cradles his or her arm in slight abduction and external rotation. It is important to assess the axillary nerve and artery, because both structures can be damaged in a dislocation. A pulse may be taken on the medial proximal humerus over the brachial artery, and the axillary nerve can be assessed by stroking the skin on the upper lateral arm to assess sensation. Because the deltoid is not only a key shoulder abductor but also contributes to shoulder flexion and extension, damage to this nerve can be devastating. In the presence of deformity that is either seen or palpated, no special tests are needed to confirm the presence of a dislocation.

Occasionally, posterior dislocations occur from a fall on or a blow to the anterior surface of the shoulder, which drives the head of the humerus posteriorly. If dislocated, the arm is carried tightly against the chest and across the front of the trunk in rigid adduction and internal rotation. The anterior shoulder appears to be flat, the coracoid process is prominent, and a corresponding bulge may be seen posteriorly (if not masked by a heavy deltoid musculature). Any attempt to move the arm into external rotation and abduction produces severe pain. Because the biceps brachii is unable to function in this position, the patient is unable to supinate the forearm with the shoulder flexed.

■ Management

Muscle spasm sets in very quickly following dislocation and makes reduction more difficult. Management of a first-time dislocation requires immediate referral to a physician. As such, in some settings, it may be necessary to activate the emergency action plan. The injury should be treated as a fracture and the arm immobilized in a comfortable position. To prevent unnecessary movement of the humerus, a rolled towel or thin pillow can be placed between the thoracic wall and humerus before applying a sling. Ice should be applied to control hemorrhage and muscle spasm.

Following reduction, the shoulder is immobilized in a sling and swathe. Traditionally, immobilization for 4 weeks followed by rehabilitation is recommended, but this protocol has not been proved to diminish the risk of recurrent instability, which is about 39%.[29] Men under the age 40 years with hyperlaxity are at the greatest risk for chronic instability following a shoulder dislocation.[29] When the patient is able to tolerate movement, ROM exercises can begin, but it is important to avoid an aggressive flexibility program in extension, abduction, and external rotation. Resisted isometric and stretching exercises can begin immediately after the acute phase has ended. Elastic band exercises below 90° of abduction can be incorporated early during the program to maintain and improve strength. Interferential current stimulation can be used to reduce inflammation, stimulate muscle reeducation, promote deep tissue circulation, and minimize fibrotic infiltration. Strength development of the lateral rotators can reduce strain on the anterior structures of the joint by pulling the humeral head posteriorly during lateral rotation of the shoulder, thus reducing anterior instability. Strong scapula stabilizers (e.g., trapezius, rhomboids, and serratus anterior) also are believed to improve anterior stability by placing the glenoid in the optimal position to perform the skill techniques required.

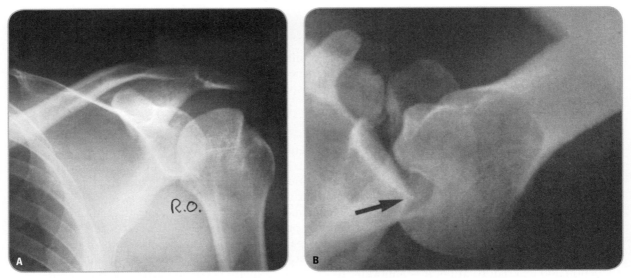

Figure 17.34. Hill-Sachs lesions. A, In this radiograph of a reduced anterior dislocation with the humeral head held in internal rotation, a Hill-Sachs compression fracture is evident. Note the posterolateral humeral head defect with a sharp, dense spine of bone running downward from the top of the humeral head toward the center of the humeral head. This line of condensation of bone is the result of an impaction fracture caused by the anterior glenoid rim. **B,** This radiograph demonstrates a subacromial posterior dislocation of the right shoulder with a large, antero-medial compression fracture defect of the humeral head, the so-called reverse Hill-Sachs sign (*arrow*).

Isokinetic internal rotation and adduction can begin within 3 to 4 weeks and advance as tolerated. More aggressive shoulder rehabilitation exercises are not typically initiated until 5 to 6 weeks after removal of the immobilization device and subsequent to achieving full ROM.

A common finding after an anterior dislocation is a **Hill-Sachs lesion** (**Fig. 17.34**). The lesion is a small defect in the articular cartilage of the humeral head caused by the impact of the humeral head on the glenoid fossa as the humerus dislocates. The lesion usually is located on the posterior aspect of the humeral head, but it may be found on the anterior portion of the humeral head following a posterior dislocation, in which it is called a reverse Hill-Sachs lesion. The lesion is used as a diagnostic tool in determining the severity of the dislocation. In patients reporting that the shoulder dislocated but spontaneously reduced, the lesion may be visible on radiographs. Although the lesion rarely is symptomatic, the condition may lead to early degeneration of the GH joint.

Chronic Dislocations

Etiology

Recurrent dislocations, or "trick shoulders," tend to be anterior dislocations that are intracapsular. The mechanism of injury is the same as that for acute dislocations. As the number of occurrences increase, however, the forces that are needed to produce the injury decrease, as do the associated muscle spasm, pain, and swelling. The patient is aware of the shoulder displacing, because the arm gives the sensation of "going dead," which is referred to as the **dead arm syndrome**. Activities in which recurrent posterior subluxations are common include the follow-through of a throwing motion or a racquet swing, the ascent phase of a push-up or a bench press, the recoil following a block in football, and certain swimming strokes.

Signs and Symptoms

Pain is the major complaint, with crepitation and/or clicking after the arm shifts back into the appropriate position. Many patients voluntarily reduce the injury by positioning the arm in flexion, adduction, and internal rotation.

Management

If the injury does not reduce, the patient should be placed in a sling and swathe, or the arm may be stabilized next to the body with an elastic wrap. Ice should be applied to control pain and inflammation. The patient should be referred immediately to a physician for reduction of the injury and further care. Following reduction, conservative treatment involves rest and immobilization, restoration of shoulder motion, and strengthening of the rotator cuff muscles. Surgery may be indicated if persistent instability occurs.

Glenoid Labrum Tears

Etiology

The glenoid labrum is a fibrocartilaginous rim that lines the glenoid fossa to better receive the humeral head. The capsule and inferior GH ligament are contiguous with the labrum at their attachment to the glenoid. Tearing of the labrum and inferior GH ligament is referred to as a Bankart lesion. The lesion is associated with recurrent anterior shoulder instability. Tears of the labrum also may result from degeneration or trauma. In many instances, the tears are asymptomatic and incidental. Longitudinal or flap tears may occur in the anterior or posterior labrum, with or without associated GH instability.

An injury to the superior labrum may begin posteriorly and extend anteriorly, disrupting the attachment of the long head of the biceps tendon to the superior glenoid tubercle (**SLAP lesion**). **Figure 17.35** demonstrates both a Bankart lesion and a SLAP lesion.

Signs and Symptoms

The patient may complain of pain, catching, or weakness, usually when the arm is overhead in an abducted and externally rotated position. The pain often is associated with clicking or popping within the joint. If a tear is the result of a dislocation or subluxation, symptoms of instability also may be present. Superior tears may be symptomatic and can be reproduced with ROM and translation testing, particularly with use of the clunk test and compression rotation test. Speed's test and Yergason test may be positive as well. Axial loading of the joint with forced internal and external rotation and the arm elevated 160° in the scapular plane with the elbow flexed (e.g., anterior impingement "crank" test) also may reproduce symptoms.[30]

Management

Treatment is based on the tear pattern and the presence or absence of GH instability. Initial conservative treatment may involve rest, anti-inflammatory drugs, and, if applicable, rehabilitation exercises. For those patients who do not respond well to conservative measures, arthroscopic debridement may be necessary.

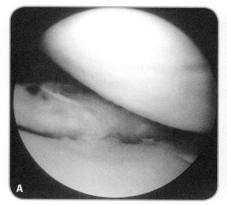
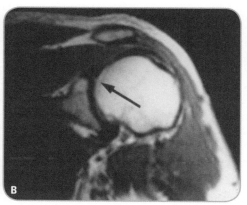
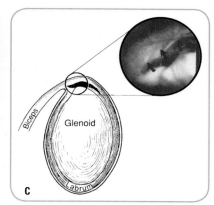

Figure 17.35. Glenoid labrum tears. A, This arthroscopic view demonstrates a detached anterior labrum (i.e., Bankart lesion). **B,** A SLAP lesion is evident at the origin of the long head of the biceps tendon. **C,** Schematic drawing and arthroscopic view of the SLAP lesion.

The soccer player with the type II AC sprain experienced the following signs and symptoms: slight elevation of the lateral clavicle; moderate swelling over the joint; moderate, palpable pain with downward pressure on the distal clavicle; palpable gap at the joint; inability to abduct the arm or horizontally adduct the arm across the chest without noticeable pain; and compromised sagittal plane stability.

OVERUSE CONDITIONS

? Why is impingement syndrome a problem for swimmers in particular?

Patients who perform repetitive overhead activities often develop anterior shoulder pain. The GH capsular ligaments are the prime stabilizers of the shoulder, especially the anteroinferior GH ligament. As muscles contract to move the arm, they create compressive and shear forces within the joint. The compression force produced by muscles acting perpendicular to the glenoid fossa stabilizes the humeral head, and the muscles acting more parallel to the glenoid produce a translational shear force. The resultant force derived from the sum of the compressive and shear forces determines the vector direction of the total joint force. A larger superior shear force produces impingement, and a larger compression force centers the humeral head in the glenoid, reducing rotator cuff impingement under the acromion.

During abduction, the strong deltoid and supraspinatus muscles pull the humeral head superiorly relative to the glenoid fossa. The remaining rotator cuff muscles must counteract this migration by producing an inferior shear force to resist the pull from the supraspinatus and deltoid muscles. If the rotator cuff tendons are weak or fatigued, they are incapable of depressing the humeral head in the glenoid fossa during overhead motions. In addition, fatigue of the infraspinatus and teres minor that resist anterior joint translation also may lead to intracapsular impingement and GH instability. The resulting compression can lead to impingement of the supraspinatus tendon and subacromial bursa between the acromion, the coracoacromial ligament, and the greater tubercle of the humerus, resulting in rotator cuff strain, impingement syndrome, bursitis, or bicipital tendinitis.

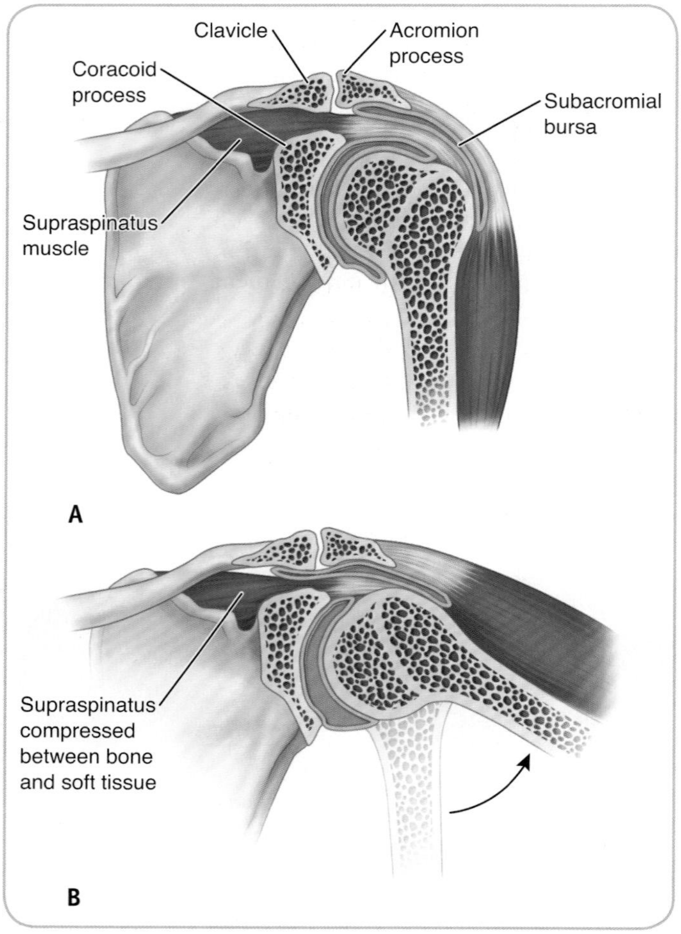

Rotator Cuff and Impingement Injuries
Etiology

Chronic rotator cuff tears to the SITS muscles result from repetitive microtraumatic episodes that primarily impinge on the supraspinatus tendon just proximal to the greater tubercle of the humerus (**Fig. 17.36**). Partial tears usually are seen in young patients, with total tears typically seen in adults older than 30 years. In older age groups, chronic tears can lead to cuff thinning, degeneration, and total rupture of the supraspinatus tendon.

Figure 17.36. Supraspinatus tendon during abduction. A, Normal position. B, Abducted position. Repetitive overhead motions can impinge the muscle or tendon between the acromion process and coracoacromial ligament, resulting in a chronic rotator cuff injury.

Impingement syndrome implies an actual, mechanical abutment of the rotator cuff and the subacromial bursa against the coracoacromial ligament and acromion. This injury is caused from the force overload to the rotator cuff and bursa that occurs during the abduction, forward flexion, and medial rotation cycle of shoulder movements. Along with injury to the supraspinatus tendon and subacromial bursa, the glenoid labrum and long head of the biceps brachii also may be injured. Impingement syndrome sometimes is called "painful arc" syndrome or "swimmer's shoulder." **Box 17.1** lists several factors that can increase the risk for an impingement syndrome.

Signs and Symptoms

Initially, pain is described as being deep in the shoulder and present at night. Activity increases the pain but only in the impingement position. As repetitive trauma continues, pain becomes progressively worse, particularly between 70° and 120° (i.e., "painful arc") of active and resisted abduction. Because forced scapular protraction leads to further impingement and pain, the patient may be unable to sleep on the involved side. Pain can be palpated in the subacromial space. If a full-thickness tear has been sustained, atrophy may be apparent in the supraspinatus or infraspinatus fossa. Depending on the extent of the injury (**Box 17.2**), positive results may be elicited in the drop arm test, empty can test, Neer shoulder impingement test, and anterior impingement test (Hawkins-Kennedy test).

Management

Initially, conservative treatment involves restricting motion below 90° of abduction, cryotherapy, NSAIDs, pain-relieving medication, 1 to 2 weeks of rest, activity modification, and occasionally, steroid injection. However, much can be accomplished through the use of therapeutic exercise and modalities. Ultrasound, electrical muscle stimulation, interferential therapy, and heat can supplement treatment and can be used to help with pain management. Overall, NSAIDs and subacromial steroid injections are effective in the short-term treatment of shoulder pain.[31] Concern exists, however, that delaying repair of a supraspinatus tear makes the eventual repair harder or even impossible; initial surgical repair generally has a good outcome.[32]

Mobility should be maintained with mild stretching exercises, particularly in external rotation at 90°, 135°, and 180° of abduction. Pendulum exercises with abduction and forward flexion up to 90°, rope-and-pulley exercises in flexion, and T-bar exercises in flexion and external rotation should be initiated early during the rehabilitation process. In addition, muscles of the rotator cuff as well as muscles that perform scapular retraction, depression, and rotation should be strengthened. In terms of strength about the shoulder, adduction should be the strongest, followed by extension, flexion,

---

BOX 17.1 Factors Contributing to Impingement Syndrome

- Excessive amount of overhead movement (i.e., overuse)
- Limited subacromial space under the coracoacromial arch and limited flexibility of the coracoacromial ligament
- Thickness of the supraspinatus and biceps brachii tendon
- Lack of flexibility and strength of the supraspinatus and biceps brachii
- Weakness of the posterior cuff muscles (e.g., infraspinatus or teres minor)
- Tightness of the posterior cuff muscles
- Hypermobility of the shoulder joints
- Imbalance in muscle strength, coordination, and endurance of the scapular muscles (e.g., serratus anterior or rhomboids)
- Shape of the acromion
- Training devices (e.g., use of hand paddles or tubing)

BOX 17.2 **Stages of Impingement Syndrome**

Stage 1

■ Condition typically is seen in individuals younger than 25 years and is reversible.

■ Localized hemorrhage and edema are present in the supraspinatus tendon.

■ Minimal pain is felt with activity, but no restriction or weakness of motion occurs.

■ Atrophy of the rotator cuff muscles may be present.

Stage 2

■ Condition typically is seen in individuals between 25 and 40 years of age.

■ Marked reactive tendinitis is present, with significant pain felt between 70° and 120° abduction.

■ Inflammation may affect the biceps brachii tendon and subacromial bursa, leading to thickening and fibrotic changes in the structures.

■ Limited ROM is found in external rotation and abduction.

■ Possible clicking sounds are heard on resisted adduction and internal rotation.

Stage 3

■ The individual has a history of chronic, long-term shoulder pain with significant weakness.

■ Rotator cuff tear usually is less than 1 cm.

■ Prominent capsular laxity with MDI is seen.

■ Noticeable atrophy of the supraspinatus and infraspinatus muscles occurs.

■ Arthroscopy may show a damaged labrum.

Stage 4

■ Rotator cuff tear is greater than 1 cm.

abduction, internal rotation, and external rotation. Exercises such as pull-ups or push-ups should be avoided during the early stages of rehabilitation, because they can impinge on the rotator cuff and complicate the condition. **Application Strategy 17.3** outlines the management of an impingement syndrome.

Swimmers present a special problem, because many strokes use adduction and internal rotation with excessive propulsion forces. Because of fatigue and lack of coordination in the scapular muscles, this motion may allow subclinical anterior subluxations to occur, resulting in damage to the glenoid labrum. This anterior lesion may be frayed but not detached, resulting in a roughened leading edge that may mechanically catch during overhead motions. As such, swimmers may feel a snapping sensation, clicking, or sense that the shoulder is "going out" when moving through the pull phase of the stroke. Occasionally, a defect or crepitus in the supraspinatus tendon may be palpated just anterior to the acromion process when the arm is extended at the GH joint. Pain also can be palpated anteriorly over the coracoacromial ligament, laterally at the insertion of the supraspinatus, posteriorly at the insertion of the infraspinatus and teres minor, or over the long head of the biceps tendon. Atrophy of the shoulder muscles with subsequent weakness in the supraspinatus and biceps brachii may be present as well. Because rest translates into detraining, other steps may need to be taken to allow continued activity. The intensity and quantity of training need to be reduced and paddle work eliminated. Stroke mechanics should be assessed to determine if changes are needed to reduce shoulder stress.

APPLICATION STRATEGY 17.3

Management of an Impingement Injury

- Use cryotherapy initially; later, replace with moist heat therapy twice a day.
- Electrical muscle stimulation, interferential current, and transcutaneous electrical nerve stimulation may be helpful for pain management.
- Use ultrasound and NSAIDs to reduce inflammation.
- Use selective rest. For 4–6 weeks, concentrate on motions that do not cause pain. Avoid abduction above 90°.
- Evaluate skill technique and correct movements that produce shoulder stress.
- Eliminate partner stretching, overhead training, and, for swimmers, use of hand paddles.
- Wand and T-bar exercises can improve sport-specific mobility but should not encourage hypermobility.
- Perform pain-free isometric and elastic band exercises at least two to three times daily to maintain muscle tone. Use low weights and high repetitions.
- Strengthen the lateral rotators (i.e., infraspinatus and teres minor) to control superior displacement of the humeral head.
- After 4–6 weeks, incorporate isokinetic exercises at high speeds and elastic band exercises in diagonal patterns.
- Begin a gradual return to activity, as long as the symptoms do not recur.

Bursitis

Etiology

Bursitis is not generally an isolated condition; rather, it is associated with other injuries, such as an impingement syndrome and preexisting degenerative changes in the rotator cuff. The large subacromial bursa is a common site of injury in swimmers and in baseball, softball, and tennis players. Located between the coracoacromial ligament and the underlying supraspinatus muscle, this bursa provides the shoulder with some inherent gliding ability. During an overhead throwing motion, this bursa can become impinged in the subacromial space.

Signs and Symptoms

Frequently, sudden shoulder pain is reported during initiation and acceleration of the throwing motion. Point tenderness can be elicited on the anterior and lateral edges of the acromion process. A painful arc exists between 70° and 120° of passive abduction. Inability to sleep, especially on the affected side, occurs because of forced scapular protraction that leads to further impingement of the bursa. Pain often is referred to the distal deltoid attachment.

Management

Standard acute protocol is followed by referral to a physician. A physician may inject a corticosteroid solution into the subacromial space to relieve the symptoms. In addition, other underlying conditions, such as a rotator cuff tear, impingement syndrome, or bicipital tendinitis, must be ruled out. Treatment is symptomatic and is the same as for a rotator cuff strain or impingement syndrome.

Bicipital Tendinitis

Etiology

Injury to the biceps brachii tendon often occurs from repetitive overuse during rapid overhead movements involving excessive elbow flexion and supination activities, such as those performed by racquet-sport players, shot-putters, baseball/softball pitchers, football quarterbacks, swimmers, and javelin throwers. Irritation of the tendon occurs as it passes back and forth in the intertubercular (bicipital) groove of the humerus. The tendon may partially sublux because of laxity of the traverse humeral ligament, a poorly developed lesser tubercle, or both. A direct blow to the tendon or tendon sheath can lead to bicipital tenosynovitis. Anterior impingement syndrome associated with overhead rotational activity also may damage the tendon.

Signs and Symptoms

Pain and tenderness is present over the bicipital groove when the shoulder is internally and externally rotated. In internal rotation, the pain stays medial; in external rotation, the pain is located in the midline or just lateral to the groove. Pain also may be elicited when the tendon is passively stretched in extreme shoulder extension with the elbow extended and the forearm pronated. Resisted supination of a flexed elbow while externally rotating the shoulder (e.g., Yergason test) increases pain, as does forward shoulder flexion of the extended, supinated elbow (e.g., Speed's test).

Management

Treatment involves restriction of rotational activities that exacerbate symptoms. Because of potential vascular impingement of the biceps tendon when the shoulder is at the side, the arm should be propped or wedged into slight abduction if immobilized in a sling. During the early stages of the condition, cryotherapy, NSAIDs, ultrasound, electrical muscle stimulation, or interferential therapy can control inflammation. Icing before and after activity should be combined with a gradual program of stretching and strengthening as soon as pain subsides. Patients experiencing bicipital tendinitis secondary to impingement should avoid horizontal abduction exercises, which can aggravate symptoms.[33]

Biceps Tendon Rupture

Etiology

Prolonged tendinitis can make the tendon vulnerable to forceful rupture during repetitive overhead motions, as commonly are seen in swimmers, or during forceful flexion activities against excessive resistance, as are seen in weight lifters or gymnasts. The rupture occurs as a result of the avascular portion of the proximal long head of the biceps tendon constantly passing over the head of the humerus during arm motion. This condition often is seen in degenerative tendons in older patients and in patients who have had corticosteroid injections into the tendon.

Signs and Symptoms

The patient often hears and feels a snapping sensation and experiences intense pain. Ecchymosis and a visible, palpable defect can be seen in the muscle belly when the patient flexes the biceps. If the muscle mass moves distally as a result of a proximal long head rupture, a "Popeye" appearance clearly is visible. Partial ruptures may produce only slight muscular deformity but are still associated with pain and weakness in elbow flexion and supination. In this case, Ludington test should help the clinician identify the presence of the rupture. Distal biceps rupture results in marked weakness with flexion and supination of the forearm.

Management

Standard acute care protocol is followed by immediate referral to a physician. Surgical repair usually is not suggested for noncompetitive patients or older patients, because return to normal physical activity can occur after completing an appropriate rehabilitation program. Surgical repair and fixation is indicated, however, for competitive patients to restore elbow flexion and forearm supination strength needed for participation in competitive sports.

Thoracic Outlet Compression Syndrome

Etiology

Thoracic outlet compression syndrome is a condition in which nerves and/or vessels become compressed in the proximal neck or axilla (**Fig. 17.37**). This condition has two clearly defined forms. One is a neurological syndrome, accounting for approximately 90% of all cases, that involves the lower trunk of the brachial plexus and is caused by abnormal nerve stretch or compression. Another is a vascular form that involves the subclavian artery and vein and is more common in men than in women.[34] Thoracic outlet compression syndrome often is aggravated in activities that require

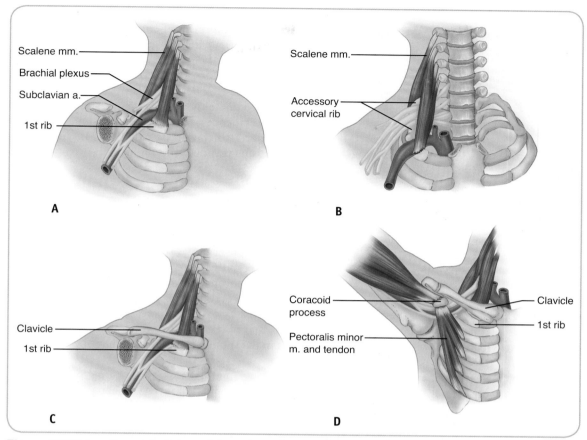

Figure 17.37. Location and etiology of thoracic outlet syndrome. A, Scalenus anterior syndrome. **B,** Cervical rib syndrome. **C,** Costoclavicular space syndrome. **D,** Hyperabduction syndrome.

overhead rotational stresses while muscles are loaded, such as weight lifting and swimming. Disorders associated with thoracic outlet syndrome include the following:

- Compression of the medial cord of the brachial plexus
- Compression of the subclavian artery and vein
- Cervical rib syndrome
- Scalenus anterior syndrome
- Hyperabduction syndrome
- Costoclavicular space syndrome
- Poor posture with drooping shoulders

Signs and Symptoms

If a nerve is compressed, an aching pain, a pins-and-needles sensation, or numbness in the side or back of the neck extends across the shoulder down the medial arm to the ulnar aspect of the hand. If compression is intermittent, due to sleeping position or muscle action, then the symptoms will also occur intermittently. Weakness in grasp and atrophy of the hand muscles also may be present in prolonged cases. If arterial or venous vessels are compressed, signs and symptoms vary depending on the specific structure being obstructed. Blockage of the subclavian vein, for example, produces edema, stiffness (especially in the hand), and venous engorgement of the arm with cyanosis (**Fig. 17.38**). If untreated, this may result in thrombophlebitis. The patient may present these signs and symptoms several hours after

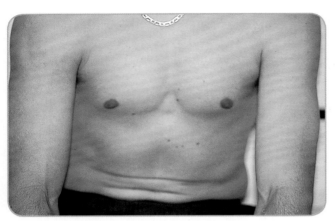

Figure 17.38. Thoracic outlet syndrome. This 20-year-old pitcher presented with "burning" pain, swelling, and erythema of the right arm. His right arm has distended veins, which stemmed from right subclavian vein thrombosis.

a bout of intense exercise. Occlusion of the subclavian artery results in a rapid onset of coolness, numbness in the entire arm, and fatigue after exertional overhead activity. The radial pulse may be obliterated while performing the Adson test, the Allen test, or the costoclavicular syndrome (military brace) test. A detailed history is needed, and it is essential to evaluate the cervical spine, shoulder, elbow, and hand for evidence of neural compression. Instability of the shoulder also should be ruled out. In addition, a postural assessment should be conducted.

Management

Immediate referral to a physician is necessary if patient presents with swelling, erythema, or distended veins for more extensive assessment to rule out serious vascular involvement. Conservative treatment involves assessing muscle strength and posture. Noted deficits should lead to an appropriate retraining program to develop strength and muscle balance in the shoulder girdle and facilitate maintenance of a corrected posture. If the condition was precipitated by a sudden increase in activity, treatment involves anti-inflammatory drugs, activity modification, and reassessment of the training program. Return to full activity may occur after ROM and strength in the shoulder musculature have been regained.

 Swimmers present a special problem with regard to impingement, because many strokes use adduction and internal rotation with excessive propulsion forces. Because of fatigue and lack of coordination in the scapular muscles, this motion may allow subclinical anterior subluxations to occur, resulting in damage to the glenoid labrum. This anterior lesion may be frayed but not detached, resulting in a roughened leading edge that may mechanically catch during overhead motions.

FRACTURES

 How can atraumatic osteolysis of the distal clavicle occur?

Most fractures to the shoulder region result from a fall on the point of the shoulder, from rolling over onto the top of the shoulder, or from indirect forces caused by falling on an outstretched arm. Clavicular fractures are more common than fractures to the scapula and proximal humerus, with nearly 80% occurring in the midclavicular region.

Clavicular Fractures

Because of the S-shaped configuration of the clavicle, it is highly susceptible to compression forces caused by a blow or fall on the point of the shoulder, a direct blow to the bone by an opponent or object, or a fall on an outstretched arm. Activities that have a high incidence of clavicular injury include ice hockey, football, the martial arts, lacrosse, gymnastics, weight lifting, wrestling, racquetball, squash, and bicycling.

Osteolysis of the Distal Clavicle

■ **Etiology**
Atraumatic osteolysis of the distal clavicle is an overuse injury resulting from repetitive microtrauma. It also has been described as a sequelae following traumatic injury to the distal clavicle

or AC joint. The condition is seen most often in weight lifting, but it also has been seen in sports where cross-training is popular and in younger patients who weight train year-round for higher level sports.[35] During repetitive activity, subsequent bone resorption causes cystic and erosive changes, and bone remodeling cannot occur because of the continual stress to the area.

■ Signs and Symptoms

Patients usually complain of a dull ache over the AC joint, which often is worse at the beginning of an exercise period. Pain and a sense of weakness during abduction and flexion of the arm also are noted. This pain and weakness may occur from weeks to years after the actual injury.[36] Palpable pain, crepitus, and swelling are present over the distal clavicle. Increased pain is experienced with horizontal adduction of the arm; any abduction of the arm greater than 90° is extremely painful. Radiographs tend to show osteopenia and lucency in the distal clavicle.

■ Management

The treatment of choice is conservative but requires patient compliance. Rest, particularly from weight training, and anti-inflammatory drugs are recommended. Surgical resection of the distal clavicle may be necessary depending on the patient's functional demands and symptoms.[35,36]

Traumatic Clavicular Fractures

■ Etiology

Nearly 80% of traumatic fractures occur in the middle third of the clavicle.[26] The sternocleido-mastoid muscle pulls the proximal bone fragment upward, allowing the distal shoulder to collapse downward and medially from the force of gravity and the pull of the pectoralis major muscle.

■ Signs and Symptoms

Swelling, ecchymosis, and a deformity may be visible and palpable at the fracture site. Greenstick fractures, which typically are seen in adolescents, also produce a noticeable deformity. Pain occurs with any shoulder motion and may radiate into the trapezius area. In older adults, fractures of the distal clavicle may involve tears of the coracoclavicular ligament, producing an increased deformity. Although rare, complications may arise if bony fragments penetrate local arteries or nerves.

■ Management

Immediate treatment involves immobilization in a sling and swathe. Following assessment by the physician, a figure eight brace or strapping often is used to pull the shoulder backward and upward for 4 to 6 weeks in young adults and for 6 or more weeks in older adults (**Fig. 17.39**). Although this immobilization prevents movement in nearly all planes, it does not prevent scapular elevation. As a result, healing may be delayed, and excessive callus formation may occur at the fracture site. This bump tends to remodel, to some degree, over a period of years but may never completely disappear. Following immobilization, gentle isometric and mobilization exercises should begin with gradual return to activity.

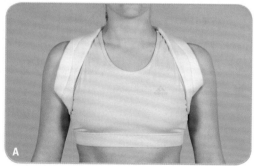

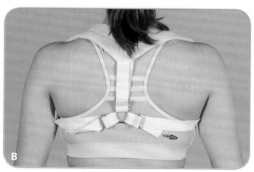

Figure 17.39. Figure eight clavicular straps. A, Anterior view. **B,** Posterior view.

Scapular Fractures

Etiology

Scapular fractures may involve the body of the scapula, spine of the scapula, acromion process, coracoid process, or GH joint. Avulsion fractures to the coracoid process result from direct trauma or from forceful contraction of the pectoralis minor or short head of the biceps brachii. Fractures to the glenoid area are associated with shoulder subluxations and dislocations. In this case, treatment is dictated by the shoulder dislocation rather than by the fracture and often requires open reduction and internal fixation or shoulder reconstruction.

Signs and Symptoms

Most fractures result in minimal displacement and exhibit localized hemorrhage, pain, and tenderness. The patient is reluctant to move the injured arm and prefers to maintain it in adduction. Arm abduction is painful. It is critical to note any signs or symptoms that would suggest an underlying pulmonary injury (e.g., pneumothorax or hemothorax).

Management

The arm should be immobilized immediately in a sling and swathe, and ice should be applied to minimize hematoma formation. The patient should be referred to a physician. Complications may arise from scarring and adhesions in the muscles overlying the scapula. Subsequently, the muscles in the region must compensate for the limited scapular motion, leading to overuse injuries. The development of adhesions in the area can be reduced with an early program of passive and active stretching exercises, usually within 2 weeks. Early mobilization also is important to avoid loss of ROM, which could lead to a frozen shoulder.

Epiphyseal and Avulsion Fractures

Etiology

Epiphyseal centers around the shoulder region remain unfused for a longer span of time than typically is seen at other epiphyseal sites. For example, the medial clavicular growth plate does not close until approximately 25 years of age, and this situation often is misdiagnosed as an SC subluxation/dislocation. The proximal humeral epiphysis does not close until 18 to 21 years of age. An epiphyseal fracture at this site, called **Little League shoulder**, often is caused by repetitive medial rotation and adduction traction forces placed on the shoulder during pitching (**Fig. 17.40**). Catchers also may sustain this fracture, because they throw the ball as hard and as often as pitchers, but with less of a windup. The injury usually occurs during the deceleration and follow-through phases of throwing or pitching.

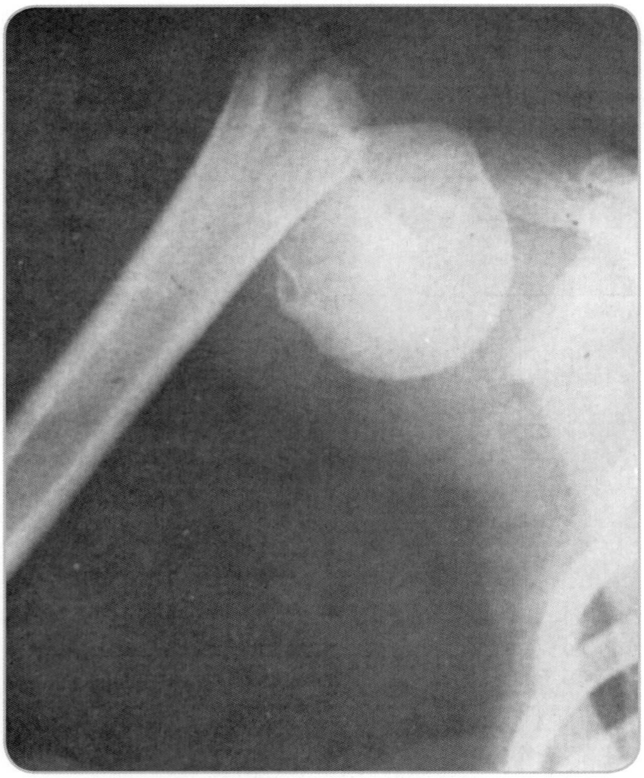

Avulsion fractures to the coracoid process can be seen in a young patient when forceful, repetitive throwing places too much stress on the growth plate. Fractures of the greater and lesser tubercle often are associated with anterior and posterior GH dislocations, respectively. When the tubercle cannot be maintained in a stable position, open reduction and internal fixation often are required.

Figure 17.40. Epiphyseal fracture to the proximal humeral growth center.

Signs and Symptoms

In an epiphyseal fracture, the patient complains of acute shoulder pain when attempting to throw hard, which if ignored may result in an acute displacement of the weakened physis. Pain may be elicited by deep palpation in the axilla. In an avulsion fracture, pain can be elicited by deep palpation over the specific bony landmark.

Management

The arm should be immobilized in a sling and swathe, and ice should be applied to control pain and swelling. Immediate referral to a physician for further care is warranted. Radiographs are necessary to view the widened epiphyseal line and demineralization. Treatment is conservative, with symptoms disappearing after 3 to 4 weeks of rest. The condition may recur if activity is resumed too quickly.

Humeral Fractures

Etiology

Humeral fractures result from violent compression forces from a direct blow, a fall on the upper arm, or a FOSH with the elbow extended. The surgical neck is the most common site for proximal humeral fractures and may display an appearance similar to that of a dislocation (**Fig. 17.41**).

Signs and Symptoms

Pain, swelling, hemorrhage, discoloration, inability to move the arm, inability to supinate the forearm, and possible paralysis may be present. The arm often is held splinted against the body.

Management

The arm should be immobilized in a sling and swathe, and ice should be applied to control pain and swelling. Immediate referral to a physician for further care is warranted. In some settings, this injury may warrant activation of the emergency action plan.

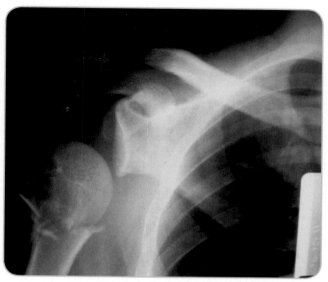

Figure 17.41. Fracture to the surgical neck of the humerus.

Up to 85% of proximal humeral fractures can be treated nonoperatively.[36] For cases in which the fracture is impacted, closed reduction allows early mobilization after 3 to 4 weeks of immobilization. Early complications of a fracture to the proximal humerus include brachial plexus injury and/or vascular injury. Late complications include shoulder stiffness, malunion, nonunion, avascular necrosis, and myositis ossificans.

 A traumatic osteolysis of the distal clavicle is an overuse injury resulting from repetitive microtrauma. It also has been described as a sequelae following traumatic injury to the distal clavicle or AC joint. During repetitive activity, subsequent bone resorption causes cystic and erosive changes, and bone remodeling cannot occur because of the continual stress imposed on the point.

REHABILITATION

? The swimmer has a painful shoulder as a result of recurrent subluxations. What areas should be the focus of a rehabilitation program for this condition?

A rehabilitation program of the shoulder must address the specific needs of the patient. The program should relieve pain and muscle tension; restore motion and balance; develop strength, endurance, and power; and maintain cardiovascular fitness. Progress within any program is dictated by the type and severity of injury, the amount of immobilization, and the supervising physician's treatment plan.

Restoration of Motion

Gentle ROM exercises, such as Codman circumduction and pendulum swings, often are used immediately after injury. The exercise is performed by making small circles and a pendulum motion in the actions of flexion and extension, and horizontal abduction and adduction. The extent of ROM should increase as pain-free motion is regained. Exercises can progress to active, assistive T-bar exercises in the supine position (**Application Strategy 17.4**). In throwing activities, the ROM needed to adequately complete the cocking phase exceeds 90° of external rotation when the arm is abducted 90°. Special attention should be focused on regaining this additional ROM but not to the point of hypermobility.

APPLICATION STRATEGY 17.4

Range of Motion Exercises for the Glenohumeral Joint

Wand and T-bar exercises. Hold the stretch for 5–10 seconds and repeat 10–20 times per session. Initially, ROM exercises can be performed two to three times daily.

1. **Supine shoulder flexion.** Grasp the wand with both hands palm-down at waist height. Raise the wand directly overhead, leading with the uninvolved arm until a stretch is felt in the involved shoulder. If an impingement syndrome is present, this exercise can be performed palm-up.
2. **Shoulder abduction.** Hold the wand with the involved arm palm-up and the uninvolved arm palm-down. With the uninvolved arm, push the wand sideward and upward toward the involved side until a stretch is felt in the involved shoulder.
3. **Shoulder adduction/horizontal adduction.** Reverse the hand positions from exercise 2. Pull the wand toward the uninvolved side until a stretch is felt in the involved shoulder.
4. **Shoulder internal/external rotation.** Keeping both palms down, abduct the shoulders and flex the elbows. Move the wand upward toward the head and then return to waist level.
5. **Shoulder horizontal abduction/adduction.** Keeping both palms down, push the wand across the body with the uninvolved arm and then pull back across the body. Do not allow the trunk to twist.
6. **Supine external rotation.** Abduct the shoulder and flex the elbow to 90°. Grip the T-bar in the hand on the involved arm. Use the opposite arm to push the involved arm into external rotation. Perform external rotation with the arm abducted at 135° and 180°.
7. **Supine internal rotation.** With the arms in the same position as in exercise 6, use the uninvolved arm to push the involved arm into internal rotation.

A rope-and-pulley system can augment active, assistive GH flexion and abduction. Shoulder shrugs performed in three directions (i.e., superior, anterior, and posterior) can increase scapular ROM.

Restoration of Proprioception and Balance

Closed chain exercises can be performed after acute inflammation has been controlled. Shifting body weight from one hand to the other may be performed on a wall, tabletop, or unstable surface, such as a foam mat or biomechanical ankle platform system (BAPS) board. Push-ups and exercises in a frontal and sagittal plane can be performed on a Pro Fitter or slide board. The dynamic stabilizers can be addressed through using a body blade, dynamic stabilizing exercises, and incorporating PNF training within the program.

Use of free weights can develop balance, coordination, and skill in moving through diagonal patterns; however, it is imperative to include transference of proprioceptive training to the actual motions. For example, pertaining to the throwing motion, this training could involve a slow, deliberate rehearsal of the throwing motion that incorporates visual feedback through the use of mirrors or videotape. As the motion is performed, biomechanical errors are corrected. Once motion has been perfected, speed of movement and distance of throw are gradually increased.

Muscular Strength, Endurance, and Power

Gentle, resisted isometric exercises often can begin immediately after injury or surgery, even while the arm is immobilized. The exercises are initiated with the GH joint in a resting position. This is followed by application of a slow, mild overload in each of the various directions of shoulder movement. A disadvantage of isometric exercise is that strength gains are relatively specific to the joint angle at which the exercise is performed; therefore, isometric contractions must be performed at multiple positions to strengthen the joint. As the patient improves, a more moderate isometric overload is applied. Finally, a higher, rapid, unexpected resistance is provided at various positions, including the end of the ROM.

When ROM approximates normal for the patient, open chain kinetic exercises can be performed in a prone, side-lying, supine, or standing position to add gravity as resistance (**Application Strategy 17.5**). A sandbag or dumbbell can be used for added resistance. The patient should complete 50 to 100 repetitions with a 1-lb weight and should not progress in resistance until 100 repetitions are achieved. Resistance should be limited to 5 lb, because this decreases the chance of rotator cuff inflammation

Rehabilitation Exercises for the Shoulder Complex

Progressive exercises should begin when pain subsides. Exercises should be controlled and focus on the line of movement.

Resistance should progress from gravity to light dumbbells or sandbags. The exercises listed in Application Strategy 17.2 should be progressively incorporated as tolerated.

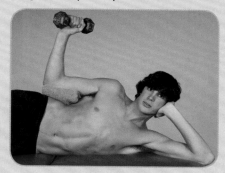

1. **Side-lying medial and lateral rotation.** Maintaining the elbow in a flexed position, perform lateral and medial rotation.

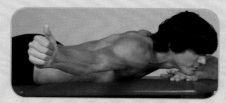

2. **Prone horizontal abduction (90°).** Positioned with the arm hanging over the table and the hand rotated outward, raise the arm and laterally rotate the humerus until it is parallel to the floor.

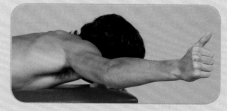

3. **Prone horizontal abduction (100°).** Positioned with the arm abducted at 100°, raise the arm and laterally rotate the humerus.

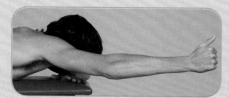

4. **Prone flexion and extension.** With the hand rotated outward as far as possible, raise the arm forward into flexion. Repeat, moving the arm into extension.

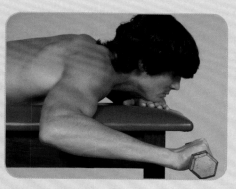

5. **Prone medial and lateral rotation.** With the shoulder abducted 90° and the elbow flexed, perform lateral and medial rotation. Repeat in the supine position.

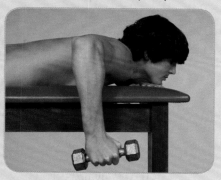

6. **Prone rows (scapular adduction).** With the shoulder abducted 90° and the elbow flexed, raise the arm off the table as if pinching the shoulder blades together. Do not raise the chest off the table.

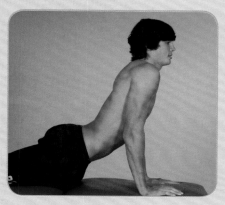

7. **Wall push-ups and press-ups.**

during the strengthening program. Careful attention should be directed to a potential painful arc of motion during concentric and eccentric contractions, because pain can further aggravate the injury. As such, the patient should work within a pain-free arc of motion with light resistance to the point of fatigue.

Muscular strength and endurance can be developed through PNF-resisted exercises in diagonal patterns to mimic functional skills or through surgical tubing used through a functional pattern. As strength improves, free-weight or machine-weight exercises for the upper body are incorporated. Many of these exercises are demonstrated in **Application Strategy 17.2.**

Plyometric exercises may involve catching a weighted ball using a quick, eccentric stretch of the muscle to facilitate a concentric contraction in throwing the ball. The exercise can progress through various one- and two-arm chest passes and overhead passes. A minitramp also can be used to do plyometric bounding push-ups.

Cardiovascular Fitness

Cardiovascular conditioning should be maintained throughout the rehabilitation program (see Chapter 13).

 Management of the swimmer's condition likely will involve rest and immobilization. As such, rehabilitation should focus on restoring shoulder motion, but it is important to avoid an aggressive flexibility program in extension, abduction, and external rotation. Strengthening exercises should progress from resisted isometric exercises to elastic band exercises below 90° of abduction. In particular, developing the strength of the lateral rotators can reduce strain on the anterior structures of the joint by pulling the humeral head posteriorly during lateral rotation of the shoulder. Strong scapula stabilizers (e.g., trapezius, rhomboids, and serratus anterior) also are believed to improve anterior stability by placing the glenoid in the optimal position to perform the required skill techniques. Isokinetic internal rotation and adduction should begin as tolerated. More aggressive shoulder rehabilitation exercises eventually should be introduced on a gradual and progressive basis.

SUMMARY

1. The shoulder complex does not function in an isolated fashion; rather, a series of joints work together in a coordinated manner to allow complicated patterns of motion. Subsequently, injury to one structure can affect other structures.

2. The throwing motion occurs in several distinct phases: windup, stride, cocking, acceleration, deceleration, and follow-through.

3. Scapulohumeral rhythm is the combined scapular and GH movement that allows coordinated shoulder motion.

4. Subsequent to the history, observation, and palpation components of an assessment, the clinician should have established a strong suspicion regarding which structures may be damaged. As such, during the physical examination component, some tests will be compulsory, whereas others will be used to confirm or exclude suspected injury or pathology. Only those tests that are absolutely necessary should be performed.

5. A moderate SC sprain is characterized by pain and swelling over the joint and an inability to horizontally adduct the arm without increased pain. The arm typically is held forward and close to the body.

6. A moderate AC sprain is characterized by an elevated distal clavicle, indicating that the coracoclavicular ligament and the AC ligaments have been torn. The patient typically has a depressed or drooping shoulder.

7. GH instability may be classified as anterior, posterior, inferior, or multidirectional. Anterior instability indicates injury to the middle and inferior GH ligaments and may have an associated Bankart lesion. MDI often is associated with pain and/or clicking during simple tasks.

8. Anterior GH dislocations are more common than posterior dislocations. The injured arm often is stabilized against the body as it is held in slight abduction and external rotation.

9. A Hill-Sachs lesion may occur with an anterior dislocation; a reverse Hill-Sachs lesion may occur with a posterior dislocation. A SLAP lesion is a superior labral tear that may disrupt the attachment of the long head of the biceps tendon and may occur with or without associated GH instability.

10. Impingement syndromes involve an abutment of the supraspinatus tendon and subacromial bursa under the coracoacromial ligament and acromion process. The glenoid labrum and long head of the biceps brachii also may be injured.

11. Thoracic outlet compression syndrome may involve compression of the lower trunk of the brachial plexus or the subclavian artery and vein. If a nerve is compressed, an aching pain or numbness may extend across the shoulder to the ulnar aspect of the hand. If arterial or venous vessels are compressed, then coolness, numbness in the entire arm, and fatigue occur after exertional, overhead activity.

12. The surgical neck is the most common site for proximal humeral fractures in adults. Adolescents, however, have a high degree of proximal humeral epiphyseal fractures because of repetitive medial rotation and adduction traction forces that are placed on the shoulder during pitching motions.

13. Pain may be referred to the shoulder from other areas of the body, particularly the heart, lungs, visceral organs, and cervical spine region.

14. Injuries that should be immediately referred to a physician include the following:

   ■ Obvious deformity suggesting a suspected fracture, separation, or dislocation

   ■ Significant loss of motion or weakness in the myotomes

   ■ Joint instability

   ■ Abnormal sensations in either the segmental dermatomes or peripheral cutaneous patterns

   ■ Absent or weak pulse distal to the injury

   ■ Any significant, unexplained pain

15. A rehabilitation program should focus on reduction of pain and spasm; restoration of motion and balance; development of strength, endurance, and power; and maintenance of cardiovascular fitness. The patient should have bilateral strength, flexibility, and muscular endurance, as well as an appropriate cardiovascular level, before returning to participation in sport and physical activity. Whenever possible, protective equipment or padding should be used to prevent reinjury.

APPLICATION QUESTIONS

1. A 20-year-old volleyball player reports to the athletic training room complaining of pain in the right arm every time the arm is abducted above 90°. What questions should be asked as part of an injury assessment for this patient? The pain and swelling associated with the condition appear to be confined to the anterior shoulder. In performing the palpation component of the injury assessment, what structures should be palpated and in which order? What specific factors should be noted? Why?

2. A 19-year-old freestyle swimmer reports to the athletic training room with shoulder pain that has been bothersome for the past 2 weeks. Following the history and inspection components of an assessment, you suspect a shoulder impingement injury. What limitations in ROM would be present if the swimmer has a shoulder impingement injury? If the supraspinatus is injured, what special test(s) would confirm the condition?

3. During a match, a high school wrestler falls on an outstretched arm and is in obvious severe pain and discomfort. Your assessment reveals an anterior displacement of the GH joint. How should this condition be managed?

4. A catcher on a high school baseball team complains of sharp shoulder pain when attempting to throw out a runner stealing second base. Palpation elicits pain in the axilla region and mild discomfort in the anterior shoulder region. What injury should be suspected? How might this injury be managed?

5. A 16-year-old gymnast lost her balance on a dismount from the beam and fell on the point of her right shoulder. Observation reveals that the involved shoulder is sagging downward and forward. The gymnast is holding the arm close to her side with the other arm's hand. There is a visible lump in the midclavicular region. What injury should be suspected? How should this injury be managed?

6. A 26-year-old male patient reports to the orthopedic clinic complaining of shoulder pain. He has been playing recreational softball for the past 2 months and his right shoulder feels loose. Pain increases during the deceleration phase of the throwing motion. As a college football player, he sustained two right shoulder anterior dislocations. The patient has GH instability in addition to a labral tear. How would you differentiate between a Bankart lesion and a SLAP lesion?

7. A soccer player fell on an outstretched arm and is now complaining of pain on the top of the shoulder. It appears that the distal clavicle is somewhat elevated. There is increased pain over the AC joint with horizontal adduction of the arm across the chest and with shoulder flexion. What structures may be involved in this injury? How might you manage this injury?

8. A 20-year-old volleyball player reports to the athletic training room complaining of pain in the right arm every time the arm is abducted above 90°. What questions should be asked to develop a history of the injury? The pain and swelling associated with the condition appear to be confined to the anterior shoulder. In performing the palpation component of the injury assessment, what structures should be palpated and in which order? What specific factors should be noted? Why?

9. A 58-year-old female has participated in badminton competitions in conjunction with the Senior Olympics. A physician diagnosed her with a painful shoulder subsequent to impingement syndrome. The physician has directed you to develop a rehabilitation program for this patient. What priorities will you establish in rehabilitating this injury and returning the patient to full functional status?

REFERENCES

1. Lintner D, Noonan TJ, Kibler WB. Injury patterns and biomechanics of the athlete's shoulder. *Clin Sports Med.* 2008;27(4):527–551.
2. Wolf BR, Ebinger AE, Lawler MP, et al. Injury patterns in Division I collegiate swimming. *Am J Sports Med.* 2009;37(10):2037–2042.
3. Reeser JC, Joy EA, Porucznik CA, et al. Risk factors for volleyball-related shoulder pain and dysfunction. *PM R.* 2010;2(1):27–36.
4. Halloran L. Wrestling injuries. *Orthop Nurs.* 2008;27(3):189–194.
5. Kelly BT, Barnes RP, Powell JW, et al. Shoulder injuries to quarterbacks in the National Football League. *Am J Sports Med.* 2004;32:328–331.
6. Macdonald PB, Lapointe P. Acromioclavicular and sternoclavicular joint injuries. *Orthop Clin North Am.* 2008;39(4):535–545.
7. Colegate-Stone T, Allom R, Singh R, et al. Classification of the morphology of the acromioclavicular joint using cadaveric and radiological analysis. *J Bone Joint Surg Br.* 2010;92(5):743–746.

8. Simovitch R, Sanders B, Ozbaydar M, et al. Acromioclavicular joint injuries: diagnosis and management. *J Am Acad Orthop Surg.* 2009;17(4):207–219.

9. Costic RS, Vangura A Jr, Fenwick JA, et al. Viscoelastic behavior and structural properties of the coracoclavicular ligaments. *Scand J Med Sci Sports.* 2003;13:305–310.

10. Crosbie J, Kilbreath SL, Dylke E. The kinematics of the scapulae and spine during a lifting task. *J Biomech.* 2010;43(7):1302–1309.

11. Escamilla RF, Andrews JR. Shoulder muscle recruitment patterns and related biomechanics during upper extremity sports. *Sports Med.* 2009;39(7):569–590.

12. Fleisig GS, Escamilla RF, Andrews JR. Biomechanics of throwing. In: Zachazewski JE, Magee DJ, Quillen WS, eds. *Athletic Injuries and Rehabilitation.* Philadelphia, PA: WB Saunders; 1996:352–353.

13. Ouellette H, Labis J, Bredella M, et al. Spectrum of shoulder injuries in the baseball pitcher. *Skeletal Radiol.* 2008;37(6):491–498.

14. Hall SJ. *Basic Biomechanics.* 6th ed. Dubuque, IA: McGraw-Hill; 2011.

15. Kendall FP, McCreary EK, Provance PG, et al. *Muscles: Testing and Function with Posture and Pain.* 5th ed. Baltimore, MD: Lippincott Williams & Wilkins; 2005.

16. Starkey C, Brown SD. *Orthopedic & Athletic Injury Examination Handbook.* 3rd ed. Philadelphia, PA: FA Davis; 2015.

17. Walton J, Mahajan S, Paxinos A, et al. Diagnostic values of tests for acromioclavicular joint pain. *J Bone Joint Surg Am.* 2004;86-A(4):807–812.

18. Magee DJ. *Orthopedic Physical Assessment.* St. Louis, MO: Elsevier Health Sciences; 2014.

19. Chronopoulos E, Kim TK, Park HB, et al. Diagnostic value of physical tests for isolated chronic acromioclavicular lesions. *Am J Sports Med.* 2004;32(3):655–661.

20. Gulick D. *Ortho Notes: Clinical Examination Pocket Guide.* 2nd ed. Philadelphia, PA: FA Davis; 2009.

21. Cleland J. *Orthopedic Clinical Examination: An Evidence-Based Approach for Physical Therapists.* Carlstadt, NJ: Icon Learning Systems; 2005.

22. Wong M. *Pocket Orthopaedics: Evidence-Based Survival Guide.* Sudbury, MA: Jones & Bartlett; 2010.

23. Park HB, Yokota A, Gill HS, et al. Diagnostic accuracy of clinical tests for the different degrees of subacromial impingement syndrome. *J Bone Joint Surg Am.* 2005;87(7):1446–1455.

24. Lee CK, Itoi E, Kim SJ, et al. Comparison of muscle activity in the empty-can and full-can testing positions using 18 F-FDG PET/CT. *J Orthop Surg Res.* 2014;9:85.

25. Asplund C, Pollard ME. Posterior sternoclavicular joint dislocation in a wrestler. *Mil Med.* 2004;169(2):134–136.

26. Bicos J, Nicholson GP. Treatment and results of sternoclavicular joint injuries. *Clin Sports Med.* 2003;22(2):359–370.

27. Schrumpf MA, Maak TG, Delos D, et al. The management of anterior glenohumeral instability with and without bone loss: AAOS exhibit selection. *J Bone Joint Surg Am.* 2014;96:e12.

28. Owens BD, Campbell SE, Cameron KL. Risk factors for posterior shoulder instability in young athletes. *Am J Sports Med.* 2013;41(11):2645–2649.

29. Olds M, Ellis R, Donaldson K, et al. Risk factors which predispose first-time traumatic anterior shoulder dislocations to recurrent instability in adults: a systematic review and meta-analysis. *Br J Sports Med.* 2014;49(14):913–922.

30. Wang DH. New exam for glenoid labral tears. *Phys Sportsmed.* 1997;25(2):15.

31. Trojian T, Stevenson JH, Agrawal N. What can we expect from nonoperative treatment options for shoulder pain? *J Fam Pract.* 2005;54(3):216–223.

32. Boileau P, Brassart N, Watkinson DJ, et al. Arthroscopic repair of full-thickness tears of the supraspinatus: does the tendon really heal? *J Bone Joint Surg Am.* 2005;87(96):1229–1240.

33. Patton WC, McCluskey GM III. Biceps tendinitis and subluxation. *Clin Sports Med.* 2001;20(3):505–529.

34. Samarasam I, Sadhu D, Agarwal S, et al. Surgical management of thoracic outlet syndrome: a 10-year experience. *ANZ J Surg.* 2004;74(6):450–454.

35. Kocher MS, Waters PM, Micheli LJ. Upper extremity injuries in the paediatric athlete. *Sports Med.* 2000;30(2):117–135.

36. Ryan RS, Munk PL. Radiology for the surgeon. Musculoskeletal case 33. Post-traumatic osteolysis of the clavicle. *Can J Surg.* 2004;47(5):373–374.

18

Upper Arm, Elbow, and Forearm Conditions

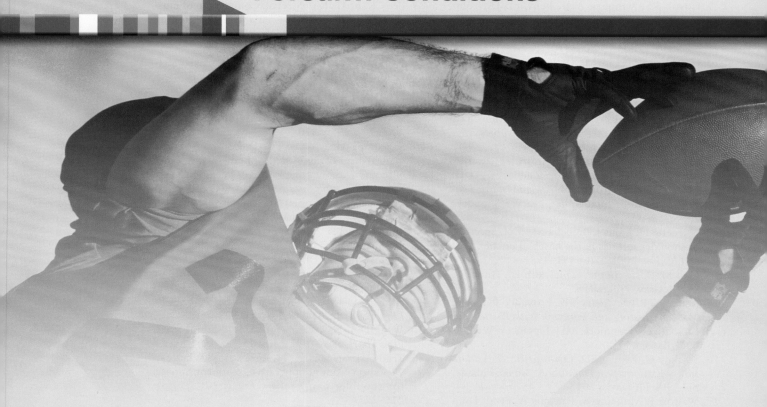

STUDENT OUTCOMES

1. Identify the important bony and soft-tissue structures in the upper arm, elbow, and forearm.

2. Describe the major motions at the elbow and list the muscles that produce them.

3. Explain the general principles used to prevent injuries to the shoulder.

4. Describe the forces that produce the loading patterns responsible for common injuries to the upper arm, elbow, and forearm.

5. Describe a thorough assessment of the elbow region.

6. List the common acute injuries and conditions sustained in the upper arm, elbow, and forearm regions by physically active individuals.

7. Describe the soft-tissue pathology in the upper arm, elbow, and forearm regions resulting from overuse.

8. Explain the management strategies for common injuries and conditions of the upper arm, elbow, and forearm.

9. Describe the various types of fractures found at the elbow and explain their management.

10. Explain the general principles and techniques used in developing a rehabilitation exercise program for the elbow region.

INTRODUCTION

The arms perform lifting and carrying tasks, cushion the body during collisions, and lessen body momentum during falls. In many sports, performance is contingent on the ability of the arms to effectively swing a racquet or club or the hands to position for throwing and catching. In collision sports such as football and rugby and in combative events such as judo and karate, acute elbow injuries are the most commonly occurring injuries.[1] Sports that involve high-speed activities such as skiing, skating, and cycling, as well as sports that require the athlete to perform at heights, such as gymnastics, pole vault, and high jump, also see a higher number of acute injuries of the elbow, wrist, and hand.[1] Muscular weakness and imbalance, decreased proprioception, inadequate muscle length and flexibility, improper conditioning, and training errors, as well as poor biomechanics, all contribute to developing chronic elbow, wrist, and hand injuries.[2,3]

This chapter begins with a review of anatomy and an overview of the kinematics and kinetics of the upper arm, elbow, and forearm. A discussion concerning prevention of injury is followed by the injury assessment process. Information regarding common injuries to the upper arm, elbow, and forearm is presented, followed by examples of rehabilitation exercises.

ANATOMY OF THE ELBOW

Although the elbow generally may be thought of as a simple hinge joint, the elbow actually is categorized as a trochoginglymus joint that encompasses three articulations: the humeroulnar, humeroradial, and proximal radioulnar joints.[4] The bony structure of the elbow and forearm is displayed in **Figure 18.1**. Several strong ligaments bind these articulations together, and a single-joint capsule surrounds all three. Twenty-three muscles associated with the elbow provide dynamic stability.[4]

Humeroulnar Joint

The humeroulnar joint at the elbow is a hinge joint. It is the articulation of the trochlea of the humerus with the reciprocally shaped trochlear fossa of the ulna. Motion capabilities primarily are flexion and extension. In some individuals, particularly women, however, a small amount (i.e., 5° to 15°) of hyperextension is allowed. The joint is most stable in the close-packed position of extension.

Humeroradial Joint

The humeroradial joint, which is lateral to the humeroulnar joint, is formed between the spherical capitellum of the humerus and the proximal radius. It is a gliding joint, with motion restricted to the sagittal plane by the adjacent humeroulnar joint. The close-packed position is with the elbow flexed at 90°, and the forearm is supinated approximately 5°.

Proximal Radioulnar Joint

The annular ligament binds the head of the radius to the radial notch of the ulna, forming the proximal radioulnar joint. It is a pivot joint that permits forearm pronation and supination to occur as the radius rolls medially and laterally over the ulna (**Fig. 18.2**). The close-packed position is at 5° of forearm supination.

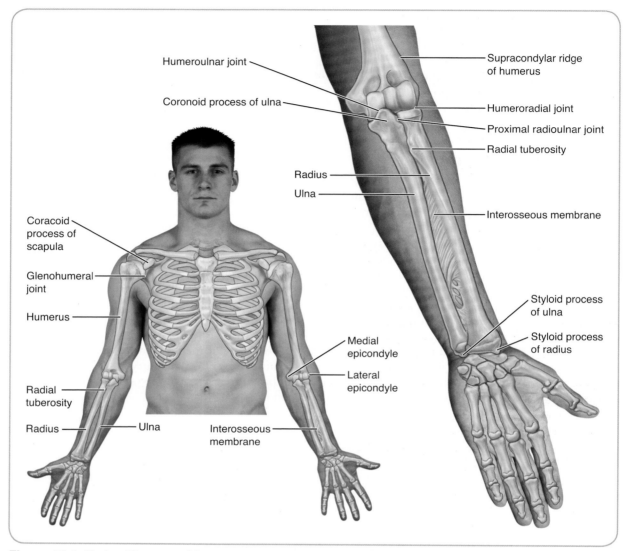

Figure 18.1. Skeletal features of the upper arm, elbow, and forearm.

Carrying Angle

The angle between the longitudinal axes of the humerus and the ulna when the arm is in anatomical position is known as the carrying angle. The angle is so named because it causes the forearm to angle away from the body when a load is carried in the hand. Given, however, that loads typically are carried with the forearm in a neutral rather than a fully supinated position, the functional significance of the carrying angle is questionable. Nevertheless, the size of the carrying angle at the elbow is one of the skeletal differences between females and males and is attributed to differences in the shape of the trochlea. When the elbow is fully extended and the forearm fully supinated, the carrying angle ranges from approximately 10° to 15° in adults and generally is greater in females than in males. The carrying angle changes with skeletal growth and maturity and is always greater on the side of the dominant hand.[5]

Ligaments of the Elbow

The elbow is reinforced by capsuloligamentous structures that are thickenings of the capsule. These form the medial and lateral ligamentous complexes (**Fig. 18.3**). The medial (ulnar) collateral ligament, the most important ligament for stability of the elbow joint, is divided into three oblique bands denoted by their anatomical location—namely, anterior, transverse, and posterior. The anterior oblique band is taut throughout the elbow's full range of motion (ROM) and is the primary restraint against valgus forces. The transverse oblique band provides little, if any, support to the medial elbow. The posterior oblique band is a fan-shaped, capsular thickening that generally is taut when the elbow is flexed beyond 90°.

The lateral (radial) collateral ligament complex consists of four components: the lateral ulnar collateral, radial collateral, annular, and accessory ligaments. The radial collateral ligament, which runs from the lateral epicondyle of the humerus and terminates at the annular ligament, resists varus forces. The posterior portion of this ligament, which is referred to as the lateral ulnar collateral ligament, extends distally to the lateral ulna.

The annular ligament fits tightly around the radial head and upper portion of the neck. It permits pronation and supination of the forearm as the radius rotates, internally and externally, on the ulna. Superior and inferior oblique bands of the annular ligament attach proximally and distally to the ulna.[6] During extreme supination, the anterior fibers of the annular ligament are taut; during extreme pronation, the posterior fibers are taut. The accessory lateral collateral ligament is a superficial layer of fibers that blends with the annular ligament to insert onto the supinator tubercle of the ulna.

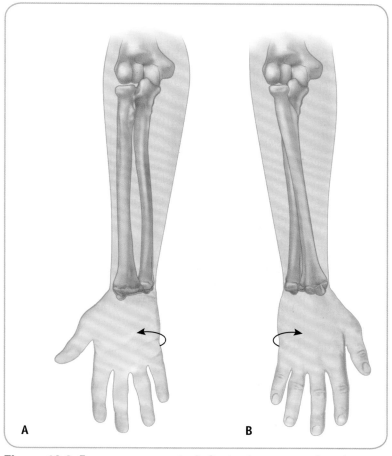

A   **B**

Figure 18.2. **Forearm movements. A,** Supination occurs when the radius and ulna are parallel to each other. **B,** Pronation involves the rotation of the radius over the ulna.

Bursae of the Elbow

Although the elbow has several small bursae, the most clinically relevant is the subcutaneous olecranon bursa located between the olecranon and the skin surface. The lubricating function of the bursa facilitates smooth gliding of the skin over the olecranon process during elbow flexion and extension.

Muscles of the Elbow

A large number of muscles cross the elbow (**Figs. 18.4** and **18.5**). Identifying the actions of these muscles is complicated by the fact that several muscles are two-joint muscles, which extend into the shoulder or the hand and fingers.

Nerves of the Elbow

The major nerves of the elbow and forearm descend from the brachial plexus and include the musculocutaneous (C5 through C7), median (C5 through T1), ulnar (C8 through T1), and radial nerves (C5 through T1) (**Fig. 18.6**). The musculocutaneous nerve provides motor supply to the flexor muscles of the anterior arm and sensory innervation to the skin of the lateral forearm. The median nerve supplies most of the flexor muscles of the anterior forearm and the skin on the palmar aspect of the hand, including the thumb, index finger, and middle finger, and the lateral half of the ring finger. The ulnar nerve provides innervation to the flexor carpi ulnaris and the medial half of the flexor digitorum profundus and to the skin on the medial border of the hand, including the little finger and the medial half of the ring finger. The radial nerve, which is the largest branch

See **Muscles of the Elbow**, available on the companion Web site at thePoint, for a summary of these muscles, including attachments, primary actions, and innervation.

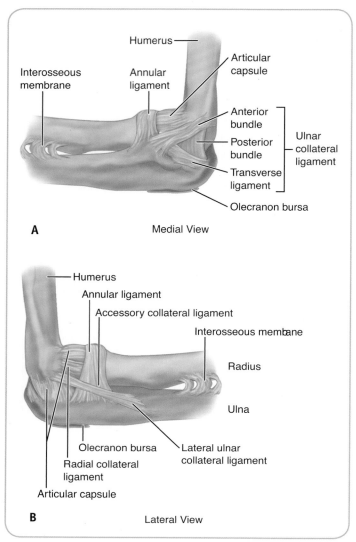

A Medial View

B Lateral View

Figure 18.3. Major ligaments and the olecranon bursa of the elbow. A, Medial view. **B,** Lateral view.

of the brachial plexus, passes anteriorly to the lateral epicondyle at the elbow and then divides into superficial and deep branches to continue along the posterolateral aspect of the forearm. The radial nerve supplies the arm and forearm extensor muscles and the skin on the posterior aspect of the arm and forearm.

Blood Vessels of the Elbow

The major arteries of the elbow and forearm region are the brachial, ulnar, and radial arteries (**Fig. 18.7**). The brachial artery courses down the medial side of the arm, providing blood supply to the flexor muscles of the arm. The deep brachial artery branches off to supply the triceps brachii. In the elbow, the brachial artery forms an anastomosis, or a network of communicating blood vessels, to supply the elbow joint. The main branch of the brachial artery crosses the anterior aspect of the elbow, where the brachial pulse can be readily palpated.

Distal to the elbow, the brachial artery splits into the ulnar and radial arteries. The ulnar artery supplies the medial forearm, and, via one of its branches, the common interosseous artery supplies the deep flexors and extensors of the forearm. The radial artery, which courses along the anterior aspect of the radius, supplies the lateral forearm muscles. Pulses can be taken for both arteries on the anterior aspect of the wrist (see **Fig. 6.3**).

KINEMATICS AND MAJOR MUSCLE ACTIONS OF THE ELBOW

The three associated joints at the elbow allow motion in two planes. Flexion and extension are sagittal plane movements that occur at the humeroulnar and humeroradial joints; pronation and supination are longitudinal rotational movements that take place at the proximal radioulnar joint.

Flexion and Extension

The elbow flexors include those muscles that cross the anterior side of the joint. The primary elbow flexor is the brachialis. Because the distal attachment of the brachialis is the coronoid process of the ulna, the muscle is equally effective when the forearm is in supination or in pronation. Another elbow flexor, the biceps brachii, has both long and short heads attached to the radial tuberosity via a single common tendon. When the forearm is supinated, the biceps contributes effectively to flexion, because it is slightly stretched. When the forearm is pronated, the muscle is less taut and, consequently, less effective. The brachioradialis, which also is an elbow flexor, is most effective when the forearm is in a neutral position (i.e., midway between full pronation and full supination). Other flexor muscles that cross the elbow are important dynamic stabilizers of the joint. In particular, the flexor carpi ulnaris and flexor digitorum superficialis provide significant stability to the medial elbow during a variety of activities, including throwing.

The triceps is the major elbow extensor. Although the three heads have separate origins, they attach to the olecranon process of the ulna through a common distal tendon. The small anconeus muscle also assists with extension at the elbow.

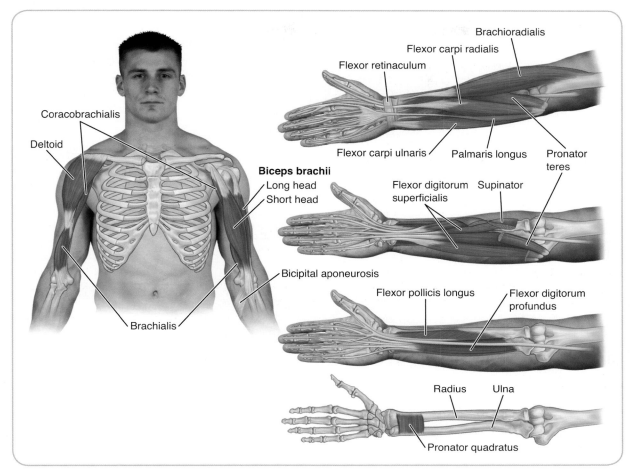

Figure 18.4. Muscles of the anterior arm and forearm.

Pronation and Supination

Pronation and supination of the forearm occur when the radius rotates around the ulna. Three radioulnar articulations exist: the proximal, middle, and distal radioulnar joints. The proximal and distal joints are pivot joints. The middle radioulnar joint is a syndesmosis, with an elastic, interconnecting membrane that permits supination and pronation but prevents longitudinal displacement of one bone with respect to the other. The primary pronator muscle is the pronator quadratus, which attaches to the distal ulna and radius. The pronator teres, which crosses the proximal radioulnar joint, assists with pronation. As the name suggests, the supinator is the muscle primarily responsible for supination. During resistance or elbow flexion, the biceps also participates in supination.

KINETICS OF THE ELBOW

Although the elbow is not considered to be a weight-bearing joint, it sustains significant loads during daily activities. For example, it has been estimated that the compressive load at the elbow reaches 300 N (67 lb) during activities such as dressing and eating, 1,700 N (382 lb) when the body is supported by the arms when rising from a chair, and 1,900 N (427 lb) when pulling a table across the floor.[7] During performance of a one-handed push-up, compression at the elbow ranges around 65% of body weight.[8] Extremely large forces are generated by muscles crossing the elbow during forceful pitching and throwing motions as well as during weight lifting and many resistance training exercises. In fact, during an activity such as pitching, valgus stress at the elbow during the late cocking

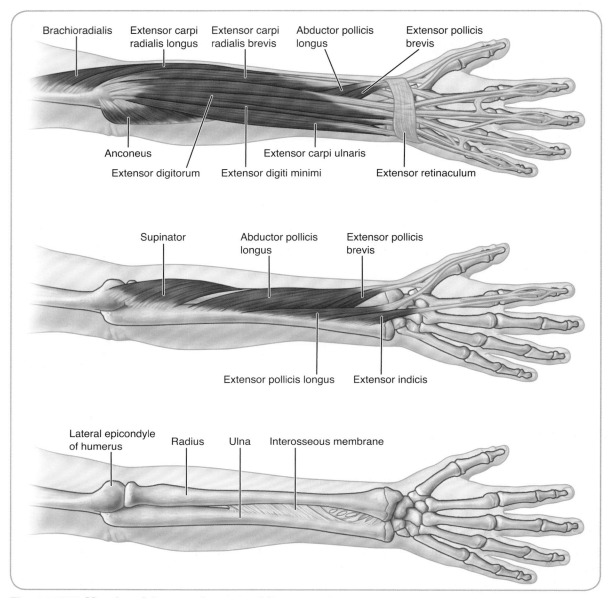

Figure 18.5. Muscles of the posterior arm and forearm.

and acceleration phases of the throw can exceed the strength of the ulnar collateral ligament, resulting in microscopic tears within it.[9] The triceps, wrist flexor–pronator muscles, and anconeus must develop tension to assist the ulnar collateral ligament in resisting the valgus load. Greater valgus loads at the elbow have been associated with higher maximum pitch velocity as well as with a sidearm delivery.[10,11] When falling onto an outstretched hand with the elbow extended, varus–valgus loads are increased 1.4 times with the arm externally rotated and 2.7 times with the arm internally rotated.[12] During the execution of many skills in gymnastics and wrestling, the elbow functions as a weight-bearing joint.

Because the attachment of the elbow extensors to the ulna is closer to the joint center than the attachments of the elbow flexors on the radius and ulna, the extensor moment arm is shorter than the flexor moment arm. This means that the elbow extensors must generate more force than the elbow flexors to produce the same amount of joint torque. This translates to greater joint compression forces during extension than during flexion, when movements with comparable speed and force requirements are executed.

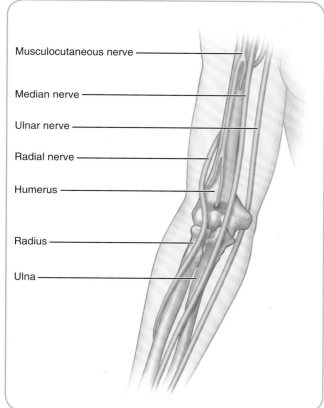

Figure 18.6. **Nerves of the elbow region.**

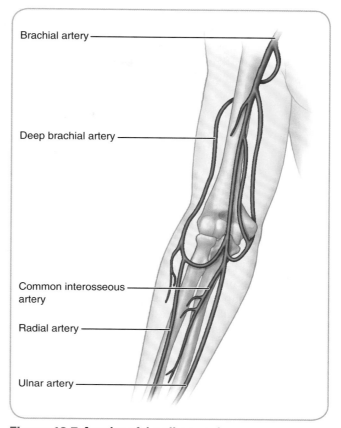

Figure 18.7. **Arteries of the elbow region.**

PREVENTION OF ELBOW CONDITIONS

The elbow often is subjected to compressive forces when the arm is placed in a position to cushion a fall or lessen the body's impact with another object. Limiting the height to which cheerleaders may stack and drop team members and the degree to which competitors in sports such as judo and wrestling may torque the elbow may contribute to a decrease in traumatic injury.[1] And while protective padding has been found to be one of the few methods for preventing some acute injuries, few sports require protective equipment at the elbow.[1] Microtraumatic forces caused by repetitive valgus and varus stresses can lead to overuse injuries, many of which are related to poor skill technique. Therefore, physical conditioning and proper skill technique are major factors in preventing injury to this region.

Early warning signs of impeding overuse injury in youth sport athletes include arm pain or soreness, fatigue, and decrease in quality or ability to throw.[13] Youth sport athletes should be encouraged to participate in only one overhead throwing sport at a time and avoid playing that one sport year round. Limiting time engaged in repetitive sport activity to no more than 16 hours per week and establishing pitching limits is thought to decrease the incidence and severity of overuse injuries for youth sport athletes.[13] Pitching limits are age-based: For pitchers between the ages of 9 and 14 years, the suggested limit is 75 pitches per game, 600 pitches per season, and between 2,000 and 3,000 pitches per year. For pitchers aged 15 to 18 years, the limit is set at 90 pitches per game with no more than two games per week.[13]

Protective Equipment

A variety of equipment types can be advantageous in preventing injury to the elbow. Because standard shoulder pads may not extend far enough to protect the upper arm, many football players attach an additional biceps pad to the shoulder pads to protect this vulnerable area. Special pads are available to protect the elbow during falls and collisions. Padded elbow sleeves or neoprene sleeves are worn in many sports to protect the olecranon from direct trauma and abrasions, particularly when playing on artificial turf. Counterforce braces, which commonly are used by participants in racquet sports, are intended to reduce muscle tensile forces that can lead to medial or lateral epicondylitis. Finally, hinged braces can add compression and support to the elbow to reduce excessive varus and valgus forces.

Physical Conditioning

The physical condition program should include a preseason and in-season component. Because throwing power and speed originates in the trunk and not the upper extremity, it is important to include exercises and training sessions that focus on neuromuscular control, balance, coordination, flexibility, and strengthening of the lower extremities.[13] This is especially true among pediatric athletes and those with a history of past injury.[13] Furthermore, when working with the youth sport athlete, the intensity, load, time, and distance the athlete is required to achieve should only be increased by about 10% each week to avoid overloading and breakdown.[13]

Many of the muscles that move the elbow also move the shoulder and wrist. Therefore, flexibility and strengthening exercises must focus on the entire arm. General flexibility exercises for the shoulder can be used in conjunction with warm-up exercises that mimic specific sport skills. For example, a tennis player may begin the warm-up session with slow, controlled forehand and backhand strokes that gradually increase in intensity. A pitcher or outfielder may begin with short, controlled throws, increasing the distance and intensity as the arm is warmed up. Strengthening exercises for the shoulder can be combined with those listed in **Application Strategy 18.1**. These exercises are designed to improve general strength in elbow flexion and extension, forearm pronation and supination, wrist flexion and extension, and radial and ulnar deviation. Physical conditioning programs should begin with light resistance and progress to a heavier resistance.

Proper Skill Technique

Nearly all overuse injuries are directly related to repetitive, throwing-type motions that produce microtraumatic tensile forces on the surrounding soft-tissue structures. Children who use a sidearm throwing motion are threefold more likely to develop problems compared with those who use a more traditional overhead technique. Movement analysis can detect improper technique in the acceleration and follow-through phase that contributes to these excessive tensile forces. High-speed photography may aid in this analysis.

Teaching sport participants the shoulder-roll method of falling is another preventive measure. Falling on an extended hand or flexed elbow is the most common mechanism for acute injuries in the upper extremity. Excessive compressive forces can be transmitted along the long axis of the bones, leading to a fracture or dislocation.

ASSESSMENT OF ELBOW CONDITIONS

 A Little League Baseball player is complaining of pain on the medial elbow during pitching. How should the assessment of this injury progress to determine the extent and severity of injury?

The elbow's primary role is to place the forearm and hand in the most appropriate position to perform efficient motion. Biomechanical errors in throwing technique at the shoulder can place additional stress at the elbow. Because use of equipment often is associated with overuse problems, it is important to determine if the individual uses a bat, racquet, field hockey or lacrosse stick, or other implement. Assessment of skill technique to rule out possible contributing factors also is advisable.

Because of the severity of the trauma, recognizing possible fractures and dislocations early in an assessment is essential. It also is important to understand that pain may be referred from the cervical region, shoulder, or wrist to the arm. As in any assessment, both arms should be fully visible to allow bilateral comparison.

 See **Application Strategy: Elbow Evaluation**, available on the companion Web site at thePoint, for a summary of the assessment of the upper arm, elbow, and forearm.

APPLICATION STRATEGY 18.1

Exercises to Prevent Injury to the Elbow Region

Begin all exercises with light resistance using dumbbells or surgical tubing.

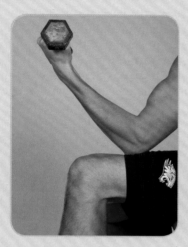

1. **Biceps curl.** Support the involved arm on the leg and fully flex the elbow. This also can be performed bilaterally in a standing position with a barbell.

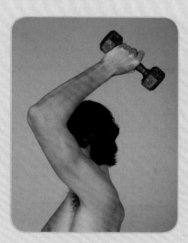

2. **Triceps curl.** Raise the involved arm over the head and extend the involved arm at the elbow. This also can be performed bilaterally in a supine or standing position with a barbell.

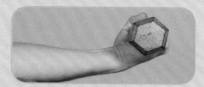

3. **Wrist flexion.** Support the involved forearm on a table or your leg with the hand off the edge. With the palm facing up, slowly do a full wrist curl and then return to the starting position.

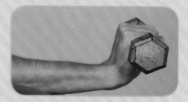

4. **Wrist extension.** Support the involved forearm on a table or your leg with the hand off the edge. With the palm facing down, slowly do a full reverse wrist curl and then return to the starting position.

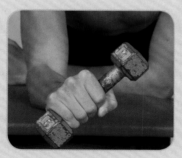

5. **Forearm pronation–supination.** Support the involved forearm on a table or your leg with the hand off the edge. With surgical tubing or a hand dumbbell, roll the forearm into pronation and then return to supination. Adjust the surgical tubing and reverse the exercise, stressing the supinators. The elbow should remain stationary.

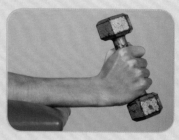

6. **Ulnar–radial deviation.** Support the involved forearm on a table or your leg with the hand off the edge. With surgical tubing or a hand dumbbell, perform ulnar deviation. Reverse directions and perform radial deviation. An alternate method is to stand with the arm at the side while holding a hammer or a weighted bar. Raise the wrist in ulnar deviation. Repeat in radial deviation.

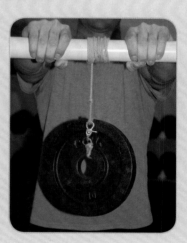

7. **Wrist curl-ups.** Exercising the wrist extensors is performed by gripping the bar with both palms facing down. Slowly wind the cord onto the bar until the weight reaches the top and then slowly unwind the cord. Reverse the hand position to work the wrist flexors.

HISTORY

> The injury assessment of the Little League Baseball player should begin with a history. What questions need to be asked to identify the cause and extent of this injury?

See **Application Strategy: Developing a History of the Injury**, available on the companion Web site at thePoint, for specific questions that should be included in an elbow evaluation.

The onset and location of symptoms are two of the most critical facts surrounding elbow trauma. This information forms the basis for determining the cause-and-effect relationship between the mechanism and the onset of injury. In gathering information about the primary complaint, questions should focus on the individual's perception of pain, weakness, or sensory changes. It also is important to note if the nature of the injury is acute or overuse. Specific questions should be asked related to equipment, technique, and recent changes in training intensity, frequency, or duration.

> The Little League Baseball player should be asked questions that address the following: when, where, and how; throwing technique and training regimen; phase of throwing motion in which pain occurs; intensity, location, and type of pain; actions that relieve pain; and any previous injury, treatment, and medication.

OBSERVATION AND INSPECTION

> The history of the Little League player reveals that an aching pain has been present for 2 to 3 days. The pain intensifies during the acceleration phase of throwing and has started to affect his performance. Explain the observation component in the ongoing assessment of the Little League player.

If the history has indicated an insidious onset of elbow trauma, the individual's full-body posture, especially of the neck and shoulder area, should be observed. In an acute injury, if the individual is in great pain or is unable or unwilling to move the elbow, the assessment should be completed in the position that is most comfortable for the individual.

Initially, the arm should be observed from an anterior position for any noticeable deformity and possible holding of the arm. If swelling is present in the joint, the individual may be unable to fully extend the elbow, resulting in a slightly flexed position. This **resting position** allows the joint to have maximal volume to accommodate intra-articular swelling. The carrying angle of the arms should be noted. A normal angle is slight valgus, with the forearm fully supinated and the elbow extended. Angles of greater than 20° are referred to as **cubital valgus**; angles of less than 10° are referred to as **cubital varus**. Baseball pitchers may exhibit cubital valgus in the throwing arm as an adaptation to repeated valgus loading during the throwing motion. The alignment of the forearm and humerus normally is fully extended, although extension beyond 0° (**cubital recurvatum**) is common, especially in females.

In the next portion of the observation, the elbow should be observed in the position of function, namely 90° of flexion, with the hand being held halfway between supination and pronation. The entire region should be assessed for symmetry and any abnormal deformity, muscle atrophy, hypertrophy, swelling, discoloration, or previous surgical incisions. In particular, the cubital fossa, which is a triangular area bounded laterally by the brachioradialis muscle and medially by the pronator teres muscle, should be inspected. The biceps brachii tendon, median nerve, and brachial artery pass through the fossa. The presence of swelling in the fossa can place pressure on the neurovascular structures as they pass through the area.

Next, the medial aspect of the arm should be inspected. The medial epicondyle of the humerus should be prominent rather than obscured by excessive swelling. The wrist flexor muscle mass should appear bilaterally equal in terms of muscle tone and mass. Atrophy of the mass may result from disuse associated with long-term tendinitis or prolonged immobilization.

Observation should then move to the lateral aspect of the arm. The wrist extensor muscle mass on the lateral aspect of the elbow also should appear bilaterally equal in terms of muscle tone and mass. Atrophy of the mass may result from disuse associated with long-term tendinitis, prolonged immobilization, or radial nerve pathology.

Finally, the arm should be observed from a posterior position. It is important to note the position of the olecranon relative to the epicondyles of the humerus. In a flexed position, the olecranon process and epicondyles should form an isosceles triangle; in an extended position, the olecranon process and epicondyles should form a straight line. The olecranon process should be clearly visible rather than obscured by excessive swelling.

Observation of the Little League player should include the following: full-body posture; carrying angle and position of function; and inspection at the site for swelling, discoloration, deformity, muscle hypertrophy, atrophy, and other signs of trauma.

PALPATION

Observation of the Little League player reveals minor swelling over the medial epicondyle. No other visible signs are apparent. Explain palpation specific to the injury sustained by the player.

The injured arm should be supported during palpation. Bilateral palpation should determine temperature, swelling, point tenderness, crepitus, deformity, muscle spasm, and cutaneous sensation. In general, palpation should move from proximal to distal, leaving the areas that are anticipated to be the most painful for last. Pulses can be taken at the radial and ulnar arteries at the wrist and at the brachial artery in the cubital fossa. The following structures should be palpated:

Anterior Palpation

1. Cubital fossa, biceps brachii tendon, median nerve, and brachial artery

2. Coracoid process and head of radius

Lateral Palpation

1. Lateral supracondylar ridge and brachioradialis muscle

2. Lateral epicondyle, common wrist extensors, and supinator muscle

3. Radial collateral ligament

4. Annular ligament and head of the radius (this is facilitated by supination and pronation of the forearm and should only be performed if no deformity is present)

Posterior Palpation

1. Triceps muscle

2. Olecranon process and olecranon fossa (this is facilitated by positioning the elbow in 45° of flexion to relax the triceps and should only be performed if no deformity is present)

3. Olecranon bursa (the skin overlying the olecranon process should be grasped, which permits palpation to note any thickening or presence of loose bodies)

4. Ulnar nerve in the cubital tunnel

5. Ulnar border distal to the styloid process at the wrist

Medial Palpation

1. Medial supracondylar ridge

2. Medial epicondyle and common wrist flexor–pronator tendons and muscles

3. Ulnar collateral ligament

 During the assessment of the Little League player, the following structures should be palpated for point tenderness, swelling, deformity, skin temperature, sensation, and other signs of trauma: medial supracondylar ridge, medial epicondyle, proximal attachment of wrist flexors and pronators, ulnar collateral ligament, ulna, olecranon, and ulnar nerve.

PHYSICAL EXAMINATION TESTS

? Palpation of the Little League player revealed point tenderness and swelling directly on the medial epicondyle. Based on the information obtained through the history, observation, and palpation, what tests should be performed as part of the physical examination of Little League player?

If a fracture or dislocation is suspected, testing should not be performed. Instead, the arm should be immobilized in an appropriate splint, and the emergency action plan should be activated. In some settings, summoning emergency medical services (EMS) may be warranted. Only those tests that are necessary to assess the current injury should be performed.

Functional Tests

The available ROM in elbow flexion–extension, forearm pronation–supination, and wrist flexion–extension should be determined. If trauma to the ulnar, median, or radial nerves is suspected, ROM testing of the thumb and fingers also should be performed.

Active Movements

The clinician should stabilize the upper arm against the body to prevent muscle substitution. As with previous assessments, bilateral comparison with the uninvolved arm is necessary. Active movements that are anticipated to be painful should be performed last to prevent painful symptoms from overflowing into the next movement.

The motions that should be assessed and the normal ROM for each are as follows:

- Flexion at the elbow (140° to 150°)

- Extension at the elbow (0° to 10°)

- Supination of the forearm (90°)

- Pronation of the forearm (90°)

- Flexion of the wrist (80° to 90°)

- Extension of the wrist (70° to 90°)

During elbow extension, it is important to recognize that some females can extend as much as 5° to 15° below the straight line. Bilateral comparison verifies whether this extra motion is normal for the individual. In performing active pronation and supination, the individual should be instructed to flex the elbow to 90° and then secure the elbow next to the body to avoid any glenohumeral motion. Goniometry measurements are demonstrated in **Figure 18.8**.

Passive Movements

If the individual is able to perform full ROM during active movements, gentle overpressure should be applied at the extremes of motion to determine end feel. The normal end feels are as follows:

- **Tissue stretch**—elbow flexion; supination; pronation
- **Tissue approximation**—shoulder adduction
- **Bone to bone**—elbow extension

Resisted Muscle Testing

The elbow should be stabilized against the body during muscle testing to prevent any muscle substitution. The testing begins with the clinician placing the muscle on a stretch. When performing the various motions, the clinician should apply gentle resistance proximal to the wrist throughout the full ROM. To avoid allowing finger flexors or extensors to assist during movement, instruct the patient to keep the thumb and fingers relaxed. Motion should be assessed several times to note any weakness or fatigue. Any sudden or jarring motions should be avoided, because this may lead to undue pain. Any lag or muscle weakness should be noted. Muscle actions that may cause extreme pain should be delayed until the final phase of muscle testing. **Figure 18.9** demonstrates motions that should be tested.

Manual Muscle Testing

If pain or weakness is found during resisted ROM, the clinician may decide to perform a manual muscle test to determine which muscle is damaged. To correctly apply the manual muscle testing techniques to the shoulder complex, the torso must be properly stabilized.[14] See **Table 18.1** for manual muscle testing procedures for the shoulder.

Stress Tests

In using stress tests, only those tests that are absolutely necessary should be performed. In moving through the tests, the clinician should begin by applying gentle stress. The force should be applied several times with increasing overpressure. The presence of pain or joint laxity should be noted.

Ulnar Collateral Ligament Stress Test (Valgus Stress Test)

Because of the amount of rotation that occurs at the shoulder, it is difficult to get an accurate valgus stress at the elbow. As such, tests should be performed at multiple angles, from full extension to 20° to 30° of flexion. When the olecranon is "unlocked" from the olecranon fossa, the ligamentous

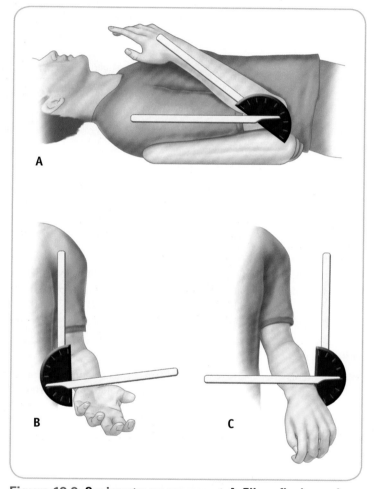

Figure 18.8. Goniometry measurement. A, Elbow flexion and extension. The fulcrum is centered over the lateral epicondyle of the humerus. The proximal arm is aligned along the humerus, using the acromion process for reference. The distal arm is aligned along the radius, using the styloid process for reference. **B, Forearm supination.** The fulcrum is centered medial to the ulnar styloid process. The proximal arm is parallel to the midline of the humerus, and the distal arm is placed across the palmar aspect of the forearm just proximal to the styloid processes of the radius and ulna. **C, Forearm pronation.** The fulcrum is centered lateral to the ulnar styloid process. The arms are placed in the same position but on the dorsal aspect of the forearm.

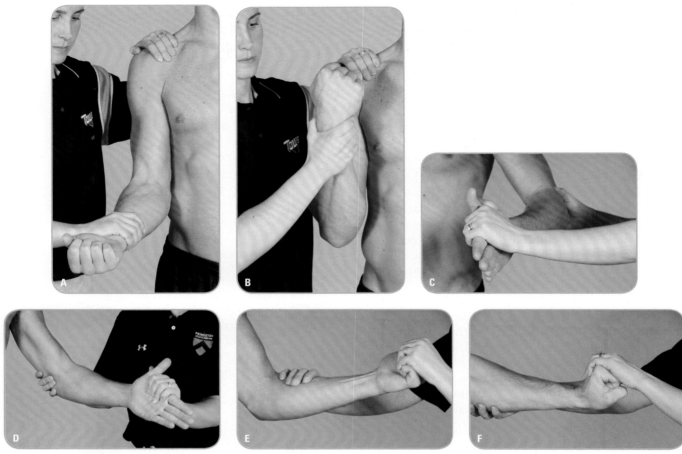

Figure 18.9. Resisted manual muscle testing for the elbow. The myotomes for each motion are listed in parentheses. **A,** Elbow flexion (C6). **B,** Elbow extension (C7). **C,** Forearm supination. **D,** Forearm pronation. **E,** Wrist flexion (C7). **F,** Wrist extension (C6).

TABLE 18.1 Manual Muscle Testing of Selected Muscles of the Elbow

MUSCLE	JOINT POSITIONING	APPLY PRESSURE
Pronator teres	The patient is supine with upper arm resting on plinth and pressed against torso, forearm pronated, and elbow in partial flexion.	To the lower forearm, above the wrist, in the direction of supination
Supinator	The patient is supine with GH and elbow joints both flexed to 90°. The forearm is supinated.	To the distal end of the forearm, just proximal to the wrist, in the direction of pronation
Biceps brachii	Patient is seated, with upper arm beside torso, and elbow flexed to 90° and supinated.	To the distal aspect of the forearm, in the direction of elbow extension
Brachioradialis	Patient is seated, with upper arm beside torso, elbow flexed to 90°, and forearm in neutral.	To the distal aspect of the forearm, in the direction of elbow extension
Brachialis	Patient is seated, with upper arm beside torso, elbow flexed to 90°, and forearm in pronation.	To the distal aspect of the forearm, in the direction of elbow extension
Triceps brachii and anconeus	Patient is supine with GH joint flexed to 90° and elbow just shy of full extension with forearm in neutral position.	To the distal aspect of the forearm in the direction of flexion

GH, glenohumeral.

For more in depth descriptions and illustrations, see Kendall FP, McCreary EK, Provance PG, et al, eds. *Muscles: Testing and Function with Posture and Pain.* 5th ed. Philadelphia, PA: Lippincott Williams & Wilkins; 2005.

structures are isolated. While the individual is seated, the arm should be stabilized and a valgus or abduction force applied to the distal forearm to stress the ulnar collateral ligament (**Fig. 18.10A**). The diagnostic value of the valgus stress test is 65% sensitivity and 50% specificity.[15] A more clinically relevant test for assessing the integrity of the ulnar collateral ligament is the moving valgus stress test.

Moving Valgus Stress Test

With 100% sensitivity and 75% specificity, the moving valgus stress test is performed with the patient either seated or standing and shoulder abducted to 90°.[16] Starting position is with the patient's elbow fully flexed while the clinician exerts moderate valgus pressure at the elbow. While keeping a valgus force at the elbow, the clinician passively moves the elbow into extension (**Fig. 18.10B**). The test is considered positive if the maneuver replicates the pain the patient experiences with activity and the pain is most intense between 70° and 120° of extension. Positive findings imply the possibility that the deep anterior bundles of the medical collateral ligament have been damaged which may lead to "chronic valgus extension overload."[16]

Radial Collateral Ligament Test (Varus Stress Test)

The radial collateral ligament test is also referred to as the varus stress test or the lateral collateral ligament stress test and is used to assess the integrity of the radial collateral (lateral) ligament of the elbow. To perform the test, the patient's arm is placed in the anatomical position while the clinician places a hand over the medial epicondyle with one hand the lateral aspect of the wrist with the other. A varus force is applied in the anatomical position and in slight flexion (**Fig. 18.10C**). Pain or gapping on the lateral aspect of the elbow implies damage to the radial collateral ligament. No data has been found on the diagnostic accuracy of this test.

Milking Test

With the patient seated and the elbow flexed at 90° and the shoulder abducted to 90°, the clinician grasps the patient's thumb and passively forces the patient's shoulder into the end range of glenohumeral external rotation. Pain at the medial elbow is considered a positive test for ulnar collateral ligament injury.

Special Tests

Several special tests can be used for detecting injury or related pathology (e.g., epicondylitis and neuritis).

Common Extensor Tendinitis Test (Cozen Test or Tennis Elbow Tests)

The Cozen test is a highly relevant clinical test for replicating pain in patients with lateral epicondylalgia, with reported 91% sensitivity.[17] The clinician stabilizes the patient's flexed elbow and palpates the lateral epicondyle. The patient is instructed to make a fist and pronate the forearm. Next, the patient

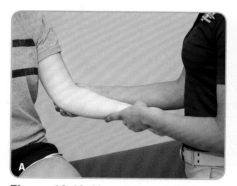 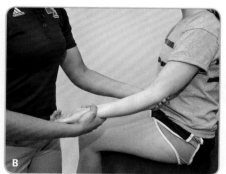 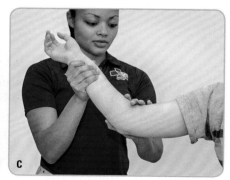

Figure 18.10. Ligamentous instability tests. A, The ulnar collateral ligament: a valgus force at multiple angles. **B,** The moving valgus stress test. **C,** The radial collateral ligament: a varus force at multiple angles.

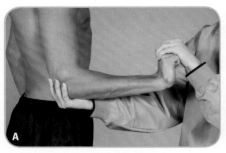 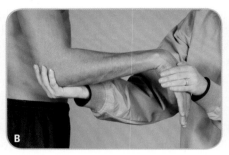 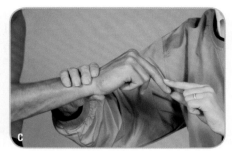

Figure 18.11. Tests for common extensor tendinitis. A, Resisted extension and radial deviation of the wrist (Cozen test). **B,** Passive stretching of the wrist extensors. **C,** Resisted extension of the extensor digitorum communis in the middle finger with the wrist extended.

attempts to radially deviate and extend the wrist while the clinician applies resistance (**Fig. 18.11A**). A positive sign is indicated if severe pain is present over the lateral epicondyle of the humerus. The same results can be elicited through passively stretching the extensor muscles by simultaneously pronating the forearm, flexing the wrist, and extending the elbow (**Fig. 18.11B**). In some cases, discomfort also can be produced by testing the extensor digitorum communis of the 3rd digit through the application of resistance distal to the proximal interphalangeal joint with the wrist extended (**Fig. 18.11C**).

Medial Epicondylitis Tests

Initially, the flexed elbow is stabilized against the body, and the forearm is supinated. The clinician palpates the medial epicondyle. Next, the clinician extends the wrist and elbow while the patient resists the movement. A positive sign is indicated by pain over the medial epicondyle of the humerus.

Tinel Sign for Ulnar Neuritis

The cubital tunnel is tapped on the posteromedial side of the elbow. A positive sign is indicated by a tingling sensation that runs down the ulnar aspect of the forearm into the medial half of the fourth finger and the entirety of the fifth finger (**Fig. 18.12**). The Tinel sign has very strong sensitivity (98%) as well as strong specificity (70%).[18]

Elbow Flexion Test for Ulnar Neuritis

This test also has high diagnostic accuracy, with 75% sensitivity and 99% specificity.[18] This test is used to identify if the ulnar nerve is entrapped in the cubital tunnel. The patient is instructed to flex the elbow completely and hold it in that position for 5 minutes. A positive test is indicated by tingling or numbness in the ulnar nerve distribution pattern of the forearm and hand.

Test for Pronator Teres Syndrome

The patient sits with the elbow flexed at 90°. The clinician strongly resists forearm pronation while the elbow is extended. A positive test is indicated by tingling or paresthesia in the median nerve distribution of the forearm and hand.

Pinch Grip Test

The patient is instructed to pinch the tip of the index finger and thumb together (**Fig. 18.13**). Normally, there should be a tip-to-tip pinch. If an abnormal pulp-to-pulp pinch is performed, the anterior interosseous nerve, which is an extension of the median nerve, may be entrapped at the elbow as it passes between the two heads of the pronator teres.

Neurological Tests

Neurological integrity can be assessed with the use of myotomes, reflexes, and cutaneous patterns, which include both segmental dermatomes and peripheral nerve patterns.

Myotomes

Isometric muscle testing should be performed in the following motions to test specific myotomes in the upper extremity:

- Scapular elevation (C4)

- Shoulder abduction (C5)

- Elbow flexion and/or wrist extension (C6)

- Elbow extension and/or wrist flexion (C7)

- Thumb extension and/or ulnar deviation (C8)

- Abduction and/or adduction of the hand intrinsics (T1)

Reflexes

Reflexes in the upper extremity include the biceps (C5 through C6), brachioradialis (C6), and triceps (C7). The patient should be relaxed, with the elbow flexed. Testing procedures are explained in **Figure 17.29**.

Cutaneous Patterns

The segmental nerve dermatome patterns for the elbow region are demonstrated in **Figure 18.14**. The peripheral nerve cutaneous patterns are demonstrated in **Figure 18.15**. Testing is performed bilaterally for altered sensation with sharp and dull touch by running the open hand and fingernails over the neck, shoulder, and anterior and posterior chest walls as well as down both sides of the arms and hands.

Activity-Specific Functional Tests

The elbow is in the middle of the upper extremity kinetic chain. Therefore, it must function properly to position the hand so that daily activities can be performed smoothly and efficiently. Activities such as combing the hair, throwing a ball, lifting an object, or pushing an object should be

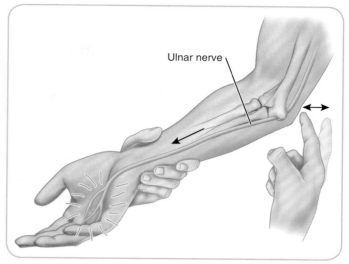

Figure 18.12. Tinel sign. Tapping over the cubital tunnel produces a tingling sensation down the ulnar nerve into the forearm and hand. A positive Tinel sign indicates ulnar nerve entrapment.

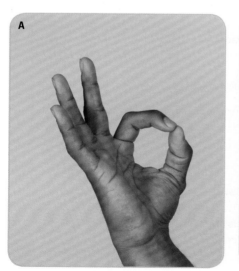
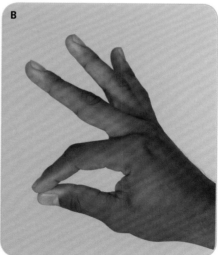

Figure 18.13. Pinch grip test. The patient is instructed to make a "O" with the thumb and forefinger. **A,** Normal tip-to-tip. **B,** Abnormal pulp-to-pulp, which signifies entrapment of the interior interosseous nerve.

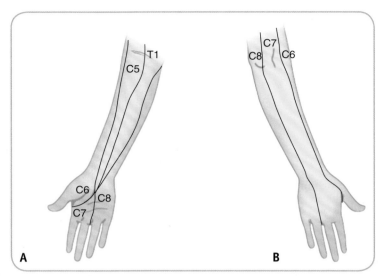

Figure 18.14. Dermatome patterns for the elbow region.
A, Anterior view. **B,** Posterior view.

performed without pain. The individual should be instructed to perform the skills that are needed to complete activities of daily living and sport-specific tasks. Each movement should be pain-free and fluid. If any of the conditions listed in **Box 18.1** are present, the individual should be referred to a physician.

 Bilateral testing of the Little League player should include active ROM, passive ROM, and resistive ROM for elbow flexion, elbow extension, pronation, supination, wrist flexion, and wrist extension; medial epicondylitis test; Tinel sign for ulnar neuritis; elbow flexion test for ulnar neuritis; pronator teres syndrome test; grip strength; and varus stress.

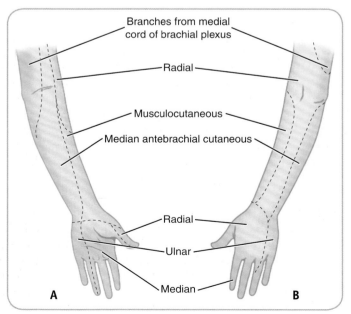

Figure 18.15. Cutaneous patterns for the peripheral nerves.
A, Anterior view. **B,** Posterior view.

> **BOX 18.1 Signs and Symptoms That Necessitate Immediate Referral to a Physician**
>
> - Possible epiphyseal or apophyseal injuries
> - Weakness in a myotome
> - Tingling or numbness in the forearm or hand
> - Gross joint instability
> - Obvious deformity suggesting a dislocation or fracture
>
> - Abnormal or absent reflexes
> - Excessive joint swelling
> - Absent or weak pulse
> - Significantly limited ROM
> - Any unexplained pain

CONTUSIONS

Following practice, a lacrosse player is complaining of pain in his right arm after being struck by another player's stick. He reports receiving several blows to the area over the past week. Palpation reveals a hardened mass of soft tissue over the distal anterior arm that is very tender and sore. Bilateral strength is good. What potentially serious condition might develop, and how should this condition be managed?

Etiology

Direct blows to the arm and forearm frequently occur in contact and collision sports. Contusions result from a compressive force sustained from a direct blow. Such injuries vary in severity according to the area and depth over which blood vessels are ruptured. Contusions occur more frequently over bony prominences.

Signs and Symptoms

Ecchymosis may be present if the hemorrhage is superficial. Significant trauma can lead to internal hemorrhage, rapid swelling, and hematoma formation that can limit ROM. Chronic blows to the anterior arm can result in the development of ectopic bone either in the belly of the muscle (i.e., **myositis ossificans**) or as a bony outgrowth (i.e., **exostosis**) of the underlying bone. The belly of the deltoid and brachialis muscles is the common site for the development of myositis ossificans after trauma. A particularly vulnerable site is just proximal to the deltoid's insertion on the lateral aspect of the humerus, where the bone is least padded by muscle tissue. Standard shoulder pads do not extend far enough to protect the area, and the edge of the pad itself may contribute to the injury. The developing mass can become painful and disabling if the radial nerve is contused, leading to transitory paralysis of the extensor forearm muscles.

Tackler's exostosis, also known as blocker's spur and commonly seen in football linemen, is not a true myositis ossificans, because the ectopic formation is not infiltrated into the muscle but, rather, is an irritative exostosis arising from the bone. A painful bony mass, usually in the form of a spur with a sharp edge, can be palpated on the anterolateral aspect of the humerus.

Management

Treatment involves standard acute care with ice, compression, and protected rest. Activity modification, nonsteroidal anti-inflammatory drugs (NSAIDs) after the first 24 to 48 hours, and a gradual, active ROM and strengthening exercise program should be initiated as tolerated. Aggressive stretching and strengthening exercises should be avoided to prevent further injury to muscle tissue.

If conservative measures do not alleviate the condition, the individual should be referred to a physician for further care, because a more serious condition may have developed. Visible radiograph changes in the muscle can be noted after 2 to 3 weeks. As the condition progresses and becomes chronic, a painful **periostitis** and **fibrositis** may develop. Surgical excision of the calcification is seldom necessary, because function usually is not impaired. If function is adversely affected, however, surgery should be delayed until the calcification is mature (usually 12 to 18 months), because it may redevelop. The area should be protected with a special pad during participation.

> The lacrosse player may be developing myositis ossificans in the brachialis muscle. Standard acute care should be followed, with referral to a physician for further assessment and possible radiography.

OLECRANON BURSITIS

> A football player has acute swelling of approximately 1 in in diameter on the proximal posterior ulna. His history reveals constant friction to the area, attributed to contact with artificial turf. What condition might be suspected, what anatomical structures are involved, and how should this condition be managed?

The subcutaneous olecranon bursa is the largest bursa in the elbow region. The superficial location predisposes the bursa to either direct macrotrauma or cumulative microtrauma by repetitive elbow flexion and extension. The bursitis can be acute or chronic, aseptic or septic. Common mechanisms of olecranon bursa injury include the following:

- A fall on a flexed elbow
- Constantly leaning on one's elbow ("student's elbow")
- Repetitive pressure and friction
- Repetitive flexion and extension
- Infection

Acute and Chronic Bursitis
Etiology
A fall on a flexed elbow can lead to an acutely inflamed bursa. Constantly leaning on one's elbow, repetitive pressure, and friction can lead to a chronic inflamed bursa.

Signs and Symptoms
The acutely inflamed bursa presents with an immediate, tender, swollen area of redness in the posterior elbow. The swelling is relatively painless. If the bursa ruptures, a discrete, sharply demarcated goose egg is visible directly over the olecranon process. Approximately half of the patients with olecranon bursitis have a history of an abrupt onset of pain and swelling; the other half have a more insidious onset over several weeks, leading to chronic inflammation. Motion is limited at the extreme of flexion as tension increases over the bursa.

Management
Acute management involves ice, rest, and a compressive wrap applied for the first 24 hours. Significant distention may necessitate aspiration followed by a compressive dressing for several days. Chronic bursitis is managed with cryotherapy, NSAIDs, and use of elbow cushions to protect the area from further insult. In long-term cases of chronic bursitis, the bursa may be aspirated or totally excised, although a risk of poor wound healing over the olecranon process exists. Corticosteroid injections also may be performed.

Septic and Nonseptic Bursitis
Etiology
Occasionally, a bursa can become infected in the absence of trauma to the area. Septic bursitis sometimes is related to seeding from an infection at a distant site, such as **paronychia**, cellulitis of the

hand, or forearm infection. Nonseptic bursitis can be caused by crystalline deposition disease or rheumatoid involvement. It has been associated with atopic dermatitis.

Signs and Symptoms

Individuals with septic bursitis are more likely to show traditional signs of infection, including malaise (lethargy), fever, pain, localized heat, restricted motion, tenderness, and swelling at the elbow. These signs and symptoms usually present within 1 week of developing symptoms. Approximately 50% of patients present with a skin lesion overlying the bursa, 92% to 100% have bursal tenderness, and 40% to 100% have peribursal cellulitis. In contrast, nonseptic bursitis is associated with an overlying skin lesion in 5% of the cases, bursal tenderness in 45% of the cases, and cellulitis in 23% to 25%.[19]

Management

An individual with an infected bursa should be referred to a physician. The physician generally aspirates the bursa and takes a sample of the fluid for culture to determine the presence of septic bursitis. Following aspiration, the elbow is immobilized in a sling, and continuous hot packs and appropriate antibiotics typically are prescribed. If an infected bursa is suspected, corticosteroids should not be injected.

> The football player has acute olecranon bursitis. Standard acute care should resolve the condition; however, the player should be closely observed for signs and symptoms of infection. Applying a pad to the area can help to prevent recurrence.

SPRAINS

> **?** A gymnast misses the vault, falls to the mat on an outstretched arm, and sustains a visible posterior dislocation of the elbow. The athlete is unwilling to move the elbow and is in extreme pain. Explain the circulatory and neurological assessment for this injury.

Collateral Ligament Sprain

Etiology

Acute tears to ligamentous and joint structures at the elbow are rare, but such injuries may occur during a fall on an outstretched hand (FOOSH), resulting in elbow hyperextension, or through a valgus/varus tensile force. Injuries arising from the application of varus and valgus forces at the elbow occur most often in sports where the hand is in contact with the ground or other players as may happen in wrestling, cheerleading, gymnastics, or rugby.[1] More commonly, however, repetitive tensile forces irritate and tear the ligaments, particularly the ulnar collateral ligament. If the ulnar collateral ligament is damaged, the ulnar nerve also may be affected.

Signs and Symptoms

The patient may describe feelings of instability and/or pain over the ulnar collateral ligament when a valgus force is applied or over the radial collateral ligament when a varus force is applied. For injury to the ulnar collateral ligament, a history of pain localized to the medial aspect of the elbow during the late cocking and acceleration phases of throwing is common. Point tenderness will be elicited over the site of injury.

Management

Treatment involves standard acute care with ice, compression, and protected rest. A brief immobilization may be necessary in acute cases. This is followed by early, protected ROM exercises to stretch the forearm flexor–pronator group and the forearm extensors.

Anterior Capsulitis

Etiology

Anterior joint pain caused by hyperextension usually is attributed to acute anterior capsulitis rather than chronic, repetitive throwing. Microtears in the capsule usually are not sufficient to cause dislocation.

Signs and Symptoms

Diffuse, anterior elbow pain presents after a traumatic episode. It is accompanied by deep tenderness on palpation, particularly on the anteromedial side. A strain to the pronator teres should be ruled out, as should entrapment of the median nerve as it courses through the pronator teres. With nerve entrapment, tingling or numbness of the thumb and index finger usually is noted.

Management

Treatment involves standard acute care with ice, compression, and protected rest. The condition is managed with immobilization for 3 to 5 days, after which active ROM exercises can begin as pain allows. Flexion contracture may result from fibrosis caused by repeated injury to the capsule.

Dislocations

Etiology

In adolescents, the most common traumatic injury to the elbow is subluxation or dislocation of the proximal radial head, often associated with an immature annular ligament. Referred to as "nursemaid's elbow" or "pulled-elbow syndrome," this condition results from longitudinal traction of an extended and pronated upper extremity, such as when a young child is swung by the arms. A small tear in the annular ligament allows the radial head to migrate out from under the annular ligament. If an individual is unable to pronate and supinate the forearm without pain, immediate referral to a physician is warranted.

Most ulnar dislocations occur in individuals younger than 20 years, with a peak incidence during the teenage years. The mechanism of injury usually is hyperextension or a sudden, violent unidirectional valgus force that drives the ulna posteriorly or posterolaterally. Approximately 60% of patients have associated fractures of the medial epicondyle, radial head, coronoid process, or olecranon process.[20] When the dislocation is associated with both radial head and coronoid fractures, it has been termed the "terrible triad of the elbow" because of the difficulties that are inherent in treatment and the consistently poor reported outcomes as compared to a simple elbow dislocation.[21] The injury also may involve disruption of the anterior capsule, tearing of the brachialis muscle, injury to the ulnar collateral ligament, and rarely, brachial artery compromise or nerve injury to the median or ulnar nerves.

Signs and Symptoms

A snapping or cracking sensation is experienced on impact, followed by severe pain, rapid swelling, total loss of function, and an obvious deformity (**Fig. 18.16**). The anterior capsule, brachialis muscle, and flexor and extensor muscle masses also may be disrupted. The arm is frequently held in flexion, with the forearm appearing shortened. The olecranon and radial head are palpable posteriorly, and a slight indentation in the triceps is visible just proximal to the olecranon. Signs and symptoms of a posterior elbow dislocation are listed in **Box 18.2**.

Nerve palsies are common, making prereduction and postreduction neurovascular examination critical. Ulnar nerve dysfunction usually is transient. If damaged, numbness will extend into the little finger. The median nerve, however, may become trapped within the joint, trapped within a healing medial epicondylar fracture, or looped anteriorly into the joint. Persistent, unexplained pain and median nerve dysfunction (e.g., finger flexor weakness or numbness in the palm of the hand) necessitate immediate reevaluation by a physician.

Activation of the emergency action plan, including summoning EMS, is warranted. Because of the risk of neurovascular injury, on-site reduction is not indicated. Additional guidelines for management of an elbow dislocation are discussed in **Application Strategy 18.2**.

Management

Reduction usually is performed under general or regional anesthesia. Early reduction minimizes the amount of muscle spasm. For cases in which the

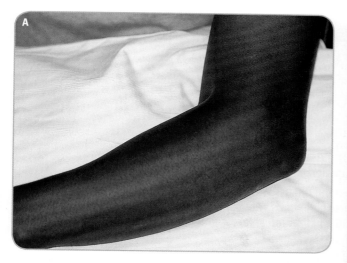

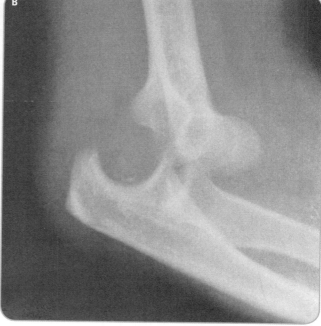

Figure 18.16. Elbow dislocation. A, Clinical view of a posterior dislocation. B, Radiograph of a typical posterior dislocation. Note that the coronoid process is adjacent to the olecranon fossa.

forearm flexors, extensors, and annular ligament have maintained their integrity with no associated fracture, limited immobilization, early ROM exercises, and proprioceptive neuromuscular facilitation exercises have proved to be quite successful. Although rare, recurrent dislocations are often related to laxity in the lateral ulnar collateral ligament of the elbow, leading to postero-lateral rotary subluxation. A recurrent dislocation in the first 6 months after initial injury is more often attributed to a missed osteochondral fracture. Elbow dislocations involving fractures of the radial head and capitellar fracture dislocations are more complex and require internal fixation.

This injury should be considered a medical emergency. The emergency action plan, including summoning EMS, should be activated.

 In assessing the dislocation sustained by the gymnast, circulatory assessment should include checking for a distal pulse, assessing skin color and temperature, and assessing capillary refill. Neurological assessment includes checking for sensation distal to the injury.

BOX 18.2 Signs and Symptoms of a Posterior Elbow Dislocation

- Snapping or cracking sensation
- Obvious deformity as the olecranon is pushed posteriorly
- Immediate, severe pain with rapid swelling, primarily on the medial aspect of the elbow
- A slightly flexed elbow is supported, if possible, by the uninjured arm.
- Pain is predominantly localized over the medial aspect of the elbow.
- Total loss of function
- Crepitation may be palpated if an associated fracture is present.

APPLICATION STRATEGY 18.2

Management Algorithm for Posterior Elbow Dislocation

1. Apply ice to reduce swelling and inflammation.
2. To rule out circulatory impairment, assess the following:
   - Radial pulse
   - Skin color
   - Blanching of the nails
3. To rule out nerve impairment, assess motor and sensory function:
   - Have the patient (if able) flex, extend, abduct, and adduct the fingers with the person looking away.
   - Stroke the palm and dorsum of the hand in several different locations with a blunt and sharp object.
   - Ask the individual to identify where you are touching and whether the object is sharp or dull.
4. Immobilize the area with a vacuum splint or other appropriate splint.
5. Take vital signs, recheck pulse and sensory functions, and treat for shock.

STRAINS

? After receiving a severe blow to the right forearm, an offensive lineman is having problems flexing his wrist and fingers. The lineman has rapid swelling, discoloration, and diminished pulse. Passive stretching of the wrist flexors increases pain. What condition should be suspected, what structures are involved, and how should this injury be managed?

Muscular strains commonly result from inadequate warm-up, excessive training past the point of fatigue, and inadequate rehabilitation of previous muscular injuries. A less common cause of strains in this area is a single, massive contraction or sudden overstretching. **Application Strategy 18.3** summarizes the management of isolated muscular strains.

APPLICATION STRATEGY 18.3

Management Algorithm for Muscular Strains

1. Control inflammation, swelling, and pain. Use ice, compression, elevation, NSAIDs, and rest if necessary.
2. Use ice, ultrasound, electrical muscle stimulation, interferential current, or thermotherapy to precede therapeutic exercise.
3. Restore ROM. (Assess flexibility at the shoulder region, because limitations may increase stress at the elbow.)
4. Perform isometric exercises throughout a pain-free ROM.
5. Progress to isotonic exercises with light resistance, building from 1 to 5 lb, throughout a pain-free range.
6. Improve neuromuscular control with closed kinetic chain exercises, such as shifting a weighted ball in the hand, press-ups, or walking on the hands in a push-up position between boxes of varying heights.
7. Add surgical tubing exercises as tolerated.
8. When pain-free, ensure adequate warm-up and gradual return to functional exercises.
9. Recommend activity modification, biomechanical analysis of skill performance, or equipment modifications.

If involved in a throwing activity, do the following:

1. Begin functional throwing with a light toss over a distance of 20–30 ft for 5 minutes and then progressing to between 15 and 20 minutes.
2. When the individual can throw for 15–20 minutes, gradually increase the distance to 150 ft.
3. When proper throwing mechanics are present, gradually increase velocity.
4. Continue a strengthening and stretching program as return to activity is initiated.

Flexor and Extensor Strains

Etiology

Repetitive tensile stresses to the elbow flexors (i.e., brachialis, biceps brachii, and brachioradialis) and pronator teres can lead to a self-limiting muscle strain, especially after an inadequate warm-up or fatigue. In rowing, excessive wrist motion during the feathering action can lead to chronic forearm tendinitis and tenosynovitis.[22] In a triceps strain, the mechanism generally is a decelerating-type injury. It has been reported in tennis and baseball players as well as in weight lifters with a history of anabolic steroid use or local steroid injections.[23]

Signs and Symptoms

Palpable pain can be elicited over the involved muscle mass. Pain increases with active and resisted motion.

Management

Treatment involves standard acute care with ice, compression, and protected rest; brief immobilization may be necessary in acute cases. Activity modification, NSAIDs, and a program of gradual active ROM and strengthening exercises should be initiated as tolerated. In rowing, special attention should be paid to improper technique, wrong-sized grips, poor rigging, and limiting rowing during wet or rough conditions, which can cause the rower to use excessive wrist motion.[21]

Rupture of the Biceps Brachii

Etiology

Approximately 97% of all biceps brachii ruptures are proximal; only 3% involve the distal attachment.[20,24] In many cases, preexisting degenerative changes in the distal tendon make it vulnerable to rupture following a sudden eccentric load (e.g., during weight lifting or trying to catch oneself during a fall). Individuals at increased risk for this injury tend to be men younger than 30 years of age with a history of using steroid medication.[21]

Signs and Symptoms

The patient may describe hearing or feeling a pop in the shoulder, upper arm, or elbow. Tenderness, swelling, and ecchymosis are visible in the antecubital fossa. The biceps tendon is not palpable, because the belly muscle retracts proximally. The individual is still able to flex the elbow and supinate the forearm, but these movements are weak when resisted. Ludington test is positive in the presence of a complete rupture.

Management

Acute treatment involves managing the patient's pain and swelling with ice, compression, and rest. Treatment for a rupture may involve a nonoperative approach or surgical repair. Some studies have found a significant loss of elbow flexion (30%) and supination (40%) strength with a nonoperative approach.[25] Although this decreased level of function may suffice for daily activities, the distal biceps tends to scar to the brachialis muscle, illuminating the normal contour of the muscle.

Surgical repair to reattach the avulsed distal biceps tendon to the radial tuberosity provides the greatest likelihood of maximal functional results and return to physical activity. Following repair, the elbow is immobilized at 90° of flexion with moderate forearm supination for 8 weeks, followed by gradual active ROM and strengthening.[20,24]

Rupture of the Triceps Brachii

Etiology

Occasionally, a direct blow to the posterior elbow or an uncoordinated triceps contraction during a fall results in an acute rupture of the tendon. In addition to the tendon rupture, 80% of all injuries involve an olecranon avulsion fracture.[12] Spontaneous ruptures of the tendon can occur, but these are rare and usually associated with systemic diseases or steroid use.

Signs and Symptoms

Pain and swelling are present over the distal attachment of the extensor mechanism on the olecranon process. A palpable defect in the triceps tendon or a step-off deformity of the olecranon may also be present. Active extension of the elbow may be weak (if a partial tear is present) or nonexistent (with a total rupture).

Management

Treatment involves standard acute care with ice, compression, and immobilization in a sling followed by immediate referral to a physician. Partial tears are treated conservatively. Surgical reattachment of the tendon onto the olecranon process is necessary in a total rupture. If an avulsion fracture of the olecranon is present, open reduction and internal fixation of the fragment are necessary. Subsequently, the elbow is immobilized in 45° of flexion for 4 weeks, followed by allowing 0° to 45° of flexion for 4 weeks and then gradual incorporation of active ROM and strengthening exercises.

Compartment Syndrome

Etiology

The deep fascia of the forearm encloses the wrist and finger flexor and extensor muscle groups in a common sheath. The two groups are separated into compartments by an interosseous membrane between the radius and ulna. The wrist and finger flexors are in the anterior compartment; the wrist and finger extensors are in the posterior compartment.

Compartment syndrome is often secondary to an elbow fracture or dislocation, crushing injury, forearm fracture, postischemic edema, or excessive muscular exertion, as in weight lifting. Hemorrhage or edema causes increased pressure within the compartment, leading to excessive pressure on neurovascular structures and tissues within the space.

Signs and Symptoms

Onset of symptoms is rapid and includes swelling, discoloration, absent or diminished distal pulse, and subsequent onset of sensory changes and paralysis. Severe pain at rest, aggravated by passive stretching of the muscles in the compartment, signals a potential problem.

Management

Treatment involves immobilization of the forearm and wrist as well as application of ice and elevation above the heart to limit pain and swelling. External compression should not be applied to the area, because the neurovascular structures already are compressed by the swelling. Immediate referral to a physician is necessary, because a fasciotomy may be needed to decompress the area.

 The football player most likely has compartment syndrome. Injury usually involves the wrist flexors, finger flexors, and median nerve. The condition warrants immediate referral to a physician.

OVERUSE CONDITIONS

 The athletic trainer for a summer tennis camp has been asked to provide suggestions to decrease the risk of lateral epicondylitis. What recommendations should be made?

The throwing mechanism discussed in Chapter 17 also can lead to overuse injuries at the elbow. During the initial acceleration phase, the body is brought forward rapidly, but the elbow and hand lag behind the upper arm. This results in a tremendous tensile valgus stress being placed on the medial aspect of the elbow, particularly the ulnar collateral ligament and adjacent tissues. As acceleration continues, the elbow extensors and wrist flexors contract to add velocity to the throw.

This whipping action produces significant valgus stress on the medial elbow and concomitant lateral compressive stress in the radiocapitellar joint (**Fig. 18.17**). Before release of the ball, the elbow is almost fully extended and is positioned slightly anterior to the trunk. During release, the elbow is flexed approximately 20° to 30°. As these forces decrease, however, the extreme pronation of the forearm places the lateral ligaments under tension. During the deceleration phase, eccentric contractions of the long head of the biceps brachii, supinator, and extensor muscles decelerate the forearm in pronation. Additional stress occurs on structures around the olecranon as pronation and extension jam the olecranon into its fossa. Impingement can occur during this jamming.

Epicondylitis is a common, chronic condition seen in activities involving pronation and supination, such as in tennis, javelin throwing, pitching, volleyball, and golf. This condition is usually referred to as a **tendinosis**, because degeneration rather than an inflammatory condition exists. A pattern of poor technique, fatigue, and overuse often is associated with this condition.

Medial Epicondylitis

Etiology

Medial epicondylitis is caused by repeated, medial tension/lateral compression (valgus) forces placed on the arm during the acceleration phase of the throwing motion.[26] The medial humeral apophyseal growth plate in the pediatric athlete is particularly vulnerable to injury and, if affected, is called Little League elbow. In a recent study of 9- to 12-year-old pitchers, medial elbow pain was found in 26%.[27] Efforts have been imposed in leagues and recreational programs to limit the number of innings pitched per game and/or the number of pitches per week and pitches per season in an attempt to decrease the incidence of medial epicondylitis in adolescents.[13]

Injury occurs when valgus forces produce a combined flexor muscle strain, ulnar collateral ligament sprain, and ulnar neuritis. The two most commonly involved tendons are the pronator teres and the flexor carpi radialis. Simultaneously, lateral compressive and shearing forces generated in the olecranon fossa can damage the lateral condyle of the humerus and radial head, leading to capitellar osteochondral injuries. Posterior stresses may lead to triceps strain, synovial impingement, olecranon fractures, or loose bodies and degenerative joint changes.

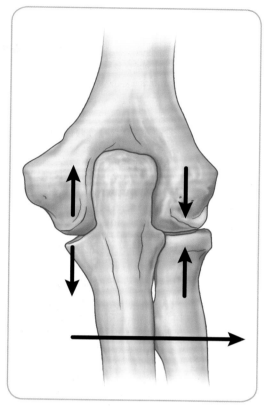

Figure 18.17. Traction–compression mechanism. An excessive valgus force can lead to both medial tensile stress and lateral compression stress, causing injury to both sides of the joint.

Signs and Symptoms

Assessment reveals swelling, ecchymosis, and point tenderness over the humeroulnar joint or the flexor/pronator origin, slightly distal and lateral to the medial epicondyle. Pain usually is severe over the medial epicondyle, extending distally 1 to 2 cm along the track of the flexor carpi radialis and pronator teres. Pain is aggravated by resisted wrist flexion and pronation and by a valgus stress applied at 20° to 30° of elbow flexion. There will be a negative Tinel sign at the cubital tunnel for ulnar neuritis. If the ulnar nerve is involved, tingling and numbness may radiate into the forearm and hand, particularly the fourth and fifth fingers.

Management

Most conditions can be managed with ice, NSAIDs, and immobilization in a sling, with the wrist in slight flexion, for 2 to 3 weeks. In cases involving apophysitis, the resting period may extend from 4 to 6 weeks with limitation or elimination of throwing.[28] Transcutaneous electric nerve stimulation (TENS), high-voltage galvanic stimulation, ultrasound, and interferential current are used to decrease pain and inflammation. Early ROM exercises and gentle, resisted isometric exercises should progress to isotonic strengthening and use of surgical tubing. Activity should not resume until the

In the adolescent, if an apophyseal fracture or an avulsion fracture of the medial epicondyle is suspected, immediate referral to a physician is warranted. In some settings, this may require activation of the emergency action plan.

individual can complete all functional tests without pain. A functional brace may limit valgus stress and allow early resumption of strenuous activities. In moderate injuries, throwing or overhead motions should be avoided for up to 6 to 12 weeks.[20]

With intra-articular injuries, ulnar nerve problems, or moderate to severe cases of pain or instability, referral to a physician is indicated. **Application Strategy 18.4** describes management of medial epicondylitis.

Common Extensor Tendinitis (Lateral Epicondylitis)

Etiology

Pain over the lateral epicondyle denotes extensor tendon overload and is the most common overuse injury in the adult elbow. The condition is typically caused by eccentric loading of the extensor muscles, predominantly the extensor carpi radialis brevis, during the deceleration phase of the throwing motion or tennis stroke. Faulty mechanics (e.g., "leading" with the elbow and off-center hits in racquet sports), poorly fitted equipment (e.g., improper grip size and improper racquet string tension), and age (i.e., 30 to 50 years of age) contribute to this condition.[20]

Signs and Symptoms

Pain is anterior or just distal to the lateral epicondyle and may radiate into the forearm extensors during and after activity. Pain initially subsides but then becomes more severe with repetition and increases with resisted wrist extension, the "coffee cup" test (i.e., pain increases while picking up a full coffee cup), and the tennis elbow test.

Management

Initial treatment should include ice, compression, NSAIDs, and rest. Grasping an object with the forearm pronated is highly discouraged until acute symptoms resolve. Rehabilitation should focus on increasing the strength, endurance, and flexibility of the extensor muscle group. If appropriate,

---

APPLICATION STRATEGY 18.4

Management Algorithm for Medial Epicondylitis

1. Limit pain and inflammation with ice, compression, NSAIDs, and rest.
2. Avoid all activities that lead to pain; immobilization may be necessary if simple daily activities cause pain.
3. Other therapies also may supplement the treatment plan, such as ice massage, contrast baths, ultrasound therapy, electrical muscle stimulation, interferential current, and friction massage over the flexor tendons.
4. Maintain ROM and strength at the wrist and shoulder.
5. Stretching exercises, within pain-free motions, should include wrist flexion–extension, forearm pronation–supination, and radial and ulnar deviation.
6. Begin with fast contractions using light resistance:

   - Perform tennis ball squeezes and other strengthening exercises within pain-free ranges.
   - Add surgical tubing as tolerated.
   - Work up to three to five sets of 10 repetitions per session before moving on to heavier resistance.
7. Incorporate early, closed chain exercises, such as press-ups, wall push-ups, or walking on the hands.
8. Add strengthening exercises for all shoulder, elbow, and wrist motions.
9. Perform a biomechanical analysis of the throwing motion to determine proper technique and make adjustments as necessary.

After return to protected activity, do the following:

1. Continue stretching exercises before and after practice.
2. Continue ice after practice to control any inflammation.
3. Return to full activity as tolerated.

Management of Common Extensor Tendinitis

1. Use ice, compression, elevation, NSAIDs, and rest to limit pain and inflammation.
2. Immobilize the wrist in slight extension to allow functional use of the hand.
3. Use cryotherapy, ultrasound, thermotherapy, electrical muscle stimulation, interferential current, and/or friction massage over the extensor tendons to reduce pain and inflammation.
4. Avoid strong gripping activities and any activities that aggravate symptoms.
5. Perform stretching exercises within pain-free motion, including wrist flexion–extension, forearm pronation–supination, and radial and ulnar deviation.
6. Perform isotonic strengthening exercises and add surgical tubing exercises as tolerated. Begin with fast contractions using light resistance.
7. Work up to three to five sets of 10 repetitions per session before moving on to heavier resistance.
8. Continue active ROM and strengthening exercises for all shoulder, elbow, and wrist motions.
9. Incorporate closed chain exercises, such as press-ups, wall push-ups, or walking on the hands.
10. Perform a biomechanical analysis of the skills to determine if improper technique may have contributed to the problem and make appropriate changes.
11. Return to full activity, as tolerated, but continue stretching exercises before and after practice. Apply ice after practice to control any inflammation.

evaluation of mechanics and equipment should be conducted. A counterforce strap placed 2 to 3 in distal to the elbow joint can limit excessive muscular tension placed on the epicondyle and usually is sufficient to eliminate symptoms. **Application Strategy 18.5** describes management of common extensor tendinitis.

Neural Entrapment Injuries

The ulnar nerve passes behind the medial epicondyle of the humerus through the cubital tunnel to rest against the posterior portion of the ulnar collateral ligament (**Fig. 18.18**). The nerve is vulnerable to compression and tensile stress, which may be caused by trauma (i.e., acute or chronic), cubital valgus deformity, irregularities within the ulnar groove, or subluxation as a result of a lax ulnar collateral ligament. The condition often is referred to as **cubital tunnel syndrome**. The individual complains of a shocking sensation along the medial aspect of the elbow, radiating as if "hitting the crazy bone." Palpation or percussion in the ulnar groove generally produces tingling and numbness down the medial aspect of the forearm into the ring and little finger (Tinel sign). Observation may reveal the disappearance of the concavity of the ulnar nerve sulcus. Because the ulnar nerve innervates several intrinsic muscles of the hand, the patient may develop gradual hand weakness, hypotrophy of the first dorsal interosseous muscle, and reduced strength of the deep 5th digit flexor and flexor carpi ulnaris, all of which result in grip and pinch weakness.[29]

The median nerve travels across the cubital fossa, passing between the two heads of the pronator teres and the two heads of the flexor digitorum

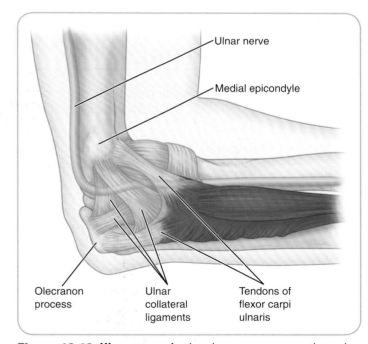

Figure 18.18. Ulnar nerve. As the ulnar nerve passes through the cubital tunnel between the ulnar collateral ligament and the olecranon fossa, it passes under the two heads of the flexor carpi ulnaris. This tendon is slack during extension, but it becomes taut during flexion, contributing to ulnar nerve compression.

Ulnar nerve

Medial epicondyle

Olecranon process

Ulnar collateral ligaments

Tendons of flexor carpi ulnaris

superficialis, to give off its largest branch, the anterior interosseous nerve. Compression may be caused by hypertrophied muscles, particularly the pronator teres, or by compression from fibrous arches near the flexor digitorum superficialis muscle, bicipital aponeurosis, or supracondylar process. It can lead to a condition called **pronator syndrome**, in which pain is felt in the anterior proximal forearm and is aggravated with pronation activities. Numbness may occur in the anterior forearm or in the middle and index fingers and thumb.

The radial nerve may be damaged during a midshaft humeral fracture. Less frequently, direct trauma or entrapment occurs at the elbow as the nerve passes anterior to the cubital fossa, pierces the supinator muscle, and runs posterior, again, into the forearm. The condition is referred to as **radial tunnel syndrome**. The terminal branch, the posterior interosseous nerve, supplies the deeper lying extensor muscles of the forearm. Symptoms of injury often mimic those of lateral epicondylitis. An aching lateral elbow pain may radiate down the posterior forearm. Significant point tenderness can be elicited over the supinator muscle, and resisted supination generally is more painful than wrist extension. Extensor weakness of the wrist, called **wrist drop**, is seen in extreme cases, but no sensory loss tends to be present.

Management

The individual should be referred to a physician immediately. Treatment for neural entrapment depends on the frequency, duration, intensity, magnitude, and cause of the problem. If recognized early, complete rest and NSAIDs can help in acute cases. If the injury is secondary to direct blows, a pad can protect the area. Occasionally, chronic nerve damage may require surgery to release any pressure or constriction on the nerve.

 The following recommendations may help to decrease the risk of lateral epicondylitis: use of a well-fitted racquet with appropriate grip size and string tension, limiting the number of single backhand strokes, increasing the strength of the wrist extensors and supinators, and performing wrist flexibility exercises.

FRACTURES

 A forearm fracture is suspected in a hockey player who was hit by an opposing player's stick. What tests can be used to determine whether a fracture is, in fact, present?

Displaced and undisplaced fractures to the humerus, radius, and ulna usually result from violent compressive forces caused by direct trauma, such as an impact with a helmet or implement, a fall on a flexed elbow or outstretched hand with or without a valgus/varus stress, or tensile forces associated with throwing. Because major nerves and vessels run along the bones, serious neurovascular injury can result from the jagged bone fragments. Fractures to the growth plates also are common in javelin throwers, gymnasts, water polo and tennis players, and adolescent baseball and softball pitchers, whereas stress fractures have been reported in gymnasts, volleyball players, and weight lifters.

Epiphyseal and Avulsion Fractures

Etiology

Because the closing growth plate of the medial epicondyle in adolescents is sensitive to tension stress, a repetitive or sudden contraction of the flexor–pronator muscle group may result in a partial or complete avulsion fracture of the medial epicondyle of the humerus. Referred to as Little League elbow, the tension stress is related to throwing curve balls and other breaking pitches that require forceful pronation. Use of this term, however, negates the fact that other individuals, such as golfers, gymnasts, javelin throwers, tennis players, bowlers, squash and racquetball players, wrestlers, and weight lifters, also are susceptible to the condition. Fracture to the secondary growth center of the lateral epicondyle is similar to a medial epicondyle fracture and is treated in a similar manner.

Signs and Symptoms

In the initial phase of the injury, the individual complains of aching during performance, but no limitations in performance and no residual pain are present. As the condition progresses, however, an aching pain during activity limits performance, and a mild postexercise ache is present. Some localized tenderness can be elicited directly over the epicondyle. In severe cases, pain can be intense, with point tenderness, swelling, and ecchymosis directly on the epicondyle.

Management

Standard acute protocol, with activity modification, is followed during the initial stages of injury. If performance is limited because of pain and if postexercise pain is present, the individual should be referred to a physician. The fracture is managed conservatively, with rest and immobilization in a sling for as little as 2 to 3 weeks. Usually, throwing is not allowed for 6 to 12 weeks. Surgery is necessary only if a valgus instability is present, the medial epicondyle is incarcerated within the elbow joint, or ulnar nerve symptoms are present.

Stress Fractures

Stress fractures to the diaphysis of the ulna can occur during intensive weight lifting. Bilateral distal radial and ulnar fractures have been found in young individuals who lift heavy weights or lose control of the barbells, resulting in added shear stress. For this reason, adolescents in a weight-lifting program should be properly instructed and supervised.

Osteochondritis Dissecans

Etiology

An unusual complication of repetitive stress to the skeletally immature elbow is osteochondritis dissecans. The mechanism is attributed to lateral compressive forces exerted during the throwing motion, which can damage the radial head, capitellum, or both. It is the leading cause of permanent elbow disability in adolescent athletes.[28] In adolescents with open growth plates (12 to 15 years of age), a focal lesion can lead to destruction of the overlying articular cartilage, with fragmentation and softening of the underlying subchondral bone. A microfracture (i.e., loose bodies) and eventual avascular necrosis lead to further joint degeneration.

An associated osteochondrosis condition, called **Panner disease**, is the most common cause of chronic lateral elbow pain, encompassing the entire capitellum in athletes younger than 10 years of age.[27] Pain is present over the lateral and anterior elbow. The pain increases with deep palpation or pronation–supination, but it quickly resolves with decreased activity. Elbow extension may be limited by 20° or more secondary to synovitis and a deformed capitellar congruity. Loose body formation is much less likely to occur in Panner disease.

Signs and Symptoms

Signs and symptoms of osteochondritis dissecans mirror Little League elbow. An insidious onset of dull, activity-related, and poorly localized pain may precede other, more severe symptoms, such as locking, decreased motion, and flexion contractures of more than 15°.[24] Swelling and tenderness are centralized over the radiocapitellar joint, and grating may be present during passive pronation and supination. The ability to fully extend the elbow may be limited.

Management

Management involves referral to a physician. Treatment is conservative with rest for 6 to 18 months. If no loose body is present, no further treatment may be needed. If a fragment is displaced, surgery may be necessary to reattach a large articular fragment or to excise a small fragment.

Displaced and Undisplaced Fractures

Supracondylar fractures, which are caused by falling on an outstretched hand, occur largely in children, with the peak incidence occurring between 4 and 8 years of age.[30] A catastrophic

The arm should be immobilized in a vacuum splint. The emergency action plan should be activated to ensure immediate transport of the patient to the nearest medical facility.

complication from this fracture is ischemic necrosis of the forearm muscles, known as **Volkmann contracture**. The brachial artery or median nerve can be damaged by the fractured bone ends, leading to major circulatory or neural impairment of the forearm and hand. As a result, the hand is cold, white, and numb. The presence of a radial or ulnar pulse does not automatically indicate adequate circulation to the forearm muscles. Severe pain in the forearm is aggravated by passive extension of the fingers. These symptoms indicate a serious problem.

Fracture of the olecranon process of the ulna results from direct trauma, such as being struck with an implement or falling on a flexed elbow. The tension of the triceps pulls the bone fragment superiorly. Because this fracture is intra-articular, it does not respond to conservative treatment and requires surgical intervention.

The head of the radius may be fractured as a result of a valgus stress that tears the ulnar collateral ligament, leading to traumatic compressive and shearing stress on the radial head. The fracture may be nondisplaced (type I), displaced (type II), or comminuted (type III). Tenderness can be elicited on palpation of the radial head, and swelling can be seen lateral to the olecranon. Flexion and extension may or may not be limited. In contrast, passive pronation and supination are both painful and restricted. There also may be an associated valgus instability of the elbow or axial instability of the forearm. A nondisplaced fracture is treated nonoperatively, with early ROM exercises to prevent joint stiffness. With more than one-third of the articular surface involved, more than 30° of angulation, or more than 3 mm of fracture gap, open reduction is recommended.[20]

The **nightstick fracture**, which is seen in football and hockey players, is caused by a direct blow to the forearm that fractures the ulna. Following closed reduction, splinting or casting for 7 to 10 days is needed to allow the initial swelling and discomfort to subside. If a radial head dislocation or a distal radial ulnar joint subluxation is present, open reduction and internal fixation are necessary.

In gymnastics, a unique forearm fracture occurs as a result of wearing leather grips with enclosed dowels. The dowels help to grip the horizontal bar. Problems arise, however, when the leather grip "catches" or grabs onto the bar and holds the hand in position, preventing the individual from continuing during a giant swing maneuver. This action causes the forearm to "wrap around" and sustain multiple fractures. Severe pain and disability with this fracture require immediate immobilization in a vacuum splint and transport to the nearest medical facility.

Fracture Management

Fractures should be suspected in all elbow and forearm injuries. In the absence of visible deformity, palpation should be used to detect the presence of deformity. If no visible or palpable deformity is present, compression, traction, and percussion can assist in determining possible fractures and are explained in **Application Strategy 18.6**. In addition, a neurological and circulatory assessment should be conducted. If the radial nerve is damaged, forearm supination and extension at the elbow, wrist, or fingers will be weak, and sensory changes may occur on the dorsum of the hand. If the median nerve is damaged, active wrist and finger flexion will be weak, and sensory changes may occur on the palm of the hand.

If the ulnar nerve is damaged, ulnar deviation and finger abduction and adduction will be weak, and sensory changes may occur on the ulnar border of the hand. The clinician should take a pulse at the wrist or the ulnar and radial arteries, or the clinician should blanch the fingernails and note capillary refill. A vacuum splint should be applied and the individual transported immediately to the nearest medical facility.

The tests to determine a possible forearm fracture include applying gentle compression along the long axis of the bone and noting any pain; encircling the distal ulna and radius with the hand, applying mild compression, and noting any pain; and performing percussion over superficial bony landmarks or using a tuning fork over the bony prominences and noting any increase in pain at the fracture site.

APPLICATION STRATEGY 18.6

Determining a Possible Fracture in the Upper Arm and Forearm in the Absence of Deformity

1. **Compression.** Palpate the region for any pain, deformity, crepitus, or loose bodies. Ask if the individual heard any cracking sounds that might indicate a possible fracture. Apply gentle compression along the long axis of the bone. Then, encircle the distal ulna and radius with your hand and give mild compression. This will produce some distraction at the proximal end of the ulna and radius. Increased pain in either position indicates a possible fracture.
2. **Distraction.** Slowly distract the bones. If pain eases, this may indicate a possible fracture. If pain increases, it indicates soft-tissue damage.
3. **Percussion.** Gently tap the superficial bony landmarks. Vibrations travel along the bone and cause increased pain at the fracture site. For example, tap the following sites:

   - **Humerus**—medial and lateral epicondyles
   - **Ulna**—olecranon process and distal styloid process
   - **Radius**—distal styloid process

4. **Tuning fork.** Tap a tuning fork and place the base on the superficial bone sites mentioned in the preceding. Increased pain indicates a possible fracture.

Any positive signs indicate a possible fracture. Immobilize the limb in a vacuum splint or other appropriate splint or sling and transport the individual to the nearest medical facility.

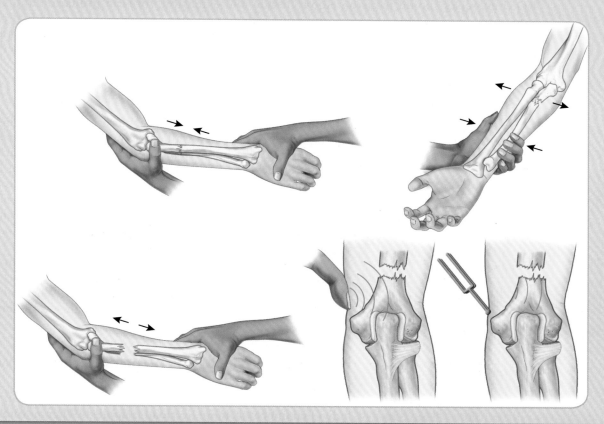

REHABILITATION

 The Little League Baseball player is diagnosed with Little League elbow. The fracture was managed conservatively with a sling for 3 weeks. When the patient begins rehabilitation, what exercises should be included in the general program?

Rehabilitation of the upper arm, elbow, and forearm must involve exercises for the entire kinetic chain, because muscles in the upper arm cross the shoulder and elbow and muscles in the forearm cross the elbow and wrist. Traumatic injuries to the elbow often require immobilization. Although the elbow is immobilized, early ROM and strengthening exercises can be conducted at the wrist, hand, and shoulder.

The management of some injuries will not require immobilization, but pain may be exacerbated by certain motions. The exercise program should focus on early mobilization in the available pain-free motions and expand to the other motions once the pain has subsided. Individuals who are involved in throwing-type activities also should include scapular stabilization exercises along with strengthening exercises for the shoulder.

The reader should refer to Chapter 17 for appropriate shoulder exercises. This section focuses only on those exercises specific to the upper arm, elbow, and forearm.

Restoration of Motion

ROM exercises should focus on elbow flexion and extension, forearm pronation and supination, wrist flexion and extension, and wrist radial and ulnar deviation. The individual can use the opposite hand to apply a low-load, prolonged stretch in the various motions to minimize joint trauma and increase flexibility (**Fig. 18.19**). The upper body ergometer also is an effective ROM tool.

Restoration of Proprioception and Balance

Closed chain exercises may be performed immediately after the acute phase of injury. Shifting body weight from one hand to the other may be performed on a wall, tabletop, or unstable surface, such as a foam mat or a biomechanical ankle platform system board. Push-ups and exercises in a frontal and sagittal plane can be performed on a Pro Fitter or slide board, if available. Step-ups can be completed on a box, stool, or StairMaster. This activity can progress to stepping up and down on boxes of differing heights, arranged so that the exercise is performed in diagonal patterns, circles, or figure eights.

As with the shoulder injury, the throwing motion should be rehearsed using mirrors or videotape. As the motion is performed, biomechanical errors at the elbow are corrected. When motion is perfected, speed of movement and distance of throw are increased gradually.

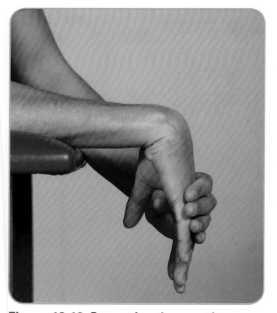

Figure 18.19. Range of motion exercises can be facilitated by using the opposite hand to apply sustained a sustained stretch.

Muscular Strength, Endurance, and Power

Gentle, resisted isometric exercises can begin immediately after injury or after surgery while the arm is still immobilized. As the individual improves, more overload is applied. When normal ROM is achieved, open kinetic chain exercises can be performed in the various motions using lightweight dumbbells; many of these exercises were demonstrated in **Application Strategy 18.1**. The individual should complete 30 to 50 repetitions using a 1-lb weight and should not progress in resistance until 50 repetitions are achieved. Wrist curls, reverse wrist curls, pronation, and supination should be performed with the forearm supported on a table. A weighted bar or hammer can be used for both radial and ulnar deviation and for pronation and supination. Another common exercise is the wrist curl-up. Using a broomstick with a light weight suspended on a 3- to 4-ft rope, the individual slowly winds the rope up around the stick and then slowly unwinds the rope. Proprioceptive neuromuscular facilitation, resisted exercises, and surgical tubing are used for concentric and eccentric loading.

Plyometric exercises may involve catching a weighted ball and using a quick, eccentric stretch of the muscle to facilitate a concentric contraction in throwing the ball. The exercise can progress through various one- and two-arm chest passes and overhead passes. A minitramp can also be used to perform plyometric bounding push-ups.

Cardiovascular Fitness

Cardiovascular conditioning should be maintained throughout the rehabilitation program. Several examples of such programs are provided in *Application Strategy: Cardiovascular-Conditioning Exercises* located on thePoint Web site.

 The Little League Baseball player should focus on restoring ROM in elbow flexion-extension, forearm pronation-supination, wrist flexion-extension, and radial and ulnar deviation. Isometric strengthening exercises should begin immediately in pain-free motions, with active exercises beginning as soon as normal ROM is achieved. The program also should include general body conditioning and strengthening exercises for the shoulder, elbow, and wrist.

SUMMARY

1. The elbow encompasses three articulations: the humeroulnar, humeroradial, and proximal radioulnar joints.

2. The medial collateral ligament is the most important ligament for stability of the elbow joint. It is divided into the anterior, transverse, and posterior oblique bands.

3. The major nerves of the elbow and forearm include the musculocutaneous, median, ulnar, and radial nerves.

4. Chronic blows to the arm can result in the development of ectopic bone, either in the belly of the muscle (myositis ossificans) or as an outgrowth (exostosis) of the underlying bone.

5. The subcutaneous olecranon bursa is the largest bursa in the elbow region. Bursitis may be acute or chronic, aseptic or septic.

6. In adolescents, the most common traumatic injury to the elbow is subluxation or dislocation of the radial head, referred to as "nursemaid's elbow" or "pulled-elbow syndrome."

7. Most ulnar dislocations occur in individuals younger than 20 years, with a peak incidence during early adolescence. The mechanism usually is hyperextension or a sudden, violent, unidirectional valgus force that drives the ulna posterior or posterolateral. Because 60% of elbow dislocations have an associated fracture, the limb should be immobilized in a vacuum splint and the individual transported immediately to the nearest medical facility.

8. Chronic injuries can result from inadequate warm-up, excessive training past the point of fatigue, inadequate rehabilitation of previous injuries, or neglect of seemingly minor conditions that progress to major complications.

9. Repetitive throwing motions place a tremendous tensile stress on the medial joint structures (i.e., medial collateral ligament, ulnar nerve, and common flexor tendons) and concomitant lateral compressive stress in the radiocapitellar joint.

10. Medial epicondylitis produces severe pain on resisted wrist flexion and pronation and with a valgus stress applied at 15° to 20° of elbow flexion.

11. Common extensor tendinitis produces severe pain on resisted wrist extension and supination and with a varus stress applied at 15° to 20° of elbow flexion.

12. Lateral compressive forces on the radiocapitellar joint can lead to osteochondritis dissecans of the skeletally immature elbow.

13. If a decision is made to refer an individual to a physician for care, the limb should be appropriately immobilized to protect the area.

14. Subsequent to the history, observation, and palpation components of an assessment, the clinician should have established a strong suspicion of the structures that may be damaged. As such, during the physical examination component, some tests will be compulsory, whereas others are used to confirm or exclude suspected injury or pathology. Only those tests that are absolutely necessary should be performed.

15. A rehabilitation program should focus on the following: reduction of pain and spasm; restoration of motion and balance; development of strength, endurance, and power; and maintenance of cardiovascular fitness. The individual should have bilateral strength, flexibility, and muscular endurance as well as an appropriate cardiovascular level before returning to participation in sport and physical activity. Whenever possible, protective equipment or padding should be used to prevent reinjury.

APPLICATION QUESTIONS

1. A high school baseball pitcher reports to the athletic training room complaining of pain on the medial elbow that began approximately 2 weeks earlier. What questions should be asked as part of an injury assessment for this individual?

2. During basketball practice, a 16-year-old male inadvertently falls and lands on a flexed elbow. What questions should be asked as part of the history component of an assessment of this injury? What factors should be addressed in the inspection/observation component of the assessment?

3. A football player is complaining of pain in his right arm during blocking drills. Palpation reveals a hardened mass within the soft tissue over the distal anterior arm. The mass is very tender and sore. Bilateral strength of the involved musculature is normal, but the pain has progressively gotten worse over the last week. What potentially serious condition might develop? How might this condition be managed?

4. A collegiate women's tennis player complains of right elbow pain that is present during and after activity, which increases during her backhand stroke. It is midseason and the condition has become worse over the past 2 weeks. How would you differentiate whether this athlete's injury is lateral epicondylitis or a chronic wrist extensor muscle strain?

5. A volleyball player is complaining of vague forearm pain aggravated during overhead spiking drills. Palpation elicits point tenderness on the proximal anterior arm. Pain increases with resisted elbow flexion and wrist ulnar deviation. What muscles are most likely involved with this condition? What additional signs or symptoms would warrant immediate physician referral?

6. A 22-year-old wrestler lands on his elbow during a match. A day later, he complains of elbow pain and tingling sensations into his forearm and hand. How would you differentiate whether this condition is cubital tunnel syndrome or radial tunnel syndrome?

7. A pole vaulter lost his grip on the pole and fell to the ground on a flexed elbow. Immediate pain and deformity is evident just proximal to the elbow. What is the probable injury? What actions are necessary to assess possible damage to the neurovascular structures of the arm?

8. What recommendations would you, as the athletic trainer for a summer tennis camp for participants in an elite youth tennis league, provide to decrease the risk of lateral epicondylitis?

9. You suspect that a high school athlete has pronator teres syndrome. How would you explain the condition and its development to the athlete and his parents?

REFERENCES

1. Steffen K, Andersen TE, Krosshaug T, et al. ECSS position statement 2009: prevention of acute sports injuries. *Euro J Sport Sci.* 2010;10(4):223–236.
2. Frisch A, Croisier JL, Urhausen A, et al. Injuries, risk factors and prevention initiatives in youth sport. *Br Med Bull.* 2009;92:95–121.
3. Lawson BR, Comstock RD, Smith GA. Baseball-related injuries to children treated in hospital emergency departments in the United States, 1994-2006. *Pediatrics.* 2009;123(6):e1028–e1034.
4. Bryce CD, Armstrong AD. Anatomy and biomechanics of the elbow. *Orthop Clin North Am.* 2008;39(2):141–154.
5. Chang CW, Wang YC, Chu CH. Increased carrying angle is a risk factor for nontraumatic ulnar neuropathy at the elbow. *Clin Orthop Relat Res.* 2008;466(9):2190–2195.
6. Sanal HT, Chen L, Haghighi P, et al. Annular ligament of the elbow: MR arthrography appearance with anatomic and histologic correlation. *AJR Am J Roentgenol.* 2009;193(2):W122–W126.
7. Rettig AC, Patel DV. Epidemiology of elbow, forearm, and wrist injuries in the athlete. *Clin Sports Med.* 1995;14(2):289–297.
8. Chou PH, Lin CJ, Chou YL, et al. Elbow load with various forearm positions during one-handed pushup exercise. *Int J Sports Med.* 2002;23(6):457–462.
9. Bowers AL, Dines JS, Dines DM, et al. Elbow medial ulnar collateral ligament reconstruction: clinical relevance and the docking technique. *J Shoulder Elbow Surg.* 2010;19(2 suppl):110–117.
10. Bushnell BD, Anz AW, Noonan TJ, et al. Association of maximum pitch velocity and elbow injury in professional baseball pitchers. *Am J Sports Med.* 2010;38(4):728–732.
11. Aguinaldo AL, Chambers H. Correlation of throwing mechanics with elbow valgus load in adult baseball pitchers. *Am J Sports Med.* 2009;37(10):2043–2048.
12. Chou PH, Lou SZ, Chen HC, et al. Effect of various forearm axially rotated postures on elbow load and elbow flexion angle in one-armed arrest of a forward fall. *Clin Biomech (Bristol, Avon).* 2009;24(8):632–636.
13. Valovich McLeod TC, Decoster LC, Loud KJ, et al. National Athletic Trainers' Association position statement: prevention of pediatric overuse injuries. *J Athl Train.* 2011;46(2):206–220.
14. Kendall FP, McCreary EK, Provance PG, et al, eds. *Muscles: Testing and Function with Posture and Pain.* 5th ed. Philadelphia, PA: Lippincott Williams & Wilkins; 2005.
15. Pandey T, Slaughter AJ, Reynolds KA, et al. Clinical orthopedic examination findings in the upper extremity: correlation with imaging studies and diagnostic efficacy. *Radiographics.* 2014;34(2):e24–e40.
16. O'Driscoll SW, Lawton RL, Smith AM. The "moving valgus stress test" for medial collateral ligament tears of the elbow. *Am J Sport Med.* 2005;33(2):231–239.
17. Dones VC III, Grimmer KA, Milanese S, et al. The sensitivity of the provocation tests in replicating pain on the lateral elbow area of participants with lateral epicondylalgia. *J Case Rep Stud.* 2014;1(1):1–15.
18. Wong MS. *Pocket Orthopaedics: Evidence-Based Survival Guide.* Sudbury, MA: Jones and Bartlett; 2010.
19. Salzman KL, Lillegard WA, Butcher JD. Upper extremity bursitis. *Am Fam Physician.* 1997;56(7):1797–1806.
20. Mehlhoff TL, Bennett JB. Elbow injuries. In: Mellion MB, Walsh WM, Madden C, et al, eds. *The Team Physician's Handbook.* 3rd ed. Philadelphia, PA: Hanley & Belfus; 2002:418–426.
21. Pugh DM, Wild LM, Schemitsch EH, et al. Standard surgical protocol to treat elbow dislocations with radial head and coronoid fractures. *J Bone Joint Surg Am.* 2004;86-A(6):1122–1130.
22. Rumball JS, Lebrun CM, Di Ciacca SR, et al. Rowing injuries. *Sports Med.* 2005;35(6):537–555.
23. Caldwell GL Jr, Safran MR. Elbow problems in the athlete. *Orthop Clin North Am.* 1995;26(3):465–485.
24. Ozyürekoğlu T, Tsai TM. Ruptures of the distal biceps tendon: results of three surgical techniques. *Hand Surg.* 2003;8(1):65–73.
25. Adirim TA, Cheng TL. Overview of injuries in the young athlete. *Sports Med.* 2003;33(1):75–81.
26. Pearl ML, Bessos K, Wong K. Strength deficits related to distal biceps tendon rupture and repair. A case report. *Am J Sports Med.* 1998;26(2):295–296.
27. Lyman S, Fleisig GS, Waterbor JW, et al. Longitudinal study of elbow and shoulder pain in youth baseball pitchers. *Med Sci Sports Exerc.* 2001;33(11):1803–1810.
28. Klingele KE, Kocher MS. Little League elbow: valgus overload injury in the paediatric athlete. *Sports Med.* 2002;32(15):1005–1015.
29. Matev B. Cubital tunnel syndrome. *Hand Surg.* 2003;8(1):127–131.
30. Platt B. Supracondylar fracture of the humerus. *Emerg Nurse.* 2004;12(2):22–29.

Wrist and Hand Conditions

STUDENT OUTCOMES

1. Identify the major bony and soft-tissue structures of the wrist and hand.

2. Describe the pathways of the median, ulnar, and radial nerves and identify the motor and sensory components of each nerve.

3. Describe the motions of the wrist and hand and identify the muscles that produce them.

4. Describe the forces that produce the loading patterns responsible for common injuries of the wrist and hand.

5. Explain the general principles used to prevent injuries to the wrist and hand.

6. Describe a thorough assessment of the wrist and hand.

7. List the common injuries and conditions sustained to the wrist and hand by physically active individuals (including sprains, dislocations, strains, tendinopathies, and nerve entrapment syndromes).

8. Describe the various types of fractures that can occur in the wrist and hand and explain their management.

9. Explain management strategies for common injuries and conditions of the wrist and hand.

10. Explain general principles and techniques used in developing a rehabilitation exercise program for the wrist and hand.

INTRODUCTION

The wrist and hand are used extensively during activities of daily living and in nearly all sport skills. Injuries to the region often result from the natural tendency to sustain the force of a fall on the hyperextended wrist. Many hand and wrist injuries also are directly related to specific sports. For example, in wrestling, football, hockey, and skiing, forced abduction of the thumb can damage the ulnar collateral ligament of the thumb, leading to an injury called a gamekeeper's thumb. Receivers in football and catchers in baseball and softball are subject to "mallet" deformity of the finger, which is caused when a ball hits the end of the finger and avulses an extensor tendon from its distal attachment. Carpal tunnel syndrome also has been reported among the physically active population in badminton, baseball, cycling, gymnastics, field hockey, racquetball, rowing, skiing, squash, tennis, and rock climbing.[1]

This chapter begins with a review of the anatomy, kinematics, and kinetics of the wrist and hand. Measures to prevent injury and assessment techniques are followed by information regarding common injuries to the wrist and hand and their management. Finally, rehabilitation exercises are found at the end of the chapter.

ANATOMY OF THE WRIST AND HAND

The wrist and hand are composed of numerous small bones and articulations. These function effectively to enable the dexterous movements performed by the hands during both daily living and sport activities.

Wrist Articulations

The wrist consists of a series of radiocarpal and intercarpal articulations (**Fig. 19.1**). Most wrist motion occurs at the radiocarpal joint. It is a condyloid joint that includes the articulation of the radius with the

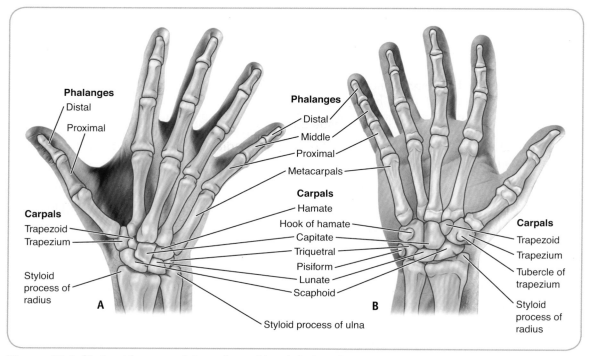

Figure 19.1. Skeletal features of the wrist and hand. A, Anterior view. **B,** Posterior view.

scaphoid, lunate, and triquetrum. The joint allows sagittal plane motions (i.e., flexion, extension, and hyper-extension) and frontal plane motions (i.e., radial deviation and ulnar deviation) as well as circumduction.

During wrist motions, the scaphoid, lunate, capitate, triquetrum, and pisiform exhibit significant nonplanar motions, with the axis of rotation for each bone shifting with the direction of the wrist movement.[2] The individual motions and interactions among these proximal carpal bones become particularly complex during the combined wrist motions, such as extension and pronation.[3] Alternately, the bones of the distal carpal row function as a single unit and are separated by gliding joints that contribute little to wrist motion. The distal carpal bones are directly linked to the motion of the third metacarpal.[4]

The distal radioulnar joint is immediately adjacent to the radiocarpal joint. The triangular fibrocartilage (TFC) is a cartilaginous disk overlying the distal ulnar head. This disk binds the end of the ulna and the radius together (i.e., head of the ulna and ulnar notch of the radius) and the distal end of the ulna and the carpal bones (i.e., lunate and triquetral bones). It makes up a portion of the TFC complex (TFCC), which acts as a stabilizer of the distal radioulnar joint. The TFCC also is the ulnar continuation of the radius, providing an articular surface for the carpal condyle. Although the ulna and radius share the articular disk, they have separate joint capsules. The volar radiocarpal, dorsal radiocarpal, radial collateral, and ulnar collateral ligaments reinforce the radiocarpal joint capsule. Its close-packed position is in extension with radial deviation.

Hand Articulations

A large number of joints are required to provide the extensive motion capabilities of the hand. Included are the carpometacarpal (CM), intermetacarpal, metacarpophalangeal (MP), and interphalangeal (IP) joints. The fingers are numbered as digits 1 through 5, with the first digit being the thumb.

Carpometacarpal and Intermetacarpal Joints

The CM joint of the thumb is a classic saddle joint. A capsule surrounding the joint serves to restrict motion. The flexion–extension axis and abduction–adduction axis at the joint are not perpendicular to each other or to the bones, and they do not intersect.[5] The articulating trapezium and metacarpal bones at the joint appear to have greater congruence, or better fit, in males than in females, which may predispose the female joint to osteoarthritis.[6]

The CM joints of the four fingers are essentially gliding joints, although some anatomists have described them as modified saddle joints. The CM and intermetacarpal joints of the fingers are mutually surrounded by joint capsules that are reinforced by the dorsal, volar, and two interosseous CM ligaments. Among these, the V-shaped interosseous ligaments are the strongest, providing very strong interconnections between the bases of the adjacent metacarpals.

Metacarpophalangeal Joints

The knuckles of the hand are formed by the MP joints. These are condyloid joints formed by the articulation of the rounded, distal heads of the metacarpals with the concave, proximal ends of the phalanges. The ends of the articulating bones at these joints are a poor fit, lending no bony stability.[7] The MP joints are each enclosed in a capsule that is reinforced by strong collateral ligaments. A dorsal ligament also merges with the MP joint of the thumb. Close-packed positions of the MP joints in the fingers and thumb are full flexion and opposition, respectively.

Interphalangeal Joints

The proximal IP (PIP) and distal IP (DIP) joints of the fingers, and the single IP joint of the thumb, are hinge joints. Subtle differences in the geometry of the articulating bone surfaces and soft-tissue restraints govern the motion capabilities at the PIP joints. An articular capsule joined by volar and collateral ligaments surrounds each IP joint. These joints are most stable in the close-packed position of full extension.

See **Major Muscles of the Hand and Fingers**, available on the companion Web site at thePoint, for a summary of the muscles, including their attachments, primary actions, and nerve innervation.

Muscles of the Wrist and Hand

Given the numerous, highly controlled, precision movements of which the hand and fingers are capable, it is no surprise that a relatively large number of muscles are responsible. Nine extrinsic muscles cross the wrist, and 10 intrinsic muscles have both of their attachments distal to the wrist. The muscles of the wrist and hand are shown in **Figures 19.2** (anterior) and **19.3** (posterior).

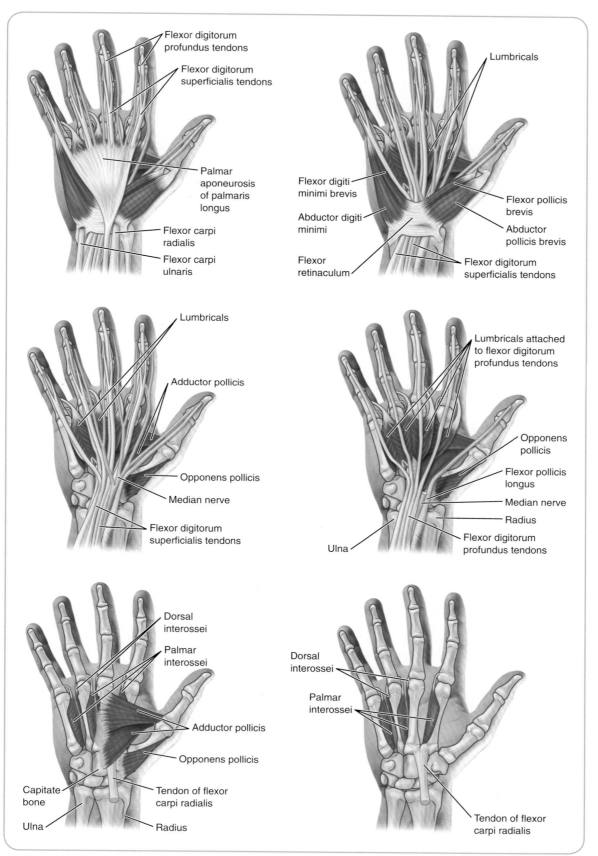

Figure 19.2. Muscles of the wrist and hand: palmar view.

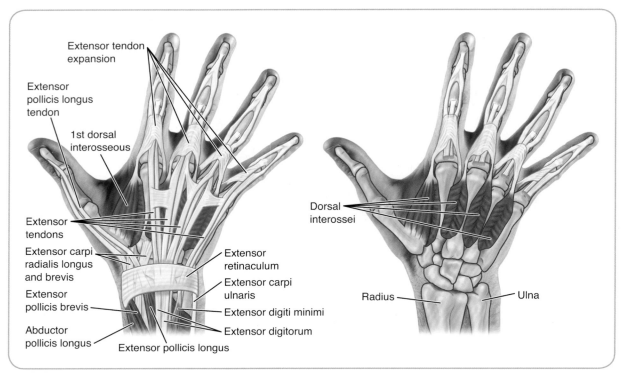

Figure 19.3. Muscles of the wrist and hand: dorsal view.

Retinacula of the Wrist

The fascial tissue surrounding the wrist is thickened into strong, fibrous bands called retinacula. They form protective passageways through which tendons, nerves, and blood vessels pass. The flexor retinaculum protects the extrinsic flexor tendons and the median nerve as they pass into the hand through the carpal tunnel on the palmar side of the wrist. Within the tunnel, the tendons are enclosed in bursal tissue and tenosynovioma. The extensor retinaculum provides a passageway for the extrinsic extensor tendons on the palmar side of the wrist.

Tendon Sheaths

The level of the metacarpal heads is the point where the flexor tendons enter a flexor tendon sheath, which is a double-walled, hollow tube sealed at both ends (**Fig. 19.4**). Filled with synovial fluid, the sheath provides low-friction gliding and nutrition for the flexor tendons. The sheath is supported by a series of retinacular thickenings called annular pulleys or cruciform pulleys, depending on their configuration. The pulleys prevent tendon bowstringing with flexion. The second (A2) and fourth (A4) annular pulleys, which are located at the proximal and middle phalanges, respectively, are the most important for preventing tendon bowstringing during active flexion.

Nerves of the Wrist and Hand

The median, ulnar, and radial nerves are major terminal branches of the brachial plexus that provide motor and sensory innervation to the wrist and hand (**Fig. 19.5**). The median nerve supplies the majority of the flexor muscles of the wrist and hand, as well as the intrinsic flexor muscles on the radial side of the palm, and cutaneous sensation to the skin on the lateral two-thirds of the palm and the dorsum of the second and third fingers. The ulnar nerve innervates the flexor carpi ulnaris, the ulnar portion of the flexor digitorum profundus, and most of the intrinsic muscles of the hand. It also provides cutaneous sensation to the fifth finger and half of the fourth finger on both the dorsal and palmar sides. The radial nerve divides into superficial and deep branches distal to the lateral epicondyle of the elbow. The superficial branch supplies the skin on the dorsum of the hand, and the deep branch innervates most of the extensor muscles of the forearm.

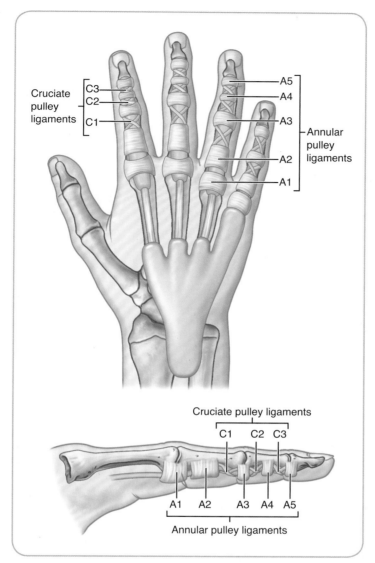

Figure 19.4. Flexor tendons, sheath, and pulley system. The tendons from the finger flexors pass through strong annular pulleys (A1 through A5), which keep the tendons and their encircling sheath closely applied to the phalanges. The thin, pliable cruciate pulleys (C1 through C3) collapse to allow full digital flexion.

Blood Vessels of the Wrist and Hand

The major vessels supplying the muscles of the wrist and hand are the radial and ulnar arteries (**Fig. 19.6**). The radial artery supplies the muscles on the radial side of the forearm as well as the thumb and index finger. The ulnar artery divides into anterior and posterior interosseous arteries to supply the deep flexor muscles and extensor muscles, respectively, of the forearm. In the palm, the radial and ulnar arteries merge to form the superficial and deep palmar arches. Another connecting branch from these arteries forms the carpal arch on the dorsal side of the wrist. Digital arteries branch from the palmar arches to supply the fingers, and branches from the carpal arch run distally along the metacarpal bones. The radial artery is superficial on the anterior aspect of the wrist. The pulse is readily palpable at this site.

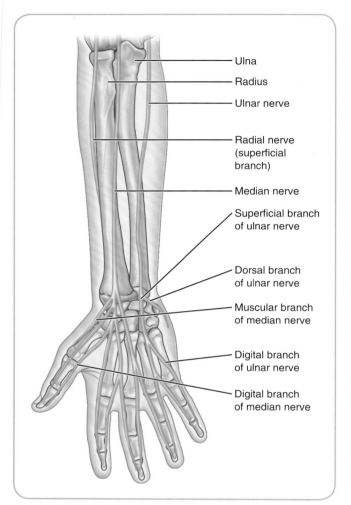

Figure 19.5. Peripheral nerve supply to the wrist and hand.

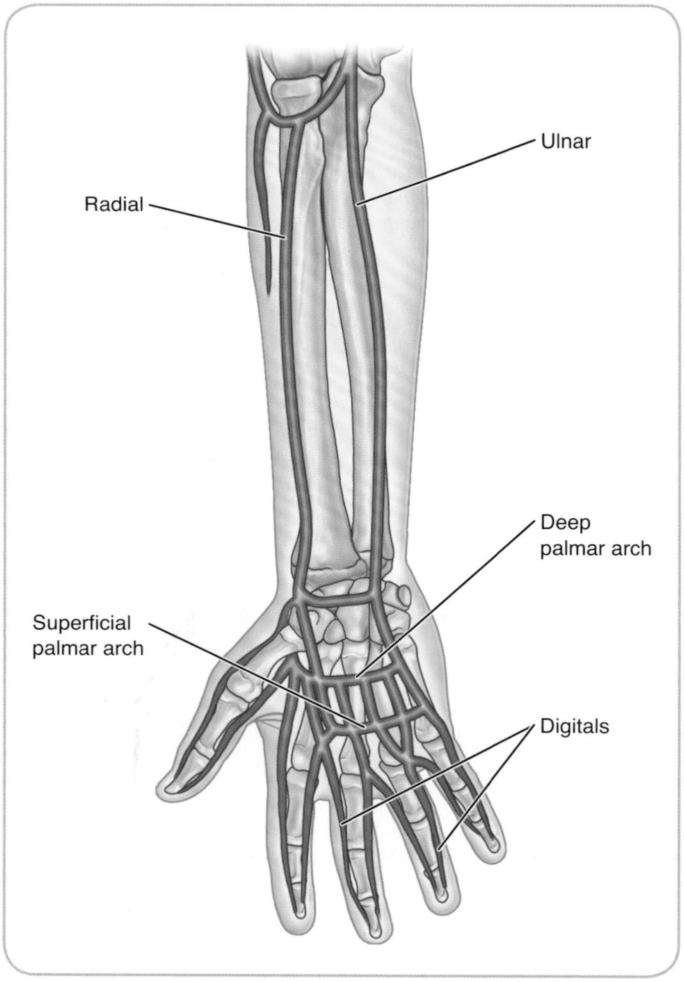

Figure 19.6. Blood supply to the wrist and hand.

KINEMATICS AND MAJOR MUSCLE ACTIONS OF THE WRIST AND HAND

The wrist is capable of both sagittal and frontal plane movements (**Fig. 19.7**). Flexion occurs when the palmar surface of the hand is moved toward the anterior forearm. Extension involves the return of the hand to anatomical position from a position of flexion, and hyperextension occurs when the dorsal surface of the hand is brought toward the posterior forearm. Movement of the hand toward the radial side of the arm is known as radial deviation; movement in the opposite direction is known as ulnar deviation. Movement of the hand through all four directions is termed circumduction.

Flexion

The major flexor muscles of the wrist are the flexor carpi radialis and flexor carpi ulnaris (**Fig. 19.2**). The palmaris longus, which often is absent in one or both forearms, contributes to flexion. The flexor digitorum superficialis and flexor digitorum profundus assist with flexion at the wrist when the fingers are completely extended, but when the fingers are in flexion, these muscles cannot develop sufficient tension to assist.

Extension and Hyperextension

The extensor carpi radialis longus, extensor carpi radialis brevis, and extensor carpi ulnaris produce extension and hyperextension at the wrist. The other posterior wrist muscles also may assist with

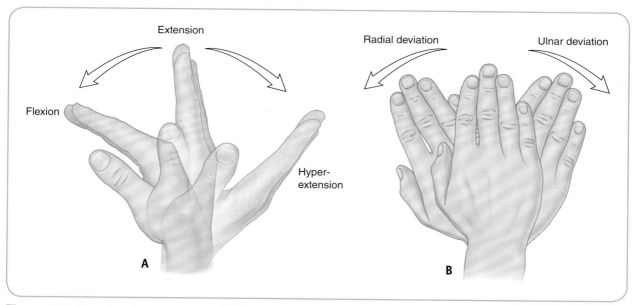

Figure 19.7. Directional movement capabilities at the wrist. A, Sagittal plane movements. **B,** Frontal plane movements.

extension movements, particularly when the fingers are in flexion. Included are the extensor pollicis longus, extensor indicis, extensor digiti minimi, and extensor digitorum (**Fig. 19.3**). When the wrist moves from full flexion to full extension, the passive tension in the extrinsic muscles causes the DIP joints to go from approximately 12° to 31° of flexion and the PIP joints from approximately 19° to 70° of flexion.[8]

Radial and Ulnar Deviation

The flexor and extensor muscles of the wrist co-operatively develop tension to produce radial and ulnar deviation of the hand at the wrist. The flexor carpi radialis and extensor carpi radialis act to produce radial deviation, and the flexor carpi ulnaris and extensor carpi ulnaris cause ulnar deviation.

Carpometacarpal Joint Motion

The CM joint of the thumb allows a large range of motion (ROM), comparable to that of a ball-and-socket joint. The fifth CM joint permits significantly less ROM, however, and only a very small amount of motion is allowed at the second through fourth CM joints because of the presence of restrictive ligaments.

Metacarpophalangeal Joint Motion

The MP joints of the fingers allow flexion, extension, abduction, adduction, and circumduction (**Fig. 19.8**). Among the fingers, abduction is defined as movement away from the middle finger and adduction as movement toward the middle finger.

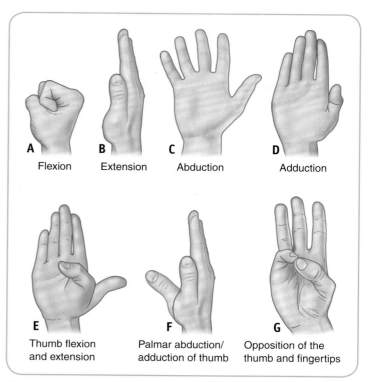

Figure 19.8. Directional movement capabilities at the fingers and thumb. A, Flexion. **B,** Extension. **C,** Abduction. **D,** Adduction. **E,** Thumb flexion and extension. **F,** Palmar abduction/adduction of the thumb. **G,** Opposition of the thumb and fingertips.

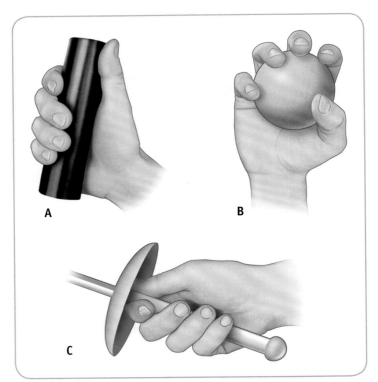

Figure 19.9. Hand grips. Muscles of the hand contract to provide several grips. **A,** Power grip. **B,** Precision grip. **C,** Fencing grip.

The MP joint of the thumb, however, functions more as a hinge joint, with the primary movements being flexion and extension.

Interphalangeal Joint Motion

The IP joints permit flexion and extension and, in some individuals, slight hyperextension. These joints are classic hinge joints.

KINETICS OF THE WRIST AND HAND

The extrinsic flexor muscles of the hand are more than twice as strong as the extrinsic extensor muscles. This should come as little surprise given that the flexor muscles of the hand are used extensively in everyday activities involving gripping, grasping, or pinching movements, whereas the extensor muscles rarely exert much force.

Three types of hand grips are predominantly used in sport activities (**Fig. 19.9**). The power grip, as typified by the baseball bat grip, is one in which the fingers and thumb are used to clamp the grip of the bat against the palm of the hand. The wrist is held in a position of ulnar deviation and slight hyperextension to increase the tension in the flexor tendons. In contrast to the power grip, the precision grip, as exemplified by the baseball grip, involves use of the semiflexed fingers and thumb to pinch the ball against the palm, with the wrist in slight hyperextension. A third grip, which is intermediate to the two previously described, is referred to as the fencing grip. Fencing requires both power and precision. The grip on the foil is essentially a power grip; however, because the thumb is aligned along the long axis of the foil handle, it enables precise control over the direction of force application. As might be expected, grip force is less with a precision grip in comparison to the palmar grips.[9]

PREVENTION OF WRIST AND HAND CONDITIONS

The very nature of many contact and collision sports places the wrist and hand in an extremely vulnerable position for injury. The hands almost always are the first point of contact to cushion the body during collisions, deflect flying objects, or lessen body impact during a fall. Falling on an outstretched hand is the leading cause of fractures and dislocations at the distal forearm, wrist, and hand. Although several pads and gloves are available, few sports require protective padding for the region.

Protective Equipment

Goalies, baseball and softball catchers, and field players in sports such as ice hockey and lacrosse are required to wear wrist and hand protection. Padded gloves prevent direct compression from a stick, puck, or ball. Several other gloves have extra padding placed at high-impact areas, aid in gripping, and protect the hand from abrasions, particularly when playing on artificial turf or a baseball or softball field. Whenever possible, protective pads and gloves should be worn during sport participation to lessen the risk of injury.

Physical Conditioning

Several muscles that move the wrist and hand cross the elbow. As such, ROM and strengthening exercises for the wrist and hand also must include exercises for the elbow (see **Application Strategy 18.1**). The exercises include elbow flexion and extension, forearm pronation and supination, wrist flexion and extension, and radial and ulnar deviation. Other exercises, such as squeezing a tennis ball or a spring-loaded grip device, can be used to strengthen the finger flexors.

The physical conditioning program should include a preseason and in-season component. Because upper extremity power and speed originates in the trunk and not the upper extremity, it is important to include exercises and training sessions that focus on neuromuscular control, balance, coordination, flexibility, and strengthening of the lower extremities.[10] This is especially true among pediatric athletes and those with a history of past injury.[11] Furthermore, when working with the youth sport athlete, the intensity, load, time, and distance the athlete is required to achieve should only be increased by about 10% each week to avoid overloading and breakdown.[10]

Proper Skill Technique

Unlike the shoulder and elbow, which is subjected to excessive stress during a throwing-type motion, the majority of wrist and hand injuries result from direct trauma. Although analysis of specific movements may detect improper technique, the analysis in many cases is incidental. An important skill technique that can prevent injury of the wrist and hand is proper instruction on the shoulder-roll method of falling. In this technique, the force of impact is dispersed over a wider area, lessening the risk for injury from direct axial loading on the extended wrist.

ASSESSMENT OF WRIST AND HAND CONDITIONS

 A cheerleader is complaining of pain over the right anatomical snuff box. How should the assessment of this injury progress to determine the extent and severity of injury?

The wrist and hand can be difficult to evaluate because of the number of anatomical structures providing motor and sensory function to the region. A thorough examination in this area often takes longer than with other joints of the body because of the multiple structures and joints that are involved. When assessing this region, two major objectives must be kept in mind. First, the injury or condition must be evaluated as accurately as possible to ensure adequate treatment. Second, the clinician must ascertain the remaining function to determine whether the individual has any incapacity in performing sport-specific skills and activities of daily living.

See **Application Strategy: Wrist and Hand Evaluation**, available on the companion Web site at thePoint.

The clinician also must keep in mind that if the mechanism of injury involves axial loading at the wrist, additional assessment may be necessary at the elbow or shoulder. Although uncommon, pain at the wrist and hand may be referred from the cervical spine, shoulder, and elbow. As such, it may be necessary to evaluate these joints before assessing the wrist and hand.

HISTORY

 The injury assessment of the cheerleader should begin with a history. What questions need to be asked to identify the cause and extent of this injury?

Questions about a wrist injury should focus on the primary complaint, past injuries, and other factors that may have contributed to the current problem (e.g., demands of the sport, changes in technique, overuse, occupational requirements, or referred pain). Questions should be asked to determine how the injury occurred, because it is important to determine if the region has been subjected to repetitive trauma, such as constant impact from a ball, racquet, bat, or stick. Current symptoms and their progression must be determined. Questions also must be asked regarding the pain (i.e., localized, general, radiating, or activities that increase or decrease pain), as should questions concerning the presence of sounds and unusual feelings. Recent changes, if any, in the training program should be noted.

Outcome assessment tools can also be incorporated into the history (subjective) portion of the examination process. When appropriate, outcome measures can be used during the initial evaluation but are most often during follow-up evaluations throughout the treatment and rehabilitation process to measure the patient's progress. The most commonly used tool is the Disabilities of the Arm, Shoulder, and Hand (DASH) questionnaire and is seen as the optimal choice to use with patients who may have multiple joints affected. If the patient is dealing with carpal tunnel syndrome, the evidence suggests that the Brigham and Women's score for carpal tunnel syndrome is a clinically useful assessment measure to use. The Patient-Rated Wrist Evaluation (PRWE) questionnaire was found to be the most responsive tool to measure outcomes in patients with a distal radius fracture.[11]

See **Application Strategy: Developing a History of the Injury**, available on the companion Web site at thePoint, for specific questions regarding the wrist and hand region.

The cheerleader should be asked questions that address the following: when, where, and how the injury occurred; current symptoms and their progression; pain (i.e., localized, general, or radiating); activities that cannot be performed because of the pain; actions or motions that replicate the pain; and previous injury, treatment, and medication.

OBSERVATION AND INSPECTION

? The history reveals falling on an outstretched hand approximately 1 month ago. The cheerleader reports that pain is more pronounced during activities that involve wrist extension. Explain the observation component in the ongoing assessment of the cheerleader.

The entire arm should be exposed for observation and inspection. Although the individual may have a wrist injury, the elbow and shoulder region also may need to be evaluated, depending on the mechanism of injury. First, the clinician should observe the position of the wrist, hand, and fingers, noting any noticeable deformity and general presentation. If swelling is present in a specific joint, the individual may be unable to fully extend that joint and may be supporting it in a slightly flexed position. If a fracture or dislocation is not present, the individual's willingness and ability to place the hand in the various positions that are requested should be observed. The functional position of the wrist, sometimes called the position of rest, is with the wrist in 20° to 35° of extension and 10° to 15° of ulnar deviation. This position allows the greatest amount of flexion of the fingers; inability to assume this position may suggest a tendon or nerve disruption.[12] The palm of the hand should be inspected for palmar creases; swelling in one or more of the hand compartments may obliterate these lines. In a bilateral comparison, the dominant hand tends to be slightly larger than the nondominant hand. The specific site of injury should be inspected for obvious abrasions, deformity, swelling, discoloration, symmetry, hypertrophy, muscle atrophy, or previous surgical incisions. Subtle skin changes may be indicative of a possible nerve injury. For example, the hand normally has moisture on it, and the absence of moisture on the distal phalanx may indicate a digital nerve injury.[12]

See **Application Strategy: Observation and Inspection of the Wrist and Hand**, available on the companion Web site at thePoint, for a summary of the observations of the wrist and hand from the dorsal and palmar views.

During the assessment of the cheerleader's injury, a general observation regarding the presentation of the hand and wrist as well as of the elbow and shoulder should be performed. In addition, the injury site should be inspected for swelling, discoloration, deformity, muscle hypertrophy or atrophy, and other signs of existing or previous trauma.

PALPATION

A bilateral comparison of the cheerleader's wrist and hand reveals no abnormal findings. Explain palpation for this injury.

If the individual is in great pain and is unable or unwilling to move the wrist or hand, the possibility of a fracture or dislocation should be determined before moving the wrist or hand. In the absence of deformity, fracture tests, including compression, percussion, vibration, and traction, should be performed. If a fracture is suspected, it should be treated accordingly. Acute care consists of ice, immobilization, and immediate referral to a physician.

The direction and sequencing for palpation should be determined by location of pain and site of injury, beginning away from the site and working toward it. Bilateral palpation can determine temperature, swelling, point tenderness, crepitus, deformity, muscle spasm, and cutaneous sensation. Temperature changes may indicate inflammation, infection, or reduction in circulation. Crepitus may indicate tenosynovitis, an irregular articular surface, or possible fracture. Circulation can be assessed by blanching the fingernails; this is performed by squeezing the nail and observing the changes in color. Initially, the nails should turn white, but color should return within 2 seconds of release. Pulses also can be taken at the radial and ulnar arteries in the wrist. The following structures should be palpated (**Figs. 19.1** to **19.4**):

Dorsal Aspect

1. Radial styloid process and tubercle of the radius

2. Styloid process of the ulna

3. Finger and thumb extensors muscles and tendons, and the thumb abductor muscles

4. The carpal bones on the dorsal and palmar aspect (should be palpated at the same time):

   - *Scaphoid*—lies distal to the radial styloid process and forms the floor of the anatomical snuff box
   - *Lunate*—lies just distal to the radial tubercle and is easily palpated during wrist flexion
   - *Triquetrum*—lies one finger's breadth distal to the ulnar styloid process
   - *Pisiform*—palpable on the medial palmar side when the wrist is slightly flexed
   - *Trapezium*—lies distal to the anatomical snuff box
   - *Trapezoid*—lies medial to the trapezium
   - *Capitate*—lies distal to the lunate and a slight indentation before the metacarpal
   - *Hamate*—lies distal to the triquetrum; the hook of the hamate is more easily palpated on the palmar aspect

5. Metacarpal bones and phalanges

6. Extensor hoods

Palmar Aspect

1. Flexor tendons

2. Carpal transverse arch that forms the carpal tunnel, and the longitudinal arch composed of the carpal bones, metacarpals, and phalanges

3. Palmar fascia and intrinsic muscles within the thenar and hypothenar muscle masses

During the assessment of the cheerleader, the bony and soft-tissue structures of the distal radius/ulna, wrist, and hand should be palpated for point tenderness, swelling, deformity, skin temperature, sensation, and other signs of trauma.

PHYSICAL EXAMINATION TESTS

> **?** Palpation reveals pain over the anatomical snuff box, and the physical examination of the injury reveals pain at the end range of passive ROM with wrist extension and ulnar deviation. Pain also is elicited during resistive ROM of those motions. What injury should be suspected, and what is the immediate management for that injury?

The wrist or hand should not be forced through any sudden motions, and caution should be used in proceeding through the physical examination. Only those tests that are necessary to assess the current injury should be performed. Tests should be performed bilaterally.

Functional Tests

The clinician should determine the available ROM in forearm pronation–supination, wrist flexion–extension, radial/ulnar deviation, finger flexion–extension, finger abduction–adduction, thumb flexion–extension, thumb abduction–adduction, and opposition of the thumb and little finger. As always, bilateral comparison is critical to distinguish normal from abnormal movement. The clinician should ask the individual to do the following:

1. Make a tight fist (flexion).

2. Straighten the fingers (extension).

3. Spread the fingers (abduction).

4. Bring the fingers together (adduction).

5. Make wrist circles (circumduction).

6. Turn hand's palm up and down (supination and pronation).

Active Movements

In determining active movements at the wrist and hand, the movements that are anticipated to be most painful should be performed last. Finger active motion usually is done in a continuous pattern of flexion and extension. It is important to note the fluidness as each digit moves throughout the ROM. If one finger does not move through the full ROM, that finger can be evaluated separately. The motions that should be assessed and the normal ROMs for each are as follows:

- Pronation/supination of the forearm (85° to 90°)

- Wrist flexion (80° to 90°)

- Wrist extension (70° to 90°)

- Radial deviation (15°)

- Ulnar deviation (30° to 45°)

- Finger flexion and extension

- Finger abduction and adduction

- Thumb flexion, extension, abduction, and adduction

- Opposition of the thumb and little finger (tip to tip)

The techniques for taking goniometry measurements of wrist flexion and extension, and of radial and ulnar deviation, are shown in **Figure 19.10**.

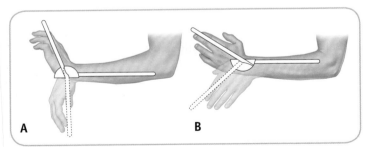

Figure 19.10. Goniometry measurement. A, Wrist flexion and extension. The fulcrum is centered over the lateral aspect of the wrist close to the triquetrum. Align the proximal arm along the lateral aspect of the ulna using the olecranon process as a reference. Then, align the distal arm along the midline of the 5th metacarpal. **B, Radial and ulnar deviation.** Center the fulcrum over the middle of the dorsum of the wrist close to the capitate. Align the proximal arm with the midline of the forearm using the lateral epicondyle as a reference. Then, align the distal arm along the midline of the third metacarpal.

Passive Movements

If the individual is unable to perform active movements in all ranges, the individual's passive movements should be assessed. Slight overpressure at the end of each motion can test the end feel of each joint. The normal end feels are as follows:

- **Tissue stretch**—movements of the wrist and finger joints

- **Bone to bone**—pronation

Resisted Muscle Testing

Active movements are tested using resisted movements throughout the full ROM. The individual can be standing or seated. The proximal joint is stabilized, and a mild resistance is applied to the distal joint. **Figure 19.11** demonstrates motions that should be tested.

Manual Muscle Testing

If pain or weakness is found during resisted ROM, the clinician may decide to perform a manual muscle test to determine which muscle is damaged. To correctly apply the manual muscle testing techniques to the wrist and hand, the elbow must be appropriately stabilized.[13] See **Table 19.1** for manual muscle testing procedures for the selected muscles of the wrist and hand.

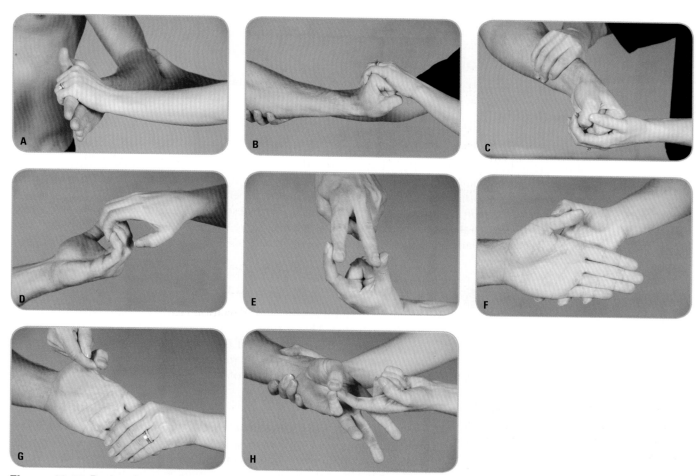

Figure 19.11. Resisted range of motion testing. A, Forearm supination and pronation. **B,** Wrist flexion and extension. **C,** Ulnar and radial deviation. **D,** Finger flexion and extension. **E,** Finger abduction and adduction. **F,** Thumb flexion and extension. **G,** Thumb abduction and adduction. **H,** Opposition.

TABLE 19.1 Manual Muscle Testing of Selected Muscles of the Wrist and Hand

MUSCLE	JOINT POSITIONING	APPLY PRESSURE
Flexor carpi ulnaris	Patient is seated with forearm in full supination and resting on table. Wrist should be flexed and deviated toward the ulna.	To the hypothenar eminence in the direction of extension and radial deviation
Flexor digitorum profundus	Patient is seated with wrist in slight extension. The clinician grasps the proximal and middle phalanges and stabilizes both joints in a neutral position while patient flexes distal phalanx.	To the palmar aspect of the distal phalanx in the direction of extension
Flexor digitorum superficialis	Patient is seated with wrist in slight extension. The clinician stabilizes the MP joint and proximal phalange in a neutral position while patient flexes the PIP joint.	To the palmar aspect of the proximal phalanx in the direction of extension
Extensor digitorum	Patient is seated with forearm pronated and wrist in neutral position. MP joints are extended with IP joints flexed.	To the dorsal aspect of the proximal phalanges in the direction of flexion

For more in depth descriptions and illustrations, see Kendall FP, McCreary EK, Provance PG, et al, eds. *Muscles: Testing and Function with Posture and Pain.* 5th ed. Baltimore, MD: Lippincott Williams & Wilkins; 2005.

Stress and Joint Play Tests

Stress and joint play tests are performed for those individuals with suspected ligament or capsule damage. Only those tests deemed to be relevant should be used, and results should be compared bilaterally.

Ligamentous Instability Test for the Wrist (Varus and Valgus Stress Test)

With the individual's elbow flexed at 90° and the forearm pronated, the clinician grips the distal forearm with one hand and the metacarpals with the other. A varus (i.e., ulnar deviation) or valgus (i.e., radial deviation) stress is applied to the wrist joint, depending on the location of pain. The test is positive when pain or laxity is present. A positive varus test (radial collateral ligament stress test) indicates damage to the radial collateral ligaments. A positive valgus (ulnar collateral ligament stress test) test indicates damage to the ulnar collateral ligament.

Ligamentous Instability Test for the Fingers (Varus and Valgus Stress Test)

The clinician stabilizes the thumb or finger with one hand proximal to the joint being tested. This is followed by applying valgus and varus stresses to the joint to test the integrity of the collateral ligaments (**Fig. 19.12**) and anteroposterior glide to stress the joint capsule. This test is used for gamekeeper's thumb and joint sprains of the fingers.

Joint Play Tests

Joint play is accessory movements that occur within a joint to facilitate proper joint motion. However, these accessory motions are not under the patient's control. Joint dysfunction is present if assessment of joint play detects hyper- or hypomobile motion. Hypermobility may be the result of sprain of the supporting ligaments or capsule. Hypomobility may be the result of adhesions, scar tissue or general capsular stiffness from chronic inflammation.[14]

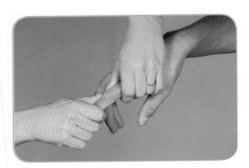

Figure 19.12. Ligament instability test. To stress the ligamentous structures around the joints, the clinician applies varus and valgus forces at the specific joint.

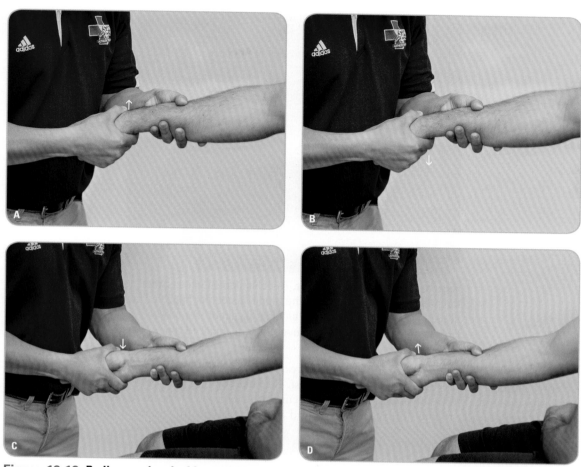

Figure 19.13. Radiocarpal and midcarpal joint play. Joint play is assessed through performing dorsal **(A)**, palmar **(B)**, radial **(C)**, and ulnar **(D)** glides of the radiocarpal joint.

■ Radiocarpal/Midcarpal Joint Play

Positive radiocarpal/midcarpal joint play suggests damage to the collateral or intercollateral ligaments or possibly to the TFCC of the wrist if hypermobility and/or pain were elicited.[15] The presence of hypomobility may indicate presence of adhesions within the joint. The test is performed with the patient in a seated position, elbow at 90° and forearm resting on the plinth (**Fig. 19.13**). The clinician stabilizes the patient at the distal aspect of the ulnar and radius and with opposite hand grasps the patient's proximal carpals. The clinician then performs a dorsal, palmar, radial, and ulnar glide to assess joint play.

■ Intercarpal Joint Play

Positive intercarpal joint play[15] tests may indicate sprain of the intercarpal ligaments or presence of scar tissue within the joint. The patient is seated, with elbow at 90° and forearm pronated. The clinician uses one hand (thumb and finger) to apply alternating palmar and dorsa forces to one carpal while using the other hand (thumb and finger) to stabilize the adjacent carpal.

Special Tests

A variety of special tests can be used for detecting injury or related pathology (e.g., muscle/tendon injury, nerve entrapment, or fracture).

Finkelstein Test

While the individual makes a fist with the thumb inside the fingers (**Fig. 19.14**), the clinician stabilizes the forearm and while the patient actively flexes the wrist in an ulnar direction. A positive Finkelstein

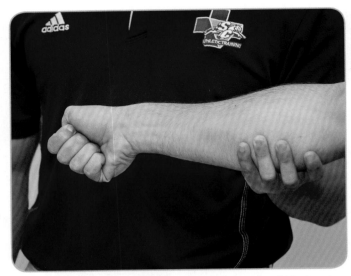

Figure 19.14. Finkelstein test. The clinician should instruct the patient to make a fist with the thumb inside the fingers. The athlete then flexes the wrist in an ulnar direction. A positive Finkelstein test produces pain over the APL and EPB tendons.

test, indicating de Quervain tenosynovitis, produces pain over the abductor pollicis longus (APL) and extensor pollicis brevis (EPB) tendons at the wrist. Because the test may be uncomfortable even for a healthy individual, false positives frequently occur with this test. All positive test results should be compared bilaterally to the uninvolved wrist and correlated with information gained through the examination process.

Phalen (Wrist Flexion) Test

Several variations on how to perform Phalen test can be found in the literature, but all agree that a positive finding implies compression of the median nerve and the presence of carpal tunnel syndrome.[14-17] The clinician instructs the individual to place the dorsum of the hands together to maximally flex the wrists and hold this position for 1 minute by gently pushing the wrists together (**Fig. 19.15A**).[17] It is important to ensure that the individual does not shrug the shoulders during the test, because this causes compression of the median branch of the brachial plexus as it passes through the thoracic outlet. An alternate position is to have the clinician apply overpressure during passive wrist flexion and hold the position for 1 minute (**Fig. 19.15B**).[15] A positive test, indicating

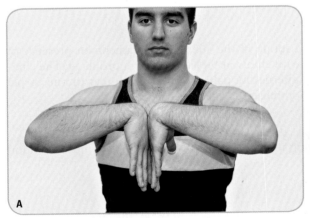
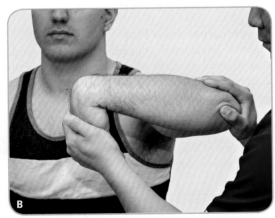

Figure 19.15. Phalen test. A, Original Phalen (wrist flexion) test indicates that the median or ulnar nerve is compressed if numbness or tingling occurs in the specific nerve distribution pattern. **B,** Modified Phalen test.

either median or ulnar nerve compression, produces numbness or tingling into the specific nerve distribution pattern: If the median nerve is compressed, sensory changes are evident in the thumb, index finger, third finger, and lateral half of the ring finger; if the ulnar nerve is compressed, sensory changes occur in the fifth finger and medial half of the ring finger.

Wrist Flexion and Median Nerve Compression Test

This test has a reported 86% sensitivity and 95% specificity, making it a very clinically useful test for detecting median nerve neuropathy. To perform the test, the patient is seated with the elbow fully extended. The wrist is flexed, and the forearm is supinated. Using the thumbs, the clinician applies a constant and even pressure over the median nerve where it passes through the carpal tunnel (**Fig. 19.16**). The test is considered positive if there is a reproduction of symptoms within 30 seconds.[16]

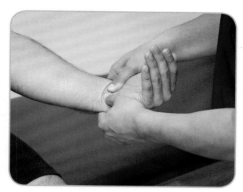

Figure 19.16. Wrist flexion and median nerve compression test.

Pinch Grip Test for Entrapment of the Anterior Interosseous Nerve

The clinician instructs the patient to pinch the tip of the index finger and thumb together (**Fig. 19.17**). If an abnormal pulp-to-pulp pinch is performed, the anterior interosseous nerve, which is an extension of the median nerve, may be entrapped at the elbow as it passes between the two heads of the pronator teres.

Scaphoid Compression Test

The scaphoid compression test is used to assist in screening in/ruling out the presence of possible scaphoid fracture. Holding the thumb of the involved hand, a longitudinal force is applied,

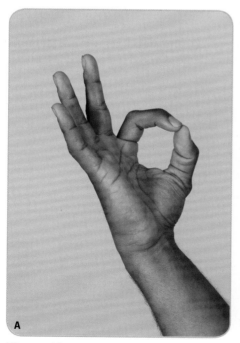
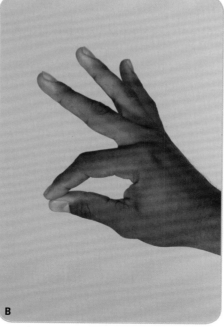

Figure 19.17. Pinch grip test. The clinician instructs the patient to make an "O" with the thumb and forefinger. **A,** Normal tip-to-tip. **B,** Abnormal pulp-to-pulp, which signifies entrapment of the interior interosseous nerve.

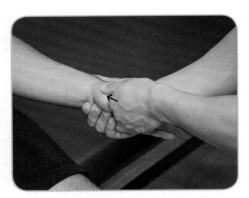

Figure 19.18. Scaphoid compression tenderness. Pain in the anatomical snuff box is positive.

compressing the metacarpal bone into the scaphoid (**Fig. 19.18**). The test is positive if painful. This test has 100% sensitivity and 80% specificity.[16]

Watson Test for Scapholunate Instability

The Watson test is used to assess instability between the scaphoid and lunate. The test has moderately strong sensitivity (69%) but poor specificity (12%).[15] Problems encountered while attempting to perform the test include eliciting significant pain when used with an acute injury and the presence of positive findings without a clinical complaint. The test is performed with the patient seated and forearm slightly pronated. The clinician applies pressure to the scaphoid with the thumb on the volar aspect. With the opposing hand, the clinician grasps the patient's metacarpals and moves the patient's wrist from ulnar deviation and slight extension into radial deviation and slight extension. Pressure is continually applied to the scaphoid.[16] A clunk and pain is considered positive.

Neurological Tests

Neurological integrity can be assessed with the use of myotomes, reflexes, and segmental dermatomes as well as peripheral nerve cutaneous patterns.

Myotomes

Isometric muscle testing to assess the myotomes should be performed in the loose-packed position and include scapular elevation (C4), shoulder abduction (C5), elbow flexion and/or wrist extension (C6), elbow extension and/or wrist flexion (C7), thumb extension and/or ulnar deviation (C8), and abduction and/or adduction of the hand intrinsics (T1).

Reflexes

Reflexes in the upper extremity include the biceps (C5–C6), brachioradialis (C6), and triceps (C7). These are discussed and demonstrated in Chapters 17 and 18.

Cutaneous Patterns

The segmental nerve dermatome patterns for the wrist and hand region are demonstrated in **Figure 19.19**. The peripheral nerve cutaneous patterns are demonstrated in **Figure 19.20**. Bilateral testing

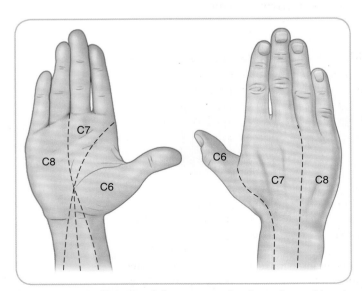

Figure 19.19. Segmental dermatomes for the wrist and hand.

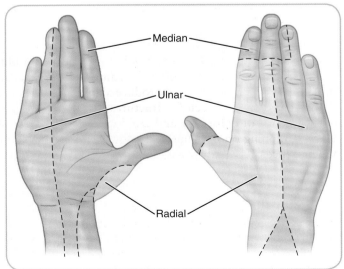

Figure 19.20. Cutaneous nerve distribution patterns for the wrist and hand.

for altered sensation should be performed using sharp and dull touch by running the open hand and fingernails over the shoulder and down both sides of the arms and hands.

Activity-Specific Functional Tests

Because the wrist, hand, and fingers are vital in performing activities of daily living, individuals should be assessed for manual dexterity and coordination. It is important to assess the abilities to hook, pinch, and grasp an object as well as activities such as combing the hair, holding a fork, brushing the teeth, or picking up a backpack. Before return to activity, the individual should be able to perform these simple functional skills in addition to having bilateral ROM and strength in the wrist and fingers. Conditions that warrant immediate referral to a physician include the following:

■ Suspected fracture or dislocation

■ Significant pain and/or excessive swelling in soft tissues or around joints

■ Joint instability

■ Loss or impairment of motion or function

■ Presence of any sensory or circulatory changes

> The assessment of the cheerleader suggests a fracture of the scaphoid. Immediate management involves ice, compression, immobilization in an appropriate splint, and immediate referral to a physician.

CONTUSIONS AND SKIN WOUNDS

> **?** In attempting to catch a pass, a football player fell and slid on the artificial turf field. He sustained an abrasion on the palmar side of one hand. What are the immediate and long-term concerns associated with cleaning this superficial wound?

Etiology

Direct impact to the hand by any object may lead to abrasions, lacerations, and puncture wounds. Although many are minor, it is always important to be alert for an underlying fracture.

Signs and Symptoms

Contusions on the back of the hand may appear as a bluish, painful discoloration. Abrasions and lacerations may involve profuse bleeding but are usually minor. Because of the loose skin covering the hand, contusions may produce significantly swelling that is disproportional to the degree of damage sustained. Screen for fractures based on the history, mechanism of injury, and palpations. The presence of deformity and crepitus support a possible fracture. If no deformity or crepitus is present, tapping on the bone or performing a long bone compression test may be used to assess for the presence of a nondisplaced fracture.

Management

Initial treatment of most closed wounds involves ice, compression, elevation, and rest. Symptoms usually disappear in 2 to 3 days. If not, the individual should be referred to a physician for follow-up care. Open wounds must be thoroughly cleansed of any foreign matter. With an abrasion, a 10-minute wash using surgical soap, a water-soluble iodine solution, and a brush can remove imbedded foreign matter. When the wound has been cleansed, an antiseptic should be applied and the wound covered with a nonocclusive dressing. The dressing should be changed daily and the wound inspected for signs of infection. If the wound appears red, swollen, or purulent or is hot and tender, immediate referral to a physician is warranted.

Completely lacerated digital vessels tend to retract, constrict, and clot, whereas partial transactions may continue to hemorrhage and may result in a traumatic aneurysm.[18] Direct pressure applied to the wound for 10 to 15 minutes with a sterile, semicompressible material should be followed by elevation of the limb above the heart and immediate transportation to the nearest medical facility. A puncture wound should be irrigated with normal saline to flush as much of the foreign material as possible from the wound. After covering the wound with a sterile dressing, the individual should be transported to a physician for further evaluation to ensure that all foreign matter has been eliminated from the wound. Although infection is the most common complication with any open wound, particularly puncture wounds, the use of prophylactic antibiotics remains controversial; however, tetanus prophylaxis is warranted when these injuries are sustained.

> The abrasion sustained by the football player should be cleansed thoroughly. Next, an antiseptic and a nonocclusive dressing should be applied. The wound should be inspected daily for signs of infection.

SPRAINS

> Following the completion of a floor routine, a gymnast reports pain in the right wrist. What signs and symptoms would suggest that the injury is a wrist sprain?

Ligamentous sprains in the wrist and hand result from either acute trauma or repetitive stress. When caused by a single episode of trauma, the severity of injury is dependent on the following:

- Characteristics of the injury force (i.e., point of application, magnitude, rate, and direction)
- Position of the hand at impact
- Relative strength of the carpal bones and ligaments

Most injuries to the region result from a compressive load applied while the hand is in some degree of extension, although hyperflexion or rotation may lead to injury. Unfortunately, because of the need to perform simple daily activities, most individuals do not allow ample time for healing. Consequently, many sprains are neglected, leading to chronic instability.

Wrist Sprains

Etiology

Axial loading on the proximal palm during a fall on an outstretched hand is the leading cause of wrist sprains. The most common ligamentous instability at the wrist occurs between the scaphoid and the lunate.[12] Gymnasts have a high incidence of dorsal wrist pain when excessive forces are exerted on the wrist, producing combined hyperextension, ulnar deviation, and intercarpal supination. These excessive forces occur during vaulting, floor exercise, and pommel horse routines. Divers who enter the water with the hands in extension, as well as skaters and wrestlers who fall on an extended hand, are also prone to this injury.

Signs and Symptoms

Assessment reveals point tenderness on the dorsum of the radiocarpal joint. A high degree of palpable pain between the distal radius and the scaphoid and lunate increases with active or passive extension. Varus, valgus, and Watson tests, as well as specific joint play tests, may be positive depending on the structure damaged.

Management

Immediate treatment involves immobilization, application of ice to reduce swelling and inflammation, and immediate referral to a physician to rule out a fracture or carpal dislocation. Subsequent management includes decreasing intensity of training; cryotherapy before and after physical activity; nonsteroidal anti-inflammatory drugs (NSAIDs); and use of an appropriate bandage, taping technique, or splint to prevent excessive hyperextension. As pain decreases, ROM exercises as well as wrist- and hand-strengthening exercises can be initiated (see **Application Strategy 18.1**).

Gamekeeper's Thumb

Etiology

Gamekeeper's thumb, an outdated term, is commonly used for the more appropriate medical term: ulnar collateral ligament sprain of the first MC joint. The thumb is exposed to more force than the fingers by virtue of its position on the hand. Integrity of the ulnar collateral ligament at the MP joint is critical for normal hand function, because it stabilizes the joint as the thumb is pushed against the index and middle finger while performing many pinching, grasping, and gripping motions. This injury is commonly seen in football, baseball/softball, and hockey as well as in skiing when the individual falls on the ski pole (skier's thumb). Tearing of the ulnar collateral ligament at the MP joint occurs when the MP joint is near full extension and the thumb is forcefully abducted away from the hand.

Signs and Symptoms

The palmar aspect of the joint is painful, swollen, and may have visible bruising with increased pain or weakness with opposition or pinching.[19] Instability is detected by replicating the mechanism of injury or by stressing the thumb in flexion and performing a valgus stress test on the joint. In partial tears, only moderate laxity is present, as is a definite end feel. In more severe cases, a soft end point or greater than a 15° difference in angular laxity compared to the uninjured thumb indicates total rupture of the ulnar collateral ligament. Bilateral comparison (as well as assessment of laxity at other major joints) helps to determine normal joint laxity for the individual.

Management

Initial treatment includes ice, compression, elevation, and referral to a physician. Many physicians will recommend X-ray evaluation prior to physical examination in order to rule out avulsion fractures, which can be displaced and unstable.[18] If no instability is present, early mobilization accompanied by cryotherapy, contrast baths, ultrasound, and NSAIDs is recommended. Strapping or taping the thumb can prevent reinjury. If joint instability is present, a thumb spica cast should be applied for 4 to 6 weeks, followed by further taping for another 3 to 6 weeks during risk activities. Severe cases require surgical repair.

Interphalangeal Collateral Ligament Sprains

Etiology

Excessive varus/valgus stress and hyperextension can damage the collateral ligaments of the fingers. Ligament failure usually occurs at its attachment to the proximal phalanx or, less frequently, in the midportion. Hyperextension of the proximal phalanx can stretch or rupture the volar plate on the palmar side of the joint (**Fig. 19.21**).

Signs and Symptoms

Even with first-degree sprains, the patient will experience stiffness, pain, and limited ROM. The patient may report presence of pain in the entire joint, and tenderness may be elicited over the injured structure when palpated. Depending on which ligament

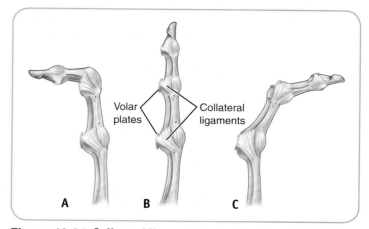

Figure 19.21. Collateral ligaments and volar plate of the fingers can be damaged in hyperextension injuries. A, Flexion. **B,** Extension. **C,** Hyperextension.

is damaged, the varus or valgus stress test may be positive. An obvious deformity may not be present unless there is a fracture or total rupture of the supporting tissues, causing a dorsal dislocation. Because rapid swelling makes assessment difficult, the clinician may utilize a tap or compression test to help assess for presence of fracture. However, a radiograph is needed to rule out an associated dislocation or fracture.

Management

Following standard acute care, a mild sprain can be treated by taping the injured finger to an adjacent finger (e.g., buddy taping). This provides some support and mobility, but such taping should not be used on an acutely swollen, painful finger because of possible constriction to the vascular flow. If more support is needed, the involved joint can be splinted in extension with a molded polypropylene splint to avoid flexion contractures.

Dislocations

Similar to many other wrist and hand injuries, dislocations often are caused by a fall on the outstretched hand or by traumatic hyperflexion, hyperextension, or rotary movement.

Distal Radioulnar Joint Injury

■ Etiology

An acute dislocation and subluxation of the distal radioulnar joint (DRUJ) can be an isolated injury or may occur in conjunction with a fracture of the radius. The mechanism of injury almost always involves hyperextension of the wrist. If an ulnar dorsal dislocation of the joint occurs, hyperpronation also is present, whereas an ulnar volar dislocation occurs in conjunction with hypersupination. Because the TFCC functions as a sling to support the ulnar border of the wrist and connects the distal ulna to the ulnar side of the radius, dislocation of the DRUJ can result in damage to some portion of this complex or its attachments.[19]

■ Signs and Symptoms

The clinical appearance of a DRUJ dislocation can vary significantly, depending on the presence or absence of an associated fracture. Generally speaking, the joint is deformed, swollen, and very painful. Swelling may be so extensive that it obscures the prominence of the ulnar head. In a dorsal dislocation, the ulnar head is more prominent dorsally. In volar dislocations, the wrist typically appears to be narrow as a result of an overlap of the distal parts of the radius and ulna. If soft-tissue swelling is not excessive, a depression may be noted near the sigmoid notch of the radius, where the ulnar head normally is located. Flexion and extension of the elbow are normal unless there is an associated fracture, but pronation and supination of the forearm are limited.[20]

■ Management

Immediate action involves immobilization of the limb in a vacuum splint and immediate transportation of the individual to a physician. The prognosis and rehabilitation program depends on the extent of tissue damage and instability. Simple DRUJ dislocations may be stabilized after the internal fixation of associated fractures and immobilized in an above-the-elbow cast. ROM exercises should be started 6 weeks after fixation.

Triangular Fibrocartilage Complex Tear

The DRUJ derives a significant amount of stability from the TFCC and the joint capsule. Therefore, the same mechanism of injury that may result in DRUJ instability may also result in TFCC tear. The TFCC is composed of five structures: (1) the articular disk, which an elongated triangular structure is resting between the ulnar/radius and lunate and triquetrum; (2) the deep and superficial layers of the subcruentum ligament; and (3) the two disk–carpal ligaments (**Fig. 19.22**). Patients with a history of falling on an outstretched hand, swinging a bat or racquet, or violently twisting their wrist and complain of wrist pain should be evaluated for the presence of TFCC injury.

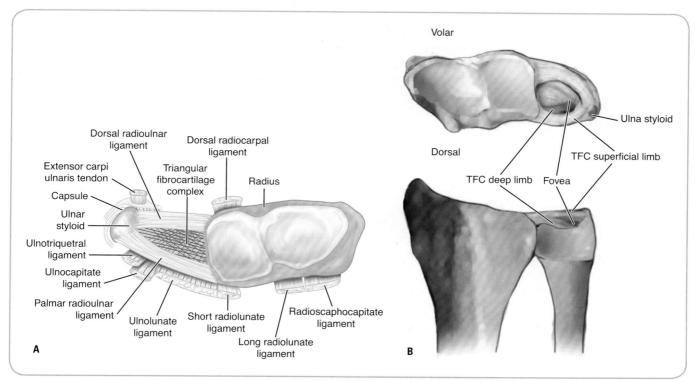

Figure 19.22. Triangular fibrocartilage complex. A, The soft-tissue structures encompassing the TFCC of the wrist stabilize the radioulnocarpal unit. The TFC proper originates from the radius medially and attaches to the base of the ulnar styloid. Fibers originating from the subsheath of the extensor carpi ulnaris dorsally cross path with fibers originating from the ulnocarpal ligaments volarly and blend with the TFC proper. **B, Distal radioulnar joint ligaments.** (The disk component of the TFCC has been removed to show the deep limbs of the radioulnar ligaments.) The volar and dorsal radioulnar ligaments are the major soft-tissue stabilizers of the DRUJ and insert onto the base of the ulnar styloid.

■ Signs and Symptoms

The patient may present with pain on the ulnar aspect of the wrist over the TFCC. Tenderness is elicited when palpating the area and may increase if palpation is performed in conjunction with passive ulnar deviation.[16] History may also reveal decreased functional use of the hand in activities such as turning doorknobs, pushing open doors, and sports-specific skills involving wrist motion. Mild swelling may be seen or palpated.

■ Management

TFCC tears may take up to 12 weeks to fully repair. Management ranges from rest and ice and anti-inflammatory medication for pain to immobilization, steroid injections, and surgical repair.[20] Therefore, it is imperative if a TFCC tear is suspected, that the patient be referred to an orthopedic physician for imaging and further evaluation.

Perilunate and Lunate Dislocation

■ Etiology

Because of the shape of the lunate and its position between the large capitate and lower end of the radius, it is particularly prone to dislocation during axial loading that causes displacement in a volar direction (**Fig. 19.23**). As force initially impacts the carpals,

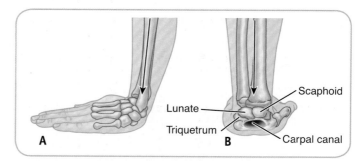

Figure 19.23. Lunate dislocation. A, The lunate can dislocate during a fall on an outstretched hand when the load from the radius compresses the lunate in a volar direction. **B,** If the bone moves into the carpal tunnel, the median nerve can become compressed, leading to sensory changes in the first and second fingers.

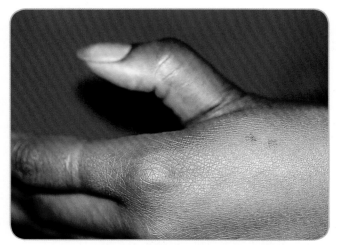

Figure 19.24. Metacarpophalangeal dislocation. The volar plates protect the anterior joint capsules of the fingers. During hyperextension, the anterior capsule and supporting ligaments can rupture, dislocating the phalanx. The resulting deformity signals a serious dislocation.

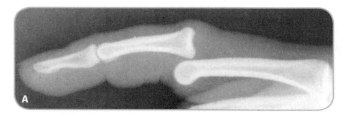

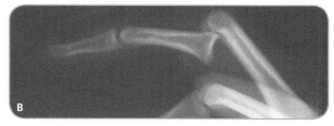

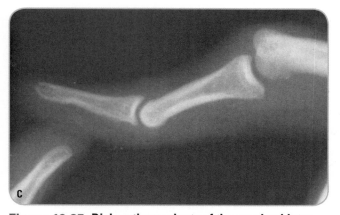

Figure 19.25. Dislocation variants of the proximal interphalangeal joint. The most common are dorsal (**A**), followed by pure volar with a central slip rupture (**B**). The least common is rotatory subluxation (**C**).

the distal row is displaced away from the lunate, resulting in the lunate resting dorsally relative to the other carpals (i.e., **perilunate dislocation**). If the force continues to extend the wrist, the dorsal ligaments rupture, relocating the carpals and rotating the lunate. The lunate then rests in a volar position relative to the other carpals (i.e., **lunate dislocation**).

■ Signs and Symptoms

The dorsum of the hand is point tender, and a thickened area on the palm can be palpated just distal to the end of the radius (proximal to the third metacarpal) if not obscured by swelling. Passive and active motion may not be painful. If the bone moves into the carpal tunnel, compression of the median nerve leads to pain, numbness, and tingling in the first and second fingers. In chronic conditions or conditions that go undiagnosed, performing the Watson test for scapholunate instability is indicated.

■ Management

Immediate action involves immobilization of the wrist in a vacuum splint and immediate transportation of the individual to a physician. Following reduction, the wrist is immobilized in moderate flexion with a silicone cast for 3 to 4 weeks. The wrist is then placed into a neutral position and protected from any wrist extension, particularly during sport participation. This condition often is overlooked until complications, such as flexor tendon contractures and median nerve palsies, arise from chronic dislocations. Repeated trauma to the lunate can lead to vascular compromise, resulting in degeneration or osteochondritis of the lunate (**Kienböck disease**). Kienböck disease should be considered if the patient presents with a painful and swollen wrist, complaining of joint stiffness and decreased ROM, decreased grip strength, and difficulty supinating.

Dislocation of the Metacarpals and Phalanges

■ Etiology

MP joint dislocations are rare but readily recognizable as a serious injury. Hyperextension or a shearing force causes the anterior capsule to tear, allowing the proximal phalanx to move backward over the metacarpal and stand at a 90° angle to the metacarpal (**Fig. 19.24**).

The most common dislocation in the body occurs at the PIP joint (**Fig. 19.25**). Because digital nerves and vessels run along the sides of the fingers and thumb, these dislocations are potentially serious. The usual mechanism of injury is hyperextension and axial compression, such as when a ball hits the end of the finger and forces it into hyperextension.

DIP dislocations usually occur dorsally and may be associated with an open wound. These individuals often reduce the injury on their own. As with MP joint dislocations, injuries to the collateral ligaments at the PIP and DIP joints can involve ruptures of the volar plate.

■ Signs and Symptoms

A swollen, painful finger is the most frequent initial complaint. Pain is present at the joint line and increases when the mechanism of injury is reproduced. With an MP dislocation, the proximal phalanx may stand at a 90° angle to the metacarpal. When the stability of an injured collateral ligament of the PIP joint exceeds 20° or has no end point on manual stress, it is considered to be a complete rupture.[21] Because of the probability of entrapping the volar plate in an IP joint, which can lead to permanent dysfunction of the finger, no attempt should be made by an untrained individual to reduce a finger dislocation.

■ Management

Immediate treatment for all dislocations involves immobilization in a wrist or finger splint, application of ice to reduce swelling and inflammation, and immediate referral to a physician for reduction of the dislocation.

If the MP joint is stable, protection with buddy taping for 2 to 3 weeks usually is sufficient. Early active ROM exercises are encouraged. In an uncomplicated dislocation of the PIP joint, the finger may be splinted in approximately 30° of flexion, with active motion being started at 10 to 14 days. Volar-displaced PIP dislocations with suspected central slip injury should have the PIP joint splinted in complete extension for 6 full weeks. During this time, active exercises of the DIP joint are imperative to maintain muscle integrity and strength of the flexor digitorum profundus and extensor mechanism. If inadequately managed, however, dislocations at the PIP joint can result in a painful, stiff finger with a fixed flexion deformity called a **coach's finger**. If the volar plate is trapped in the joint, the deformity may result in the PIP joint being held in flexion and the DIP joint in hyperextension (a pseudo-boutonnière deformity). Immobilization for a DIP joint dislocation involves splinting the DIP joint with a volar splint for approximately 3 weeks. The PIP joint can be left free so that motion can continue at this joint. Protective splinting is continued for at least 3 weeks until the finger is pain-free.

The signs and symptoms that would suggest that the gymnast has sustained a wrist sprain include excessive forces producing a hyperextension mechanism; point tenderness on the dorsum of the radiocarpal joint; point tenderness between the distal radius, scaphoid, and lunate; and pain that increases with active or passive extension.

STRAINS

While holding an opponent's jersey tightly, a basketball player felt a sharp pain in the distal phalanx of the ring finger. After releasing the jersey, the player was unable to flex the DIP joint of the ring finger. What injury should be suspected?

Muscular strains occur as a result of excessive overload against resistance or stretching the tendon beyond its normal range. In mild or moderate strains, pain and restricted motion may not be a major factor. In many injuries, muscular strains occur simultaneously with a joint sprain. The joint sprain takes precedence in priority of care, especially with an associated dislocation; as a result, tendon damage may go unrecognized and untreated.

Jersey Finger (Profundus Tendon Rupture)
Etiology

This injury typically occurs when an individual grips an opponent's jersey while the opponent simultaneously twists and turns to get away. This jerking motion may force the individual's fingers to rapidly extend, rupturing the flexor digitorum profundus tendon from its attachment on the distal phalanx. The ring finger is most commonly involved, because this finger assumes a position of slight extension relative to the other fingers, which are more flexed during the grip.

Signs and Symptoms

The individual will complain of pain and swelling at the DIP joint and report a popping sensation at the time of injury. Flexor tendon disruption is indicated by one finger lying in complete extension while others are in slight (10°) flexion at the IP joints.[18] If avulsed, the tendon can be palpated at the proximal aspect of the involved finger; it typically has a hematoma formation along the entire flexor tendon sheath and may compromise the palmar digital artery blood supply. If a portion of bone is avulsed, it may become trapped distal to the A4 pulley over the middle phalanx or distal to the A2 pulley, or it may retract all the way into the palm. Because of the avulsion, the individual is unable to flex the DIP joint against resistance.

Management

Following standard acute care, the individual should be referred to a physician. For cases in which the tendon has retracted into the palm, surgical reattachment of the tendon must be performed within 7 to 10 days (before permanent contracture occurs). Typical return to play is 6 to 12 weeks after surgery.[19]

Mallet Finger

Etiology

Mallet finger, or baseball finger, occurs when an object hits the end of the finger while the extensor tendon is taut, such as when catching a ball. The resulting forceful flexion can avulse the lateral bands of the extensor mechanism from their distal attachment, or the tendon may remain attached to an avulsed piece of bone or fracture fragment, leaving a characteristic mallet deformity (**Fig. 19.26**).

Signs and Symptoms

Unlike the jersey finger, in which the flexor tendon retracts into the proximal aspect of the finger, isolated rupture of the extensor tendon usually does not retract. Examination reveals pain, swelling, and a variable lack of active extension at the DIP joint. Dorsal bone avulsion fractures typically signify a grade III rupture of the extensor tendon. If untreated, complete tears lead to permanent DIP extensor lag.

Management

Following standard acute care, the individual should be referred to a physician for further treatment, which may involve splinting the DIP joint in complete extension for 6 to 8 weeks, with an additional 6 to 8 weeks of splinting during sport participation. Motion at the PIP and MP joints, however, is highly encouraged. Soft-tissue irritation or ulceration on the dorsum of the DIP may occur secondary to splinting; this can be avoided by keeping the splint dry and alternating its position between the dorsal and palmar aspects of the finger. Extreme hyperextension of the distal phalanx also may impair vascular supply to the tip of the finger, leading to further skin damage. If large fracture fragments are present, surgical repair may be necessary.

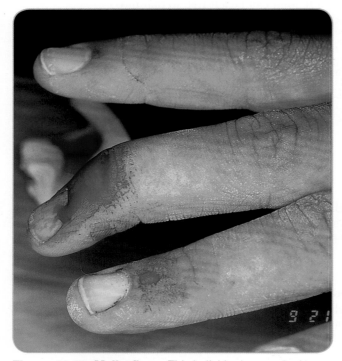

Figure 19.26. Mallet finger. This individual was asked to straighten the middle finger but was unable to extend the DIP joint, suggesting that the extensor tendon is avulsed from the attachment on the distal phalanx. The tendon also may avulse a small piece of bone, leading to an avulsion fracture.

Boutonnière Deformity

Etiology

A boutonnière deformity is caused by blunt trauma to the dorsal aspect of the PIP joint or by rapid, forceful flexion of the joint against resistance. The central slip of the extensor tendon ruptures at the middle phalanx, leaving no active extensor mechanism intact over the PIP joint. An injury to the volar plate also can lead to a flexion deformity of the PIP joint that resembles a boutonnière deformity; however, the central slip of the extensor tendon is not involved. This condition is called a **pseudo-boutonnière deformity**.

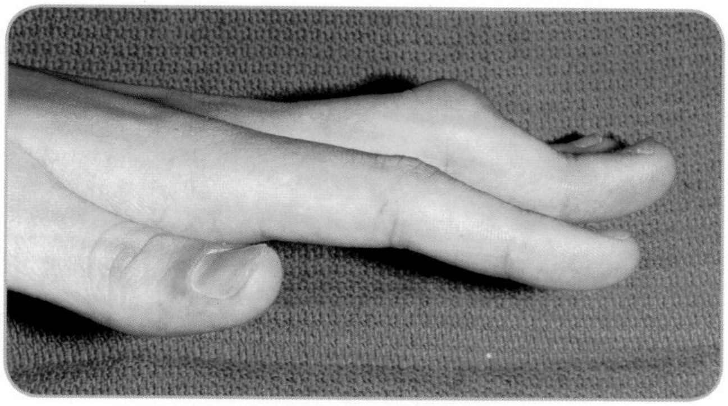

Figure 19.27. Boutonnière deformity. In a boutonnière deformity, the proximal joint flexes while the distal joint hyperextends.

Signs and Symptoms

The deformity is not usually present immediately; rather, it develops over 2 to 3 weeks, as the lateral slips move in a palmar direction and cause hyperextension at the MP joint, flexion at the PIP joint, and hyperextension at the DIP joint (**Fig. 19.27**). Because the head of the proximal phalanx protrudes through the split in the extensor hood, this condition sometimes is referred to as a "buttonhole rupture." The PIP joint is swollen and lacks full extension.

Management

Any injury that limits PIP extension to 30° or less and produces dorsal tenderness over the base of the middle phalanx should be treated as an acute tendon rupture and immediately referred to a physician. Initial treatment involves splinting the PIP joint in complete extension for 5 to 6 weeks. To avoid the development of adhesions, the DIP joint should not be immobilized.

Tendinopathies

Individuals who are involved in strenuous and repetitive training often inflame tendons and tendon sheaths in the wrist and hand. Injuries can be acute or chronic in nature, but tendons are most at risk for injury when tension is rapidly applied at an oblique angle. Tendons that are already under tension and muscles that are maximally innervated or stretched are risk factors for rupture. Overuse can lead to derangement of both the mechanical and physiological components of the normal tendon. This condition is referred to clinically as tendinitis. In comparison, when the tendon sheath is inflamed as a result of trauma, overuse, or infection, it is called **tenosynovitis** (Fig. 19.28).

Trigger Finger

Etiology

Snapping flexor tendons, or trigger finger, may be present in individuals who have multiple, severe traumas to the palmar aspect of the hand or in individuals who perform repeated movement and clenching of the fingers. It most commonly occurs in the middle or ring finger but may occur in the thumb and other fingers. Repeated trauma and inflammation lead to a thickening of the tendon sheath as it passes over the proximal phalanx. A nodule can form and grow within the thickened, synovium-lined tendon sheath that eventually prevents the tendon from sliding within the annular ligaments of the finger. The finger becomes locked in flexion when the nodule becomes too thick, or the sheath too constricted, to allow the finger to be actively reextended (**Fig. 19.29**).

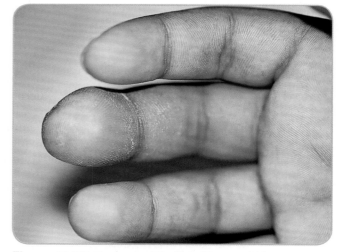

Figure 19.28. Tenosynovitis. This 13-year-old boy complained of pain in the finger for 3 days after a paronychia had been drained. Note the swelling and erythema of the distal phalanx.

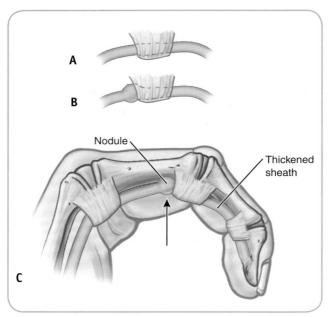

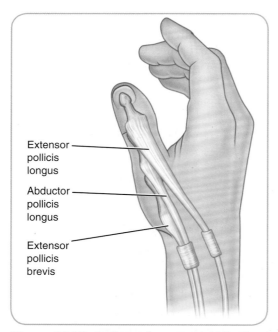

Figure 19.29. Trigger finger. A, Under normal conditions, the flexor tendons slide within the synovial sheaths under the annular ligaments at the proximal and middle phalanx. **B,** Repeated trauma can cause a nodule to form in the tendon sheath, or the sheath may become thickened. **C,** Flexion occurs, and the finger becomes locked in flexion when the nodule becomes too thick or the sheath too constricted. The finger is then unable to reextend.

Figure 19.30. de Quervain tenosynovitis. The APL and EPB share the same synovial sheath. Excessive friction among the tendons, sheath, and bony process leads to tenosynovitis of the tendons.

Signs and Symptoms

Initially, the pain may present as an aching sensation in the joint and gradually, specific areas of point tenderness may be found. As the condition progresses, a locking action usually occurs when the individual first wakes from sleep. A painful popping sensation often is perceived when the flexed PIP joint is passively returned to extension. Additional palpable crepitus may indicate an underlying systemic disease (e.g., systemic sclerosis, rheumatoid arthritis, or granulomatous infection).

Management

Treatment includes NSAIDs, resting the finger, splinting when necessary, and possible cortisone injections into the sheath. For those individuals who do not respond to a steroid injection or who prefer quick, more definitive relief, an incision proximal to the palpable nodule may be necessary to cut the annular ligament and allow the tendon to slide freely.[22]

de Quervain Tenosynovitis

Etiology

Individuals who must use a forceful grasp, combined with repetitive use of the thumb and ulnar deviation, are particularly at risk for de Quervain tenosynovitis. Sports such as tennis, golf, fly fishing, and javelin and discus throwing place a high demand on the APL and EPB. These two tendons share a single synovial tendon sheath that travels through a bony groove over the radiostyloid process and then turns sharply (as much as 105°) to enter the thumb when the wrist is in radial deviation. Tenosynovitis results from friction among the tendons, stenosing sheath, and bony process (**Fig. 19.30**). The tendons slide within the sheath not only during movements of the thumb but also during movements of the wrist with the thumb fixed, as in bowling and throwing.

Signs and Symptoms

The individual complains of pain over the radial styloid process that increases with thumb and wrist motion. Palpation reveals point tenderness over the tendons, either at or just proximal to the radial styloid, and occasionally crepitation. Movements of the thumb are painful, and snapping of the tendons may be present with some activities. Pain is reproduced in two ways: (1) by abducting the thumb against resistance and (2) by flexing the thumb and cupping it under the fingers and then flexing the wrist in ulnar deviation to stretch the thumb tendons (**Fig. 19.14**). Swelling may be present in the first dorsal compartment.

Management

Treatment is conservative with ice, rest, and NSAIDs. If symptoms are not relieved, steroid injections, immobilization with a thumb spica for 3 weeks, or both may be indicated. In severe cases, surgical decompression may be necessary.

Intersection Syndrome

Etiology

Intersection syndrome is a tendinitis or friction tendinitis in the first and second dorsal compartments. It has been described in rowers, indoor racquet players, canoeists, and weight lifters who overuse the radial extensors of the wrist by excessive curling.[23] The muscle and tendons of these two compartments traverse each other at a 60° angle at a site approximately two to three fingerbreadths proximal to the wrist joint on the dorsal aspect (i.e., 4 to 6 cm proximal to Lister tubercle). The condition also has been described as a stenosing tenosynovitis of the sheath of the second compartment (i.e., the radial extensors) at the area where it traverses the muscle bellies of the first compartment (i.e., APL and EPB).

Signs and Symptoms

Examination reveals point tenderness on the dorsum of the forearm, two to three fingerbreadths proximal to the wrist joint. Crepitation or squeaking is noted with passive or active motion. Visible swelling is present along the course of the affected tendons.

Management

Treatment consists of ice massage, rest, NSAIDs, splinting, and avoidance of exacerbating activities. A corticosteroid injection may be necessary to relieve acute symptoms. Rehabilitation should consist of ROM exercises and wrist extensor strengthening. A tenosynovectomy and a fasciotomy of the APL muscle may be necessary if conservative treatment is not effective.

Dupuytren Contracture

Etiology

For unknown reasons, nodules can develop in the palmar aponeurosis. These nodules limit finger extension and, eventually, cause a flexion deformity. The condition, known as Dupuytren contracture, is rare but can impact normal function of the fingers.

Signs and Symptoms

A fixed flexion deformity is visible, occurring more frequently on the ring or little finger. The finger cannot be extended.

Management

Because normal finger function cannot occur with the flexion deformity, the nodule causing the contracture must be surgically removed.

Ganglion Cysts

Etiology

Ganglion cysts are benign tumor masses typically seen on the dorsal aspect of the wrist, although they may occur on the volar aspect.

Signs and Symptoms

Associated with tissue sheath degeneration, the cyst itself contains a jellylike, colorless fluid of mucin and is freely mobile and palpable. Occurring spontaneously, cysts seldom cause any pain or loss of motion. Discomfort from the pressure may occur as the ganglion increases in size.

Management

Treatment is symptomatic: Aspiration, injection, and rupture of the cyst have not proved to be successful, because the condition may recur. Surgical excision remains the treatment of choice.

The mechanism of injury and the symptoms suggest that the basketball player has sustained a rupture of the profundus tendon (i.e., jersey finger). Avulsion of the tendon from the distal phalanx results in an inability to flex the DIP.

FINGERTIP INJURIES

A high school cheerleader has a mild case of paronychia. Are antibiotics required in the management of this condition?

Direct trauma to the nail bed, such as that caused when the finger is impacted by a ball, jammed into an object, or crushed when stepped on, can lead to a subungual hematoma. Infections also can occur in the nail fold, leading to a condition called paronychia.

Subungual Hematomas

Etiology

Direct trauma to the nail bed can result in blood forming under the fingernail, which is called a subungual hematoma.

Signs and Symptoms

Increasing pressure under the nail bed due to hemorrhage can lead to throbbing pain.

Management

After ruling out an underlying fracture, the finger should be soaked in ice water for 10 to 15 minutes to numb the area and reduce the bleeding under the nail bed. If the pain diminishes, it may not be necessary to drain the hematoma. This is preferable, because draining the hematoma opens an avenue for infection. If discomfort interferes with the ability to perform physical activities, however, the hematoma should be drained under the direction of a physician. This is performed by cutting a hole through the nail with a rotary drill or a no. 11 surgical blade or by melting a hole through the nail with the end of a paper clip heated to a bright red color (**Fig. 19.31**). **Application Strategy 19.1** explains the proper care for a subungual hematoma. After the blood has been drained, the area must be checked daily for signs of infection; if signs of infection are present, immediate referral to a physician is warranted.

Paronychia

Etiology

Paronychia is an infection along the nail fold. It commonly is seen with a hangnail and in individuals whose hands are frequently immersed in water.

Signs and Symptoms

The nail fold becomes red, swollen, and painful, and it can produce purulent drainage (**Fig. 19.32**).

Management

The condition is treated with warm-water soaks and germicide. In more severe cases, the physician may recommend systemic antibiotics and drainage of localized pus or may perform a partial nail resection.

Treatment of the cheerleader's paronychia should include warm-water soaks and germicide. An antibiotic is necessary only in severe cases.

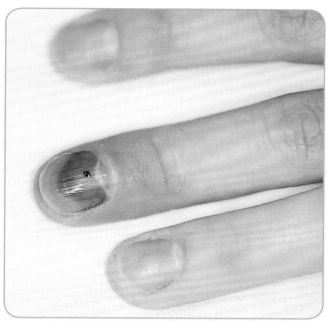

Figure 19.31. Subungual hematoma. Note the hole that was made to drain the excess blood and relieve pain.

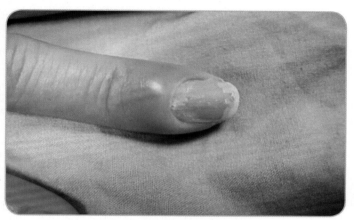

Figure 19.32. Paronychia of the right middle finger. The infection is clearly localized to the dorsal surface, although the pulp is slightly swollen because of edema.

APPLICATION STRATEGY 19.1

Management Algorithm for Subungual Hematoma[a]

To numb the area and reduce hemorrhage, do the following:

1. Soak the finger in ice water for 10–15 minutes.
2. Clean the hands thoroughly with antiseptic soap and water and apply latex gloves.
3. Cleanse the finger thoroughly with either of the following:
   - Antiseptic soap
   - An antibacterial solution
4. Make a hole through the nail. Do either of the following:
   Cut the hole, using
   - A sterile, no. 11 surgical blade or
   - A rotary drill, cleaned and disinfected with iodine solution, or
   Melt the hole with the end of a paper clip heated to bright red.
5. Have the patient exert mild pressure on the distal pulp of the finger to drive excess blood through the hole.
6. Watch carefully for signs of shock and treat accordingly by doing the following:
   - Placing the patient in a supine position
   - Elevating the feet above the level of the heart
7. Soak the finger in an iodine solution for 10 minutes.
8. Cover the phalanx with a sterile dressing and apply a protective splint.

Follow up:

1. Do not apply heat for 48 hours.
2. Check the finger daily for signs of infection; if any appear, immediately refer the patient to a physician.

[a]Because of the nature of opening a wound and the potential for subsequent infection, this procedure should be discussed with the supervising physician and documented as a standing order.

NERVE ENTRAPMENT SYNDROMES

 An ice hockey goalie complains of numbness in the little finger. He is unable to grasp a piece of paper between the thumb and index finger and has a weakness in grip strength. Inspection reveals atrophy of the hypothenar mass. What condition should be suspected, and how should this condition be managed?

Nerve entrapment syndromes, or compressive neuropathies, can be subtle and often are overlooked. They occur in activities such as bowling, cycling, karate, rowing, baseball/softball, field hockey, lacrosse, rugby, weight lifting, handball, and wheelchair athletics. Mechanisms of injuries most commonly involve repetitive compression, contusion, or traction. A compressive neuropathy also may be caused by anatomical structures such as anomalous muscles or vessels, fibrous bands, osteofibrous tunnels, or muscle hypertrophy. Pathological structures, such as ganglia, lipomas, osteophytes, aneurysms, and localized inflammation, also can compress a nerve. This discussion of compressive neuropathies is limited to those found in the distal forearm, wrist, and hand (**Box 19.1**).

Median Nerve Entrapment

The median nerve lies medial to the brachial artery in the cubital fossa and passes distally between the two heads of the pronator teres. The nerve divides at the distal margin to form the anterior interosseous nerve to supply the flexor pollicis longus, flexor digitorum superficialis to the index and middle digits, and pronator quadratus. The main trunk of the median nerve continues distally beneath the fibrous arch of the flexor digitorum superficialis. The palmar cutaneous branch supplies sensation to the volar wrist, thenar eminence, and palm. The median nerve continues through the carpal tunnel beneath the flexor retinaculum to supply sensation to the palm and the radial three and one-half digits. The deep motor branch supplies the abductor pollicis brevis, opponens pollicis, superficial head of the flexor pollicis brevis, and two lateral lumbricales.

Anterior Interosseous Nerve Syndrome

■ Etiology

Seen sporadically, anterior interosseous nerve syndrome can occur after a set of strenuous or repetitive elbow motion exercises. Structurally, there may be compression of the nerve by fibrous bands from the deep head of the pronator teres or flexor digitorum superficialis, affecting any or all of the muscles innervated by the nerve. Because the nerve has no sensory cutaneous portion, however, no sensory changes occur.

■ Signs and Symptoms

The individual presents in one of two ways:

1. **Acute onset:** The individual suddenly loses use of the flexor pollicis longus and index finger profundus tendons.

2. **Slow, insidious onset:** Gradual weakening of these muscles becomes apparent, with weakness during heavy activity.

BOX 19.1 Nerve Entrapment Syndromes

Median Nerve
- Anterior interosseous syndrome
- Carpal tunnel syndrome

Ulnar Nerve
- Ulnar tunnel syndrome
- Cyclist's palsy
- Bowler's thumb

Radial Nerve
- Distal posterior interosseous nerve syndrome
- Superficial radial nerve entrapment

Examination reveals weakness or loss of flexion of the IP joint of the thumb and DIP joint of the index finger. The individual characteristically is unable to make a circle with the index finger and thumb (i.e., pinch grip test).

■ Management

Initial treatment involves splinting the extremity and avoiding heavy activity. If no return of function is noted after 6 months, surgical intervention and decompression of the nerve may be necessary.

Carpal Tunnel Syndrome

■ Etiology

The floor of the carpal tunnel is formed by the volar wrist capsule, with the roof formed by the transverse retinacular ligament traveling from the hook of the hamate and pisiform on the lateral side to the volar tubercle of the trapezium and tuberosity of the scaphoid on the medial side. This unyielding tunnel accommodates the median nerve, finger flexors in a common sheath, and flexor pollicis longus in an independent sheath (**Fig. 19.33**). Any irritation of the synovial sheath covering these tendons can produce swelling or edema that puts pressure on the median nerve.

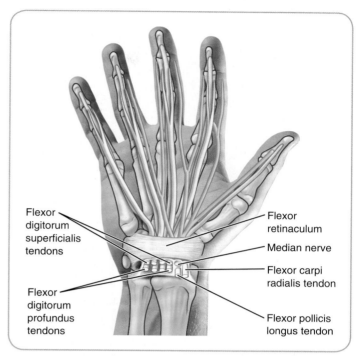

Figure 19.33. Carpal tunnel. The flexor tendons of the fingers pass through the carpal tunnel in a single synovial sheath.

Carpal tunnel syndrome (CTS) is the most common compression syndrome of the wrist and hand, although it is not commonly seen in the physically active population. Movement of tendons and nerves during prolonged, repetitive hand movements may contribute to the development of CTS.[24] In addition, CTS may be caused by direct trauma or anatomical anomalies. It typically is seen in the dominant extremity. Sporting activities that predispose an individual to CTS include those that involve repetitive or continuous flexion and extension of the wrist, such as cycling, throwing sports, racquet sports, archery, and gymnastics. Etiologies for CTS other than traumatic causes include infectious origins (e.g., diphtheria, mumps, influenza, pneumonia, meningitis, malaria, syphilis, typhoid, dysentery, tuberculosis, and gonococcus) and metabolic causes (e.g., hypothyroidism, diabetes, rheumatoid arthritis, gout, vitamin deficiency, heavy metal poisoning, and carbon monoxide poisoning).[25]

■ Signs and Symptoms

A common sign is pain that awakens the individual in the middle of the night but that often is relieved by "shaking out the hands" (known as a positive "flick"). Pain, numbness, tingling, or a burning sensation may be felt only in the fingertips on the palmar aspect of the thumb, index, and middle finger. Generally, only one extremity is affected. Grip and pinch strength may be limited. A common complaint is difficulty manipulating coins. Symptoms are reproduced when direct compression is applied over the median nerve in the carpal tunnel for approximately 30 seconds. Although a positive Phalen maneuver is a classic clinical sign of the syndrome, diminished sensitivity to pain and weak thumb abduction are more predictive of abnormal nerve conduction.[26]

■ Management

Individuals with suspected CTS should be referred to a physician for care. Immobilization in slight wrist extension with a dorsal splint is used to rest the wrist for up to 3 to 5 weeks, particularly at night when symptoms occur. Cold, NSAIDs, or, in some situations, diuretics can initially reduce swelling and pain in the area caused by tenosynovitis. Use of a compression wrap should be avoided, however, because this adds additional compression on the already impinged structures. More than half of the individuals with this condition respond well to conservative treatment, although symptoms may

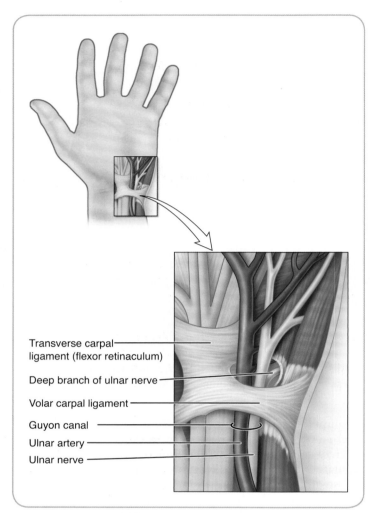

Transverse carpal ligament (flexor retinaculum)

Deep branch of ulnar nerve

Volar carpal ligament

Guyon canal

Ulnar artery

Ulnar nerve

Figure 19.34. Impingement of the ulnar nerve. The ulnar nerve can become impinged in the tunnel of Guyon as it runs under the ligament between the hamate and pisiform.

recur, necessitating a corticosteroid injection into the canal. Long-term benefits from corticosteroid injections, however, may not include symptomatic relief as compared to a properly applied splint.[27] In cases that do not respond well to conservative treatment, surgical decompression or carpal tunnel release can be necessary.

Ulnar Nerve Entrapment

The ulnar nerve passes through the ulnar groove posterior to the medial epicondyle to enter the cubital tunnel formed by the aponeurosis and two heads of the flexor carpi ulnaris. The nerve continues distally between the flexor digitorum profundus dorsally and the flexor carpi ulnaris palmarly. The palmar cutaneous nerve arises in the midforearm to supply the proximal hypothenar eminence. The dorsal cutaneous nerve arises 5 to 8 cm proximal to the ulnar styloid and supplies the dorsum of the ulnar side of the hand. In the wrist, the nerve courses between the hook of the hamate and pisiform and then passes through the Guyon canal to move distally into the fingers (**Fig. 19.34**). The superficial branch supplies the overlying palmaris brevis and then becomes entirely sensory to supply the hypothenar eminence and the ring and small fingers. The deep branch curves around the hook of the hamate to supply the ulnar intrinsics, ending its terminal branch in the first dorsal interossei.

Ulnar Tunnel Syndrome

■ Etiology
Compression of the ulnar nerve may occur as the nerve enters the ulnar tunnel or as the deep branch curves around the hook of the hamate and traverses the palm. This condition frequently is seen in cycling and racquet sports and in baseball/softball catchers, hockey goalies, and handball players who experience repetitive compressive trauma to the palmar aspect of the hand. Distal ulnar nerve palsy also may be seen as push-up palsy, following fractures of the hook of the hamate, or as a result of a missed golf shot or baseball swing.

■ Signs and Symptoms
The lesion may present with motor, sensory, or mixed symptoms. Coincident involvement of the median nerve is common. The individual complains of numbness in the ulnar nerve distribution, particularly in the little finger, and is unable to grasp a piece of paper between the thumb and index finger. Slight weakness in grip strength and atrophy of the hypothenar mass also may be present. Tapping just distal to the pisiform bone produces a tingling sensation that radiates into the little finger and ulnar aspect of the ring finger; although this method is highly sensitive in eliciting a response, it is not very specific.[16]

■ Management
Treatment involves splinting, NSAIDs, and avoidance of any precipitating activity. If symptoms do not disappear within 6 months of conservative treatment, surgical decompression of the Guyon canal may be necessary.

Cyclist's Palsy

■ Etiology

Cyclist's palsy, which also is linked to ulnar nerve entrapment, occurs when a biker leans on the handlebars for an extended period of time.

■ Signs and Symptoms

Swelling in the hypothenar area will be present. Symptoms mimic those of the more serious ulnar nerve entrapment syndrome, but they usually disappear rapidly after completion of the ride.

■ Management

Properly padding the handlebars, wearing padded gloves, varying hand position, and properly fitting the bike to the rider can greatly reduce the incidence of this condition.

Bowler's Thumb

■ Etiology

Bowler's thumb involves compression of the ulnar digital sensory nerve, on the medial aspect of the thumb in the web space, while gripping the ball. Constant pressure on this spot can lead to scarring in the area. The radial digital nerve of the index finger is similarly at risk in racquet sports.

■ Signs and Symptoms

Numbness, tingling, or pain may develop on the medial aspect of the thumb. The individual may have swelling or thickening over the medial palmar aspect at the base of the thumb. Although no true motor involvement is present, grip strength may be decreased secondary to pain. Athletic trainers develop similar symptoms from excessive use of dull scissors or from added pressure on the thumb as one cuts through thick tape jobs or pads.

■ Management

Treatment depends on the stage of injury. Because the predominant cause is inflammatory in nature, treatment is directed at reducing inflammation. Cryotherapy, immobilization with a molded plastic thumb guard, NSAIDs, and, if necessary, a corticosteroid injection usually are successful in relieving symptoms.

Radial Nerve Entrapment

The radial nerve bifurcates near the radiocapitellar joint to become the posterior interosseous and superficial radial nerves. The posterior interosseous nerve travels between the two heads of the supinator, around the proximal radius, and under the forearm extensors to supply the terminal articular branches to the wrist. The superficial radial nerve travels underneath the brachioradialis to become subcutaneous in the distal forearm and supply sensation to the dorsoradial portion of the hand, including the first web space and the proximal phalanges of the first three digits. The most common compressive neuropathy of the radial nerve, which occurs at the radial tunnel, is discussed in Chapter 18.

Distal Posterior Interosseous Nerve Syndrome

■ Etiology

Compression of the distal posterior interosseous nerve occurs as it passes dorsally over the distal radius and enters the wrist capsule. Gymnasts are particularly prone to this injury because of repetitive and forceful wrist dorsiflexion.

■ Signs and Symptoms

The individual usually complains of a deep, dull ache in the wrist that is reproduced with forceful wrist extension or deep palpation of the forearm with the wrist in flexion. Because the condition often can be confused with carpal instability, ganglions, and wrist sprains, the clinician should perform several tests for carpal stability.

■ Management

If the condition does not improve following standard acute care and activity modification, referral to a physician for further treatment is warranted.

Superficial Radial Nerve Entrapment

■ Etiology
The superficial branch of the radial nerve can be compressed at the wrist as it pierces the deep fascia to become subcutaneous between the tendons of the extensor carpi radialis longus and brachioradialis. This constriction is made worse by sports that require repeated pronation and supination, such as batting, throwing, and rowing; by gloves that are strapped too tight; or by the use of tight wristbands.

■ Signs and Symptoms
The individual complains of burning pain, sensory changes, and night pain over the dorsoradial aspect of the wrist, hand, dorsal thumb, and index finger. The absence of pain with wrist motions can rule out a tendinitis-, arthritis-, or impingement-type syndrome.

■ Management
If the condition does not improve following standard acute care and activity modification, referral to a physician is warranted.

 The ice hockey goalie may have ulnar tunnel syndrome. Treatment involves splinting, NSAIDs, and avoidance of any precipitating activity. If symptoms do not disappear within 6 months of conservative treatment, surgical decompression of the Guyon canal may be necessary.

FRACTURES OF THE WRIST AND HAND

? A volleyball player appears to have sustained a boxer's fracture. What is the immediate management of this injury?

Fractures of the distal ulna and radius and of the carpal bones usually are caused by axial loading when an individual falls on an outstretched hand. The majority are simple and nondisplaced. Subsequent to the advent of external orthoses, many fractures can be immobilized adequately to allow individuals to continue with regular sport participation. Specific rules governing special protective equipment, however, require that braces, casts, or any unyielding substances on the elbow, forearm, wrist, or hand be padded on all sides so as not to endanger other players. When the fracture has reached a stage at which external support is no longer necessary during daily activities, it may be advantageous to wear a splint during sport participation.

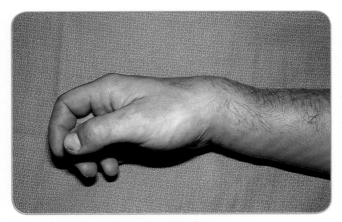

Figure 19.35. Clinical view of a Colles fracture.

Distal Radial and Ulnar Fractures

Etiology

Fractures to the distal radius and ulna present a special problem. In adolescents, epiphyseal and metaphyseal fractures are common. These fractures usually heal without residual disability. In older individuals, one or both bones may be fractured, or one bone may be fractured with the other bone dislocated at the elbow or wrist joint. A **Colles fracture** occurs within 1.5 in of the wrist joint and results in a "dinner-fork" deformity when the distal segment displaces in a dorsal and radial direction (**Fig. 19.35**). A reverse of this fracture is the **Smith fracture**, which tends to move toward the palmar aspect (volar). A **Monteggia fracture** is characterized by a fracture of the proximal third of the ulna accompanied by a dislocation of the radial head. In a **Galeazzi fracture**,

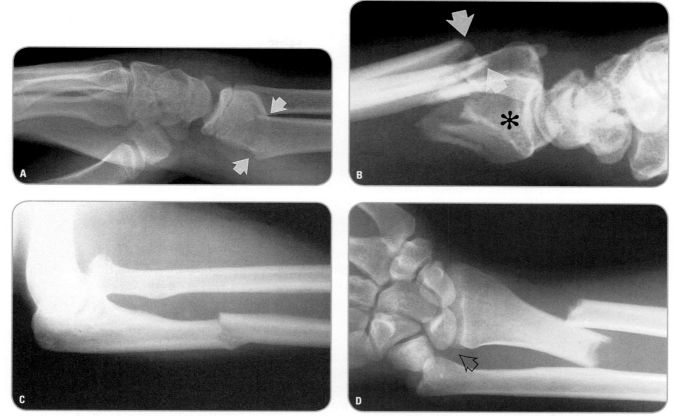

Figure 19.36. Forearm fractures. A, Colles fracture. The extra-articular distal radial fracture is associated with a fracture of the base of the ulnar styloid. **B, Smith fracture.** This type of fracture is characterized by a transverse fracture of the distal radius, with volar and proximal displacement of the distal radial fragment. **C, Monteggia fracture.** This type of fracture is characterized by a fracture of the proximal third of the ulna, accompanied by a dislocation of the radial head. **D, Galeazzi fracture.** The distal radioulnar dislocation is secondary to the marked shortening of the radius caused by the severe ulnar displacement and dorsal angulation of the distal radial fragment.

the distal radioulnar dislocation is secondary to the marked shortening of the radius caused by the severe ulnar displacement and dorsal angulation of the distal radial fragment. **Figure 19.36** demonstrates the four common fractures of the forearm.

Signs and Symptoms

In adolescents, fractures of the growth plate may present with the distal fragment being dorsally displaced. Other signs and symptoms associated with traumatic fractures include intense pain, swelling, deformity, and a false joint. Swelling and hemorrhage may lead to circulatory impairment, or the median nerve may be damaged as it passes through the forearm.

Management

Immediate immobilization in a vacuum splint and a careful neurovascular evaluation of the hand should be followed by immediate referral to a physician. In many instances, open reduction and internal fixation with rigid plates and screws are necessary to restore function.

Stress Fracture of the Distal Radial Epiphyseal Plate (Gymnast's Wrist)

Etiology

The distal radial epiphyseal plate is the classic location for the stress injury commonly called "gymnast's wrist." In contrast to other growth-plate overuse syndromes in adolescents, this fracture is caused by compression. Repetitive performances on the pommel horse and uneven bars cause excessive wrist loading, leading to pain over the dorsum of the wrists. Pain increases as the wrist is carried into maximum dorsiflexion, such as occurs in vaulting, tumbling, and beam work.

Signs and Symptoms

Diffuse tenderness typically is present over the dorsum of the midcarpal area. Pain increases with the extremes of wrist motion. Edema, discoloration, and clinical instability generally are not present. The distal ulnar epiphysis also may be involved.

Management

Treatment involves splinting, NSAIDs, and avoidance of the offending exercises until the individual is asymptomatic. Complete resolution of symptoms may require 3 to 6 months or longer. A dorsal block splint may be beneficial for practice and competition to avoid extremes of wrist extension.

Carpal Fractures

The small bones of the wrist greatly enhance the mobility of the hand. Of the eight bones, only the scaphoid and lunate articulate with the radius; therefore, these two bones transmit the entire force of a fall on an outstretched hand to the forearm.

Scaphoid Fractures

Etiology

Scaphoid fractures account for more than 70% of all carpal bone injuries in the general population and are the most common wrist bone fracture in physically active individuals.[28] Peak incidence is between 12 and 15 years of age.[29] In many cases, the individual falls on the wrist, has normal radiographs, and is discharged with the diagnosis of a wrist sprain and without further care. Several months later, however, the individual continues to experience persistent wrist pain. Radiographs at this time may reveal an established nonunion fracture of the scaphoid (**Fig. 19.37A**). Because of a poor blood supply to the area, aseptic necrosis (death of the tissue) is a common complication with this fracture.

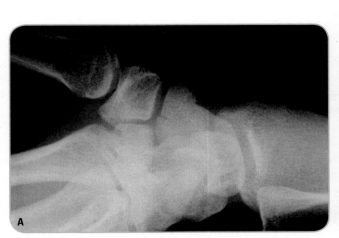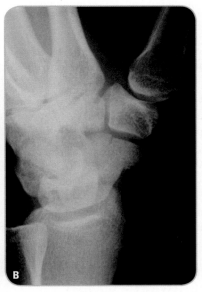

Figure 19.37. Scaphoid fracture. A, Radiograph of a scaphoid fracture. Nonunion fractures occur when the area has a poor blood supply. **B,** The scaphoid forms the floor of the anatomical snuff box. It is bounded by the EPB medially and by the extensor pollicis longus laterally. Increased pain during palpation in this region indicates a possible fracture to the scaphoid bone.

Signs and Symptoms

Assessment reveals a history of falling on an outstretched hand. Pain is present during palpation of the anatomical snuff box (**Fig. 19.37B**), which lies directly over the scaphoid, or with inward pressure along the long axis of the first metacarpal bone. Pain increases during wrist extension and radial deviation.

Management

Treatment involves ice, compression, immobilization in an appropriate splint, and immediate referral to a physician. Nondisplaced scaphoid fractures can be immobilized in a thumb spica cast, with the wrist in slight radial deviation. The cast is changed at 2-week intervals to ensure proper molding around the forearm until union occurs.[29] Follow-up radiographs are obtained at 3- to 4-week intervals to monitor healing and detect signs of delayed union, nonunion, malunion, or avascular necrosis. Some fractures may take several weeks or months to heal; during this time, the individual may participate with a padded, short-arm thumb cast or silicone cast. Displaced scaphoid fractures are secured with internal fixation.

Lunate Fracture/Kienböck Disease

Etiology

Of the carpal bones, the lunate has the largest area, proportionately, of cartilage surface; however, a true lunate fracture is rare in sports. These fractures are difficult to identify and diagnose; therefore, some may be overlooked. Because a large portion of the lunate is cartilage and cancellous bone, the amount of pain associated with a fracture to this area is minimal. Avascular necrosis of the lunate, however, which also is known as **Kienböck disease**, is common if the vascular pathway is disrupted. Its cause has yet to be determined, but it is thought to arise from repetitive trauma or an unrecognized lunate fracture. Kienböck disease should be considered if the patient presents with a painful and swollen wrist, complaining of joint stiffness and decreased ROM, decreased grip strength, and difficulty supinating.

Signs and Symptoms

A history of trauma may or may not be present. The individual usually complains of dorsal wrist pain, swelling, and weakness of the wrist associated with use. If left untreated, Kienböck disease can result in chronic tenderness, pain, and swelling over the lunate as well as in decreased grip strength and weakness during wrist extension. Pain during passive extension of the third finger is a common characteristic with this condition.

Management

Treatment involves ice, compression, immobilization in an appropriate splint, and immediate referral to a physician. Early radiographs are needed to ascertain the correct diagnosis. The preferred treatment is early surgical intervention.

Hamate Fracture

Etiology

Direct impact to the hamate may lead to a nonunion fracture. This typically occurs when an individual strikes a stationary object with a racquet or club in full swing. Once fractured, the ligamentous insertions of the transverse carpal ligament, pisohamate ligament, short flexor, and opponens digiti minimi act to displace the fragment and prevent union.

Signs and Symptoms

Physical examination reveals tenderness over the hypothenar muscle mass. Painful abduction of the small finger against resistance is present, as is decreased grip strength.

Management

Treatment involves ice, compression, immobilization in an appropriate splint, and immediate referral to a physician. Radiographs and tomograms using a carpal tunnel view with the wrist in extension confirm the diagnosis. Care usually is symptomatic, with a protective orthosis worn for 4 to 6 weeks (until tenderness subsides). It may be 2 to 3 months before a racquet or bat will feel comfortable in the hand again.

Triquetrum Fractures

Etiology

Fractures of the triquetrum are fairly common. An avulsion fracture is believed to be caused by sudden wrist flexion or sudden, forceful impingement of the ulnar styloid into the dorsum of the triquetrum. The ulna tends to shear a portion of bone away from the triquetrum. This type of fracture occurs when pressure is put on the wrist during a fall and the wrist is hyperextended and deviated to the ulnar side.

Signs and Symptoms

The individual usually reports a history of acute wrist dorsiflexion injury or direct trauma to the wrist area. Pain in the dorsal wrist is present over the triquetrum.

Management

Treatment involves ice, compression, immobilization in an appropriate splint, and immediate referral to a physician. Immobilization in a short-arm cast with mild extension of the wrist for 4 to 6 weeks is the treatment of choice. Some fractures may become nonunion and require surgical excision.

Metacarpal Fractures

Uncomplicated fractures of the metacarpals result in severe pain, swelling, and deformity. Unique fractures at the base of the first metacarpal may involve a simple intra-articular fracture (i.e., Bennett fracture) or a comminuted fracture (i.e., **Rolando fracture**). A unique fracture involving the neck of the 4th or 5th metacarpal is called a boxer's fracture, and it occurs when an individual punches an object with a closed fist, leading to rotation of the head of the metacarpal over the neck.

Uncomplicated Fractures

■ Etiology

Axial compression on the hand can lead to a fracture dislocation of the proximal end of the metacarpal. This often goes undetected, however, because edema obscures the extent of injury. Fractures of the shaft of the metacarpal are more easily recognized.

■ Signs and Symptoms

Increased pain and a palpable deformity are present in the palm of the hand directly over the involved metacarpal. Gentle percussion and compression along the long axis of the bone increase pain at the fracture site (**Application Strategy 19.2**). These same techniques can be used to detect possible fractures in the carpals and phalanges.

■ Management

Fractures should be immobilized in the position of function, with the palm face down and the fingers slightly flexed. Ice should be applied to reduce hemorrhage and swelling; an elastic compression bandage should not be applied to a swollen hand, because it may lead to increased distal swelling in the fingers. The fingernails must remain uncovered so that circulation can be periodically assessed. The individual should be referred immediately to a physician for further assessment.

Bennett Fracture

■ Etiology

A Bennett fracture is an articular fracture of the proximal end of the first metacarpal and usually is associated with a dislocation. It typically is caused by axial compression, as occurs when a punch is thrown with a closed fist or the individual falls on a closed fist. The pull of the APL tendon at the base of the metacarpal displaces the shaft proximally. A small medial fragment, however, is held in

APPLICATION STRATEGY 19.2

Determining a Possible Fracture to a Metacarpal

1. Palpate for pain along the shaft of the bone.
2. Apply compression along the long axis of the bone. A positive sign occurs if pain is felt at the injury site.
3. Apply percussion or vibration at the end of the bone. A positive sign occurs if pain is felt at the injury site.
4. Apply distraction at the end of the bone. A positive sign occurs if pain is decreased; increased pain may indicate a ligamentous injury.

Head of 2nd metacarpal

Head of 2nd metacarpal

Head of 2nd metacarpal

place by the deep volar ligament, leading to a fracture dislocation (**Fig. 19.38**).

■ Signs and Symptoms

Pain and swelling are localized over the proximal end of the first metacarpal, but deformity may or may not be present. Inward pressure exerted along the long axis of the first metacarpal elicits increased pain at the fracture site.

■ Management

Acute care consists of ice, compression, immobilization in a wrist splint, and immediate referral to a physician. The preferred treatment for this fracture is closed reduction and percutaneous pinning for less than 3 mm of fracture displacement and open reduction and fixation for greater displacements.

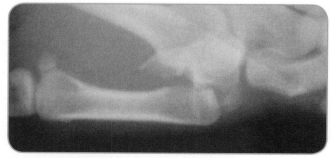

Figure 19.38. Bennett fracture. A Bennett fracture usually is associated with a dislocation of the MP joint of the thumb. An avulsion fracture, however, occurs when a segment of the metacarpal is held in place by the deep volar ligament.

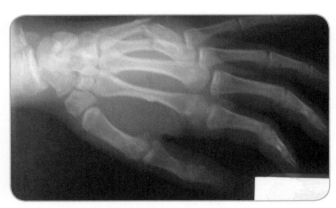

Figure 19.39. Boxer's fracture. These fractures usually involve the 4th and 5th metacarpals.

Rolando Fracture

■ Etiology

Similar to a Bennett fracture, a Rolando fracture involves only an intra-articular fracture of the first metacarpal, with no dislocation. The potential for serious complications is significantly increased, however, because it tends to be more comminuted.

■ Signs and Symptoms

Pain and swelling are localized over the proximal end of the first metacarpal. Deformity is more apparent than with a Bennett fracture. Inward pressure exerted along the long axis of the first metacarpal elicits increased pain at the fracture site.

■ Management

Acute care consists of ice, compression, immobilization in a wrist splint, and immediate referral to a physician. Open reduction and internal fixation with multiple Kirschner wires may be necessary for excellent results. When the fracture is accurately reduced and fixated, complete healing leads to excellent joint ROM; however, because the joint surface was involved in the fracture, arthritic symptoms may eventually develop.

Boxer's Fracture

■ Etiology

Fractures involving the distal metaphysis or neck of the 4th or 5th metacarpals are commonly seen in young males involved in punching activities, hence, the name boxer's fracture (although the fracture rarely occurs in boxers) (**Fig. 19.39**). The fracture typically has an apex dorsal angulation and is inherently unstable secondary to the deforming muscle forces and the frequent volar comminution.

■ Signs and Symptoms

Sudden pain, inability to grip objects, rapid swelling, and possible deformity are present. Palpation reveals tenderness and pain over the fracture site as well as possible crepitus and bony deviation. Delayed ecchymosis is common. Pain increases with axial compression of the involved metacarpal and percussion.

■ Management

Acute care consists of ice, compression, immobilization in a wrist splint, and immediate referral to a physician. Closed reduction is followed by immobilization in a splint for 4 to 6 weeks, followed by early ROM exercises.

Phalangeal Fractures

Etiology

Fractures of the phalanges are very common in sport participation, and these fractures can be difficult to manage. They may be caused by having the fingers stepped on or impinged between two hard objects, such as a football helmet and the ground, or by hyperextension that may lead to a fracture dislocation (**Fig. 19.40**).

Signs and Symptoms

Increased pain is present with circulative compression around the involved phalanx. Gentle percussion and compression along the long axis of the bone increase pain at the fracture site. Particular attention should be given to a possible fracture of the middle and proximal phalanges.

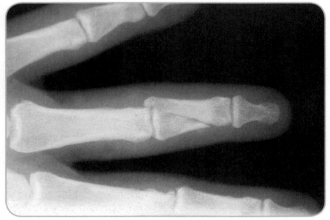

Figure 19.40. Phalangeal fracture. This fracture demonstrates a shearing pattern in the diaphysis.

These fractures tend to have marked deformity because of the strong pull of the flexor and extensor tendons. The four fingers move as a unit. Failure to maintain the longitudinal and rotational alignments of the fingers can lead to long-term disability in grasping or manipulating small objects in the palm of the hand. This deformity often results in one finger overlapping another when a fist is made.

Management

Acute care involves ice to reduce pain and swelling. While the hand is immobilized in a full-wrist splint, gauze pads or a gauze roll are placed under the fingers to produce approximately 30° of finger flexion and reduce the pull of the flexor tendons. The individual should be referred immediately to a physician. Immobilization depends on the type of fracture and its location and may vary from 2 to 4 weeks.

> Immediate management for the suspected boxer's fracture includes ice, compression, immobilization in a wrist splint, and immediate referral to a physician.

REHABILITATION

> A scaphoid fracture can take several weeks or months to heal. What exercises could be included during this period to help the cheerleader maintain her fitness?

Injuries to the wrist and hand often require immobilization; however, early ROM and strengthening exercises should be conducted at the elbow and shoulder. Many of the exercises for the wrist and hand are discussed and demonstrated in Chapter 18, because they often are combined with rehabilitation of the elbow.

Restoration of Motion

Immobilization typically results in joint contractures and stiffness in the fingers. Therefore, active ROM exercises should begin as soon as possible. In the acute phase, exercises can be performed using cryokinetic techniques. Ice immersion is alternated with active ROM exercises. The individual can use the opposite hand to apply a low-load, prolonged stretch in the various motions to minimize joint trauma and increase flexibility. As inflammation decreases, a warm whirlpool or paraffin bath may be used to facilitate motion.

Restoration of Proprioception and Balance

Closed chain exercises may involve shifting body weight from one hand to the other on a wall, table-top, or unstable surface, such as a foam mat or biomechanical ankle platform system (BAPS) board. Push-ups and step-ups on a box, stool, or StairMaster also can be used. Precision techniques to restore dexterity can be performed by picking up and manipulating the following objects:

1. Coins of different thicknesses

2. Playing cards

3. Small objects of different shapes

4. Large, light objects

5. Large, heavy objects

In addition, the individual can tear tape, use scissors to cut paper, or juggle balls of different sizes.

Muscular Strength, Endurance, and Power

Once the ROM approximates what is normal for the individual, open chain kinetic exercises are performed in the various motions using lightweight dumbbells. Many of these exercises are listed and explained in **Application Strategy 18.1**. The individual should complete 30 to 50 repetitions with a 1-lb weight and should not progress in resistance until 50 repetitions have been achieved. Using a table to support the forearm, wrist curls, reverse wrist curls, pronation, and supination can be performed. Wrist curl-ups using a light weight suspended from a broomstick on a 3- to 4-ft rope can be used to increase strength in the wrist flexors and extensors. A weighted bar or hammer can be used for radial and ulnar deviation and for pronation and supination. Proprioceptive neuromuscular facilitation (PNF)-resisted exercises, surgical tubing, or strong rubber bands can be used in all motions for concentric and eccentric loading. Gripping exercises using a tennis ball or putty can be combined with pinching small and large objects. Plyometric exercises may involve catching a weighted ball in a single hand and throwing it straight up and down or using a minitramp to do bounding push-ups.

Cardiovascular Fitness

Cardiovascular conditioning should be maintained throughout the rehabilitation program. Several examples of such programs are provided at thePoint.

 The cheerleader should engage in general body conditioning and strengthening exercises. Only those exercises that aggravate the condition are contraindicated.

SUMMARY

1. Most wrist motion occurs at the radiocarpal joint. The TFC is the cartilaginous disk that acts as a stabilizer of the DRUJ and serves as the ulnar continuation of the radius.

2. The CM joint of the thumb is a classic saddle joint that allows it to have more motion than the CM joints of the other four digits.

3. Retinacular tissue is found throughout the hand and forms protective passageways through which tendons, nerves, and blood vessels pass.

4. Most injuries to the wrist are a result of axial loading on the proximal palm during a fall on an outstretched hand.

5. Excessive varus/valgus stress and hyperextension can damage the collateral ligaments of the fingers. Failure of a ligament usually occurs at its attachment to the proximal phalanx or, less frequently, in the midportion.

6. The most common dislocation in the body occurs at the PIP joint. Because digital nerves and vessels run along the sides of the fingers and thumb, dislocation can be serious if it is reduced by an untrained individual.

7. Muscular strains occur as a result of excessive overload against resistance or stretching the tendon beyond its normal range. Ruptures of a muscle tendon may cause the tendon to retract, necessitating surgical reattachment of the tendon in its proper position.

8. Chronic overuse of a tendon can lead to tendinitis or friction tendinitis in one or more of the dorsal tunnels. Treatment usually consists of ice, rest, NSAIDs, splinting, and avoidance of exacerbating activities.

9. CTS is the most common compression syndrome of the wrist and hand. It is characterized by pain and numbness that wakes the individual in the middle of the night and that often is relieved by shaking the hands.

10. Compression of the ulnar nerve leads to weakness in grip strength, atrophy of the hypothenar mass, and loss of sensation over the little finger.

11. If pain is present during palpation of the anatomical snuff box or with inward pressure along the long axis of the first metacarpal bone, a fracture of the scaphoid should be suspected.

12. Any injury that impairs the function of the hand or fingers should be referred to a physician. The area should be immobilized to prevent further damage, ice applied to control hemorrhage and swelling, and the individual transported in an appropriate manner.

APPLICATION QUESTIONS

1. A softball catcher was hit in the throwing hand by the bat of the hitter. Observation reveals immediate swelling over the 5th metacarpal of the affected hand. What areas should be addressed in the palpation component of an assessment of this injury? What special tests should be performed in assessing this injury?

2. A cheerleader reports to the athletic training room complaining of wrist pain. She fell the previous day on an outstretched hand while performing a back flip. Observation reveals minor swelling but no discoloration or deformity. Palpation reveals sharp pain in the anatomical snuff box. What injury should be suspected? How might the condition be managed?

3. A long-distance cyclist complains of bilateral numbness in the little finger and medial half of the ring finger and an inability to adduct the little finger. The individual cannot recall an incident that could have caused this condition but states that the training distance has significantly increased this past week. What possible factors are involved in this condition? What suggestions can be made to alleviate the symptoms yet permit this cyclist to continue training?

4. You are providing athletic training coverage for a Senior Olympics event. During a softball game, a 58-year-old male pitcher sustains a blow to the end of his finger off a line drive hit. Initially, the pitcher reports pain to the area, which is visibly swollen. The pitcher is confident that it's "just a jammed finger." How would you respond to this scenario?

5. A shot putter pinched a finger under the shot, causing blood to accumulate under the fingernail. The fingertip is extremely painful from the increasing pressure. What factor(s) should be considered in deciding whether or not to relieve the pressure?

6. A football player had his hand stepped on by another player. Immediate pain and a cracking sensation were felt in the palm of the hand. Observation reveals noticeable swelling on the dorsum of the hand. Palpation of the 3rd metacarpal and percussion on the distal end of the third finger cause increased pain. What injury should be suspected? How should the hand be immobilized?

7. While attempting a jump maneuver, a skateboarder loses his balance. The 16-year-old male falls on an outstretched hand. How would you differentiate whether this injury is a perilunate dislocation or a lunate dislocation?

8. A hockey player complains of thumb pain and instability. You suspect an ulnar collateral ligament tear. What tests should be performed to confirm your suspicion?

9. In preparation for tennis season, which begins in 8 weeks, a 45-year-old recreational tennis player would like to strengthen the muscles in her wrist and hand. What exercises would you recommend? Why?

REFERENCES

1. Dimeff RJ. Entrapment neuropathies of the upper extremity. *Curr Sports Med Rep.* 2003;2(5):255–261.
2. Foumani M, Strackee SD, Jonges R, et al. In-vivo three-dimensional carpal bone kinematics during flexion-extension and radio-ulnar deviation of the wrist: dynamic motion versus step-wise static wrist positions. *J Biomech.* 2009;42(16):2664–2671.
3. Upal MA. Carpal bone kinematics in combined wrist joint motions may differ from the bone kinematics during simple wrist motions. *Biomed Sci Instrum.* 2003;39:272–277.
4. Kobayashi M, Berger RA, Linscheid RL, et al. Intercarpal kinematics during wrist motion. *Hand Clin.* 1997;13(1):143–149.
5. Chang LY, Pollard NS. Method for determining kinematic parameters of the in vivo thumb carpometacarpal joint. *IEEE Trans Biomed Eng.* 2008;55(7):1897–1906.
6. Yao J, Park MJ. Early treatment of degenerative arthritis of the thumb carpometacarpal joint. *Hand Clin.* 2008;24(3):251–261.
7. Dumont C, Ziehn C, Kubein-Meesenburg D, et al. Quantified contours of curvature in female index, middle, ring, and small metacarpophalangeal joints. *J Hand Surg Am.* 2009;34(2):317–325.
8. Su FC, Chou YL, Yang CS, et al. Movement of finger joints induced by synergistic wrist motion. *Clin Biomech (Bristol, Avon).* 2005;20(5):491–497.

9. de Freitas PB, Jaric S. Force coordination in static manipulation tasks performed using standard and non-standard grasping techniques. *Exp Brain Res.* 2009;194(4):605–618.

10. Valovich McLeod TC, Decoster LC, Loud KJ, et al. National Athletic Trainers' Association position statement: prevention of pediatric overuse injuries. *J Athl Train.* 2011;46(2):206–220.

11. Changulani M, Okonkwo U, Keswani T, et al. Outcome evaluation measures for wrist and hand: which one to choose? *Int Orthop.* 2008;32(1):1–6.

12. Daniels JM II, Zook EG, Lynch JM. Hand and wrist injuries: part I. Nonemergent evaluation. *Am Fam Physician.* 2004;69(8):1941–1948.

13. Kendall FP, McCreary EK, Provance PG, et al, eds. *Muscles: Testing and Function with Posture and Pain.* 5th ed. Baltimore, MD: Lippincott Williams & Wilkins; 2005.

14. Magee DJ. *Orthopedic Physical Assessment.* 6th ed. St. Louis, MO: Elsevier Saunders; 2014.

15. Starkey C, Brown SD. *Orthopedic & Athletic Injury Examination Handbook.* 3rd ed. Philadelphia, PA: FA Davis; 2015.

16. Wong MS. *Pocket Orthopaedics: Evidence-Based Survival Guide.* Sudbury, MA: Jones and Bartlett; 2010.

17. Abraham MK, Scott S. The emergent evaluation and treatment of hand and wrist injuries. *Emerg Med Clin North Am.* 2010;28(4):789–809.

18. Daniels JM II, Zook EG, Lynch JM. Hand and wrist injuries: part II. Emergent evaluation. *Am Fam Physician.* 2004;69(8):1949–1956.

19. Coel R. Hand injuries in young athletes. *Athl Ther Today.* 2010;15(4):42–45.

20. Wijffels M, Brink P, Schipper I. Clinical and nonclinical aspects of distal radioulnar joint instability. *Open Orthop J.* 2012;6:204–210.

21. Kato N, Nemoto K, Nakajima H, et al. Primary repair of the collateral ligament of the proximal interphalangeal joint using a suture anchor. *Scand J Plast Reconstr Surg Hand Surg.* 2003;37(2):117–120.

22. Finsen V, Hagen S. Surgery for trigger finger. *Hand Surg.* 2003;8(2):201–203.

23. Rumball JS, Lebrun CM, Di Ciacca SR, et al. Rowing injuries. *Sports Med.* 2005;35(6):537–555.

24. Ugbolue UC, Hsu WH, Goitz RJ, et al. Tendon and nerve displacement at the wrist during finger movements. *Clin Biomech (Bristol, Avon).* 2005;20(1):50–56.

25. Holm G, Moody LE. Carpal tunnel syndrome: current theory, treatment, and the use of B6. *J Am Acad Clin Nurse Pract.* 2003;15(1):18–22.

26. Viera AJ. Management of carpal tunnel syndrome. *Am Fam Physician.* 2003;68(2):265–272.

27. Sevim S, Dogu O, Camdeviren H, et al. Long-term effectiveness of steroid injections and splinting in mild and moderate carpal tunnel syndrome. *Neurol Sci.* 2004;25(2):48–52.

28. McNally C, Gillespie M. Scaphoid fractures. *Emerg Nurse.* 2004;12(1):21–25.

29. Kocher MS, Waters PM, Micheli LJ. Upper extremity injuries in the paediatric athlete. *Sports Med.* 2000;30(2):117–135.

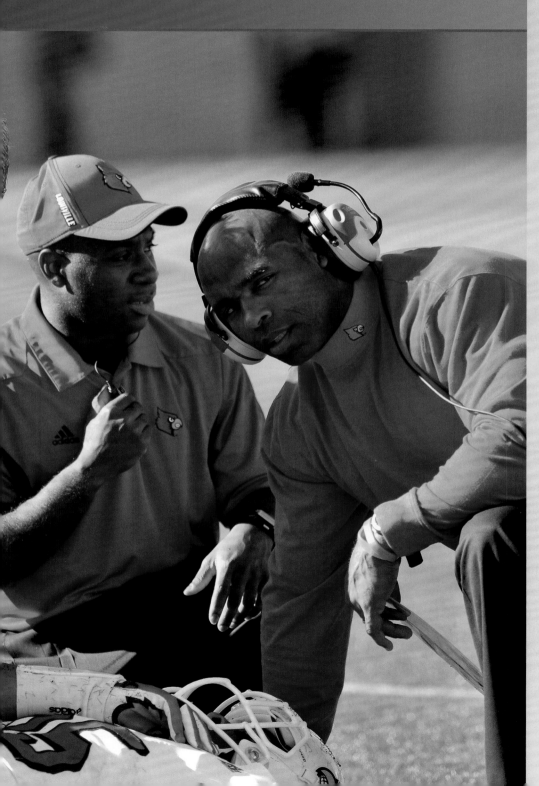

Conditions to the Axial Region

20

Head and Facial Conditions

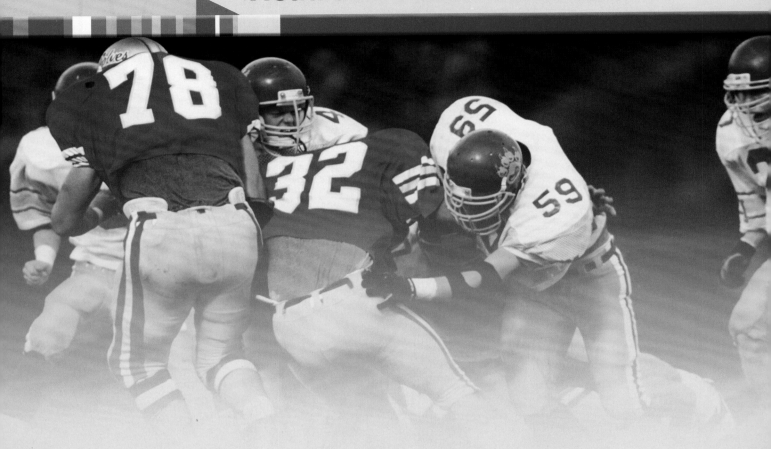

STUDENT OUTCOMES

1. Locate the major bony and soft-tissue structures of the head and facial region.

2. Explain the importance of wearing protective equipment to prevent injury to the head and facial region.

3. Describe the forces responsible for cranial injuries.

4. Identify the signs and symptoms associated with a possible skull fracture.

5. Recognize the critical signs and symptoms that indicate a focal or diffuse cranial injury.

6. Describe how the evaluation and management of a focal cranial injury differs from how a diffuse cranial injury is managed.

7. Explain why baseline concussion testing is important for making an accurate and efficient diagnosis in an acute situation.

8. List the components of the baseline concussion testing protocol.

9. Explain how to use the Sport Concussion Assessment Tool 3 (SCAT3), Vestibular/Ocular Motor/Reflex Screening (VOMS/VORS), and cranial nerve assessments.

10. Summarize the steps of the graduated return to play protocols for patients recovering from concussion and explain the value of using this protocol.

11. Identify the signs and symptoms associated with a possible facial fracture.

12. Describe the signs and symptoms of epistaxis, deviated septum, and fractured nose.

13. Describe the differences in managing a loose versus a fractured or dislocated tooth.

14. Recognize common external and internal ear conditions and explain their management.

15. Describe the use of an otoscope to assess nose and ear conditions.

16. Identify the signs and symptoms of serious nasal, ear, or eye injuries that warrant immediate referral to a physician.

17. Describe the evaluation of an eye injury and the use of an ophthalmoscope.

INTRODUCTION

The head and facial area are frequent sites for minor injuries, including lacerations, contusions, and mild concussions. However, the incidence of facial injuries, eye, ear, and dental injuries are significantly decreased when protective equipment is worn. Although intracranial injuries have been associated with sport-related fatalities, increased standards for protective equipment and rule changes that prohibit leading with the head for contact as well as the development and use of the face mask have significantly decreased the incidence of injuries since the mid-1970s. Although face masks, properly fitting helmets, and mouth guards may decrease the incidence of catastrophic brain injury, there is little evidence to support that protective equipment decreases the risk of concussion.[1]

This chapter begins with a general anatomical review of the head and facial region. Discussion concerning preventive measures is followed by information regarding the mechanisms of injury most commonly linked to cranial injuries. The signs, symptoms, and management of the more common focal and diffuse cranial injuries are discussed, followed by steps to include in a thorough assessment of a head injury. Within the discussion on the importance of conducting baseline concussion assessments, information is presented on the Sport Concussion Assessment Tool 3 (SCAT3), cranial nerve assessment, vital sign assessment, mental status assessment, and the value of comparing pre- and postinjury assessment findings to make decisions regarding management and return to participation decisions. The final section discusses the more common facial, nasal, ear, and eye injuries and their management.

ANATOMY OF THE HEAD AND FACIAL REGION

> **?** While playing racquetball, a 40-year-old man collides with the back wall of the court and hits his head. He sustains a superficial cut to the back of the head that is bleeding profusely. What anatomical structures are likely to have been injured, and is this a potentially serious injury?

This review focuses on the brain and its coverings; the facial area, including the eyes, ears, and nose; and the nerve and blood supply to the region. Although the numerous muscles of the face and jaw enable speaking, chewing, and facial expression, these muscles are not commonly involved in injuries attributed to participation in sport and physical activity and, therefore, are not discussed.

Bones of the Skull

The skull is composed primarily of flat bones that interlock at immovable joints called sutures (**Fig. 20.1**). The bones that form the portion of the skull referred to as the cranium protect the brain.

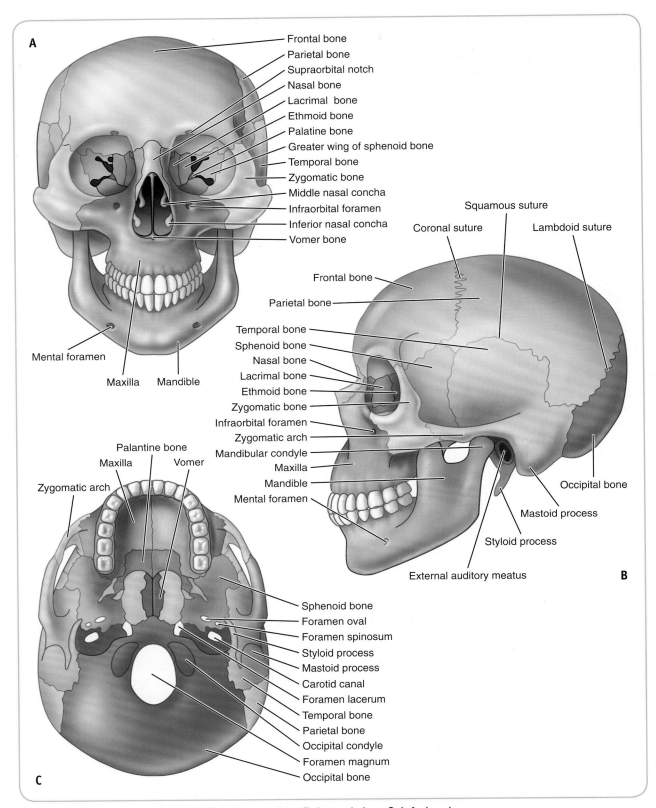

Figure 20.1. The bones of the skull. A, Frontal view. **B,** Lateral view. **C,** Inferior view.

The thin bones of the cranium include the frontal, occipital, sphenoid, and ethmoid bones as well as two parietal and two temporal bones. The material properties and thickness of the cranial bones vary, with the strongest being the occipital bone and the weakest being the temporal bones. The facial bones provide the structure of the face and form the sinuses, orbits of the eyes, the nasal cavity, and the mouth; these bones include the paired maxilla, zygomatic, palatine, nasal, lacrimal, vomer, and inferior nasal concha bones, along with the bridge and mandible. The large opening at the base of the skull that sits atop the spinal column is called the foramen magnum.

The Scalp

The scalp is composed of three layers: the skin, the subcutaneous connective tissue, and the pericranium. The protective function of these tissues is enhanced by the hair and by the looseness of the scalp, which enable some dissipation of force when the head sustains a glancing blow. The scalp and face have an extensive blood supply; as a result, superficial lacerations tend to bleed profusely.

The Brain

The four major regions of the brain are the cerebral hemispheres, diencephalon, the brainstem, and the cerebellum. The entire brain and spinal cord are enclosed in three layers of protective tissue known collectively as the meninges (**Fig. 20.2**). The outermost membrane is the dura mater, which is a thick, fibrous tissue containing the dural sinuses that act as veins to transport blood from the brain to the jugular veins of the neck. The arachnoid mater is a thin membrane internal to the dura mater; it is separated from the dura mater by the subdural space. Beneath the arachnoid mater is the subarachnoid space, which is filled with cerebrospinal fluid (CSF) and contains the largest of the blood vessels supplying the brain. The arachnoid mater is connected to the inner pia mater by web-like strands of connective tissue. The dura mater and arachnoid mater are rather loose membranes; in comparison, the pia mater is in direct contact with the cerebral cortex and contains numerous small blood vessels.

The Eyes

The eye is a hollow sphere, approximately 2.5 cm (1 in) in diameter in adults (**Fig. 20.3**). The anterior eye surface receives protection from the eyelids, eyelashes, and the attached conjunctiva. The conjunctiva lines the eyelid and the external surface of the eye and secretes mucus to lubricate the external eye. The lacrimal glands, which are located above the lateral ends of the eyes, continually release tears across the eye surface through several small ducts. The lacrimal ducts, which are located at the medial corners of the eyes, serve as drains for the moisture. These ducts funnel the moisture into the lacrimal sac and, eventually, into the nasal cavity.

The eye is surrounded by three protective tissue layers called tunics. The outer tunic is a thick, white connective tissue called the sclera and forms the "white of the eye." The cornea, which is found in the central anterior part of the sclera, is clear to permit the passage of light into the eye. The choroid, or the middle covering, is a highly vascularized tissue that usually appears blue or brown on the anterior eye and contains the pupil. The inner protective layer is the retina, which contains light-sensitive photoreceptor cells that stimulate nerve endings to provide sight.

The Nose

The nose is composed of bone and hyaline cartilage. The roof is formed by the cribriform plate of the ethmoid bone. The nasal bones form the bridge of the nose. Inferiorly, the lateral walls are shaped by the superior and middle conchae of the ethmoid bone, the vertical plates of the palatine bones, and the inferior nasal conchae (**Fig. 20.4**). The nasal cavity is separated into right and left halves by the nasal septum, which is made of cartilage and can be deviated or fractured if struck by a blunt object. A deviated septum can complicate the assessment and treatment of soft-tissue injuries.

The Ear

The ear is divided into three major areas: the outer ear (auricle and external auditory canal), the middle ear (tympanic membrane), and the inner ear (labyrinth) (**Fig. 20.5**). Assisting the middle and

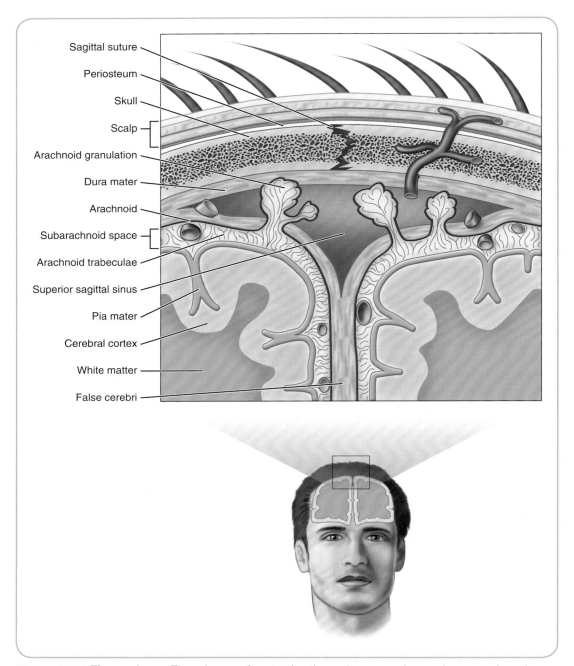

Figure 20.2. **The meninges.** Three layers of protective tissue, known as the meninges, enclose the brain and spinal cord.

inner ear in the process of hearing and equalizing pressure between the two areas is the eustachian tube, a canal that links the nose and middle ear.

Nerves of the Head and Face

Twelve pairs of cranial nerves emerge from the brain. These nerves have motor functions, sensory functions, or both. The cranial nerves are numbered and named according to their functions and are listed in **Table 20.1.**

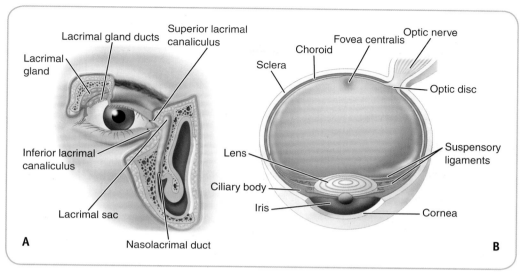

Figure 20.3. The eye. A, The lacrimal structures of the eye. **B,** Internal structures of the eye globe.

Blood Vessels of the Head and Face

The major vessels supplying the head and face are the common carotid and vertebral arteries (**Fig. 20.6**). The common carotid artery ascends through the neck on either side to divide into the external and internal carotid arteries just below the level of the jaw. The external carotid arteries and their branches supply most regions of the head external to the brain. The middle meningeal artery supplies the skull and dura mater; if this artery is damaged, serious epidural bleeding can result. The internal carotid arteries send branches to the eyes and supply portions of the cerebral hemispheres

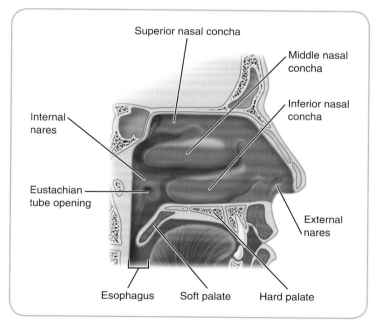

Figure 20.4. The nose. The nose is composed of bone and cartilage.

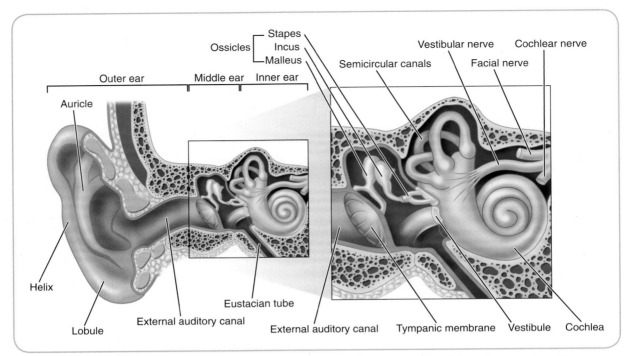

Figure 20.5. The ear. The ear is divided into three major areas: the outer ear (auricle and external auditory canal), the middle ear (tympanic membrane), and the inner ear (labyrinth).

TABLE 20.1 The Cranial Nerves

NUMBER	NAME	SENSORY	MOTOR FUNCTION	ASSESSMENT
I	Olfactory	X (smell)	Sense of smell	Identify familiar odors (chocolate, coffee).
II	Optic	X (vision)	Vision	Test visual fields: Snellen chart (blurring or double vision).
III	Oculomotor	X	Control of some of the extrinsic eye muscles	Test pupillary reaction to light.
IV	Trochlear	X	Control of the remaining extrinsic eye muscles	Perform upward and downward gaze.
V	Trigeminal	X (general sensation)	Sensation of the facial region and movement of the jaw muscles	Touch face to note difference in sensation. Clench teeth; push down on chin to separate jaws.
VI	Abducens	X	Control of lateral eye movement	Perform lateral and medial gaze.
VII	Facial	X (taste)	Control of facial movement, taste, and secretion of tears and saliva	Smile and show the teeth. Close eyes tight.
VIII	Vestibulocochlear	X (hearing and balance)	Hearing and equilibrium (acoustic)	Identify the sound of fingers snapping near the ear. Balance and coordination (stand on one foot).
IX	Glossopharyngeal	X (taste)	Taste, control of the tongue and pharynx, and secretion of saliva	Gag reflex; ask the athlete to swallow.
X	Vagus	X (taste)	Taste and sensation to the pharynx, larynx, trachea, and bronchioles	Gag reflex; ask athlete to swallow or say "Ah."
XI	Accessory	X	Control of movements of the pharynx, larynx, secretion of saliva	Resisted shoulder shrug
XII	Hypoglossal	X	Control of tongue movements	Stick out the tongue.

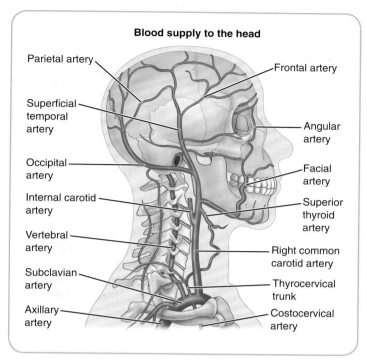

Figure 20.6. Blood supply to the head. The common carotid and vertebral arteries are the major vessels supplying blood to the brain.

and the parietal and temporal lobes of the cerebrum. The left and right vertebral arteries and their branches supply blood to the posterior region of the brain.

 Because the scalp and face have an extensive blood supply, superficial lacerations of the head tend to bleed profusely. Given the mechanism of injury, however, it is important to rule out cerebral trauma or skull fracture. If no signs of a cerebral trauma or skull fracture (discussed later in this chapter) are present, the scalp injury is not serious as long as bleeding is controlled.

PREVENTION OF HEAD AND FACIAL INJURIES

 A high school athletic director is faced with making budget cuts. He requests justification for purchasing mouth guards for teams other than football (i.e., soccer, basketball, lacrosse, and field hockey). Provide a rationale for ensuring that athletes in any sport involving contact should be provided with mouth guards.

The most important preventive measure for the head and facial area is the use of protective equipment. Many sports, such as baseball/softball, competitive bicycling, fencing, field hockey, football, ice hockey, lacrosse, and wrestling, require some type of head or facial protective equipment for participation. When used properly, protective equipment can protect the head and facial area from accidental or routine injuries, but no clinical evidence has definitively determined that use of protective equipment can prevent concussions.[1] Protective equipment cannot prevent all injuries. To minimize injuries, equipment must be properly fitted, clean, in good condition, and used in the manner for which it was designed.

Protective equipment may include a helmet, face guard, mouth guard, eyewear, ear wear, and a throat protector. Helmets protect the cranial portion of the skull by absorbing and dispersing impact forces, thereby reducing cerebral trauma. Face guards protect and shield the facial region. Mouth guards have been shown to reduce dental and oral soft-tissue injuries, jaw fractures, and temporomandibular joint (TMJ) injuries. Eyewear, ear wear, and throat protectors reduce injuries to their respective regions. Chapter 3 provides information regarding protective equipment for the head and face.

 A properly fitted mouth guard can help to prevent dental and oral soft-tissue injuries, and it also can help to reduce the incidence of jaw fractures and TMJ injuries.

CRANIAL INJURY MECHANISMS

? Explain the mechanism for a contrecoup cerebral injury.

The occurrence of a skull fracture or intracranial injury is dependent on the material properties of the skull, the thickness of the skull in the specific area, the magnitude and direction of impact, and the size of the impact area. Direct impact causes two phenomena to occur—namely, deformation and acceleration. When a blow impacts the skull, the bone deforms and bends inward, placing the inner border of the skull under tensile strain while the outer border is compressed (**Fig. 20.7A**). If the impact is of sufficient magnitude and the skull in the region of impact is thin, a skull fracture occurs at the site where tensile loading occurs. In contrast, if the skull is thick and dense enough at the area of impact, it may sustain inward bending without fracture. A fracture then may occur some distance from the impact zone in a region where the skull is thinner (**Fig. 20.7B**).

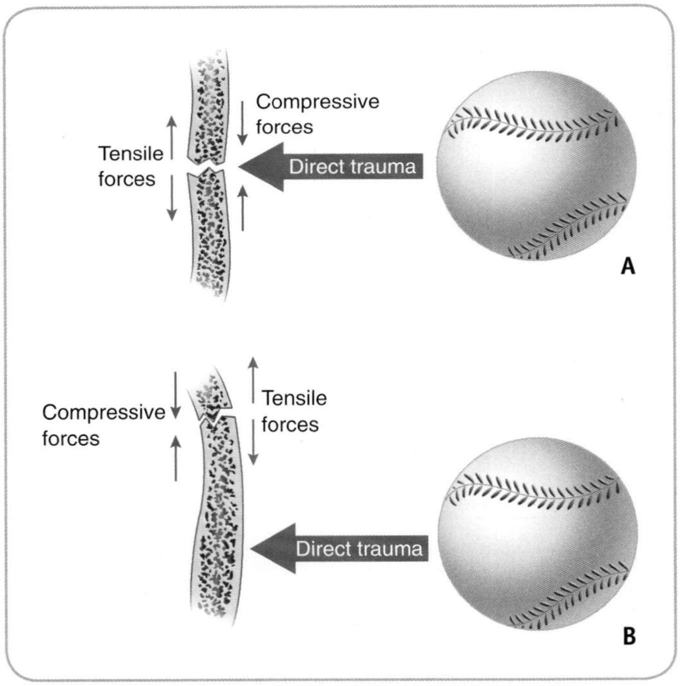

On impact, shock waves pass through the skull to the brain, causing it to accelerate. This acceleration can lead to shear, tensile, and compression strains within the brain substance, with shear being the most serious. Axial rotation coupled with acceleration can lead to **contrecoup injuries** (**Fig. 20.8**), which are injuries located away from the actual impact site.

Cerebral trauma can lead to **focal injuries**, involving only localized damage (i.e., epidural, subdural, or intracerebral hematomas), or **diffuse injuries**, involving widespread disruption and damage to the function and/or structure of the brain. Although diffuse injuries account for only one-quarter of the fatalities caused by head trauma, they tend to be a more prevalent cause of long-term neurological deficits. If cerebral injuries are recognized and treated immediately, the severity can potentially be limited to the initial structural damage; however, if other factors, such as ischemia, hypoxia, cerebral swelling, and hemorrhaging around the brain occur, additional damage and possible neurological dysfunction result. Therefore, an accurate assessment of head injuries is essential to ensure prompt medical attention to rule out serious underlying problems that may complicate the original injury. A conscious, ambulatory patient should not be considered to have only a minor injury

Figure 20.7. Mechanical failure in bone. When a blow impacts the skull, the bone deforms and bends inward, placing tensile stress on the inner border of the skull. **A,** If an impact is of sufficient magnitude and the skull is thin in the region of the impact, a skull fracture occurs at the impact site. **B,** If the skull is thick and dense enough at the area of impact, it may sustain bending without fracture; however, the fracture may occur some distance from the impact zone, in a region where the skull is thinner.

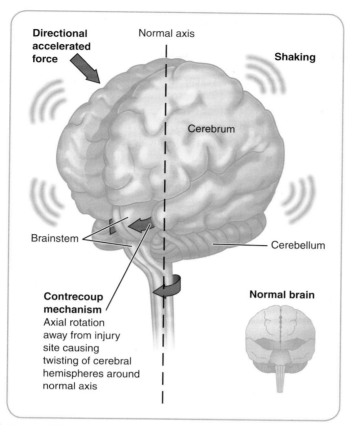

Figure 20.8. **A contrecoup injury.** Axial rotation coupled with acceleration can result in a contrecoup injury.

but, rather, should be assessed continually to determine if posttraumatic signs or symptoms indicate a more serious underlying condition.

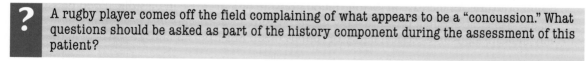

The mechanism for a contrecoup cerebral injury can be illustrated by this example: A football running back is sprinting downfield when he collides with an opposing player and is knocked backward, his head striking the ground. The running back's body and brain are moving in the same direction when an opposing force causes his brain to accelerate within the skull in the opposite direction. The injury occurs not at the site of contact with the ground but on the opposite side of the brain.

ASSESSMENT OF CRANIAL CONDITIONS

 A rugby player comes off the field complaining of what appears to be a "concussion." What questions should be asked as part of the history component during the assessment of this patient?

Any patient who receives a blow or any significant acceleration–deceleration type of force to the head should be evaluated thoroughly. Because significant head trauma may also cause neck injury, it should always be assumed that a cervical injury is present until cleared. Methods of assessing the cervical spine and cervical spine pathology are covered in the next chapter, Chapter 21. Although information presented in this chapter focuses on assessing the head in real-life situations, information presented in this chapter and in Chapter 21 are used simultaneously to assist the clinician in conducting the assessment. For matters of clarity, these components are presented separately. In addition, because of the complexity of assessing a cranial injury, additional thought questions and answers are provided throughout this section.

In approaching a patient who has sustained trauma to the head or face, the clinician should first conduct a primary survey to establish the status of the patient's airway, breathing, and circulation (ABCs). Next, assess the patient's level of consciousness using methods described in **Table 7.1** and begin immediately observing for indications of trauma to the head such as posturing, abnormal pupils, raccoon eyes or Battle sign (see **Figs. 7.1** to **7.3**), or the presence of CSF in blood coming from the nose or ears. If the patient is face down, the head and neck should be stabilized and the patient should be log rolled into a supine position while continuing to stabilize the cervical spine. Any mouth guard, dentures, or partial plates should be removed to prevent occlusion of the airway. Rescue breathing and cardiopulmonary resuscitation should be initiated as needed, and the emergency action plan (EAP) should be implemented.

Vital Signs

It is imperative to begin conducting a vital sign assessment as quickly as possible to establish a baseline of information that can be rechecked periodically to determine if the patient's status is improving or deteriorating. Vital signs include pulse, respiration, blood pressure, and body temperature. With head trauma, however, body temperature is not as critical as the other signs. Any abnormal variations, presented in **Table 7.2**, such as a falling pulse rate, rising blood pressure, or irregular breathing, indicate increasing intracranial pressure.

1. **Pulse**

   - *Small, weak pulse*—Pulse pressure is diminished, and the pulse feels weak and small; causes include decreased stroke volume and increased peripheral resistance.

   - *Short, rapid, weak pulse*—indicates heart failure or shock

   - *Slow, bounding pulse*—indicates increasing intracranial pressure

   - *Accelerated pulse*—A rapid pulse (i.e., 150 beats per minute) may indicate pressure on the base of the brain.

2. **Respiration**

   - *Slow breathing (bradypnea)*—Breathing at less than 12 breaths per minute indicates increased intracranial pressure.

   - *Cheyne-Stokes breathing*—Periods of deep breathing alternating with periods of apnea (no breathing) indicates brain damage.

   - *Ataxic (Biot's) breathing*—Characterized by unpredictable irregularity; breaths may be shallow or deep and stop for short periods, indicating respiratory depression and brain damage typically at the medullary level.

   - *Apneustic breathing*—Characterized by prolonged inspirations unrelieved by attempts to exhale, which indicates trauma to the pons.

3. **Blood pressure:** An increase in systolic blood pressure or a decrease in diastolic blood pressure indicates rising intracranial pressure. Low blood pressure rarely occurs in a head injury; however, it may indicate a possible cervical injury or serious blood loss from an injury elsewhere in the body.

4. **Pulse pressure:** The normal difference between diastolic and systolic pressure is approximately 40 mm Hg. A pulse pressure greater than 50 mm Hg indicates increased intracranial bleeding.

History and Mental Status Testing

Information obtained during the history will assist the clinician in sequencing the different components of the assessment process. When dealing with a potential head injury, assessing mental status beyond the level of consciousness (AVPU, A/OX4, GCS) is often a part of the history-taking process (see **Table 7.1**). The patient may initially appear confused with memory loss and may have a heightened distractibility, an inability to maintain a coherent stream of thought, and an inability to carry out a sequence of goal-directed movements. The confusion and memory dysfunction may be immediate after injury, or it may be a delayed process, taking several minutes to fully evolve. The clinician should note the presence of slurred speech, difficulty in constructing sentences, or an inability to understand commands. The following examples may be used to gather the history of the injury and test the mental status of the injured participant:

1. **Orientation and mechanism of injury:** Ask the patient about the time, place, and situation. Attempt to determine the mechanism of injury (i.e., was the patient struck by a moving object such as ball, bat, knee or did the patient collide with another player, or fall with the head striking the ground).

2. **Loss of consciousness (LOC):** Although less than 10% of all concussions result in an LOC,[1] patients who have sustained an epidural hematoma often will have an initial LOC followed by a lucid period before declining. It is important to determine if the patient is totally unresponsive, confused, or disoriented. If LOC occurred, it is important to note whether it occurred immediately on direct impact or whether the person progressed to unconsciousness. In addition, the length of time of unconsciousness should be recorded. The patient's response to painful stimuli (e.g., squeezing the trapezius, pinching soft tissue between the thumb and index finger in the axilla, knuckle to the sternum, or squeezing the Achilles tendon) or positive results from pathological reflex testing (see **Table 7.2**) should be noted. The occurrence of a seizure also should be noted.

3. **Symptoms:** A headache is one of the most reported symptoms (86%) with a concussion[2,3]; however, progressive headaches indicate increasing intracranial pressure and signal danger. It is important to note if the patient is experiencing nausea, because intracranial pressure can stimulate the reflex onset of nausea and vomiting. If this symptom is present, it indicates a fairly serious intracranial injury. Other common symptoms that may be reported include dizziness, confusion, disorientation, blurred vision, amnesia, neck pain, and fatigue.[4] The patient may also report visual disturbances such as an increased sensitivity to light (photophobia) or "seeing stars or lights" as time of injury and an increased sensitivity to sound.

4. **Memory:** Assessment of memory should include question to assess for the presence of both **anterograde** (events after the point of injury) and **retrograde** (events prior to the point of injury) amnesia. Assessing anterograde amnesia may be conducted by asking the patient to describe events from the time of injury to the current point in time. Retrograde amnesia can be assessed by asking the patient to describe the events leading up to the event that caused the injury. Other options include naming three words or identify three objects for the patient and then ask the person to recall these words or objects. Every 5 minutes, ask the patient to do so again. Additionally, ask the patient to recall recent newsworthy events or provide details of the current activity (e.g., plays, moves, strategies).

5. **Concentration:** Recite three digits and ask the patient to recite them backward. Move to four digits and then to five digits (e.g., 3-1-7, 4-6-8-2, and 5-3-0-7-4). Ask the patient to list the months of the year in reverse order.

6. **Behavior:** The patient's behavior, attitude, and demeanor may change after head trauma. This may present as irrational and inappropriate behavior, belligerence, or verbal or physical abuse directed at others.

 The rugby player should be questioned regarding how the injury occurred, location, type, and intensity of pain and to determine if any LOC occurred. Next, it is important to see if the patient is confused, disoriented, dizzy, or nauseous or has a headache, blurred vision, ringing in the ears, sensitivity to light or sound, or feels out of it. Does the patient remember what happened before and after the injury occurred? The ability to concentrate is included during the history-taking process and involves providing the patient with a set of serial items and asking them to recite the items back to you in reverse order.

Observation and Inspection

> **?** In the continued assessment of this patient, what should be included in the physical exam portion of the evaluation?

An observation of facial expression and function should be performed throughout the evaluation (**Table 20.1**). The following areas and conditions should be assessed in the observation component of the evaluation:

1. **Leakage of CSF:** CSF is a clear, colorless fluid that protects and cushions the brain and spinal cord. A basilar skull fracture may result in blood and CSF leaking from the ear. A fracture to the cribriform plate in the anterior cranial area may result in blood and CSF leaking from the nose.

2. **Signs of trauma:** Discoloration around the eyes (raccoon eyes) and behind the ears (Battle sign) may indicate a skull fracture. A depression, elevation, or bleeding may indicate a skull fracture, laceration, or hematoma. Snoring, which may result from a fracture to the anterior cranial floor, should be noted.

3. **Skin color:** Skin color and the presence of moisture or sweat should be assessed. If shock is developing, the skin may appear ashen or pale and may be moist and cool.

4. **Loss of emotional control:** Irritability, aggressive behavior, or uncontrolled crying for no apparent reason indicates cerebral dysfunction.

Palpation

Palpation can help to determine possible skull or facial fractures. The clinician should palpate for point tenderness, crepitus, depressions, elevations, swelling, blood, or changes in skin temperature. The following sites should be palpated:

1. Scalp and hair

2. Base of the skull (occiput), external ear, and periauricular area

3. TMJ

4. Cervical spinous processes

5. Hyoid bone and cartilages

6. Mandible

7. Maxilla

8. Teeth

9. Zygomatic arch (cheek)

10. Frontal bone and entire eye orbit

11. Nasal bones and nasal cartilage

Neurological Tests

Tests should be used that assess the upper motor neuron function of the brain through coordination, sensation, and agility and should include a combination of cognition, postural stability, and self-reported symptoms. An evaluation of myotomes and dermatomes is not an effective tool in assessing cranial injuries because they address lower motor neuron function associated with the spinal column and spinal nerves.

1. **Cranial nerve assessment:** The integrity of the cranial nerves can be assessed quickly by sense of smell, vision, eye tracking, smiling, clenching the jaw, hearing, balance, sense of taste, speaking, and strength of shoulder shrugs (**Table 20.1**).

2. **Pupil abnormalities:** Pupils are equal and reactive to light (PEARL). A dilated pupil on one side may indicate a subdural or epidural hematoma. Dilated pupils on both sides indicate a severe cranial injury with death imminent. The clinician should ask the patient to look up, down, and diagonally (i.e., move from an upper left gaze to a lower right gaze; upper right gaze to a lower left gaze). The coordinated and fluid motion of both eyes should be noted. The patient should be asked about blurred or double vision or the presence of "stars" or flashes of light on impact. Blurred or double vision, abnormal oscillating movements of the eye (**nystagmus**), or uncoordinated gross movement through the cardinal planes indicate a disturbance of the cranial nerves that innervate the eyes and eye muscles.

3. **Babinski reflex:** The patient should be lying down with the eyes closed and the leg held in a slightly elevated and flexed position. A pointed object is stroked along the plantar aspect of the foot. A normal sign is for the toes to curl downward in flexion and adduction (**Fig. 20.9A**). An abnormal Babinski sign suggests an upper motor neuron lesion and is demonstrated by the extension of the big toe and abduction (splaying) of the other toes (**Fig. 20.9B**).

4. **Strength:** A bilateral comparison of grip strength should be performed by having the clinician place the hands inside the patient's hands and then asking the patient to squeeze.

5. **Neuropsychological assessments**

   ■ **Standardized Assessment of Concussion:** SCAT3[1,5,6] is an abbreviated neurocognitive test designed for medical personnel in evaluating athletes aged 13 years and older for potential concussion. A modified Child-SCAT3 should be used for children aged 5 to 13 years of age.[6] SCAT3 (**Fig. 20.10**) evaluates four key mental functions (orientation, immediate memory, concentration, and delayed recall) as well as balance (Modified Balance Error Scoring System testing) and symptoms (graded symptoms score). The graded symptom checklist has been recommended by the National Athletic Trainers' Association,[1] the Zurich International Conference on Concussion in Sport,[6] and the American Academy of Pediatrics[7] for use during the initial evaluation of a head injury. The SCAT3 is designed for use in assessing the presence of concussion and is useful only for sideline evaluations and follow-up assessment within the first 24 hours.[1]

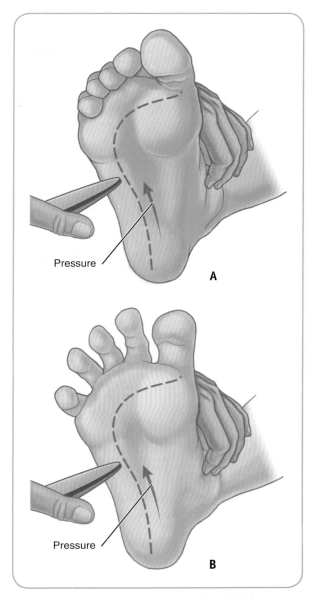

Figure 20.9. The Babinski reflex. The clinician strokes the bottom of the foot along the lateral border, moving distally into the middle of the foot and over the ball of the foot. **A,** A normal sign is the toes curling under (flexing). **B,** An abnormal sign shows the toes splaying.

   ■ **Paper-and-pencil tests:** A number of assessment tools focus on verbal learning, verbal scanning, attention, concentration, short-term memory, visual perception and tracking, and general brain function. These include the Hopkins Verbal Learning Test (John Hopkins University, Baltimore, MD), Trail Making Test A & B (Reitan Neuropsychology Laboratory, Tucson, AZ), Wechsler Digit Span Test (Psychological Corporation, San Antonio, TX), Stroop Color-Word Interference Test (Stoelting Co, Wood Dale, IL), Symbol Digit Modalities Test (Western Psychological Services, Los Angeles, CA), and Controlled Oral Word Association Test (COWAT; Psychological Assessment Resources, Inc, Odessa, FL).[8] However, the SCAT2/3 are the mostly used.

SCAT3™

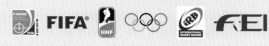

Sport Concussion Assessment Tool – 3rd Edition

For use by medical professionals only

Name	Date / Time of Injury:	Examiner:
	Date of Assessment:	

What is the SCAT3?[1]

The SCAT3 is a standardized tool for evaluating injured athletes for concussion and can be used in athletes aged from 13 years and older. It supersedes the original SCAT and the SCAT2 published in 2005 and 2009, respectively[2]. For younger persons, ages 12 and under, please use the Child SCAT3. The SCAT3 is designed for use by medical professionals. If you are not qualified, please use the Sport Concussion Recognition Tool[1]. Preseason baseline testing with the SCAT3 can be helpful for interpreting post-injury test scores.

Specific instructions for use of the SCAT3 are provided on page 3. If you are not familiar with the SCAT3, please read through these instructions carefully. This tool may be freely copied in its current form for distribution to individuals, teams, groups and organizations. Any revision or any reproduction in a digital form requires approval by the Concussion in Sport Group.
NOTE: The diagnosis of a concussion is a clinical judgment, ideally made by a medical professional. The SCAT3 should not be used solely to make, or exclude, the diagnosis of concussion in the absence of clinical judgement. An athlete may have a concussion even if their SCAT3 is "normal".

What is a concussion?

A concussion is a disturbance in brain function caused by a direct or indirect force to the head. It results in a variety of non-specific signs and/or symptoms (some examples listed below) and most often does not involve loss of consciousness. Concussion should be suspected in the presence of **any one or more** of the following:

- Symptoms (e.g., headache), or
- Physical signs (e.g., unsteadiness), or
- Impaired brain function (e.g. confusion) or
- Abnormal behaviour (e.g., change in personality).

SIDELINE ASSESSMENT

Indications for Emergency Management

NOTE: A hit to the head can sometimes be associated with a more serious brain injury. Any of the following warrants consideration of activating emergency procedures and urgent transportation to the nearest hospital:

- Glasgow Coma score less than 15
  Deteriorating mental status
  Potential spinal injury
- Progressive, worsening symptoms or new neurologic signs

Potential signs of concussion?

If any of the following signs are observed after a direct or indirect blow to the head, the athlete should stop participation, be evaluated by a medical professional and **should not be permitted to return to sport the same day** if a concussion is suspected.

Any loss of consciousness?	Y N
"If so, how long?"	
Balance or motor incoordination (stumbles, slow/laboured movements, etc.)?	Y N
Disorientation or confusion (inability to respond appropriately to questions)?	Y N
Loss of memory:	Y N
"If so, how long?"	
"Before or after the injury?"	
Blank or vacant look:	Y N
Visible facial injury in combination with any of the above:	Y N

1 Glasgow coma scale (GCS)

Best eye response (E)	
No eye opening	1
Eye opening in response to pain	2
Eye opening to speech	3
Eyes opening spontaneously	4

Best verbal response (V)	
No verbal response	1
Incomprehensible sounds	2
Inappropriate words	3
Confused	4
Oriented	5

Best motor response (M)	
No motor response	1
Extension to pain	2
Abnormal flexion to pain	3
Flexion / Withdrawal to pain	4
Localizes to pain	5
Obeys commands	6

Glasgow Coma score (E + V + M)	of 15

GCS should be recorded for all athletes in case of subsequent deterioration.

2 Maddocks Score[3]

"I am going to ask you a few questions, please listen carefully and give your best effort."
Modified Maddocks questions (1 point for each correct answer)

What venue are we at today?	0	1
Which half is it now?	0	1
Who scored last in this match?	0	1
What team did you play last week / game?	0	1
Did your team win the last game?	0	1
Maddocks score		of 5

Maddocks score is validated for sideline diagnosis of concussion only and is not used for serial testing.

Notes: Mechanism of Injury ("tell me what happened"?):

_____

_____

_____

_____

Any athlete with a suspected concussion should be REMOVED FROM PLAY, medically assessed, monitored for deterioration (i.e., should not be left alone) and should not drive a motor vehicle until cleared to do so by a medical professional. No athlete diagnosed with concussion should be returned to sports participation on the day of Injury.

© 2013 Concussion in Sport Group

Figure 20.10. The Sport Concussion Assessment Tool 3 (SCAT3).

BACKGROUND

Name: _____ Date: _____

Examiner: _____

Sport/team/school: _____ Date/time of injury: _____

Age: _____ Gender: ☐ M ☐ F

Years of education completed: _____

Dominant hand: ☐ right ☐ left ☐ neither

How many concussions do you think you have had in the past? _____

When was the most recent concussion? _____

How long was your recovery from the most recent concussion? _____

Have you ever been hospitalized or had medical imaging done for ☐ Y ☐ N
a head injury?

Have you ever been diagnosed with headaches or migraines? ☐ Y ☐ N

Do you have a learning disability, dyslexia, ADD/ADHD? ☐ Y ☐ N

Have you ever been diagnosed with depression, anxiety ☐ Y ☐ N
or other psychiatric disorder?

Has anyone in your family ever been diagnosed with ☐ Y ☐ N
any of these problems?

Are you on any medications? If yes, please list: ☐ Y ☐ N

SCAT3 to be done in resting state. Best done 10 or more minutes post excercise.

SYMPTOM EVALUATION

3 ### How do you feel?

"You should score yourself on the following symptoms, based on how you feel now".

	none	mild		moderate		severe	
Headache	0	1	2	3	4	5	6
"Pressure in head"	0	1	2	3	4	5	6
Neck Pain	0	1	2	3	4	5	6
Nausea or vomiting	0	1	2	3	4	5	6
Dizziness	0	1	2	3	4	5	6
Blurred vision	0	1	2	3	4	5	6
Balance problems	0	1	2	3	4	5	6
Sensitivity to light	0	1	2	3	4	5	6
Sensitivity to noise	0	1	2	3	4	5	6
Feeling slowed down	0	1	2	3	4	5	6
Feeling like "in a fog"	0	1	2	3	4	5	6
"Don't feel right"	0	1	2	3	4	5	6
Difficulty concentrating	0	1	2	3	4	5	6
Difficulty remembering	0	1	2	3	4	5	6
Fatigue or low energy	0	1	2	3	4	5	6
Confusion	0	1	2	3	4	5	6
Drowsiness	0	1	2	3	4	5	6
Trouble falling asleep	0	1	2	3	4	5	6
More emotional	0	1	2	3	4	5	6
Irritability	0	1	2	3	4	5	6
Sadness	0	1	2	3	4	5	6
Nervous or Anxious	0	1	2	3	4	5	6

Total number of symptoms (Maximum possible 22) _____

Symptom severity score (Maximum possible 132) _____

Do the symptoms get worse with physical activity? ☐ Y ☐ N

Do the symptoms get worse with mental activity? ☐ Y ☐ N

☐ self rated ☐ self rated and clinician monitored

☐ clinician interview ☐ self rated with parent input

Overall rating: If you know the athlete well prior to the injury, how different is the athlete acting compared to his/her usual self?

Please circle one response:

no different	very different	unsure	N/A

Scoring on the SCAT3 should not be used as a stand-alone method to diagnose concussion, measure recovery or make decisions about an athlete's readiness to return to competition after concussion. Since signs and symptoms may evolve over time, it is important to consider repeat evaluation in the acute assessment of concussion.

COGNITIVE & PHYSICAL EVALUATION

4 ### Cognitive assessment
Standardized Assessment of Concussion (SAC)[4]

Orientation (1 point for each correct answer)

What month is it?	0	1
What is the date today?	0	1
What is the day of the week?	0	1
What year is it?	0	1
What time is it right now? (within 1 hour)	0	1
Orientation score		of 5

Immediate memory

List	Trial 1		Trial 2		Trial 3		Alternative word list		
elbow	0	1	0	1	0	1	candle	baby	finger
apple	0	1	0	1	0	1	paper	monkey	penny
carpet	0	1	0	1	0	1	sugar	perfume	blanket
saddle	0	1	0	1	0	1	sandwich	sunset	lemon
bubble	0	1	0	1	0	1	wagon	iron	insect
Total									

Immediate memory score total _____ of 15

Concentration: Digits Backward

List	Trial 1	Alternative digit list		
4-9-3	0 1	6-2-9	5-2-6	4-1-5
3-8-1-4	0 1	3-2-7-9	1-7-9-5	4-9-6-8
6-2-9-7-1	0 1	1-5-2-8-6	3-8-5-2-7	6-1-8-4-3
7-1-8-4-6-2	0 1	5-3-9-1-4-8	8-3-1-9-6-4	7-2-4-8-5-6
Total of 4				

Concentration: Month in Reverse Order (1 pt. for entire sequence correct)

Dec-Nov-Oct-Sept-Aug-Jul-Jun-May-Apr-Mar-Feb-Jan   0   1

Concentration score _____ of 5

5 ### Neck Examination:

Range of motion   Tenderness   Upper and lower limb sensation & strength

Findings: _____

6 ### Balance examination

Do one or both of the following tests.

Footwear (shoes, barefoot, braces, tape, etc.) _____

Modified Balance Error Scoring System (BESS) testing[5]

Which foot was tested (i.e. which is the **non-dominant** foot) ☐ Left ☐ Right

Testing surface (hard floor, field, etc.) _____

Condition

Double leg stance:		Errors
Single leg stance (non-dominant foot):		Errors
Tandem stance (non-dominant foot at back):		Errors

And/Or

Tandem gait[6,7]

Time (best of 4 trials): _____ seconds

7 ### Coordination examination
Upper limb coordination

Which arm was tested: ☐ Left ☐ Right

Coordination score _____ of 1

8 ### SAC Delayed Recall[4]

Delayed recall score _____ of 5

Figure 20.10. The Sport Concussion Assessment Tool 3 (SCAT3). *(continued)*

INSTRUCTIONS

Words in *Italics* throughout the SCAT3 are the instructions given to the athlete by the tester.

Symptom Scale

"You should score yourself on the following symptoms, based on how you feel now".

To be completed by the athlete. In situations where the symptom scale is being completed after exercise, it should still be done in a resting state, at least 10 minutes post exercise.
For total number of symptoms, maximum possible is 22.
For Symptom severity score, add all scores in table, maximum possible is 22 x 6 = 132.

SAC[4]

Immediate Memory

"I am going to test your memory. I will read you a list of words and when I am done, repeat back as many words as you can remember, in any order."

Trials 2 & 3:

"I am going to repeat the same list again. Repeat back as many words as you can remember in any order, even if you said the word before."

Complete all 3 trials regardless of score on trial 1 & 2. Read the words at a rate of one per second.
Score 1 pt. for each correct response. Total score equals sum across all 3 trials. Do not inform the athlete that delayed recall will be tested.

Concentration
Digits backward

"I am going to read you a string of numbers and when I am done, you repeat them back to me backwards, in reverse order of how I read them to you. For example, if I say 7-1-9, you would say 9-1-7."

If correct, go to next string length. If incorrect, read trial 2. **One point possible for each string length.** Stop after incorrect on both trials. The digits should be read at the rate of one per second.

Months in reverse order

"Now tell me the months of the year in reverse order. Start with the last month and go backward. So you'll say December, November ... Go ahead"

1 pt. for entire sequence correct

Delayed Recall

The delayed recall should be performed after completion of the Balance and Coordination Examination.

"Do you remember that list of words I read a few times earlier? Tell me as many words from the list as you can remember in any order."

Score 1 pt. for each correct response

Balance Examination

Modified Balance Error Scoring System (BESS) testing[5]

This balance testing is based on a modified version of the Balance Error Scoring System (BESS)[5]. A stopwatch or watch with a second hand is required for this testing.

"I am now going to test your balance. Please take your shoes off, roll up your pant legs above ankle (if applicable), and remove any ankle taping (if applicable). This test will consist of three twenty second tests with different stances."

(a) Double leg stance:

"The first stance is standing with your feet together with your hands on your hips and with your eyes closed. You should try to maintain stability in that position for 20 seconds. I will be counting the number of times you move out of this position. I will start timing when you are set and have closed your eyes."

(b) Single leg stance:

"If you were to kick a ball, which foot would you use? [This will be the dominant foot] Now stand on your non-dominant foot. The dominant leg should be held in approximately 30 degrees of hip flexion and 45 degrees of knee flexion. Again, you should try to maintain stability for 20 seconds with your hands on your hips and your eyes closed. I will be counting the number of times you move out of this position. If you stumble out of this position, open your eyes and return to the start position and continue balancing. I will start timing when you are set and have closed your eyes."

(c) Tandem stance:

"Now stand heel-to-toe with your non-dominant foot in back. Your weight should be evenly distributed across both feet. Again, you should try to maintain stability for 20 seconds with your hands on your hips and your eyes closed. I will be counting the number of times you move out of this position. If you stumble out of this position, open your eyes and return to the start position and continue balancing. I will start timing when you are set and have closed your eyes."

Balance testing – types of errors

1. Hands lifted off iliac crest
2. Opening eyes
3. Step, stumble, or fall
4. Moving hip into > 30 degrees abduction
5. Lifting forefoot or heel
6. Remaining out of test position > 5 sec

Each of the 20-second trials is scored by counting the errors, or deviations from the proper stance, accumulated by the athlete. The examiner will begin counting errors only after the individual has assumed the proper start position. **The modified BESS is calculated by adding one error point for each error during the three 20-second tests. The maximum total number of errors for any single condition is 10.** If a athlete commits multiple errors simultaneously, only one error is recorded but the athlete should quickly return to the testing position, and counting should resume once subject is set. Subjects that are unable to maintain the testing procedure for a minimum of **five seconds** at the start are assigned the highest possible score, ten, for that testing condition.

OPTION: For further assessment, the same 3 stances can be performed on a surface of medium density foam (e.g., approximately 50 cm x 40 cm x 6 cm).

Tandem Gait[6,7]

Participants are instructed to stand with their feet together behind a starting line (the test is best done with footwear removed). Then, they walk in a forward direction as quickly and as accurately as possible along a 38mm wide (sports tape), 3 meter line with an alternate foot heel-to-toe gait ensuring that they approximate their heel and toe on each step. Once they cross the end of the 3m line, they turn 180 degrees and return to the starting point using the same gait. A total of 4 trials are done and the best time is retained. Athletes should complete the test in 14 seconds. Athletes fail the test if they step off the line, have a separation between their heel and toe, or if they touch or grab the examiner or an object. In this case, the time is not recorded and the trial repeated, if appropriate.

Coordination Examination

Upper limb coordination
Finger-to-nose (FTN) task:

"I am going to test your coordination now. Please sit comfortably on the chair with your eyes open and your arm (either right or left) outstretched (shoulder flexed to 90 degrees and elbow and fingers extended), pointing in front of you. When I give a start signal, I would like you to perform five successive finger to nose repetitions using your index finger to touch the tip of the nose, and then return to the starting position, as quickly and as accurately as possible."

Scoring: 5 correct repetitions in < 4 seconds = 1
Note for testers: Athletes fail the test if they do not touch their nose, do not fully extend their elbow or do not perform five repetitions. **Failure should be scored as 0.**

References & Footnotes

1. This tool has been developed by a group of international experts at the 4th International Consensus meeting on Concussion in Sport held in Zurich, Switzerland in November 2012. The full details of the conference outcomes and the authors of the tool are published in The BJSM Injury Prevention and Health Protection, 2013, Volume 47, Issue 5. The outcome paper will also be simultaneously co-published in other leading biomedical journals with the copyright held by the Concussion in Sport Group, to allow unrestricted distribution, providing no alterations are made.

2. McCrory P et al., Consensus Statement on Concussion in Sport – the 3rd International Conference on Concussion in Sport held in Zurich, November 2008. British Journal of Sports Medicine 2009; 43: i76-89.

3. Maddocks, DL; Dicker, GD; Saling, MM. The assessment of orientation following concussion in athletes. Clinical Journal of Sport Medicine. 1995; 5(1): 32 – 3.

4. McCrea M. Standardized mental status testing of acute concussion. Clinical Journal of Sport Medicine. 2001; 11: 176 – 181.

5. Guskiewicz KM. Assessment of postural stability following sport-related concussion. Current Sports Medicine Reports. 2003; 2: 24 – 30.

6. Schneiders, A.G., Sullivan, S.J., Gray, A., Hammond-Tooke, G. & McCrory, P. Normative values for 16-37 year old subjects for three clinical measures of motor performance used in the assessment of sports concussions. Journal of Science and Medicine in Sport. 2010; 13(2): 196 – 201.

7. Schneiders, A.G., Sullivan, S.J., Kvarnstrom. J.K., Olsson, M., Yden. T. & Marshall, S.W. The effect of footwear and sports-surface on dynamic neurological screening in sport-related concussion. Journal of Science and Medicine in Sport. 2010; 13(4): 382 – 386

Figure 20.10. The Sport Concussion Assessment Tool 3 (SCAT3). *(continued)*

ATHLETE INFORMATION

Any athlete suspected of having a concussion should be removed from play, and then seek medical evaluation.

Signs to watch for

Problems could arise over the first 24 – 48 hours. The athlete should not be left alone and must go to a hospital at once if they:

- Have a headache that gets worse
- Are very drowsy or can't be awakened
- Can't recognize people or places
- Have repeated vomiting
- Behave unusually or seem confused; are very irritable
- Have seizures (arms and legs jerk uncontrollably)
- Have weak or numb arms or legs
- Are unsteady on their feet; have slurred speech

Remember, it is better to be safe.
Consult your doctor after a suspected concussion.

Return to play

Athletes should not be returned to play the same day of injury.
When returning athletes to play, they should be **medically cleared and then follow a stepwise supervised program,** with stages of progression.

For example:

Rehabilitation stage	Functional exercise at each stage of rehabilitation	Objective of each stage
No activity	Physical and cognitive rest	Recovery
Light aerobic exercise	Walking, swimming or stationary cycling keeping intensity, 70 % maximum predicted heart rate. No resistance training	Increase heart rate
Sport-specific exercise	Skating drills in ice hockey, running drills in soccer. No head impact activities	Add movement
Non-contact training drills	Progression to more complex training drills, eg passing drills in football and ice hockey. May start progressive resistance training	Exercise, coordination, and cognitive load
Full contact practice	Following medical clearance participate in normal training activities	Restore confidence and assess functional skills by coaching staff
Return to play	Normal game play	

There should be at least 24 hours (or longer) for each stage and if symptoms recur the athlete should rest until they resolve once again and then resume the program at the previous asymptomatic stage. Resistance training should only be added in the later stages.

If the athlete is symptomatic for more than 10 days, then consultation by a medical practitioner who is expert in the management of concussion, is recommended.

Medical clearance should be given before return to play.

Scoring Summary:

Test Domain	Score		
	Date: _____	Date: _____	Date: _____
Number of Symptoms of 22			
Symptom Severity Score of 132			
Orientation of 5			
Immediate Memory of 15			
Concentration of 5			
Delayed Recall of 5			
SAC Total			
BESS (total errors)			
Tandem Gait (seconds)			
Coordination of 1			

Notes:

_____
_____
_____
_____
_____
_____
_____
_____
_____
_____
_____
_____
_____
_____
_____

CONCUSSION INJURY ADVICE

(To be given to the **person monitoring** the concussed athlete)

This patient has received an injury to the head. A careful medical examination has been carried out and no sign of any serious complications has been found. Recovery time is variable across individuals and the patient will need monitoring for a further period by a responsible adult. Your treating physician will provide guidance as to this timeframe.

If you notice any change in behaviour, vomiting, dizziness, worsening headache, double vision or excessive drowsiness, please contact your doctor or the nearest hospital emergency department immediately.

Other important points:

- Rest (physically and mentally), including training or playing sports until symptoms resolve and you are medically cleared
- No alcohol
- No prescription or non-prescription drugs without medical supervision. Specifically:
  · No sleeping tablets
  · Do not use aspirin, anti-inflammatory medication or sedating pain killers
- Do not drive until medically cleared
- Do not train or play sport until medically cleared

Clinic phone number _____

Patient's name _____

Date / time of injury _____

Date / time of medical review _____

Treating physician _____

Contact details or stamp

Figure 20.10. The Sport Concussion Assessment Tool 3 (SCAT3).

■ **Computerized neuropsychological tests:** Recently, a number of computerized neuropsychological tests have been developed to test patients who have sustained a concussion. Advantages in administering these tests include the ability to conduct, store, retrieve, and compare baseline values with postinjury values.[9] Examples of the more common tests include the Concussion Assessment and Cognitive Testing, Automated Neuropsychological Assessment Metrics (ANAM) (National Rehabilitation Hospital, Assistive Technology and Neuroscience Center, Washington, DC), CogSport Axon (CogState Ltd, Victoria, Australia), Concussion Resolution Index (CRI) (HeadMinder, Inc, New York, NY), Concussion Vital Signs, and the Immediate Postconcussion Assessment and Cognitive Testing (ImPACT; University of Pittsburg Medical Center, Pittsburgh, PA).[1] Each of the computerized tests has published data on test–retest reliability, and all have demonstrated deficits in concussed athletes compared with their baseline assessments.[10–13]

6. **Coordination and balance**

■ **Finger-to-nose test:** The purpose of the finger-to-nose (FTN) test is to assess voluntary muscle control and upper limb coordination.[14] In order for coordinated movement to occur, there must be integration of proprioceptive information coming from the limb and going to the brain, primarily the cerebellum. The information is processed and return information is sent back to the limb, directing movement quality, speed, and accuracy. If the cerebellum has been damaged, smooth motion does not occur. The FTN test has been used to measure temporal coordination in poststroke patients.[14] The method described for performing the FTN test on poststroke patients is similar to the method described in the SCAT3. When used with poststroke patients, patients completed the test twice, once with eyes open and once with eyes closed, and the starting position is with hands on knees.[14] According to the SCAT3 protocol, to perform the FTN test, the patient is in a seated position with arm flexed at 90° and fully extended. The patient is instructed to touch his or her nose five consecutive times but must return to the starting position after each nose touch. The action is timed. The clinician should note if the patient accurately touches his or her nose and whether or not the patient returns arms fully to the starting position between each attempts (**Fig. 20.11**). The patient receives a

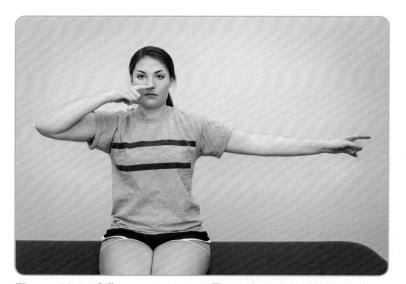

Figure 20.11. A finger-to-nose test. The patient should be seated with the eyes open and shoulders flexed to 90° with arms fully extended, stretched out in front of the patient's body. The clinician instructs the patient to touch the index finger to the nose five consecutive times, returning to the starting position between each nose touch. An inability to perform this test indicates physical disorientation and a lack of coordination and should preclude reentry to activity.

TABLE 20.2 Modified Balance Error Scoring System[a]

STANCE/CRITERIA	NUMBER OF ERRORS	MAXIMUM ERRORS ALLOWED
Double-leg stance (narrow stance; feet together): Patient should have his or her hands on the hips and eyes closed.		10
Single-leg stance (standing on nondominant foot with the dominant leg held in approximately 30° of hip flexion and 45° of knee flexion): Patient should have his or her hands on the hips and eyes closed.		10
Tandem stance (standing heel to toe with nondominant foot in back, and weight on nondominant foot): Patient should have his or her hands on the hips and eyes closed.		10
Total Scores		30

Balance Testing—Types of Errors[5]

1. Hands lifted off iliac crest
2. Opening eyes
3. Step, stumble, or fall
4. Moving hip into >30° abduction
5. Lifting forefoot or heel
6. Remaining out of test position >5 seconds

Each of the 20-second trials is scored by counting the errors, or deviations from the proper stance, accumulated by the athlete. The clinician will begin counting errors only after the patient has assumed the proper start position. *The modified Balance Error Scoring System is calculated by adding 1 error point for each error during the three 20-second tests. The maximum total number of errors for any single condition is 10.* If an athlete commits multiple errors simultaneously, only one error is recorded but the athlete should quickly return to the testing position, and counting should resume once subject is set. Subjects that are unable to maintain the testing procedure for a minimum of *5 seconds* at the start are assigned the highest possible score, 10, for that testing condition.[5]

[a]This test is based on a modified version of the original Balance Error Scoring System test and is a component of the SCAT3.[5,15,16] To administer the test, the clinician will need a device that measures time in seconds.

score of 1 if the patient is able to perform five correct repetitions in less than 4 seconds. The patient fails the test and receives a score of 0 if the patient does not touch his or her nose, does not fully extend the elbow, or cannot perform five repetitions successfully.[5]

- ■ **Modified Balance Error Scoring System (BESS):** Designed to assess impairment of balance and coordination in the physically active population, this test assesses balance using three different stances on two different types of surfaces. The BESS has been found to have moderate to good reliability in detecting large balance deficits in patients with concussion or fatigue.[15] The *modified BESS* has been found to have greater reliability than the original BESS and is more easily and quickly administered.[15,16] The assessment involves three different stances (**Table 20.2**) with each stance being completed twice, once while standing on a firm surface and again while standing on a foam surface for a total of six trials (**Fig. 20.12**). The battery of tests is performed before the start of participation in an activity or sport (e.g., as part of the preparticipation examination) to establish a baseline of information. Following head injury, the modified BESS can be administered on site or in an office/clinic setting to compare the current results with the initial findings.

Determination of Findings

Protocols for caring for patients with suspected cranial injury should be included within the organization's policy and procedures as well as a component of the EAP. If the patient is not in a crisis situation, an evaluation of vital signs, mental status, symptoms check, and neurological tests should be completed every 5 to 7 minutes to determine the progress of the condition. If the patient has been evaluated by a physician on site and the signs and symptoms linger but appear to be minor, it is essential to ensure ongoing monitoring of the patient. An individual close to the injured party, such as

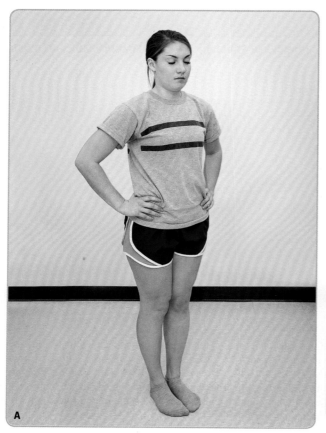

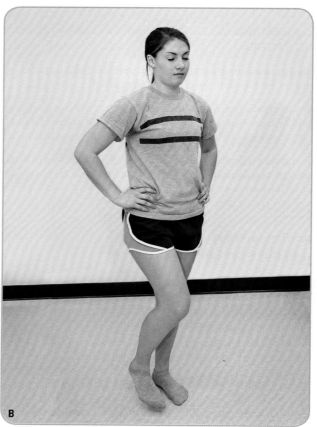

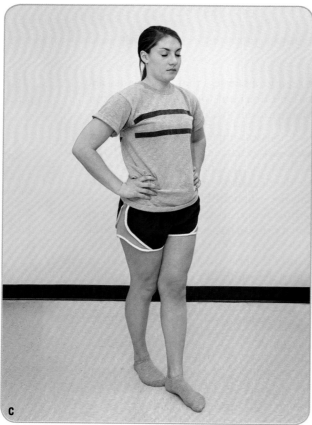

Figure 20.12. The Modified Balance Error Scoring System. This test involves three different stances (**A,** double leg; **B,** single leg; and **C,** tandem leg), each completed once while standing on a firm surface.

APPLICATION STRATEGY 20.1

Cranial Injury Evaluation

Determine the initial level of consciousness.

1. If unconscious or altered level of conscious and/or complaining of neck pain or findings consistent with cervical spine injury:
   a. Stabilize head and neck.
   b. Check ABCs.
   c. Remove equipment.
   d. Activate the emergency plan, including summoning EMS if necessary.
   e. Take and monitor vital signs (i.e., pulse, respiration, and blood pressure).
   f. Babinski reflex
2. If conscious with no complaints of neck pain or findings consistent with cervical spine injury:
   a. Take history and assess mental status:
      - Orientation (e.g., time, place, person, and situation-mechanism of injury)
      - Concentration (e.g., count digits backward or recite the months of the year in reverse order)
      - Memory (e.g., names of teams in previous contests, recall of three words and three objects, recent newsworthy events, or details of the contest)
      - Symptoms (e.g., headache, nausea, or tinnitus, pain)
   b. Observation and inspection
      - Leakage of CSF
      - Signs of trauma (e.g., deformity, body posturing, or discoloration around the eyes and behind the ears)
      - Loss of emotional control (e.g., irritability, aggressiveness, or uncontrolled crying)
   c. Palpate bony and soft-tissue structures for point tenderness, crepitus, depressions, elevations, swelling, blood, or changes in skin temperature.
   d. Neurological examination
      - Cranial nerve assessment
      - Pupil abnormalities (e.g., pupil size, response to light, eye movement, nystagmus, or blurred or double vision)
      - Strength
      - Neuropsychological assessments (SCAT3)
      - Coordination and balance (e.g., finger-to-nose test, gait, error scoring system) (SCAT3)
3. If patient presents with normal findings after repeated assessment over period of time, administer external provocation tests and monitor for onset or return or increase of symptoms.
   a. External provocative test
      - 40-yard sprint
      - Five sit-ups
      - Five push-ups
      - Five knee bends
   b. Take vital signs, and recheck every 5–7 minutes.

a parent, spouse, or roommate, should be informed of the injury and be told to look for problematic signs, including changes in behavior, unsteady gait, slurring of speech, a progressive headache or nausea, restlessness, mental confusion, or drowsiness. These danger signs should be fully explained to the observer and provided on an information sheet.

Application Strategy 20.1 summarizes an assessment of a cranial injury.

 Once history reveals the potential that the patient may have sustained a brain injury, vital signs should be assessed at once and the patient inspected for signs of skull and brain trauma. A cranial nerve assessment and assessment of mental status should be conducted followed by administering the SCAT3.

SCALP INJURIES

In attempting to keep a ball from going out of bounds, a basketball player collides with the bleachers. As the athletic trainer approaches the player, she notices bleeding from the scalp. Explain the immediate management of this injury.

The scalp is the outermost anatomical structure of the cranium and the first area of contact in head trauma. The scalp is highly vascular and bleeds freely when compromised, making it a frequent site for soft-tissue injuries.

Etiology

Blunt trauma or penetrating trauma often leads to scalp abrasions, lacerations, contusions, or hematomas between the layers of tissue.

Signs and Symptoms

The patient will report being hit on the head. Bleeding can be profuse and may mask serious underlying conditions; therefore, damage to the brain and spine should be cleared through history taking and if needed, physical examination.

Management

The primary concern with any scalp injury is to control bleeding, prevent contamination, and assess for a possible skull fracture. In keeping with universal precautions, latex gloves should be worn during the management of any open wound. Mild direct pressure should be applied to the area with sterile gauze until the bleeding has stopped. The wound should be inspected for any foreign bodies or signs of a skull fracture. If a skull fracture is ruled out, the wound should be cleansed with surgical soap or saline solution and covered with a sterile dressing, and the patient should be referred to a physician for possible suturing.

Abrasions and contusions should be treated with gentle cleansing, topical antiseptics, and ice to control hemorrhage. Hematomas, or "goose eggs," involve a collection of blood between the layers of the scalp and the skull. Crushed ice and a pressure bandage should be used to control hemorrhage and edema. If the condition does not improve in 24 hours, the patient should be referred to a physician.

In managing the bleeding scalp, it would be appropriate for the athletic trainer to hand sterile gauze to the patient and direct the patient to apply gentle pressure to the area while the athletic trainer puts on latex gloves. Once gloved, the athletic trainer should inspect the area and continue to apply pressure until the bleeding has stopped. If a skull fracture is ruled out, the area should be cleansed with surgical soap or saline solution and covered with a sterile dressing. Depending on the nature of the wound, referral to a physician may be required for possible suturing.

SKULL FRACTURES

While driving toward the basket, a basketball player is undercut. She falls sideways and strikes her head sharply on the floor. The patient complains of an intense headache, disorientation, and blurred vision. Might these signs and symptoms indicate that a possible skull fracture may be present?

Etiology

When a severe blow to the head occurs, a skull fracture should always be suspected. Skull fractures may be linear (i.e., in a line), comminuted (i.e., in multiple pieces), depressed (i.e., fragments driven

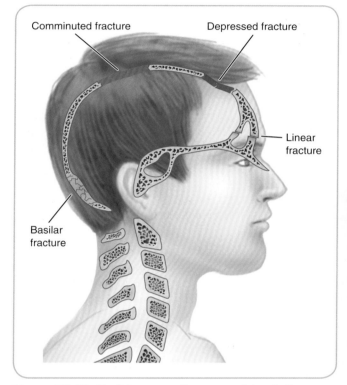

Figure 20.13. Skull fractures. Fractures of the skull are categorized as linear, comminuted, depressed, or basilar.

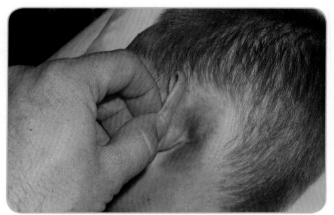

Figure 20.14. Battle sign. Superficial ecchymosis over the mastoid process.

internally toward the brain), or basilar (i.e., involving the base of the skull) (**Fig. 20.13**). Often, however, it is difficult to detect the presence of a deep scalp hematoma. With a break in the skin adjacent to the fracture site and a tear in the underlying dura mater, a patient has a high risk of bacterial infection into the intracranial cavity, which can result in **septic meningitis**.

Signs and Symptoms

Depending on the fracture site, different signs may appear (**Box 20.1**). For example, a fracture at the eyebrow level may travel into the anterior cranial fossa and sinuses, leading to discoloration around the eyes (**raccoon eyes**). Bony fragments may damage the optic or olfactory cranial nerves, leading to blindness or a loss of smell. A basilar fracture above and behind the ear may lead to a **Battle sign**, which is a discoloration that can appear within minutes behind the ear (**Fig. 20.14**). In some cases, blood or CSF may leak from the nose or ear canal. Identification of the type of leaking fluid

---

BOX 20.1 Possible Signs and Symptoms of a Skull Fracture

- Visible deformity (do not be misled by a "goose egg" [a fracture may be under the site])
- Bleeding or clear fluid (CSF) from the nose and/or ear
- Deep laceration or severe bruise to the scalp
- Loss of smell
- Palpable depression or crepitus

- Loss of sight or major vision disturbances
- Unequal pupils
- Unconsciousness for more than 2 minutes after direct trauma to the head
- Discoloration under both eyes (raccoon eyes) or behind the ear (Battle sign)

APPLICATION STRATEGY 20.2

Evaluation and Management of a Suspected Skull Fracture

Evaluation

1. Stabilize the head and neck.
2. Check the ABCs.
3. Take vital signs (i.e., pulse, respiration, and blood pressure).
4. Observe for the following:

   - Swelling or discoloration around the eyes or behind the ears
   - Blood or CSF leaking from the nose or ears
   - Pupil size, pupillary response to light, and eye movement
5. Palpate for depressions, blood, and crepitus. Palpate cervical vertebrae for associated neck injury.

Management

1. Activate the emergency plan, including summoning EMS.
2. Cover any open wounds with a sterile dressing but do not apply pressure to the area.
3. Elevate the upper body and head if there is no evidence of shock or of neck or spinal injury. If such evidence is present, keep the patient lying flat.
4. Treat for shock.
5. Recheck vital signs and symptoms every 5 minutes until EMS arrives.

---

can be assessed by gently absorbing some of it with a gauze pad and then observing the pad for possible separation of clear fluid from blood. This action is called "targeting," or the "halo test," and it is important to note that this test is not always reliable. A hearing loss or facial paralysis also may be present. A fracture to the temple region may damage the meningeal arteries, causing epidural bleeding between the dura mater and the skull (epidural hematoma). This can be life-threatening and is discussed in more detail in the Focal Cerebral Conditions.

Management

A skull fracture can be life-threatening. If any of the signs and symptoms mentioned in **Box 20.1** becomes apparent, activate the emergency plan. **Application Strategy 20.2** summarizes management of a suspected skull fracture.

Signs that indicate a possible skull fracture include deformity, unequal pupils, discoloration around both eyes or behind the ears, bleeding or CSF leaking from the nose and/or ear, and any loss of sight or smell. The basketball player did not exhibit any of these red flags. Even so, the patient should be thoroughly evaluated for head trauma. If any of the signs appear during the assessment, the emergency plan should be activated.

FOCAL CEREBRAL CONDITIONS

? After colliding with a fellow lacrosse player, a player complains of a headache and dizziness. Following 15 minutes of ice application to the region, the patient complains of increasing headache, dizziness, and nausea. There also is increased mental confusion. What do these symptoms indicate, and how should this injury be managed?

Focal cerebral injuries usually result in a localized collection of blood or hematoma. The skull has no room for additional accumulation of blood or fluid; as such, any additional foreign matter within the cranial cavity increases pressure on the brain, leading to significant alteration in neurological function. Depending on the location of the accumulated blood relative to the dura mater, these hematomas are classified as epidural (outside the dura mater) or subdural (deep to the dura mater). A cerebral contusion also is classified as a focal injury; however, no mass-occupying lesion is associated with this condition.

Epidural Hematoma

Etiology

An epidural hematoma is very rare during sport participation. Typically, the condition is caused by a direct blow to the side of the head and almost always is associated with a skull fracture (**Fig. 20.15A**). If the middle meningeal artery or its branches are severed, the subsequent arterial bleeding leads to a "high-pressure" epidural hematoma. The middle meningeal vein also may be damaged, leading to a more insidious onset of symptoms.

Signs and Symptoms

The patient may experience an initial LOC at the time of injury, followed by a lucid interval during which the patient feels relatively normal and asymptomatic. Within 10 to 20 minutes, however, a gradual decline in mental status occurs as the hematoma outside the brain reaches a critical size and compresses the underlying brain. Other signs and symptoms may include increased headache, drowsiness, nausea, and vomiting, as well as a decreased level of consciousness; an ipsilateral dilated pupil on the side of the hematoma; and subsequently, contralateral weakness and decerebrate posturing (see **Fig. 7.1**). This triad of symptoms, however, is only present in one-third of patients with epidural hematomas.[17]

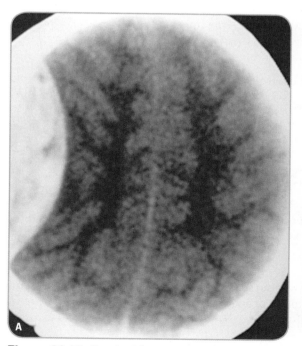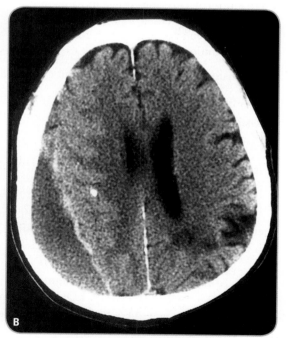

Figure 20.15. Cerebral hematomas. A, This epidural hematoma resulted from a fracture that extended into the orbital roof and sinus area, leading to rapid hemorrhage in the right frontal lobe of the brain. **B,** The subdural hematoma on the right side of the brain is fairly evident. A chronic subdural hematoma can be seen on the left side of the brain.

Management

Activation of the emergency plan, including summoning emergency medical services (EMS), is warranted. The clinician should continue to maintain the ABCs, assess vital signs, and treat for shock. This condition may require immediate surgery to decompress the hematoma to control arterial bleeding.

Subdural Hematoma

Etiology

A subdural hematoma is approximately threefold more frequent than an epidural hematoma and is the leading cause of catastrophic death in football players.[17] Hemorrhage occurs when the bridging veins between the brain and the dura mater are torn. It is caused by acceleration forces of the head rather than by the impact of the force. A subdural hematoma may be classified as either acute, which presents 48 to 72 hours after injury, or chronic (**Fig. 20.15B**), which occurs in a later time frame with more variable clinical manifestations, and either simple or complicated. In a simple subdural hematoma, blood collects in the subdural space, but no underlying cerebral injury occurs. Complex subdural hematomas are characterized by contusions of the brain's surface and associated cerebral swelling that increase intracerebral pressure. The mortality rate for simple subdural hematomas is approximately 20%, whereas complicated subdural hematomas have a mortality rate of 50%.[18]

Signs and Symptoms

In a simple subdural hematoma, the patient is less likely to be rendered unconscious. These patients seldom demonstrate deterioration in the level of consciousness, and fewer than 15% have a lucid interval. **In a complicated subdural hematoma, the patient typically is knocked out and remains unconscious.** Signs and symptoms of increasing intracranial pressure include the following:

- Pupillary dilation and retinal changes on the affected side
- Irregular eye tracking or eye movement
- Severe headache
- Nausea and/or vomiting
- Confusion and/or drastic changes in emotional control
- Progressive or sudden impairment of consciousness
- Rising blood pressure
- Falling pulse rate
- Irregular respirations
- Increased body temperature

Signs and symptoms may not become apparent for hours, days, or even weeks after injury, subsequent to the clot absorbing fluid and expanding.

Activation of the emergency plan, including summoning EMS, is warranted. The clinician should continue to maintain the ABCs, assess vital signs, and treat for shock.

Management

The early diagnosis of a subdural hematoma is essential for a successful recovery. LOC implies a poor prognosis, with an overall mortality rate of 35% to 50%.[19]

Cerebral Contusion

A cerebral contusion is a focal injury, but a mass-occupying lesion is not present. Instead, a microhemorrhage, cerebral infarction, necrosis, and edema of the brain occur. This condition is visible on a computed tomographic (CT) scan as an area of high-density blood interspersed with brain tissue.

Etiology

Cerebral contusions most often occur as a result of an acceleration–deceleration mechanism from the inward deformation of the skull at the impact site. For example, an acceleration force is generated when another patient or an object (e.g., a ball or hockey puck) hits a patient's head. In this situation, the site of maximal injury usually is at the point of impact (i.e., coup injury). In comparison, deceleration forces are generated when a patient's head strikes the ground, and the subsequent site of maximal injury is opposite the point of impact (i.e., contrecoup injury). Injury results from the brain rebounding against the skull or from a vacuum phenomenon existing within the parenchyma at that location. The contrecoup lesions lead to hemorrhage in the cerebral tissue directly opposite the impact site, typically at the inferior surfaces of the frontal and temporal lobes. Although the contusion can occur in any portion of the cortex, brainstem, or cerebellum, these lobes, because of the close anatomical relationship between bony ridges and the frontal lobes, are particularly susceptible to this type of injury. The injury may be limited to small, localized areas or may involve large, extensive areas.

Signs and Symptoms

Clinical signs and symptoms vary greatly, depending on the location, number, and extent of the hemorrhagic lesions. A cerebral contusion injury may evolve over hours or days after the injury. The patient may present with essentially normal function or may experience any type of neurological deterioration, including coma. Frequently, behavioral or mental status changes are present because of the involvement of the frontal or temporal lobes.[20] A danger flag (red flag) exists when a patient has a normal neurological examination but persistent symptoms such as headaches, dizziness, or nausea occurs.

Management

Activation of the emergency plan, including summoning EMS, is warranted. The clinician should continue to maintain the ABCs, assess vital signs, and treat for shock.

> Increasing dizziness, headache, nausea, and mental confusion are red flags that indicate serious intracranial hemorrhage. The management of this condition involves activating the emergency plan (including summoning EMS), monitoring vital signs, and treating for shock.

DIFFUSE CEREBRAL CONDITIONS

> **?** After colliding with an opponent, a high school football player was momentarily stunned, "saw stars," and had blurred vision for approximately 30 seconds. After 3 or 4 minutes, the patient reported feeling much better, except for a slight headache. Can this patient return to activity?

Diffuse cerebral injuries involve trauma to widespread areas of the brain rather than to one specific site. The range of these injuries can vary from mild to severe, involving the impairment of neural function, structural damage, or both.

Cerebral Concussions

Etiology

In November 2001, the First International Symposium on Concussion in Sport was held in Vienna[21] to provide recommendations to improve the safety and health of athletes who suffer concussive injuries. Several issues were discussed, including protective equipment, epidemiology, and basic and clinical science, grading systems, cognitive assessment, and management. A second international symposium in 2004, held in Prague,[22] subsequently defined sport-related concussions as a complex pathophysiologic process affecting the brain, induced by traumatic biomechanical forces. In 2008, the Third International Conference on Concussion in Sport, held in Zurich,[23] sought to revise and update recommendations from the first two symposia. The Fourth International Symposium on Concussion in Sport was held in Zurich in 2012[6] and further revised the SCAT and graduated return to play protocols. The science and our understanding of concussions continue to evolve; therefore, the management of return-to-play (RTP) decisions remains the realm of clinical judgment for each individual patient.

Definition of Concussion

Although some professionals use the terms concussion and mild traumatic brain injury (mTBI) interchangeably, this is not recommended. Concussions are considered a subset of traumatic brain injury and should never be referred to as "ding" or "bell ringer."[1,6] The Fourth International Symposium on Concussion in Sport defined concussion as "a brain injury and is a complex pathophysiological process affecting the brain, induced by biomechanical forces."[6] With concussions, certain common features incorporate clinical, pathological, and biomechanical injury constructs that may be used to further define the nature of a concussive head injury and include the following[1,6,21–23]:

- Concussions may be caused by a direct blow to the head, face, neck, or elsewhere on the body with an impulsive force that can be transmitted to the head. These injuries typically result in the rapid onset of short-lived impairment of neurological function that resolves spontaneously. In some cases, the onset of impairment may take longer.[6]

- Neuropathologic changes may occur, but the acute clinical symptoms typically reflect a functional disturbance rather than a structural injury.

- Concussions may or may not involve an LOC but instead may lead to a gradient of clinical symptoms that are associated with grossly normal structural neuroimaging studies.

- Resolution of the clinical and cognitive symptoms usually follows a sequential course. The injury may cause an immediate and transient impairment of neural function, such as alteration of consciousness and disturbance of vision and equilibrium. Under normal conditions, the brain balances a series of electrochemical events in billions of brain cells. When the brain is shaken or jarred, brain function can be disrupted temporarily without causing injury or damage to brain tissue. For example, mild trauma can result in an interruption of cerebral function. Signs and symptoms range from mild to moderate and are transient and reversible. This can be attributed to the minimal damage to soft-tissue structures. As the impact magnitude increases with an acceleration injury, both cerebral function and structural damage may occur, resulting in more serious signs and symptoms. These include varying degrees of LOC, headache, confusion, memory loss, nausea, **tinnitus**, pupillary changes, dizziness, and loss of coordination.

Classification of Concussions

Although more than 16 different classification schemes attempt to define the various degrees of brain dysfunction in cerebral concussions, current best practices do not recommend using a concussion grading scale to base concussion management.[1,6] Instead, once a diagnosis of concussion has been made, management should be based on the patient's individual findings. The majority (80% to 90%) of concussions resolve in a short (7- to 10-day) period, although the recovery time frame may be longer in children and adolescents.[1,6] It is critical to understand that no two concussions are identical, nor will the signs and symptoms be the same. Each injury will vary depending on the magnitude of force to the head, the level of metabolic dysfunction, the tissue damage and duration of time needed to recover, the number of previous concussions, and the time between injuries.

Baseline Measurements

Information obtained postinjury is more meaningful when there is baseline data for comparison. Athletes at high risk for sustaining a concussion should have baseline testing done prior to the onset of the competitive season. For athletes who have a history of concussions as well as adolescent athletes, baseline testing should occur annually.[1] Baseline testing should include clinical history and

TABLE 20.3 Concussion Baseline Testing Protocol Sample

COMPONENT	SAMPLE TESTING/QUESTIONS
History	1. How many concussions have you had? 2. What is the time span in which you experienced your concussions? 3. What was the longest amount of time it took for all symptoms to resolve? 4. Did you ever lose consciousness? If so, how long? 5. Did you ever experience seizures? 6. Do you ever or are you currently experiencing any of these symptoms? 　a. Headache, nausea, vomiting, dizziness, ringing in the ears, blurred vision 　b. Dizziness, memory loss, confusion, feeling in fog, disoriented, fatigued 　c. Difficulty sleeping or altered sleeping patterns, change in personality
Physical and neurological assessment	1. Vital sign assessment 2. Cranial nerve assessment 3. VOMS[25]
Motor control	1. Modified BESS test 2. FTN test
Neurocognitive function	1. SCAT3 (sections 4 and 8) 2. The ImPACT test

The SCAT3 can be used in entirety to obtain baseline measurements.

symptoms, physical and neurological assessment, and motor control and neurocognitive function.[1,6] A sample concussion baseline assessment protocol is presented in **Table 20.3**.

Signs and Symptoms

The 2012 Zurich panel agreed that the diagnosis of a concussion will involve the assessment of a range of clinical manifestations in five categories: symptoms, physical, emotional, cognitive, and sleep (**Table 20.4**).[6] A headache is one of the most reported symptoms (86%) with a concussion.[2,3] LOC occurs in less than 10% of concussions but does indicate that further imaging and intervention is necessary.[2] Amnesia is another important indicator of a more serious injury. In a recent study, it was found that males reported more cognitive symptoms, such as amnesia and confusion/disorientation, more frequently than did females. Females, on the other hand, reported more neurobehavioral and somatic symptoms, such as drowsiness and sensitivity to noise.[24] The patient should be assessed for **retrograde** (before the event) and **anterograde** (after the event) amnesia by asking questions about events before and after the injury. Other signs and symptoms that may become apparent are similar to depression, anxiety, and attention-deficit disorders. It is recommended that the patient should be monitored at 5-minute intervals from the time of injury until the condition is rectified or the patient is referred for further care.[3]

TABLE 20.4 Clinical Manifestations of Concussion

SYMPTOMS	PHYSICAL	EMOTIONAL	COGNITIVE	DISORDERED SLEEP
Headache Nausea Vomiting	LOC Balance problems Visual problems Fatigued Photophobia Sensitivity to noise	Irritability Sadness More emotional Nervousness	Feeling like in a "fog" Dazed or stunned Feeling slowed down Difficulty concentrating Difficulty remembering Forgetful of recent information Confused about recent events Answers questions slowly Repeats questions	Insomnia Drowsiness Sleeping more than usual Sleeping less than usual Difficulty falling asleep

External Provocative Tests

For patients who report no symptoms, it may be appropriate to use external provocative tests. If the assessment has already determined a possible intracranial injury, the patient should not be subjected to these tests. External provocative tests require the patient to perform exertional activities, such as running or push-ups. Any appearance of associated symptoms (e.g., headaches, dizziness, nausea, unsteadiness, photophobia, blurred or double vision, loss of emotional control, or mental status changes) is abnormal.

- 40-yard sprint

- Five jumping jacks

- Five sit-ups

- Five push-ups

- Five knee bends

Management

Because many of the signs and symptoms of concussion are similar to those of cerebral hematomas and contusions, these more acute life-threatening conditions must be ruled out. If cerebral hematoma or contusion is suspected at any time during the assessment and monitoring process, or cannot be clearly ruled out, the EAP should be activated and the patient monitored for ABCs until EMS arrives and care is transferred.

For the patient with a suspected concussion, the patient should be removed from play and examined immediately using standard emergency management principles, including the assessment of the cervical spine and cranial nerves to identify any cervical spine or vascular intracerebral injuries.[6] Once the immediate first aid is administered, a detailed clinical assessment of signs and symptoms should be made using the SCAT3 or a similar tool, such as Maddocks questions, or the Standardized Assessment of Concussion (SAC) (**Fig. 20.10**).[1,5,6]

A brief **Vestibular/Ocular Motor Screening (VOMS) Assessment** has also been found to be a clinically useful tool for detecting sport-related concussions.[25] VOMS is designed to assess for presence of vestibular and ocular motor deficits by comparing onset and intensity of patient symptoms pre- and posttesting. Five motions or domains are tested: (1) smooth pursuit, (2) horizontal and vertical **saccades**, (3) convergence, (4) horizontal vestibular ocular reflex (VOR), and (5) visual motion sensitivity (VMS). Patients are asked to rate their symptoms on a scale of 0 (none) to 10 (severe) after each assessment to see if the motion/actions provoke symptoms. Patients are questioned on the following symptoms: headache, dizziness, nausea, and fogginess. Onset or increase in symptoms suggests presence of vestibular/ocular motor deficits associated with a concussion. VOMS can be used as part of the battery of baseline tests for acute evaluation and follow evaluation. Positive findings suggest that the patient may benefit from having vestibular ocular therapy as part of the overall treatment plan.[25] The suspected diagnosis of a concussion should include one or more of the following domains[6]:

- Symptoms: somatic (e.g., headache), cognitive (e.g., feeling "like in a fog"), and/or emotional symptoms (e.g., extremes of emotion or unstable)

- Physical signs (e.g., LOC, amnesia, visual problems)

- Behavior changes (e.g., irritability, sadness)

- Cognitive impairment (e.g., slowed reaction times, difficulty concentrating)

- Sleep disturbance (e.g., drowsiness)

If any of these signs and symptoms is present, a concussion should be suspected. The patient is removed from participation and evaluated by a physician or athletic trainer. The diagnosis of concussion is made through the clinical evaluation and supported by assessment tools, such as the SCAT3.[1,6] The patient should be monitored for the initial few hours postinjury. During this time, vital signs and assessment of mental status, neurological function, and symptoms should be checked at regular intervals for deterioration in status.[6] The patient is not allowed to return to participation on the day of injury.[1]

Patients who have been diagnosed with a concussion should be instructed to avoid ingesting or taking any medications or substances that may impair cognitive function and neurological recovery.[1] During the acute stages of recovery (the first 24 to 48 hours), the patient is instructed to avoid physical exertion and cognitive load and instead should be encouraged to rest. It is important to eat well and stay hydrated. The patient will also need academic accommodation during the healing process because cognitive load can delay the healing process and exacerbate symptoms.[1]

Return-to-Play Protocol

The foundation of concussion management is physical and cognitive rest until symptoms resolve and then a graduated program of exertion is conducted prior to medical clearance and RTP. Most patients will recover spontaneously over several days, but each must be reminded that both a physical and cognitive rest is required. Activities that require focus and concentration (e.g., academic work, video games, text messaging) may exacerbate symptoms and delay recovery. RTP following a concussion should follow a stepwise process, as outlined in **Table 20.5**. With this progression, the patient can proceed to the next level if asymptomatic at the current level. Generally speaking, each level should take approximately 24 hours so that the patient can move through the protocol in about 1 week once asymptomatic at rest and with provocative exercise.

In some sport settings with physicians experienced in concussion management and with sufficient resources (e.g., access to neuropsychologists, consultants, neuroimaging), as well as access to immediate sideline neurocognitive assessment, RTP may be more rapid. The same basic principles still require full clinical and cognitive recovery before consideration of RTP. This is supported by the American Academy of Neurology, U.S. Team Physician Consensus Statement, and National Athletic Trainers' Association position statement.[8,16] For individuals younger than the age of 18 years, it is recommended that a more conservative approach be taken.[6,12]

Posttraumatic Headaches

Etiology

Posttraumatic vascular headaches can be confused with a simple concussion or a postconcussive headache. A vascular headache is a result of vasospasm and does not usually occur with impact but rather develops shortly afterward.

TABLE 20.5 Graduated Return-to-Play Protocol

REHABILITATION STAGE	FUNCTIONAL EXERCISE AT EACH STAGE OF REHABILITATION	OBJECTIVE OF EACH STAGE
1. Active recovery	Symptom limited physical and cognitive rest; biking in darkened room, low intensity, no resistance, looking forward with no head motion	Recovery
2. Light aerobic exercise	Walking, swimming, or stationary cycling, keeping intensity <70% of maximum predicted heart rate; no resistance training	Increase heart rate
3. Sport-specific exercise	Skating drills in ice hockey, running drills in soccer, no head impact activities	Add movement
4. Noncontact training drills	Progression to more complex training drills (e.g., passing drills in football and ice hockey); may start progressive resistance training	Exercise, coordination, and cognitive load
5. Full-contact practice	Following medical clearance, participate informal training activities	Restore athlete's confidence; coaching staff assesses functional skills
6. Return to play	Normal game play	

From McCrory P, Meeuwisse WH, Aubry M, et al. Consensus statement on concussion in sport: the 4th International Conference on Concussion in Sport held in Zurich, November 2012. *Br J Sports Med.* 2013;47:250–258.

Signs and Symptoms

Symptoms, such as a localized area of blindness, may follow the appearance of brilliantly colored, shimmering lights (scintillating scotoma). Posttraumatic migraine headaches, also referred to as a footballer's migraine, have been reported in soccer players after repetitive heading of the ball. In addition, migraines are characterized by recurrent attacks of severe headache with sudden onset, with or without visual or gastrointestinal problems.

Management

This patient should be immediately referred to a physician for further evaluation and care.

Postconcussion Syndrome

Etiology

Postconcussion syndrome (PCS) may develop after any concussion and tends to occur more frequently in women than in men.[26,27] There is a normal course of symptom persistence after any concussion, which is generally followed by a gradual resolution. The difference between postconcussive *symptoms* and postconcussive *syndrome* is the length of symptom persistence. A myriad of cognitive, physical, or emotional impairments may last for several weeks to months after injury. The extended duration of symptoms is thought to be related to altered neurotransmitter function.

Signs and Symptoms

Physical symptoms of PCS include headache, vertigo, fatigue and low energy, sleep disturbance, nausea, vision changes, tinnitus, dizziness, light, and photophobia. Cognitive symptoms include slowed thinking and response time, mental fogginess, poor concentration, distractibility, trouble with learning and memory, disorganization, and problem-solving difficulties. Behavioral symptoms may include depression, anxiety, panic attacks, irritability, personality changes, increased emotionality, clinginess, apathy, increased sensitivity to alcohol, and lowered frustration tolerance.[28] Some of these symptoms may predispose the patient to second-impact syndrome.

Management

The patient can undergo magnetic resonance imaging (MRI) or CT, but the scan generally is normal in the initial and the follow-up evaluation. No definitive treatment exists other than independent symptomatic measures to control the symptoms. When available, patients with PCS should be referred to an experienced neuropsychologist for evaluation. Computerized neuropsychiatric testing may be helpful as a tool for RTP decisions, and with persisting symptoms, traditional neuropsychiatric testing can be considered. Medications may be beneficial in some cases. A physician and neuropsychologist should supervise the level of activity and should prohibit the patient from returning to activity until symptoms resolve both at rest and on exertion. A trial off of any medications for PCS is essential to be certain the patient has truly become asymptomatic and has a symptom-free interval before RTP.[1,29]

Second-Impact Syndrome

Etiology

Second-impact syndrome (SIS), a type of diffuse brain injury, is precipitated by an earlier event where a patient sustains a concussion which is unresolved. If, while in this postconcussive state, the patient receives a second blow to the head, SIS may result. Diffuse cerebral swelling and brainstem herniation occur.[30] This cascade of events can occur in 3 to 5 minutes from the time the patient receives the subsequent blow.[31]

Signs and Symptoms

With the initial injury, visual, motor, or sensory changes occur, and the patient may have difficulty with thought and memory. Before these symptoms resolve, which may take days or even weeks, the patient returns to activity and sustains a second head trauma. This second trauma may be relatively minor and does not have to be the result of direct contact. Following the trauma, the patient may appear to be stunned but often completes the current action or play and, in some cases, can walk unassisted. As the vascular engorgement within the cranium increases intracranial pressure, the brainstem becomes compromised. Subsequently, the patient collapses with rapidly dilating pupils, progressing to a loss of eye movement, coma, and respiratory failure. The usual interval from second impact to brainstem failure is short (typically 2 to 5 minutes).

Management

Management involves an immediate activation of the emergency care plan, including summoning EMS, and maintenance of basic life support. The first step in providing appropriate care is recognizing that the patient has sustained a traumatic brain injury and immediate activation of the EAP and summoning EMS is imperative. For patients with a Glasgow Coma Scale of less than 9 and an SpO_2 level of less than 90%, supplemental oxygen should be administered while waiting for EMS to arrive.[32] Otherwise, maintain open airway, monitor LOC and ABCs, assess vital signs, and treat for shock.

During efforts to prevent SIS, it is imperative that any patient who complains of a headache, light-headedness, visual disturbances, or other neurological symptoms not be allowed to participate in any physical activity with the potential for head trauma until totally asymptomatic.

 The patient was momentarily stunned, "saw stars," and had blurred vision. This is not uncommon in a simple concussion. A lingering headache should signal caution, however, and return to activity should not be permitted. This patient should be carefully watched for increased headache intensity, unsteady gait, nausea, photophobia, or mood swings, which dictate immediate evaluation by a physician.

FACIAL CONDITIONS

? A hockey player was taking a shot on goal when his stick hit the jaw of the player guarding him. That player skated off the ice and was bleeding from the mouth and unable to close the jaw. He is having difficulty articulating his words. Explain the palpation of this condition. What type of injury should be suspected, and why?

Injuries to the cheek, nose, lips, and jaw are very common in sports that involve moving projectiles (e.g., sticks, balls, bats, racquets), in contact sports (e.g., football, rugby, ice hockey), and in sports that involve collisions with objects (e.g., diving, skiing, ice hockey, swimming). Many of these injuries can be prevented by wearing properly fitted face masks and mouth guards. Because the facial area has a vast arterial system, lacerations bleed freely and rapid swelling often hides the true extent of injury. **Box 20.2** identifies the signs and symptoms of serious facial injuries that warrant further examination by a physician.

BOX 20.2 Facial Red Flags Requiring Further Examination by a Physician

- Obvious deformity or crepitus
- Irregular eye movement or failure to accommodate to light
- Appearance of a long face
- Malocclusion of the teeth
- Increased pain on palpation

Facial Soft-Tissue Conditions

Etiology

Facial injuries are very common in contact and collision sports. Contusions, which are the most commonly encountered facial injury, usually result from blunt trauma.[33] Blunt trauma can be caused by a direct compressive force with a sharp object, such as hockey puck or another player's elbow or head.

Signs and Symptoms

As in scalp injuries, facial injuries are painful and bleed freely.

Management

Facial contusions, abrasions, and lacerations are managed in the same manner as those located elsewhere on the body. Ice is applied to control swelling and hemorrhage. If an abrasion or laceration is present, the wound should be cleansed with sterile saline, an antibiotic ointment should be used, and an occlusive dressing of gauze or tape should be applied. Tissue adhesive (e.g., DERMABOND) is recommended for the closure of simple lacerations, rather than butterfly bandages or Steri-Strips, particularly where there is not a point of high skin tension. The area can then be protected with sterile gauze and tape. The patient can return to participation, but at the conclusion of the event, the patient should see a physician to determine if sutures are needed. Lacerations older than 12 hours should not be sutured but, rather, should be allowed to heal by secondary intention because of the increased risk of wound infection.[34] Larger and more complicated injuries, such as those with jagged edges or damage to nerves, veins, or bony structures, should be referred immediately to a physician.

Temporomandibular Joint Conditions

Etiology

The TMJ is a sliding hinge joint that is stabilized by ligaments and is separated into upper and lower compartments by a fibrocartilage meniscus. Injury occurs when a blow to the mandible transmits the force to the condyles. Injuries may involve intracapsular bleeding (hemarthrosis), inflammation of the capsular ligaments (capsulitis), meniscal displacement, subluxation/dislocation of the condyles, or fracture.

Signs and Symptoms

Common signs and symptoms include an inability to open the mouth (normal opening = 40 mm or 1.6 in), deviation of the jaw to the side of the injury on opening, pain on opening and biting, malocclusion (change in bite), joint noise (i.e., clicking, popping, crepitus), or an inability to close the mouth.[33]

Management

A crushed ice pack should be placed over the area to control swelling. The clinician may elect to temporarily immobilize the jaw with an elastic bandage wrapped under the chin and over the top of the head. Subsequent management of TMJ injuries often involves refraining from opening the mouth for 7 to 10 days and eating a soft diet. Anti-inflammatory medication may assist in reducing pain and inflammation. During the acute period, lifting of heavy weights should be restricted.

Facial Fractures

Direct impact can fracture the facial bones, including the mandible (jaw), the maxilla (upper jaw), the zygomatic bone (cheek), or nasal bones. The most common fractures occur to the nasal bones, followed by the zygomatic bone and the mandible, respectively.[35]

Zygomatic Fractures

■ **Etiology**

Besides forming the cheekbone, the zygoma forms a portion of the eye orbit and orbital rim, serves as an attachment point for the masseter muscle, and forms the outer facial frame. As such, fractures can affect the vision, the function of the jaw, and cosmetically, the width of the face.[36] Fractures to the zygomatic bone are typically caused by a direct blow to the arch, such as when being hit by a hockey puck or hockey stick.

■ Signs and Symptoms

Direct impact to the zygomatic bone results in a flat or depressed appearance of the cheek. Swelling and periorbital ecchymosis about the eye may occlude vision and hide damage to the orbit. Occasionally, the eye on the side of the fracture may appear to be sunken, or the eye opposite the fracture may appear to be raised. Double vision is common, and paresthesia or anesthesia (numbness) may be present on the affected cheek.

■ Management

A crushed ice pack should be placed over the area to control swelling, but it is important to avoid pressure or compression over the fracture site. The patient should be referred immediately to a physician. In most cases, the condition can easily be reduced surgically and may not require internal fixation. An exception occurs when the fracture involves the eye orbit and surgical repair becomes more extensive. Healing usually occurs within 6 to 8 weeks. Special facial protection should be worn for 3 to 4 months. A complication of this condition includes blurred vision over an extended period. As such, patients in activities requiring eye–hand coordination may not return to the previous level of participation for some time.

Mandibular Fractures

■ Etiology

Direct trauma to the lower jaw, often seen in contact sports, can lead to a mandibular fracture. Because of the sharp angles and little padding, this bone is particularly at risk for injury.

■ Signs and Symptoms

Mandibular fractures present with swelling, malocclusion, numbness in the distribution of the inferior alveolar nerve (lower lip), and intraoral lacerations.[36] This injury seldom occurs as an isolated, single fracture; it more often is a double fracture or a fracture dislocation. The most common fracture sites are the mandibular angle and condyles, which lead to malocclusion (**Fig. 20.16**). Because the articulation of words is impossible, changes in speech are apparent. Oral bleeding may occur even though a mouth guard is properly fitted and worn. Pain, discoloration, swelling, and facial distortion may be present. The patient is unable to maintain a firm bite on a tongue depressor placed in the mouth (**Fig. 20.17**).

■ Management

It is important with this type of fracture for the clinician to maintain an open airway, because the tongue may occlude the airway. Management involves dressing any open wounds and immobilizing the jaw with an elastic bandage wrapped under the chin and over the top of the head. A crushed ice pack may be placed over the area to control swelling; however, pressure or compression over the fracture site should be avoided. The patient should be referred immediately to a physician.

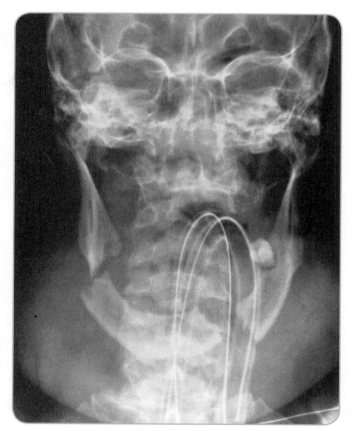

Figure 20.16. A mandibular fracture. The most common site for a mandibular fracture is near the angle of the jaw, which leads to malocclusion of the teeth.

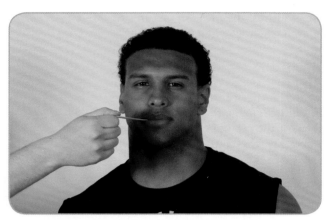

Figure 20.17. The tongue blade test. In a suspected mandibular fracture, a tongue blade (tongue depressor) is placed in the patient's mouth. The patient is instructed to hold the blade in place as the clinician rotates or twists the blade. A positive sign is the inability to hold a firm bite on the blade or increased pain on movement of the blade.

Repair involves internal fixation (i.e., wiring the jaw closed) or using bone plates, which may allow some patients to return to sport participation. During the healing period, a high-protein, high-carbohydrate liquid diet is required. A weight loss of 5% to 10% is not uncommon. Mild activities such as stationary bicycling, swimming, and the use of light weights to maintain muscle tone and conditioning are recommended.

Maxillary Fractures

■ Etiology

Fractures of the maxilla are classified according to fracture patterns described by René Le Fort and are based on the most superior level of the fracture site (**Fig. 20.18**). Most fractures result from very high-impact forces, such as a hockey stick or an opponent's elbow. The more serious fractures can lead to airway obstruction and generally require hospitalization. This injury ranks as the fourth most common facial fracture.

■ Signs and Symptoms

If the upper jaw or midface is fractured, the maxilla may be mobile, giving the appearance of a longer face. Nasal bleeding, ecchymosis in the cheek or buccal region, malocclusion, nasal deformity, or a flattening and splaying of the naso-orbital region may be present.

■ Management

Treatment involves maintaining the airway. A forward-sitting position allows for adequate drainage of saliva and blood. A crushed ice pack may be placed over the area to control swelling, but it is important to avoid pressure or compression over the fracture site. The patient should be referred immediately to a physician. Although reduction and internal fixation often are used to immobilize the region, extensive surgery and possible secondary reconstruction occasionally are necessary to treat the condition.

 Because the patient is bleeding, universal precautions should be followed during palpation of the maxilla, the mandible, the zygomatic bone, the nasal bone, and the TMJ. As indicated by the apparent malocclusion and inability to close the jaw, the hockey player may have a fractured jaw.

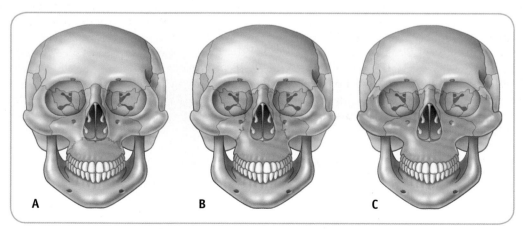

Figure 20.18. Maxillary fractures. Fractures to the maxilla may involve separation of the palate (Le Fort Fracture I) **(A)**, may extend into the nasal region (Le Fort Fracture II) **(B)**, or may involve complete craniofacial dissociation (Le Fort Fracture III) **(C)**.

NASAL CONDITIONS

 A basketball player received a lateral blow to the nose from an opposing player's elbow. The nose is bleeding and has a flattened appearance. What signs and symptoms indicate that this patient needs to be referred immediately to a physician?

Nasal injuries are common in sports during which protective face guards are not worn. Epistaxis, deviated septums, and nasal fractures are common injuries to the nasal region. **Box 20.3** identifies the signs and symptoms of nasal conditions that warrant further examination by a physician.

Epistaxis

Etiology

Epistaxis, or nosebleed, is a relatively common injury and is reported to occur in up to 60% of the general population. Although somewhat distressing for the patient, less than 10% of adult patients require definitive medical attention.[37] Anterior bleeds are far more common and may be caused from any the following[38]:

- Picking the nose (most common)
- Facial trauma secondary to blunt facial impact or motor vehicle collision ✳
- Mucosal hyperemia secondary to allergic or viral rhinitis
- Presence of a foreign body (if bleed is accompanied by purulent discharge)
- Chronic excoriation secondary to chronic intranasal drug use

Signs and Symptoms

Anterior bleeding originates from superficial blood vessels on the anterior septum known as the Kiesselbach plexus. Posterior bleeding generally arises from the posterior nasal cavity via branches of the sphenopalatine arteries, leading to significant hemorrhage. Posterior epistaxis may be asymptomatic or may present insidiously as nausea, hematemesis, anemia, hemoptysis, or melena.[37]

Management

Most nosebleeds stop spontaneously after applying mild pressure at the nasal bone for 5 to 15 minutes. The patient should be mouth breathing and leaning forward. Ice can be applied to the dorsum of the nose to reduce bleeding, or ice can be applied to the back of the neck, which activates the mammalian dive reflex, thereby causing peripheral vasoconstriction.[37] A nasal plug, or pledget, may be used but seldom is needed; if used, however, the plug can be coated with topical astringents or soaked with vasoconstrictors, such as tannic acid or a 1% phenylephrine hydrochloride solution (as long as the patient is not allergic to them). The plug should extend externally for at least half an inch. If bleeding continues for more than 5 minutes despite manual pressure and ice, the patient should be referred to a physician.

Patients should be instructed not to blow their nose following significant bouts of epistaxis. Recurrent bouts may need to be treated with nasal cauterization, chemically with silver nitrate sticks, or with electrocautery under local anesthesia.

BOX 20.3 Nasal Red Flags Requiring Further Examination by a Physician

- Bleeding or CSF from the nose
- Nosebleed that does not stop within 5 minutes
- Loss of smell
- Foreign objects that cannot be removed easily
- Nasal deformity or fracture

Deviated Septum

Etiology

The nasal septum is the partition between the right and left sides of the nose. A deviated septum may be congenital and asymptomatic; however, nasal trauma, such as a nasal fracture or lateral compression on the nasal region, can displace the septum, leading to difficulty breathing. Under normal circumstances, when a patient closes one nostril and attempts to breathe through the other, that nostril closes during inhalation, and breathing is unobstructed. Expiration should be easy and smooth.

Signs and Symptoms

The most obvious sign is a consistent difference in airflow between the two sides of the nose when one nostril is blocked. Inspection with an otoscope can confirm the presence of a deviated septum. If trauma was involved in the injury, a septal hematoma may be visible through the otoscope (**Application Strategy 20.3**).

Management

If a deviated septum is suspected, the patient should be referred to a physician for further care. Surgery often is indicated to drain a septal hematoma and repair the deviated septum; this may involve reshaping the nasal cartilage and bone (i.e., septoplasty or submucous resection). Correction of a deviated septum usually does not change the outer appearance of the nose.

Nasal Fractures

Etiology

The nose is the most prominent facial feature and is the most commonly fractured bone in the adult face.[39] Persistent or profuse bleeding may indicate a complex nasal fracture with an injury to the ethmoid artery that requires direct visualization.

APPLICATION STRATEGY 20.3

Use of an Otoscope to Inspect the Nose and Ear

To inspect the nose:

1. Use the largest ear speculum available. Tilt the patient's head back and insert the speculum gently into the vestibule of each nostril, avoiding contact with any sensitive area. Hold the otoscope handle to one side to avoid the patient's chin to improve your mobility.
2. Direct the speculum posteriorly and then upward in small steps while visualizing the inferior and middle concha bullosa, the nasal septum, and the narrow nasal passage between them. Some asymmetry of the two sides is normal.
3. Check the nasal mucosa that covers the septum and the concha bullosa for any swelling, bleeding, or exudate. Note any deviation, inflammation, or perforation of the septum.

To inspect the ear:

1. Using the largest ear speculum that the canal will accommodate, position the patient's head so that you can see comfortably through the instrument.
2. To straighten the ear canal, gently pull the auricle upward, backward, and slightly away from the head. Movement of the auricle and external ear ("tug test") is painful in acute *otitis externa* (inflammation of the ear canal) but not in *otitis media* (inflammation of the middle ear). Tenderness behind the ear may be present in otitis media.
3. Holding the otoscope handle between the thumb and fingers, brace the hand against the patient's face. Insert the speculum gently into the ear canal, directing it somewhat down and forward and through the hairs, if any.
4. Inspect the ear canal for any discharge, foreign bodies, redness of the skin, or swelling. Cerumen, which varies in color and consistency from yellow and flaky to brown and sticky or even to dark and hard, may partially or entirely block the view.
5. Inspect the eardrum, noting its color and contour.

Adapted from Bickley LS, Szilagyi PG. *Bates' Guide to Physical Examination and History Taking*. Philadelphia, PA: Lippincott Williams & Wilkins; 2007.

Signs and Symptoms

Epistaxis is almost always present, and the nose may appear to be flattened and lose its symmetry, particularly with a lateral force. Because of its prominence, the nose is particularly susceptible to lateral displacement.[39] Severity can range from a slightly depressed, greenstick fracture (seen in adolescents), to total displacement and/or disruption in the bony and cartilaginous parts of the nose. The nasal airway can be obstructed with bony fragments, or the fracture can extend into the cranial region and cause a loss of CSF. There may be crepitus over the nasal bridge and ecchymosis under the eyes.

Management

If the only injury is to the nose, the patient should be evaluated to ensure that no septal hematoma (i.e., blood from an acute injury that accumulates beneath the septal perichondrium) has formed, which would require immediate referral to a physician for incision and drainage. The nose should then be viewed by standing behind and above the patient while looking down an imaginary line to determine if the nose is centered. Using a small mirror, the injured patient should look at the nose to determine if it appears to be normal. Treatment involves controlling bleeding, applying ice to limit swelling and hemorrhage, and referring the patient to a physician for further examination. A custom acrylic face shield, a helmet with face mask, or other protective device should be worn during contact sports for 4 weeks after injury.[33] **Application Strategy 20.4** provides guidelines for the assessment and care of a nasal injury.

 Signs and symptoms that indicate a serious nasal injury include excessive bleeding or CSF from the nose, a loss of smell, nasal deformity or fracture, or a nosebleed that does not stop within 5 minutes. If present, the patient should be referred immediately to a physician.

APPLICATION STRATEGY 20.4

Evaluation and Management of a Nasal Injury

1. Check ABCs. Bony fragments may occlude the airway.
2. Determine responsiveness.
3. Check for signs of a concussion and/or skull fracture.
4. History
   - Primary complaint (e.g., pain, dizziness, disorientation, nausea, vision disturbances, or tinnitus)
   - Mechanism of injury
   - Disability from injury (e.g., inability to breathe through one side of nose)
5. Observation and inspection
   - Obvious deformity or abnormal deviation
   - Bleeding and/or CSF from the nose
   - Check pupil size, pupillary response to light, eye movement, nystagmus, or blurred or double vision, which may indicate an associated cranial injury
   - Abnormal breathing rate and pattern
   - Stand behind the patient and look down an imaginary line to see if the nose is deviated.
6. Palpation
   - Palpate the two nasal bones with the forefinger and thumb (checking for swelling, depressions, crepitus, mobility, etc.).
   - Check the internal structures of the nasal area for any abnormalities.
7. After bleeding is controlled, inspect the internal structures for any abnormalities.
8. Apply ice to control the hemorrhage and refer the patient to a physician for further care.

ORAL AND DENTAL CONDITIONS

 Following a collision during a high school soccer game, an athlete complains of significant pain after being hit in the mouth. The inside of the upper lip is bleeding, and one tooth is intruded. How should this injury be managed?

The most commonly injured tooth is the maxillary central incisor, which is positioned front and center and receives 80% of all dental trauma.[40] During sport and physical activity, nearly all such injuries are preventable through regular use of mouth protectors. Mouth protectors prevent injury to the lips, teeth, cheek, tongue, mandible, neck, TMJ, and brain by absorbing shock, spreading impact, cushioning the contact between the upper and lower jaws, and keeping the upper lip away from the incisal edges of the teeth. Although certain sports (e.g., football, boxing, field hockey, lacrosse) require mouth guards, few coaches or league officials require these devices in other contact and collision sports. **Box 20.4** identifies the signs and symptoms of oral and dental conditions that warrant further examination by a physician.

Periodontal Disease

Etiology

Periodontal disease (gum disease) ranges from **gingivitis**, or mild inflammation of the gums, to **periodontitis**, or inflammation of the deeper gum tissues that normally hold the teeth in place. Approximately 80% of American adults have some form of gum disease. Gingivitis usually is caused by bacteria that irritate the gums, leading to swelling and bleeding. Bacteria, along with minerals in the saliva, form tartar (calculus), which provides an environment for additional bacteria to accumulate and irritate the gums. If left unchecked, gingivitis can lead to the more serious form of gum disease, periodontitis. This long-term infection eventually can result in loss of the teeth. Thorough daily brushing, regular flossing, and frequent professional cleaning can reduce the risk of developing serious gingivitis.

Signs and Symptoms

Initial signs of gingivitis include tender, swollen, or bleeding gums, particularly when the teeth are brushed. There also may be a change in color of the gums from pink to dusky red. Plaque, which is the soft, white form of salivary salts, protein, and bacteria that covers the teeth and leads to gingivitis, is not readily visible. Signs and symptoms of periodontitis may include swollen or recessed gums; an unpleasant taste in the mouth; bad breath; tooth pain, especially when eating hot, cold, or sweet foods; loose teeth; change in the bite; and drainage or pus around one or more teeth.

Management

Gingivitis usually clears after a professional cleaning by a dentist or hygienist, followed by proper daily oral hygiene. The cleaning removes tartar and plaque from the teeth, which eliminates the source of irritation to the gums, allowing the gums to heal. If gingivitis has progressed to periodontitis, more extensive treatment is necessary; the dentist may try to remove the pockets of bacteria between the

---

BOX 20.4 Oral and Dental Red Flags Requiring Further Examination by a Physician

- Lacerations involving the lip, outer border of the lip, or tongue
- Any individual complaining of a persistent toothache or sensitivity to heat and cold
- Loose teeth either laterally displaced, intruded, or extruded

- Inability to close the jaw
- Chipped, cracked, fractured, or dislodged teeth
- Malocclusion of the teeth

gums and teeth and may recommend antibiotics. Other nonsurgical treatments may include scaling, sometimes done with an ultrasonic device, to remove tartar and bacteria from the tooth surfaces and beneath the gums. A technique known as root planing is used to smooth the root surfaces, discouraging further accumulation of tartar. In advanced stages of periodontitis, surgery may be necessary.

Dental Caries (Tooth Decay)

Etiology

Dental caries, also known as tooth decay and cavities, are caused primarily by plaque. When plaque collects and hardens, tartar is formed. Bacteria within the plaque contain acids that begin to dissolve the tooth enamel. These problems can cause openings in the tooth enamel, which then allow bacteria to infect the center of the tooth (the pulp). This condition can be accelerated by ingesting acid-rich foods or foods that are high in sugar and starch. Combined with poor oral hygiene, this condition can lead to a painful tooth cavity. If neglected, the infection can spread from the pulp to the root of the tooth and, finally, to the bones supporting the tooth. An **abscessed tooth** is a painful infection at the root of a tooth or between the gum and a tooth. Although primarily caused by severe tooth decay, the condition also can result from gingivitis or trauma to the tooth, such as when a tooth is broken or chipped.

Signs and Symptoms

A tooth with a cavity typically presents with pain during chewing and sensitivity to hot or cold foods and beverages. If a tooth abscess is present, a throbbing pain or a sharp or shooting pain is common. Other symptoms may include fever, a bitter taste in the mouth, bad breath, swollen neck glands, general discomfort, uneasiness or ill feeling, redness and swelling of the gums, a swollen area of the upper or lower jaw, or an open, draining sore on the side of the gum. If the root of the tooth dies as a result of infection, the toothache may stop. This does not mean the infection has healed, however; the infection remains active and continues to spread and destroy tissue. If any symptoms are present, the patient should be referred immediately to a dentist.

Management

In mild tooth decay, the dentist scrapes the region and applies a filling. If a more serious condition is present, a radiograph may be obtained to assess the presence of a tooth abscess and bone erosion. To eliminate infection, the abscess may need to be drained via a procedure known as a root canal. Root canal surgery also may be recommended to remove any diseased root tissue after the infection has subsided; subsequently, a crown may be placed over the tooth. The tooth also may be extracted, allowing drainage through the socket. A third way to drain the abscess is by an incision into the swollen gum tissue. Antibiotics are prescribed to help fight the infection. Warm saltwater rinses and over-the-counter pain-reducing medications can be used to relieve pain and discomfort associated with an abscessed tooth.

Mouth Lacerations

Etiology

Trauma to the facial region can lead to lacerations of the lips, tongue, or internal buccal cavities. Most lacerations are minor and treated the same as in other lacerations.

Signs and Symptoms

Bleeding is often profuse. The lacerated tissue may appear swollen with jagged edges.

Management

Management involves applying direct pressure to stop the bleeding, cleaning the area with a saline solution, applying Steri-Strips if needed, and covering the wound with a dry, sterile dressing. Lacerations that extend completely through the lip or that involve the outer lip or large tongue lacerations require special suturing. A badly scarred tongue can affect taste and can interfere with speech

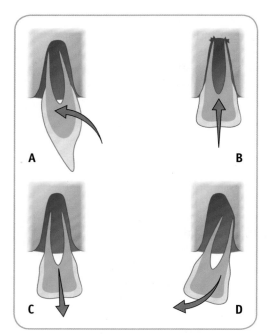

Figure 20.19. Loose teeth. Loose teeth may involve partial displacement **(A)**, intrusion **(B)**, extrusion **(C)**, or avulsion **(D)**. _put back into mouth, save ligament_

patterns. Tongue lacerations require careful cleansing with water or a mouthwash to avoid infection and referral to a physician for possible suturing. The patient should not be permitted to return to participation until the wound is healed. If sutures are applied, protection is continued for at least 7 days.

Loose, Subluxated, or Luxated Teeth

Etiology

Direct trauma to the mouth can lead to a loose, a subluxated, or a luxated tooth. Many injuries to the dental area can be prevented by wearing a mouth guard.

Signs and Symptoms

A loosened tooth may be partially displaced, intruded, extruded, or avulsed (**Fig. 20.19**). In many cases, oral bleeding may also be present.

Management

When the tooth has been displaced outwardly or is laterally displaced, the clinician should try to place the tooth back into its normal position without forcing it. Teeth that are intruded should be left alone; any attempt to move the tooth may result in a permanent loss of the tooth or damage to any underlying permanent teeth. The patient should be referred to a dentist immediately. A dental radiograph can rule out damage under the gum line and ensure the tooth is properly replaced. The damaged tooth is then splinted to the surrounding teeth for 2 to 3 weeks. Teeth that have been totally avulsed from their sockets often can be located in the patient's mouth or on the ground. These teeth can be saved, but time is of the essence. A dislocated tooth should be held by the crown. It is important not to rub the tooth or remove any dirt. If the tooth is rinsed in milk or saline and replaced intraorally in the tooth socket within 30 minutes, the prognosis for a successful replanting is 90%. It should be noted that tap or drinking water can damage the periodontal ligament cells on the root surface and compromise implantation procedures. Implantation that occurs after 2 hours results in a 95% failure rate.[40] Semirigid fixation for 7 to 10 days may be followed by root canal therapy. Contact drills and competition are restricted during this period of time, and an appropriate face or mouth guard should be worn to prevent further injury.

Fractured Tooth

Etiology

As in other facial injuries, direct trauma can fracture a tooth. Use of a protective mouth guard can reduce the incidence of dental fractures. With any dental injury, a concussion or other head or neck injury should be ruled out.

Signs and Symptoms

Fractures may occur through the enamel, dentin, pulp, or root of the tooth. Fractures involving the enamel cause no symptoms and can be smoothed by the dentist to prevent further injury to the lips and the inner lining of the oral cavity. Fractures extending into the dentin cause pain and increased sensitivity to cold and heat. Fractures exposing the pulp or root of the tooth lead to severe pain and sensitivity.

Management

The patient should be referred to a dentist who will apply a sedative dressing over the exposed area and, later, will attach a permanent, composite resin crown. Fractures exposing the pulp involve more extensive dental work. If the pulp exposure is small, a pulp-capping procedure, whereby calcium hydroxide is placed on the area, can bridge the exposed area and, if successful, can eliminate the need for a root canal. Another treatment involves removing a portion of the pulp in the root canal, leaving the uninjured pulp in the root. This has been successful in younger patients whose roots have not yet fully formed. The final method of treatment is a total root canal.

 The clinician should not attempt to move the intruded tooth, because the action could result in a permanent loss of the tooth or damage to any underlying permanent teeth. The patient should be referred immediately to a dentist.

EAR CONDITIONS

 A wrestler was not wearing protective headgear during practice. He is now complaining about a burning, aching sensation on the outer ear. It appears to be somewhat inflamed and sensitive to touch, but no swelling is apparent. How should this injury be managed, and what signs might indicate a more serious problem?

Several conditions may affect the ear. Foreign bodies in the ear usually are harmless and easily removed with a speculum. Trauma to the ear can lead to auricular hematoma, and an infection of the ear can lead to localized inflammation of the auditory canal (**otitis externa**), impacted cerumen, swimmer's ear (**otitis media**), or a tympanic membrane rupture. **Box 20.5** identifies the signs and symptoms of ear conditions that warrant further examination by a physician.

External Ear Conditions

Etiology

Auricular hematoma, or cauliflower ear, is a relatively minor injury caused when repeated blunt trauma pulls the cartilage away from the perichondrium. A hematoma forms between the perichondrium and cartilage of the ear and compromises blood supply to the cartilage, leading to a painful and throbbing injury. This condition, which is common in wrestlers, can be prevented by wearing proper headgear.

Signs and Symptoms

The outer ear will appear red, puffy, and swollen. If left untreated, the hematoma forms a fibrosis in the overlying skin, leading to necrosis of the auricular cartilage that results in the characteristic cauliflower ear appearance (**Fig. 20.20**).

Management

Immediate treatment involves icing the region to reduce pain and swelling. An ice pack should be applied for 20 minutes. If the swelling is still present, the hematoma must be aspirated by a physician to avoid pressure and permanent cartilage damage. Once aspirated, a pressure dressing should be applied for 7 to 14 days. The patient should not take aspirin or nonsteroidal anti-inflammatory drugs for several days; however, antibiotics are recommended for 7 to 10 days because of a high risk for

---

BOX 20.5 Ear Red Flags Requiring Further Examination by a Physician

- Bleeding or CSF from the ear canal
- Feeling of fullness in the ear; vertigo
- Bleeding or swelling behind the ear (Battle sign)
- Foreign body in the ear that cannot be easily removed
- Hematoma or swelling that removes the creases of the outer ear
- Popping or itching in the ear
- Tinnitus or hearing impairment
- Pain when the ear lobe is pulled

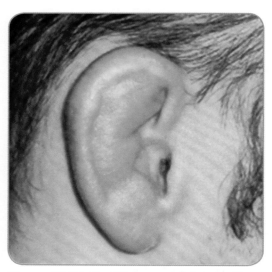

Figure 20.20. Cauliflower ear deformity. The hematoma results in the skin being pulled away from the ear cartilage.

infection.[33] It is imperative that the patient wear protective headgear to prevent reoccurrence.

Internal Ear Conditions
Etiology

A blow to the ear, pressure changes (as seen in diving and scuba diving), and infection may injure the external auditory meatus and eardrum. Although typically seen in water sports, damage to the internal ear may occur in any sport, such as in soccer when a player is hit on the ear by a ball.

Signs and Symptoms

A patient with an internal ear condition may experience intense pain in the ear, a feeling of fullness, nausea, tinnitus, dizziness, or hearing loss.

Management

The patient should be evaluated immediately by a physician. Most minor ruptures of the eardrum heal spontaneously; larger ruptures may require surgical repair.

Impacted Cerumen
Etiology

Cerumen, or ear wax, is produced by the ceruminous glands, which are modified apocrine glands in the external auditory canal. Cerumen is a sticky substance thought to trap insects and foreign material in the ear canal. In many patients, the ear is naturally cleansed as the cerumen dries and then falls out of the external auditory canal. In others, however, cerumen builds up excessively and becomes compacted, a condition that can impair hearing.

Signs and Symptoms

Impacted cerumen causes some degree of hearing loss or muffled hearing. Pain generally is not present because no infection is present.

Management

Removal of the excess ear wax can be accomplished by irrigating the ear canal with warm water. A cotton tip applicator should not be used because this may increase the impaction or damage the eardrum. If irrigation is not successful, referral to a physician is necessary to remove the cerumen with a curette.

Otitis Externa
Etiology

Otitis externa is a bacterial infection that involves the lining of the external auditory canal. Because of its prevalence among patients who participate in water activities, it is commonly called swimmer's ear. Otitis externa frequently occurs in patients who fail to dry the ear canal after being in water, resulting in a change of the pH of the ear canal's skin.

Signs and Symptoms

In acute conditions, pain is the predominant symptom. In chronic cases, such as those seen with excessive use of a cotton swab, itching is a more common complaint, with discomfort and pain being secondary. There may or may not be a discharge of pus. Gentle pressure around the external auditory opening and pulling on the pinna causes increased pain. If left untreated, the infection can spread to the middle ear, causing balance disturbances or hearing loss. Commercial ear plugs may not be helpful in preventing this condition.

Management

Custom ear plugs from an audiologist or otolaryngologist may be necessary. The condition also can be prevented by using ear drops to dry the canal. The majority of ear drops contain an acidifying agent, either aluminum acetate or vinegar. An effective homemade remedy is equal parts of white vinegar (acetic acid), 70% alcohol, and water. One or two drops after water exposure or showering is the standard recommendation. If no improvement is seen, the patient should be referred to a physician, who may prescribe drops containing broad-spectrum antibiotics.

Otitis Media

Etiology

Localized infections of the middle ear (**otitis media**) often occurs secondary to upper respiratory infections. These infections often are caused by bacteria, but they also may be caused by viruses. Bacterial and viral infections have the same signs and symptoms.

Signs and Symptoms

When the mastoid area is pressed, the patient will complain of pain and a sense of fullness in the ear. Swelling of the mucous membranes may cause a partial or complete block of the eustachian tube (the connection between the middle ear and the pharynx), resulting in the inhibition of hearing. The tympanic membrane may appear red and bulging. Serous otitis often is associated with otitis media and an upper respiratory infection; an amber-colored or bloody fluid is seen through the eardrum and is associated with complaints of ears popping.

Management

A physician may prescribe an antibiotic for 10 days if there is an infection, or decongestants may be used to shrink the swollen mucous membranes. If the middle ear of a patient with otitis media is completely filled with fluid, air travel should be discouraged. If the ear is filled with fluid and air and the eustachian tube is not working properly, the air bubbles will expand on ascent and contract on descent. Both ascent and descent cause severe pain and may rupture the eardrum. In addition, rupture of the membranes separating the middle ear from the inner ear could occur, with catastrophic results. Therefore, air travel is not recommended until the middle ear has returned to normal appearance and function.

Tympanic Membrane Rupture

Etiology

The tympanic membrane vibrates when sound waves strike it, starting the process of converting sound waves into nerve impulses that travel to the brain. Damage to the eardrum interrupts the hearing process and may impair hearing. The eardrum also acts as a barrier to keep outside material, such as bacteria, from entering the middle ear. A ruptured (perforated) eardrum is a tear or a hole in the eardrum, which can allow bacteria to more easily reach the middle ear and cause infection. A ruptured eardrum may be caused by an infection (e.g., otitis media); direct trauma (e.g., being slapped or being hit by a ball on the external ear); changes in pressure (e.g., rapid ascent or descent in a plane or underwater); loud, sudden noises (e.g., explosion); or foreign objects in the ear (e.g., cotton swab or bobby pin pushed too far into the ear canal).

Signs and Symptoms

A ruptured eardrum initially can be very painful. Other signs and symptoms include sharp, sudden ear pain or discomfort; tinnitus; clear, pus-filled, or bloody drainage from the ear; sudden decrease in ear pain followed by drainage; and hearing loss. Use of an otoscope may identify the damaged area.

Management

The patient should be referred immediately to a physician for further care. Most small-to-moderate perforations of the tympanic membrane heal without treatment within a few weeks, although some may take months. If the tear or hole in the eardrum does not heal by itself, treatment may involve an eardrum patch or surgery. Closing the perforation is essential to prevent water from entering the ear while showering, bathing, or swimming, which could cause middle ear infections. Hearing is improved, and any tinnitus is diminished. Repair of the perforation also prevents the development of a skin cyst in the middle ear (cholesteatoma), which can cause chronic middle ear infections and damage the ear structure.

 Ice should be placed on the wrestler's ear to control swelling. If any hemorrhage or edema between the perichondrium and cartilage appears to flatten the wrinkles or creases of the ear, the patient should be referred immediately to a physician for follow-up care. Protective ear wear should be worn by all wrestlers at every practice and during competitions.

EYE CONDITIONS

 While moving through the circuit training area in an exercise facility, an adult exerciser received a significant blow to the eye from another exerciser's elbow. What signs and symptoms indicate a serious condition?

The eyes are exposed daily to potential trauma and injury, yet many eye injuries could be prevented by wearing protective eyewear. This is especially true in racquetball and squash, in which players are confined to a limited space with swinging racquets and balls traveling at high speeds. Patients who require corrective lenses should use strong plastic or semirigid rubber frames and impact-resistant lenses. If glasses are not required, the American Academy of Pediatrics and the American Academy of Ophthalmology recommend that protective eyewear and/or face masks should be worn during participation in sports with a high risk of injury.[41] Sport participants with only one good eye should consult an ophthalmologist to determine what mandatory protective eyewear should be worn to prevent further injury. **Box 20.6** identifies the signs and symptoms of eye conditions that necessitate further examination by a physician.

Periorbital Ecchymosis

Etiology

The eye globe is well protected within the orbital rim, but in many sports, the external eye region is susceptible to direct trauma from flying implements, balls, and competitor's elbows. The area is highly vascular and, when impacted, can produce capillary bleeding into the tissue spaces.

Signs and Symptoms

Impact forces can cause significant swelling and hemorrhage into the surrounding eyelids. This discoloration is called **periorbital ecchymosis**, or, more commonly, a black eye. The impact can also lead to subconjunctival hemorrhage or faulty vision.

BOX 20.6 Eye Red Flags Requiring Further Examination by a Physician

- Visual disturbances or loss of vision
- Blood in the anterior chamber
- Unequal pupils or bilateral, dilated pupils
- Embedded foreign body
- Irregular eye movement or failure to adjust to light

- Individual complaining of floaters, light flashes, or a "curtain falling over the eye"
- Severe ecchymosis and swelling (raccoon eyes)
- Itching, burning, watery eye that appears pink
- Suspected corneal abrasion or corneal laceration
- Displaced contact lens that cannot be easily removed

Management

Trauma to the eye requires inspection for obvious abnormalities, palpation of the orbit for a possible orbital fracture, and assessment of pupillary response to light by shining a concentrated light beam into the eye and noting the bilateral rate of constriction. The ability of a patient to focus clearly on an object must be assessed. The anterior chamber of the eye should be inspected for any obvious bleeding (see "Hemorrhage into the Anterior Chamber" section). Treatment involves controlling the swelling and hemorrhage by using crushed ice or ice water in a latex surgical glove; it is essential that the glove does not have rosin or other powdered substances on it. Because of possible leakage, chemical ice bags should not be used. This condition requires referral to an ophthalmologist for further examination to rule out an underlying fracture or injury to the globe.

Foreign Bodies

Etiology

Dust or dirt in the eye is a frequent occurrence in all sports. At times, the debris can be potentially dangerous.

Signs and Symptoms

Foreign debris in the eyes can lead to intense pain and tearing. The patient may attempt to remove the substance by rubbing the eye or tearing the eye to flush the object out. Depending on the pain level, the patient may resist any attempt to open the eyelids to view the eye.

Management

The foreign body, if not embedded or on the cornea, should be removed and the eye should be inspected for any scratches, abrasions, or lacerations (**Application Strategy 20.5**).

A foreign object that is impaled or embedded should not be touched, and removal should not be attempted. Activation of the emergency plan is warranted, including summoning EMS. Medically trained patients will stabilize the object and provide rigid protection for the orbit. In the cornea, a fluorescein stain may reveal the object's location, and topical anesthetics may be necessary to facilitate the physician's examination.

Sty

Etiology

A sty (hordeolum) is an infection of the sebaceous gland at the edge of the eyelid and is typically caused by *Staphylococcus* bacteria. Blepharitis is an inflammation of the eyelash follicle along the edge of the eyelid. A sty may be brought on by improper or incomplete removal of eye makeup, use of outdated or infected cosmetics, poor eyelid hygiene, inflammatory diseases of the eyelid, stress, and hormonal changes.

APPLICATION STRATEGY 20.5

Removing a Foreign Body from the Eye

1. Examine the lower lid by gently pulling the skin down below the eye. Ask the patient to look up and inspect the lower portion of the globe and eyelid for any foreign object.
2. Examine the upper lid by asking the patient to look downward.
3. Grasp the eyelashes and pull downward.
4. Place a cotton-tipped applicator on the outside portion of the upper lid.
5. Pull the lid over the applicator and hold the rolled lid against the upper bony ridge of the orbit.
6. Remove the foreign body with a sterile, moist gauze pad. If you are unable to successfully remove the foreign object, patch both eyes with a sterile, oval gauze pad (without adding pressure), and refer the patient to a physician for immediate care.

Signs and Symptoms

The condition presents as a red nodule that will progress into a painful pustule within a few days. The nodule will be tender to the touch and may elicit a scratchy sensation on the eyeball. There may also be crusting of the eyelid margins, burning in the eye, droopiness of the eyelid, blurred vision, and mucous discharge in the eye.

Management

Treatment involves the application of warm, moist compresses. If the pustule does not improve within 2 days, physician referral is required because a prescription topical ointment may be necessary.

Conjunctivitis (Pinkeye)

Etiology

Conjunctivitis is an inflammation, often resulting from chlorine irritation or bacterial infection of the conjunctiva.

Signs and Symptoms

The condition leads to itching, burning, and watering of the eye, causing the conjunctiva to become inflamed and red and giving a "pink eye" appearance.

Management

This bacterial condition can be highly infectious, so the patient should be referred immediately to a physician for medical treatment.

Corneal Lacerations

Etiology

A corneal laceration is a partial- or full-thickness injury to the cornea. A partial-thickness injury does not violate the globe of the eye (abrasion). A full-thickness injury penetrates completely through the cornea, causing a ruptured globe. Lacerations to the cornea are caused by sharp objects, such as fingernails, darts, skate blades, or broken glass.

Signs and Symptoms

With an abrasion, there is a sudden onset of pain, tearing, and photophobia. Blinking and movement of the eye only aggravate the condition. An examination may not reveal a foreign object, but the patient continues to complain that something is in the eye. With a laceration, severe pain, discomfort, decreased visual acuity, or distortion or displacement of the pupil is present. The pupil should be inspected for symmetry with the opposite eye. Lacerations of the cornea often penetrate iris tissue, causing distortion and displacement of the pupil.

Management

With an abrasion, the initial management involves covering the eye with a dry, sterile dressing. A corneal abrasion is best seen by using a fluorescein dye strip. Soft contact lenses should be removed before applying the dye, because these lenses absorb the dye and can be ruined. The orange color of the dye is augmented by using a blue light, which changes the orange dye to a bright green and illuminates the abrasion. Treatment usually involves a topical ointment, such as 2% homatropine, to reduce pain, relax ciliary muscle spasms, and prevent secondary bacterial infection. It may be advantageous to wear an eye patch for 24 to 48 hours. If used, the patch must be tight enough to ensure that the lids are closed beneath the patch and firm enough to prevent the lids from opening and closing.

If a laceration is suspected, any pressure on the globe should be avoided to prevent extrusion of the intraocular contents. The eye should be covered using a protective shield with the pressure exerted on the bony orbit, not on the soft tissue. This condition warrants immediate referral to a physician. The patient should be moved in either a supine or an upright position. (Avoid a prone or head-down position.) As such, it may be necessary to activate the emergency plan, including summoning EMS, for transportation to the nearest medical facility.

Subconjunctival Hemorrhage

Etiology

Direct trauma also can lead to **subconjunctival hemorrhage**. It is often referred to as red eye. The condition is seen more common in patients with high blood pressure or in those taking blood thinners.

Signs and Symptoms

Several small capillaries rupture, making the white sclera of the eye appear red, blotchy, and inflamed. This condition is not as serious as it may appear to be.

Management

This relatively harmless condition requires no treatment and resolves spontaneously in 1 to 3 weeks. If blurred vision, pain, limited eye movement, or blood in the anterior chamber is present, however, immediate referral to an ophthalmologist is warranted.

Hemorrhage into the Anterior Chamber

Etiology

Hemorrhage into the anterior chamber (**hyphema**) usually results from blunt trauma caused by a small ball (e.g., squash or racquetball), hockey puck, stick (e.g., field hockey or ice hockey), or a swinging racquet (e.g., squash or racquetball). The small size of the object enables it to fit within the confines of the eye orbit, thereby inflicting direct damage to the eye.

Signs and Symptoms

Initially, a red tinge in the anterior chamber may be present, but within a few hours, blood begins to settle into the anterior chamber, giving a characteristic meniscus appearance (**Fig. 20.21**). Frequently, it occurs in microscopic quantities, and visual acuity may not be affected. Such bleeding indicates that an intraocular injury has occurred, however, and the source of the bleeding must be identified to prevent recurrent bleeding, which can lead to both massive and destructive results.

Management

Both eyes should be patched. Because this condition necessitates immediate referral to a physician, it may be necessary to activate the emergency plan, including summoning EMS, so that the patient can be transported in a semireclining or a seated position. The condition requires hospitalization, bed rest, bilateral patching of the eyes, and sedation. The initial hemorrhage usually resolves in a few days, with good prognosis for full recovery.

Detached Retina

Etiology

Damage to the posterior segment of the eye can occur with or without trauma to the anterior segment. A detached retina occurs when fluid seeps into the retinal break and separates the neurosensory retina from the retinal epithelium. This can occur days or even weeks after the initial trauma.

Signs and Symptoms

Detachment almost always begins at the retinal periphery, resulting in a positive scotoma (a blind spot perceived by the patient) at the edge of the visual field. As the detachment progresses and the scotoma enlarges, the patient frequently describes the condition with phrases like "a curtain fell over my eye" or "I keep seeing flashes of lights going on and off." An ophthalmoscope may be used to view the optic disc and retinal vessels (**Application Strategy 20.6**).

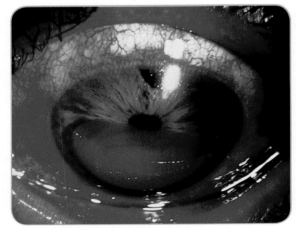

Figure 20.21. Hyphema. Blood in the anterior chamber of the eye signals a serious eye injury.

APPLICATION STRATEGY 20.6

Using the Ophthalmoscope

1. Darken the room. Switch on the ophthalmoscope light and turn the lens disc until you see the large round beam of white light. Shine the light on the back of your hand to check the type of light, its desired brightness, and the electrical charge of the ophthalmoscope.
2. Turn the lens disc to the zero diopter (a diopter is a unit that measures the power of a lens to converge or diverge light). In the zero diopter setting, the lens neither converges nor diverges light. Keep your finger on the edge of the lens disc so you can turn the disc to focus the lens while examining the fundus.
3. Hold the ophthalmoscope in the right hand to examine the right eye, and in the left hand to examine the left eye. This prevents bumping the patient's nose and provides more mobility and a closer range for visualizing the fundus. There may be some initial difficulty using the nondominant eye to view the fundus, but this should pass with practice.
4. Hold the ophthalmoscope firmly braced against the medial aspect of your bony orbit, with the handle tilted laterally at about a 20° slant from the vertical. Check to make sure you can see clearly through the aperture. Instruct the patient to look slightly up and over your shoulder at a point directly ahead on the wall.
5. Place yourself about 15 in away from the patient and at an angle 15° lateral to the patient's line of vision. Shine the light beam on the pupil and look for the orange glow in the pupil, the *red reflex*. Note any opacity interrupting the red reflex.
6. Place the thumb of your other hand across the patient's eyebrow. (This technique helps keep you steady but is not essential.) Keeping the light beam focused on the red reflex, move in with the ophthalmoscope on the 15° angle toward the pupil until you are very close to it, almost touching the patient's eyelashes.

Try to keep both eyes open and relaxed, as if gazing into the distance, to help minimize any fluctuating blurriness as your eyes attempt to accommodate.

It may be necessary to lower the brightness of the light beam to make the examination more comfortable for the patient, to avoid *hippus* (spasm of the pupil), and to improve your observations.

Adapted from Bickley LS, Szilagyi PG. *Bates' Guide to Physical Examination and History Taking.* Philadelphia, PA: Lippincott Williams & Wilkins; 2007.

Management

If a detached retina is suspected, both eyes should be patched. Immediate referral to an ophthalmologist is required, because surgery often is necessary.

Orbital Blowout Fracture

Etiology

A blowout fracture is caused by the impact from a blunt object (one usually larger than the eye orbit). On impact, forces drive the orbital contents posteriorly against the orbital walls. This sudden increase in intraorbital pressure is released in the area of least resistance, typically the inferior orbital floor (roof of the maxillary sinus). The medial orbital wall may also be involved. The result is that the globe descends into the defect in the floor.

Signs and Symptoms

An examination may reveal **diplopia**, absent eye movement, numbness on the side of the fracture below the eye, and a recessed, downward displacement of the globe. The lack of eye movement becomes evident when the patient is asked to look up and only one eye is able to move (**Fig. 20.22**).

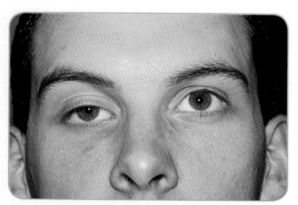

Figure 20.22. Orbital blowout fracture. An orbital fracture can entrap the inferior rectus muscle, leading to an inability to elevate the eye.

Management

Ice should be applied to the area to limit swelling; however, do not add additional compression or pressure over the suspected fracture site. The patient should be referred immediately to a physician. Tomograms or radiographs are necessary to confirm a fracture, and surgery may be indicated to repair the defect in the orbital floor.

Displaced Contact Lens

Hard contact lenses can slow the progression of **myopia** (nearsightedness). In sports, however, soft contact lenses are preferred, both because eye accommodation and adjustment time are less and because the lenses can be easily replaced and worn for longer periods of time.

Hard contact lenses frequently are involved in corneal abrasions. Foreign objects get underneath the lens and damage the cornea, or the cornea may be injured while putting in or taking out the lens. If irritation is present, the lens should be removed and cleaned. In an eye injury, patients may be able to remove the lens themselves. Pain or photophobia may preclude them from doing this, however, and it may become necessary to assist them. **Application Strategy 20.7** demonstrates a full assessment of an eye injury.

 Dilated pupils, any abnormal eye movement, throbbing pain or headache, and vision disturbances such as diplopia, sensitivity to light, and loss of all or part of a field of vision indicate a serious eye injury that warrants immediate referral.

APPLICATION STRATEGY `20.7`

Eye Evaluation

1. Check ABCs.
2. Determine responsiveness.
3. History
   - Determine primary complaint. Ask about the level of pain, discomfort, extent of voluntary eyelid movement, and extent of vision.
   - Determine mechanism of injury. Objects larger than the eye orbit may lead to orbital fracture. Objects smaller than the eye orbit may lead to direct trauma to the eye globe. Did the trauma result from blunt trauma, a sharp object, or a projectile?
4. Observation and inspection
   - Look for obvious deformity or abnormal deviation in the surrounding eye orbit.
   - Observe ecchymosis and extent of swelling in the eyelids and surrounding tissue. If the eyelid is swollen shut and the patient cannot voluntarily open it, do not force it open, which may cause further damage.
   - Observe any bleeding from deep lacerations of the eyelid.
   - Observe the level of both pupils and the eye globe for anterior or posterior displacement, presence of any corneal lacerations, and bleeding in the anterior chamber.
   - Inspect pupil size, accommodation to light, and sensitivity to light with a penlight.
5. Palpation
   - Carefully palpate the bony rim of the eye orbit and cheek bone for any swelling, depressions, crepitus, or mobility.
   - Control any bleeding.
6. Special tests
   - Determine the eye vision. Compare the vision of the uninjured eye to the injured eye. Is it blurred or sensitive to light? Does the patient have double vision? Can the patient distinguish how many fingers you are holding up in all four quadrants of vision? Can the patient distinguish objects that are close from objects that are far away?
   - Determine eye movement. Move your finger through the six cardinal planes of vision. Do the eyes move in a coordinated manner? If one eye moves upward and the other remains in a stationary position, the inferior rectus muscle may be entrapped because of an orbital fracture.
   - Vision disturbances, such as persistent blurred vision, diplopia, sensitivity to light, loss of all or part of a field of vision, dilated pupils, any abnormal eye movement, and throbbing pain or headache, indicate a serious eye injury that warrants immediate referral.

SUMMARY

1. Wearing protective equipment can significantly reduce the incidence and severity of head and facial injuries.

2. Minor injuries, such as nosebleeds, contusions, abrasions, lacerations, and minor concussions, can be handled easily on the field by the clinician. If complications arise or the condition does not improve within a reasonable amount of time, the clinician should immediately consult a physician about the injury.

3. Signs that indicate a possible skull fracture include deformity, unequal pupils, discoloration around both eyes or behind the ears, bleeding or CSF leaking from the nose and/or ear, and any loss of sight or smell.

4. Signs or symptoms of increasing intracranial pressure following head trauma include a severe headache, pupil irregularity or irregular eye tracking, confusion or progressive or sudden impairment of consciousness, rising blood pressure and falling pulse rate, and drastic changes in emotional control.

5. Signs and symptoms of a concussion include headache, dizziness or vertigo, lack of awareness of surroundings, nausea and vomiting, deteriorating level of consciousness, disturbance of vigilance with heightened distractibility, inability to maintain coherent thought patterns, and inability to carry out a sequence of goal-directed movements.

6. Patients who have sustained a concussion should not return to play the same day but instead should follow stepwise graduated RTP protocol.

7. Injuries that indicate increasing intracranial pressure, memory dysfunction, or gross observable poor coordination require immediate referral to a physician.

8. Fractures to the facial bones often result in malocclusion.

9. The nose is particularly susceptible to lateral displacement from trauma. Simultaneously, the trauma also may lead to a concussion.

10. When a loose tooth has been displaced outwardly or laterally, the clinician should try to place the tooth back into its normal position without forcing it. Teeth that are intruded should be left alone; any attempt to move the tooth may result in a permanent loss of the tooth. The patient should be referred to a dentist immediately.

11. A dislocated tooth should be located, rinsed in milk or a saline solution, and replaced intra-orally within the tooth socket. The patient should be seen by a dentist within 30 minutes for replacement of the tooth.

12. Cauliflower ear is common in wrestlers but is completely preventable by wearing proper headgear at all times when on the mat.

13. Otitis externa is a bacterial infection involving the lining of the external auditory meatus, commonly called swimmer's ear. Otitis media is a localized infection of the middle ear.

14. A foreign body in the eye, if not embedded or on the cornea, should be removed and the eye should be inspected for any scratches, abrasions, or lacerations.

15. Direct trauma to the eye can lead to corneal laceration, rupture of the globe, hemorrhage into the anterior chamber, detached retina, or orbital fracture. Loss of visual acuity, abnormal eye movement, diplopia, numbness below the eye, or a downward displacement of the globe should signal a serious condition. The patient should be referred to an ophthalmologist immediately.

APPLICATION QUESTIONS

1. Concussions are graded after the resolution of all symptoms and dysfunction. Do you think this is advantageous or problematic? Why? (Provide a justification for your response.)

2. A field hockey player has been hit in the head with a ball. The athlete is conscious but dazed. What questions should be asked as part of the history component of an on-the-field evaluation?

3. During hitting practice, a foul tip strikes the head of a baseball player standing near the dugout. The history and observation components of the assessment reveal the following: The skin is not broken; the patient is complaining of an intense headache, disorientation, and blurred vision; and the patient cannot recall what happened. In the continued assessment of this condition, is it advisable to perform neurological testing immediately or only if new symptoms develop and existing symptoms becomes worse? Why?

4. In a collision with the shortstop, a 17-year-old base runner received an elbow to the side of the head. The player was dazed and removed from the game. Following 15 minutes of ice application to the region, the patient complains of an increasing headache, nausea, and sensitivity to sunlight. She is lethargic and disoriented. What do these symptoms indicate? How will you manage this injury?

5. You are a high school athletic trainer. One of your annual goals is to actively engage coaches, parents, and athletes in assisting with the identification and management of concussions. What strategies could you employ to accomplish this goal?

6. Following a collision during a tackle, an 18-year-old football player remains down on the field. When you reach the athlete, he is conscious, but it is not clear if he momentarily lost consciousness and has since regained it. How would you differentiate between a simple and a complicated subdural hematoma?

7. A 21-year-old female lacrosse player stepped in front of an opposing player who was taking a shot on goal and was struck on the jaw by the ball. Although she was wearing a mouth guard, bleeding from the mouth is apparent and she is unable to close the jaw with the teeth in their proper alignment. What injury should be suspected? How should the condition be managed?

8. A 16-year-old third baseman covering a hit was struck on the side of the nose when the ball bounced upward unexpectedly. His nose is bleeding and appears to be swollen at the bridge of the nose. What signs and symptoms would indicate that this patient needs to be referred immediately to a physician?

9. A 20-year-old wrestler was not wearing protective headgear during practice. He is now complaining about a burning, aching sensation on the outer ear. Upon inspecting the ear, you notice that the area is somewhat inflamed and sensitive to touch, but no swelling is apparent. How should this condition be managed? What signs or symptoms might indicate a more serious problem?

10. An 18-year-old collegiate basketball player was struck in the mouth by an elbow. The inside of the upper lip is bleeding. There are at least three loose teeth, and one tooth appears to be broken in half. How should this injury be managed?

REFERENCES

1. Broglio SP, Cantu RC, Gioia GA, et al. National Athletic Trainers' Association position statement: management of sport concussion. *J Athl Train.* 2014;49(2):245–265.

2. Guskiewicz KM, Weaver NL, Padua DA, et al. Epidemiology of concussion in collegiate and high school football players. *Am J Sports Med.* 2000;28(5):643–650.

3. Guskiewicz KM, Bruce SL, Cantu RC, et al. National Athletic Trainers' Association position statement: management of sport-related concussion. *J Athl Train*. 2004;39(3):280–297.

4. Blinman TA, Houseknecht E, Snyder C, et al. Postconcussive symptoms in hospitalized pediatric patients after mild traumatic brain injury. *J Pediatr Surg*. 2009;44(6):1223–1228.

5. McCrory P, Meeuwisse W, Aubry M, et al. Sport concussion assessment tool—3rd edition: SCAT3. *Br J Sports Med*. 2013;47:259–262.

6. McCrory P, Meeuwisse WH, Aubry M, et al. Consensus statement on concussion in sport: the 4th International Conference on Concussion in Sport held in Zurich, November 2012. *Br J Sports Med*. 2013;47:250–258.

7. Halstead ME, Walter KD; and the Council on Sports Medicine and Fitness. American Academy of Pediatrics. Clinical report—sport-related concussion in children and adolescents. *Pediatrics*. 2010;126(3):597–615.

8. Guskiewicz KM. Concussion in sport: the grading-system dilemma. *Athl Ther Today*. 2001;6(1):18–27.

9. Notebaert AJ, Guskiewicz KM. Current trends in athletic training practice for concussion assessment and management. *J Athl Train*. 2005;40(4):320–325.

10. Nakayama Y, Covassin T, Schatz P, et al. Examination of the test-retest reliability of a computerized neurocognitive test battery. *Am J Sports Med*. 2014;42(8):2000–2005.

11. Schatz P, Pardini JE, Lovell MR, et al. Sensitivity and specificity of the ImPACT test battery for concussion in athletes. *Arch Clin Neuropsychol*. 2006;21(1):91–99.

12. Segalowitz SJ, Mahaney P, Santesso DL, et al. Retest reliability in adolescents of a computerized neuropsychological battery used to assess recovery from concussion. *NeuroRehabilitation*. 2007;22(3):243–251.

13. Kontos AP, Braithwaite R, Dakan S, et al. Computerized neurocognitive testing within 1 week of sport-related concussion: meta-analytic review and analysis of moderating factors. *J Int Neuropsychol Soc*. 2014;20(3):324–332.

14. Johansson G. *Clinical and Kinematic Assessments of Upper Limb Function in Persons With Post-Stroke Symptoms* [dissertation]. Umea, Sweden: Department of Community Medicine and Rehabilitation, Physiotherapy, Umea University; 2015. http://umu.diva-portal.org/smash/get/diva2:812649/FULLTEXT01.pdf. Accessed November 13, 2015.

15. Bell DR, Guskiewicz KM, Clark MA, et al. Systematic review of the balance error scoring system. *Sports Health*. 2011;3(3):287–295.

16. Hunt TN, Ferrara MS, Bornstein RA, et al. The reliability of the modified balance error scoring system. *Clin J Sport Med*. 2009;19(6):471–475.

17. Ghiselli G, Schaadt G, McAllister DR. On-the-field evaluation of an athlete with a head or neck injury. *Clin Sports Med*. 2003;22(3):445–465.

18. Logan SM, Bell GW, Leonard JC. Acute subdural hematoma in a high school football player after 2 unreported episodes of head trauma: a case report. *J Athl Train*. 2001;36(4):433–436.

19. Putukian M, Madden CC. Head injuries. In: Mellion MB, Walsh WM, Madden C, et al, eds. *The Team Physician's Handbook*. Philadelphia: Hanley & Belfus; 2002. Pages 354–364.

20. Bailes JE, Hudson V. Classification of sport-related head trauma: a spectrum of mild to severe injury. *J Athl Train*. 2001;36(3):236–243.

21. Aubry M, Cantu R, Dvorak J, et al. Summary and agreement statement of the First International Conference on Concussion in Sport, Vienna, 2001. Recommendations for the improvement of safety and health of athletes who may suffer concussive injuries. *Phys Sportsmed*. 2002;30(2):57–63.

22. McCrory P, Johnston K, Meeuwisse W, et al. Summary and agreement statement of the Second International Conference on Concussion in Sport, Prague, 2004. *Phys Sportsmed*. 2005;33(4):29–44.

23. McCrory P, Meeuwisse W, Johnston K, et al. Consensus statement on concussion in sport: the 3rd International Conference on Concussion in Sport held in Zurich, November 2008. *J Athl Train*. 2009;44(4):434–448.

24. Frommer LJ, Gurka KK, Cross KM, et al. Sex differences in concussion symptoms of high school athletes. *J Athl Train*. 2011;46(1):76–84.

25. Mucha A, Collins MW, Elbin RJ, et al. A brief vestibular/ocular motor screening (VOMS) assessment to evaluate concussions: preliminary findings. *Am J Sports Med*. 2014;42(10):2479–2486.

26. Dick RW. Is there a gender difference in concussion incidence and outcomes? *Br J Sport Med*. 2009;43(suppl 1):i46–i50.

27. McCauley SR, Boake C, Levin HS, et al. Postconcussional disorder following mild to moderate traumatic brain injury: anxiety, depression, and social support as risk factors and comorbidities. *J Clin Exp Neuropsychol*. 2001;23(6):792–808.

28. Jotwani V, Harmon KG. Postconcussion syndrome in athletes. *Curr Sport Med Rep*. 2010;9(1):21–26.

29. Jordan BD. The clinical spectrum of sport-related traumatic brain injury. *Nat Rev Neurol*. 2013;9(4):222–230.

30. Bey T, Ostick B. Second impact syndrome. *West J Emerg Med*. 2009;10(1):6–10.

31. Kolb JJ. How a cautious approach to TBI patients may help reduce the incidents of second impact syndrome. *J Emerg Med Serv*. 2014;39(1).

32. DeWall J. Evidence-based guidelines for adult traumatic brain injury care. *J Emerg Med Serv*. 2015;35(4).

33. Romeo SJ, Hawley CJ, Romeo MW, et al. Facial injuries in sports: a team physician's guide to diagnosis and treatment. *Phys Sportsmed.* 2005;33(4):45–53.

34. Onate JA, Guskiewicz KM, Riemann BL, et al. A comparison of sideline versus clinical cognitive test performance in collegiate athletes. *J Athl Train.* 2000;35(2):155–160.

35. Iida S, Kogo M, Sugiura T, et al. Retrospective analysis of 1502 patients with facial fractures. *Int J Oral Maxillofac Surg.* 2001;30(4):286–290.

36. Reehal P. Facial injury in sport. *Curr Sports Med Rep.* 2010;9(1):27–34.

37. Young TK, Hall R. The occasional management of epistaxis. *Can J Rural Med.* 2010;15(2):70–74.

38. Alter H. Approach to the adult with epistaxis. http://www.uptodate.com/patients/content/topic.do?topicKey=~2056/corp_da3. Accessed October 10, 2015.

39. Tu HK, Davis LF, Nique TA. Maxillofacial injuries. In: Mellion MB, Walsh WM, Madden C, et al, eds. *The Team Physician's Handbook.* Philadelphia, PA: Hanley & Belfus; 2002. Pages 388–396.

40. Woodmansey KF. Athletic mouth guards prevent orofacial injuries. *J Am Coll Health.* 1997;45(4):179–182.

41. American Academy of Pediatrics and American Academy of Ophthalmology. Policy statement: protective eyewear for young athletes. *Pediatrics.* 2004;113(3):619–622.

Cervical and Thoracic Spinal Conditions

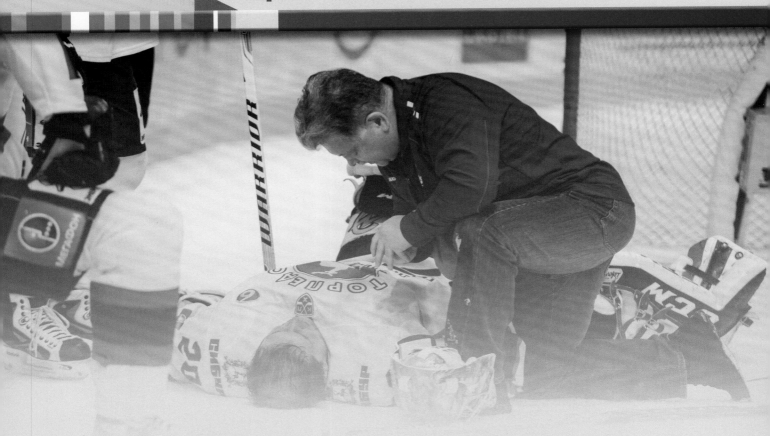

Ivica Drusany / Shutterstock.com

STUDENT OUTCOMES

1. Locate and explain the functional significance of the bony and soft-tissue structures of the cervical and thoracic regions of the spine.

2. Describe the motion capabilities in the cervical and thoracic regions of the spine.

3. Identify the factors that contribute to mechanical loading on the cervical and thoracic regions of the spine.

4. Describe specific strategies in activities of daily living to reduce stress in the cervical and thoracic regions.

5. Identify the anatomical variations that can predispose individuals to cervical and thoracic injuries.

6. Explain the measures used to prevent injuries to the cervical and thoracic spinal regions.

7. Describe a thorough assessment of the cervical and thoracic spinal regions.

8. Describe the common injuries and conditions found in the cervical and thoracic regions.

9. List the rehabilitative exercises for the cervical and thoracic spinal regions.

INTRODUCTION

The spine is a complex linkage system that transfers loads between the upper and lower extremities, enables motion of the trunk in all three planes, and protects the delicate spinal cord. Most injuries to the neck and upper back are relatively minor, consisting of contusions, muscle strains, and ligament sprains. Acute spinal fractures and dislocations in this region are extremely serious, however, and can lead to paralysis or death. Sport-related spinal cord injury account for 9.2% of all spinal cord injuries reported between 2010 and 2013.[1] The highest incidence of catastrophic spinal cord injury occurs in American football.[2] Prompt and accurate on-site assessment is essential for optimizing the outcomes of these potentially devastating injuries.[3]

This chapter begins with a review of the intricate anatomical structures that make up the cervical and thoracic regions of the spine, followed by a discussion of the kinematics and kinetics of these regions. A discussion concerning the identification of anatomical variations that may predispose individuals to cervical and thoracic spinal conditions leads into the strategies used to prevent injury. Assessment techniques used in examining the cervical and thoracic spine region are presented followed by information regarding common injuries sustained within these regions of the spinal column during participation in sport and physical activity. Finally, examples of general rehabilitation exercises for the cervical and thoracic regions are provided.

ANATOMY OF THE CERVICAL AND THORACIC SPINE

The five regions of the spine—namely, the cervical, thoracic, lumbar, sacral, and coccygeal regions—are structurally and functionally distinct. The spine includes four normal curves (**Fig. 21.1**). As viewed from the side, the thoracic and sacral curves are convex posteriorly, and the lumbar and cervical curves are concave posteriorly. These curves constitute posture and can be modified by a host of factors, including heredity, disease, and forces acting on the spine. Abnormal spinal curves are referred to as curvatures. Please refer back to Chapter 8 for a discussion of exacerbated curvature of the thoracic region.

Cervical and Thoracic Spinal Column and Vertebrae

The human body has 7 cervical vertebrae and 12 thoracic vertebrae (**Figs. 21.2** and **21.3**). A typical vertebra consists of a body, a hollow ring known as the vertebral arch, and several bony processes (see **Fig. 21.3**). The superior and inferior articular processes mate with the articular processes of adjacent vertebrae to form the **facet joints**. The right and left pedicles have notches on their superior and inferior borders that provide openings between adjacent pedicles and are called intervertebral foramina. The spinal nerves pass through these foramina. The spinous and transverse processes serve as handles for muscle attachments. Forming a stacked column, the neural arches, posterior sides of the bodies, and intervertebral disks form a protective passageway for the spinal cord and associated blood vessels. The thinnest part of the neural arch is called the **pars interarticularis**. The pars region of the vertebrae is susceptible to stress fractures.

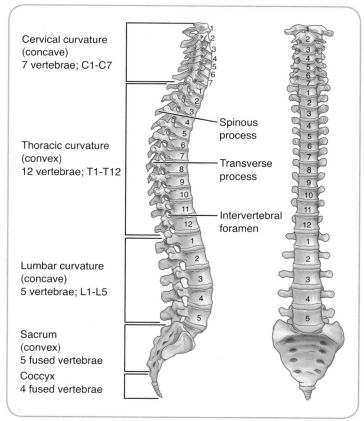

Cervical curvature (concave)
7 vertebrae; C1-C7

Thoracic curvature (convex)
12 vertebrae; T1-T12

Lumbar curvature (concave)
5 vertebrae; L1-L5

Sacrum (convex)
5 fused vertebrae

Coccyx
4 fused vertebrae

Spinous process

Transverse process

Intervertebral foramen

Figure 21.1. Vertebral column. Four characteristic curves of the spine can be viewed from the lateral aspect.

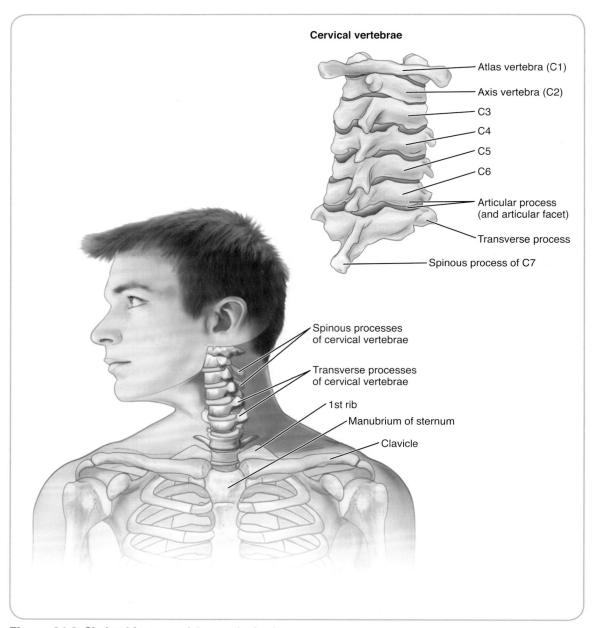

Cervical vertebrae

Atlas vertebra (C1)

Axis vertebra (C2)

C3

C4

C5

C6

Articular process (and articular facet)

Transverse process

Spinous process of C7

Spinous processes of cervical vertebrae

Transverse processes of cervical vertebrae

1st rib

Manubrium of sternum

Clavicle

Figure 21.2. Skeletal features of the cervical spine.

The 1st cervical vertebra is called the **atlas,** because it bears the weight of the head. Articulating with the occipital condyles, the atlanto-occipital joint permits the nodding of the head (see **Fig. 21.2**). The atlas does not have a body or a spinous process. Instead, it has anterior and posterior arches and a thick, lateral mass. The 2nd cervical vertebra, or **axis,** is characterized by a toothlike process called the dens or odontoid process, which projects upward from its body. This process is held in place against the inner surface of the atlas by the transverse ligament. This joint allows the head to rotate and pivot on the neck. The transverse processes of the cervical vertebrae have a foramen (**transverse foramen**), through which the vertebral artery, vein, and a plexus of sympathetic nerves pass. The spinous processes of the cervical vertebrae C2 through C6 often are bifid. The 7th cervical vertebra, or vertebra prominens, has a large spinous process with a somewhat bulbous tip.

The thoracic vertebrae have extra facets (costal facets) on the transverse processes and the body for articulation with the ribs (see **Fig. 21.3**). The spinous processes of the thoracic vertebrae tend to be

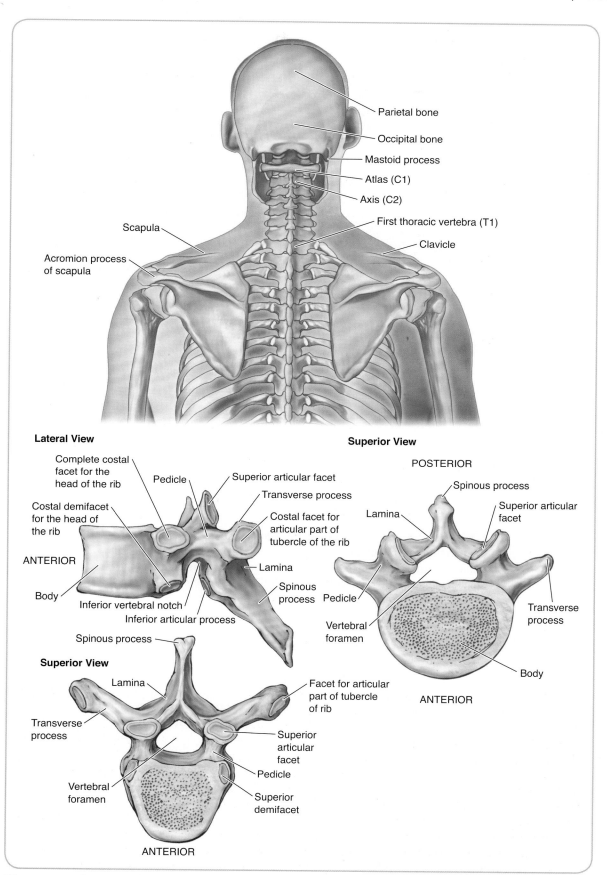

Figure 21.3. Skeletal features of posterior cervical and thoracic spine.

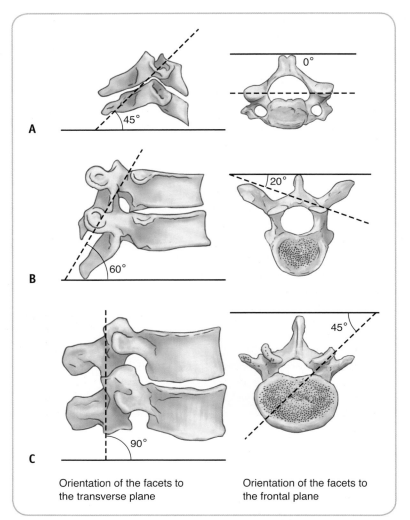

Orientation of the facets to the transverse plane

Orientation of the facets to the frontal plane

Figure 21.4. Approximate orientations of the facet joints. The facet joint orientation in both the sagittal plane (lateral view) and transverse plane (superior view) shifts progressively throughout the length of the spinal column. **A,** Cervical vertebrae (C3–C7). **B,** Thoracic vertebrae. **C,** Lumbar vertebrae.

long and slender, and they direct markedly downward so that they overlap each other. Those of the lower thoracic vertebrae are broader and directed more posteriorly, in this respect being transitional between typical thoracic and typical lumbar vertebrae.

Vertebral size progressively increases from the cervical region down through the lumbar region. This serves a functional purpose because when the body is in an upright position, each vertebra must support the weight of the trunk positioned above it as well as that of the arms and head. The size and angulation of the vertebral processes also vary throughout the spinal column. This changes the orientation of the facet joints, which limit range of motion (ROM) in the different spinal regions (**Fig. 21.4**).

Within the cervical, thoracic, and lumbar regions, any two adjacent vertebrae and the soft tissues between them are collectively referred to as a **motion segment**. The motion segment is referred to as the functional unit of the spine (**Fig. 21.5**).

Intervertebral Disks

Fibrocartilaginous disks provide cushioning between the articulating vertebral bodies. The intervertebral disk consists of a thick ring of fibrous cartilage referred to as the **annulus fibrosus**, which surrounds a gelatinous material known as the **nucleus pulposus**. The disks have a dual function: They serve as shock absorbers and allow the spine to bend. Because the disks receive no blood supply, they must rely on changes in posture and body position to produce a pumping action that brings in nutrients and flushes out metabolic waste products with an influx and outflux of fluid. Because maintaining a fixed body position curtails this pumping action, sitting in one position for a long period of time can negatively affect disk health.

Ligaments of the Spine

A number of ligaments support the spine (**Fig. 21.6**). Anterior and posterior longitudinal ligaments connect the vertebral bodies of the motion segments. The supraspinous ligament attaches to the spinous processes throughout the length of the spine and is enlarged in the cervical region, where it is known as the ligamentum nuchae (or "ligament of the neck"). Another major ligament, the ligamentum flavum, connects the pedicles of adjacent vertebrae. This ligament contains a high proportion of elastic fibers that keep it constantly in tension, contributing to spinal stability. The interspinous ligaments, intertransverse ligaments, and ligamentum flava link the spinous processes, transverse processes, and laminae of adjacent vertebrae, respectively.

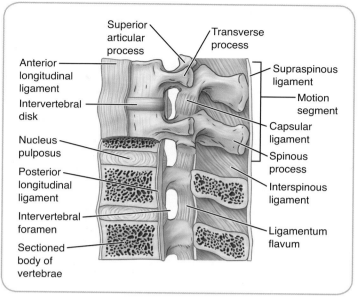

Figure 21.5. Motion segment of the spine. A motion segment includes two adjacent vertebrae and the intervening soft tissues. It is considered to be the functional unit of the spine.

Muscles of the Cervical and Thoracic Regions of the Spine and Trunk

The muscles of the neck and trunk are paired, with one on the left and one on the right side of the body (**Figs. 21.7** and **21.8**). These muscles produce lateral flexion and/or rotation of the trunk when they act unilaterally and trunk flexion or extension when they act bilaterally. Collectively, the primary movers for back extension are called the erector spinae muscles.

See **Muscles of the Spine**, found on the companion Web site at thePoint, for the attachments, actions, and innervations of the major muscles of the upper trunk.

Spinal Cord and Spinal Nerves

The brain and spinal cord make up the central nervous system. The spinal cord extends from the brainstem to the level of the 1st or 2nd lumbar vertebrae. Like the brain, the spinal cord is encased in the three meninges. The spinal cord serves as the major neural pathway for conducting sensory impulses to the brain and motor impulses from the brain. It also provides direct connections between sensory and motor nerves inside the cord, enabling reflex activity. Deep tendon reflexes are used consistently during injury assessment to determine possible spinal nerve damage. Exaggerated, distorted, or absent reflexes indicate damage to the nervous system, often before other signs are apparent.

Thirty-one pairs of spinal nerves emanate from the cord, including 8 cervical and 12 thoracic. Many of the spinal nerves converge (combine) and diverge (separate) to form a complex network of interjoining nerves, called a nerve plexus.

The Cervical Plexus

The cervical plexus consists of the ventral rami of spinal nerves C1 through C4. These nerves innervate muscles of the neck, shoulder, and diaphragm (phrenic nerves, C3 through C5) and supply sensation for the skin of the ear, neck, and upper chest. The plexus lies lateral in relation to the first three cervical vertebrae, ventrolateral to the levator scapulae and scalenus medius, and deep

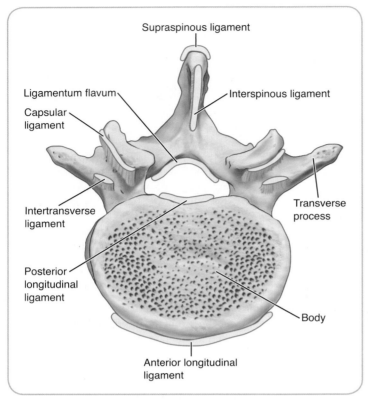

Figure 21.6. Superior view of the ligaments of the vertebral column.

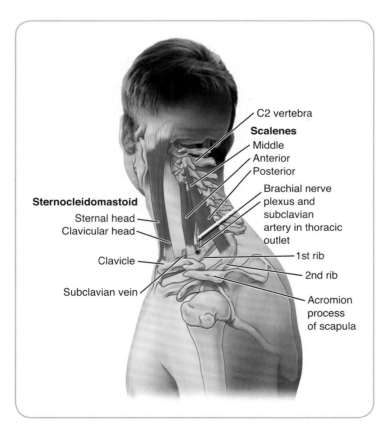

Figure 21.7. Muscles of the neck: lateral view.

to the sternocleidomastoid muscle. Impingement of the plexus results in headaches, neck pain, and breathing difficulties and most often results from pressure on the nerves by the suboccipital and sternocleidomastoid muscles.

The Brachial Plexus

The shoulder region and upper extremity receive sensory and motor innervation from the brachial plexus, which originates from the C5 through T1 nerve roots. These nerve roots converge and diverge to form three trunks, followed by three divisions, and then by three cords. This complex structure terminates in distal branches that form the musculocutaneous, median, ulnar, axillary, and radial nerves, which innervate the arm, forearm, and hand (**Fig. 21.9**). The C5 and C6 nerve roots form the upper trunk, the C7 forms the middle trunk, and the C8 and T1 form the lower trunk. Each trunk then divides into anterior and posterior divisions. The posterior divisions converge to form the posterior cord. The anterior divisions of the upper and middle trunk form the lateral cord, whereas the anterior division of the lower trunk forms the medial cord.

The posterior cord branches into the axillary and radial nerves, which innervate the shoulder, elbow, wrist, and finger extensors. Placing the arm in anatomical position, the lateral half of the medial cord joins with the medial half of the lateral cord to form the large median nerve that innervates most of the wrist and finger flexors. The remaining portion of the medial cord terminates at the ulnar nerve, which innervates the flexor carpi ulnaris and the intrinsic muscles of the hand. The remaining portion of the lateral cord terminates at the musculocutaneous nerve, which innervates the main elbow flexors. Minor branches from the medial and lateral cords innervate the pectoral muscles and cutaneous nerves on the medial arm and forearm. Variations in the length and quality of the components of the brachial plexus often occur, adding to its complexity.[4]

Blood Vessels

The largest blood vessels coursing through the neck are the common carotid arteries (**Fig. 21.10**). The common carotid arteries divide into external and internal carotid arteries, which provide the major blood supply to the brain, head, and face. The vertebral arteries, which are located in the posterior neck, are a source of blood supply for the spinal cord.

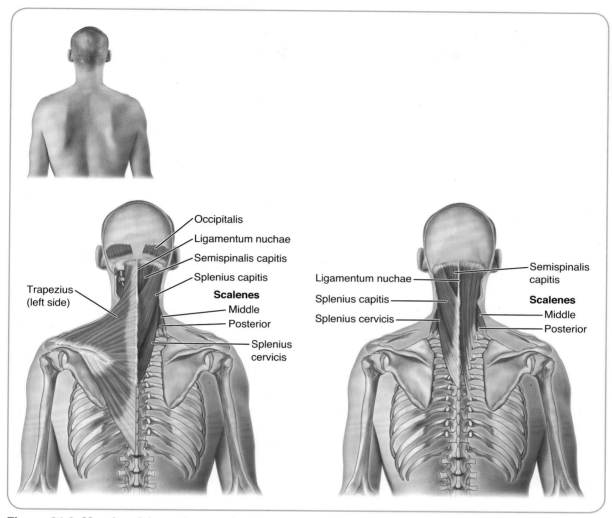

Figure 21.8. Muscles of the neck: posterior view.

KINEMATICS AND MAJOR MUSCLE ACTIONS OF THE CERVICAL AND THORACIC SPINE

Kinematics is the study of the spatial and temporal aspects of motion, which translates to movement, form, or technique. Evaluation of the kinematics of a particular movement can provide information about the timing and sequencing of movement, which can then yield important clues for injury prevention. This section describes the kinematics of the cervical and thoracic spine and identifies the muscles responsible for specific movements.

The vertebral joints enable motion in all planes of movement and permit circumduction. The motion allowed between any two adjacent vertebrae is small, so spinal movements always involve a number of motion segments. The ROM allowed at each motion segment is governed by anatomical constraints, which vary throughout the cervical, thoracic, and lumbar regions of the spine.

Flexion, Extension, and Hyperextension

Spinal flexion is anterior bending of the spine in the sagittal plane, with extension being the return to anatomical position from a position of flexion. When the spine is extended backward past anatomical position in the sagittal plane, the motion is termed **hyperextension**. The active sagittal plane motion capability of the motion segments at different levels of the spine varies, with approximately

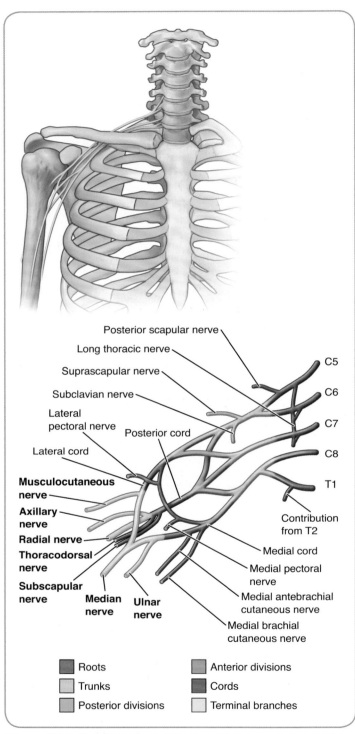

Posterior scapular nerve

Long thoracic nerve

Suprascapular nerve

Subclavian nerve

Lateral pectoral nerve

Posterior cord

Lateral cord

Musculocutaneous nerve

Axillary nerve

Radial nerve

Thoracodorsal nerve

Subscapular nerve

Median nerve

Ulnar nerve

C5

C6

C7

C8

T1

Contribution from T2

Medial cord

Medial pectoral nerve

Medial antebrachial cutaneous nerve

Medial brachial cutaneous nerve

▣ Roots	▣ Anterior divisions
▣ Trunks	▣ Cords
▣ Posterior divisions	▣ Terminal branches

Figure 21.9. Brachial plexus. The brachial plexus is formed by the segmental nerves C5–T1.

137° cumulatively allowed in the cervical region in adolescents and approximately 127° in young and middle-aged adults.[5]

Sagittal plane motion in the thoracic region is restricted by the rib cage, with a flexion–extension capability of only approximately 4° in the upper thoracic segments, of approximately 6° in the mid-thoracic segments, and of up to 12° in the two lower thoracic segments.[5] The ROM for spinal hyperextension is approximately 22° in the thoracic region.[5]

Lateral Flexion and Rotation

Movement of the spine away from anatomical position in a lateral direction in the frontal plane is termed lateral flexion. In the thoracic region, the cumulative ROM for lateral flexion to each side is approximately 31°, with 50° to 52° permitted in the cervical region.[5,6] Spinal rotation capability is greatest in the cervical region, with cumulative rotational ROM between the base of the skull and C7 of approximately 143° and 151° in adolescents and young adults, respectively.[6] In the thoracic region, approximately 9° of rotation is permitted among the upper six motion segments; however, from T7 to T8 downward, the ROM in rotation progressively decreases.[5]

KINETICS OF THE SPINE

Kinetics is the study of the forces associated with motion. Because force ultimately is the cause of injury, understanding the kinetics pertaining to the spine is an important foundation for understanding mechanisms of injury.

Forces acting on the spine include body weight, tension in the spinal ligaments and paraspinal muscles, intra-abdominal pressure, and any applied external loads. When the body is in an upright position, the major form of loading on the spine is axial. In this position, body weight, the weight of any load held in the hands, and the tension in the surrounding ligaments and muscles contribute to spinal compression. Although most of the axial compression load on the spine is borne by the vertebral bodies and disks, the facet joints also assist with load bearing. When the cervical spine is in hyperextension, the facet joints may bear up to approximately 30% of the load.

Effect of Loading

The primary axial load on the cervical spine during nonimpact situations is caused by the weight of the head. Holding the head in other than an upright position tends to elevate the tension required of the cervical paraspinal muscles. The compression load on the thoracic spine is affected by the weight of the body positioned above the thoracic spine and by the weight of any load held in the hands.

External loads generally create more compression on the thoracic spine than do changes in body position.

Effect of Impact

For individuals participating in high-speed collision and contact sports, impact forces are an inherent risk in terms of potential spinal injuries. Because the ROM in the cervical spine is greatest in flexion, a head position of extreme flexion generates the largest bending movement. When combined with axial compression loading, this generates the leading mechanism of injury for severe cervical spine injuries. For example, when a football tackle is executed with the head in a flexed position, the cervical spine is aligned in a segmented column and is subjected to both large compressional forces, generated by the cervical muscles, and axial impact forces (**Fig. 21.11**). Impact causes loading along the longitudinal axis of the cervical vertebrae, leading to compression deformation. The intervertebral disks can absorb some energy initially; however, as continued force is exerted, further deformation and buckling occurs, leading to failure of the intervertebral disks, cervical vertebrae, or both (**Fig. 21.12**). The potential results include subluxation, disk herniation, facet dislocation, or fracture dislocation at one or more spinal levels. Axial loading of the cervical spine is significantly associated with increased risk of fracture during injuries.[7] In soccer, heading the ball does not typically cause traumatic injury, but players may develop degenerative changes to the cervical spine earlier than the normal population because of the repetitive stress.[8]

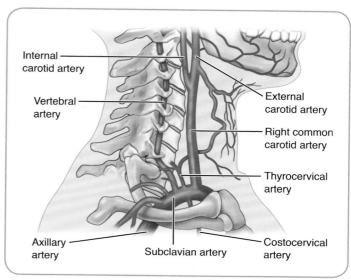

Figure 21.10. Blood vessels to the spine. Cervical vertebrae receive a large portion of their blood supply from the vertebral artery, a branch of the subclavian artery.

ANATOMICAL VARIATIONS PREDISPOSING INDIVIDUALS TO SPINAL CONDITIONS

Mechanical stress derived from lateral spinal muscle imbalances or from sustaining repeated impact forces can cause back pain and/or injury. Excessive spinal curvatures can be congenital or acquired through weight training or sport participation. Please refer to Chapter 8 for a discussion on excessive spinal curvatures.

PREVENTION OF SPINAL CONDITIONS

Although most of the load on the spine is borne by the vertebral bodies and disks, the facet joints assist with some load bearing. Protective equipment can prevent some injuries to the cervical and thoracic regions; however, physical conditioning plays a more important role in preventing injuries to the overall region.

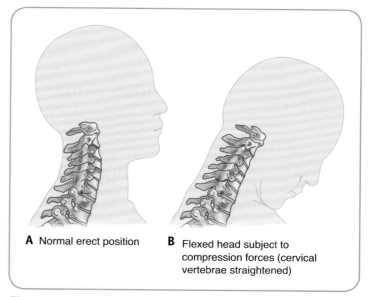

Figure 21.11. Axial loading. A, In a normally erect position, the cervical spine is slightly extended. **B,** When a football tackle is executed with the head flexed at about 30°, the cervical vertebrae are aligned in a column and subjected to compression forces, generated by the cervical muscles, and to axial loading.

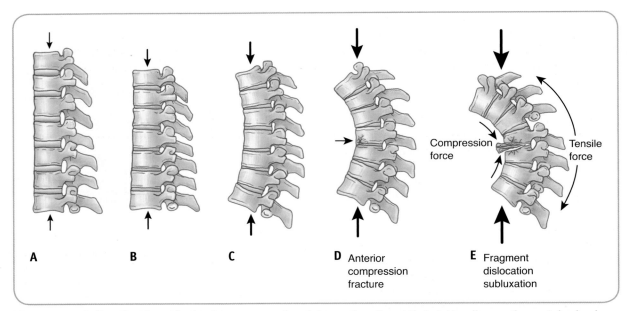

Figure 21.12. Results of cervical spine compression deformation. A and **B,** Axial loading on the vertebral column causes compressive deformation of the intervertebral disks. **C,** Angular deformation and buckling occurs as the load continues and the maximum compression deformation is reached. **D** and **E,** Continued force results in an anterior compression fracture, subluxation, or dislocation.

Protective Equipment

Several pieces of equipment can be used to protect the spine. In the cervical region, a neck roll or posterolateral pad made of a high, thick, and stiff material can be attached to shoulder pads to limit excessive motion of the cervical spine. Such restraints have been shown to reduce the incidence of repetitive burners and stingers; however, they also may increase the risk of cervical spine injuries by limiting the natural flexibility of the neck. In the upper body, shoulder pads extend over and protect the upper thoracic region. Rib protectors composed of air-inflated, interconnected cylinders can protect a limited region of the thoracic spine. Many of these protective devices are discussed and demonstrated in Chapter 3.

Physical Conditioning

Strengthening of the back muscles is imperative to stabilize the spinal column. Strengthening exercises for the cervical region may involve isometric contractions, manual resistance, or weight training with free weights or specialized machines. Exercises should include neck flexion, extension, lateral flexion, and rotation as well as scapular elevation. Stabilization of the cervical spine is particularly important for wrestlers and football lineman, who are consistently subjected to extremes of motion at the neck. Exercises to strengthen the thoracic region should involve back extension, lateral flexion, and rotation; abdominal strengthening; and exercises for the lower trapezius and latissimus dorsi.

Normal ROM is essential in stabilizing the spine and preventing injury. If warranted, stretching exercises should be used to promote and maintain normal ROM in the cervical and thoracic regions.

Proper Skill Technique

Proper skill technique is vital in preventing spinal injuries. Helmets are designed to protect the cranial region from injury but do not prevent axial loading on the cervical spine. It is critical that proper techniques be taught and reinforced in an effort to reduce the potential for injury. Since the 1976 rule change banning spearing in high school football, a large reduction in the incidence of catastrophic spinal injuries has occurred. In 2004, the National Athletic Trainers' Association (NATA) published a position statement strongly discouraging head-down contact and spearing in tackle football whether intentional or unintentional.[9] As part of the position statement, the NATA highly recommended that officials enforce the existing rules to further reduce the incidence of head-down contact.

ASSESSMENT OF SPINAL CONDITIONS

 Before the start of an afternoon practice, a college field hockey player reports to the athletic training room with a "stiff neck." She reports that she did not experience any neck pain or discomfort during or after practice the previous day.

Injury assessment of the spine is complex and cannot be rushed. In a traumatic episode, if a fully conscious person is not experiencing severe pain, spasm, or tenderness, it is rare that the individual has sustained a significant spinal injury. More likely, the individual has experienced a minor injury, such as a muscular strain or sprain. Even so, it is essential that injury assessment be performed in a deliberate manner, taking as much time as necessary.

See **Application Strategy: Cervical Spine Injury Evaluation**, available on the companion Web site at thePoint, for a summary of the assessment procedure.

The severity of pain and the presence or absence of neurological symptoms, neck spasm, and tenderness can indicate whether spinal involvement should be suspected. When in doubt, it should be assumed that a severe spinal injury is present, and the emergency care plan should be activated. Once a significant physical finding indicates possible nerve involvement, protective equipment should be removed and the patient immobilization with immediate transportation to the nearest medical facility is warranted, regardless of whether a total assessment is completed.[10] **Box 21.1** identifies several signs and symptoms that necessitate activating the emergency care plan and, potentially, summoning emergency medical services (EMS).

For cases in which the individual walks into an examination room complaining of neck or upper back pain, it is relatively safe to assume that a serious spinal injury is not present. The assessment that follows focuses on a cervical and thoracic spinal assessment in a conscious individual. Specific information related to an acute injury is included where appropriate.

HISTORY

 What basic information needs to be obtained from the field hockey player as part of the history component of this injury assessment?

BOX 21.1 Red Flags That Warrant Immobilization and Immediate Referral to a Physician

- Severe pain, point tenderness, or deformity along the vertebral column
- Pain radiating into the extremities
- Trunk or abdominal pain that may be referred from the visceral organs
- Loss or change in sensation anywhere in the body
- Paralysis or inability to move a body part
- Any injury for which you are uncertain about the severity or nature
- Diminished or absent reflexes
- Muscle weakness in a myotome

See **Application Strategy: Developing a History for a Cervical Spine Injury**, available on the companion Web site at thePoint, for general questions related to a spinal injury.

A history of the injury should include information regarding the primary complaint, mechanism of injury, characteristics of the symptoms, disability resulting from the injury, previous injuries to the area, and any family history that may have some bearing on the specific condition. In a spinal injury, questions should be asked about the location of pain (i.e., localized or radiating), type of pain (i.e., dull, aching, sharp, or burning), presence of sensory changes (i.e., numbness, tingling, or absence of sensation), and possible muscle weakness or paralysis. If the injury is to the neck, questions should be asked to determine any long- and short-term memory loss, which may indicate an associated concussion or subdural hematoma. It is important to note the length of time it takes the individual to respond to the questions.

> In attempting to determine the cause and extent of injury, the field hockey player should be asked questions pertaining to the primary complaint (i.e., what, when, and how questions), mechanism of injury (e.g., potential mechanism the previous day), characteristics and onset of symptoms (i.e., nature, location, severity, or disability), unusual sensation, and related medical history (i.e., past injuries/treatment).

OBSERVATION AND INSPECTION

? The field hockey player cannot recall a specific mechanism of injury but states that she was involved in a collision during practice the previous day. She reports pain and stiffness on the left side of the neck upon waking up this morning, which has continued throughout the day. She does not report any previous history of injury to the cervical spine, and no evidence of sensory or motor deficits is found. What specific factors should be observed and inspected in the ongoing assessment of the field hockey player, and is it appropriate to perform a scan examination?

See **Application Strategy: Postural Assessment of the Cervical and Upper Thoracic Spine**, available on the companion Web site at thePoint, for specific postural factors to observe in the head and spinal region.

Observation should begin as soon as the clinician sets eyes on the individual. Body language can signal pain, disability, and muscle weakness. It is necessary to note the individual's willingness or ability to move, general posture, ease in motion, and general attitude. Clothing and protective equipment may prevent visual observation of abnormalities in the spinal alignment. As such, the individual should be suitably dressed so that the back is as exposed as possible; for girls and women, a bra, halter top, or swimsuit can be worn. Observation should begin with a postural assessment, progress through a scan examination and gait analysis, and end with an inspection of the injury site. Please refer to Chapter 8 for a full discussion on posture and gait assessment techniques.

Scan Examination

Active movement should not be performed when pain is present over the vertebrae or when motor/sensory deficits are present. If that is not the case, a scan examination can be used to assess general motor function (**Application Strategy 21.1**). It can potentially rule out injury at other joints that may be overlooked because of intense pain or discomfort at the primary injury site. Active movement of the spine may be included in this step and need not be repeated with functional tests. It is important to note any hesitation in moving a body part or preference for using one side over the other.

Injury Site Inspection

Local inspection of the injury site should include observation for deformity, swelling, discoloration, muscle spasm, atrophy, hypertrophy, scars that might indicate previous surgery, and general skin condition. It is important to note any altered coloration of the skin, ulcers, or vein distention as evidence of upper limb ischemia.

Scan Examination for a Cervical Spine Injury

The athletic trainer should instruct the athlete to perform the skills listed in the following. During these movements, observe for signs of pain, hesitation to move a body part, or abnormal movement. If these signs are present, complete a more thorough evaluation of the affected body part, and if necessary, immobilize the area and refer the athlete to a physician for further care.

- Touch the chin to the chest.
- Lean sideways and do lateral flexion of the trunk.
- Look up at the ceiling while keeping the back straight.
- While placing a hand on a table for support,

  - Turn the head sideways in both directions.
  - Do a single straight-leg raise forward, backward, and sideways.
  - Try to touch each ear to the shoulder.
  - Rotate the trunk sideways while keeping the hips stabilized.
  - Flex the knee.
  - Lean forward and touch the toes.
  - Rise up on the toes.
  - Look up at the ceiling with hyperextension of the trunk.
  - Balance on the heels.

Gross Neuromuscular Assessment

With an acute injury, a posture and scan examination is not possible; however, it is beneficial to perform a neuromuscular assessment before palpation to detect any motor and/or sensory deficits. The individual should not be moved but, rather, asked to perform submaximal, bilateral hand squeeze, and ankle dorsiflexion. These two actions assess the cervical and lumbar spinal nerves, respectively. Muscle weakness and/or diminished sensation over the hands and feet indicate a serious injury. If any deficits are noted, the emergency plan, including summoning EMS, should be activated. If no deficits are noted, it does not rule out possible neurological involvement or fracture. Therefore, palpation should be done with the individual maintained in the position in which he or she was found.

 Observation should note the individual's willingness or ability to move, general posture, ease in motion, and general attitude. Observation should begin with a postural assessment, progress through a scan examination and gait analysis, and end with an inspection of the injury site.

PALPATION

? A postural examination reveals a slight head tilt to the left side, with the chin pointed toward the opposite shoulder. An inspection of the area reveals no abnormal findings. Because the patient is experiencing pain on the left side and not over the vertebrae, a scan examination is performed and reveals limited ROM on the involved side because of pain. Describe the appropriate progression of the palpation component in the assessment of the field hockey player.

With injuries that do not involve neural damage, fracture, or dislocation, palpation can proceed in the following manner. Bony and soft-tissue structures are palpated to detect temperature, swelling, point tenderness, trigger points, deformity, crepitus, muscle spasm, and cutaneous sensation. Palpation may be done in a seated, standing, supine, or prone position. To relax the neck and spinal

TABLE 21.1 Surface Landmarks on the Back

VERTEBRA	BONY LANDMARK
C2	One finger's breadth inferior to the mastoid process
C6	Posterior to the cricoid cartilage
C7 and T1	Prominent spinous processes in neck
T2	Top of scapula
T4	Base of spine of scapula
T7	Inferior angle of scapula
T12	Lowest floating rib
L4	Top of iliac crest
L5	Demarcated by bilateral dimples
S2	Level of posterior superior iliac spines

muscles, the individual should lie on a table. When the clinician is palpating posterior neck structures, the individual should be supine. The clinician should reach around the neck with both hands and palpate either side of the spine with the fingertips. Muscle spasms in the erector spinae, sternocleidomastoid muscles, scalene muscles, and/or upper trapezius may indicate dysfunction of the cervical spine. In palpating the thoracic region, the individual should be prone. A pillow or blanket should be placed under the hip region to tilt the pelvis back and relax the lumbar curvature. Muscle spasm in the lower erector spinae, lower trapezius, serratus posterior, quadratus lumborum, latissimus dorsi, or gluteus maximus may indicate dysfunction of the thoracic or lumbar spine. Surface landmarks can facilitate palpation (**Table 21.1**); the following structures should be palpated:

Anterior Aspect

1. Hyoid bone, thyroid cartilage, 1st cricoid ring, and trachea

2. Sternocleidomastoid muscle, manubrium, clavicle, and supraclavicular fossa

3. Sternum, ribs, and costal cartilage

4. Abdomen and inguinal area. Note any abnormal tenderness or masses indicating internal pathology that is referring pain to the spinal region.

Posterior Aspect

1. External protuberance of the occiput

2. Mastoid processes

3. Spinous processes. The spinous processes of C2, C6, and C7 are the most prominent. Note any tenderness, crepitus, or deviation from the norm. A noticeable discrepancy can indicate a fracture or vertebral subluxation. Pain and tenderness without positive findings on muscle movement may indicate that the problem is not musculoskeletal in origin.

4. Facet joints. The facet articulations are approximately a thumb's breadth (2 to 3 cm or 0.8 to 1.2 in) to either side of the spinous process. Point tenderness, especially with extension and rotation to the same side, suggests facet joint pain. In the thoracic area, it is difficult to palpate these joints because of the overlying musculature. Muscle spasm and tenderness may indicate pathology in

the gallbladder (spasm on the right side around the 8th and 9th costal cartilages), spleen (spasm at the left side at the level of ribs 9 to 11), and kidneys (posterior spasm at the level of ribs 11 to 12).

5. Interspinous and supraspinous ligaments, ligamentum flavum, paraspinal muscles, and quadratus lumborum. Trigger points of the paraspinal and shoulder girdle regions refer pain to a more distal area. Tender points that increase with muscular contraction indicate a localized muscle strain. An area that is tender to palpation but not painful during muscle contraction may indicate referred pain from another area.

6. Scapula, trapezius, latissimus dorsi, and paravertebral muscles. Tightness or spasms in the paravertebral muscles increases lordosis in the lumbar spine.

Lateral Aspect

1. Transverse process of cervical vertebrae

2. Lymph nodes and carotid arteries. The lymph nodes will only be palpable if they are swollen. The nodes are palpated along the line of the sternocleidomastoid muscle, and the carotid pulse may be palpated between the sternocleidomastoid muscle and the trachea.

3. Temporomandibular joints, mandible, and parotid glands. The parotid gland lies over the angle of the mandible. If the gland is swollen, it is palpable as a soft, boggy structure.

 Both bony and soft-tissue structures should be palpated to determine the presence of swelling, spasm, and crepitus as well as to detect point tenderness, temperature, or trigger points.

PHYSICAL EXAMINATION TESTS

 Palpation of the field hockey player reveals spasm in the musculature on the involved side. What tests should be performed in the ongoing assessment of the field hockey player?

It is imperative to work slowly through the different tests because injuries to the spinal region can be very complex. If, at any time, movement leads to increased acute pain, change in sensation, or if the individual resists moving the spine, a significant injury should be assumed to exist. As such, the emergency plan should be activated, including summoning EMS.

Functional Tests

Goniometry measurements of the spine are not typically taken because of the difficulty in measuring individual regional motions. Completion of gross movement patterns is adequate to determine normal ROM. Further assessment can be conducted if motion is limited.

Active Movement

If active movement of the spine was conducted during the scan examination, it need not be repeated. The individual's willingness to perform the movement as well as the smoothness and completeness of the movement should be noted. It is important to determine whether pain, spasm, or stiffness block the full ROM. Movements to the left and right should be compared bilaterally, and cervical and thoracic movement should be tested in the standing position. Spinal movements include the following:

1. Cervical flexion (80° to 90°)

2. Cervical extension (70°)

3. Lateral cervical flexion (left and right; 20° to 45°)

4. Cervical rotation (left and right; 70° to 90°)

5. Forward thoracic trunk flexion (20° to 45°)

6. Thoracic trunk extension (25° to 45°)

7. Lateral trunk flexion (left and right; 20° to 40°)

8. Trunk rotation (35° to 50°)

Passive Range of Motion

Passive movement should not be performed in an individual with an acute injury when motor and sensory deficits are present. These deficits may indicate a spinal injury, and any movement could be catastrophic. In performing passive motion, the individual is placed in a supine position. The cervical region is moved passively through the various movements. The normal end feel for the cervical spine is tissue stretch in all four movements. Thoracic passive movement seldom is performed in a gross fashion. Individual movement may be tested by palpating over and between the spinous processes of the lower cervical and upper thoracic spines as the patient performs the motions. Normal motion between the spinous processes include flexion (move apart), extension (move together), rotation (one side moves forward, and the other moves back), and lateral flexion (one side moves apart, and one side moves together). The normal end feels for thoracic movements also are tissue stretch.

Resisted Muscle Testing

Resisted movement is performed throughout the full ROM in the same movements as active muscle testing. It is important to stabilize the hip and trunk during cervical testing to avoid muscle substitution. This can be accomplished by having the individual in the seated position and the clinician using one hand to stabilize the shoulder or thorax while the other hand applies manual overpressure. When testing the thoracic region, the weight of the trunk stabilizes the hips. The individual should be instructed not to allow the clinician to move the body part that is being tested. Maximal force must be applied when testing the major muscle groups to detect early weakness. By repetitively loading the resisting muscle with rapid, consecutive impulses, more subtle weakness can be detected. The assessed cervical and thoracic movements are demonstrated in **Figures 21.13** and **21.14**, respectively.

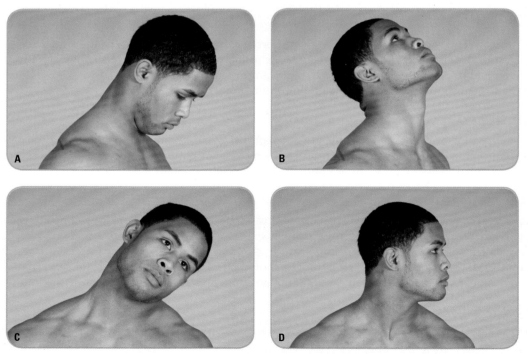

Figure 21.13. Active movements of the cervical spine. A, Flexion. **B,** Extension. **C,** Lateral flexion. **D,** Rotation.

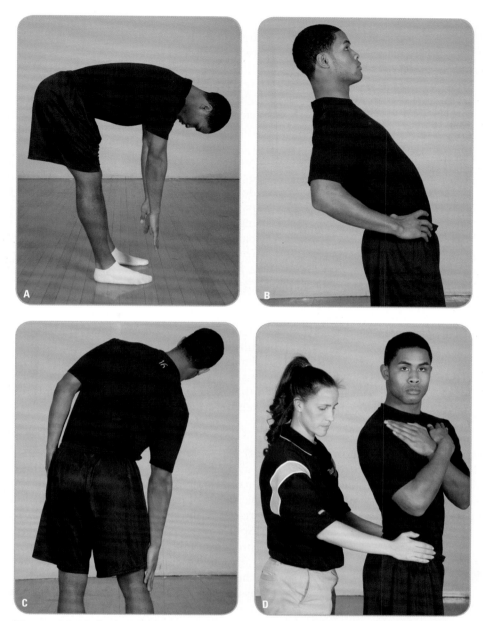

Figure 21.14. Active movements of the thoracic region. A, Flexion. **B,** Extension. **C,** Lateral flexion. **D,** Rotation.

Stress and Functional Tests

Several stress tests can be used in spinal assessment. Only those deemed to be relevant should be performed. If any increased pain or change of sensation occurs, the individual should be immobilized, and the emergency plan should be activated, including summoning EMS.

Cervical Spine Tests

■ Brachial Plexus Traction Test

This test should not be performed until the possibility of bony trauma has been ruled out. While standing behind the patient, the athletic trainer passively flexes the patient's head to one side while applying a downward pressure on the opposite shoulder (**Fig. 21.15**). If pain increases or radiates into the upper arm that is being depressed, it indicates stretching of the brachial plexus. If pain increases

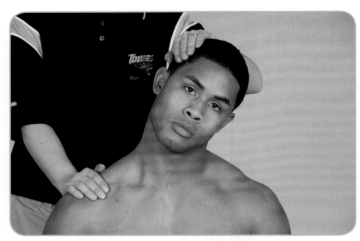

Figure 21.15. Brachial plexus traction test. The clinician applies downward pressure during lateral bending away from the involved shoulder while simultaneously depressing the involved shoulder. Radiating pain or a burning sensation indicates injury to the brachial plexus. If pain increases on the side toward the lateral bending, it indicates irritation or compression of the nerve roots between two vertebrae.

on the side toward the lateral bending, it indicates irritation or compression of the nerve roots between two vertebrae.

■ Cervical Compression Test

The compression test can detect pressure on a cervical nerve root as a result of degeneration or narrowing of a neural foramen. This test should not be performed if any suspicion of vertebral fracture is present. While the patient is sitting on a stable chair or table, the clinician applies compression straight down on the patient's head (**Fig. 21.16**). Increased pain or altered sensation is a positive sign, indicating pressure on a nerve root. The distribution of the pain and altered sensation can indicate which nerve root is involved. The cervical compression test is a highly sensitivity (83%) test with low specificity (34%).[11]

■ Cervical Distraction Test

This test is performed by having the clinician place one hand under the patient's chin and the other hand around the occiput and then slowly lifting the head (**Fig. 21.17**). The test is positive if pain decreases or is relieved as the head is lifted; this indicates that pressure on the nerve root is relieved. Pain that is increased with distraction indicates ligamentous injury. The cervical distraction test has a reported poor sensitivity (43% to 44%) but strong specificity (90% to 98.5%).[11,12]

■ Spurling Test (Foraminal Compression Test)

The Spurling test[13] was first introduced in 1944 as a clinical assessment tool for diagnosing cervical nerve pathology. Since that time, many variations have appeared in the literature. The description included within this text is thought to elicit higher levels of pain, levels of paresthesia, and pain distribution patterns than other variations and, therefore, is the recommended technique.[13] Because the Spurling test is a provocation test, a progressed approach should be taken.

The patient is placed in a seated position while the patient's neck is passively extended. The patient is questioned for presence, type, location, and intensity of pain. If none present, the clinician then laterally bends the neck while still keeping it in extension. The patient is questioned for presence, type, location, and intensity of pain. If no pain is reported, an axial load is then applied with extension and lateral bending (**Fig. 21.18**). If this position, with or without pressure, reproduces radiating pain into the upper limb, a nerve root impingement caused by a narrowing of the neural foramina is suggested. The distribution of the pain and altered sensation can indicate which nerve root is involved. The sensitivity for Spurling is 55% with 92% specificity.

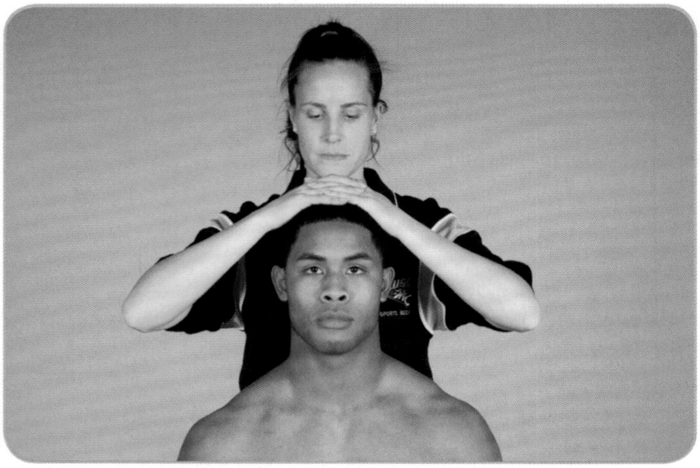

■ Shoulder Abduction Test

A positive shoulder abduction test occurs when the patient has a relief of symptoms associated with nerve root compression. This test is also known as

Figure 21.16. Compression test. The neck should be in a neutral position. The clinician carefully pushes straight down on the patient's head. Increased pain or altered sensation is a positive sign, indicating pressure on a nerve root. The test also can be performed with the neck slightly flexed to one side.

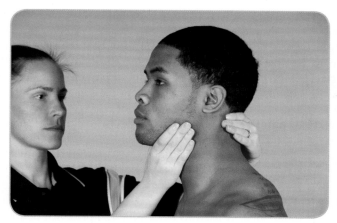

Figure 21.17. Distraction test. The clinician lifts the head slowly. The test is positive if pain is decreased or relieved as the head is lifted, indicating that pressure on the nerve root is relieved. Pain that increases with distraction indicates ligamentous injury.

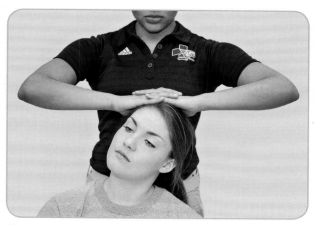

Figure 21.18. Spurling test. The clinician passively extends and laterally bends the neck. If no symptoms are reported, the clinician carefully applies downward pressure on the patient's head. Increased pain indicates cervical nerve root involvement.

the shoulder abduction relief test or Bakody test.[14] The patient may be seated or standing and is asked to abduct the shoulder, resting the hand on the top of the head (**Fig. 21.19**). A decrease in symptoms may indicate a nerve root compression, possibly resulting from a herniated disk, epidural vein compression, or nerve root compression, usually in the C4–C5 or C5–C6 areas. A patient may also perform this maneuver without being prompted to because it provides a relief from symptoms. The shoulder abduction test has moderate (43%) sensitivity and strong (90%) specificity.[11,12]

■ Upper Limb Tension Test

This test is used to assess for the presence of cervical radiculopathy due to mechanical factors such as impingement or entrapment of the nerve. A positive test occurs if the patient experiences pain, tingling, or numbness; therefore, the patient should be questioned at each step of the test for onset of symptoms. To begin with, the patient is supine with the patient's arm at side, forearm pronated, elbow flexed, and wrist and fingers in a comfortable position. Neck should be laterally flexed to opposite side. Between each step, the clinician should hold the patient in the position described for 6 seconds before progressing to next step. Test is completed when symptoms appear.

To assess the median nerve, the clinician passively depresses the patient's shoulder and maintains shoulder depression throughout test. The shoulder is abducted to 110°, and the elbow is placed in full extension. The forearm is then supinated with wrist, fingers, and thumb extended.

To assess the radial nerve, the clinician passively depresses the patient's shoulder and maintains shoulder depression throughout test. The shoulder is abducted to 10°, and the elbow is moved into full extension. The forearm is pronated with wrist flexed and ulnar deviated. The fingers and thumb are then flexed, followed by laterally rotating the shoulder.

To assess the radial nerve, the clinician passively depresses the patient's shoulder and maintains shoulder depression throughout test. The shoulder is medially rotated and elbow placed in full extension. Wrist and fingers are flexed.

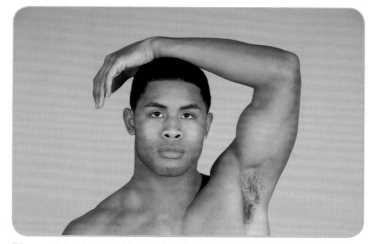

Figure 21.19. Shoulder abduction test. The patient actively abducts the arm and places the hand on top of the head. If symptoms are relieved, a nerve root compression or herniated disk may be present.

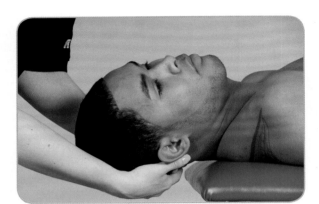

Figure 21.20. Vertebral artery test. While supporting the patient's head, the clinician passively extends, laterally flexes, and rotates the head, then holds this position for 30 seconds. If the patient becomes dizzy, confused, nauseated, or has abnormal eye movement, the patient should be referred immediately to a physician to determine if the vertebral artery is occluded.

■ Vertebral Artery Test

The patient should be supine. The clinician is seated at the head of the patient and supports the occiput in both hands. The clinician passively extends and laterally flexes and rotates the cervical spine in the same direction and then holds the position for 30 seconds (**Fig. 21.20**). If the patient experiences any dizziness, confusion, abnormal movement of the eyes (nystagmus), unilateral pupil changes, or nausea, occlusion of the cervical vertebral artery should be suspected, and the patient should be referred to a physician immediately, without performing additional tests.

■ Valsalva Test

Valsalva maneuver is used to determine the presence of space-occupying lesions (e.g., herniated disk, tumor, or osteophytes). While supine, the individual is asked to take a deep breath and then hold it while bearing down, as if moving the bowels. Caution should be used with this test, however, because the maneuver increases intrathecal pressure, which can slow the pulse, decrease venous return, and increase venous pressure, each of which may cause fainting. A positive test is indicated by increased pain.

Thoracic Spine Tests

Spring Test for Facet Joint Mobility

Hypomobility of the vertebrae, especially at the facet joint, may be assessed with the spring test (**Fig. 21.21**). With the patient prone, the clinician stands over the patient with the thumbs placed over the spinous process to be tested. The clinician carefully pushes the spinous process anteriorly, feeling for a springing of the vertebrae. The test is positive if pain is elicited or if the vertebra does not move ("spring").

Thoracic Outlet Test

Adson test, military brace test, and Allen test are used to assess for the presence of thoracic outlet syndrome (TOS). These tests are described in Chapter 17.

Neurological Tests

Because trauma to the brain or spinal cord can be reflected in **hyperreflexia**, muscle weakness, loss of sensation, and ataxia, several tests should be performed to assess for upper and lower motor neuron lesions. Upper quarter neurological screening tests for trauma to the C5–T1 nerve roots, whereas lower quarter neurological screening tests the L1–S2 nerve roots. In addition, loss of bowel and bladder control can be a sign of upper motor neuron lesions. Neurological integrity can be assessed through special tests, myotomes, reflexes, segmental dermatomes, and peripheral nerve cutaneous patterns.

Upper Motor Neuron Tests

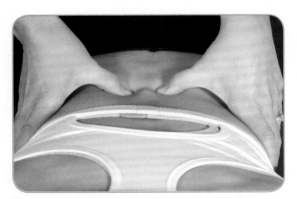

Figure 21.21. Facet joint spring test. While placing the thumbs directly over the spinous process, the clinician carefully pushes the spinous process anteriorly, feeling for the springing of the vertebrae. If pain is elicited or the vertebra is hypomobile, facet joint pathology is present.

■ Oppenheim Test

The patient should be supine. Using the edge of his or her fingernail, the clinician strokes the crest of the anteromedial tibia (**Fig. 21.22**). A positive sign is extension of the big toe and abduction (splaying) of the other toes or hypersensitivity to the test and suggests an upper motor neuron lesion.

■ Babinski Test

The patient should be supine, with the eyes closed and the leg held in a slightly elevated and flexed position. A pointed object is stroked along the plantar aspect of the foot (see **Fig. 20.9**). A normal sign is for the toes to curl downward in flexion and adduction. A positive sign is extension of the big toe and abduction (splaying) of the other toes, which suggests an upper motor neuron lesion.

■ Hoffmann Sign

The **Hoffman sign** is the upper limb equivalent of the Babinski test. The clinician holds the patient's middle finger and briskly flicks the distal phalanx. A positive sign occurs if the interphalangeal joint of the thumb of the same hand flexes.

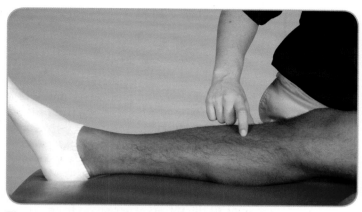

Figure 21.22. Oppenheim test. The patient is supine. The clinician runs a fingernail along the crest of the anteromedial tibia. A positive test result is seen when the great toe extends and the other toes splay or when the patient reports hypersensitivity to the test.

Myotomes

Isometric muscle testing is performed in the neck and upper extremities to test specific myotomes (**Table 21.2**). Myotomes were originally discussed in Chapter 6. Maximal force should be applied when testing the major muscle groups to detect weakness.

Reflexes

Repetitive tapping of the reflexes may show a gradual decline in the reflex response not otherwise noted with a single tap. Absent or decreased reflexes are not necessarily pathological, especially in individuals who have well-developed muscles. Upper limb reflexes can be increased by having the individual perform an isometric contraction, such as squeezing the knees together during the test. Reflexes in the upper extremity include the biceps (C5–C6), brachioradialis (C6), and triceps (C7). Asymmetry between sides should raise suspicion of an abnormality.

TABLE 21.2 Myotomes Used to Test Selected Nerve

NERVE ROOT SEGMENT	ACTION TESTED
C1–C2	Neck flexion[a]
C3 and cranial nerve XI	Lateral neck flexion[a]
C4 and cranial nerve XI	Shoulder elevation
C5	Shoulder abduction
C6	Elbow flexion and/or wrist extension
C7	Elbow extension and/or wrist flexion
C8	Thumb extension and/or ulnar deviation
T1	Finger abduction and adduction
L5	Demarcated by bilateral dimples
S2	Level of posterior superior iliac spines

[a]These myotomes should not be performed if a cervical fracture or dislocation is suspected, because they may cause serious damage or even death.

Cutaneous Patterns

The wide variation of dermatomal innervation and the subjectivity of the test make it less useful than motor or reflex testing; however, the test is useful to check for a sensory loss in a peripheral nerve distribution if an upper limb peripheral nerve entrapment is suspected. The segmental nerve dermatome patterns and peripheral nerve cutaneous patterns were shown in **Figure 6.7**. Bilaterally testing for altered sensation with sharp and dull touch is performed by running the open hand and fingernails over the head, neck, back, thorax, abdomen, and upper and lower extremities (front, back, and sides). The patient is asked if the sensation feels the same on one body segment as compared to the other.

Referred Pain

Pain can be referred to the thoracic spine from various abdominal organs. **Figure 6.1** shows cutaneous areas of the thorax where pain from visceral organs is referred.

Activity-Specific Functional Testing

Before returning to sport/activity, the individual must have a normal neurological examination with pain-free ROM, normal bilateral muscle strength, cutaneous sensation, and reflexes. Axial head compression can be performed on the sideline as an additional safety check. If pain is present, the individual should not return to sport/activity. The sport/activity-specific functional tests that should be performed include walking, bending, lifting, jogging, running, figure eight running, carioca running, and sport/activity-specific skills. Tests must be performed pain-free and with unlimited movement.

 The testing component of an assessment should include functional testing, stress testing, special tests, neurological testing, and activity-specific functional testing. Given the findings (i.e., history, observation, inspection, and palpation) pertaining to the field hockey player, a "wry" neck (torticollis) should be suspected. Functional testing (i.e., active, passive, and resisted ROM) is warranted.

CERVICAL SPINE CONDITIONS

 The major concern with cervical injuries is the potential involvement of the spinal cord and nerve roots. What specific signs and symptoms of a cervical injury suggest neural involvement and, as such, a potentially catastrophic injury?

The relatively small size of the cervical vertebrae, combined with the nearly horizontal orientation of the cervical facet joints, makes the cervical spine the most mobile region of the spinal column. As such, this area is especially vulnerable to injury.

Torticollis

Etiology

Torticollis, or scoliosis of the cervical spine, is a deformity of the neck in which the head tilts toward one shoulder and, simultaneously, the chin rotates toward the opposite shoulder. It is a symptom as well as a disease, and it has a host of underlying pathologies. Torticollis can be divided into two types: congenital and acquired. Infants who are born with torticollis appear to be healthy at delivery but, within 2 to 8 weeks, develop soft-tissue swelling over an injured sternocleidomastoid. Injury may result from birth trauma or intrauterine malpositioning (breech positioning).

In children, acquired torticollis may result from trauma or be secondary to infection of the throat, pharynx, or cervical adenitis. In adults, the condition may result from a muscular strain, viral infection, psychogenic etiology, vertebral or clavicular fractures, or traumatic unilateral facet subluxation or impingement.

The common "**wry neck**" as a result of a muscular strain often follows exposure to cold air currents or, occasionally, sleeping with the neck in an abnormal position, which leads to painful, tender cervical muscles. The individual maintains the head in a position toward the side of the involved muscle to provide for a potential state of relaxation of that muscle. A ligamentous or capsular injury occurs when the neck is completely extended, flexed, or rotated and the individual turns the head abruptly, which exceeds the yield point of the tissues. This results in a rotary subluxation when one or more pairs of facets move beyond their normal ROM. As a result of this excess motion, the articular surfaces lose their physical relationship and are "jammed" together, with resultant separation of the anatomically opposite joints. As a result of capsular tearing and stretching as well as impingement along with traumatic edema of the synovium and capsular tissue, unilateral narrowing of the intervertebral foramen, and resultant pain, occurs.

Signs and Symptoms

The patient presents with the head tilted to one side and the chin pointed toward the opposite shoulder. For example, if the head tilts right and the chin points left, the muscles on the right side are affected. Subsequently, ROM is limited. In addition, a palpable lump or swelling may be found in the involved muscle.

Management

In acquired torticollis, symptoms usually resolve spontaneously within 2 weeks. Treatment is symptomatic and consists of cryotherapy, heat, massage, supportive cervical collar, muscle relaxants, interferential muscle stimulation, and analgesics. ROM exercises should allow normal motion to be regained relatively quickly. Continued care will enhance the ability of the individual to resume normal activities.

Cervical Sprains

Etiology

Cervical sprains typically occur at the extremes of motion or in association with a violent muscle contraction or external force. Injury can occur to any of the major ligaments traversing the cervical spine as well as to the capsular ligaments surrounding the facet joints. Minor activity, such as maintaining the head in an uncomfortable posture or sleeping position, also can produce sprains of the neck.

Signs and Symptoms

Symptoms include pain, stiffness, and restricted ROM, but no neurological or osseous injury exists. The cervical distraction test may be negative because instead of relieving pain, the test will elicit pain as the soft tissues are stretched. Unlike cervical strains, the symptoms of a severe sprain can persist for several days.

Management

Initial treatment includes rest, cryotherapy, prescribed nonsteroidal anti-inflammatory drugs (NSAIDs), and use of a soft cervical collar for support. Follow-up treatment may involve continued cryotherapy or superficial heat, gentle stretching, and isometric exercises. Return to competition should not occur until the individual is free of neck pain, with and without axial compression, and when ROM and neck strength are normal. This decision should be made collaboratively with the physician.

Cervical Strains

Etiology

Cervical strains usually involve the sternocleidomastoid or upper trapezius, although the scalenes, levator scapulae, and splenius muscles may be involved as well. The same mechanisms that cause cervical sprains also cause cervical strains, and in many instances, both injuries occur simultaneously.

Signs and Symptoms

Symptoms include pain, stiffness, and restricted ROM. Palpation reveals muscle spasm and increased pain during active contraction or passive stretching of the involved muscle.

Management

Cryotherapy, prescribed NSAIDs, gentle stretching and isometric exercises of the involved muscle, and use of a soft cervical collar for support facilitate symptoms subsiding within 3 to 7 days. Follow-up treatment may involve continued cryotherapy or superficial heat as well as strengthening the neck muscles through appropriate resistance exercise. Return to competition should not occur until the individual is free of neck pain, with and without axial compression, and when ROM and neck strength are normal. This decision should be made collaboratively with the physician.

Cervical Spinal Stenosis

Etiology

Structural spinal stenosis is defined as a narrowing of the sagittal canal diameter of 14 mm or less, and may be congenital, acquired, and asymptomatic. In athletes, the condition is often secondary to degenerative osteophyte formation, which narrows the canal and is referred to as acquired stenosis rather than congenital stenosis.[15]

Individuals may remain asymptomatic until a direct blow to the forehead (forced hyperextension) or occiput (hyperflexion) produces neurological signs. Lateral blows causing rapid lateral flexion with or without rotation also can lead to acute symptoms. The most commonly affected cervical segments are C5 and C6.

Signs and Symptoms

On impact, the individual may develop immediate quadriplegia with sensory changes or motor deficits in both arms, either legs, or all four extremities. Sensory changes may include burning pain, numbness, tingling, or total loss of sensation. Motor changes may include weakness or complete paralysis, with arm weakness being greater than leg weakness, secondary to contusion (bruising) of the central portion of the spinal cord (central cord syndrome). The changes are *always bilateral, differentiating this condition from a nerve root injury*, which is always unilateral. The episode may be transient, with full recovery in 10 to 15 minutes, although in some cases, complete recovery does not occur for 36 to 38 hours.[16] This condition often is called a **neurapraxia**, because neural changes are only temporary.

Management

Structural spinal stenosis may be discovered during routine radiographs, but a magnetic resonance image often is needed to determine the presence of functional stenosis. An individual who has had an episode of structurally related cervical spinal neurapraxia, with or without transient quadriplegia, is not necessarily predisposed to permanent neurological injury. Individuals with developing spinal stenosis or spinal stenosis associated with congenital abnormalities have returned safely to participation. A growing number of physicians, however, have concluded that individuals who have functional stenosis of the cervical spine with associated cervical spine instability, or acute or chronic intervertebral disk disease, should be advised to discontinue participation in contact sports.

Because of the serious nature of this injury, the emergency plan, including summoning EMS, should be activated. This condition requires that equipment be removed and the patient immobilized on a vacuum mattress or scoop stretcher with the head secured to the immobilization device.[10]

Spear Tackler's Spine

Etiology

Flexion of the neck, as seen in spear tackling, produces a straightened cervical spine that acts like a segmental column, predisposing the spine to permanent neurological injury with further axial loading. Spear tackler's spine originally was described in 1993, after a review of data from the

National Football Head and Neck Injury Registry.[17] The registry reported that four athletes who suffered permanent neurological injury had the following common characteristics:

- Developmental narrowing of the cervical spinal canal

- Straightening or reversal of the normal cervical lordotic curve

- Preexisting minor posttraumatic radiographic evidence of bony or ligamentous injury

- History of using spear-tackling techniques

Signs and Symptoms

As with any catastrophic neck injury, the individual may develop immediate pain with sensory changes and motor deficits distal to the injury site. Sensory changes may include burning pain, numbness, tingling, or total loss of sensation. Motor changes may include weakness or complete paralysis. Dermatome and myotome testing will reveal deficits with the distribution patterns aligning with C1–C7 nerve root levels.

Management

Prompt assessment involves a primary survey for unconsciousness, airway, breathing, and circulation. Further evaluation for consciousness should determine the level of extremity numbness, weakness, neck pain, and painful dysesthesias or paresthesias. If the patient is unable to move all or any limbs or has gross weakness, numbness, or significant pain upon palpation of the cervical spine, immediate use of in-line stabilization and activation of EMS is indicated.[10] It is recommended that, in the case of a football injury, the helmet and shoulder pads should be removed and the patient placed on a rigid immobilization device such as a scoop stretcher of vacuum mattress and secured to the device.[10]

Because of the serious nature of this injury, the emergency plan, including summoning EMS, should be activated. This patient requires transport using a rigid immobilization device that includes appropriately immobilizing and securing the head and neck.[10]

Spinal Cord Injury

Etiology

Spinal cord injury as a result of hyperflexion, hyperextension, or rotation of the spinal column can lead to different degrees of motor and sensory loss. Primary injury is caused essentially by trauma (e.g., contusion to the cord or nerve roots, laceration from bony fragments due to a fracture or dislocation of the vertebrae) and results in hemorrhagic changes that lead to ischemia and necrosis. Secondary injury results from various chemical and vascular changes.

Most spinal cord injuries affect the cervical and higher thoracic regions. When the cord is injured, there is a sudden loss of conduction due to the migration of potassium ions from inside the cells into the extracellular spaces. This is associated with a transient loss of somatic and autonomic reflex activity below the level of neurological damage and is called spinal shock. This translates into hypotension, bradycardia, and loss of thermoregulation due to the passive dilation of dermal blood vessels and consequent inability to maintain body heat and the loss of sweat gland activity. These cardiovascular changes are called neurogenic shock and are typically seen 4 to 6 hours after injury in patients with cord lesions above T6. Spinal and neurogenic shock can last between 48 hours and 6 weeks postinjury.[18]

According to the American Spinal Injury Association (ASIA), complete spinal cord injury involves the most sacral segments of the cord, S4 and S5. Incomplete injuries do not involve these segments and can lead to a diagnosis of four classic cord syndromes: anterior cord syndrome, posterior cord syndrome, central cord syndrome, and Brown-Séquard syndrome.[19]

Signs and Symptoms

Spinal cord injuries can result in various levels of paralysis in motor function or sensory loss. With a complete lesion, in which the spinal cord has been totally severed, there will be a complete loss of all motor function and sensation below the level of injury. Recovery of significant function below the level of injury is highly unlikely. With an incomplete lesion, the four classic syndromes present with their own predicable signs and symptoms.

Anterior cord syndrome typically results from damage to the anterior two-thirds of the spinal cord but can also include damage to the anterior spinal artery. Ischemia leads to variable loss of motor function and loss of pain and temperature sensation below the level of injury. Sensitivity to light touch, deep pressure, vibration, and proprioception are preserved. Individuals with this diagnosis have a 10% to 20% potential of motor recovery.[19]

Posterior cord syndrome is very rare and involves the posterior third of the spinal cord, known as the dorsal column. This region is sensory in nature and provides pathways for transmitting impulses relating to light touch, deep pressure, vibration and proprioception, and kinesthetic awareness. If injury occurs here, the senses are lost, but motor function and sense of pain and temperature are preserved.

The *Brown-Séquard syndrome* involves a hemisection of the spinal cord with loss of ipsilateral motor function and contralateral pain and temperature caused by a penetrating injury, for example, from bony fragments, a knife, or gun. Although this classic condition is rarely seen, most patients present with Brown-Séquard-plus syndrome, characterized by some motor weakness on one side of the body and decreased pain and temperature on the opposite side. Recovery from this syndrome is very likely, with 75% to 90% of patients being able to walk independently after rehabilitation.[19]

The most commonly observed incomplete spinal cord injury is the *central spinal cord syndrome*. This condition results in incomplete loss of motor function, with upper extremity weakness being more pronounced than lower extremity weakness. This disproportionate weakness is thought to be the result of hemorrhagic and ischemic injury to the corticospinal tracts because of their somatotopic arrangement. Fibers of cervical nerves that innervate the upper extremities are arranged more medially than those subserving function to the lower extremities.[15] This syndrome usually involves the cervical region of the spinal cord and tends to affect older people with cervical spondylosis who have experienced hyperextension injuries.[19] Cervical cord syndrome has good potential for recovery, especially in younger patients.[20]

Management

As with any catastrophic injury, suspected spinal injuries must be handled with extreme caution and care. Immediate activation of EMS is important. Automated external defibrillator (AED), oxygen, and other emergency response equipment should be readily accessible if needed. Prompt recognition and proper management must ensure that excessive movement does not exacerbate any initial damage to the spine, thereby reducing any chance of secondary injury. An assessment of the primary survey to determine level of consciousness, airway, breathing, and circulation is needed to identify any life-threatening injury. If no life-threatening injury is present, a neurological screening should be conducted to determine the presence of any extremity numbness, painful dysesthesias or paresthesias, weakness, and neck pain. If it is determined that the patient is unconscious, or complains of numbness, weakness, paralysis, or neck pain, the individual should be immediately stabilized and transported for further testing and diagnosis.

Cervical Disk Injuries

Etiology

Less common than lumbar disk injuries, cervical disk injuries usually affect older, physically active individuals. The primary mechanisms involve sustained, repetitive cervical compression, axial loading, or hyperflexion injuries during contact sports. Disk disease may be classified as either soft- or hard-disk disease. Soft-disk herniation refers to an acute process in which the nucleus pulposus herniates through the posterior annulus, resulting in signs and symptoms of cord or nerve root compression. In sports participation, acute cervical disk herniations are thought to result from uncontrolled lateral bending of the neck.[20] In contrast, hard-disk disease refers to a more chronic, degenerative process, with a diminished disk height and the formation of marginal osteophytes. The condition usually begins early in life and proceeds through a series of defined steps preceding most, if not all, symptomatic disk herniations.

Signs and Symptoms

Individuals with degenerative disk disease and acute disk herniations usually present with varying degrees of neck or arm pain that may radiate into the shoulder or arm. Pain often is exacerbated by Valsalva maneuvers (e.g., breath holding, straining, or coughing) and neck movement. Spurling maneuver (i.e., turning the head with the neck extended) often reproduces sharp radicular pain into the affected extremity in the distribution of the compressed nerve root. If the spinal cord is compressed, a positive Babinski sign often is present. Severe cases may involve complete loss of motor function below the level of injury, including arm and leg paralysis. Symptoms in the physically active population tend to be more pronounced because of the demands of their sport.

Management

Suspected disk herniations should be referred for physician evaluation and are confirmed through MRI. Initial treatment for the majority of all herniated cervical disk injuries is nonoperative. Treatment consists of rest, immobilization in a cervical collar for 1 to 3 days, activity modification, anti-inflammatory medication, cervical traction, and occasionally, therapeutic injections.[21]

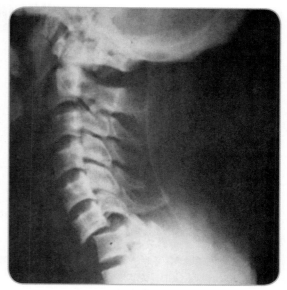

Figure 21.23. Cervical fracture dislocation. The mechanism of axial loading and violent neck flexion can result in a cervical fracture dislocation.

Therapeutic exercise may be instituted as symptoms improve, emphasizing isometric strengthening and cervical ROM, followed by sport/activity-specific exercises and drills. The individual may return to sport/activity participation once he or she is asymptomatic and has regained full strength and mobility.

Cervical Fractures and Dislocations

Etiology

Unsafe practices, such as diving into shallow water, spearing in football, or landing on the posterior neck during gymnastic or trampoline activities, can lead to cervical fractures and dislocations from the axial loading and violent neck flexion (**Fig. 21.23**). Some fractures, such as those of the spinous process or unilateral laminar fractures, may require only immobilization in a cervical collar. Others, such as a bilateral pars interarticularis fracture of C2 ("hangman fracture"), may require a cervical collar or halo vest immobilization.

Signs and Symptoms

In sports, serious injuries commonly occur at the 4th, 5th, and 6th cervical vertebrae. Because neural damage can range from none to complete severance of the spinal cord, there is a range of accompanying symptoms (**Box 21.2**). Painful palpation over the spinous processes, muscle spasm, or palpable defect indicates a possible fracture or dislocation. Radiating pain, numbness, weakness in a myotome, paralysis, and loss of bladder or bowel control are all critical signs of neural damage. If a unilateral cervical dislocation is present, the neck is visibly tilted toward the dislocated side, with muscle tightness resulting from stretch on the convex side and muscle slack on the concave side.

Management

Because spinal cord damage can lead to paralysis or death, a suspected unstable neck injury should be treated as a medical emergency. An unstable neck injury should be suspected in an unconscious individual, an individual who is awake but has numbness and/or paralysis, and in a neurologically intact individual who has neck pain or pain with neck movement. Without moving the head or neck out of alignment, light cervical traction should be applied while

Because of the serious nature of this injury, the emergency plan, including summoning EMS, should be activated. In-line stabilization is maintained until patient's head is secured to rigid immobilization device.

BOX 21.2 Red Flags Indicating a Possible Cervical Spine Injury

- Pain over the spinous process, with or without deformity
- Paralysis or inability to move a body part
- Unrelenting neck pain or muscle spasm
- Absent or weak reflexes
- Abnormal sensations in the head, neck, trunk, or extremities
- Loss of bladder or bowel control
- Muscular weakness in the extremities
- Mechanism of injury involving violent axial loading, flexion, or rotation of the neck
- Loss of coordinated movement

---

the neck is being stabilized, and airway, breathing, and circulation (ABCs) should be assessed for any life-threatening situation.

> Critical signs of neural damage include sensory changes (i.e., burning pain, numbness, tingling, or total loss of sensation), motor changes (i.e., weakness in a myotome, complete paralysis), and loss of bladder or bowel control are critical signs of neural damage.

BRACHIAL PLEXUS CONDITIONS

While throwing a two-handed overhead pass, a basketball player is hit on the right arm. The arm is forced into excessive external rotation, abduction, and extension. The player experiences an immediate burning pain and a prickly sensation that radiates down the arm and into the hand as well as an inability to raise the arm. What injury should be suspected, and is this a serious injury?

The brachial plexus is a complex neural structure that innervates the upper extremity and that typically is damaged in two manners (**Fig. 21.24**). A stretch injury may be caused when a tensile force leads to forceful, downward traction of the clavicle while the head is distracted in the opposite direction, such as when an individual is tackled and subsequently rolls onto the shoulder with the head turned to the opposite side. A stretch injury also may occur when the arm is forced into excessive external rotation, abduction, and extension. The injury usually affects the upper trunk (C5, C6) of the brachial plexus, which leads to a sensory loss or paresthesia in the thumb and index finger. A second mechanism of injury involves compression of the fixed plexus between the football shoulder pad and the superior medial scapula, where the brachial plexus is most superficial. This site, called the **Erb point**, is located 2 to 3 cm above the clavicle at the level of the transverse process of the C6 vertebra.

Brachial plexus injuries are graded in three levels (**Table 21.3**). Grade I represent neurapraxia, the mildest lesion. A neurapraxia is a localized conduction block that causes temporary loss of sensation and/or loss of motor function from selective demyelination of the axon sheath without true axonal disruption. Recovery usually occurs within days to a few weeks. Grade II are axonotmesis injuries that produce significant motor and mild sensory deficits that last for at least 2 weeks. Axonotmesis disrupts the axon and myelin sheath, but it leaves the epineurium intact. Axonal regrowth occurs at a rate of 1 to 2 mm per day; full or normal function usually is restored. Grade III are neurotmesis

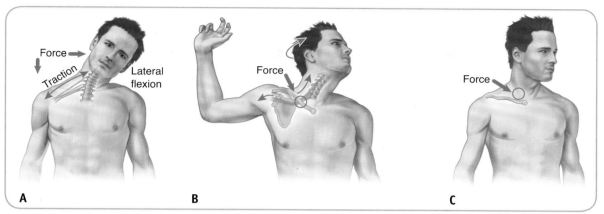

Figure 21.24. Common mechanisms of a brachial plexus stretch. A, A blow to the head causing lateral flexion and shoulder depression may lead to a traction injury to the upper trunk of the brachial plexus. **B,** An injury also can occur when a blow to the supraclavicular region causes lateral flexion with rotation and extension of the cervical spine away from the blow. **C,** Compression over the Erb point, representing the most superficial passage of the brachial plexus, also can lead to pain and paresthesia radiating into the upper extremity.

injuries, which disrupt the endoneurium. These severe injuries have a poor prognosis, with motor and sensory deficit persisting for up to 1 year. Surgical intervention often is necessary to avoid poor or imperfect regeneration.

Acute Brachial Plexus Injury

Etiology

Traumatic injuries are most often caused by forceful separation of the neck from the shoulder. These injuries are commonly seen in motorcycle accidents but may also be seen in falls, industrial accidents, and penetrating and sport-related injuries.[22]

Signs and Symptoms

The individual notices an immediate, severe, burning pain and prickly paresthesia that radiates from the supraclavicular area down the arm and into the hand, hence, the nickname "burner" or "stinger." Pain usually is transient and subsides in 5 to 10 minutes, but tenderness over the supraclavicular area and shoulder weakness may persist for hours or even days after the injury. Often, the individual tries to shake the arm to "get the feeling back." Muscle weakness is evident in actions involving shoulder abduction and external rotation. Palpation over Erb point may elicit tenderness or reproduction of symptoms. Neurovascular screening may reveal deficits in C5–T1 nerve root levels, and the brachial plexus traction test may be positive. There should be no tenderness to palpation of the cervical spine.

GRADE	INJURY	SIGNS	PROGNOSIS
I	Neurapraxia	Temporary loss of sensation and/or loss of motor function	Recovery within a few days to a few weeks
II	Axonotmesis	Significant motor and mild sensory deficits	Deficits last at least 2 weeks. Regrowth is slow, but full or normal function usually is restored.
III	Neurotmesis	Motor and sensory deficits persist for up to 1 year.	Poor prognosis Surgical intervention often is necessary.

TABLE 21.3 Classifications of Brachial Plexus Injury

Management

When weakness is present, the individual should be removed from activity. A brief nerve root screening should be performed. The myotomes should be tested bilaterally:

■ Shoulder abduction for the C5 nerve root

■ Elbow flexion for C6

■ Elbow extension for C7

■ Thumb extension for C8

■ Finger abduction and adduction for T1

For patients with no known history of a brachial plexus injury and how experiences an acute episode for the first time, the patient should not be allowed to return to activity until the following criteria for return to play has been met:

■ No neck pain, arm pain, or dysesthesia (impairment of sensation)

■ Full pain-free ROM in the neck and upper extremity

■ Normal strength on manual muscle testing as compared to preseason measurements

■ Normal deep tendon reflexes

■ Negative brachial plexus traction test

It also is imperative to follow the individual closely with a postactivity examination and with successive examinations for several days to detect any recurrence of weakness.

Treatment may involve ice massage to the upper trapezius and shoulder to decrease pain and inflammation of a secondary muscle strain. A sling may be necessary, particularly for individuals with weakness in the rotator cuff muscles.

Following a grade II or III brachial plexus injury, strength training is contraindicated during early rehabilitation, because immature motor end plates may be damaged during resistance training. ROM exercises for the cervical spine should begin in the supine position and progress to a seated position. Isometric strengthening exercises can progress to diagonal flexion and extension and then to exercises using machines or free weights. When shoulder ROM is near normal in all planes, closed chain strengthening should be initiated, with progression into isotonic and isodynamic exercise. Scapulothoracic motion should be smooth and isolated, avoiding any muscle substitution. Concentric and eccentric strengthening exercises should be conducted in external and internal rotation (45° abduction), adduction, and extension.

Chronic Recurrent Cervical Nerve Root Neurapraxia

Etiology

Chronic recurrent cervical nerve root neurapraxia involves neck extension with ipsilateral lateral deviation. Also known as chronic burner syndrome, the condition has been associated with cervical canal stenosis, reversal of lordosis, disk disease, foraminal stenosis, and a positive Spurling sign suggesting that the injury may be due to the compression mechanism of dorsal nerve roots within the intervertebral foramina.[22]

Signs and Symptoms

Chronic burners are characterized by more frequent acute episodes that may not produce areas of numbness. Muscle weakness in the shoulder muscles may develop hours or even days after the initial injury and may result in a dropped shoulder or visible atrophy of the shoulder muscles.

Management

These individuals should be examined after activity, during the week, and again the following week, because weakness may not become apparent until days after the initial injury. Initial treatment follows the same parameters of acute burners. In football, the use of lifters, a supplemental pad at the base of the neck, or a modified A-frame shoulder pad supplemented by a cervical collar attached to the posterior aspect of the shoulder pads may limit excessive lateral neck flexion and extension to prevent reoccurrence. This patient should be sent to an orthopedic physician for examination to assist in identification of possible anatomical causes of the condition.

Suprascapular Nerve Injury

Etiology

The suprascapular nerve also may be damaged with the same mechanisms. This nerve innervates the supraspinatus, infraspinatus, and glenohumeral joint capsule. During motions such as those in pitching, spiking, or overhead serving, extreme velocity and torque forces generated during the cocking, acceleration, and release phases subject this nerve and its adjoining artery to rapid stretching.

Signs and Symptoms

Both the supraspinatus and infraspinatus muscles may appear to be weak and atrophied. Infraspinatus wasting usually is more apparent, however, because it is not hidden under the trapezius muscle. Because the supraspinatus and infraspinatus are not functioning properly, other problems, such as rotator cuff tendinitis, impingement syndrome, bicipital tenosynovitis, or bursitis of the shoulder, may be present and overshadow this condition.

Management

If an individual with chronic shoulder problems does not respond well to standard treatment, the individual should be referred to a physician for further evaluation. Once identified, the condition responds well to a ROM and strengthening program.

 The basketball player experienced a brachial plexus stretch injury. The paresthesia (i.e., burning and prickling) and muscle weakness should resolve in a few minutes, at which time the individual can return to activity. If neurological symptoms persist, the individual should not be allowed to return to activity and referral to a physician is warranted.

THORACIC SPINE CONDITIONS

 A 15-year-old, butterfly-stroke swimmer is complaining of localized pain and tenderness in the midback region over the thoracic spine. The pain came on gradually and only hurts during execution of the stroke. Fracture tests are negative. What other condition(s) might be suspected?

The protective rib cage limits movement in the thoracic motion segments; however, the thoracolumbar junction is a region of potentially high stress during flexion–extension movements of the trunk. Injuries to this area may include contusions, strains, sprains, fractures, and apophysitis.

Thoracic Contusions, Strains, and Sprains

Etiology

Direct blows to the back during contact sports frequently yield contusions to the muscles in the thoracic region. Such injuries range in severity but generally are characterized by pain, ecchymosis, spasm, and limited swelling.

Signs and Symptoms

Thoracic sprains and strains result from either overloading or overstretching muscles in the region through violent or sustained muscle contractions. Painful spasms of the back muscles serve as a protective mechanism to immobilize the injured area and may develop as a sympathetic response to sprains. The presence of such spasms, however, makes it difficult to determine whether the injury is actually a sprain or a strain. Dramatic improvement in a thoracic sprain can be seen in 24 to 48 hours. In contrast, severe strains may require 3 to 4 weeks to heal.

Management

Initial treatment consists of cryotherapy, NSAIDs, and activity modification. Follow-up management may include application of superficial heat, ultrasound, massage, and appropriate stretching and resistance exercise as needed to recondition the individual.

Thoracic Spinal Fractures and Apophysitis

Etiology

The rib cage stabilizes and limits motion in the thoracic spine and, in doing so, lessens the likelihood of injury to this area. Thoracic fractures tend to be concentrated at the lower end of the thoracic spine, in the transitional region between the thoracic and lumbar curvatures. The majority of fractures are caused by axial loading, flexion, or rotation.[23]

Large compressive loads, such as those sustained during heavy weight lifting, head-on contact in football or rugby, or landing on the buttock area during a fall, can fracture the vertebral end plates or lead to a wedge fracture, which is named after the shape of the deformed vertebral body (**Fig. 21.25A**). Females with osteopenia, a condition of reduced bone mineralization, are particularly susceptible to these fractures. More commonly, compressive stress during small, repetitive loads in an activity such as running leads to a progressive compression fracture of a weakened vertebral body.

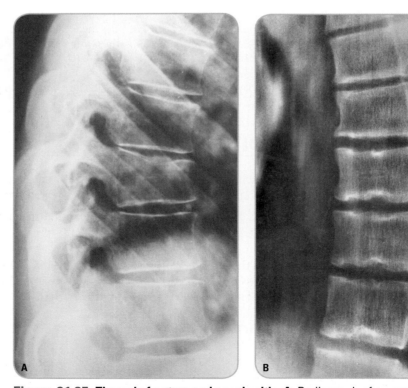

Figure 21.25. Thoracic fracture and apophysitis. A, Radiograph of a compression wedge fracture in the thoracic region as a result of several compressed motion segments. **B,** Scheuermann disease occurs when end plate changes lead to erosion in the anterior vertebral body, which drives a herniated disk forward into the body. In this radiograph, several end plate changes can be seen leading to erosion of the vertebral bodies.

Another leading cause of thoracic fractures among adolescents and young adults is **Scheuermann disease**. This condition, which appears to be related to mechanical stress, involves degeneration of the epiphyseal end plates of the vertebral bodies and typically includes at least three adjacent motion segments. The vertebral end plates have a wavy appearance, and the intervertebral disk spaces are narrowed. If the end plate is sufficiently compromised, additional compression from axial and flexion overload forces cause prolapse of the intervertebral disk into the vertebral body (**Fig. 21.25B**). The result is a decrease in spinal height and an accentuation of the thoracic curve, leading to kyphosis. Onset typically occurs in the late juvenile period, from 8 to 12 years of age; more severe fixed deformities are seen in individuals from 12 to 16 years of age. The condition is twice as common in girls as in boys. A high incidence of Scheuermann disease has been documented among gymnasts, trampolinists, cyclists, wrestlers, and rowers. Following referral to a physician, treatment involves modification of activity in proportion to the pain. Stretching exercises for the shoulder, neck, and back muscles should be coupled with strengthening the abdominal and spinal extensor muscles. If the kyphosis continues to progress, bracing may be included with the exercise program.

Repeated flexion–extension of the thoracic spine can cause inflammation of the apophyses, which are the growth centers of the vertebral bodies. Like Scheuermann disease, apophysitis is a progressive condition that is characterized by local pain and tenderness. After referral to a physician, treatment for apophysitis includes elimination of the flexion–extension stress as well as strengthening abdominal and other trunk muscles.

Signs and Symptoms

As with any fracture, pain and muscle guarding are present in the region of the fracture site.

Management

Referral to a physician is warranted. Stable injuries, such as uncomplicated compression fractures, may be treated in an orthosis with a halo ring support at the physician's discretion. Braces may not be necessary as the rib cage and sternum, if intact, will splint the spinal column fractures due to high thoracic compression. Unstable fractures may necessitate surgical intervention.

 The swimmer may have developed apophysitis because of the repeated flexion-extension motions that are executed during the butterfly stroke. This individual should be referred to a physician for follow-up examination.

REHABILITATION

Rehabilitation programs must be developed on an individual basis and address the specific needs of the individual. Exercises to relieve pain related to postural problems may not address pain related to an acute injury; therefore, a variety of exercises are listed in this section to allow selection of those most appropriate for the individual. The program should relieve pain and muscle tension; restore motion and balance; develop strength, endurance, and power; and maintain cardiovascular fitness. Patient education also is critical in teaching the skills and techniques that are needed to prevent recurrence.

Relief of Pain and Muscle Tension

Maintaining a prolonged posture can lead to discomfort. This can be avoided by doing active ROM exercises to relieve stress on supporting structures, promote circulation, and maintain flexibility. For example, exercises, including neck flexion, extension, lateral flexion and rotation, shoulder rolls, and glenohumeral circumduction, can be beneficial for relieving tension in the cervical and upper thoracic region. Conscious relaxation training can relax an individual who generally is tense or release tension in specific muscle groups, such as the upper trapezius. Grade I and II mobilization exercises can be initiated early in the program to relieve pain and stretch tight structures to restore accessory movements to the joints.

Restoration of Motion

Flexibility exercises and mobilization techniques can be used to increase the ROM of specific structures in the cervical and thoracic spine. Flexibility exercises can include passive and active stretching techniques. The intensity and duration of the exercise will vary relative to the site of the inflamed tissue. Examples of ROM exercises for the cervical spine are illustrated in **Application Strategy 21.2.**

Joint mobilization techniques for the cervical and thoracic spine can be used to restore motion. As a general rule, grade III and IV mobilization exercises can begin as soon as pain and muscle guarding are relieved.

APPLICATION STRATEGY 21.2

Flexibility Exercises for the Cervical Spine

- Flexibility exercises can be performed actively and passively to increase ROM in the cervical spine. A stretch should be held for approximately 20 seconds, and the action repeated four or five times. The patient should feel a slight stretch in the absence of any pain.
- The motions of cervical flexion (**A**), extension (**B**), lateral flexion (**C**), and rotation (**D**) should be performed as necessary. Stretching exercises can be performed in a seated position and should begin with the patient in a position of axial extension (i.e., with the chin tucked and the neck straight).
- Initially, the exercises should be performed actively. Additional stretching can be provided by having the patient or the clinician use his or her hands to apply light pressure as the motion reaches its end range. Again, it is important that the motion be free of pain.
- Joint mobilization techniques also can be used to improve flexibility; however, specific techniques for the cervical spine are not within the scope of this textbook.

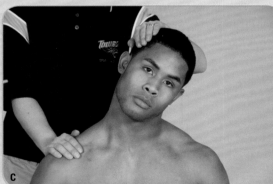

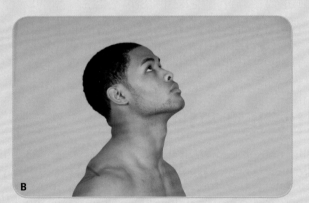

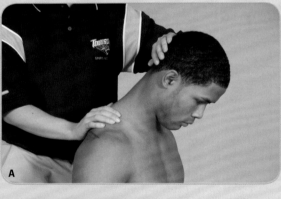

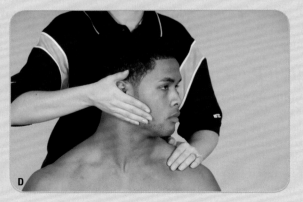

Restoration of Proprioception and Balance

Restoring proprioceptive awareness of balanced posture and positioning is essential for maintaining normal alignment of the spine. Proprioceptive exercises should be initiated at the same time as the strengthening program. Exercises for the cervical and thoracic spines should focus on patient awareness of correct alignment and active control of posture.

Muscular Strength, Endurance, and Power

Isometric contractions to strengthen the neck musculature can progress to manual resistance, self-resistance, and commercial machines as available and tolerated. In addition, functional exercises specific to the needs of the individual are advantageous. For example, neck strength is particularly important for wrestlers and football linemen, who need added stability and strength in the cervical region.

Cardiovascular Fitness

In selecting exercises to maintain and improve cardiovascular fitness, one should be aware of the potential problems with specific exercises. For example, aquatic exercises offer a variety of benefits, but a cervical spine injury could be aggravated by performing the freestyle stroke. Specifically, the continuous cervical rotation may have an adverse effect on the cervical spine. In a similar manner, cycling as a means of aerobic training could present problems depending on the type of bike that is used. A bike that enables an upright position typically would be more appropriate, because less stress is transmitted to both the cervical and thoracic spine as compared with other bikes.

SUMMARY

1. The spine is a linkage system that transfers loads between the upper and lower extremities, enables motion in all three planes, and protects the delicate spinal cord. Although most injuries to the back are relatively minor and can be managed successfully using the PRICE principles (protect, restrict activity, ice, compression, and elevation), spinal fractures and nerve conditions do occur.

2. Two adjacent vertebrae and the soft tissues between them are collectively referred to as a motion segment. The motion segment is the functional unit of the spine. The intervertebral disk is a fibrocartilaginous disk that provides cushioning between the articulating vertebral bodies.

3. The interspinous ligaments, intertransverse ligaments, and ligamentum flava link the spinous processes, transverse process, and laminae, respectively, of adjacent vertebrae. Collectively, the primary movers for back extension are called the erector spinae muscles.

4. The spinal cord extends from the brainstem to the level of the 1st or 2nd lumbar vertebrae. Thirty-one pairs of spinal nerves emanate from the cord, with the distal bundle of spinal nerves known as the cauda equina.

5. Anatomical variations in the cervical and thoracic regions that can predispose an individual to spinal injuries include kyphosis and scoliosis.

6. Functional spinal stenosis is defined as a loss of cerebrospinal fluid (CSF) around the cord or, in more extreme cases, as a deformation of the spinal cord. The cervical segments most commonly affected are C5 and C6.

7. Signs and symptoms that indicate a serious cervical spine injury include pain over the spinous process, with or without deformity; unrelenting neck pain or muscle spasm; abnormal sensations in the head, neck, trunk, or extremities; muscular weakness in the extremities; paralysis or inability to move a body part; and absence of weak reflexes.

8. Because spinal cord damage can lead to paralysis or death, a suspected unstable neck injury should be treated as a medical emergency. The emergency care plan should be activated, including summoning EMS.

9. Brachial plexus injuries are graded in three levels:

- *Neurapraxia injuries*—temporary loss of sensation and/or loss of motor function that recovers within 2 weeks

- *Axonotmesis injuries*—significant motor and mild sensory deficits that last for at least 2 weeks

- *Neurotmesis injuries*—severe motor and sensory deficits that persist for up to 1 year with poor prognosis

10. Thoracic fractures tend to be concentrated at the lower end of the thoracic spine. Large compressive loads can lead to a wedge fracture, or Scheuermann disease can lead to degeneration of the epiphyseal end plates of the vertebral bodies, causing the intervertebral disk to prolapse into the vertebral body.

11. Assessment of a spinal injury should begin with a thorough history of the injury and include neurological tests to determine possible nerve involvement. The severity of pain and the presence or absence of neurological symptoms, neck spasm, and tenderness can indicate when backboard and neck stabilization are needed.

12. If, at any time, an individual complains of acute pain in the spine, change in sensation anywhere on the body, or resistance to moving the spine, a significant injury should be assumed and the emergency care plan activated, including summoning EMS.

13. A rehabilitation program should focus on reduction of pain and spasm; restoration of motion and balance; development of strength, endurance, and power; and maintenance of cardiovascular fitness.

APPLICATION QUESTIONS

1. After being tackled, a football player comes off the field shaking his left arm. What questions should be asked as part of an injury assessment for this individual?

2. Following completion of the history and palpation components of an assessment for a neck injury sustained by a wrestler, you suspect injury to the sternocleidomastoid and/or upper trapezius. What findings from the testing component of the assessment would confirm your suspicion?

3. A 14-year-old male football athlete was involved in a spearing collision during a game that you were covering as an athletic trainer. He complains of neck pain and is unable to move without increasing the radiating pain. How would you differentiate between an acute cervical disk herniation and a cervical fracture?

4. A high school football player reports to practice with a neck roll attached to his shoulder pads. The athlete's father purchased the neck roll and told his son to wear it. How would you respond to this situation? Are there any concerns associated with the use of a neck roll?

5. You are providing athletic training services for practice sessions in association with the annual state all-star football game. In your capacity as a volunteer athletic trainer, what signs and symptoms involving injury to the cervical spine would you identify as "red flags" that warrant summoning of EMS?

6. A volleyball player reports to the athletic training room with a "stiff" neck. The individual does not recall an injury but rather reports that she noticed the stiffness upon awakening this morning. The athlete's head appears to be slightly tilted to the right side, and ROM is limited in right (R) lateral flexion and R cervical rotation. Should this individual be permitted to practice with or without restrictions? Explain your response.

7. Following a collision with another player, an 18-year-old ice hockey player skates to the bench and reports neck pain. How would you differentiate between a cervical strain and a cervical sprain? How would you manage each condition?

8. Following an assessment of a 12-year-old female gymnast, you suspect Scheuermann disease and have recommended that she see her family physician. How would you explain this condition to the parents of the gymnast?

9. The high school at which you are employed as an athletic trainer does not have a strength and conditioning coach. The wrestling coach asks you for suggestions regarding strengthening exercises to prevent neck injuries for the members of the wrestling team. What types of exercises would you recommend?

REFERENCES

1. National Spinal Cord Injury Statistical Center. *Spinal Cord Injury: Facts and Figures at a Glance.* Birmingham, AL: University of Alabama; 2013:2.

2. Swartz EE, Boden BP, Courson RW, et al. National Athletic Trainers' Association position statement: acute management of the cervical spine-injured athlete. *J Athl Train.* 2009;44(3):306–331.

3. Banerjee R, Palumbo MA, Fadale PD. Catastrophic cervical spine injuries in the collision sport athlete, part 1: epidemiology, functional anatomy, and diagnosis. *Am J Sports Med.* 2004;32(4):1077–1087.

4. Leinberry CF, Wehbé MA. Brachial plexus anatomy. *Hand Clin.* 2004;20(1):1–5.

5. Moskovich R. Biomechanics of the cervical spine. In: Nordin M, Frankel VH, eds. *Basic Biomechanics of the Musculoskeletal System.* 3rd ed. Philadelphia, PA: Lippincott Williams & Wilkins; 2001. Pages 256–285.

6. Tommasi DG, Foppiani AC, Galante D, et al. Active head and cervical range of motion: effect of age in healthy females. *Spine (Phila Pa 1976).* 2009;34(18):1910–1916.

7. Thompson WL, Stiell IG, Clement CM, et al. Association of injury mechanism with the risk of cervical spine fractures. *CJEM.* 2009;11(1):14–22.

8. Kartal A, Yildiran I, Senköylü A, et al. Soccer causes degenerative changes in the cervical spine. *Eur Spine J.* 2004;13(1):76–82.

9. Heck JF, Clarke KS, Peterson TR, et al. National Athletic Trainers' Association position statement: head-down contact and spearing in tackle football. *J Athl Train.* 2004;39(1):101–111.

10. National Athletic Trainers' Association. 2015 update: executive summary from the task force on the appropriate prehospital management of the spine-injured athlete. http://www.nata.org /sites/default/files/Executive-Summary-Spine -Injury-updated.pdf. Accessed November 9, 2015.

11. Starkey C, Brown SD. *Orthopedic and Athletic Injury Examination Handbook.* Philadelphia, PA: FA Davis; 2015.

12. Wong M. *Pocket Orthopaedics: Evidence-Based Survival Guide.* Sudbury, MA: Jones & Bartlett; 2010.

13. Anekstein Y, Blecher R, Smorgick Y, et al. What is the best way to apply the Spurling test for cervical radiculopathy? *Clin Orthop Relat Res.* 2012;470(9):2566–2572.

14. Miller KJ. The shoulder abduction test for cervical radicular pathology. *Dynamic Chiropractic.* 2014;32(3):1–5.

15. Bailes JE, Petschauer M, Guskiewicz KM, et al. Management of cervical spine injuries in athletes. *J Athl Train.* 2007;42(1):126–134.

16. Moore J, Rice EL, Moore JM. Neck injuries. In: Mellion MB, Walsh WM, Madden C, et al, eds. *Team Physician's Handbook.* 3rd ed. Philadelphia, PA: Hanley & Belfus; 2005. Pages 365–372.

17. Torg JS, Sennett B, Pavlov H, et al. Spear tackler's spine. An entity precluding participation in tackle football and collision activities that expose the cervical spine to axial energy inputs. *Am J Sports Med.* 1993;21(5):640–649.

18. Sheerin F. Spinal cord injury: causation and pathophysiology. *Emerg Nurse.* 2005;12(9): 29–38.

19. Kirshblum S, Donovan W. Neurological assessment and classification of traumatic spinal cord injury. In: Kirshblum S, Campagnolo D, DeLisa JE, eds. *Spinal Cord Medicine.* Philadelphia, PA: Lippincott Williams & Wilkins; 2011.

20. Torg JS, Ramsey-Emrhein JA. Cervical spine and brachial plexus injuries: return-to-play recommendations. *Phys Sportsmed.* 1997;25(7): 61–88.

21. Gregory J, Cowey A, Jones M, et al. The anatomy, investigations and management of adult brachial plexus injuries. *Orthop Trauma.* 2009;23(6):420–432.

22. Chao S, Pacella MJ, Torg JS. The pathomechanics, pathophysiology and prevention of cervical spinal cord and brachial plexus injuries in athletics. *Sports Med.* 2010;40(1):59–75.

23. Vialle LR, Vialle E. Thoracic spine fractures. *Injury.* 2005;36(suppl 2):B65–B72.

Lumbar Spinal Conditions

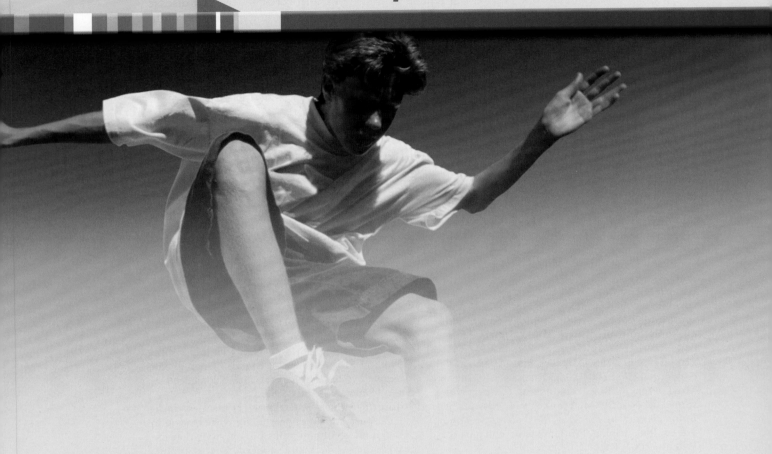

STUDENT OUTCOMES

1. Locate and explain the functional significance of the bony and soft-tissue structures of the lumbar spine.

2. Describe the motion capabilities of the lumbar spine.

3. Identify the factors that contribute to mechanical loading on the spine.

4. Describe specific strategies in activities of daily living to reduce spinal stress in the lumbar region.

5. Identify anatomical variations that can predispose individuals to lumbar spine injuries.

6. Explain the measures used to prevent injuries to the lumbar spinal region.

7. Describe a thorough assessment of the lumbar spine.

8. Describe the common injuries and conditions of the lumbar spine and low back area in physically active individuals.

9. Identify rehabilitative exercises for the lumbar region.

INTRODUCTION

Low back pain is a widespread problem that affects both the athletic and nonathletic populations. In the adult population, low back pain is the leading cause of job-related disability and time loss.[1] Over 80% of adults will report having had episodes of low back pain at some point in their life. Low back pain affects both men and women. Most low back pain is short-term, lasting from a few days to about 12 weeks. Chronic or long-term low back pain refers to pain lasting longer than 12 weeks.[1] About 10% to 15% of youth sport athletes will report having episodes of low back pain.[2] Although the main causes of low back pain in athletes are musculotendinous strains and ligamentous sprains, chronic or recurring pain often is a symptom of lumbar disk degeneration or stress injuries to the bony articulations of the lumbar spine.[3] Pain emanating from the lumbar disks most commonly affects the low back, buttocks, and hips and may result from progressive damage to the annular fibers, particularly the pain fibers that reside in the outer third of the annulus.[4] Low back problems are especially common in equestrian sports, weight lifting, ice hockey, gymnastics, diving, football, wrestling, and aerobics.

This chapter begins with a review of the anatomical structures in the lumbar spine, followed by a discussion of the kinematics and kinetics of the region. Identification of anatomical variations that may predispose individuals to lumbar spinal conditions leads to strategies used to prevent injury. Assessment techniques used in assessing lumbar spine pathologies are presented, followed by information regarding common injuries sustained within the lumbar spine during participation in sports and physical activities. This chapter concludes with examples of general rehabilitation exercises and a summary of topics covered.

ANATOMY OF THE LUMBAR SPINE

As mentioned in Chapter 21, the lumbar and sacral regions of the spine are anatomically and functionally unique. Normal lumbar curvature is concave and sacral curvature is convex from the posterior perspective.

Lower Spinal Column

The lower spinal column, which forms a convex curve anteriorly, includes five lumbar, five fused sacral, and four small, fused coccygeal vertebrae (**Fig. 22.1**). The sacrum articulates with the ilium to form the sacroiliac (SI) joint.

Supporting the weight of the head, trunk, and upper extremities, the lumbar vertebral bodies have larger articulating surface areas and greater depth than those of any other spinal region. In addition, the orientation of the facet joints varies in comparison to the cervical and thoracic spines (see **Fig. 21.4**). Information concerning the general structures of the spinal vertebrae and intervertebral disks is presented in Chapter 21.

Ligaments of the Lumbar Spine and Trunk

General information regarding the spinal ligaments is presented in Chapter 21. Specific to the lumbar spine, several ligaments, including the iliolumbar ligaments, posterior SI ligaments, sacrospinous ligament, and the sacrotuberous ligament, are responsible for maintaining its articulation with the sacrum (**Fig. 22.2**).

Muscles of the Lumbar Spine and Trunk

The muscles of the trunk are paired, with one on the left side and one on the right side of the body (**Fig. 22.3**). These muscles produce lateral flexion and/or rotation of the trunk when acting unilaterally and trunk flexion or extension when acting bilaterally. Collectively, the primary movers for back extension are called the erector spinae muscles.

See **Muscles of the Lumbar Spine**, available on the companion Web site at thePoint, for the attachments, actions, and innervations of the major muscles of the lumbar region.

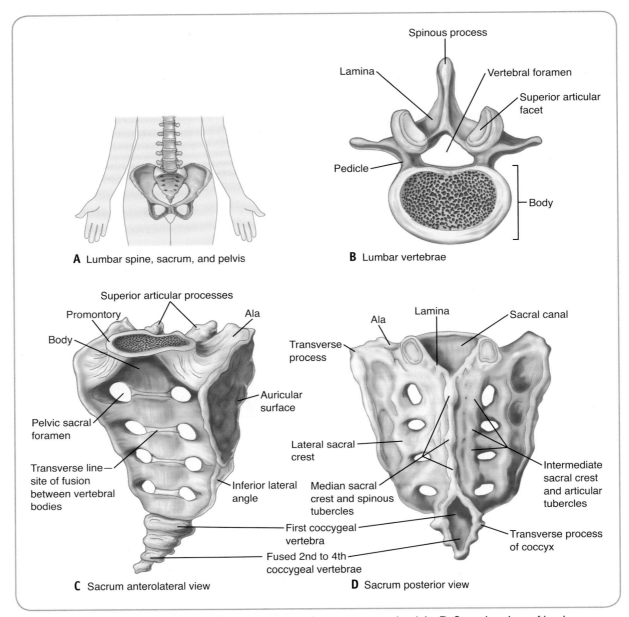

Figure 22.1. Bones of the lumbar region. A, Lumbar spine, sacrum, and pelvis. **B,** Superior view of lumbar vertebra. **C,** Anterolateral view of sacrum and coccyx. **D,** Posterior view of sacrum and coccyx.

Spinal Cord and Spinal Nerves

The lumbar plexus and sacral plexus are prominent in the lower trunk. The distal end of the spinal cord, at approximately L1–L2, includes a bundle of spinal nerves that extends downward through the vertebral canal and is known collectively as the cauda equina, after its resemblance to a horse's tail.

The Lumbar Plexus

Supplying the anterior and medial muscles of the thigh region is the lumbar plexus, formed by the T12 through L5 nerve roots (**Fig. 22.4**). The posterior branches of the L2 through L4 nerve roots form

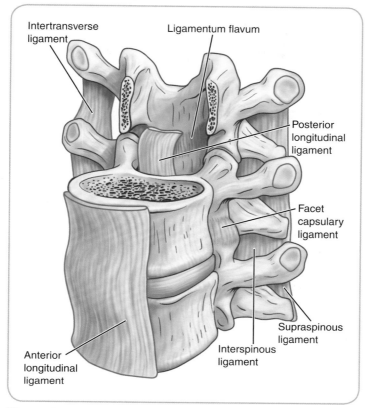

Figure 22.2. Ligaments of the lumbar spine.

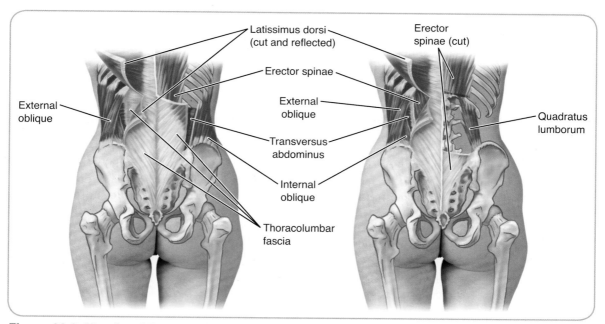

Figure 22.3. Muscles of the low back.

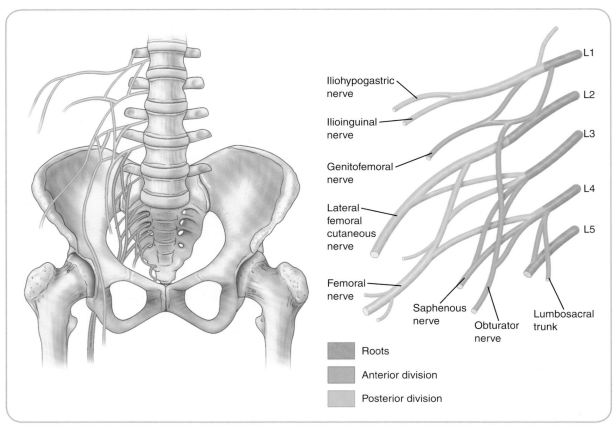

Figure 22.4. Lumbar plexus. The lumbar plexus is formed by the segmental nerves T12 through L5. The lower portion of the plexus merges with the upper portion of the sacral plexus to form the lumbosacral trunk.

the femoral nerve, innervating the quadriceps, whereas the anterior branches form the obturator nerve, innervating most of the adductor muscle group.

The Sacral Plexus

A portion of the lumbar plexus (L4–L5) forms the lumbosacral trunk and courses downward to form the upper portion of the sacral plexus (**Fig. 22.5**). This plexus supplies the muscles of the buttock region and, through the sciatic nerve, the muscles of the posterior thigh and entire lower leg. The sciatic nerve is composed of two distinct nerves, the tibial nerve and the common peroneal nerve. The tibial nerve, formed by the anterior branches of the upper five nerve roots, innervates all the muscles on the posterior leg with the exception of the short head of the biceps femoris. The common peroneal nerve, formed by the posterior branches of the upper four nerve roots, innervates the short head of the biceps femoris and then divides in the vicinity of the head of the fibula into the deep peroneal nerve and the superficial peroneal nerve. These nerves innervate the anterior compartment of the lower leg and lateral compartments of the lower leg, respectively.

KINEMATICS AND MAJOR MUSCLE ACTIONS OF THE LUMBAR SPINE

The vertebral joints enable motion in all planes of movement as well as circumduction. Because the motion allowed between any two adjacent vertebrae is small, spinal movements always involve

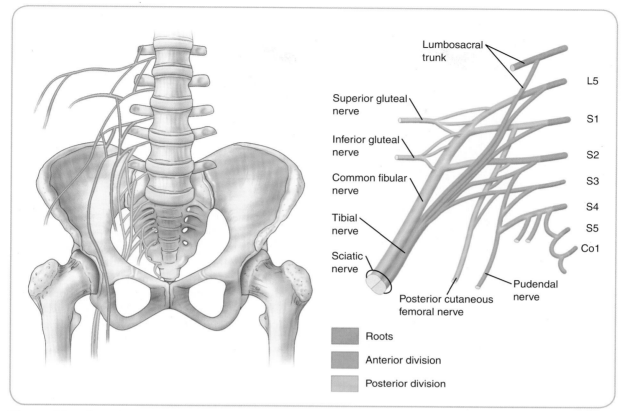

Figure 22.5. Sacral plexus. The sacral plexus is formed by the segmental nerves L4 through S5. This plexus innervates the lower leg, ankle, and foot via the tibial and common peroneal nerves.

a number of motion segments. The range of motion (ROM) allowed at each motion segment is governed by anatomical constraints that vary through the lumbar region of the spine.

Flexion, Extension, and Hyperextension

The flexion–extension capability of the lumbar spine is cumulatively approximately 83°, with more motion allowed at the L2–L3 motion segment and progressively diminishing through L4–L5.[5,6] It is important to avoid confusing spinal flexion with hip flexion or with forward pelvic tilt, although all three motions occur during an activity such as touching the toes. Hip flexion (see **Figs. 16.15A** and **16.16D**) consists of anteriorly directed, sagittal plane rotation of the femur with respect to the pelvic girdle (or vice versa), and forward pelvic tilt (see **Fig. 16.13A**) is anteriorly directed movement of the anterior superior iliac spine (ASIS) with respect to the pubic symphysis.

When the spine is extended backward past anatomical position in the sagittal plane, the motion is termed **hyperextension**. The ROM for spinal hyperextension is considerable in the lumbar region, ranging as high as 21° at L5 through S1. The cumulative ROM for hyperextension is 54° in the lumbar region. Lumbar hyperextension is required in many sport skills, including several swimming strokes, the high jump and pole vault, wrestling, and numerous gymnastic skills. Repeated, extreme lumbar hyperextension is associated with increased risk of spondylolysis, a stress fracture of the pars interarticularis region of the spine.[7]

Lateral Flexion and Rotation

Movement of the spine away from anatomical position in a lateral direction in the frontal plane is termed lateral flexion. In the lumbar region, the cumulative ROM for lateral flexion to one side

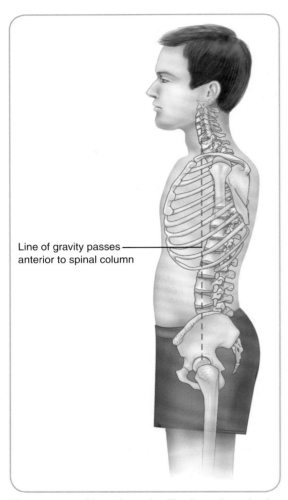

Line of gravity passes
anterior to spinal column

Figure 22.6. Line of gravity. The line of gravity for the head and trunk passes anterior to the spinal column during upright standing. The moment arm for head/trunk weight at any given vertebral joint is the perpendicular distance between the line of gravity and the spinal column.

is approximately 18°.[5] Spinal rotation capability is small in the lumbar region, with only approximately 2° of motion allowed because of the interlocking of the articular processes.[6] The lumbosacral joint permits approximately 5° of rotation. Images depicting lumbar ROM are provided later in the chapter during the assessment discussion.

KINETICS OF THE LUMBAR SPINE

As discussed in Chapter 21, forces acting on the spine include body weight, tension in the spinal ligaments and paraspinal muscles, intra-abdominal pressure, and any applied external loads. When the body is upright, the major form of loading on the spine is axial, and the lumbar spine supports the weight of the body segments above it. Although most of the axial compression load on the spine is borne by the vertebral bodies and disks, the facet joints, when the spine is in hyperextension, may bear as much as approximately 30% of the load. Under significant compressive loading, such as during a heavy lifting task, increases in intra-abdominal pressure occur that may help to stiffen the trunk to prevent the spine from buckling.[8] When the paraspinal muscles are fatigued, there are increased levels of co-contraction, which also help to stiffen the spine and increase spinal stability.[9]

The Effect of Body Position

One factor that can dramatically affect the load on the lumbar spine is body position. When the body is in an upright position, the line of gravity passes anterior to the spinal column (**Fig. 22.6**). As a result, the spine is under a constant, forward bending moment. As the trunk is progressively flexed, the line of gravity shifts farther away from the spine. The farther the line of gravity from the spine, the larger the moment arm for body weight and the greater the bending moment generated. To maintain body position, this moment must be counteracted by tension in the back muscles. The more tension that is required to maintain body position, the greater the compression load on the spine. Lifting with the trunk being erect minimizes the tension requirement for the lumbar muscles, because the moment arm for body weight is minimized. For the same reason, holding the load as close to the trunk as possible during lifting and carrying minimizes the load on the back.[10,11] In comparison to the load that is present during upright standing, compression on the lumbar spine increases with sitting, increases more with spinal flexion, and increases still further with a slouched sitting position (**Fig. 22.7**). When carrying a load, forces acting on the spine increase with walking, with carrying the load at shoulder height, and with asymmetric lifting.[10,11] **Box 22.1** lists guidelines for preventing lumbar spinal stress during the performance of daily activities.

Effect of Movement Speed

Another factor that affects loading of the lumbar spine is body movement speed. Executing a lift in a very rapid, jerking fashion dramatically increases compression and shear forces on the lumbar spine as well as tension in the paraspinal muscles.[12] This is one reason why isotonic resistance training exercises should be performed in a slow, controlled fashion.

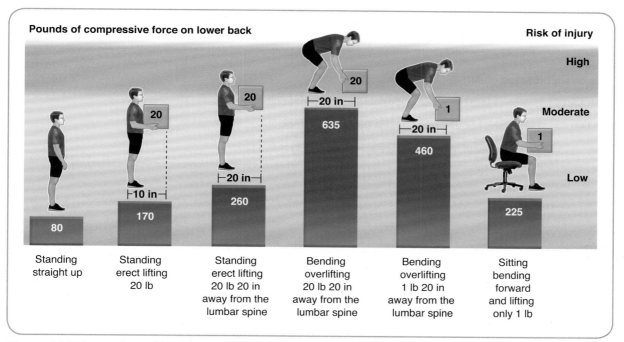

Figure 22.7. Comparison of load placed on lumbar spine in different body positions.

ANATOMICAL VARIATIONS PREDISPOSING INDIVIDUALS TO SPINAL CONDITIONS

Mechanical stress derived from lateral spinal muscle imbalances or from sustaining repeated impact forces can cause back pain and/or injury. Excessive spinal curvatures can be congenital or acquired through weight training or sports participation. Defects in the pars interarticularis of the neural arch can be caused by mechanical stress, also placing a patient at risk for serious spinal injury. Excessive spine curvature and postural abnormalities were discussed in Chapter 8 and should be reviewed at this time in relations to predisposing individuals to spinal conditions.

PREVENTION OF SPINAL CONDITIONS

Although most of the load on the spine is borne by the vertebral bodies and disks, the facet joints assist with some load bearing. Protective equipment can prevent some injuries to the spinal region; however, physical conditioning plays a more important role in preventing injuries to this area. In addition, because the low back is subjected to a variety of stresses as part of normal daily activities, an awareness of proper posture is essential in minimizing the risk of injury.

Protective Equipment

Weight-training belts, abdominal binders, and other similar lumbar/sacral supportive devices support the abdominal contents, stabilize the trunk, and potentially can assist in preventing spinal deformity and damage. These devices place the low back in a more vertical lifting posture, decrease lumbar lordosis, limit pelvic torsion, and lessen axial loading on the spine by increasing intra-abdominal pressure, which in turn reduces compressive forces in the vertebral bodies. Many of these protective devices are discussed in Chapter 3.

BOX 22.1 Preventing Low Back Injuries in Activities of Daily Living

Sitting

- Sit on a firm, straight-backed chair.
- Place the buttocks as far back into the chair as possible to avoid slouching.
- Sit with the feet flat on the floor, not extended and/or raised on a stool.
- Avoid sitting for long periods of time, particularly with the knees fully extended.

Driving

- Place the seat forward so that the knees are level with the hips and you do not have to reach for the pedals.
- If the left foot is not working the pedals, place it flat on the floor.
- Keep the back of the seat in a nearly upright position to avoid slouching.

Standing

- If you must stand in one area for an extended time,
  - Shift body weight from one foot to the other.
  - Elevate one foot on a piece of furniture to keep the knees flexed.
  - Perform toe flexion and extension inside the shoes.
  - Hold the chin up, keep the shoulders back, and relax the knees.
  - Avoid arching the back.

Lifting and Carrying

- Use a lumbosacral belt or have assistance when lifting heavy objects.
- To lift an object,
  - Place the object close to the body.
  - Bend at the knees, not the waist, and keep the back erect.
  - Tighten the abdominal muscles and inhale before lifting the object.
  - Exhale during the lift.
  - Do not twist while lifting.
- To carry a heavy object,
  - Hold the object close to the body at waist level.
  - Carry the object in the middle of the body, not to one side.

Sleeping

- Sleep on a firm mattress. If needed, place a sheet of 0.75-in plywood under the mattress.
- Sleep on the side and place pillows between the legs.
- When sleeping supine, place pillows under the knees. Avoid sleeping in the prone position.
- Avoid sleeping with the arms extended overhead.

Physical Conditioning

Strengthening of the back muscles is imperative to stabilize the spinal column. Exercises to strengthen the low back area should involve back extension, lateral flexion, and rotation. In addition, it is important to strengthen the abdominal muscles to maintain appropriate postural alignment.

Normal ROM also is essential in stabilizing the spine and preventing injury. If warranted, stretching exercises should be used to promote and maintain normal ROM. In particular, it is advantageous to ensure maximal motion in lateral flexion, forward flexion, and rotation.

Proper Skill Technique

Poor posture during walking, sitting, standing, lying down, and running may lead to chronic low back strain or sprains. Cases of postural deformity should be assessed to determine the cause, and an appropriate exercise program should be developed to address the deficits.

Lifting techniques also can affect spinal loading. Executing a lift in a very rapid, jerking fashion dramatically increases compression and shear forces on the spine as well as tension in the paraspinal muscles. For this reason, isotonic resistance exercises should always be performed in a slow, controlled fashion. Breathing technique should be emphasized as well. Specifically, it is desirable to inhale deeply as a lift is initiated and exhale forcefully and smoothly at the end of the lift. Use of a supportive weight-training belt and a spotter also can potentially reduce the chance of injury to the lumbar region during heavy weight lifting.

ASSESSMENT OF LUMBAR SPINAL CONDITIONS

? A 17-year-old cheerleader reports to the athletic training room complaining of aching pain during trunk flexion that is aggravated with resisted hyperextension that produces sharp, shooting pains into the low back and down the posterior leg. How should the assessment of this injury progress to determine the extent and severity of injury?

Injury assessment of the lumbar spine is difficult and complex. In the event of an acute injury with possible nerve involvement, immobilization and immediate transportation to the nearest medical facility is warranted, regardless of whether a total assessment is completed. **Box 22.2** identifies several red flags that warrant immobilization and immediate referral to a physician.

When the patient walks into the examination room and complains of low back pain, it is relatively safe to assume that a serious spinal injury is not present. Most of the examination will involve differentiating symptoms, including distinguishing the presence of radicular symptoms into the leg from a space-occupying lesion or herniated disk, from other conditions, such as a strain, sprain, or facet problem more likely to cause localized low back pain. Even after a detailed and methodical assessment,

---

BOX 22.2 Red Flags That Warrant Immobilization and Immediate Referral to a Physician

- Severe pain, point tenderness, or deformity along the vertebral column
- Pain radiating into the extremities
- Trunk or abdominal pain that may be referred from the visceral organs
- Loss or change in sensation anywhere in the body
- Paralysis or inability to move a body part
- Any injury in which uncertainty exists regarding the severity or nature
- Diminished or absent reflexes
- Muscle weakness in a myotome

See **Application Strategy: Lumbar Spinal Injury Evaluation**, available on the companion Web site at thePoint, for a summary of the assessment procedure.

a definitive determination of the source of pain may not be obvious. As such, referral to a physician for advanced testing and assessment may be necessary.

The assessment that follows focuses on a lumbar assessment for a conscious individual. Specific information related to an acute injury is included where appropriate.

HISTORY

? The injury assessment of the cheerleader should begin with a history. What questions need to be asked to identify the cause and extent of injury?

A history of the injury should include information regarding the primary complaint, mechanism of injury, characteristics of the symptoms, disability resulting from the injury, previous injuries to the area, and family history that may have some bearing on this specific condition. In cases of lumbar spinal injury, questions should be asked about the location of pain (i.e., localized or radiating), type of pain (i.e., dull, aching, sharp, burning, or radiating), presence of sensory changes (i.e., numbness, tingling, or absence of sensation), and possible muscle weakness or paralysis. It also is important to determine the length of time the problem has been present. Acute back pain usually lasts 3 to 4 days. Subacute back pain lasts up to 12 weeks, however, and chronic back pain can extend longer than 3 months.[1]

See **Application Strategy: Developing a History for a Spinal Injury**, available on the companion Web site at thePoint, for general questions related to a lumbar spinal injury.

The cheerleader should be asked questions that would assist in determining the cause and extent of injury. Questions should address the primary complaint (i.e., what, when, and how questions), mechanism of injury, location of pain (i.e., localized or radiating), type of pain (i.e., dull, aching, sharp, burning, or radiating), presence of sensory changes (i.e., numbness, tingling, or absence of sensation) and possible muscle weakness, unusual sensations (i.e., sound or feelings), onset of symptoms, related medical history, and past injuries/treatment.

OBSERVATION AND INSPECTION

? The 17-year-old cheerleader has been participating in cheerleading for 5 years. The primary complaint is an aching pain during trunk flexion that is aggravated with resisted hyperextension that produces sharp shooting pains into the low back and down the posterior aspect of the right leg. The cheerleader reports the condition has been present for 2 weeks, and she cannot recall a traumatic episode that may have caused the condition. Would it be appropriate to do a scan examination to rule out other painful areas, and what specific factors should be observed to identify the injury?

The observation component of an assessment should be initiated as soon as the clinician sees the patient. Body language can signal pain, disability, and muscle weakness. It is important to note the individual's willingness or ability to move, general posture, ease in motion, and general attitude.

See **Application Strategy: Postural Assessment of the Low Back Region**, available on the companion Web site at thePoint, for specific postural factors to observe in the head and spinal region.

Clothing and protective equipment may prevent visual observation of abnormalities in the spinal alignment. As such, the patient should be suitably dressed so that the back is as exposed as possible; for girls and women, a bra, halter top, or swimsuit can be worn. The observation should begin with a postural assessment, progress through a scan examination and gait analysis, and end with an inspection of the injury site. Postural and gait assessments were discussed in Chapter 8.

Inspection of the Injury

Local inspection of the injury site should include observation for deformity, swelling, discoloration, muscle spasm, atrophy, hypertrophy, scars that might indicate previous surgery, and the general skin condition. A step deformity in the lumbar spine may indicate a spondylolisthesis (**Fig. 22.8**).

Gross Neuromuscular Assessment

During an acute on-site injury assessment, a posture assessment and scan may not be possible. It is beneficial, however, to perform a neuromuscular assessment prior to palpation to detect any motor and/or sensory deficits. This can be done without moving the patient by having the person perform a submaximal, bilateral hand squeeze and ankle dorsiflexion. These two actions assess the cervical and lumbar spinal nerves, respectively. Muscle weakness and/or diminished sensation over the hands and feet indicate a serious injury. If any deficits are noted, the emergency care plan, including summoning emergency medical services (EMS), should be activated. If no deficits are noted, it does not rule out possible neurological involvement or fracture. Therefore, the palpation should be done with the patient maintained in the position found.

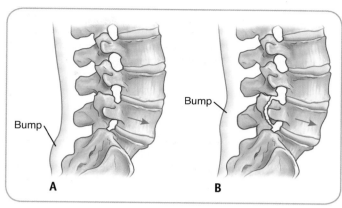

Figure 22.8. Step deformity in the lumbar spine. A step deformity occurs when the spinous process of one vertebra is more prominent than the vertebra below or above it. **A,** Spondylitis. **B,** Spondylolisthesis.

 During a scan examination, trunk flexion and extension produced a dull pain in the low back. Lateral flexion to the right caused sharp pain to radiate into the right buttock and posterior leg. Gait analysis showed a shortened stride on the right side. Visual inspection showed no abnormalities. The injury is confined to the low back region.

PALPATION

 What specific structures need to be palpated to determine if the injury is of bony or soft-tissue origin, and can neural involvement be ruled out during the palpation?

Bony and soft-tissue structures are palpated to detect temperature, swelling, point tenderness, deformity, crepitus, muscle spasm, and cutaneous sensation. In injuries that do not involve neural damage, fracture, or dislocation, palpation can proceed with the patient in a supine position. The umbilicus lies at the level of the L3–L4 disk space and is the center point for the intersection of the abdominal quadrants. Using careful deep palpation, the clinician may be able to palpate the anterior aspects of the L4, L5, and S1 vertebrae, disks, and accompanying anterior longitudinal ligament. The abdomen also should be palpated for pain and muscle spasms that may be responsible for referred pain into the lumbar region from internal organs. The inguinal area, iliac crest, and symphysis pubis also can be palpated for signs of infection (e.g., enlarged lymph nodes), hip pointers, apophysitis, or osteitis pubis.

When moving into the prone position, a pillow or blanket should be placed under the hip region to tilt the pelvis back and relax the lumbar curvature. Muscle spasm in the lower erector spinae, lower trapezius, serratus posterior, quadratus lumborum, latissimus dorsi, or gluteus maximus can indicate dysfunction of the thoracic or lumbar spine. The following surface landmarks in the lumbar region can facilitate palpation:

- L4—top of iliac crest
- L5—demarcated by bilateral dimples
- S2—level of posterior superior iliac spine (PSIS)

In palpating the spinous processes of the lumbar spine, particular attention should be noted at the L4, L5, and S1 levels. A visible or palpable dip or protrusion can indicate spondylolisthesis (**Fig. 22.8**). If the fingers are moved laterally 2 to 3 cm (0.8 to 1.2 in), the facet joints can be palpated for signs of pathology. Because of their depth, it may be difficult to palpate the joints; however, a spasm in the overlying paraspinal muscles can be palpated. The spinous processes of the sacrum also can be palpated. Because no interposing soft-tissue spaces are between them, they may be harder to distinguish. The S2 spinous process is at the level of a line drawn between the two PSIS ("posterior dimples"). In moving to the PSIS, the clinician can palpate the iliac crest for signs of injury and then palpate the gluteal muscles for pain, spasm, or possible nodules. Having the patient flex the hip at 90° allows easier palpation of the ischial tuberosity, greater trochanter, and sciatic nerve, which is located midway between the ischial tuberosity and greater trochanter. Finally, the piriformis muscle should be palpated deep to the gluteal muscles for pathology. The following structures should be palpated:

The Anterior Aspect

1. **Umbilicus and abdominal area.** Note any abnormal tenderness or masses indicating internal pathology that is referring pain to the spinal region.

2. **Inguinal area.** Palpate for possible hernia, infection (enlarged lymph nodes), or other pathology.

3. **Iliac crest, ASIS, and symphysis pubis.** Palpate for pain, tenderness, or defect indicating pathology (e.g., avulsion fracture, hip pointer, apophysitis, or osteitis pubis).

The Posterior Aspect

1. **Spinous processes of the lumbar vertebrae.** Note any tenderness, crepitus, or presence of a step-off deformity (i.e., one vertebra is more anterior than the one below it). This indicates spondylolisthesis, which most commonly is seen between the L4 and L5 or the L5 and S1 vertebrae. Pain and tenderness without positive findings on muscle movement may indicate that the problem is not musculoskeletal in origin.

2. **Facet joints.** The facet articulations are approximately a thumb's breadth to either side of the spinous process. Point tenderness at these sites, especially with extension and rotation to the same side, suggests facet joint pain.

3. **Interspinous and supraspinous ligaments, paraspinal muscles, and quadratus lumborum.** Trigger points within specific muscles may refer pain to a more distal area. Tender points that increase with muscular contraction indicate a localized muscle strain. An area that is tender to palpation but is not painful during muscle contraction may indicate referred pain from another area.

4. **Iliac crest, PSIS, and sacrum.** The interspace between L4 and L5 lies at the same level as the top of the iliac crest. The S2 spinous process lies in the middle of a line drawn between the PSIS. Palpate for pain, tenderness, and other pathology (e.g., hip pointer or apophysitis).

5. **Ischial tuberosity, sciatic nerve, and greater trochanter.** Flex the hip to 90° for easier palpation of these structures. The sciatic nerve is located midway between the ischial tuberosity and greater trochanter (**Fig. 22.9**).

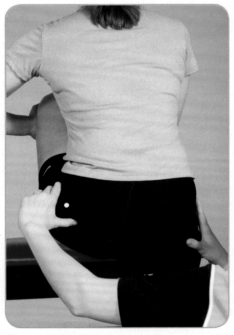

Figure 22.9. Sciatic nerve. To palpate the sciatic nerve, flex the hip, and locate the ischial tuberosity and greater trochanter. The sciatic nerve may be palpated at the midpoint. It is designated here by the *white dot*.

The palpation component of the assessment of the cheerleader should include bony and soft tissues of the lumbar region (i.e., spinous processes of the lumbar vertebrae; facet joints; interspinous and supraspinous ligaments, paraspinal muscles, and quadratus lumborum; iliac crest, PSIS, and sacrum; and ischial tuberosity, sciatic nerve, and greater trochanter). Palpation also should include anterior structures (i.e., umbilicus and abdominal area, iliac crest, and ASIS).

Because the cheerleader is younger than 18 years, palpation can only be performed with permission from the parent or guardian. It also is important to recognize that the cheerleader may feel uncomfortable being touched by a health care provider of the opposite gender. If a same-gender clinician is not available, the evaluation should be observed by a third party (e.g., another clinician, parent, or guardian).

PHYSICAL EXAMINATION TESTS

? In the palpation component of the assessment of the cheerleader, point tenderness was elicited in the low back region between the L3 and S1 vertebrae, with increased pain in the L4–L5 region. A muscle spasm was present on either side of the lumbar region. Pain also was elicited with palpation midway between the ischial tuberosity and greater trochanter. Based on the information obtained through the history, observation, and palpation, what tests should be performed to determine nerve root impingement, and what tests should be conducted as part of a neurological assessment of the cheerleader's condition?

It is imperative to work slowly through the tests that are used to assess low back conditions, because injuries to the lumbar region can be very complex. If, at any time, movement leads to increased acute pain or change in sensation, or if the patient resists moving the spine, a significant injury should be assumed and the emergency plan should be activated.

Functional Tests

The completion of gross movement patterns in a standing position is adequate to determine normal and pain-free ROM. Further assessment can be conducted if motion is limited or the patient is unwilling to do the movements.

Active Movement

If active movement of the spine was conducted during the scan examination, it need not be repeated. The individual's willingness to perform the movement should be noted. It is important to note if movement is fluid and complete or if pain, spasm, or stiffness blocks the full ROM. The presence of a painful arc, particularly a lightning-like pain, present during forward flexion and extension should be noted as well. This often indicates a space-occupying lesion (e.g., herniated disk), but it also may be caused by instability. Movements to the left and right should be compared bilaterally. The ROM listed usually is the summation of the entire lumbar spine, not just at one level, along with hip movement. Basic active movements of the lumbar spine (**Fig. 22.10**) include the following:

1. Forward trunk flexion (40° to 60°)

2. Trunk extension (20° to 35°)

3. Lateral trunk flexion (left and right; 15° to 20°)

4. Trunk rotation done in a standing and sitting position (3° to 18°)

Because spinal injuries seldom occur during a single motion, combined motions of the spine should be included in the examination. These movements include lateral flexion in flexion, lateral

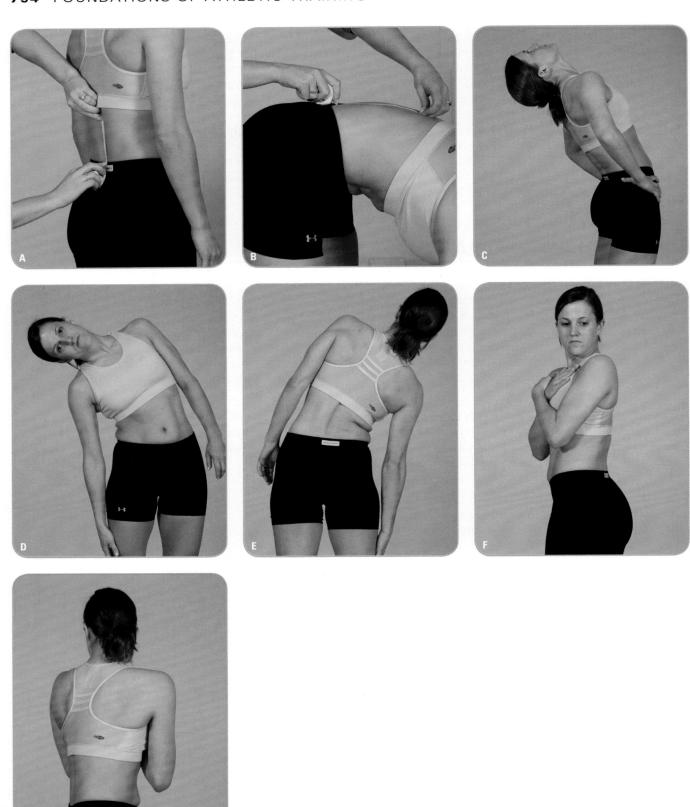

Figure 22.10. Active movements of the lumbar spine. A and **B,** Measuring forward flexion with a tape measure. **C,** Extension. **D** and **E,** Lateral flexion. **F,** Rotation (standing). **G,** Rotation (sitting).

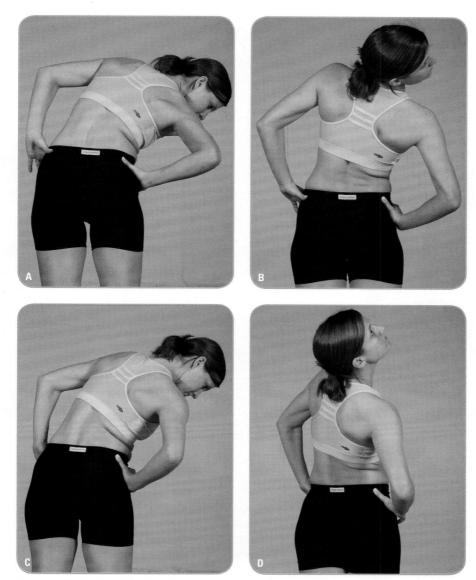

Figure 22.11. Combined active movements. A, Lateral flexion in flexion. **B,** Lateral flexion in extension. **C,** Rotation and flexion. **D,** Rotation and extension.

flexion in extension, flexion and rotation, and extension and rotation (**Fig. 22.11**). These movements may lead to signs and symptoms different from the basic motions and are indicated if these motions reproduce the patient's symptoms. For example, extension and rotation are more likely to reproduce symptoms in a facet syndrome compared with only extension or only rotation.

Passive Range of Motion

Passive movements are difficult to perform in the lumbar region. If active movements are full and pain-free, gentle overpressure may be applied as the patient reaches the full range of active motion.[13] Extreme care must be exercised in applying the overpressure, because the upper body weight is already being applied to the lumbar joints by virtue of gravity (i.e., compressive forces) and their position (i.e., shear forces). While sustaining the position at the end of the ROM for 10 to 20 seconds, the patient should be asked if the symptoms increase. Likewise, if symptoms increased during the active combined movements, these movements should be repeated, but only after the patient has completed the basic movements. The normal end feels for the lumbar movements are tissue stretch.[13]

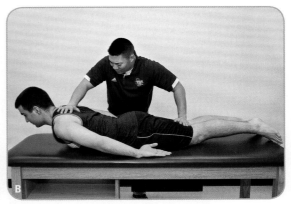

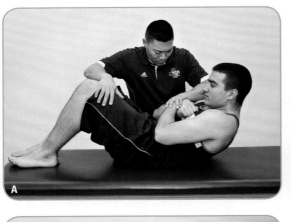

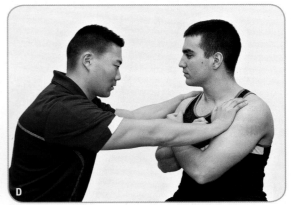

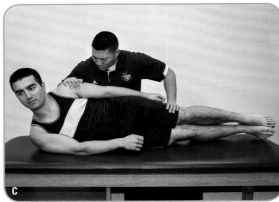

Figure 22.12. Resisted isometric movements of the lumbar spine. A, Flexion. **B,** Extension. **C,** Lateral flexion. **D,** Rotation to the right.

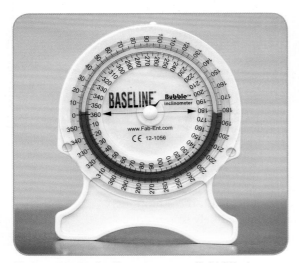

Figure 22.13. Inclinometers are fluid filled measurement instruments that use gravity's effect to measure joint position and motion. Because universal goniometers and inclinometers use different systems to measure joint motion, it is recommended that the two not be used interchangeably. (From Norkin CC, White DJ. *Measurement of Joint Motion: A Guide to Goniometry.* 4th ed. Philadelphia, PA: FA Davis; 2009.)

Resisted Muscle Testing

Resisted movement is initially performed in a neutral position with the patient seated to stabilize the hip. The patient is instructed to not allow the clinician to move the body part being tested by applying a maximal isometric contraction in flexion, extension, lateral flexion, and rotation. By repetitively loading the patient's resisting muscle with rapid, consecutive impulses, more subtle weakness can be detected. Lumbar movements to be tested are shown in **Figure 22.12.**

Goniometry

Goniometry measurements of the spine are difficult to assess when using a universal goniometer. Spinal motion is less difficult to measure when using an inclinometer (**Fig. 22.13**).[14] The American Medical Association recommends using double inclinometers for assessing spinal ROM.[15] However, the most reliable method for measuring lumbar ROM is radiography.[14] Table 22.1 provides directions for using inclinometers to measure lumbar ROM: flexion (**Fig. 22.14**), extension (**Fig. 22.15**), and lateral bending (**Fig. 22.16**).[16]

Stress and Functional Tests

Several stress tests can be used in a spinal assessment. Only those deemed to be relevant should be performed. Because many of

TABLE 22.1 Measuring Lumbar Range of Motion Using Inclinometers

MOTION	1. Lumbar flexion (approximately 60° degrees) 2. Lumber extension (ranges from 20° to 38°, depending on age and gender) 3. Lumber lateral flexion (approximately 25°–30°)
STARTING POSITION	Patient in standing
INCLINOMETER PLACEMENT	Two inclinometers are needed. The upper inclinometer is placed over the *spinous process of T12*, and the second inclinometer is placed over the *sacrum at the S2* level. In the starting position, both inclinometers should be set at the zero position.
PATIENT INSTRUCTIONS	1. "Please bend forward as far as possible while keeping knees straight." 2. "Please bend backward as far as possible." 3. "Please bend to the side but do not rotate your trunk. Please keep both feet flat on the ground and knees straight."
ENDING POSITION	1. Flexion 2. Extension 3. Lateral flexion
MEASURING RANGE OF MOTION	Subtract the degrees recorded on the sacral inclinometer from the degrees recorded on the inclinometer at the T12 level.
MOTION	1. Thoracolumbar lateral flexion 2. Thoracolumbar rotation
STARTING POSITION	1. Patient in standing 2. Patient in forward flexion
INCLINOMETER PLACEMENT	Two inclinometers are needed. The upper inclinometer is placed over the *spinous process of T1* and the second inclinometer is placed over the sacrum at the *S2 level*. In the starting position, both inclinometers should be set at the zero position.
PATIENT INSTRUCTIONS	1. "Please bend to the side as far as possible, keeping both feet flat on ground and knees straight." 2. "Please rotate trunk as far as possible without moving out of extension."
ENDING POSITION	1. Laterally flexed 2. Lateral rotation
MEASURING RANGE OF MOTION	Subtract the degrees recorded on the sacral inclinometer from the degrees recorded on the inclinometer at the T1 level.

Adapted from Norkin CC, White DJ. *Measurement of Joint Motion: A Guide to Goniometry.* 4th ed. Philadelphia, PA: FA Davis; 2009.

these tests are designed to put stress on neurological tissue, they often cause pain or discomfort, which may be bilateral. For a test to be positive, however, the patient's symptoms must be reproduced; otherwise, the test is considered to be negative. Tests are grouped on the basis of patient position.

Lumbar Tests in a Seated Position

■ Slump Test

This test is a neural tension test designed to assess potential lumbar nerve root irritation. While in a seated position on an examining table, the patient is instructed to "slump" so that the spine flexes and the shoulders sag forward. Initially, the clinician maintains the position of the patient's head in a neutral position (**Fig. 22.17A**). The presence of any symptoms that are produced by the slump should be noted. If no symptoms are present, the patient flexes the neck and the clinician places pressure on the shoulders of the patient (**Fig. 22.17B**). If no symptoms are produced, slight overpressure of neck flexion is applied by the clinician (**Fig. 22.17C**). If no symptoms are elicited, one of the patient's knees is passively extended, and the foot of the same leg is passively dorsiflexed, to see if any symptoms occur (**Fig. 22.17D**).

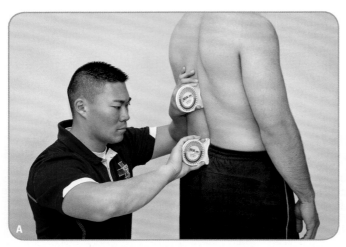
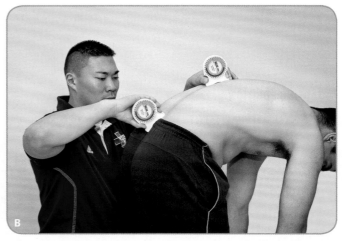

Figure 22.14. Using inclinometer to measure active lumbar flexion. A, Starting position with double inclinometers placed over the spinous process of T12 and second inclinometer over the sacrum at the S2 level. **B,** Ending position.

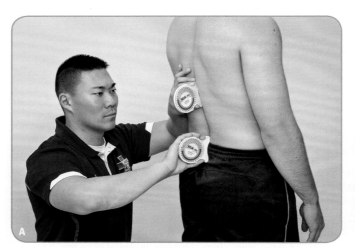
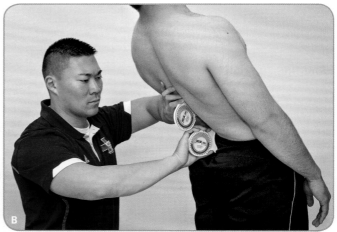

Figure 22.15. Using inclinometer to measure active lumbar extension. A, Starting position with double inclinometers placed over the spinous process of T12 and second inclinometer over the sacrum at the S2 level. **B,** Ending position.

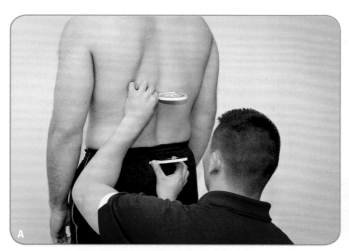
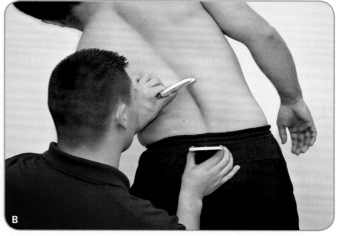

Figure 22.16. Using inclinometer to measure active lumbar lateral flexion. A, Starting position with double inclinometers placed over the spinous process of T12 and second inclinometer over the sacrum at the S2 level. **B,** Ending position.

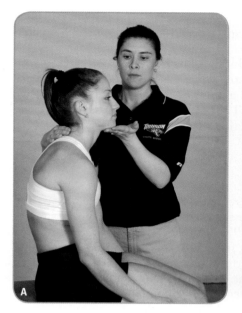
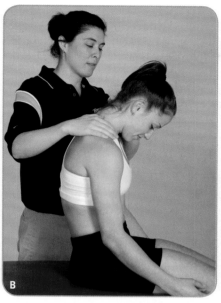
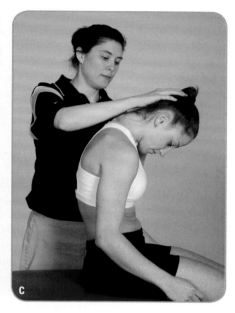
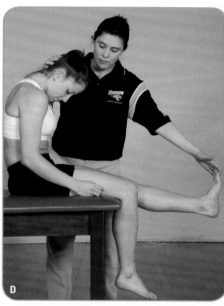
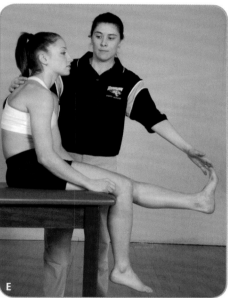

Figure 22.17. Slump test. The test is performed in several stages. **A,** While sitting on a table, the clinician asks the person to "slump" so that the spine flexes and the shoulders sag forward while the clinician holds the head in a neutral position. **B,** If no symptoms are present, the clinician applies light pressure, pushing down on the shoulders while the patient holds the head in a neutral position. **C,** If no symptoms are produced, overpressure is applied to the cervical spine. **D,** If no symptoms occur, the clinician passively extends one of the patient's knees and dorsiflexes the ankle of the same leg. **E,** The patient is instructed to extend the neck. The test is considered to be positive if symptoms of sciatic pain are reproduced, indicating impingement of the dura and spinal cord or nerve roots.

If no symptoms are reported, the patient is asked to extend the neck. The presence or lack of symptoms should be noted (**Fig. 22.17E**). This process is repeated with the opposite leg. A test is positive if symptoms of sciatic pain are reproduced, indicating impingement of the dura and spinal cord or nerve roots. The pain usually is produced at the site of the lesion. Specificity scores for the slump test range from 55% to 73% with sensitivity scores ranging from 42% to 83%.[17,18] The wide range of scores may be attributed to the fact that many modifications have been made to the slump test, with different sequencing order as well as altering whether the patient is actively or passively engaged in the motions.

■ Valsalva Test

The Valsalva maneuver is used to determine the presence of space-occupying lesions (e.g., herniated disk, tumor, or osteophytes). While seated, the patient is asked to take a deep breath and hold it while bearing down, as if moving the bowels. It is important for the clinician to exercise caution with this test, because the maneuver increases intrathecal pressure, which can slow the pulse, decrease venous return, and increase venous pressure, each of which actions may cause fainting. A positive test is indicated by increased pain radiating from low back. The Valsalva maneuver has very strong sensitivity (95%) as well as strong specificity (73%), making this a clinically useful test.[17]

Lumbar Tests in a Supine Position

■ Straight Leg Raising Test

Also known as Lasègue test, this examination is used to differentiate the source of the patient's pain: SI joint pain, irritation of the sciatic nerve, disk herniation, or tight hamstrings. Although the straight leg raising (SLR) test has had sensitivity ratings as high as 97%,[18] other sources state it as low as 33%.[17,19] Specificity findings seem to be varying also, ranging from 57% to 87%.[17–19] This variability may be due to the many modifications that are made when performing the SLR and calls into question the clinical usefulness of this test.[20] Therefore, it is important to obtain a solid history and consider findings discovered through inspection and palpation combined with the findings from the SLR test.

The test should be performed in stages, and at each stage, asking the patient for presence of pain and to describe the type and location of the pain being experienced. To perform the SLR test, the patient is placed in a relaxed, supine position with the hip medially rotated and the knee extended. The clinician should grasp the individual's heel with one hand and place the other on top of the patella to prevent the knee from flexing. The leg is passively and slowly raised until the patient complains of pain or tightness. Ask the patient to describe the location and type of pain being felt. The leg is then lowered until the pain is relieved. The leg should not be lowered further. Next, the clinician passively dorsiflexes the patient's foot and again asks the patient for presence, location, and type of pain experienced. If no pain is experienced, further modification includes asking the patient to flex the neck onto the chest while the clinician continues to dorsiflex the foot (**Fig. 22.18**).

If the patient does not experience pain until between 70° and 90° of hip flexion, with no neurological symptoms, the pain may be caused by SI joint dysfunction. Pain that is experienced prior to reaching 70° of hip flexion originates in the lumbar spine and radiates may suggest presence of disk involvement. If pain is experienced at 30° of hip flexion and originates in the buttock area, SI nerve irritation should be suspected.

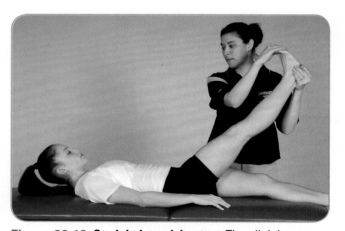

Figure 22.18. Straight leg raising test. The clinician passively flexes the patient's hip while keeping the knee extended until pain or tension is felt. Next, the leg is lowered slowly until the pain or tension disappears. Next, the clinician dorsiflexes the ankle. If no pain occurs, patient is asked to flex the neck, while the clinician continues to passively dorsiflex the ankle.

Pain that is reproduced when the ankle is passively dorsiflexed helps to rule out tight hamstrings as the cause of the pain. Passive dorsiflexion places tension on the dural sheath by stretching it. Pain in the hamstring region that is relieved by lowering the leg and that is not reproduced with passive ankle dorsiflexion suggests tight hamstrings.

■ Well Straight Leg Raising Test

The well SLR test differs from the previous test in that the unaffected leg is raised. A positive sign is pain on the side opposite the leg being raised, indicating a space-occupying lesion (e.g., a herniated intervertebral disk).

■ Bowstring Test (Tension or Popliteal Pressure Sign)

The bowstring or tension sign test is designed to assess tension or pressure on the sciatic nerve and is a modification of the SLR test. The clinician passively flexes the patient's hip while maintaining full knee extension until the patient complains of pain. Ask the patient to describe the type of pain experienced and the location. If pain is experienced, the clinician then flexes the knee slightly (20°), reducing the symptoms. Thumb or finger pressure is then exerted over the tibial portion of the sciatic nerve as it passes through the popliteal space to reestablish the painful radiating symptoms (**Fig. 22.19**). Replication of tenderness or radiating pain is a positive sign for sciatic nerve irritation.

■ Brudzinski Test

This test is similar to the SLR test, but the movements are actively performed by the patient. The patient is supine, with the hands cupped behind the head (**Fig. 22.20A**). The test is positive if the patient complains of neck and low back discomfort and attempts to relieve the meningeal irritation by involuntarily flexing the knees and hips. Positive findings suggest possible dural sheath irritation.

■ Kernig Test

This test can aid in identifying the presence of a bulging disk, nerve root impingement, inflammation of the dural sheath, or irritation of the meninges. In Kernig's position, the patient lies supine, with the hip flexed and the knee extended (**Fig. 22.20B**). Pain in the head, neck, or lower back suggests meningeal irritation, which may indicate presence of meningitis. If the pain is relieved when the patient flexes the knee, it is considered to be a positive test, indicating meningeal irritation, nerve root involvement, or dural irritation. The Brudzinski and Kernig tests may be done either separately or together.

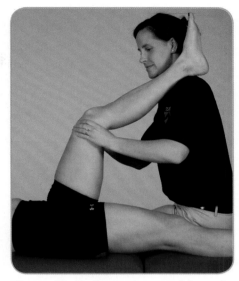

Figure 22.19. Bowstring test. After pain results in an SLR test, the clinician flexes the knee slightly (20°) to reduce the symptoms. Thumb pressure is then exerted in the popliteal area to reproduce the painful radicular symptoms.

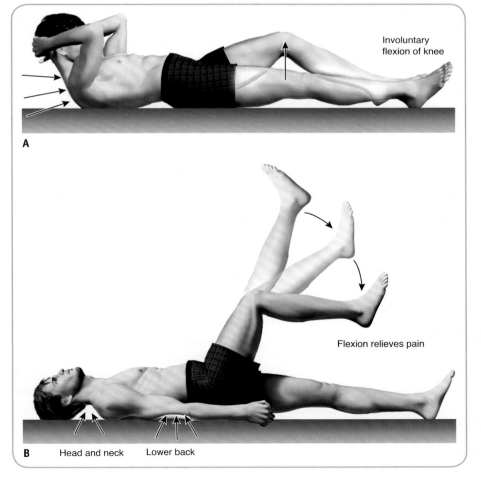

A — Involuntary flexion of knee

B — Head and neck — Lower back — Flexion relieves pain

Figure 22.20. Brudzinski and Kernig tests. A, In Brudzinski test, the individual lays supine and dorsiflexes the neck. **B,** In Kernig test, the individual actively flexes the hip, with the knee extended. The test is considered to be positive if knee extension leads to head, neck, or low back pain that is relieved with knee flexion.

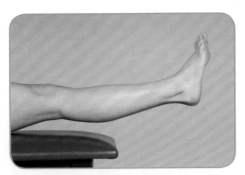

Figure 22.21. Milgram test. The patient is instructed to raise both legs 2–6 in and hold the position for 30 seconds. The test is considered to be positive if the affected limb or limbs cannot be held for 30 seconds or if symptoms are reproduced in the affected limb.

■ Milgram Test

This test attempts to increase intrathecal pressure, resulting in an increased bulge of the nucleus pulposus, primarily in the lumbar spine. The patient lies supine, simultaneously lifts both legs off the table by 2 in to 6 in, and holds this position for 30 seconds (**Fig. 22.21**). The test is considered to be positive if the affected limb or limbs cannot be held for 30 seconds or if symptoms are reproduced in the affected limb. This test should be performed with caution, because it places a high stress load on the lumbar spine.

■ Piriformis Syndrome Tests

Because the piriformis muscle may impinge or entrap the sciatic nerve, symptoms associated with piriformis syndrome are similar to symptoms experienced by patients with lumbar disk herniation. Therefore, it is important to distinguish the cause of the patient's sciatic pain so that proper treatment is provided.

Pace Sign and FAIR Test

When performing the FAIR (flexion, adduction, and internal rotation) test, recreation of symptoms is referred to as a positive **pace sign**. To perform the **FAIR** test, the patient is placed in a supine or recumbent position (**Fig. 22.22**). The clinician passively moves the limb of the affected side into 60° of hip flexion with the knee flexed to an angle of 60° to 90°. The hip of the affected side is then internally rotated and adducted, applying a downward pressure at the end range of the maneuver. The hip of the noninvolved side should be stabilized throughout the process. A positive pace sign implies that the pain may be caused by the piriformis syndrome.[21] The FAIR test has been found to be a clinically useful test for identifying piriformis syndrome with a reported 88% sensitivity and 83% specificity.[22]

Piriformis Muscle Stretch Test

However, there are many different piriformis muscle stretch tests described within the literature, often with the same name, but with varying techniques described.[21] The description that follows is the one most frequently used to describe the piriformis muscle stretch test. The patient lies

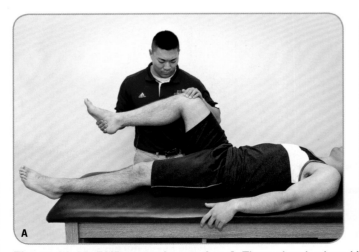
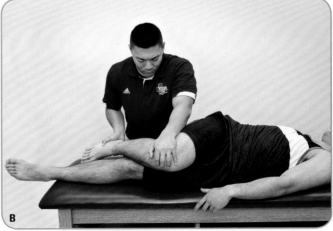

Figure 22.22. FAIR test and pace sign. A, The patient is placed in supine position, and the clinician passively moves the limb of the affected side into 60° of hip flexion with the knee flexed to an angle of 60° to 90°. **B,** The hip of the affected side is then internally rotated and adducted, applying a downward pressure at the end range of the maneuver. Reproduction of symptoms (pace sign) indicates a positive finding.

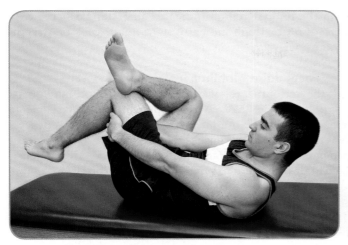

Figure 22.23. Piriformis muscle stretch test. Starting in a supine position, the patient slightly flexes the hip and knee of the uninvolved side. The ankle of the involved side is placed on the knee of the uninvolved side. The patient then passively (using both hands) pulls the thigh of the uninvolved leg to his or her chest, thereby stretching the piriformis and lateral rotators of the involved side. Reproduction of pain is a positive finding.

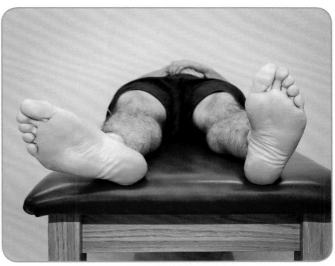

Figure 22.24. Piriformis sign. View the patient from a caudal or feet first perspective. The presence of external rotation of the lower extremity present only on the involved side in an otherwise relaxed patient is a positive finding.

supine, with the knees flexed and the feet flat on the table. The foot/ankle of the affected leg is crossed and placed on top of the unaffected knee. The patient grasps the uninvolved knee and pulls to the chest (**Fig. 22.23**). The test is positive if symptoms are reproduced. Be aware that it is also the same maneuver one would use to *stretch* the piriformis muscle and is therefore also a therapeutic exercise.

Piriformis Sign

A positive piriformis sign indicates that the piriformis and lateral rotators are excessively tight. To assess for the presence of a piriformis sign, place the patient in a supine position. View the patient from a caudal or feet-first perspective. The presence of external rotation of the lower extremity present only on the involved side in an otherwise relaxed patient is a positive finding (**Fig. 22.24**).[21]

Lumbar Tests in a Prone Position

■ Femoral Nerve Stretch Test

This test is used to assess nerve root lesions at the L2, L3, or L4 level. The femoral nerve stretch test (FNST) has been found to be one of the most reliable (88% to 100%) clinical test in screening for midlumbar nerve root impingement and has a reported 97% sensitivity.[18,23] This test is also referred to as the prone knee bend test, although some variation between the two tests does exist. The description that follows is specific to the FNST. The patient is prone, and the knee is passively flexed until the foot rests against the buttock, or until the onset of symptoms, making sure the hip is not rotated. If the knee cannot be flexed beyond 90° because of a pathological condition, passive extension of the hip, with the knee flexed as much as possible, is performed (**Fig. 22.25**).

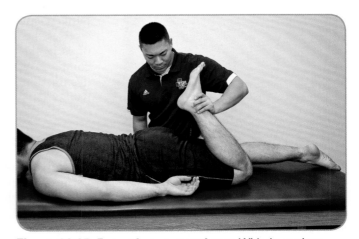

Figure 22.25. Femoral nerve stretch test. With the patient prone, the clinician passively flexes the knee as far as possible toward the buttocks. Unilateral pain in the lumbar area, buttock, and/or posterior thigh may indicate an L2 or L3 nerve root lesion.

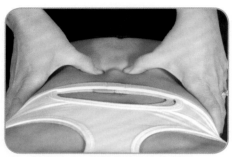

Figure 22.26. Facet joint spring test. While placing the thumbs directly over the spinous process, the clinician carefully pushes the spinous process anteriorly, feeling for the springing of the vertebrae. If pain is elicited or the vertebra is hypomobile, facet joint pathology is present.

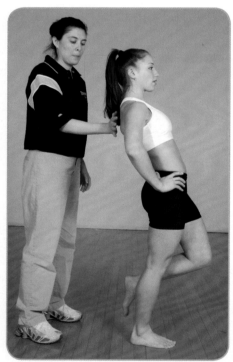

Figure 22.27. Single-leg stance test. The clinician needs to stand behind the patient to support the shoulder region as the patient balances on one leg and then hyperextends the spine. A test is positive when pain is evoked in the back when the opposite leg is raised, indicating a pars interarticularis stress fracture. Bilateral pars fractures result in pain when either leg is lifted.

Unilateral pain in the lumbar region indicates an L2 or L3 nerve root lesion. Pain in the anterior thigh indicates tight quadriceps or stretching of the femoral nerve.

■ Spring Test for Facet Joint Mobility

Hypomobility of the vertebrae, especially at the facet joint, may be assessed with the spring test (**Fig. 22.26**). With the patient prone, the clinician stands over the patient with the thumbs placed over the spinous process to be tested. The clinician carefully pushes the spinous process anteriorly, feeling for a springing of the vertebrae. The test is considered to be positive if pain is elicited or if the vertebra does not move ("spring").

Lumbar Tests in a Standing Position

■ Single-Leg Stance Test

This test can aid in the assessment of spondylolysis, spondylolisthesis, and SI joint irritation. The patient stands on one leg and extends the spine while balancing on the single leg (stork position) (**Fig. 22.27**). The clinician stands nearby providing support for the patient and may aid in providing overpressure at an end ROM. The test is then repeated with the opposite leg. If pain is elicited when the opposite leg is lifted, a unilateral lesion to the pars interarticularis should be suspected; if pain is elicited when either leg is lifted, a bilateral pars interarticularis fracture should be suspected. If rotation is combined with extension and pain results, possible facet joint pathology is indicated on the side to which rotation occurs. The single-leg stance test (also known as stork test) has good interrater reliability (88% to 100%) and both moderate sensitivity (55%) and sensitivity (46% to 68%).[17]

■ Quadrant Test

This test can screen for various pathologies of the lumbar spine, such as dural irritation, facet joint compression, and SI joint dysfunction. The clinician stands behind the patient. The patient extends the spine while the clinician controls the movement by stabilizing the patient's shoulders. If needed, the clinician may use his or her shoulder to support the weight of the patient's head. Overpressure is applied in extension while the patient laterally flexes and rotates toward the painful side. This movement pattern causes maximum narrowing of the intervertebral foramen and stresses the facet joints on the side where rotation occurs. The presence of radicular pain suggests impingement of the lumbar nerve roots. In comparison, localized pain is indicative of facet joint pathology; SI joint dysfunction would be suggested if pain is specific to the area of the PSIS (**Fig. 22.28**).

Lumbar Tests for Malingering

■ Hoover Test

Because the assessment of lumbopelvic disorders is difficult to perform objectively, the Hoover test is used to determine if the patient is a malingerer. The clinician's hands cup each heel of the supine patient while the legs remain relaxed on the examining table (**Fig. 22.29**). The patient is then asked to lift one leg off the table while keeping the knees straight, as in an active SLR test. If the patient does not lift the leg or the clinician does not feel pressure under the opposite heel, the patient may not be trying to lift the leg or may be a malingerer. Pressure under the normal heel increases, however, if the lifted limb is weaker because of the increased effort to lift the weak leg. A bilateral comparison then is made to determine any differences.

Neurological Tests

Injury to the lumbar region and spinal cord can be reflected in **hyperreflexia**, muscle weakness, loss of sensation, and ataxia. Several tests should be performed to assess lower motor neuron lesions. Lower quarter neurological screening tests the L1–S2 nerve roots. Neurological integrity can be assessed through special tests, segmental dermatomes, myotomes, reflexes, and peripheral nerve cutaneous patterns.

Cutaneous Patterns

The wide variation of dermatomal innervation and the subjectivity of the test make it less useful than motor or reflex testing. The segmental nerve dermatome patterns and peripheral nerve cutaneous patterns are demonstrated in **Figure 6.7**. Testing should be performed bilaterally.

Myotomes

Isometric muscle testing is performed in the upper and lower extremities to test specific myotomes (**Table 22.2**). These were originally discussed in Chapter 6. The ankle movements should be performed with the knee flexed approximately 30°, especially if the patient is complaining of sciatic pain, because full dorsiflexion is considered to be a provocative maneuver for stretching neurological tissue. Similarly, a fully extended knee increases the stretch on the sciatic nerve and may result in false signs, such as weakness that results from pain rather than from pressure on the nerve root.

Reflexes

Repetitive tapping of the reflexes may show a gradual decline in the reflex response not otherwise noted in a single tap. Absent or decreased reflexes are not necessarily pathological, especially in individuals who have well-developed muscles. Upper limb reflexes can be increased by having the patient perform an isometric contraction, such as squeezing the knees together during the test. In the lower extremity,

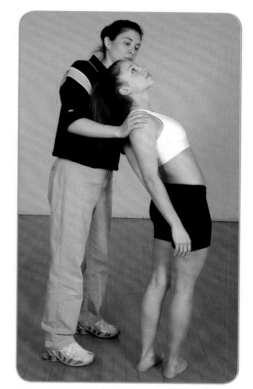

Figure 22.28. Quadrant test. The patient extends the spine while the clinician controls the movement by holding the shoulders. The clinician applies overpressure in extension while the patient laterally flexes and rotates toward the painful side. This movement is continued until symptoms are reproduced or the end of the ROM is reached.

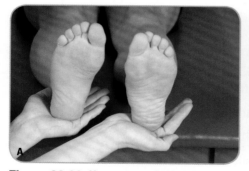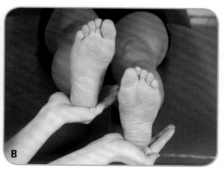

Figure 22.29. Hoover test. A, Under normal conditions, when an individual tries to elevate one leg, the action is accompanied by downward pressure on the opposite leg. **B,** When the individual attempts to elevate the "weak" leg but the opposite (asymptomatic) leg does not "help," at least some of the weakness probably is feigned.

TABLE 22.2 Myotomes Used to Test Selected Nerves

NERVE ROOT SEGMENT	ACTION TESTED
L1–L2	Hip flexion
L3	Knee extension
L4	Ankle dorsiflexion
L5	Toe extension
S1	Plantar flexion of the ankle, foot eversion, and hip extension
S2	Knee flexion

the two major reflexes are the patella (L3–L4) and Achilles tendon (S1) (**Table 22.3**). Asymmetry between sides should raise suspicion of an abnormality.

Referred Pain

Pain can be referred to the thoracic spine from various abdominal organs. **Figure 6.1** demonstrates the area that the pain is commonly referred to in the torso.

Activity-Specific Functional Testing

Before a return to play, the patient must have a normal neurological exam, with pain-free ROM and normal bilateral muscle strength, cutaneous sensation, and reflexes. If pain is present, the patient should not return to competition. Sport-specific functional tests that should be performed include walking, bending, lifting, jogging, running, figure eight running, carioca running, and sport-specific skills. All must be performed pain-free and with unlimited movement.

 In assessing the cheerleader, the special tests that are used to determine nerve root impingement may include Valsalva test, Milgram test, Hoover test, slump test, SLR test, well SLR test, bilateral SLR test, Brudzinski test, Kernig test, tension (bowstring) test, FNST, and single-leg stance test. Performing all tests may not yield more usable information than utilizing a few clinically relevant tests. When deciding which battery of tests to use, consideration should be given to the patient's age, activity level, degree of distress, dysfunction, and pain. Neurological testing for the cheerleader should include myotomes, reflexes, and dermatomes.

TABLE 22.3 Deep Tendon Reflexes in the Lower Extremity

REFLEX	SEGMENTAL LEVELS
Patellar	L2, L3, and L4
Posterior tibial	L4 and L5
Medial hamstring	L5 and S1
Lateral hamstring	S1 and S2
Achilles	S1 and S2

CONDITIONS OF THE LUMBAR SPINE

> **?** What criteria should be used to determine whether a patient who reports low back pain should be referred to a physician?

The lumbar spine must support the weight of the head, trunk, and arms as well as any load held in the hands. In addition, the two lower lumbar motion segments (i.e., L4–L5 and L5–S1) provide a large ROM in flexion–extension. As such, it is not surprising that mechanical abuse often results in episodes of low back pain or that the lower lumbar disks are injured more frequently than any others in the spine. Many patients will sustain injury that may respond positively to conservative treatment, but it is important to determine which patients need to be referred for diagnostic testing and imaging and those that do not.

Lumbar Contusions, Strains, and Sprains

Etiology

An estimated 75% to 80% of the population experiences low back pain stemming from mechanical injury to muscles, ligaments, or connective tissue. Common causes of low back pain are presented in **Box 22.3**. Although low back pain typically strikes adults, nearly 30% of children experience low back pain up to the age of 16 years.[24] Several known pathologies may cause low back pain, but reduced spinal flexibility, repeated stress, and activities that require maximal extension of the lumbar spine are most associated with chronic low back pain.

Muscle strains may result from a sudden extension action with trunk rotation on an overtaxed, unprepared, or underdeveloped spine. Chronic strains may stem from improper posture, excessive lumbar lordosis, flat back, or scoliosis.

Signs and Symptoms

Pain and discomfort can range from diffused to localized. Pain associated with lumbar contusions, strains, and sprains does not radiate into the buttocks or posterior thigh and show no signs of neural involvement, such as muscle weakness, sensory changes, or reflex inhibition. If a muscle strain is present, pain will increase when the structure is passively stretched and with active concentric contraction. Ruling in the presence of a contusion, strain, or sprain usually also involves ruling out disk or nerve involvement. Tests such as the Valsalva maneuver, the straight leg raise, single-leg stance, and quadrant test should be negative in that there is no onset of neurological symptoms, and if pain is produced, it will be localized to the facet joint, ligament, or muscle that has been injured.

Management

Acute protocol is followed to control pain and hemorrhage. In the initial treatment phase, patients with low back pain have responded well to cryotherapy, nonsteroidal anti-inflammatory drugs (NSAIDs), and muscle relaxant medication.[2] However, there is concern regarding the potential side effects of using these medications as well as the potential for violating guidelines regarding banned

---

BOX 22.3 Causes of Low Back Pain

- Muscle strains and sprains
- Spinal infections (e.g., tuberculosis)
- Sciatica
- Neoplastic tumor (i.e., primary or metastatic)
- Protruded or herniated disk

- Ankylosing spondylitis (arthritis of the spine)
- Pathological fracture
- Benign space-occupying lesions
- Disk space infections
- Abdominal aortic aneurysm

substances for athletes participating in National Collegiate Athletic Association (NCAA) sporting events.[2] Following cold treatment, superficial heat and spinal manipulation therapy have been found to be strongly supported in the literature as very effective in treating low back conditions that do not involve the disks or nerve roots.[2] Any treatment plan selected should be designed to address the cause of the pain. For example, a weak core resulting in poor posture may be the underlying cause of the patient's pain, and thus, the therapeutic exercise program should address strengthening the core and focusing on posture training.

Low Back Pain in Runners

Etiology

Many runners develop muscle tightness in the hip flexors and hamstrings. Tight hip flexors tend to produce a forward body lean, which leads to anterior pelvic tilt and hyperlordosis of the lumbar spine (see **Fig. 16.13A**). Because the lumbar muscles develop tension to counteract the forward bending moment of the entire trunk when the trunk is in flexion, these muscles are particularly susceptible to strain. Coupled with tight hamstrings, a shorter stride often emerges.

Signs and Symptoms

Symptoms include localized pain that increases with active and resisted back extension, but radiating pain and neurological deficits are not present. During postural assessment, anterior pelvic tilt and hyperlordosis of the lumbar spine also may be observed. When assessing the patient's passive ROM, limited and restricted ROM may be noted with pathological end feel found. Gait analysis may reveal a forward lean and shortened gait pattern.

Management

Treatment focuses on avoiding excessive flexion activities and a sedentary posture (**Box 22.4**). Flexion causes the mobile nucleus pulposus to shift posteriorly and press against the annulus fibrosus at its thinnest, least buttressed place. In most cases, this just leads to pain, but in others, it may lead to a herniated disk. In addition, physical activity is necessary to pump fluid through the spinal disks to keep them properly hydrated; by interfering with this process, immobility can prolong pain.

BOX 22.4 Reducing Low Back Pain in Runners

- Wear properly fitted shoes that control heel motion and provide maximum shock absorption.
- Increase flexibility at the hip, knee, ankle plantar flexors, and trunk extensors.
- Increase strength in the abdominal and trunk extensor muscles.
- Avoid excessive body weight.
- Warm up before and after running.
- Run with an upright stance rather than with a forward lean.
- Avoid excessive side-to-side sway.
- Run on even terrain and limit hill work. Avoid running on concrete.
- Avoid overstriding to increase speed because this increases leg shock.
- Gradually increase distance, intensity, and duration. Do not increase any parameter more than 10% in 1 week.
- If orthotics are worn and pain persists, check for wear and rigidity.
- Consider alternatives to running, such as cycling, rowing, or swimming.

Ice, NSAIDs, muscle relaxants, transcutaneous electrical nerve stimulation (TENS), and electrical muscle stimulation may be used to reduce pain and inflammation. Lumbar stabilization exercises can be combined with extension exercises, progressive activity, and early mobilization. Aerobic exercise, such as walking, swimming, or biking, should be included in all programs. If symptoms do not improve within a week, the patient should be referred to a physician to rule out a more serious underlying condition. In an effort to decrease the incidence of low back pain, training techniques should allow for the adequate progression of distance and intensity and should include extensive flexibility exercises for the hip and thigh region.

Myofascial Pain

Etiology

Myofascial pain is referred pain that emanates from a myofascial trigger point, which is a hypersensitive, localized nodule within a taut band of muscle tissue and its surrounding fascia. When compressed or palpated, pain is produced in a predictable distribution of referred pain. In the lumbar area, the piriformis muscle and quadratus lumborum are common trigger point sites associated with extended sitting, standing, running, and walking activities. The piriformis, in particular, can impact the sciatic nerve as it courses through, above, or below the muscle on its path into the posterior leg. Individuals who slip unexpectedly and catch themselves also can irritate the trigger points.

Signs and Symptoms

Aggravation of the piriformis can lead to referred pain in the SI area, the posterior hip, and the upper two-thirds of the posterior thigh. Aching and deep pain increases with activity or with prolonged sitting with the hip adducted, flexed, and internally rotated. If the sciatic nerve is impinged, pain and possible changes in sensation may extend into the leg. Piriformis syndrome is described at length in Chapter 16. If the patient's pain is originating from the piriformis, a trigger point may be palpable within the piriformis and the FAIR test; the piriformis muscle stretch test should be positive. The piriformis sign and pace sign may or may not be present.[21]

Referred pain from the quadratus lumborum (QL) often gives a false sign of a disk syndrome and often is overlooked as a source of low back pain. The superficial fibers can refer a sharp, aching pain to the low back, iliac crest, or greater trochanter or can extend it to the abdominal wall. The deep fibers may refer pain to the SI joint or lower buttock region. Pain increases during lateral bending toward the involved side, while standing for long periods of time, and during coughing or sneezing. To screen for myofascial pain originating from the QL, carefully observe the patient while in a prone position. The iliac crest on the involved side may appear elevated due to spasm of the QL. During palpation, assess for the presence of a trigger point. Activation of the trigger point will recreate the patient's symptoms.

Management

Trigger point treatment involves stretching the involved muscle back to its normal resting length as a way to relieve the irritation that led to the initial pain. The patient should be placed in a comfortable position on the uninvolved side if the piriformis is involved or prone if the QL is involved. Three potential techniques can be used. One technique involves the application of pressure slowly and progressively over the trigger point. Pressure is maintained until the tenderness is gone. Another technique involves ice massage applied over the length of the muscle and then over the referred pain pattern. The ice is applied in longitudinal, parallel strokes in only one direction while a passive stretch is applied progressively to the involved muscle. The third technique involves a deep-stroking massage over the length of the muscle, moving in a distal to proximal direction. As the massage continues, the taut band should relax, the tender nodules soften, and the pain decrease.

Facet Joint Pathology

Etiology

Throughout the longitudinal axis of the spine, three distinct anatomical columns can be defined at any spinal motion segment—namely, the anterior, middle, and posterior columns. The posterior

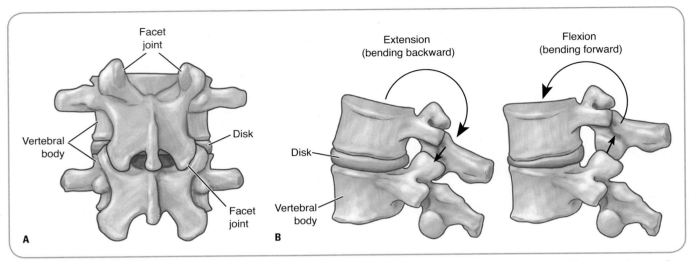

Figure 22.30. Posterior column of the spine. A, Normal facet orientation. **B,** Stress placed on facets during flexion and extension.

column contains the pars interarticularis, facet joints, and spinous processes and is supported by the ligamentum flavum and interspinous ligaments (**Fig. 22.30A**). The facet joint is a synovial joint richly innervated via the medial branch of the posterior primary rami of at least two adjacent spinal nerves. The facet joint capsules act as passive restraints against excessive lumbar rotation and flexion and serve as a protective mechanism for the intervertebral disk (**Fig. 22.30B**).

Lumbar facet pathology may involve subluxation or dislocation of the facet, but more often, the facet pain is due to facet joint syndrome (i.e., inflammation), or degeneration of the facet itself (i.e., arthritis). **Facet syndrome** is characterized by pain, soreness, and stiffness that increase with active extension and in periods of prolonged sitting. Some patients only experience pain or discomfort in the morning. The exact pathophysiology is unclear. Theories include possible mechanical irritation of the nearby nerve root, chemical irritation arising from the inflammatory process (e.g., capsular and synovial inflammation), meniscoid entrapment, synovial impingement, joint subluxation, chondromalacia facette, mechanical injury to the joint's capsule, and restriction to normal articular motion from soft or articular causes.

Signs and Symptoms

Signs and symptoms can include nonspecific low back, hip, and buttock pain with a deep and achy quality. The pain may radiate into the posterior thigh, but it does not radiate below the knee. Some patients describe their pain as being worse in the morning, aggravated by rest and hyperextension, and relieved by repeated motion. Flattening of lumbar lordosis may be visible. Point tenderness may be elicited to a unilateral or bilateral paravertebral area. Pain often is exacerbated by trunk rotation, stretching into full extension, lateral bending toward the involved side, and with torsion. Sensory alternations usually are absent unless the nerve root is secondarily involved.

Limited flexibility of the pelvic musculature can directly impact the mechanics of the lumbosacral spine. If facet joint pathology is present, an abnormal pelvic tilt and rotation of the hip secondary to tight hamstrings, hip rotators, and quadratus may be or may not be evident. Palpation may reveal increased tension of the musculature in the area of the dysfunction as well as increased tenderness. The spring test may be positive for restricted motion. Typically, resisted ROM testing is normal; however, a subtle weakness in the erector spinae and hamstring muscles may contribute to pelvic tilt abnormalities. This subtle weakness may be appreciated with trunk, pelvic, and lower extremity extension asymmetry. If facet hypertrophy narrows the neural foramen, causing nerve root impingement, an SLR test may elicit a positive response. Typically, this maneuver is normal.

Management

If facet joint syndrome is suspected, conservative treatment options should result in improved patient outcomes. The initial treatment should focus on education, relative rest, pain relief, and maintenance of positions that provide comfort, exercises, and some modalities. Therapeutic exercises should include instruction regarding proper posture and body mechanics in activities of daily living that protect the injured joints, reduce symptoms, and prevent further injury. Positions that cause pain should be avoided. Modalities such as superficial heat and cryotherapy may help to relax the muscles and reduce pain. In addition, medications such as NSAIDs can be advantageous. Spinal manipulation and mobilization also can be used to reduce pain. Once the painful symptoms are controlled during the acute phase of treatment, stretching and strengthening exercises of the lumbar spine and associated muscles can be initiated. If the patient does not respond to conservative therapies, the patient should be referred for radiographs or magnetic resonance imaging. The facet may also be injected with an anesthetic, which should result in reduction of symptoms.

Lumbar Spinal Stenosis

Etiology

Lumbar spinal stenosis (LSS) involves narrowing of the spinal canal with cord or nerve impingement resulting in symptoms of radiculopathy or pseudoclaudication. The narrowing can occur in the vertebral canal, the lateral recess, or the neuroforamina. The condition may further be subdivided into central or lateral stenosis that can occur focally or diffusely throughout several spinal levels. Stenosis may also be divided by its etiology into the following groups: degenerative, spondylolisthetic, iatrogenic (postsurgical), posttraumatic, and metabolic (Paget disease). The degenerative form is most common (**Fig. 22.31**).[25]

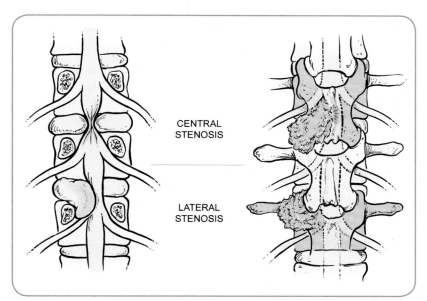

Figure 22.31. Spinal stenosis. Central stenosis (top, left, and right) usually develops at the disk level from a bulging disk with facet joint overgrowth from the inferior articular process of the lumbar vertebrae and thickening and redundancy of the ligamentum flavum. Lateral stenosis (bottom, left, and right) includes both the lateral recess and foraminal stenosis resulting from overgrowth from the superior articular process of the vertebra and other degenerative changes similar to those of central stenosis. Lateral recess stenosis affects the spinal nerve root at the disk level.

Signs and Symptoms

LSS is seen more often in older patients but should be a consideration for patients who have a long history of participating in sports that require extended periods of flexion into extension movements, such as football linemen. Symptoms gradually appear and worsen over time. Typical symptoms of LSS are leg pain, with or without back pain, which is aggravated by walking. Other symptoms include one or a combination of the following: pain and/or numbness in the lower extremities, and neurogenic claudication (pain and numbness with walking), which occurs secondary to narrowing of the spinal canal, nerve root canal, or intervertebral foramina.[26] The patient may describe a relief of symptoms when sitting or leaning forward. Standing and extension may increase severity of symptoms. Because symptoms extend into the leg when walking and are aggravated by walking, peripheral vascular disease should be considered as a differential diagnosis for LSS. Whereas symptoms associated with LSS will decrease when seated or with forward leaning, pain originating from peripheral vascular disease dissipates only when the patient stops activity.[26] Physical examination alone does not yield a conclusive lumbar stenosis diagnosis. Therefore, if LSS is suspected, the patient should be referred for a conclusive diagnosis using imaging studies from a magnetic resonance imaging scan or a computed tomographic scan with myelogram (using an X-ray dye in the spinal sack fluid).

Management

To date, there is a dearth of evidence-based research on the most effective treatment of LSS. Individuals with mild symptoms respond well to conservative treatment, which may involve analgesics, therapeutic exercise, treadmill walking, ultrasound, or epidural steroid injections. Surgical treatment is suggested in patients with severe symptoms of LSS.

Sciatica

Etiology

Sciatica, an inflammatory condition of the sciatic nerve, is classified in terms of four levels of severity, each with its own management strategy (**Box 22.5**). The condition can be caused by a herniated disk, annular tear, myogenic or muscle-related disease, spinal stenosis, facet joint arthropathy, or compression of the nerve between the piriformis muscle.

 See **Signs and Symptoms of Sciatica**, available on the companion Web site at thePoint, for the common signs and symptoms that accompany the various etiologies of sciatica.

Signs and Symptoms

If related to a herniated disk, radiating leg pain is greater than back pain and increases with sitting and leaning forward, coughing, sneezing, and straining. Pain is reproduced during an ipsilateral SLR test (see **Fig. 22.18**).

In an annular tear, back pain is more prevalent and is exacerbated with SLR. Morning pain and muscular stiffness that worsens if chilled or when the weather changes (arthritic-like symptoms) are characteristic of myogenic or muscle-related disease. Pain typically radiates into the buttock and thigh region.

BOX 22.5 Classification and Management of Sciatica

- **Sciatica only:** No sensory or muscle weakness. Modify activity appropriately and develop rehabilitation and prevention program. Any increased pain requires immediate reevaluation.

- **Sciatica with soft signs:** Some sensory changes, mild or no reflex change, normal muscle strength, and normal bowel and bladder function. Remove from sport participation for 6–12 weeks.

- **Sciatica with hard signs:** Sensory and reflex changes, and muscle weakness caused by repeated, chronic, or acute condition. Normal bowel and bladder function. Remove from participation for 12–24 weeks.

- **Sciatica with severe signs:** Sensory and reflex changes, muscle weakness, and altered bladder function. Consider immediate surgical decompression.

If LSS is present, back and leg pain develop after the patient walks a limited distance and concomitantly increase as the distance increases. Pain is not reproduced with an SLR test, but it can be reproduced with prolonged spine extension, which is relieved with spine flexion. If a facet joint is involved, pain is localized over the joint on spinal extension and is exacerbated with ipsilateral lateral flexion. If the sciatic nerve is compressed by the piriformis muscle, pain increases during internal rotation of the thigh.

Management

Referral to a physician is necessary to check for a potentially serious underlying condition. Under normal circumstances, bed rest usually is not indicated, although side lying with the knees flexed may relieve symptoms. Lifting, bending, twisting, and prolonged sitting and standing aggravate the condition and, therefore, should be avoided. When asymptomatic, abdominal and extensor muscle strengthening exercises can begin, with a gradual return to activity. If symptoms resume, however, activity should cease, and the patient should be referred back to the physician. Occasionally, extended rest is needed for symptoms to resolve totally, and if a significant disk protrusion is present, surgery may be indicated.

Conditions of the Lumbar Disk

Etiology

Prolonged mechanical loading of the spine can lead to microruptures in the annulus fibrosus, resulting in degeneration of the disk (**Fig. 22.32**). Bulging or protruded disks refer to some eccentric accumulation of the nucleus with slight deformity of the annulus. When the eccentric nucleus produces a definite deformity as it works its way through the fibers of the annulus, it is called a **prolapsed disk**. It is called an **extruded disk** when the material moves into the spinal canal, where it runs the risk of impinging on adjacent nerve roots. Finally, with a **sequestrated disk**, the nuclear material has separated from the disk itself and, potentially, can migrate. The most commonly herniated disks are the lower two lumbar disks at L4–L5 and L5–S1, followed by the two lower cervical disks. Most ruptures move in a posterior or posterolateral direction as a result of torsion and compression, not just compression.

Signs and Symptoms

Because the intervertebral disks are not innervated, the sensation of pain does not occur until the surrounding soft-tissue structures are impinged. When compression is placed on a spinal nerve of the sciatic nerve complex (L4–S3), sensory and motor deficits are reflected in the myotome and dermatome patterns associated with the nerve root (**Fig. 22.33**). In addition, an alteration in tendon reflexes is apparent. A disk need not be completely herniated to give symptoms, which include sharp pain and muscle spasms at the site of herniation that often shoot down the sciatic nerve into the lower extremity. The patient may walk in a slightly crouched position, leaning away from the side of the lesion. Forward trunk flexion may exacerbate symptoms while active extension relieves symptoms. The Valsalva maneuver, the straight leg rise test (see **Fig. 22.18**), bowstring test (see **Fig. 22.19**), and the Brudzinski/Kernig (see **Fig. 22.20**) may exacerbate pain and increase distal symptoms. Significant signs indicating the need for

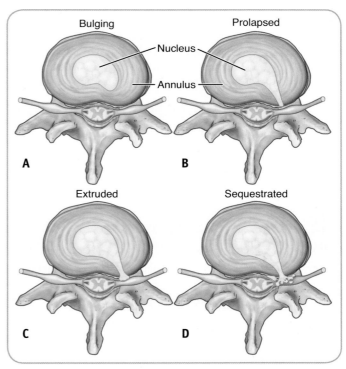

Figure 22.32. Herniated disks. Herniated disks are categorized by severity as an eccentrically loaded nucleus progressively moves from **(A)** protruded, **(B)** prolapsed, and **(C)** extruded, culminating in **(D)** sequestrated when the nuclear material moves into the canal to impinge on the adjacent spinal nerves.

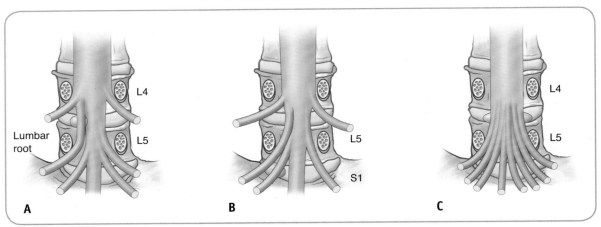

Figure 22.33. Possible effects on the spinal cord and spinal nerves according to the level of herniation.
A, Herniation between L4 and L5 compresses the L5 nerve root. **B,** Herniation between L5 and S1 can compress the nerve root crossing the disk (S1) and the nerve root emerging through the intervertebral foramina (L5).
C, A posterior herniation at the L4–L5 level can compress the dura mater of the entire cauda equina, leading to bowel and bladder paralysis.

immediate referral to a physician include muscle weakness, sensory changes, diminished reflexes in the lower extremity, and abnormal bladder or bowel function. **Table 22.4** outlines physical findings associated with disk herniation in the low back region.

Management

In mild cases, treatment consists of minimizing load on the spine by avoiding activities that involve impact, lifting, bending, twisting, and prolonged sitting and standing. Painful muscle spasms can be eliminated with ice and/or heat, the administration of prescribed NSAIDs and/or muscle relaxants, ultrasound, TENS, passive exercise, and gentle stretching. Following the resolution of spasms and acute pain, rehabilitation should include spine and hamstring flexibility, spinal strength and stabilization exercises, and functional stabilization control in sports and daily activities.

Lumbar Fractures and Dislocations

Etiology

Transverse or spinous process fractures are caused by extreme tension from the attached muscles or from a direct blow to the low back during participation in contact sports, such as football, rugby,

TABLE 22.4 Physical Findings Associated with a Herniated Disk			
SIGNS AND SYMPTOMS	**L3–L4 (L4 ROOT)**	**L4–L5 (L5 ROOT)**	**L5–S1 (S1 ROOT)**
Pain	Lumbar region and buttocks	Lumbar region, groin, and SI area	Lumbar region, groin, and SI area
Dermatome and sensory loss	Anterior midthigh over patella and medial lower leg to great toe	Lateral thigh, anterior leg, top of foot, and middle three toes	Posterior lateral thigh and lower leg to lateral foot and fifth toe
Myotome weakness	Ankle dorsiflexion	Toe extension (extensor hallux)	Ankle plantar flexion (gastrocnemius)
Reduced deep tendon reflex	Quadriceps	Medial hamstrings	Achilles tendon
SLR test	Normal	Reduced	Reduced

soccer, basketball, hockey, and lacrosse. These fractures often lead to an additional injury of the surrounding soft tissues but are not as serious as compression fractures. Compression fractures more commonly involve the L1 vertebra at the thoracolumbar junction.

Hyperflexion, or jack-knifing of the trunk, crushes the anterior aspect of the vertebral body. The primary danger with this injury is the possibility of bony fragments moving into the spinal canal and damaging the spinal cord or spinal nerves. Because of the facet joint orientation in the lumbar region, dislocations occur only when a fracture is present. Fracture dislocations resulting from sports participation are rare.

Signs and Symptoms

Symptoms include localized, palpable pain that may radiate down the nerve root if a bony fragment compresses a spinal nerve. Because the spinal cord ends at approximately the L1 or L2 level, fractures of the lumbar vertebrae below this point do not pose a serious threat but, rather, should be handled with care to minimize potential nerve damage to the cauda equina. Confirmation of a possible fracture is made with a radiograph or CT scan.

Management

Conservative treatment consists of initial bed rest, cryotherapy, and minimizing mechanical loads on the low back until symptoms subside, which may take 3 to 6 weeks.

Pars Interarticularis Fractures

The pars interarticularis is the weakest bony portion of the vertebral neural arch, the region between the superior and inferior articular facets. Fractures in this region are termed spondylolysis and spondylolisthesis (**Fig. 22.34**). Although some pars defects may be congenital, they also may be caused by mechanical stress from axial loading of the lumbar spine during repeated weight loading in flexion, hyperextension (i.e., back arching), and rotation. These repetitive movements cause a shearing stress to the vertebrae, resulting in a stress fracture.

Fractures of the pars interarticularis may range from hairline to complete separation of the bone. A bony defect in spondylolysis tends to occur at an earlier age, typically before 8 years of age, yet often does not produce symptoms until 10 to 15 years of age. The fracture may heal with less periosteal callus and tends to form a fibrous union more often than fractures at other sites.

A bilateral separation in the pars interarticularis, called **spondylolisthesis**, results in the anterior displacement of a vertebra with respect to the vertebra below it (**Fig. 22.35**). The most common site for this injury is the lumbosacral joint (L5 through S1), with 90% of the slips occurring at this level. Spondylolisthesis often is diagnosed in children between the ages of 10 and 15 years and is more common in boys than in girls. High-degree slips, however, are seen more commonly in females than in males.[27] Unlike most stress fractures, spondylolysis and spondylolisthesis do not typically heal with time but, rather, tend to persist, particularly in cases with no interruption in participation in sport and physical activity. Those who are particularly susceptible to this condition include female gymnasts, interior football linemen, weight lifters, volleyball players, pole vaulters, wrestlers, and rowers.

Although most spondylitic conditions are asymptomatic, low back pain and associated neurological symptoms are likely to occur when the underlying cause is repeated mechanical stress. The patient may complain

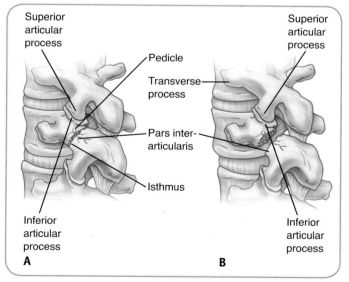

Figure 22.34. Spondylolysis and spondylolisthesis.
A, Spondylolysis is a stress fracture of the pars interarticularis.
B, Spondylolisthesis is a bilateral fracture of the pars interarticularis accompanied by anterior slippage of the involved vertebra.

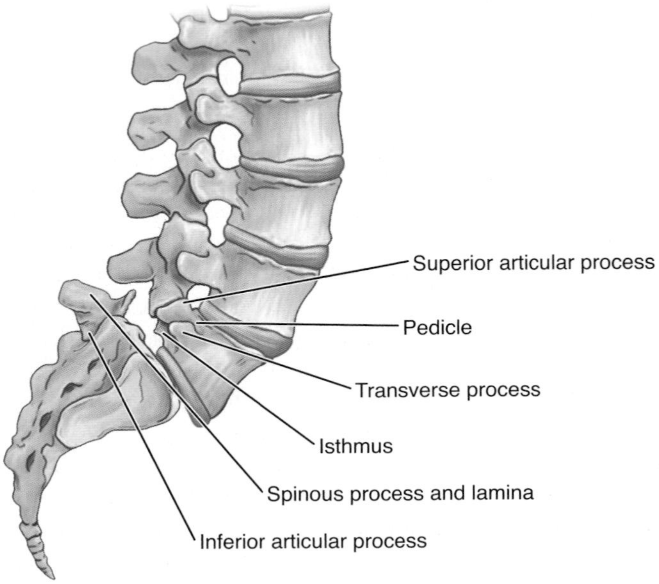

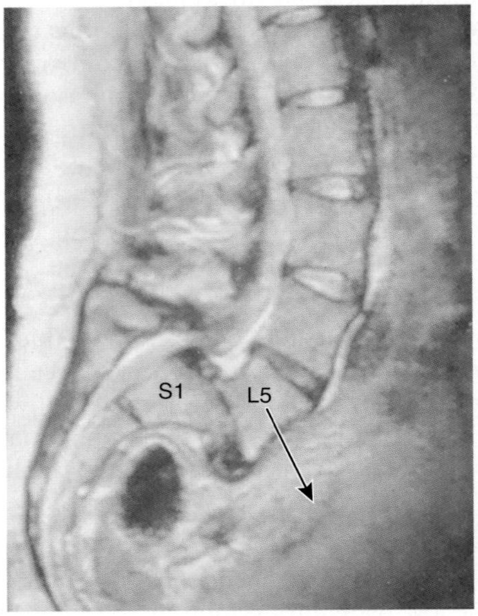

Figure 22.35. Spondylolisthesis. This magnetic resonance imaging scan of spondylolisthesis demonstrates an anterior shift of the L5 vertebra.

of unilateral, dull backache aggravated by activity, usually hyperextension and rotation. Standing on one leg and hyperextending the back aggravates the condition. Demonstrable muscle spasm occurs in the erector spinae muscles or hamstrings, leading to flattening of the lumbosacral curve, but no sciatic nerve symptoms usually are present. Pain may radiate into the buttock region or down the sciatic nerve if the L5 nerve root is compressed. This patient should be referred to a physician.

Slippage is measured by dividing the distance the superior vertebral body has displaced forward onto the inferior by the anteroposterior dimensions of the inferior vertebral body. In mild cases (i.e., slippage of 0% to 25%), modifications in training and technique can permit the patient to continue to participate in physical activity. In moderate cases (i.e., slippage from 25% to 50%), however, most physicians do not begin active rehabilitation until the patient has been asymptomatic for 4 weeks. Following that period, the focus of rehabilitation is the development of flexibility in the hamstrings and gluteal muscles, combined with strengthening the abdomen and back extensors. If the slip is greater than 50%, the patient presents with flat buttocks, tight hamstrings, and alterations in gait and a palpable step-off deformity may be present at the level of the defect. This patient should be excluded from participation in contact sports unless the condition is asymptomatic and absence of continued slippage has been documented.

If a fracture or dislocation is suspected, the emergency plan, including summoning EMS for transport to the nearest medical facility, should be activated.

If assessment of a low back injury reveals signs of nerve root involvement (i.e., sensory or motor deficits and diminished reflexes) or disk injury, physician referral is warranted.

SACRUM AND COCCYX CONDITIONS

? A 40-year-old man initiated a training program to improve his cardiovascular fitness. His workout for the past month has consisted of running on a treadmill. Over the past week, he began to develop pain in the sacral region during his workout. The pain has now become so persistent and chronic that it hurts to sit for an extended period of time. What injury may be present, and what recommendations can be made to this person relative to caring for the injury?

Because the sacrum and coccyx are essentially immobile, the potential for mechanical injury to these regions is dramatically reduced. In many cases, injuries result from direct blows and stress on the SI joint.

Sacroiliac Joint Sprain

Etiology

Sprains of the SI joint may result from a single traumatic episode that involves bending and/or twisting, repetitive stress from lifting, a fall on the buttocks, excessive side-to-side or up-and-down motion during running and jogging, running on uneven terrain, suddenly slipping or stumbling forward, or wearing new shoes or orthoses. The injury may irritate or stretch the sacrotuberous or sacrospinous ligament, or it may lead to an anterior or posterior rotation of one side of the pelvis relative to the other. Hypermobility results from rotation of the pelvis. During healing, the joint on the injured side may become hypermobile, allowing the joint to subluxate in either an anterior- or posterior-rotated position.

Signs and Symptoms

Symptoms may involve unilateral, dull pain in the sacral area that extends into the buttocks and posterior thigh. On observation, the ASIS or PSIS may appear to be asymmetrical when compared bilaterally. A leg length discrepancy may be present, but muscle spasm is not often seen. Standing on one leg and climbing stairs may increase the pain. Forward bending reveals a block to normal movement, with the PSIS on the injured side moving sooner than on the uninjured side. Lateral flexion toward the injured side increases pain, as do straight leg raises beyond 45°.

Management

Treatment for SI sprains includes cryotherapy, prescribed NSAIDs, and gentle stretching to alleviate stiffness. As the conditions improves, flexibility, pelvic stabilization exercises, mobilization of the affected joint, and strengthening exercises for the low back should be initiated.

Coccygeal Conditions

Etiology

Direct blows to the region can produce contusions and fractures of the coccyx.

Signs and Symptoms

Pain resulting from a fracture may last for several months. Prolonged or chronic pain in the region also may result from irritation of the coccygeal nerve plexus. This condition is termed coccygodynia.

Management

Treatment for coccygeal pain includes analgesics, use of padding for protection, and a ring seat to alleviate compression during sitting.

 This patient has probably irritated the SI joint from repeated stress while running on the treadmill. This patient should ice the region to control inflammation and pain and should stretch the low back and buttock region. A detailed assessment (including a gait analysis while running) should be performed to determine the potential cause of the injury so that a proper rehabilitation program and, subsequently, an appropriate cardiovascular conditioning regimen can be developed.

REHABILITATION

? The findings from the special tests and neurological testing revealed increased pain in the right lumbar region on resisted trunk extension, lateral flexion, and rotation to the right; diminished quadriceps reflex on the right side; muscle weakness apparent with knee extension and ankle dorsiflexion; and pain elicited down the right leg during an SLR test. These signs and symptoms suggest the possibility of sciatica resulting from an extruded disk at the L4 level.

The cheerleader was seen by a physician who prescribed NSAIDs, muscle relaxants, and rest until the symptoms subside. When the patient begins rehabilitation, what exercises should be included in the general program?

Rehabilitation programs must be developed on a patient basis and address the specific needs of the patient. Exercises to relieve pain related to postural problems may not address sciatic pain. Therefore, a variety of exercises are listed in this section to allow selection of those that are appropriate for the patient. The program should relieve pain and muscle tension; restore motion and balance; develop strength, endurance, and power; and maintain cardiovascular fitness. Patient education also is critical in teaching the skills and techniques that are needed to prevent recurrence.

Relief of Pain and Muscle Tension

Maintaining a prolonged posture can lead to discomfort. This can be avoided by doing active ROM exercises to relieve stress on supporting structures, to promote circulation, and to maintain flexibility. For example, in the lower thoracic and lumbar region, exercises such as back extension, side bending in each direction, spinal flexion (avoiding hip flexion), trunk rotation, and walking a short distance may relieve discomfort in the lumbar region. With nerve root compression injuries, however, extension exercises may increase discomfort and may be contraindicated. In some cases, conscious relaxation training can relax a patient who generally is tense or release tension in specific muscle groups. In addition, grade I and II mobilization exercises can be initiated early in the program to relieve pain and stretch tight structures to restore accessory movements to the joints.

Restoration of Motion

Once pain and muscle guarding are relieved, grade III and IV mobilization exercises can begin. In addition to mobilization exercises, flexibility and ROM exercises also can be initiated. Flexion exercises stretch the lumbar fascia and back extensors, open the intervertebral foramen and facet joints to reduce nerve compression, relieve tension on lumbar vertebrae caused by tight hip flexors, and increase intra-abdominal pressure by strengthening the abdominals. Examples of flexion exercises (**Application Strategy 22.1**) include the single- and double-knee to the chest stretches, hamstring stretch, hip flexor stretch, lateral rotator stretch, crunch curl-ups, and diagonal crunch curl-ups. Exercises to stretch the upper thoracic and pectoral region; trunk rotators and lateral flexors; and hip adductors, abductors, extensors, and medial and lateral rotators also should be added to improve flexibility. Other exercises include bringing both knees to the chest and gently rocking back and forth in a cranial/caudal direction and, in a standing position, shifting the hips from one side to another; lateral trunk flexion; and rotation exercises. Flexion-based exercises should be avoided if hypermobility or instability is suspected or if the maneuvers increase low back pain.

Extension exercises improve spinal mobility, reduce load on the intervertebral disks, strengthen the back extensors, and allow self-mobilization of the motion segments. Back extension exercises described in **Application Strategy 22.1** include prone extension exercises, beginning with raising to the elbows and then to the hands, the alternate arm and leg lift, double-arm and leg lift, and alternate arm and leg extension on all fours. Other extension exercises may include prone single-leg hip extension and double-leg hip extension while holding onto a table, beginning with the knee or knees flexed and then with the knee or knees extended.

Pelvic and abdominal stabilizing exercises are used to teach a patient to place the hip in a neutral position to maintain the spine in the most comfortable position and control the forces that are exerted during repetitive microtrauma. During each exercise, the patient concentrates on maintaining the hip in a neutral position by contracting and relaxing the abdominal muscles. During functional activities, the patient can initiate stabilization contractions before starting any movement. This presets the posture and can reduce stress on the back. Many of these exercises are demonstrated in **Application Strategy 22.2**. Pelvic tilt maneuvers can help to reduce the degree of lumbar lordosis and, initially, can be performed with bent-knees standing, straight leg standing, and sitting.

Restoration of Proprioception and Balance

Proprioception and balance are regained through lower extremity closed chain exercises. For example, squats, leg presses, lunges, or exercises on a StairMaster, Pro Fitter, or slide board can restore proprioception and balance in the hip and lower extremity. Stabilization exercises on all fours and

APPLICATION STRATEGY 22.1

Flexibility and Strength Exercises for the Lumbar Region

Flexibility Exercises

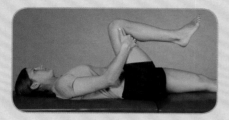

1. **SI angle knee-to-chest stretch.** In a supine position, pull one knee toward the chest with the hands. Keep the back flat. Switch to the opposite leg and repeat.

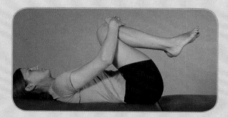

2. **Double-knee-to-chest stretch.** In a supine position, pull both knees to the chest with the hands. Keep the back flat.

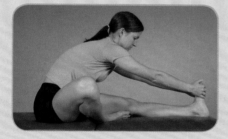

3. **Hamstring stretch, seated position.** Place the leg to be stretched straight out, with the opposite foot tucked toward the groin. Reach toward the toes until a stretch is felt.

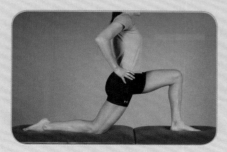

4. **Hip flexor stretch (lunge).** Extend the leg to be stretched behind you. Place the contralateral leg in front of you. While keeping the back straight, shift your body weight forward.

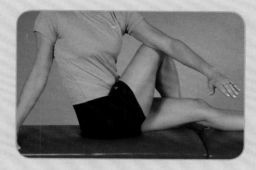

5. **Lateral rotator stretch, seated position.** Cross one leg over the thigh and place the elbow on the outside of the knee. Gently stretch the buttock muscles by pushing the bent knee across the body while keeping the pelvis on the floor.

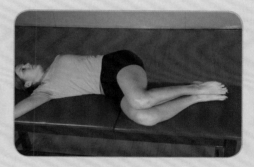

6. **Lower trunk rotation stretch.** In a supine position, rotate the flexed knees to one side, keeping the back flat and the feet together.

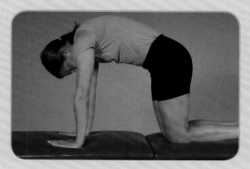

7. **Angry cat stretch (posterior pelvic tilt).** Kneel on all fours, with the knees hip-width apart. Tighten the buttocks and arch the back upward while lowering the chin and tilting the pelvis backward. Relax the buttocks and allow the pelvis to drop downward and forward.

(continued)

Strengthening Exercises

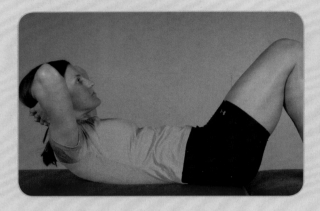

1. **Crunch curl-up.** In a supine position with the knees flexed, flatten the back, and curl up to elevate the head and shoulders from the floor. Alternate exercises include diagonal crunch curl-ups and hip crunches.

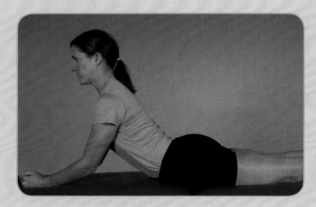

2. **Prone extension.** In a prone position, rise up on the elbows. Progress to rising up onto the hands.

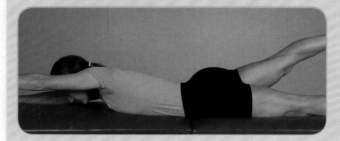

3. **Alternate arm and leg lift.** In a fully extended prone position, lift one arm and the opposite leg off the surface at least 3 in. Repeat with the opposite arm and leg.

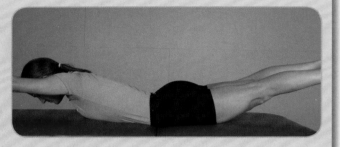

4. **Double-arm and leg lift.** In a fully extended prone position, lift both arms and legs off the surface at least 3 in. Hold and return to starting position.

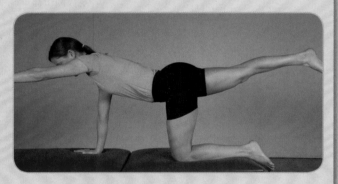

5. **Alternate arm and leg extension on all fours.** Kneel on all fours; raise one leg behind the body while raising the opposite arm in front of the body. Ankle and wrist weights may be added for additional resistance.

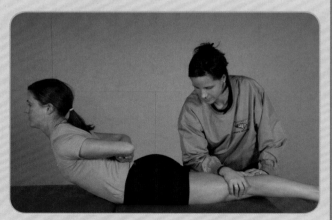

6. **Back extension.** Use a back extension machine or have another individual stabilize the feet and legs. Raise the trunk into a slightly hyperextended position.

Pelvic Stabilization and Abdominal Strengthening Exercises

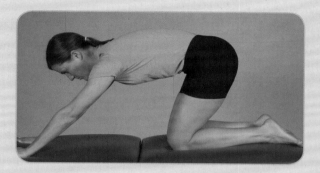

1. **Stabilization in a neutral position.** With the back in a neutral position, slowly shift forward over the arms, adjusting pelvic position as you move. A tendency exists to "sag" the back; therefore, progressively tighten and relax the abdominal muscles during forward movement and backward movement, respectively.

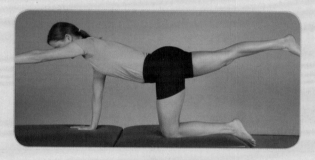

2. **Stabilization in "two-point" position.** Balance on the right leg and left arm. Slowly move forward and back without losing a neutral position. Switch to the opposite arm and leg.

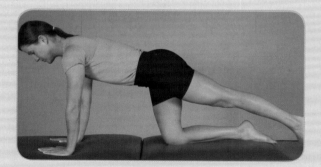

3. **Leg exercise.** Without arching the back, lift one leg out behind you. Do not lift the foot more than a few inches from the floor. A variation is to move a flexed knee sideways, away from the body and then back to the original position.

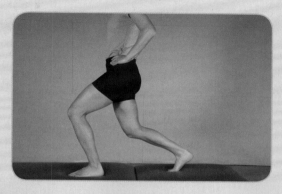

4. **Half-knee to stand (lunges).** Move to a standing position while maintaining a neutral hip position. Push evenly with both legs. Repeat several times and then switch the forward leg.

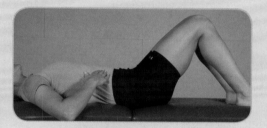

5. **Pelvic tilt.** With the hips and knees bent and the feet on the floor, do an isometric contraction of the abdominal muscles (posterior pelvic tilt) and hold. Using the phrase "tuck the stomach in" may convey the correct motion. Then, arch the back by doing an anterior pelvic tilt. Alternate between the two motions until the individual can control pelvic motion.

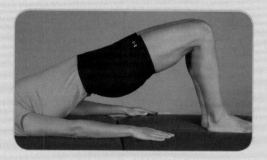

6. **Bridging.** Keeping the back in a neutral position, raise the hips and back off the floor (contract the abdominal muscles to hold the position). Hold for 5–10 seconds, drop down, and relax. Repeat. Variations include adding pelvic tilt exercises, lifting one leg off the floor (keeping the back in neutral position), and combining pelvic tilts and one-leg lift with bridging.

use of surgical tubing through functional patterns also can restore proprioception and balance. These exercises should be performed in front of a mirror or videotaped, if possible, so that the patient can observe proper posture and mechanics. In addition, constant verbal reinforcement from the supervising clinician can maximize feedback.

Muscular Strength, Endurance, and Power

Abdominal strengthening exercises, such as those described in **Application Strategy 22.2**, should begin with pelvic tilts and progress to crunch curl-ups and diagonal crunch curl-ups to reduce functional lordosis. Progressive prone extension exercises and resisted back extension exercises can increase strength in the erector spinae.

Cardiovascular Fitness

Aquatic exercises are very beneficial, because buoyancy can relieve the load on sensitive structures. Deep water allows the patient to exercise all muscle groups through a full ROM without the pain associated with gravity. Performing sport-specific skills against water resistance can apply an equal and uniform force to the muscles, similar to that in isokinetic strengthening. With low back pain, an upper body ergometer, stationary bicycle, StairMaster, or slide board may be incorporated as tolerated. Jogging can begin after all symptoms have subsided.

 As acute symptoms subside, pain and muscle tension should be relieved. The following exercises should be included in the rehabilitation program for the cheerleader: stretching of the piriformis, gluteals, and hamstrings, which should be combined with extension exercises to strengthen the back extensors; stretching of the abdominals; and a reduction of pressure on the intervertebral disks; and stabilization exercises, including abdominal strengthening, and strengthening of the medial rotators of the hip through proprioceptive neuromuscular facilitation and Thera-Band exercises. As strength is regained, functional activities can be incorporated, with a gradual return to full activity.

SUMMARY

1. Anatomical variations in the low back region that can predispose a patient to spinal injuries include lordosis, sway back, flat back, and pars interarticularis fractures, which can lead to spondylolysis or spondylolisthesis.

2. Runners are particularly prone to low back pain resulting from tight hip flexors and hamstrings. Symptoms include localized pain that increases with active and resisted back extension, but radiating pain and neurological deficits are not present. Anterior pelvic tilt and hyperlordosis of the lumbar spine also may be present.

3. Sciatica may be caused by a herniated disk, annular tear, myogenic or muscle-related disease, spinal stenosis, facet joint arthropathy, or compression of the nerve between the piriformis muscle.

4. The most commonly herniated disks are the lower two lumbar disks at L4–L5 and L5–S1, followed by the two lower cervical disks. Most ruptures move in a posterior or posterolateral direction as a result of torsion and compression.

5. The assessment of a spinal injury should begin with a thorough history of the injury and should include neurological tests to determine possible nerve involvement. The severity of pain and the presence or absence of neurological symptoms, spasms, and tenderness can indicate when a backboard and stabilization are needed.

6. If, at any time, a patient complains of acute pain in the spine, mentions a change in sensation anywhere on the body, a careful and thorough examination should be conducted prior to moving the patient to determine if activation of EMS is warranted.

7. A rehabilitation program should focus on reducing pain and spasms; restoring motion and balance; developing strength, endurance, and power; and maintaining cardiovascular fitness.

APPLICATION QUESTIONS

1. A 21-year-old cross-country runner reports to the athletic training room with low back pain. What questions should be asked concerning the runner's training and conditioning regimen?

2. A 24-year-old female high jumper is complaining of pain in the low back and SI region that is aggravated by flexion and hyperextension of the trunk during jumping. What questions should be asked to develop a thorough medical history of this individual?

3. A 21-year-old track and field athlete reported to the athletic training room complaining of low back pain. He is a shot put thrower and says that the twisting motion of the throw causes pain in his low back that is sharp and shooting. How would you differentiate between an SI joint sprain and sciatica? What other possible conditions must be considered?

4. A 15-year-old female gymnast reported to the clinic complaining of low back pain. The pain has increased over the past 2 weeks, particularly during activities involving lumbar hyperextension. Based on the history, inspection, and palpation components of an assessment, you suspect spondylosis. What findings from the testing component of an assessment would confirm your suspicion?

5. A 30-year-old male recreational basketball player reports to the orthopedic clinic complaining of low back pain. Your assessment suggests facet joint pathology. How should this condition be managed?

6. A 45-year-old professional golfer is complaining of low back pain. Your assessment suggests a herniated disk. How would you differentiate between involvement of the L3–L4 (L4) root and the L4–L5 (L5) root?

7. A distance runner complains of pain when sitting for long periods of time, which increases when leaning forward. Pain is also present when running up hills and when running on concrete. The pain has started to radiate into the posterior leg. What indicators would suggests that this patient needs to be referred to a physician for follow-up care?

8. In using some of the equipment in the weight room, the athletes are expected to move weight plates from the floor and place them on machines. What instructions would you provide to the athletes to reduce the incidence of low back injury while moving the weight plates?

9. An 18-year-old male lacrosse player has chronic low back pain. What flexibility exercises would you recommend to decrease the pain?

REFERENCES

1. National Institute of Neurological Disorders and Stroke. *Back Pain Fact Sheet*. Bethesda, MD: Office of Communications and Public Liaison, National Institute of Neurological Disorders and Stroke, National Institutes of Health. NIH publication 15-5161. http://www.ninds.nih.gov/disorders/backpain/detail_backpain.pdf. Published August 3, 2015. Accessed October 25, 2015.

2. Petering RC, Webb C. Treatment options for low back pain in athletes. *Sports Health*. 2011; 3(6):550–555.

3. Bono CM. Low-back pain in athletes. *J Bone Joint Surg Am*. 2004;86(2):382–396.

4. Anderson MW. Lumbar discography: an update. *Semin Roentgenol*. 2004;39(1):52–67.

5. Bible JE, Biswas D, Miller CP, et al. Normal functional range of motion of the lumbar spine during 15 activities of daily living. *J Spinal Disord Tech*. 2010;23(2):106–112.

6. Li G, Wang S, Passias P, et al. Segmental in vivo vertebral motion during functional human lumbar spine activities. *Eur Spine J*. 2009;18(7):1013–1021.

7. Tallarico RA, Madom IA, Palumbo MA. Spondylolysis and spondylolisthesis in the athlete. *Sports Med Arthrosc*. 2008;16(1):32–38.

8. Cholewicki J, Juluru K, McGill SM. Intra-abdominal pressure mechanism for stabilizing the lumbar spine. *J Biomech*. 1999;32(1):13–17.

9. Grondin DE, Potvin JR. Effects of trunk muscle fatigue and load timing on spinal responses during sudden hand loading. *J Electromyogr Kinesiol*. 2009;19(4):e237–e245.

10. Holtermann A, Clausen T, Aust B, et al. Risk for low back pain from different frequencies, load mass and trunk postures of lifting and carrying among female healthcare workers. *Int Arch Occup Environ Health*. 2013;86(4):463–470.

11. Hoozemans MJ, Kingma I, de Vries WH, et al. Effect of lifting height and load mass on low back loading. *Ergonomics*. 2008;51(7):1053–1063.

12. Marras WS, Knapik GG, Ferguson S. Loading along the lumbar spine as influence by speed, control, load magnitude, and handle height during pushing. *Clin Biomech (Bristol, Avon)*. 2009;24(2):155–163.

13. Magee DJ. *Orthopedic Physical Assessment*. 6th ed. Philadelphia, PA: WB Saunders; 2014.

14. Norkin CC, White DJ. *Measurement of Joint Motion: A Guide to Goniometry*. 4th ed. Philadelphia, PA: FA Davis; 2009.

15. American Medical Association. *Guides to the Evaluation of Permanent Impairment*. 6th ed. Chicago, IL: American Medical Association; 2009.

16. MacDermid JC, Arumugam V, Vincent JI, et al. Reliability of three landmarking methods for dual inclinometry measurements of lumbar flexion and extension. *BMC Musculoskelet Disord*. 2015;16:121.

17. Starkey C, Brown SD. *Orthopedic and Athletic Injury Examination Handbook*. Philadelphia, PA: FA Davis; 2015.

18. Wong M. *Pocket Orthopaedics: Evidence-Based Survival Guide*. Sudbury, MA: Jones & Bartlett; 2010.

19. Capra F, Vanti C, Donati R, et al. Validity of the straight-leg raise test for patients with sciatic pain with or without lumbar pain using magnetic resonance imaging results as a reference standard. *J Manipulative Physiol Ther*. 2011; 34(4):231–238.

20. Scaia V, Baxter D, Cook C. The pain provocation-based straight leg raise test for diagnosis of lumbar disc herniation, lumbar radiculopathy, and/or sciatica: a systematic review of clinical utility. *J Back Musculoskelet Rehabil*. 2012;25(4):215–223.

21. Boyajian-O'Neill LA, McClain RL, Coleman MK, et al. Diagnosis and management of piriformis syndrome: an osteopathic approach. *J Am Osteopath Assoc*. 2008;108(11):657–664.

22. Fishman LM, Dombi GW, Michaelsen C, et al. Piriformis syndrome: diagnosis, treatment, and outcome—a 10-year study. *Arch Phys Med Rehabil*. 2002;83(3):295–301.

23. Suri P, Rainville J, Katz JN, et al. The accuracy of the physical examination for the diagnosis of midlumbar and low lumbar nerve root impingement. *Spine (Phila Pa 1976)*. 2011;36(1):63–73.

24. Duggleby T, Kumar S. Epidemiology of juvenile low back pain: a review. *Disabil Rehabil*. 1997; 19(12):505–512.

25. Englund J. Lumbar spinal stenosis. *Curr Sports Med Rep*. 2007;6(1):50–55.

26. Goren A, Yildiz N, Topuz O, et al. Efficacy of exercise and ultrasound in patients with lumbar spinal stenosis: a prospective randomized controlled trial. *Clin Rehabil*. 2010;24(7):623–631.

27. Kalichman L, Kim DH, Li L, et al. Spondylolysis and spondylolisthesis: prevalence and association with low back pain in the adult community-based population. *Spine (Phila Pa 1976)*. 2009;34(2):199–205.

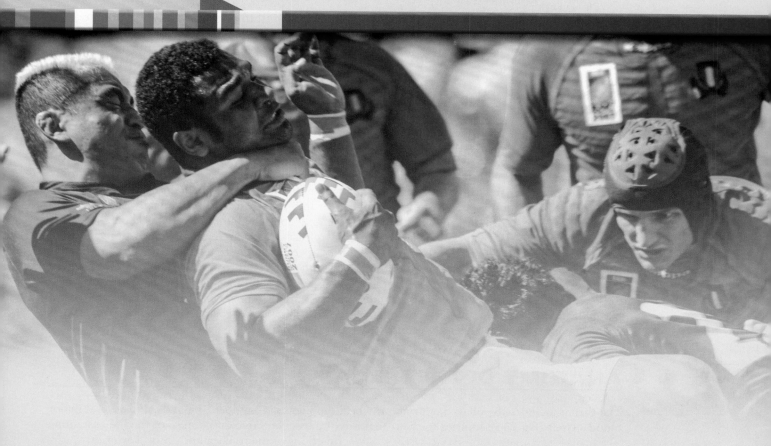

STUDENT OUTCOMES

1. Identify the important bony and soft-tissue structures of the throat, thorax, and viscera.

2. List the primary and accessory organs in the female and male reproductive systems.

3. Identify the primary organs located in each quadrant of the abdominopelvic region.

4. Explain the effects of hormones on the human body.

5. Describe measures to prevent injuries to the throat, thorax, and viscera.

6. Describe the assessment of the throat, thorax, and visceral regions.

7. Analyze and interpret urinalyses findings.

8. Describe the signs and symptoms of superficial injuries of the throat, chest wall, and abdominal wall and explain the management of these injuries.

9. Describe internal complications of the thoracic area, occurring spontaneously or as a result of direct trauma, that can lead to a life-threatening situation.

10. Describe the signs and symptoms of sternal and rib fractures and explain the management of these injuries.

11. Describe the signs and symptoms of intra-abdominal injuries and explain the management of these injuries.

12. Identify injuries and conditions of the genitalia related to participation in sports and physical activity.

13. Describe the management procedures for acute injury of the throat, thorax, and viscera.

INTRODUCTION

Torso injuries occur in nearly every sport, particularly those involving sudden deceleration and impact. Injuries to the reproductive organs, however, are rare, particularly in females. Although protective equipment and padding are available to protect the anterior throat, thorax, and viscera, only football, men's lacrosse, ice hockey, fencing, catchers in baseball and softball, and goalies in lacrosse and field hockey require specific safety equipment for this vital region. Approximately 2% of all athletic injuries affect the abdomen, with the most commonly injured abdominal organs being the spleen, liver, and kidney.[1] Most injuries are superficial and are easily recognized and managed. Some injuries, however, may involve the respiratory and circulatory system, leading to a life-threatening situation.

This chapter begins with a review of the anatomy of the anterior throat, thorax, and viscera, followed by a brief discussion on the prevention of injuries. A step-by-step assessment is presented to help determine the extent and seriousness of the injury. Common injuries are then presented, followed by internal complications that result from trauma or spontaneous rupture. Because rehabilitation of the region usually is included with other body regions, specific exercises for the thorax and visceral region are not discussed.

ANATOMY OF THE THROAT

The throat includes the pharynx, larynx, trachea, esophagus, a number of glands, and several major blood vessels (**Fig. 23.1**). Injuries to the throat are of particular concern because of the life-sustaining functions of the trachea and carotid arteries.

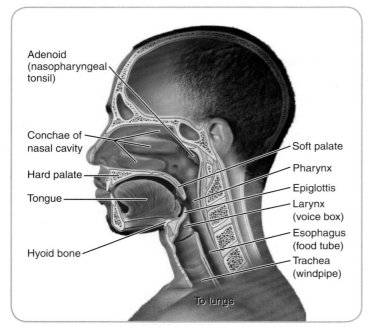

Adenoid (nasopharyngeal tonsil)

Conchae of nasal cavity

Hard palate

Tongue

Hyoid bone

Soft palate

Pharynx

Epiglottis

Larynx (voice box)

Esophagus (food tube)

Trachea (windpipe)

To lungs

Figure 23.1. The throat region. A lateral cross-sectional view.

Pharynx, Larynx, and Esophagus

The pharynx, commonly known as the throat, connects the nasal cavity and mouth to the larynx and esophagus. The pharynx lies between the base of the skull and the 6th cervical vertebra. The laryngeal prominence on the thyroid cartilage that shields the front of the larynx is known as the Adam's apple. A specialized, spoon-shaped cartilage, called the epiglottis, covers the superior opening of the larynx during swallowing to prevent food and liquids from entering. If a foreign body does slip past the epiglottis, the cough reflex is initiated, and the foreign body normally is ejected back into the pharynx. The larynx also contains the vocal cords, which are two bands of elastic connective tissue surrounded by mucosal folds. When expired air from the lungs passes over the vocal cords, sound is able to be produced.

The hyoid bone, the only bone of the body that does not articulate directly with any other bone, lies just inferior to the mandible in the anterior neck.

It is anchored by the narrow stylohyoid ligaments to the styloid processes of the temporal bones, and it serves as an attachment point for neck muscles that raise and lower the larynx during swallowing and speech.

The esophagus carries food and liquids from the throat to the stomach. It is a muscle-walled tube that originates from the pharynx in the midneck and follows the anterior side of the spine. The body of the esophagus is divided into cervical, thoracic, and abdominal regions. The esophagus is pinched together at both the upper and lower ends by muscles referred to as sphincters. The co-ordinated action of the esophageal walls propels food into the stomach. The esophageal sphincters maintain a barrier against reverse movement of the esophageal contents into the pharynx and gastric fluids into the esophagus. When the esophagus is empty, the tube is collapsed.

Trachea

The trachea extends inferiorly from the larynx through the neck into the midthorax, where it divides into the two right and left bronchial tubes. The tracheal tube is formed by C-shaped rings of hyaline cartilage that are joined by fibroelastic connective tissue. Smooth muscle fibers of the trachealis muscle form the open side of the "C" and allow the expansion of the posteriorly adjacent esophagus as swallowed food passes. Contraction of the trachealis muscle during coughing can dramatically reduce the size of the airway and, in doing so, increases the pressure inside the trachea to promote the expulsion of mucus.

Blood Vessels of the Throat

The largest blood vessels coursing through the neck are the common carotid arteries (**Fig. 23.2**). The common carotid arteries, which provide the major blood supply to the brain, head, and face, divide into external and internal carotid arteries at the level of the Adam's apple. Branches from the carotid arteries include the superior thyroid arteries, the facial artery, and the lingual artery; these arteries supply the thyroid and larynx, the face and sinuses, and the mouth and tongue, respectively. Several arteries branch from the left and right subclavian arteries and course upward through the posterior side of the neck, including the costocervical trunk, the thyrocervical trunk, and the vertebral artery.

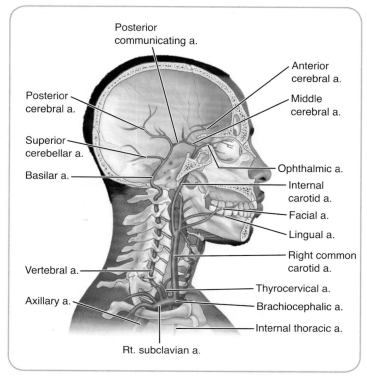

Figure 23.2. The arterial supply to the neck and throat region.

ANATOMY OF THE THORAX

The thoracic cavity, or chest cavity, lies anterior to the spinal column and extends from the level of the clavicle down to the diaphragm. The major organs of the thorax are the heart and lungs. These organs are not commonly injured. However, internal complications caused by direct trauma or spontaneous damage can necessitate emergency action.

Thoracic Cage and Pleura

The thorax includes the sternum, ribs, costal cartilages, and thoracic vertebrae. These structures form a protective cage around the heart and lungs (**Fig. 23.3**). The sternum consists of the manubrium, which articulates with the 1st and 2nd ribs; the body, which articulates with the 2nd through 7th ribs; and the xiphoid process, a trapezoidal projection composed of hyaline cartilage that ossifies around 40 years of age. The costal cartilages of the first seven pairs of ribs attach directly to the sternum. The costal cartilages of ribs 8 through 10 attach to the costal cartilages of the immediately superior ribs. The last two rib pairs are known as floating ribs, because they do not attach anteriorly to any other structure.

The thoracic cavity is lined with a thin, double-layered membrane called the pleura. The pleural cavity is a narrow space between the pleural membranes that is filled with pleural fluid secreted by the membranes, which enables the lungs to move against the thoracic wall with minimal friction during breathing. A further discussion on the anatomy of the lungs is provided in Chapter 26.

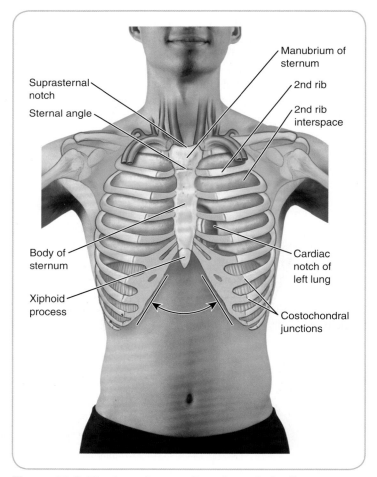

Figure 23.3. The thoracic cage. Note that only the first seven pairs of ribs articulate anteriorly with the sternum through the costal cartilages.

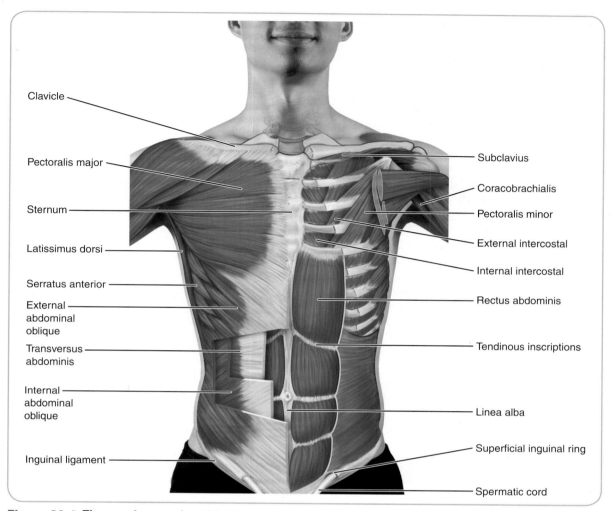

Clavicle

Pectoralis major

Sternum

Latissimus dorsi

Serratus anterior

External
abdominal
oblique

Transversus
abdominis

Internal
abdominal
oblique

Inguinal ligament

Subclavius

Coracobrachialis

Pectoralis minor

External intercostal

Internal intercostal

Rectus abdominis

Tendinous inscriptions

Linea alba

Superficial inguinal ring

Spermatic cord

Figure 23.4. The anterior muscles of the trunk.

Muscles of the Thorax

The muscles of the thoracic region and the muscles of respiration are shown in **Figures 23.4** and **23.5**. The major respiratory muscle is the diaphragm, a powerful sheet of muscle that completely separates the thoracic and abdominal cavities. During relaxation, the diaphragm is dome-shaped. During contraction, it flattens, increasing the size of the thoracic cavity. In turn, this increase in cavity volume causes a decrease in intrathoracic pressure, resulting in inhalation of air into the lungs.

See **Muscles of the Thorax**, found on the companion Web site at thePoint, for a summary of the muscles of the thoracic region and the muscles of respiration, including their attachments, primary actions, and nerve innervation.

ANATOMY OF THE VISCERAL REGION

The visceral region includes the organs and vessels between the diaphragm and the pelvic floor and can be divided into four quadrants: right upper quadrant, left upper quadrant, left lower quadrant, and right lower quadrant (**Fig. 23.6**). Specific structures are located within each quadrant and are presented in **Table 23.1** and **Figure 23.7**. The peritoneal space includes the diaphragm, liver, spleen, stomach, and transverse colon. A portion of the cavity is covered by the bony thorax. The retroperitoneal space, which is the region behind the peritoneum and pelvis, includes the aorta, vena cava, pancreas, kidneys, ureters, and portions of the duodenum and colon. The pelvic organs and vessels include the rectum, bladder, uterus, and iliac vessels. The abdomen contains both solid and hollow organs. The solid

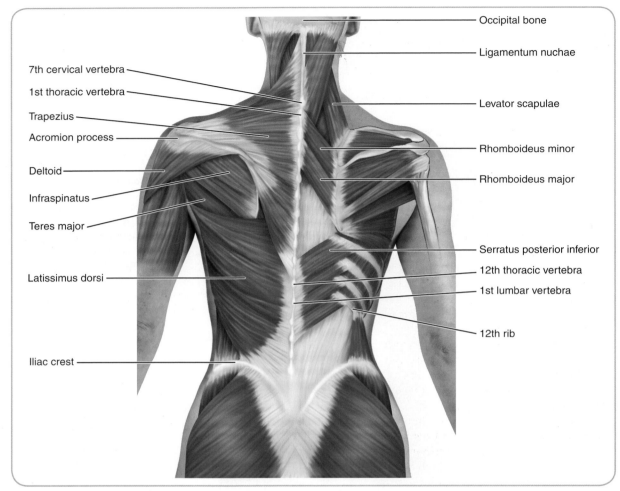

7th cervical vertebra

1st thoracic vertebra

Trapezius

Acromion process

Deltoid

Infraspinatus

Teres major

Latissimus dorsi

Iliac crest

Occipital bone

Ligamentum nuchae

Levator scapulae

Rhomboideus minor

Rhomboideus major

Serratus posterior inferior

12th thoracic vertebra

1st lumbar vertebra

12th rib

Figure 23.5. The posterior muscles of the trunk.

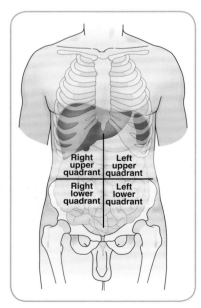

Figure 23.6. Quadrants of the abdominopelvic region.

organs include the spleen, liver, pancreas, kidneys, and adrenal glands. The hollow organs include the stomach, gallbladder, small and large intestines, bladder, and ureters. The pelvic girdle protects the lower abdominal organs.

Pelvic Girdle and Abdominal Cavity

The pelvic girdle, or pelvis, consists of the sacrum, ilium, ischium, and pubis. The joints between these bones are fused in adults, and as such, no movement is allowed. The pelvis forms a protective basin around the internal organs of the abdomen, and it transfers loads between the spine and lower extremity through the hip joint. The pelvis also provides a mechanical link between the upper and lower extremities. Its primary role is to stabilize the lower trunk while motion occurs in the extremities.

Visceral Organs

The stomach is a J-shaped bag positioned between the esophagus and small intestine. Food is stored in the stomach for approximately 4 hours, during which time hydrochloric acid secreted in the stomach breaks it down into a paste-like substance known as **chyme**. The chyme then moves into the small intestine, where it is progressively absorbed. A few substances, including water, electrolytes, aspirin, and alcohol, are absorbed into the bloodstream across the stomach lining without full digestion.

The small intestine is approximately 2 m (6 ft) in length and is responsible for most of the digestion and absorption of food as it is propelled through the

TABLE 23.1 Abdominopelvic Quadrants: Important Organs

QUADRANT	ORGANS
Lower left quadrant (LLQ)	Descending colon, sigmoid colon, left ovary, left fallopian tube, left ureter
Left upper quadrant (LUQ)	Stomach, spleen, left lobe of liver, body of pancreas, left kidney, left adrenal gland, parts of transverse and descending colon
Right upper quadrant (RUQ)	Liver, gall bladder, duodenum, pancreas, right kidney
Right lower quadrant (RLQ)	Cecum, appendix, ascending colon, right ovary and fallopian tube, right ureter

organ by waves of alternate circular contraction and relaxation by a process called **peristalsis**. This process takes approximately 3 to 6 hours. During the next 12 to 24 hours, water and electrolytes are further absorbed from the stored material in the large intestine, or colon. Mass peristaltic movements pass through the intestines several times per day to move the feces to the rectum.

The vermiform appendix protrudes from the large intestine in the right lower quadrant of the abdomen. It can become a protected environment for the accumulation of bacteria, leading to inflammation of the appendix, or appendicitis.

The liver, which is located in the upper right quadrant under the diaphragm, produces bile, a greenish liquid that helps break down fat in the small intestine. The liver also absorbs excess glucose from the bloodstream and stores it, in the form of glycogen, for later use. Additional functions of the liver include processing fats and amino acids, manufacturing blood proteins, and detoxifying certain poisons and drugs. These functions can be severely impaired by alcohol abuse, which can result in cirrhosis of the liver. **Hepatitis** is inflammation of the liver caused by a viral infection, which also can reduce the liver's efficiency. The gallbladder functions as an accessory to the liver by storing concentrated bile on its way to the small intestine.

The spleen, which is the largest of the lymphoid organs, performs four vital functions:

1. Cleansing the blood of foreign matter, bacteria, viruses, and toxins

2. Storing excess red blood cells for later reuse, and releasing others into the blood for processing by the liver

3. Producing red blood cells in the fetus

4. Storing blood platelets

The pancreas secretes most of the digestive enzymes that break down food in the small intestine. It also secretes the hormones insulin and glucagon, which lower and elevate blood sugar levels, respectively.

The kidneys filter and cleanse the blood. They are vital for filtering out toxins, metabolic wastes, drugs, and excess ions and excreting them from the

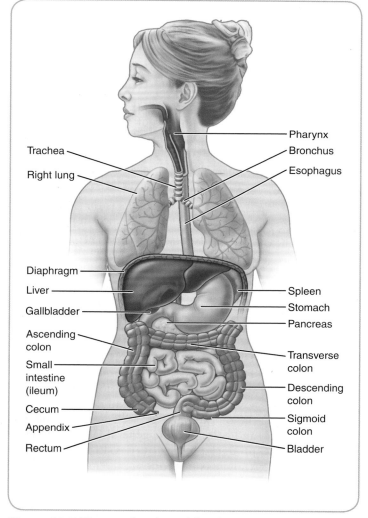

Figure 23.7. The anterior view of the visceral organs.

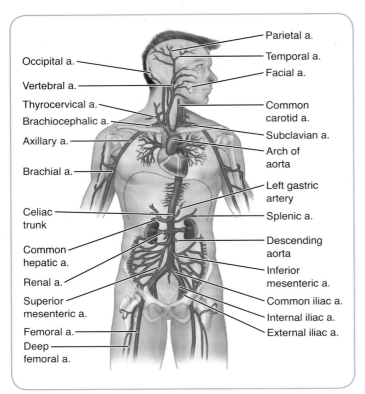

Parietal a.
Occipital a.
Temporal a.
Facial a.
Vertebral a.
Thyrocervical a.
Brachiocephalic a.
Common carotid a.
Axillary a.
Subclavian a.
Arch of aorta
Brachial a.
Left gastric artery
Celiac trunk
Splenic a.
Common hepatic a.
Descending aorta
Renal a.
Inferior mesenteric a.
Superior mesenteric a.
Common iliac a.
Internal iliac a.
Femoral a.
External iliac a.
Deep femoral a.

Figure 23.8. The arterial system of the trunk.

body in urine. The kidneys also return needed substances, such as water and electrolytes, to the blood. The ureters connect the kidneys to the urinary bladder, which is an expandable sac that stores urine.

Blood Vessels of the Trunk

The major blood vessel of the trunk is the aorta, with its numerous branches (**Fig. 23.8**). The left and right coronary arteries branch from the ascending aorta to supply the heart muscle. The first arterial branch from the aortic arch is the brachiocephalic artery, which splits into the right common carotid artery and right subclavian artery. The second and third branches from the aortic arch are the left common carotid artery and the left subclavian artery, respectively. The thoracic aorta yields 10 pairs of intercostal arteries to supply the muscles of the thorax, the bronchial arteries to the lungs, the esophageal artery to the esophagus, and the phrenic arteries to the diaphragm. The distal portion of the descending aorta becomes the abdominal aorta. The first branch of the abdominal aorta is the celiac trunk, which forms the left gastric artery to the stomach, the splenic artery to the spleen, and the common hepatic artery to the liver. Other branches of the abdominal aorta include the superior and inferior mesenteric arteries to the small intestine and the first half of the large intestine, the renal arteries to the kidneys, the ovarian arteries in females, and the testicular arteries in males. The distal portion of the abdominal aorta divides into the common iliac arteries, which further divide into the internal iliac artery to supply the organs of the pelvis, and the external iliac artery, which enters the thigh to become the femoral artery.

See **Muscles of the Pelvic Girdle**, found on the companion Web site at thePoint, for a summary of the locations, primary functions, and innervations of the major muscles of the pelvic girdle.

Muscles of the Pelvic Girdle

As is the case throughout the neck and trunk, muscles in the pelvic region are named in pairs, with one located on the left and the other on the right side of the body. These muscles cause lateral flexion or rotation when they contract unilaterally, but they contribute to spinal flexion or extension when bilateral contractions occur.

ANATOMY OF THE GENITALIA

The reproductive organs of the female and male include the primary and accessory sex organs. The primary sex organs—the ovaries and testes—produce gametes (specifically, ovum and sperm, respectively) that, when joined together, develop into a fetus. Important sex hormones influence sexual differentiation and development of secondary sex characteristics and, in the female, regulate the reproductive cycle. The sex hormones predominantly are produced by the primary sex organs and belong to the general family known as **steroids**. In the female, estrogen and progesterone are produced by the ovaries. In the male, the adrenal cortex and testes produce hormones collectively known as **androgens**, the most active being testosterone. The accessory sex organs transport, protect, and nourish the gametes after they leave the ovaries and testes. In females, the accessory sex organs include the fallopian tubes, uterus, vagina, and vulva. In males, the accessory sex organs include the epididymis, ductus deferens, seminal vesicles, prostate gland, bulbourethral glands, scrotum, and penis.

Female Reproductive System

The female reproductive system includes the ovaries, which produce ova (female eggs); the fallopian tubes, which transport, protect, and nourish the ova; the uterus, which provides an environment for development of the fertilized embryo; and the vagina, which serves as the receptacle for sperm (**Fig. 23.9**). These structures are protected by the pelvic girdle and seldom are injured during participation in sport and physical activity.

The ovarian cycle begins at puberty with the release of an ovum, or egg, from the ovary. The ovum, which is released at ovulation, travels through a fallopian tube to the uterus, where it embeds itself in the uterine wall. The menstrual cycle lasts anywhere from 28 to 40 days, involves a repeated series of changes within the lining of the uterus, and is controlled by the ovarian cycle. Menses, or menstrual flow, is a phase in the menstrual cycle that lasts 3 to 6 days; during this time, the thickened vascular walls of the uterus, the unfertilized ovum, and blood from the damaged vessels of the endometrium are discharged.

The hormones estrogen and progesterone are produced by the ovaries. **Estrogens** help to regulate the menstrual cycle and influence the development of female physical sex characteristics, such as the appearance of breasts, pubic and axillary hair, increased subcutaneous fat (particularly in the hips and breasts), and widening of the pelvis. Estrogens also are responsible for the rapid growth spurt seen in girls between the ages of 10 and 13 years. This growth is short-lived, however, because increased levels of estrogen cause early closure of the epiphyses of long bones, in turn causing females to reach their full height between the ages of 15 to 18 years. In contrast, males may continue to grow until the age of 19 to 21 years. **Progesterones** are responsible for regulating the menstrual cycle and stimulating the development of the uterine lining in preparation for pregnancy.

The external genital organs of the female are known as the vulva, or pudendum. The outer rounded folds, referred to as the labia majora, protect the vestibule into which the vagina and urethra open.

Male Reproductive System

The male reproductive system includes the testes, which produce spermatozoa; a number of ducts that store, transport, and nourish the spermatozoa; several accessory glands that contribute to the formation of semen; and the penis, through which urine and semen pass (**Fig. 23.10**). **Testosterone**, which is the primary androgen produced by the testes, stimulates the growth and maturation of the internal and external genitalia at puberty and is responsible for sexual motivation. Secondary sex characteristics that are testosterone-dependent include the appearance of pubic, axillary, and facial hair; enhanced hair growth on the chest or back; and a deepening of the voice as the larynx enlarges. Androgens also increase bone growth, bone density, and skeletal muscle size and mass.

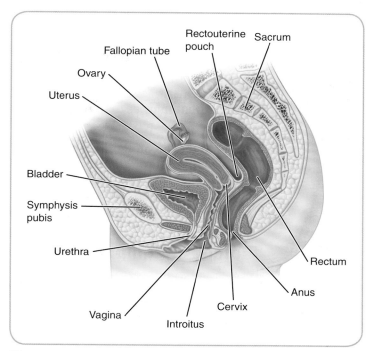

Figure 23.9. **A median section of the female pelvis.**

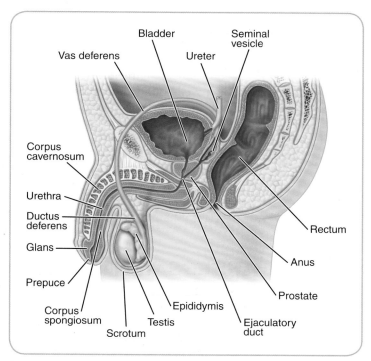

Figure 23.10. **A median section of the male pelvis.**

PREVENTION OF INJURIES TO THE THROAT, THORAX, AND VISCERA

 The throat, thorax, and viscera are vulnerable to direct impact injuries. This region is such a critical area that injuries can be life threatening. What measures can be taken to prevent injuries to this region?

Injuries to the throat, thorax, and abdomen occur in nearly every sport, yet few sports require protective equipment for all players. In sports where high-velocity projectiles are present, throat and chest protectors are required only for specific player positions (e.g., catcher or goalie). As with other body regions, protective equipment, in combination with a well-rounded physical conditioning program, can reduce the risk of injury. Although proper skill techniques can prevent some injuries, this is not a major factor in this region.

Protective Equipment

Face masks with throat protectors are required for fencing participants, baseball/softball catchers, and field hockey, ice hockey, and lacrosse goalies. Many of these athletes wear an extended pad attached to the mask to protect the throat region.

Many participants in collision and contact sports wear full chest and abdominal protection. In young baseball and softball players (younger than 12 years of age), it has been suggested that all infield players wear chest protectors. Adolescent rib cages are less rigid, placing the heart at greater risk from a direct impact. Although there are many commercially made wall protectors for use by youth lacrosse and baseball athletes, it is important to remember that no chest wall protectors have yet been found to be effective in preventing commotio cordis.[2] In this age group, more baseball and softball deaths occur from impacts to the chest than to the head.

Shoulder pads can protect the upper thoracic region, and rib protectors can provide protection against rib, upper abdominal, or low back contusions. Body suits made of mesh with pockets can hold rib and hip pads to protect the sides and back.

The male genitalia are more susceptible to injury than the female genitalia. Protective cups can protect the penis and scrotum from injury. Sport bras can provide added support to reduce excessive vertical and horizontal breast motion during exercise. Protective equipment is illustrated and discussed in Chapter 3.

Physical Conditioning

Flexibility and strengthening of the torso muscles should not be an isolated program; rather, it should include a well-rounded conditioning program for the back, shoulder, abdomen, and hip regions. Range of motion (ROM) and strengthening exercises should include both open and closed kinetic chain activities. Exercises for the thorax and abdominal region are included in the chapters on Pelvic, Hip, and Thigh Conditions, Shoulder Conditions, Cervical and Thoracic Spinal Conditions, and Lumbar Spinal Conditions.

 Injuries to the throat, thorax, and viscera can be prevented by wearing appropriate protective equipment. Physical conditioning should include a well-rounded flexibility and strengthening program for the shoulder, back, abdominal, and hip regions.

ASSESSMENT OF THROAT, THORAX, AND VISCERAL CONDITIONS

 During practice, a 20-year-old football player was struck in the abdomen with a helmet and experienced a sudden onset of abdominal pain in the upper left quadrant. How should the assessment of this injury progress to determine the extent and severity of injury?

The injury assessment for thoracic and visceral injuries should focus on vital signs and the history of the injury. Chest or abdominal trauma, although initially appearing to be superficial and minor, can mask an internal hemorrhage and swelling that can seriously compromise the function of vital organs. An individual's condition can slowly deteriorate and become a life-threatening condition. Although general observation and palpation can confirm the possibility of a serious underlying condition, an understanding of the history of the injury and constant monitoring of vital signs strengthen the assessment.

The clinician should assess consciousness, respiration, and circulation. If the individual is having difficulty breathing, anxiety and panic may make the task more difficult. If a spinal injury has been ruled out, the individual should be placed in a supine position, with the knees flexed, to facilitate breathing. The airway should be open and clear of any blood or vomitus. The trachea should be in the middle of the throat and should not move during respirations. If breathing does not return to normal within a minute or two, the emergency medical plan, including summoning emergency medical services (EMS), should be activated. It is always better to have EMS en route during the assessment than to wait and see if the condition gets better. Several conditions can intensify in severity with time, thereby seriously compromising the health of the injured party. The clinician should record vital signs so that a baseline of information is established. Methods for assessing level of consciousness, airway, breathing, vital sign assessment, and clearing the patient of potential cervical spine injury were presented in Chapter 7.

As is the case with an acute abdominal injury, water and food should not be given to the individual. Not only can the condition be aggravated, any food or fluid in the gastrointestinal tract will make the surgery, if necessary, more dangerous. While waiting for EMS to arrive, the vital signs should be monitored frequently and the individual should be treated for shock.

See **Application Strategy: Thorax and Visceral Region Evaluation**, available on the companion Web site at thePoint, for a summary of the assessment of the thorax and visceral regions.

HISTORY

? The assessment of the football player's injury should begin with a history. The mechanism of injury and the site of the trauma have already been identified. What additional questions need to be asked as part of the on-field assessment of this injury?

Because few special tests are available for the region, the clinician must rely heavily on information provided in the history. Injuries to the ribs, costal cartilage, or abdominal muscles usually produce tenderness at the site of injury. Abdominal pain may indicate a serious abdominal injury, but it also can be a symptom in conditions as minor as precompetition anxiety. The issue is not to draw a distinction between acute and nonacute pain but, rather, to draw one between possible surgical and nonsurgical conditions. Because pain tolerance can vary, every complaint of thoracic or abdominal pain must be assessed.

The clinician should gather information regarding the primary complaint, the mechanism of injury, and the characteristics of the symptoms. Pain that is sudden in onset, severe or explosive, progressive, continuous, and lasts more than 6 hours generally indicates a serious internal problem that necessitates surgical intervention. Persistent pain that awakens the person or that occurs during relative inactivity also is a red flag. Pain that is gradual, mild-to-moderate, intermittent, recurrent, occurs after exercise or eating, or resolves partially or completely in less than 6 hours indicates a less serious condition that favors a nonsurgical diagnosis.[3] **Table 23.2** identifies some common nonmusculoskeletal sources of abdominal pain and the typical signs and symptoms that are associated with each condition. The patient should be referred for additional examination if any of the conditions listed in **Table 23.2** are suspected.

The clinician should ask questions about previous injuries to the area that may have some bearing on this specific condition. It is important to remember that some conditions, such as a ruptured spleen, can delay hemorrhage for hours, days, or even weeks after the initial trauma. Other injuries with an acute onset may have signs and symptoms that subside only to recur later. Questions should be asked about activities that aggravate the pain. Coughing, sneezing, rapid movements, and

TABLE 23.2 Common Nonmusculoskeletal Sources of Abdominal Pain

CONDITION	SIGNS AND SYMPTOMS
Appendicitis (acute)	Inflammation of the appendix resulting in constant pain; progresses in severity; begins in the outer umbilical region; moves to the right lower quadrant; nausea, vomiting, and loss of appetite; low-grade fever
Cholecystitis (acute)	Inflammation of the gallbladder, resulting in constant pain in the right upper quadrant; onset often follows a meal; nausea and vomiting; tenderness in the right upper quadrant and right shoulder; splinting on the right side
Perforated peptic ulcer	Perforated stomach ulcer resulting in a sudden onset of pain in the midepigastric region that spreads and is aggravated by movement; individual is reluctant to move and appears acutely ill; rigid abdomen; grunting respiration; absent bowel sounds
Ectopic pregnancy	Pregnancy in the fallopian tube, which results in a tubal rupture causing a sudden, severe, and persistent pain, generally following a missed or abnormal period; typically epigastric; often associated with hypotension and tachycardia
Ovarian cyst	An abnormal cystic tumor of the ovary that usually is benign; constant pain with a sharp, sudden onset; usually in the ipsilateral lower area of the abdomen below the umbilicus; may have nausea and vomiting following the pain
Pelvic inflammatory disease	Chronic inflammation of the pelvis caused by multiple infections, including chlamydia and gonorrhea, resulting in pain at the end of or shortly after a normal menstrual period; bilateral lower quadrant pain aggravated by manipulation of the cervix; rarely, nausea and vomiting; possible cervical discharge; fever
Urinary calculus	Pain location changes with the movement of the urinary stone and may radiate to the testicle or groin of the involved side; pain is very severe; individual cannot get comfortable

walking, especially down stairs, can cause peritoneal irritation. Musculoskeletal pain often is relieved by changing position.

 See **Application Strategy: Developing a History for a Thoracic or Abdominal Injury**, found on the companion Web site at thePoint, for specific questions that can be asked for chest and abdominal injuries.

In younger athletes who are sexually active, females experience abdominal pain twice as often as males of the same age. Males, however, tend to have a higher incidence of conditions necessitating surgical intervention. Pain that is sudden in onset and follows an abnormal menstrual period might stem from an ectopic pregnancy, which would constitute a medical emergency. Pain that occurs shortly after a normal menstrual period, is bilateral, and is accompanied by fever and abdominal pain but not nausea and vomiting suggests pelvic inflammatory disease.

 During the on-field assessment of the football player, the mechanism of injury and the location of trauma have been identified. The clinician should ask questions related to the location and type of pain (including pain in areas other than the injured site) and the presence of any dizziness, nausea, weakness, numbness, or other unusual feelings.

OBSERVATION AND INSPECTION

 During the history, the individual reports pain in his upper chest and left shoulder. He also complains of feeling weak and light-headed. What factors should be observed and inspected as part of the ongoing on-field assessment of this injury?

An observation of body position can give an indication regarding the site, nature, and severity of injury. For example, in an acute thoracic injury, the individual may lean toward the injured side, using an arm or a hand to stabilize the region. In an acute abdominal injury, the individual typically lies on the injured side and brings the knees toward the chest to relax the abdominal muscles. Facial expressions can confirm the individual's hesitation to perform any movement because of severe pain. A chest expansion can reveal the rate and depth of respirations.

Inspection

The individual should be sufficiently undressed so that the site of injury can be observed. An inspection should include the neck, back, chest, abdomen, and groin, with any deformity, edema, bruising, ecchymosis, and skin color being noted. A deformity may indicate a sternal or rib fracture, costochondral separation, or muscle rupture. An abrasion or localized bruising on the chest wall could suggest a possible rib fracture or internal complication. Diffuse bruising in the axilla and chest wall may indicate a ruptured pectoralis major. A bruise or ecchymosis in the umbilical area (i.e., **Cullen sign**) indicates intraperitoneal bleeding. A distention in the abdomen may indicate an internal hemorrhage. Pale, cold, and clammy skin is associated with shock. Cyanosis, or a bluish tinge to the skin, indicates a lack of oxygen resulting from internal pulmonary or cardiac problems. Coughing up bright red or frothy blood indicates a severe lung injury. Vomitus containing blood that looks like used coffee grounds indicates that blood has been swallowed and partially digested.

The rate and depth of respirations should be noted, particularly if the individual has any difficulty catching his or her breath. If the condition is only transitory (e.g., the "wind has been knocked out"), breathing and color should quickly return to normal. An individual with an internal injury tends to use rapid and shallow breaths, because deep breathing increases pain. The clinician should observe the symmetric rise and fall of the chest; any abnormal motion may indicate a fractured rib or pneumothorax. If breathing does not quickly return to normal or the individual's condition rapidly deteriorates, the injury should be considered significant, and the emergency medical plan, including summoning EMS, should be activated.

See **Application Strategy: Observation and Inspection of the Thorax and Viscera**, found on the companion Web site at thePoint, for specific observations that can help to determine the extent and severity of thoracic or abdominal injuries.

Auscultation and Percussion

If auscultation or percussion is used in the assessment, both should be completed before palpation. Because the visceral organs are interconnected by connective tissue, any palpation in the abdomen moves the internal organs and, as such, can produce inaccurate or false sounds.

Auscultation is used to listen for the presence or absence of sounds in the body and should precede any physical contact with the individual to prevent the alteration of peristalsis by physical stimulation. A stethoscope usually has two heads: the bell and the diaphragm. The bell is used to detect low-pitched sounds, whereas the diaphragm is better at detecting higher pitched sounds. When using the bell of the stethoscope, light pressure should be applied to maintain contact with the skin surface. Firm pressure is applied when using the diaphragm to keep it pressed tightly to the skin. Because the bell or diaphragm must always be in contact with the skin, listening through clothing is never acceptable. It may take 2 to 3 minutes in each area to adequately evaluate the nature and character of the underlying conditions, particularly with bowel sounds.

Auscultation of the Lungs

In the thorax, the flow of air should be heard throughout the various regions of each lung (**Fig. 23.11**). Because most breath sounds are high-pitched, the diaphragm is used to evaluate lung sounds. Individuals who should be evaluated include those with the following signs and symptoms (**Box 23.1**)[3]:

- Shortness of breath or dyspnea
- Cough with or without a bloody sputum
- Pleuritic pain
- A resting respiratory rate greater than 22 breaths per minute
- Cyanosis or finger clubbing

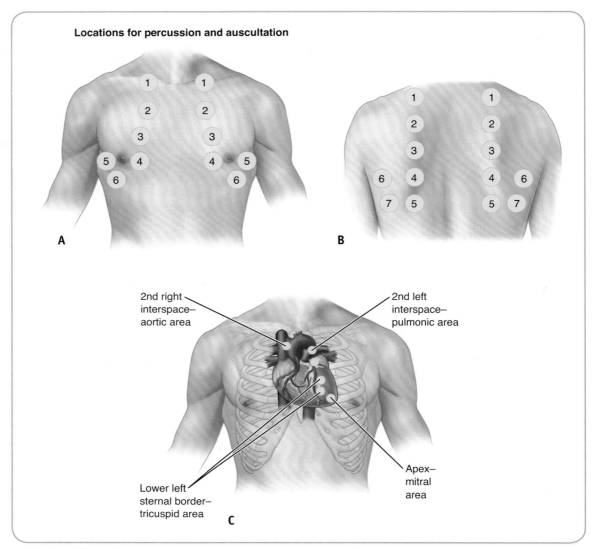

Locations for percussion and auscultation

Figure 23.11. Auscultation. An auscultation is performed with a stethoscope to listen at various sites for air exchange in the lobes of the lungs. **A,** Anterior view. **B,** Posterior view. **C,** Cardiac sounds also can be auscultated over four specific sites.

BOX 23.1 Signs and Symptoms Indicating the Need for Lung Auscultation

- Shortness of breath or dyspnea (could indicate conditions such as pneumonia, pneumothorax, asthma, or heart failure)

- Cough with or without a bloody sputum (could indicate pneumonitis, bronchitis, fibrotic lung disease, or bronchial carcinoma)

- Pleuritic pain (could indicate acute inflammation of the pleural surface, herpes zoster involving the intercostal nerves, or rib fracture)

- A resting respiratory rate of greater than 22 breaths per minute

- Cyanosis or finger clubbing (could indicate several pulmonary diseases, including chronic suppurative disease or pulmonary carcinoma)

TABLE 23.3 Characteristics of Normal Breath Sounds

	DURATION OF SOUNDS	INTENSITY OF EXPIRATORY SOUND	PITCH OF EXPIRATORY SOUND	LOCATIONS WHERE NORMALLY HEARD
Vesicular	Inspiratory sounds last longer than expiratory ones	Soft	Relatively low-pitched	Over most of both lungs
Bronchovesicular	Inspiratory and expiratory sounds are about equal	Intermediate	Intermediate-pitched	Often in the 1st and 2nd interspaces anteriorly and between the scapulae
Bronchial	Expiratory sounds last longer than inspiratory ones	Loud	Relatively high-pitched	Over the manubrium, if heard at all
Tracheal	Inspiratory and expiratory sounds are about equal	Very loud	Relatively high-pitched	Over the trachea in the neck

From Bickley LS, Szilagyi PG. *Bates' Guide to Physical Examination and History Taking.* Philadelphia, PA: Lippincott Williams & Wilkins; 2003:227; with permission.

The patient should be instructed to breathe deeply through an open mouth. The clinician should listen for at least one full breath at each site, moving from one side to the other and comparing symmetric areas of the lungs. The intensity of breath sounds should be noted. Breath sounds usually are louder in the lower posterior lung fields and may vary from area to area. Characteristics of normal breath sounds are summarized in **Table 23.3**. Abnormal sounds are summarized in **Table 23.4**.[4]

TABLE 23.4 Abnormal Breath Sounds

SOUND	CHARACTERISTICS
Crackles	May result from abnormalities of the lungs (e.g., pneumonia, fibrosis, or early congestive heart failure) or the airways (e.g., bronchitis or bronchiectasis)
Fine crackles	Soft, high-pitched, and very brief (5–10 msec). They sometimes are compared to rubbing dry strands of hair together between the thumb and finger close to the ear.
Coarse crackles	Somewhat louder than fine crackles, lower in pitch, and not quite so brief (20–30 msec)
Wheezes	Relatively high-pitched (~400 MHz or higher) and has a hissing or shrill quality. Wheezing suggests narrowed airways, as in asthma, bronchitis, chronic obstructive pulmonary disease, and congestive heart failure.
Rhonchi	Relatively low-pitched (~200 MHz or lower) and have a rumbling or snoring quality. They usually are caused by the passage of air through bronchi obstructed by thick mucus.
Stridor	A wheeze that is entirely or predominantly inspiratory. It often is louder in the neck than over the chest wall, and it indicates partial obstruction of the larynx or trachea.
Pleural rub	Inflamed or roughened pleural surfaces momentarily grate against each other and are delayed by friction, producing creaking sounds known as a pleural rub or pleural friction rub. Pleural rubs resemble crackles acoustically but usually are confined to a relatively small area of the chest wall and typically are heard in both phases of respiration.
Mediastinal crunch	A series of precordial crackles synchronous with heartbeat, not with respiration. They are best heard in the left lateral position (Hamman sign) and are caused by mediastinal emphysema.
Absence of sounds	May be caused by pleural effusion, pneumothorax, tension pneumothorax, hemothorax, or traumatic asphyxia

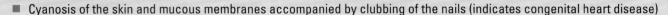

BOX 23.2 Signs and Symptoms Indicating the Need for Heart Auscultation

■ Cyanosis of the skin and mucous membranes accompanied by clubbing of the nails (indicates congenital heart disease)

■ Any signs of Marfan syndrome

■ Palpitations or a history of syncope, angina, and fatigue

■ Rapid pulse (tachycardia) of more than 100 beats per minute at rest

■ Slow pulse (bradycardia) of less than 40 beats per minute at rest

■ Unusual and severe dyspnea after routine exercise

■ Sustained arterial hypertension

■ Retrosternal pain brought on by exertion but relieved with rest

■ Traumatic chest injuries that could cause cardiac injury

Auscultation of the Heart

A normal cardiac cycle consists of two sounds, often called "lub-dub," which is caused by the blood flowing against the valves as they close. Individuals who should have the heart evaluated include those listed in **Box 23.2**.

An abnormal sound is called a murmur and is produced by turbulent energy in the walls of the heart and blood vessels. Obstruction to flow, or flow from a narrow to a larger diameter vessel, produces the turbulence, which sets up motion currents that strike the walls and produce vibrations that can be heard with a stethoscope. Murmurs also can be produced when a large volume of blood is flowing through a normal opening. Murmurs may be described as "blowing," "rumbling," or "harsh." If abnormal sounds such as a click, snap, or a murmur are present, the individual should be referred to a physician.

The diaphragm of the stethoscope is more effective in detecting the relatively high-pitched sounds of S_1 (i.e., first sound) and S_2 (i.e., second sound), the murmurs of aortic and mitral regurgitation, and pericardial friction rubs. The bell of the stethoscope is more sensitive to the low-pitched sounds of S_3 and S_4 and the murmur of mitral stenosis.

The clinician should be on the right side of the patient with the individual recumbent and the head and chest elevated to 45°. This position allows the clinician to observe chest movements associated with cardiac function as well as to place the stethoscope head correctly during auscultation. Some clinicians begin at the apex; others prefer to start at the base (i.e., upper margins of the heart). Either pattern is satisfactory.

Four classic sites are used to determine cardiac sounds (see **Fig. 23.11**):

1. Aortic (second intercostal space, right sternal border)

2. Pulmonic (second intercostal space, left sternal border)

3. Tricuspid (left lower sternal border)

4. Mitral (cardiac apex)

After listening to each site, the clinician should instruct the patient to roll partly onto the left side, which positions the left ventricle closer to the chest wall. In this position, the clinician should place the bell lightly on the apical impulse. Finally, the patient should be instructed to sit up, lean forward, exhale completely, and stop breathing in expiration; this position accentuates aortic murmurs that otherwise might go undetected.

Auscultation of the Abdomen

In the abdomen, auscultation can determine bowel motility. It is important to listen to the abdomen before performing percussion or palpation, because these maneuvers may alter the frequency of bowel sounds.

The diaphragm of the stethoscope should be placed gently on the abdomen, assessing each of the four quadrants shown in **Figure 23.6**. Bowel sounds should be noted relative to their frequency and character. Normal bowel sounds consist of clicks and gurgles, occurring at an estimated frequency of 5 to 34 per minute.[5] Hyperperistalsis with rushes, cramps, and diarrhea suggests gastroenteritis.

Percussion

Percussion typically is used over a bony structure to determine a possible fracture, but it also can be used in the chest and abdominal region to indicate internal complications. The clinician should place their nondominant hand on the patient's abdomen over the various internal organs. This is followed by the clinician using the second and third finger of the dominant hand to tap on the distal interphalangeal joint of the middle finger of the nondominant hand. The tapping should be performed as a quick rapid motion (**Fig. 23.12**). The tone indicates if the organ is hollow (tympanic) or solid (full).

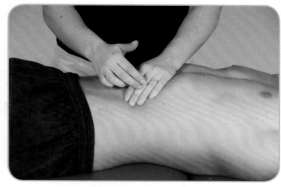

Figure 23.12. Percussion. Percussion is used in the abdominal region to indicate internal complications and should be performed before palpation.

In the chest, the same sites used during auscultation are percussed and bilaterally compared. Dullness replaces resonance when fluid or solid tissue replaces air-containing lung tissue. Because pleural fluid usually sinks to the inferior pleural space (i.e., posteriorly in a supine patient), only a very large effusion can be detected anteriorly. The heart normally produces an area of dullness to the left of the sternum from the 3rd to 5th interspace.

In the abdomen, the four quadrants are tested to assess the distribution of tympany and dullness. Tympany usually predominates because of gas in the gastrointestinal tract, but fluid and feces may produce normal, scattered areas of dullness. It is important to note any large, dull areas that may indicate an enlarged organ and any facial expressions to indicate any discomfort.

Hypoperistalsis, or a silent abdomen, could indicate a serious underlying problem, such as an obstruction or an internal hemorrhage. Immediate referral to the nearest medical facility is warranted. Activation of the emergency plan, including summoning EMS, is warranted. While waiting for EMS to arrive, the clinician should maintain the airway, assess vital signs, and treat for shock as necessary.

 Note the football player's willingness or ability to move, ease in motion, and general attitude. The inspection should include viewing the chest and abdomen, with any deformity, edema, bruising, ecchymosis, and skin color being noted.

PALPATION

 The general attitude of the football player indicates that he is uncomfortable and in pain. No abnormal findings are apparent by inspection. As part of the ongoing on-field assessment of this injury, what areas should be palpated?

It is important to begin palpation away from the painful area so that pain will not be carried over into other areas. Palpation begins with gentle circular motions, feeling for deformity, crepitus, swelling, rigidity, muscle guarding, or tenderness. The patient should be in a supine position with the knees flexed for more comfort.

The trachea should be palpated during breathing to ensure that it does not move, because movement may indicate a tension pneumothorax. The clinician should palpate the clavicle, sternum, costochondral cartilage, and ribs, moving in an anterior-to-posterior direction and noting any pain, deformity, or crepitus. The left anterior rib cage should be palpated for an enlarged spleen. The spleen may be more prominent if the patient raises his or her arms above the head. While palpating the posterior rib cage, the clinician should locate the approximate position of the kidneys. The left kidney is well protected by the posterolateral rib cage; the right kidney rests more inferior.

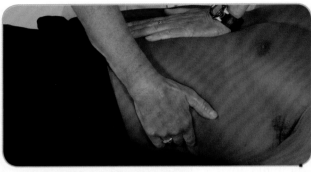
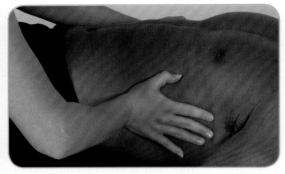

Figure 23.13. **Compression of the rib cage in a supine position. A,** Anteroposterior compression for rib fracture. **B,** Lateral compression for costochondral separation.

Possible rib fractures and costochondral separations are assessed with gentle pressure applied to the sternum and vertebrae in an anteroposterior direction (**Fig. 23.13A**). This action causes the rib cage to bow out laterally. Lateral compression on the sides of the rib cage causes strain on the costochondral junctions (**Fig. 23.13B**). Compression should begin superiorly and move down, in an inferior direction, until the entire area is covered. Pain at a specific site indicates a positive sign.

The fingernails can be blanched to determine normal capillary refill. Certain cardiac or pulmonary conditions may result in cyanosis of the nail beds, fingers, and toes.

An examination of the abdomen begins by gently stroking the area. An underlying peritoneal irritation causes a light touch to be perceived as a disagreeable sensation, referred to as **dysesthesia**, and suggests a serious underlying condition. Palpation should be performed using the flat part of several fingers, with both hands moving in small, circular motions (**Fig. 23.14**). It is important to avoid poking or making sudden moves, because this may cause the individual to jerk and tighten the muscles. Palpation should begin away from the injured site and should move across the abdomen in a straight line. Any muscle guarding or rigidity should be noted. Muscle guarding that cannot be voluntarily relaxed may indicate internal peritoneal hemorrhage. It is important to palpate for tenderness, muscle resistance, and superficial masses or deficits in the continuity of the abdominal wall. Deeper palpation can detect rigidity, swelling, or masses. Rebound tenderness at the **McBurney point** is indicative of appendicitis (**Fig. 23.15**). The rebounding pain is caused when the inflamed appendix is impacted by the viscera returning to the normal position. This phenomenon, however, also can occur with peritonitis.

The focus of the palpation of the injury to the football player should be the upper left quadrant, but it is important to palpate the entire abdomen. The palpation should assess point tenderness, swelling, deformity, rebound pain, spasms, and rigidity.

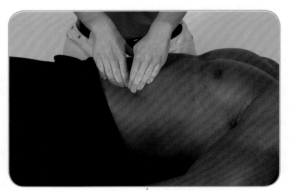

Figure 23.14. **Palpation of the abdomen.** The clinician should use the flat part of several fingers and move both hands in small, circular motions.

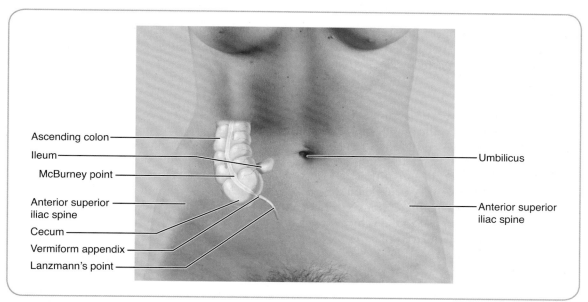

Figure 23.15. McBurney point. This point is the location where the base of the appendix is most commonly found. It is in the right lower quadrant about one-third of the distance from the anterior superior iliac spine to the umbilicus. Rebound tenderness over McBurney point suggests the presence of appendicitis. Another cause of appendicitis can be an interruption of the blood supply to the appendix. Lanzmann point is a tender point in appendicitis that is situated on a line between the two anterior superior iliac spines, 5 to 6 cm from the right spine and 2 cm below McBurney point.

PHYSICAL EXAMINATION TESTS

The palpation reveals rigidity over the upper left quadrant. An assessment of vital signs indicates the following: blood pressure is 96/70 mm Hg, pulse is weak at 96 beats per minute, and the skin is cool and clammy. What injury should be suspected, and how should this condition be managed?

Very few special tests are available for the thorax and visceral area. Most of the information must be gathered during the history, observation, and palpation phase of the assessment. If the condition is not serious and a muscular strain is suspected, active, passive, and resisted muscle testing can be performed. Neck and trunk motion include flexion, extension, lateral flexion, and rotation. The clinician should note the individual's willingness to perform the motion, ease of motion, and bilateral comparison of motions when applicable.

Vital Signs

It is important to note pulse rate and rhythm, blood pressure, temperature, and respiratory rate and characteristics. The pulse usually is taken at the carotid artery; however, a pulse also can be taken at the radial, femoral, or brachial arteries. A normal pulse rate for a physically active individual ranges between 60 and 100 beats per minute, depending on when the pulse is taken. The pulse rate is higher, for example, if taken immediately after exercise. Highly conditioned individuals tend to have lower pulse rates.

Respirations should range between 12 and 20 breaths per minute, with highly conditioned individuals falling into the lower range. Rapid, shallow breaths may indicate internal injury or shock. Deep, quick breaths may indicate asthma or pulmonary obstruction. Noisy, raspy breaths may indicate a partial airway obstruction.

Any sputum should be checked for the presence of blood. Pink or bloody sputum indicates internal bleeding and should be treated as a serious condition.

Painful abdominal conditions frequently are reflected in the vital signs as tachycardia, tachypnea, and elevated temperature. With conditions that involve the upper abdomen or lower lobes of the lung, respiration may be rapid, shallow, painful (grunting), or splinted. Hypotension may result from gastrointestinal bleeding, dehydration, or vagal stimulation.

Urinalysis

Urinalysis is a common test that uses chemically treated dipsticks to provide fast, general results for such information as specific gravity, pH, and levels of leukocytes, nitrate, protein, glucose, ketones, urobilinogen, bilirubin, and blood in the urine (**Fig. 23.16**). In conducting a urinalysis, the patient should be instructed to clean and rinse the external urethra. In collecting the specimen, the patient should be told to direct the initial flow of urine into the toilet bowl before directing it into a clean specimen cup. One to 2 oz of urine should be collected. The clinician should insert the dipstick into the fluid following the manufacturer's recommended immersion times, and the color produced on the dipstick is then matched to the values provided by the manufacturer. Normal and abnormal urinalysis findings are presented in **Table 23.5**.

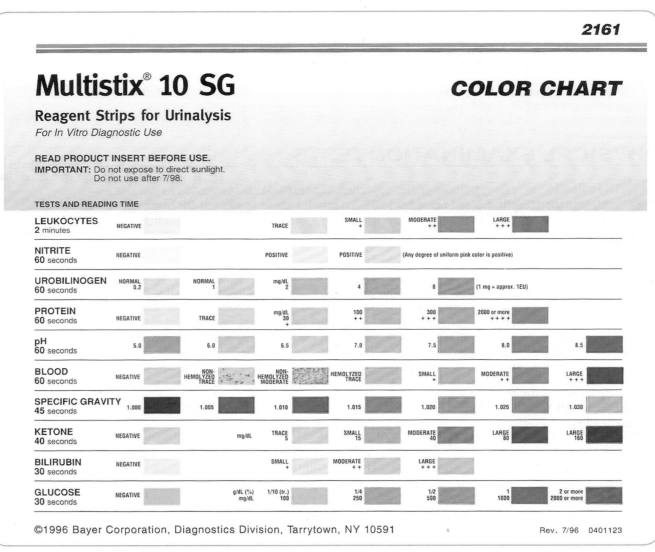

Figure 23.16. Urinalysis chart for chemical dipstick testing. After dipping the stick into the urine in accordance with manufacturer's protocol, the color produced on the dipstick is then matched to the values provided by the manufacturer.

TABLE 23.5 Normal and Abnormal Urinalysis Results

COMPONENT	NORMAL FINDINGS	ABNORMAL FINDINGS AND POTENTIAL CAUSES
Appearance	Color is a light yellow to a dark amber color.	Cloudy urine may indicate infection.
Odor	Odorless	Fruity odor may indicate presence of ketone bodies.
Leukocytes (WBC)	Normal is 0.	Elevated levels suggest possible infection in urinary tract or kidneys.
Nitrates	Normal is 0.	Elevated levels suggest possible UTI.
Urobilinogen	Normal range is 3.2–16.0.	Greater levels suggest liver disease. Lower levels may suggest jaundice.
Protein	Normal is 0 to trace.	Greater than trace indicates possible rhabdomyolysis, pregnancy, renal disease, and congestive heart failure.
Ph	Normal range is 4.5–7.2, with 6.0 average.	*Lower levels* indicate possible acidosis, dehydration, or diabetic ketoacidosis; creates an environment conducive to developing kidney stones. *Higher levels* indicate possible UTI, pyloric obstruction, or kidney dysfunction.
Blood (hemoglobin)	Normal is 0.	Elevated levels can occur due to diseases of the kidney and urinary tract, trauma, medications, or strenuous exercise.
Specific gravity	Normal values: 1.005–1.025	*Low specific gravity (<1.005)* is characteristic of diabetes or kidney infection. *High specific gravity (>1.035)* suggests possible dehydration, liver failure, or shock.
Ketones	Normal is 0 to trace.	Greater than trace ketones is also associated with diabetes but may occur with starvation and after bouts of vomiting and diarrhea.
Bilirubin	Normal is 0.	Presence of any amount of bilirubin is early indicator of liver disease.
Glucose	Normal is 0 to trace.	Greater than trace glucose may be the result of ingesting large glucose-rich foods that "spill" glucose into the urine but is also associated with diabetes.

WBC, white blood cell; *UTI*, urinary tract infection.

Neurological Test

Neurological tests in the thorax and abdomen are somewhat limited. Dermatomes vary and often overlap. Although the dermatomes tend to follow the ribs, the absence of only one dermatome may not lead to a loss in sensation. Sites for referred pain can indicate the origin of injury and are illustrated in **Figure 6.1**. Myotome testing includes finger abduction and adduction (T1) and hip flexion (L1–L2). No other myotome testing exists for the axial region. In addition, no deep tendon reflexes exist for the region, although it always is appropriate to test the deep tendon lumbar and sacral reflexes (i.e., patellar reflex and Achilles reflex).

 Based on the on-field assessment of the football player, a splenic injury should be suspected. As such, activation of the emergency plan, including summoning EMS, is warranted. While waiting for EMS to arrive, the clinician should maintain the airway, assess vital signs, and treat for shock as necessary.

THROAT CONDITIONS

 During a rebound attempt, a basketball player is struck in the anterior neck with an elbow. The player is coughing and having difficulty swallowing. What injury should be suspected? How should the situation be managed?

 Activation of the emergency plan, including summoning EMS, is warranted. While waiting for EMS to arrive, the clinician should apply firm, direct pressure over the wound. The clinician also should maintain the airway, assess vital signs, and treat for shock as necessary.

Neck Lacerations

Etiology

Although uncommon, lacerations to the neck can occur. In ice hockey, for example, a skater may attempt to leap over another player who is down on the ice. The edge of the skate blade may slice the down player. Bicycle accidents (neck striking the handlebars) and falls (neck striking an object) are more likely to occur in children, whereas motor vehicle, minibike, snowmobile, water jet ski, or all-terrain vehicle accidents occur in adolescents and adults.

Signs and Symptoms

If the trauma is sufficiently deep, it can damage the jugular vein or carotid artery on the lateral side of the neck.

Management

Immediate control of the hemorrhage is imperative. In addition to blood loss, air may be sucked into the vein and carried to the heart as an air embolism. Such an embolism can be fatal.

Contusions and Fractures

Etiology

Contusions and fractures to the trachea, larynx, and hyoid bone can occur during hyperextension of the neck. In this position, the thyroid cartilage (Adam's apple) becomes prominent and vulnerable to direct impact forces. In rare instances, these injuries can be fatal as a result of the extravasation of blood into the laryngeal tissues, leading to airway edema and asphyxia resulting from obstruction.

 With significant trauma, activation of the emergency plan, including summoning EMS, is warranted. In these cases, it is important to consider an associated injury to the cervical spine. The clinician also should maintain the airway, assess vital signs, and treat for shock as necessary.

If the patient recovers on-site, observation should continue throughout the day to note the presence of any delayed respiratory problems. **Application Strategy 23.1** explains the management of tracheal and laryngeal injuries.

Signs and Symptoms

Immediate symptoms include hoarseness, dyspnea (difficulty breathing), coughing, difficulty swallowing (dysphagia), laryngeal tenderness, and an inability to make high-pitched "e" sounds. Significant trauma to the region can result in severe pain, laryngospasm, and acute respiratory distress (**Box 23.3**). Laryngospasm occurs when the adductor muscles of the vocal cords pull together in a shutter-like fashion and the upper surface of the vocal cords closes over the top, causing complete obstruction. The individual may recover on site, leave the area, and return home, only to have increasing respiratory problems en route. As the internal hemorrhage and swelling increases, the occlusion becomes more complete, and the individual's breathing becomes more difficult. Panic and anxiety can increase respiration and, in doing so, compound the problem. Swelling usually is maximal within 6 hours but may occur as late as 24 to 48 hours after injury. Cyanosis and a loss of consciousness may occur with a complete occlusion.

APPLICATION STRATEGY 23.1

Management Algorithm for Tracheal and Laryngeal Injuries

If severe anterior throat trauma has occurred:

Assume a possible spinal injury and treat accordingly.

Ensure an open airway:

- If needed, use the jaw-thrust maneuver to achieve a chin-up position.
- Apply ice to control swelling, if appropriate.

If an obvious deformity is present in the pharynx:

Manually straighten the airway.

If a major laceration is present:

- Control hemorrhage with firm, manual pressure.
- Maintain pressure during assessment.
- Loosen any restrictive clothing.
- To reduce panic or anxiety, talk calmly to the patient, providing assurance that you are there to help.
- Treat for shock and monitor vital signs until EMS arrives.

Management

In an effort to diminish panic and anxiety resulting from the sudden inability to breathe, the clinician should immediately reassure the patient. The clinician should help the patient to focus on his or her breathing rate.

 Activate the emergency medical plan, including summoning EMS.

 The basketball player struck in the anterior neck could have a contusion or fracture to the trachea, larynx, or hyoid bone. In an effort to diminish panic and anxiety because of the sudden inability to breathe, the clinician should immediately reassure the patient. An open airway should be maintained, and the patient should be asked to focus on the breathing rate. In cases involving severe anterior neck trauma or spasm, it is important to consider an associated injury to the cervical spine. If breathing does not return to normal in a few minutes, activation of the emergency medical plan, including summoning EMS, is warranted.

BOX 23.3 Signs and Symptoms Indicating Tracheal and Laryngeal Injuries

- Mild bruising and redness
- Shortness of breath
- Pain and point tenderness
- Subcutaneous crepitation
- Difficulty swallowing or coughing
- Spasmodic coughing

- Hoarseness or loss of voice[a]
- Laryngospasm[a]
- Presence of hemorrhage with blood-tinged sputum[a]
- Loss of contour of the Adam's apple (thyroid cartilage)[a]
- Cyanosis or respiratory distress

[a]A "red flag" that necessitates activation of EMS.

THORACIC CONDITIONS

In an effort to improve his cardiovascular fitness, a healthy, 35-year-old man began a supervised running program. He has been running for 3 weeks and occasionally experiences a stitch in the side while running. A physician has advised him that the condition is not serious and has suggested that he attempt to run through the pain. What techniques can be used to alleviate the pain while running?

Thoracic injuries frequently are caused by sudden deceleration and impact, which can lead to compression and a subsequent deformation of the rib cage. The extent of damage depends on the direction, the magnitude of force, and the point of impact. For example, a glancing blow may bruise the chest wall, whereas a baseball that strikes the ribs directly may fracture a rib and drive the bony fragments internally, causing subsequent lung or cardiac damage. **Box 23.4** identifies signs and symptoms that indicate a serious thoracic condition.

Stitch in the Side

Etiology

Potential causes include trapped colonic gas bubbles, localized diaphragmatic hypoxia with spasm, liver congestion with stretching of the liver capsule, and poor conditioning.

Signs and Symptoms

A stitch in the side refers to a sharp pain or spasm in the chest wall, usually on the lower right side, during exertion.

Management

The frequency of a stitch usually diminishes as an individual's level of aerobic conditioning improves. Attempts can be made to run through the pain by the following:

- Forcibly exhaling through pursed lips
- Breathing deeply and regularly
- Leaning away from the affected side
- Stretching the arm on the affected side over the head as high as possible

Breast Conditions

Excessive breast motion during activity can lead to soreness, contusions, and nipple irritation. Although breast conditions usually are associated with women, men also may have conditions of the breast and nipples inducting contusion, gynecomastia, and nipple irritation.

BOX 23.4 Red Flags Indicating a Serious Thoracic Condition

- Shortness of breath or difficulty breathing
- Deviated trachea or trachea that moves during breathing
- Anxiety, fear, confusion, or restlessness
- Distended neck veins
- Bulging or bloodshot eyes
- Suspected rib or sternal fracture

- Severe chest pain aggravated by deep inspiration
- Abnormal chest movement on affected side
- Coughing up bright red or frothy blood
- Abnormal or absent breath sounds
- Rapid, weak pulse
- Low blood pressure
- Cyanosis

Contusions

■ Etiology

Excessive breast motion or direct trauma can lead to hemorrhage and edema formation in the breast tissue. Moderate-to-severe contusions to the breast may produce fat necrosis or a hematoma formation, both of which are painful and may result in the formation of a localized breast mass. The appearance of these lesions on a mammogram may be indistinguishable from that of a malignant tumor. Direct trauma should be recorded on a woman's permanent medical record to avoid any erroneous conclusions when reading a future mammogram.

■ Signs and Symptoms

In mild contusion, hemorrhage and edema may be present in the soft tissue of the breast. In moderate contusion, a painful hematoma may be present.

■ Management

Immediate management of a breast contusion includes the application of ice and external support to the area.

Nipple Irritation

■ Etiology

Nipple irritation commonly is seen in distance runners. Two commonly seen conditions are called runner's nipples and cyclist's nipples. **Runner's nipples** are associated with friction over the nipple area. **Cyclist's nipples** are caused by the combined effects of perspiration and wind chill.

■ Signs and Symptoms

With runner's nipples, the shirt rubs over the nipples causing friction, which can lead to abrasions, blisters, or bleeding. In cyclist's nipples, the nipples become cold and painful. Each condition can persist for several days.

■ Management

The initial treatment of runner's nipples involves cleansing the wound, applying an antibiotic ointment, and covering the wound with a nonadhering, sterile gauze pad. Infection secondary to the injury may involve the entire nipple region or may extend into the breast tissue and necessitate referral to a physician. This condition can be prevented by applying petroleum-based products and adhesive bandages over the nipples. The initial treatment for cyclist's nipples is to warm the nipples after completion of the event to prevent irritation. This condition can be prevented by wearing a windproof jacket.

Gynecomastia

■ Etiology

Gynecomastia is an excessive development of the male breast tissue, often accompanied by pain or sensitivity. The condition usually is bilateral and is more prevalent in adolescent males, particularly those taking anabolic steroids. Other causes include testicular, pituitary, and adrenal pathologies.

■ Sign and Symptoms

Symptoms associated with the condition include nipple soreness, tenderness to pressure, and increased susceptibility to irritation through friction from a shirt.

■ Management

Typically, the condition is physiological and resolves spontaneously in 6 to 12 months. Occasionally, surgical removal of extra breast tissue may be indicated for cosmetic reasons or for a biopsy specimen to rule out malignancy.

Strain of the Pectoralis Major Muscle

Etiology

Strains of the pectoralis major muscle can occur in a variety of activities, including power lifting (particularly while bench pressing), boxing, and wrestling. The mechanism of injury usually is indirect, resulting from extreme eccentric muscle tension. A rupture results when the actively contracting muscle is overburdened by a load or an extrinsic force that exceeds tissue tolerance. A strain of the pectoralis major also can result from direct trauma involving a sudden deceleration maneuver, such as when punching in boxing or blocking with an extended arm in football.

Ruptures are seen almost exclusively in men between 20 and 40 years of age.[6] A higher incidence of this injury is seen with anabolic steroid abuse.[7,8] Steroid use causes muscle hypertrophy and an increase in power secondary to rapid strength gain not accompanied by a concomitant increase in tendon size.

Signs and Symptoms

An audible pop, snap, or tearing sensation usually is accompanied by immediate, marked pain and weakness. The pain often is described as an aching or fatigue-like pain rather than a sharp pain. If the proximal attachment ruptures, the muscle retracts toward the axillary fold, causing it to appear enlarged. Swelling and ecchymosis are limited to the anterior chest wall. If the distal attachment is ruptured, the muscle bulges medially into the chest region, causing the axillary fold to appear thin. Swelling and ecchymosis occur on the anterior chest wall and upper arm. Shoulder motion is limited by pain. Horizontal adduction and internal rotation of the shoulder are weak and accentuate the deformity.

Management

Treatment depends on the extent of damage and follows the standard protocol for muscle strains. If the strain is mild or moderate, the subsequent treatment should focus on control of the inflammation, protected ROM exercises, and gradual strengthening. When ROM has been achieved, the individual's strength, endurance, and power can be restored.

Rupture of the muscle can require surgical intervention. Surgical treatment has been performed successfully following delays as long as 5 years after the injury; however, the best results are achieved with prompt recognition and surgery.[7,9]

Costochondral Injury

Etiology

Costochondritis and costochondral sprains may occur during a collision with another object or as a result of a severe twisting motion of the thorax, such as during the sweep motion in rowing.[10] This action can sprain or separate the costal cartilage where it attaches to the sternum or where the anterior margin of the rib attaches to the anterior end of the costal cartilage, thus putting pressure on the intercostal nerve lying between it and the rib above (**Fig. 23.17**). Slipping rib syndrome, as it sometimes is called, more frequently involves the 10th rib, followed by the 9th or 8th rib. The onset of symptoms may be insidious, occurring long after the initial trauma.[11]

Signs and Symptoms

The individual may hear or feel a pop. The initial localized sharp pain may be followed by intermittent stabbing pain for several days. Pain may slowly decrease in intensity, but sharp clicks may occur during bending maneuvers as the displaced cartilage overrides the bone. A visible deformity and localized pain can be palpated at the involved joint. The pain can be reproduced either by hooking the fingers under the anterior costal

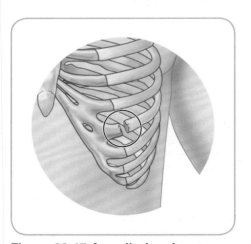

Figure 23.17. An undisplaced costochondral separation. The costal cartilage separates from the site at which the anterior margin of the rib attaches to the anterior end of the costal cartilage.

margin and by pulling the rib cage anteriorly or by adducting the arm on the affected side coupled with rotation of the head toward the affected side.[10] More severe sprains produce pain during deep inhalation and can refer the pain to the epigastric region or the spine.

Management

The standard acute protocol should be followed to reduce pain and inflammation. The individual should be referred to a physician for further assessment. The discomfort usually resolves itself with 3 or 4 weeks of rest and anti-inflammatory medication, but it may persist for 9 to 12 weeks. Occasionally, a physician may choose to inject the site with steroid medication to relieve chronic pain.

Sternal Fractures

Etiology

The sternum rarely is fractured in sports, but such an injury may occur as a result of rapid deceleration and high impact into an object or acute flexion that causes the upper fragment to displace anteriorly over the lower fragment. The fracture itself is not significant; however, the incidence of an associated intrathoracic injury is high. The most common site of fracture is the body of the sternum, with most fractures transverse.[12]

Signs and Symptoms

A sternal fracture causes an immediate loss of breath. Localized pain is present, with pressure over the sternum, and is aggravated by deep inspiration if the fracture is incomplete. If the fracture is complete, a palpable defect is present, and pain occurs during normal respiration. Because of the anatomical location, any suspected fracture should be assessed for underlying injury, such as cardiac contusion, injury of internal mammary vessels, retrosternal and mediastinal hematoma, and pulmonary laceration or contusion.[8]

> If a sternal fracture is suspected, the emergency plan, including summoning EMS, should be activated. Observation in the hospital with a cardiac monitor often is necessary because of the high incidence of associated intrathoracic trauma. While waiting for EMS to arrive, the clinician should maintain the airway, assess vital signs, and treat for shock as necessary.

Management

The treatment of an undisplaced sternal fracture is nonoperative. Rest and pain control with analgesics is recommended. Surgical repair utilizing wiring, plates, and screws is used for unstable injuries, displaced factures, and uncontrollable pain and associated injuries that complicate pulmonary or cardiac function. Other cases involving persistent pain, nonunion, or malunion with deformity may also require surgical intervention.[12]

Rib Fractures

Etiology

Stress fractures to the ribs can result from an indirect force, such as a violent muscle contraction. They typically occur at the rib's weakest point (i.e., where it changes direction or has the smallest diameter). Opposing contractions of the scalene muscles and upper digitations of the serratus anterior muscle may fracture the 1st rib at its thinnest segment where the subclavian artery crosses, as is seen in weight lifting or baseball pitching. Anterolateral stress fractures of the 4th and 5th ribs have been reported in golfers and rowers because of excessive action of the serratus anterior muscle.[8,9] Violent muscle contractions also are known to cause fractures to the floating ribs or avulsion fractures to the lower three ribs. In particular, the external oblique muscles often are involved.

Rib fractures are the most common thoracic injury as a result of blunt trauma.[13] The force usually is applied in the anteroposterior plane, leading to fractures at the posterior angles of the 5th through 9th ribs. Nondisplaced fractures are more common than displaced. If the fracture is displaced, the clinician should conduct an internal injury assessment. If a fracture occurs to the lower two ribs, there may be associated damage to the kidneys, liver, or spleen. Splenic trauma has been reported in up to 20% of left lower rib fractures, and liver trauma has been reported in up to 10% of right lower rib fractures.[10]

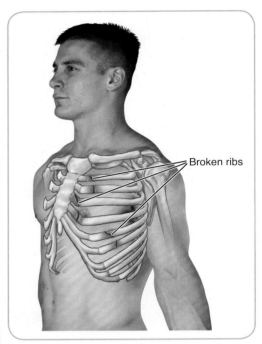

Figure 23.18. An undisplaced fractured rib.

If three or more ribs are fractured indicating presence of a flail chest, or signs and symptoms suggesting internal injury are present, the emergency plan, including summoning EMS, should be activated. While waiting for EMS to arrive, the clinician should maintain the airway, assess vital signs, and treat for shock as necessary.

Signs and Symptoms

Intense localized pain over the fracture site is aggravated by deep inspiration, coughing, or chest movement (**Fig. 23.18**). In many cases, the individual takes shallow breaths and leans toward the fracture site, stabilizing the area with a hand to prevent excessive movement of the chest to ease the pain. A visible contusion and palpable crepitus may be present at the impact site. If the fracture has displaced and punctured a lung, the patient may cough up blood, especially bright red or frothy blood. A stethoscope should be used to listen for abnormal or absent breath sounds in the lungs. The rate and depth of respirations should be recorded. Manual compression of the rib cage in an anteroposterior direction and in a lateral compression produces pain over the fracture site (see **Fig. 23.13**). If any signs of respiratory distress, cyanosis, or shock appear, a thorough assessment for an underlying visceral injury should be conducted. **Box 23.5** identifies other signs and symptoms indicating a possible sternal or rib fracture.

Management

Treatment involves standard acute protocol. A 6-in elastic bandage can be wrapped around the thorax with circular motions distal to the injury site, or a sling and swathe may be used to immobilize the chest if pain is intense or multiple fractures are suspected. If one or two ribs are fractured, the individual should be referred to a physician immediately.

Pain tends to be most severe during the first 3 to 5 days following injury and ultimately disappears after 3 to 6 weeks. Depending on the fracture site, the presence of a displaced or nondisplaced fracture, and the number of ribs involved, it may be necessary to refrain from participation in sports and physical activities until healing is complete. Strapping or taping to reduce chest movement is not recommended, because it may aggravate the condition. With a simple fracture, a flak jacket or rib vest can be worn to protect the area from reinjury.

BOX 23.5 Signs and Symptoms Indicating a Possible Sternal or Rib Fracture

- History of direct blow, compression of the chest, or violent muscle contraction

- Individual may lean toward the fractured side, stabilizing the area with a hand to prevent movement of the chest

- Localized discoloration or swelling over the fracture site

- Visible, slight step deformity

- Palpable pain and crepitus at the fracture site

- Increased pain on deep inspiration

- Increased pain on trunk rotation and lateral flexion away from the fracture site

- Increased pain on manual compression of the rib cage in an anteroposterior direction or with lateral compression

- Shallow breathing

- Cyanosis

- Rapid, weak pulse and low blood pressure with multiple fractures; with a fracture that has damaged intercostals, vessels, and nerves; or if the lung or pleural sac has been penetrated

The male runner could attempt the following: exhaling forcibly through pursed lips, breathing deeply and regularly, leaning away from the affected side, or stretching the arm on the affected side over the head as high as possible.

INTERNAL COMPLICATIONS

 During preseason volleyball practice, a player experiences hyperventilation while sprinting. What is the management of this condition?

Several conditions may alter breathing and cardiac function. Hyperventilation is associated with an inability to catch one's breath and, in most instances, is not a serious problem. Direct trauma to the thorax can lead to serious underlying problems, although these conditions are rare in sport participation. Among the more serious complications are pulmonary contusion, pneumothorax, tension pneumothorax, hemothorax, and heart contusions.

Hyperventilation
Etiology

Hyperventilation often is linked to pain, stress, or trauma in sport participation. Other causes may include altitude, asthma, pulmonary embolus, left ventricular failure, aspirin, alcohol withdrawal, anxiety or panic, or central nervous system lesions.[14] The respiratory rate increases during activity. Rapid, deep inhalations draw more oxygen into the lungs. Conversely, long exhalations result in too much carbon dioxide being exhaled.

Signs and Symptoms

Signs and symptoms include an inability to catch one's breath, numbness in the lips and hands, spasm of the hands, chest pain, dry mouth, dizziness, and occasionally, fainting. Inspiratory difficulty or frequent sighing may also be present.

Management

It is important to calm the individual because panic and anxiety can complicate the condition. Treatment involves concentrating on slow inhalations through the nose and exhalations through the mouth until the symptoms have stopped. Although breathing into a paper bag has proved to be quite successful in restoring the oxygen–carbon dioxide balance, many individuals find it to be embarrassing. Breathing into a paper bag is not needed except in severe cases.

Lung Injuries
Etiology

Injury to the lungs can range from a contusion to a life-threatening situation. Nonpenetrating chest trauma is rare in sport participation. Forces transmitted through the thorax, as in landing on a football or a body slam onto the hard ground, cause blood and protein to leak into the alveoli and interstitial spaces, leading to pulmonary collapse. Penetrating chest trauma, due to a fractured rib or a penetrating wound to the chest (e.g., a stab wound), can result in a laceration of lung tissue.

Signs and Symptoms

Common signs and symptoms of pulmonary **contusions** include chest pain, rapid breathing, shortness of breath, rales, and coughing. Breathing may be compromised, and hypoxia may appear 2 to 4 hours after trauma. The condition may go undetected until the individual coughs up blood or has other problems, such as a pneumothorax, rib fracture, or subcutaneous emphysema.

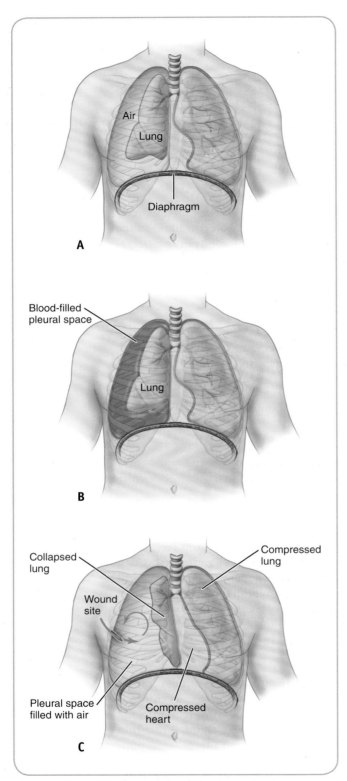

Figure 23.19. The internal complication to the lungs.
A, Pneumothorax. **B,** Hemothorax. **C,** Tension pneumothorax. Each condition can become life threatening if the lung collapses.

A **pneumothorax** is a condition whereby air is trapped in the pleural space, causing a portion of a lung to collapse. Although the etiology of a pneumothorax can vary, the two most common types are spontaneous and nonspontaneous. Spontaneous pneumothorax occurs unexpectedly, with or without an underlying disease. Risk factors include male gender, cigarette smoking, and an asthenic physiognomy.[15] In particular, 20- to 30-year-old males who are tall, lean, and have a long and narrow chest appear to be at increased risk. Other pulmonary conditions that may lead to a spontaneous pneumothorax include asthma, cystic fibrosis, emphysema, and pneumonia.[16] In a spontaneous pneumothorax, pain can stop abruptly after onset, leading to a delay in treatment. Dyspnea and chest discomfort gradually increase until the individual finally seeks medical care. In some cases, symptoms may flare up suddenly, producing acute pain localized to the side of the pneumothorax and difficulty in breathing.

Nonspontaneous, or traumatic, pneumothorax ranks second only to rib fractures as the most common sign of chest injury and can be seen in 40% to 50% of patients with chest trauma.[15] Air is allowed to escape into the pleural cavity with each inhalation, thus preventing the lung from expanding fully (**Fig. 23.19A**). The most common symptoms of a traumatic pneumothorax are dyspnea, cyanosis, severe chest pain on the affected side, deviation of the trachea, and decreased or absent breath sounds over the affected area with hyperresonance to percussion (**Box 23.6**).[17] Other symptoms may include asymmetric chest expansion, confusion, fatigue, anxiety, restlessness, and a decrease in blood pressure. Pain may be referred to the shoulder tip, across the chest, or over the abdomen. If not recognized and treated promptly, the condition can develop into tension pneumothorax.

A **hemothorax** involves the loss of blood, rather than air, into the pleural cavity (**Fig. 23.19B**). Fractured ribs may tear lung tissue and blood vessels in the chest or chest cavity. The individual usually presents with severe pain, hypoxia, decreased breath sounds unilaterally or bilaterally, dyspnea, tachypnea, and dullness to percussion over the affected side.[17] The individual may cough up frothy blood. As the condition deteriorates, the signs and symptoms of shock appear, including hypotension, decreased venous return, and cyanosis. The neck veins may be flat, secondary to hypovolemia, or distended because of the mechanical effects of intrathoracic pressure. Tracheal deviation and/or a mediastinal shift are classic signs caused by the contents of the thoracic cavity shifting away from the accumulation of blood as a result of the increased intrathoracic pressure.[17]

A **tension pneumothorax** occurs when air or blood progressively accumulates in the pleural space during inspiration and cannot escape on expiration.

The pleural space expands with each breath, displacing the mediastinum to the opposite side. This displacement compresses the heart, the uninjured lung, the thoracic aorta, and the vena cava, causing a decrease in blood return to the right side of the heart, thereby decreasing cardiac output (**Fig. 23.19C**). Signs and symptoms include chest pain, tracheal deviation away from the tension pneumothorax, respiratory distress, unilateral absence of breath sounds on the affected side, hypotension, and circulatory compromise leading to cyanosis and possibly death.[13,17] Asymmetric chest wall movement may be visible, as may be distended neck veins.

Traumatic asphyxia results from direct, massive trauma to the thorax. Classic symptoms include a bluish tinge over the neck and facial regions, subconjunctival hemorrhage, ecchymosis, and minute hemorrhagic spots on the face. A loss of vision also has been reported as a result of retinal edema, but such a loss may improve within hours or days.

Management

Each of these conditions is considered a medical emergency, and the patient should be transported to the nearest hospital as quickly as possible. The individual should be kept calm, quiet, and seated while focusing on controlled breathing until the ambulance arrives.

Activation of the emergency plan, including summoning EMS, is warranted. While waiting for EMS to arrive, the clinician should maintain the airway, assess vital signs, and treat for shock as necessary.

Cardiac Injuries

Direct trauma to the upper left chest can compress the heart between the sternum and spine. Blunt trauma may lead to **cardiac tamponade** or cause **commotio cordis**. Other more insidious heart conditions that impact sport participants are heart murmurs and athletic heart syndrome.

Sudden death due to cardiac anomalies is defined as an event that is nontraumatic and unexpected and occurs either instantaneously or within minutes of an abrupt change in an individual's previous clinical state. For individuals younger than 35 years of age, the most common cause is **hypertrophic cardiomyopathy**, with a higher frequency seen in male athletes as compared with females.[16] Other causes of sudden death include abnormalities in the coronary arteries, aortic rupture associated with Marfan syndrome, and mitral valve prolapse. In individuals older than 35 years of age, the most common cause is ischemic coronary artery disease. Because of the complexity of sudden death, it is discussed in greater detail in Chapter 25.

Heart Contusion and Cardiac Tamponade

■ Etiology

Blunt chest trauma can compress the heart between the sternum and spine, leading to blunt cardiac injury or **heart contusion** (formally called myocardial contusion). The symptoms associated with heart contusions range from moderate to severe. Because it lies directly posterior to the sternum, the right ventricle often is injured. Red blood cells and fluid leak into the surrounding tissues and, in doing so, decreases circulation to the heart muscle. This action leads to localized cellular damage and necrosis of the heart tissue.[18] Cardiac tamponade is caused by the same mechanism.

Cardiac tamponade occurs when massive blunt trauma ruptures the myocardium or lacerates a coronary artery, which leads to an increased volume of blood or edematous exudate into the pericardial sac. As blood and fluid fill the pericardial sac, the tension limits venous inflow and diastolic filling, and cardiac output is diminished. The heart is unable to fill and/or pump effectively, and without early recognition and treatment, cardiac arrest occurs.[18]

■ Signs and Symptoms

Heart contusion will result in shortness of breath, chest and heart pain, weakness, and fatigue. Symptoms will range in severity. Decreased cardiac output secondary to arrhythmias, or irregular heartbeats, are of major concern. Shock may be present. In serious cases, the Beck triad may be present to signify possible cardiac tamponade (i.e., venous pressure elevation is apparent through distended neck veins, decreased arterial pressure [hypotension], muffled heart tones). Although heart contusion may be slow to present all symptoms, with cardiac tamponade, the individual collapses within seconds and goes into respiratory arrest.

■ Management

An ambulance should be summoned immediately for transport to the nearest hospital. The athletic trainer should treat the individual for shock and be prepared to do cardiopulmonary resuscitation (CPR) if vital signs are absent. In many cases, resuscitation is unsuccessful even if given immediately after the injury. This may result from structural cardiac disruption caused by the trauma.

Activation of the emergency plan, including summoning EMS, is warranted. While waiting for EMS to arrive, the clinician should maintain the airway and, if necessary, initiate breathing and chest compressions.

Commotio Cordis

Commotio cordis results when the heart is struck at the beginning of the T wave in the cardiac cycle and disrupts the electrical impulses that control normal heart rhythm.[18] The leading mechanism of injury was from a projectile striking the chest, including baseballs, softballs, hockey pucks, and lacrosse balls. Commotio cordis is described in detail in Chapter 24. Unlike cardiac tamponade, the patient collapses almost instantaneously upon impact due to ventricular tachycardia. The most effective treatment is immediate application of an automatic external defibrillator, although commotio cordis usually is a fatal event.

Heart Murmur

■ Etiology

Heart murmurs are distinguished from normal heart sounds by their longer duration. They are attributed to turbulent blood flow and may be benign or diagnostic of valvular heart disease. Murmurs are most often caused by defective heart valves. A stenotic heart valve has an abnormally narrowed valvular orifice that cannot open completely and obstructs blood flow, as in *aortic stenosis*. A valve may also be unable to close completely, as in *aortic regurgitation*, which is blood leaking backward through the valve when it should be closed. Murmurs also can be caused by conditions such as pregnancy, fever, thyrotoxicosis (a diseased condition resulting from an overactive thyroid gland), or anemia.

■ Signs and Symptoms

A diastolic murmur occurs when the heart muscle relaxes between beats. A systolic murmur occurs when the heart muscle contracts. Continuous murmurs are heard through the cardiac cycle and may present as a clicking, whooshing, or swishing noise heard through auscultation with a stethoscope. Systolic murmurs are graded by intensity (loudness) from 1 to 6. A grade 1 is very faint, heard only with a special effort. A grade 6 is extremely loud and can be heard with a stethoscope slightly removed from the chest.

■ Management

All heart murmurs should be assessed by a physician for a medical diagnosis to determine the source of the murmur and any underlying pathology. This is done through auscultation, chest X-rays, and echocardiograms. If the murmur does not indicate heart disease, sports participation is allowed with no restrictions.

Because hyperventilation can produce panic and anxiety, the clinician should initially attempt to calm the volleyball player. Next, the clinician should encourage the patient to concentrate on his or her breathing. Specifically, the patient should be instructed to inhale slowly through the nose and exhale through the mouth until breathing returns to normal. Breathing into a paper bag has proven to be quite successful in restoring the oxygen–carbon dioxide balance associated with hyperventilation, but this technique can be embarrassing for the patient and is not necessary except in severe cases.

ABDOMINAL WALL CONDITIONS

? Following a blow to the abdomen, a high school ice hockey player experiences dyspnea. A solar plexus contusion is suspected. How should the condition be managed?

The muscles of the abdominal wall are strong and powerful yet also flexible enough to absorb impact. Consequently, injuries to the abdominal wall usually are minor; however, some conditions, such as a contusion to the solar plexus and hernias, can affect sports participation.

Skin Contusions

Etiology

Blunt trauma can result in a minor contusion or damage to internal organs.

Signs and Symptoms

Simple contusions to the abdominal wall are evident by tenderness over the area of impact, pain during active contraction of the abdominal muscles, and the absence of referred pain. Any case involving blunt trauma requires an assessment to rule out internal injury. Information specific to intra-abdominal conditions is provided later in this chapter.

Management

The management of a simple contusion includes the application of ice and compression to limit the hemorrhage. A pressure dressing may be applied if a large hematoma forms.

Muscle Strains

Etiology

Muscle strains are caused by direct trauma, sudden twisting, or a sudden hyperextension of the spine. The rectus abdominis is the most commonly injured muscle. Complications arise when the epigastric artery or intramuscular vessels are damaged, leading to a rectus sheath hematoma. Nearly 80% of hematomas occur below the umbilicus.

Signs and Symptoms

Sudden abdominal pain, nausea, vomiting, marked tenderness, swelling, and muscle guarding may be present. Straight leg raising or hyperextension of the back increases the pain. A palpable mass may or may not be present; if a mass is present, it becomes fixed with contraction of the muscle. Other signs include a bluish discoloration around the periumbilical region 72 hours after injury (Cullen sign) and pain with resisted trunk or hip flexion.[8]

 If internal injury is suspected, activation of the emergency plan, including summoning EMS, is warranted. While waiting for EMS to arrive, the clinician should maintain the airway, assess vital signs, and treat for shock as necessary.

Management

Treatment consists of ice, rest, and the use of nonsteroidal anti-inflammatory drugs for the first 36 to 48 hours. Local heat and whirlpools can be used after

48 to 72 hours with activity modification until the hematoma and soreness resolve. Activities such as twisting, turning, trunk flexion, or sudden stretching should be avoided until painful symptoms subside.

Solar Plexus Contusion ("Wind Knocked Out")

Etiology

A blow to the abdomen with the muscles relaxed is referred to as a solar plexus punch. Although the true cause of the breathing difficulty is unknown, it is thought to be caused by diaphragmatic spasm and a transient contusion to the sympathetic **celiac plexus**.

Signs and Symptoms

The blow results in an immediate inability to catch one's breath (dyspnea). Fear and anxiety may complicate the condition.

Management

The assessment should include a thorough airway analysis. Any mouth guard or partial dental plates should be removed. Any restrictive equipment and clothing around the abdomen should be loosened, and the individual should be instructed to flex his or her knees toward the chest. Although it may seem paradoxic, the individual should be instructed to take a deep breath and hold it. This action should be repeated until normal breathing is restored. Another method for restoring normal breathing is to instruct the individual to whistle. This action forces the diaphragm to relax. Because a severe blow may lead to an intra-abdominal injury, an assessment should be performed to rule out an internal injury.

Hernias

Etiology

A **hernia**, which is a protrusion of the abdominal viscera through a weakened portion of the abdominal wall, can be either congenital or acquired. Congenital hernias are present at birth and may be related to family history. Acquired hernias occur after birth and may be aggravated by a direct blow, strain, or abnormal intra-abdominal pressure, such as that exerted during heavy weight lifting. The three most common hernias are indirect, direct, and femoral (**Fig. 23.20**).

An indirect inguinal hernia is the most common type of hernia in young athletes. A weakness in the peritoneum around the deep inguinal ring allows the abdominal viscera to protrude through the ring into the inguinal canal and, occasionally, even extend into the scrotum. This weakness in the peritoneum typically is not present in women. Large indirect hernias may reduce spontaneously, because they cannot extend easily into the inguinal canal. Direct hernias, which tend to be more common in men older than 40 years of age, result from a weakness in an area of fascia bounded by the rectus abdominis muscle, the inguinal ligament, and the epigastric vessels. Femoral hernias, more commonly seen in women, allow the abdominal viscera to protrude through the femoral ring into the femoral canal, compressing the lymph vessels,

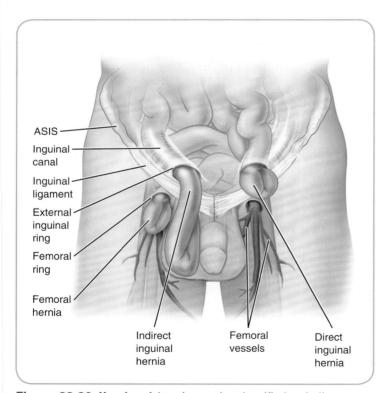

ASIS
Inguinal canal
Inguinal ligament
External inguinal ring
Femoral ring
Femoral hernia

Indirect inguinal hernia
Femoral vessels
Direct inguinal hernia

Figure 23.20. Hernias. A hernia may be classified as indirect **(A)**, in which the small intestine extends into the scrotum; direct **(B)**, in which the small intestine extends through a weakening in the internal inguinal ring; or femoral **(C)**, in which the small intestine protrudes posterior to the inguinal ligament and medial to the femoral artery. *ASIS*, anterior superior iliac spine.

connective tissue, and femoral artery and vein. The herniation presents as a mass that is inferolateral to the pubic tubercle and medial to the femoral artery and vein.

The danger of a hernia lies in continued trauma to the weakened area during falls, blows, or increased intra-abdominal pressure exerted during activity. The hernia can twist on itself and produce a strangulated hernia, which can become gangrenous.

Signs and Symptoms

Symptoms vary, but in most cases, the first sign of a hernia is a visible, tender swelling and an aching feeling in the groin. Some hernias are asymptomatic until the preparticipation examination, when the physician palpates the protrusion by invaginating the scrotum with a finger. Protrusion of the hernia increases with coughing.

Management

Most hernias require surgical repair. Individuals with an indirect hernia repair can begin walking, mild upper extremity exercises, and bicycling within 6 weeks of surgery. A return to noncontact sports participation can occur in 7 weeks, and a return to contact sports can occur within 8 to 10 weeks.

Repair of direct inguinal and femoral hernias is more extensive. Strenuous activities are prohibited for 3 weeks postsurgery. A return to noncontact sports can occur in 8 weeks, and a return to contact sports can occur in 12 weeks. Activities that stretch or pull the abdominal muscles should be avoided. Recommended activities include swimming, biking, and weight training for the upper extremities.

In some situations, an individual with a hernia that has not been repaired can participate in non-contact sports. Surgical repair is recommended to prevent recurrent, irreducible hernias, however, which can lead to a small bowel obstruction.

The ice hockey player experiencing dyspnea following a blow to the abdomen is believed to have sustained a solar plexus contusion. The management of this condition includes assessing the airway for obstruction, removing any mouth guard or dental apparatus, loosening restrictive equipment around the abdomen, and having the patient flex his knees toward his chest. If breathing does not return to normal within a few minutes, the emergency plan, including summoning EMS, should be activated.

INTRA-ABDOMINAL CONDITIONS

A 22-year-old lacrosse player was struck in the abdomen with an opponent's stick. She experienced a sudden onset of abdominal pain in the upper right quadrant. She also reported pain to the inferior angle of the right scapula. What injury should be suspected, and how should this condition be managed?

Trauma to the abdomen can lead to severe internal hemorrhage if organs or major blood vessels are lacerated or ruptured. Injuries can be open or closed, with closed injuries typically caused by blunt trauma. If damaged, hollow viscera can leak their contents into the abdominal cavity, causing severe hemorrhage, **peritonitis**, and shock. Many signs and symptoms indicating an intra-abdominal injury, regardless of the organ involved, are similar in nature (**Box 23.7**). Variations arise in the area of palpable pain and the site of referred pain.

Acute management of suspected intra-abdominal injuries also is very similar, regardless of the injured organ. Initially, the clinician should keep the individual relaxed while assessing the airway, breathing, and circulation. If necessary, the emergency medical plan, including summoning EMS, should be activated. While waiting for EMS to arrive, the individual should be placed in a supine position with the knees flexed to relax the low back and abdominal muscles. The vital signs should be monitored regularly, and the individual should be treated for shock. **Application Strategy 23.2** summarizes the acute management of intra-abdominal injuries.

BOX 23.7 **Common Signs and Symptoms of Intra-abdominal Pathology**

- Abdominal pain
- Abdominal tenderness and/or rigidity
- Presence of rebound tenderness
- Abdominal distention
- Absent or diminished bowel sounds

- Nausea and/or vomiting
- Hematuria
- Fever
- Shock

Splenic Rupture

Etiology

Although the spleen rarely is injured in sport participation, certain systemic disorders, such as infectious mononucleosis, can enlarge this organ, making it vulnerable to injury. The spleen is the most commonly injured abdominal organ and is the most frequent cause of death from abdominal blunt trauma in sports.[8] Subsequent to trauma, the spleen can lose blood very rapidly because of its vascularity; however, the spleen can splint itself and stop hemorrhaging. This may appear to be advantageous, but it actually is problematic because the splinting is not sufficient and a delayed hemorrhage can be produced days, weeks, or even months later after a seemingly minor jarring motion.

An individual who has infectious mononucleosis should be disqualified from contact and strenuous noncontact sports and physical activity for at least 3 weeks. After 3 weeks, a return to strenuous noncontact sports and physical activity is acceptable if the individual feels up to the activity, the spleen is nonpalpable, and the liver function tests are normal. If the spleen remains palpable or the liver function tests are abnormal, contact sports and activities are contraindicated for an additional week or longer.[19]

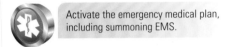 Activate the emergency medical plan, including summoning EMS.

APPLICATION STRATEGY **23.2**

Management Algorithm for Suspected Intra-abdominal Injuries

In case of vomiting:

Roll the person on the side to allow drainage.

Make certain the airway remains open.

Control any external hemorrhage with pressure and a sterile dressing.

Lay the patient supine:

- Keep the knees flexed to relax the abdominal muscles.
- Do not extend the legs or elevate the feet.

Record vital signs:

- Respiratory rate and depth (rapid, shallow breathing indicates shock)
- Pulse rate and strength (rapid, weak pulse indicates shock)
- Blood pressure (a marked drop in both readings indicates shock)
- Pupillary response to light (lackluster, dilated pupils indicates shock)

Do not give anything by mouth to the patient.

Treat for shock and monitor vital signs until EMS arrives.

Signs and Symptoms

Indications of a splenic rupture include a history of blunt trauma to the left upper quadrant and a persistent, dull pain in the upper left quadrant, left lower chest, and left shoulder, which is referred to as the **Kehr sign**. This referred pain, which is seen in nearly 60% of patients with a splenic injury, is caused by irritation of the diaphragm innervated by the phrenic nerves, which arise from the ventral rami of segments C3–C5.[20] The free blood also can irritate the right side of the diaphragm, in which case pain is referred to the dermatome patterns in the right shoulder. Symptoms at the time of injury include nausea, cold and clammy skin, and signs of shock.

Management

Treatment usually involves nonoperative intravenous therapy, strict bed rest, and intensive monitoring of vital signs. Because the spleen is essential to the body's immune system function, it is important to protect the individual by administering additional immunizations and considering the needs of an immunocompromised system. Physical activities should be restricted for at least 2 weeks. A return to vigorous physical activity is not recommended until 2 to 3 months after injury. If surgical repair is indicated, a minimum period of 3 months is needed for the abdominal musculature to heal and regain adequate strength before a return to vigorous activity. Most physicians recommend a 6-month interval after a splenectomy before an individual returns to contact sports.

If splenic injury is suspected, activation of the emergency plan, including summoning EMS, is warranted. While waiting for EMS to arrive, the clinician should maintain the airway, assess vital signs, and treat for shock as necessary. Refer to **Application Strategy 23.2** for further management procedures.

Liver Contusion and Rupture

Etiology

A direct blow to the upper right quadrant can contuse the liver. As with the spleen, systemic diseases, such as hepatitis, can enlarge the liver, thus making it more susceptible to injury.

If a liver injury is suspected, activation of the emergency plan, including summoning EMS, is warranted. While waiting for EMS to arrive, the clinician should maintain the airway, assess vital signs, and treat for shock as necessary.

Signs and Symptoms

Significant palpable pain, point tenderness, hypotension, and shock are indicative of liver trauma. In addition, pain may be referred to the inferior angle of the right scapula.

Management

An individual with a liver contusion should be referred immediately to a physician for diagnosis and treatment. An individual with an enlarged liver (i.e., hepatomegaly) should avoid contact sports until the liver has returned to its normal size or is nonpalpable. If lacerated, the liver is capable of massive bleeding; however, the bleeding typically stops by the time the wound is exposed during surgery. For this reason, there has been an increasing trend toward nonoperative management.[21] Refer to **Application Strategy 23.2** for further management procedures.

Appendicitis

Etiology

The vermiform appendix is a pouch extending from the cecum (see **Fig. 23.7**). If it becomes obstructed (e.g., with hardened fecal material), venous circulation can become impaired, leading to increased bacterial growth and the formation of pus. The resulting inflamed appendix, a condition called **appendicitis**, can lead to ischemia and gangrene. If the appendix ruptures, feces and bacteria are sprayed over the abdominal contents, causing peritonitis.

The patient needs to be referred for examination. In some cases, such as the presence of shock, vomiting, and diarrhea, activation of the emergency plan, including summoning EMS, is warranted. While waiting for EMS to arrive, the clinician should maintain the airway, assess vital signs, and treat for shock as necessary. Refer to **Application Strategy 23.2** for further management procedures.

Signs and Symptoms

Abdominal pain 2 to 7 days prior to the actual presentation of the condition is the most common symptom of acute appendicitis. Often, there is a history of classic migratory pain (initial periumbilical or epigastric pain) localizing to the right lower quadrant.[22] Rebound pain can be elicited at the McBurney point (**Fig. 23.15**), which is one-third the distance between the anterior superior iliac spine and the umbilicus. Other symptoms that may be present include a loss of appetite, nausea, vomiting, diarrhea, and low-grade fever.

Management

If the patient presents with symptoms consistent with more advanced stages, such as the presence of shock, vomiting, and diarrhea, the individual should be referred immediately to an acute medical facility. Surgical intervention is often required to remove the appendix.

Renal and Genitourinary Conditions

The kidneys are located in the retroperitoneal upper lumbar area of the abdomen. The upper third of the right kidney and upper half of the left kidney are located under the 12th rib. Posteriorly, the organs are protected by the psoas, paravertebral, and latissimus dorsi muscles and are encased in pericapsular fat. Despite this protection, the kidneys can be injured when the body is extended and the abdominal muscles are relaxed, such as when a receiver leaps to catch a pass. The ureters run along the posterior peritoneal wall and are at risk for injury where they cross the bony rim of the pelvis. The bladder lies with the pelvis and is more vulnerable to injury when full. Several chronic and acute conditions can affect these organs.

Kidney Contusion

■ Etiology

The kidney may be injured as a result of a direct blow or a contrecoup injury from a high-speed collision. Because the kidney normally is distended by blood, an external force can cause an abnormal extension of the engorged kidney. The degree of renal injury depends on the extent of the distention and on the angle and magnitude of the blow.

■ Signs and Symptoms

The individual may complain of pain, tenderness, and **hematuria**. Pain can be referred posteriorly to the low back region, to the sides of the buttocks, and anteriorly to the lower abdomen. Hypovolemic shock may result from extensive bleeding.

■ Management

Treatment involves applying ice to control inflammation and pain, treating for shock, and if needed, transporting the individual to the nearest medical facility. A radiograph or computed tomographic scan may be used to determine the extent of the injury. Most injuries are handled conservatively, with rest and fluid management. Spontaneous healing and a return of normal renal function can be expected. Individuals, who have a solitary kidney, especially when the kidney is pelvic, iliac, polycystic, or anatomically abnormal, should be counseled about the increased risk of injury. Although contact sports place the remaining kidney at very little risk, participation in contact or collision sports should be individually assessed. Use of a flak jacket or other customized padding may reduce the incidence of injury during contact or impact sports.

Kidney Stones

■ Etiology

Some substances filtered by the kidneys (especially calcium, oxalate, uric acid, and cystine) have a tendency to form crystals. Other substances (e.g., citrate and magnesium) help to prevent crystal formation. When these substances are not in balance, the urine becomes too concentrated, acidic, or alkaline, and crystals can form. Risk factors for this condition include a family history of kidney stones, being a white male between 20 and 40 years of age, certain diseases (e.g., gout, chronic urinary tract infections [UTIs], cystic kidney disease, hyperparathyroidism, renal tubular acidosis, and cystinuria), certain medications (e.g., diuretics), having only one kidney, eating a diet high in protein and low in fiber, a lack of adequate water intake, and living a sedentary lifestyle. In some cases, however, the exact cause of kidney stones may be unknown (i.e., idiopathic nephrolithiasis).

There are four main types of kidney stones, each stemming from a different cause:

- **Calcium stones.** Most kidney stones are formed from calcium (85% in men; 65% in women).[20] These stones may result from large amounts of vitamin D, which may cause the body to absorb too much calcium; drugs, such as thyroid hormones and some diuretics; certain cancers; overactive parathyroid glands; and some kidney conditions.

- **Uric acid stones.** As the name suggests, these stones are formed from uric acid, a byproduct of protein metabolism. A diet high in meat may cause excess amounts of uric acid in the urine. These stones also have been attributed to chemotherapy treatment.

- **Struvite stones.** Found mainly in women, struvite stones almost always are the result of chronic UTIs caused by bacteria that secrete specific enzymes. These enzymes increase the amount of ammonia in the urine, which makes up the crystals in struvite stones. These stones often are large and have a characteristic stag's horn shape, which can cause serious damage to the kidneys.

- **Cystine stones.** These stones represent approximately 1% of kidney stones. They form in people with a hereditary disorder that causes the kidneys to excrete excessive amounts of certain amino acids (cystinuria).

Over time, these crystals may combine to form a small, hard mass. In some cases, this mass or stone breaks off and passes into the ureter, eventually traveling to the bladder for expulsion.

■ Signs and Symptoms

Individuals may be asymptomatic until the kidney stone is large enough (>7 mm) to cause a blockage or infection. Then, an intense, colicky pain begins suddenly and intensifies over 15 to 30 minutes. The pain usually starts in the back or flank, just below the edge of the ribs, and moves anteriorly toward the groin as the stone moves down the ureter toward the bladder. If the stone stops moving, the pain may stop. Other signs and symptoms may include bloody, cloudy, or foul-smelling urine; nausea; vomiting; a persistent urge to urinate; and, if an infection is present, fever and chills.

■ Management

Treatment varies depending on the type of stone and on the cause. Individuals may be able to move the stone through the urinary tract simply by drinking as much as 2 to 3 quarts of water per day and by staying physically active. If the stones are too large to pass on their own or cause bleeding, kidney damage, or an ongoing UTI, surgical intervention with an extracorporeal shock wave lithotripsy may be necessary. Extracorporeal shock wave lithotripsy uses shock waves to break the stones into small crystals, which can then be passed in the urine. Following treatment, it may take several months for all the stone fragments to pass.

Urinary Tract Infections

■ Etiology

A UTI describes any infection that begins in the urinary system. Although many cases are simply painful and annoying, the condition can become a serious health problem if the infection spreads to the kidneys. Although any structure in the genitourinary system can be infected, most infections occur in the lower tract.

Cystitis (inflammation of the bladder) and **urethritis** (inflammation of the urethra) are the most common UTIs. Most cases are caused by *Escherichia coli*, which ascend the urinary tract from the opening in the urethra. The bacteria also may be introduced during urinary tract catheterization. In addition, urethritis can be caused by sexually transmitted organisms, such as *Chlamydia trachomatis* and *Neisseria gonorrhoeae*, which are the agents of chlamydia and gonorrhea, respectively. Women are 10 times more likely than men to have ascending UTIs, except when compared to men older than 50 years of age, largely because women have a shorter urethra. Sexually active women also are more susceptible to cystitis, because sexual intercourse enhances bacterial transfer from the urethra into the bladder.

■ Signs and Symptoms

Signs and symptoms may not be indicative regarding the severity of the condition. Some individuals may present with very few symptoms yet have significant **bacteriuria**. An individual with cystitis may complain of pain during urination (i.e., **dysuria**), urinary frequency and urgency, and pain superior to the pubic region. Cloudy, bloody, or foul-smelling urine also may be noted. An individual with urethritis may present similar symptoms, with the exception that the quality of the urine often is not affected. Other symptoms, such as high fever, shaking, chills, nausea, vomiting, and low back pain, may indicate a simultaneous upper UTI of the kidney (i.e., **acute pyelonephritis**). Urinalysis may reveal elevated levels of leukocytes, nitrates, and higher pH levels.

■ Management

Referral to a physician is necessary because a urine culture is required to identify the organism responsible for the infection. Subsequently, medication in the form of antibiotics and sulfa drugs is prescribed to treat the infection. Symptoms usually will clear within a few days of treatment, but it is critical to take the entire course of medication to ensure that the infection is completely eradicated. A longer course of antibiotic treatment may be recommended with recurrent UTIs. In addition, increased clear fluid intake may be recommended to promote urinary outflow. Analgesics, urinary antiseptics, and antispasmodics also may be prescribed for the relief of pain and bladder spasms.

Hematuria

■ Etiology

Blood in the urine (i.e., **hematuria**) can be macroscopic, gross, or microscopic. The condition may be caused by a direct kidney injury, bladder contusion, UTI, drug or medication use, "march" or foot-strike hemolysis, infection, sickle cell disease, rhabdomyolysis, or preexisting pathology. Nontraumatic renal hematuria, referred to as athletic pseudonephritis, is characterized by decreased renal blood flow that leads to ischemia in the kidney and the subsequent passage of red blood cells. Traumatic renal hematuria involves obvious direct contact or indirect trauma from repetitive jarring during running or jumping. Traumatic bladder hematuria is believed to result from repetitive contact of the posterior bladder wall against the base of the bladder. Most participants in sports and physical activity void before activity. Running with an empty bladder increases the risk of gross hematuria (i.e., visible blood in the urine) because no fluid cushion exists between the posterior wall and the base of the bladder. This condition commonly is seen in long-distance runners, hence the name runner's bladder. Hematuria caused by running resolves within 24 to 48 hours of rest.

■ Signs and Symptoms

Massive external trauma associated with pelvic fractures can seriously damage the bladder, leading to lower abdominal pain and tenderness. Bruising in the lower abdominal region may be visible. Palpation may reveal abdominal tenderness, muscle guarding, or rigidity. An individual with a bladder contusion is able to void, and gross or microscopic hematuria is present. An individual with a bladder rupture usually is unable to void, and a specimen obtained by a catheter reveals blood in the pelvic cavity.

■ Management

Physically active individuals with benign hematuria secondary to exercise may continue to be active but should be encouraged to drink quantities of clear fluids before, during, and after exercise to avoid dehydration. Small amounts of urine should be maintained in the bladder during exercise to cushion against repetitive trauma. If gross or microscopic hematuria persists, referral to a physician is necessary. Additional tests may be necessary to rule out serious underlying conditions, such as renal disease, sickle cell anemia, and urine cytology.

Proteinuria

■ Etiology

In the kidney, blood filtration occurs primarily in the glomeruli, which are microscopic, raspberry-shaped tangles of blood vessels. The glomeruli permit small molecules, such as waste products, to escape from the bloodstream into the urine for removal from the body while keeping larger molecules, such as useful proteins, in circulation. Normal protein excretion is 30 to 45 mg per day. Elevated levels of protein, primarily albumin, are thought to occur in as many as 70% of competitive athletes after exertion.[23] Other conditions that may lead to elevated protein levels include dehydration, heat-related illness, fever, emotional stress, inflammatory conditions, some acute illnesses (e.g., diabetes, hypertension, and some kidney diseases), orthostatic (postural) disorder, pregnancy, and regular high-protein diets.

Excessive protein in the urine (≥150 mg per day) may indicate early signs of renal disease. In the United States, diabetes is the leading cause of end-stage renal disease. In both type 1 and type 2 diabetes, the first sign of deteriorating kidney function is minute amounts of albumin in the urine, a condition called **microalbuminuria**. As kidney function declines, levels of albumin in the urine increase, and microalbuminuria becomes full-fledged proteinuria.

Hypertension is the second leading cause of end-stage renal disease and, if not controlled, can progress to renal failure. African Americans in the age range of 20 to 49 years are 20-fold more likely than their white counterparts to develop hypertension-related kidney failure. Other groups at risk for proteinuria are American Indians, Hispanic Americans, Pacific Islander Americans, older people, and overweight people.[24] People with a family history of kidney disease should have their urine tested regularly.

■ Signs and Symptoms

Albumin functions to retain fluid in the blood by acting like a sponge to soak up fluid from body tissues. Because the protein has been excreted, blood can no longer soak up enough fluid, leading to noticeable swelling in the hands, feet, abdomen, or face. Large amounts of protein in the urine may cause it to look foamy in the toilet. More commonly, however, no signs or symptoms are noticeable.

■ Management

Testing a urine sample with a chemically treated dipstick is the only way to determine the amount of protein in the urine. In the absence of protein, the dipstick panel is yellow; proteins in the solution interfere with the dye–buffer combination, causing the panel to turn green. Exertional proteinuria usually reads 2+ to 3+ by dipstick measurement within 30 minutes of exercise but clears in 24 to 48 hours. Evidence suggests a direct relationship between the intensity of exercise and the amount of proteinuria.[23] False-positive results can occur under the following conditions:

■ Alkaline urine (pH >7.5)

■ Dipstick immersed too long

■ Highly concentrated urine

■ Gross hematuria

■ Presence of penicillin, sulfonamides, or tolbutamide

■ Presence of pus, semen, or vaginal secretions

False-negative results can occur with dilute urine and when the urinary proteins are nonalbumin or of low molecular weight.[24,25] Because the results of urine dipstick analysis are a crude estimate for the urine protein concentration, individuals with positive findings should be referred to a physician for a more complete evaluation. More sensitive tests for protein or albumin in the urine are recommended for individuals at risk of kidney disease, especially those with diabetes. If a laboratory test shows high levels of protein, the test should be repeated 1 to 2 weeks later. If the second test also shows high levels, additional tests should be conducted to evaluate kidney function.

A physician may prescribe an angiotensin-converting enzyme inhibitor or an angiotensin-receptor blocker for an individual with diabetes or hypertension. These drugs have been found to protect kidney function even more than other drugs that provide the same level of blood pressure control. A restriction of dietary salt and protein intake also may be recommended.[24]

The lacrosse player had a history of direct trauma to the upper right quadrant of the abdomen. In addition to pain at the site of the trauma, she reported pain to the inferior border of the right scapula. This history suggests a possible liver contusion or rupture. This condition warrants activation of the emergency medical plan, including summoning EMS.

INJURIES AND CONDITIONS OF THE GENITALIA

? While attempting to tag a sliding base runner, a baseball player was struck in the groin by an opponent's foot. He immediately fell to the ground and drew his knees to the chest while grasping the genital region. What possible conditions can occur as a result of direct trauma to the genitalia? What signs and symptoms indicate that an immediate referral to a physician is warranted?

The male genitalia are more susceptible to injury than female genitalia because several structures are external to the body and, as such, are exposed to direct trauma. Protective cups can protect the penis and scrotum from injury. Direct trauma can damage the penis, urethra, and scrotum, which holds the testes. In addition, congenital variations in testicular suspension make certain individuals susceptible to torsion of the testicle.

Male Genital Injuries

Direct trauma to the groin can cause severe pain and dysfunction to the testes and penis. Lacerations are rare, but swelling and hemorrhage inside the scrotal sac can occur. As part of the follow-up management of an injury to the male genital organs, the individual should be instructed to perform a periodic self-assessment for pain and swelling and be provided with guidelines on seeking further medical care if necessary.

Penile Injuries

■ Etiology
Superficial wounds to the penis may involve a contusion, abrasion, laceration, avulsion, or penetrating wound. In addition, the urethra can be damaged. Cyclists may develop transient paresthesia of the penis as a result of pressure on the pudendal nerve.

■ Signs and Symptoms
Extreme pain and discomfort will be present, with associated bleeding from the wound.

■ Management
Most injuries resolve without specific treatment. Superficial bleeding should be controlled by applying a cold compress. Referral to a physician is only necessary if the hemorrhage persists or if swelling impairs the function of the urethra, leading to an inability to void. Adjusting the saddle height, tilt, and number of cycling bouts usually resolves the condition. Rising up on the pedals also can relieve pressure temporarily.

Scrotal Injuries

■ Etiology
Blunt scrotal trauma can cause a contusion, hematoma, torsion, dislocation, or rupture of a testicle. If the tunica vaginalis ruptures, the vascular and tubercle components of the testes can be seriously damaged.

■ Signs and Symptoms
Direct trauma to the groin can compress the testicles against the pelvis, leading to a nauseating, painful condition. Immediate internal hemorrhage, effusion, and muscle spasms may occur.

Occasionally, blunt trauma leads to swelling in the tunica vaginalis (**traumatic hydrocele**) (**Fig. 23.21A**). In 9% to 19% of men, the plexus of veins on the posterior testicle can become engorged, constituting a **varicocele**. These lesions may be described as "a bag of worms" adjacent to the testicle and cord (**Fig. 23.21B**). If the plexus ruptures in response to blunt trauma, blood rapidly accumulates in the scrotum, leading to a **hematocele**. In nearly 50% of patients with traumatic hematocele, testicular rupture also is present. Pain is not a good indicator of which structure is damaged. Swelling and hemorrhage inside the scrotal sac can enlarge the sac to the size of a tennis ball or grapefruit. Each condition can lead to irreparable testicular damage if an evaluation and treatment by a physician is delayed.

An individual with torsion of a testicle may or may not have a history of trauma. Congenital variations in the testicular suspension can cause rotational twisting of the vascular pedicle and spermatic cord, producing varying degrees of circulatory compromise (**Fig. 23.21C**). This condition typically is seen at or around puberty, manifesting itself after physical activity. Groin pain may develop gradually or rapidly, and it sometimes occurs with associated nausea and vomiting. Immediate referral to a physician is necessary if correction of the condition is to be successful. A high-resolution ultrasound is used to determine if the blood supply is absent in the testicle as well as the extent and severity of the injury. Recovery is nearly 100% if corrected within 6 to 8 hours.

A scrotal mass also can be indicative of testicular cancer, which is the most common malignancy in males from 16 to 35 years of age. Males with an undescended or partially descended testicle are at higher risk than others for developing testicular cancer. The first sign of a mass is a slightly enlarged testicle that has a change in its consistency. The mass is separate from the cord and epididymis. In many cases, a dull ache or a sensation of dragging and heaviness is present in the lower abdomen or groin. The diagnosis is established using ultrasound or transillumination with a bright light. Early detection and surgical treatment yields an excellent survival rate.

■ Management
A testicular spasm can be relieved by placing the individual on his back and flexing his knees toward the chest (**Fig. 23.22**). Another method to reduce testicular spasm involves lifting the individual a few inches off the ground and then dropping him to the ground. As the pain subsides, a cold compress should be placed on the scrotum to reduce swelling and hemorrhage. Treatment for swelling inside the scrotal sac involves aspiration of fluid and an injection of a solution to toughen the involved tissues. Symptoms disappear in 85% to 90% of the cases with this treatment. Suspected testicular cancer should be immediately referred to a physician as the condition is highly treatable when diagnosed early.

Female Genital Injuries
Etiology

Injuries to the vulva usually are caused by trauma associated with a fall, straddling, or penetration resulting in forced perineal stretching because of sudden leg abduction. These injuries have occurred in a variety of activities, including gymnastics, water skiing, snowmobiling, motorcycling, bicycling, sledding, cross-country skiing, and horseback riding.

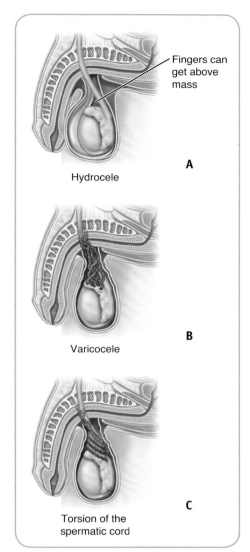

Fingers can get above mass

Hydrocele **A**

Varicocele **B**

Torsion of the spermatic cord **C**

Figure 23.21. Testicular injury.
A, Hydrocele. **B,** Varicocele. **C,** Spermatic cord torsion around the tunica vaginalis.

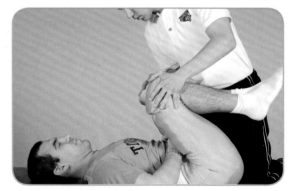

Figure 23.22. Relieving a testicular spasm. The patient should lie on his back and flex the knees toward the chest until pain is relieved.

Signs and Symptoms

A hematoma can result from a direct impact to the genital region. If the trauma is great enough, the pubic symphysis may also be injured, leading to osteitis pubis.

Management

Nearly all injuries are easily treated by the application of ice, mild compression, and bed rest. Occasionally, high-speed water skiing injuries result in water being forced under high pressure into the vulva and vagina, leading to a rupture of the vaginal walls. The water also can be forced through the uterus and fallopian tubes, leading to localized pelvic peritonitis. These injuries are easily preventable by wearing a neoprene wetsuit or nylon-reinforced suit.

 Direct trauma to the groin can lead to a laceration, scrotal contusion, hematoma, torsion, dislocation, or rupture of the testicles. If persistent pain or swelling of the testicles occurs, the patient should seek immediate medical attention.

SUMMARY

1. Severe blunt trauma to the anterior neck region, thorax, and viscera can have devastating effects that lead to serious ventilatory and circulatory compromise.

2. Blows to the throat may result in severe pain, laryngospasm, and acute respiratory distress.

3. A stitch in the side is a sharp pain or spasm in the chest wall, usually on the lower right side. Several strategies can be used to enable the affected individual to run through the pain.

4. Severe blunt trauma to the breast should be documented on a woman's permanent medical record to avoid misreading a mammogram.

5. A strain of the pectoralis major muscle involves an actively contracting muscle that is overburdened by a load or extrinsic force that exceeds tissue tolerance. If muscle fibers have been ruptured, resisted horizontal adduction and internal rotation of the shoulder are weak and accentuate the deformity.

6. Signs and symptoms indicating a possible internal thoracic condition include the following:

   - Shortness of breath or difficulty breathing

   - Severe chest pain aggravated by deep inspiration

   - Abnormal chest movement

   - Abnormal or absent breath sounds

7. A hernia is a protrusion of abdominal viscera through a weakened portion of the abdominal wall and can be either congenital or acquired. An indirect inguinal hernia is the most common hernia in young athletes.

8. Signs and symptoms indicating a possible intra-abdominal condition include the following:

   - Severe abdominal pain

   - Nausea or vomiting

   - Distended abdomen

   - Tenderness, rigidity, or muscle spasm

   - Rebound pain

■ Absence of bowel sounds

■ Blood in the urine or stool

9. Certain injuries may not develop until hours, days, or even weeks later. As such, the presumption of possible intrathoracic or intra-abdominal injuries with any blunt trauma necessitates a complete assessment.

10. Assessment of injury to the thorax and visceral region should focus on the vital signs and history of the injury.

11. Observation, palpation, and sites of referred pain can confirm suspicions of an existing internal injury.

12. If at any time, signs and symptoms indicate an intrathoracic or intra-abdominal injury, the emergency medical plan, including summoning EMS, should be activated. The vital signs should be monitored every 5 to 7 minutes to determine if the individual's condition is improving or deteriorating.

13. If on-site recovery occurs, the individual should still be provided with information identifying the signs and symptoms that could develop later and indicate that the condition is getting worse. The individual also should be provided with instructions for seeking medical assistance.

APPLICATION QUESTIONS

1. During a collision, an ice hockey player is struck in the anterior neck by the blade of another player's skate. Blood is spurting from the region. What is the first thing that you should do? How would you manage this condition?

2. During a collision in a bike race, a rider fell forward onto the handlebars and is now complaining of sharp pain on the lower right side of the rib cage, aggravated by deep breathing, coughing, and palpation over the injured site. During the assessment, you notice that he is coughing up bright red blood. What injuries might be present? How would you manage this condition?

3. A 20-year-old football player was struck in the abdomen with a helmet and experienced a sudden onset of abdominal pain in the upper left quadrant. What questions should be asked to develop a history of this injury? What structures would you palpate first? Last? What specific factors should be noted during the palpations?

4. You are a high school athletic trainer. During preseason volleyball practice, a 16-year-old female begins to hyperventilate during sprinting drills. How would you manage this condition? If the initial management does not result in a return to normal breathing within several minutes, what actions would you then take?

5. A 22-year-old male was performing a bench press with the weight at 80% of his one repetition max. During the third repetition of the second set, he felt a snapping sensation over his right upper chest wall. He is also complaining of an aching, fatigue-like pain in his arm and chest. In looking at the chest wall, what factors might you be looking for to suggest a potential injury? What muscle tests could be done to determine a possible pectoralis major muscle strain?

6. In attempting an overhead hit in volleyball, an athlete experiences a sharp pain in the midabdominal region. There is no visible swelling or discoloration and no radiating pain. In palpating this injury, what are you feeling for? Are there any special tests to determine if this injury is an abdominal strain?

7. A 21-year-old female gymnast finished practice an hour ago but is now complaining of vague chest discomfort and shortness of breath. She is also experiencing pain on the top of the right shoulder. Her pulse is somewhat elevated but you are not sure if that is due to anxiety or an

injury. Following the history component of the assessment, you suspect a pulmonary complication because of pain on deep inspiration. However, you are not sure if it is superficial or internal. What factors can you observe that might provide information to help determine if there is an injury to the chest wall or an internal complication?

REFERENCES

1. Finch CF. The risk of abdominal injury to women during sport. *J Sci Med Sport.* 2002;5(1):46–54.
2. Maron BJ, Estes NA III. Commotio cordis. *N Engl J Med.* 2010;362(10):917–927.
3. Bergman RT. Assessing acute abdominal pain: a team physician's challenge. *Phys Sportsmed.* 1996;24(4):72–82.
4. Bickley LS, Szilagyi PG. *Bates' Guide to Physical Examination and History Taking.* Philadelphia, PA: Lippincott Williams & Wilkins; 2012.
5. McChesney JA, McChesney JW. Auscultation of the chest and abdomen by athletic trainers. *J Athl Train.* 2001;36(2):190–196.
6. Beloosesky Y, Grinblat J, Hendel D, et al. Pectoralis major rupture in a 97-year-old woman. *J Am Geriatr Soc.* 2002;50(8):1465–1467.
7. Dodds SD, Wolfe SW. Injuries to the pectoralis major. *Sports Med.* 2002;32(14):945–952.
8. Chang CJ, Graves DW. Athletic injuries of the thorax and abdomen. In: Mellion MB, Walsh WM, Madden C, et al, eds. *Team Physician's Handbook.* Philadelphia, PA: Hanley & Belfus; 2002:441–459.
9. de Castro Pochini A, Ejnisman B, Andreoli CV, et al. Pectoralis major muscle rupture in athletes: a prospective study. *Am J Sports Med.* 2010;38(1):92–98.
10. Rumball JS, Lebrun CM, Di Ciacca SR, et al. Rowing injuries. *Sports Med.* 2005;35(6):537–555.
11. Udermann BE, Cavanaugh DG, Gibson MH, et al. Slipping rib syndrome in a collegiate swimmer: a case report. *J Athl Train.* 2005;40(2):120–122.
12. Raghunathan R, Porter K. Sternal fractures. *Trauma.* 2009;11(2):77–92.
13. Golden PA. Thoracic trauma. *Orthop Nurs.* 2000;19(5):37–45.
14. Gardner WN. Hyperventilation. *Am J Respir Crit Care Med.* 2004;170(2):105–106.
15. Baumann MH, Noppen M. Pneumothorax. *Respirology.* 2004;9(2):157–164.
16. Robinson PD, Cooper P, Ranganathan SC. Evidence-based management of paediatric primary spontaneous pneumothorax. *Paediatr Respir Rev.* 2009;10(3):110–117.
17. Yamamoto L, Schroeder C, Morley D, et al. Thoracic trauma: the deadly dozen. *Crit Care Nurs Q.* 2005;28(1):22–40.
18. Smith D. Chest injuries, what the sports physical therapist should know. *Int J Sports Phys Ther.* 2011;6(4):357–360.
19. Moeller JL. Contraindications to athletic participation: cardiac, respiratory, and central nervous system conditions. *Phys Sportsmed.* 1996;24(8):47–58.
20. Eckert KL. Penetrating and blunt abdominal trauma. *Crit Care Nurs Q.* 2005;28(1):41–59.
21. Ray R, Lemire JE. Liver laceration in an intercollegiate football player. *J Athl Train.* 1995;30(4):324–326.
22. Lee SL, Ho HS. Acute appendicitis: is there a difference between children and adults? *Am Surg.* 2006;72(5):409–413.
23. Burroughs KE, Hilts MJ. Renal and genitourinary problems. In: Mellion MB, Walsh WM, Madden C, et al, eds. *Team Physician's Handbook.* Philadelphia, PA: Hanley & Belfus; 2002.
24. Carroll MF, Temte JL. Proteinuria in adults: a diagnostic approach. *Am Fam Physician.* 2000;62(6):1333–1340.
25. Wilson LA. Urinalysis. *Nurs Stand.* 2005;19(35):51–54.

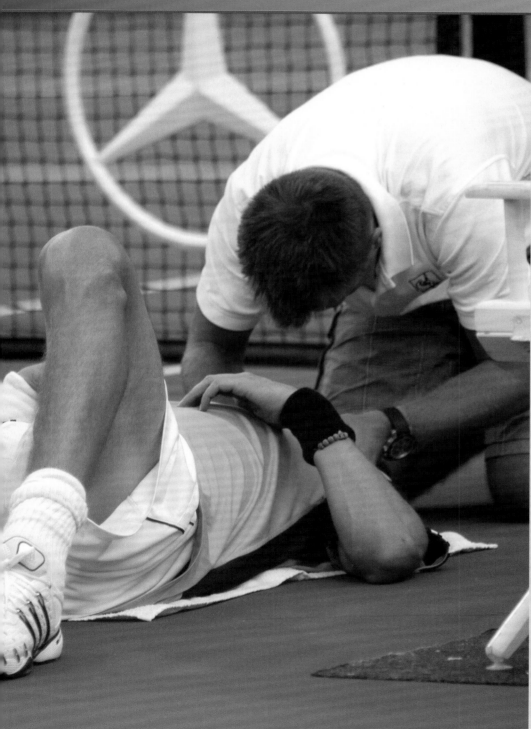

Systemic Conditions and Special Considerations

Cardiovascular Disorders

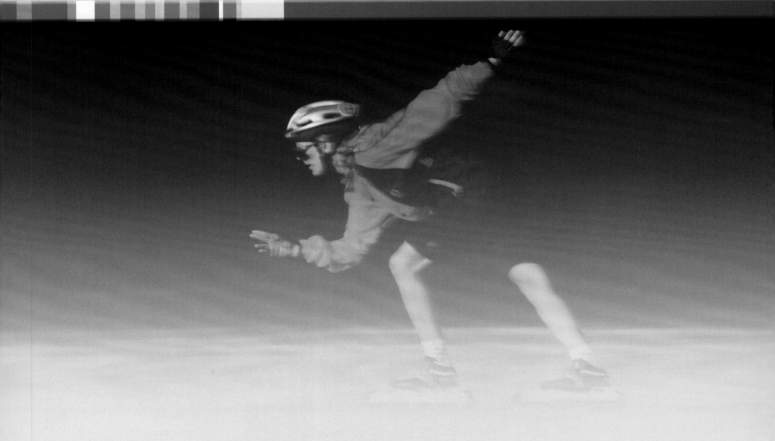

STUDENT OUTCOMES

1. Describe the signs and symptoms of anemia and explain the potential impact of this blood disorder on sport and physical activity performance.

2. Explain the methods for minimizing the effects of anemia on sport and physical activity performance.

3. Identify the early signs of hemophilia and describe the treatment of this condition.

4. Describe Reye syndrome and the strategies for preventing it.

5. Describe the physiological causes, signs, symptoms, and management of syncope.

6. Describe the basic physiological principles, signs, symptoms, and management of shock.

7. Identify the four stages of hypertension and state the predisposing factors or diseases that place an individual at risk for developing hypertension.

8. Identify medications that can adversely elevate blood pressure.

9. Identify the factors and conditions that can lead to hypotension.

10. Describe the management of hypertension and hypotension.

11. Identify the epidemiological factors and basic physiological principles associated with sudden death in the physically active population.

12. Identify the cardiac-related causes of sudden death in individuals younger than and older than 30 years.

13. List the risk factors for coronary artery disease and Marfan syndrome.

14. Identify the noncardiac conditions that can lead to sudden death.

15. Describe the two-tiered approach that is used during a preparticipation physical examination to identify risk factors associated with sudden death.

16. Explain the ethical, legal, and practical considerations that affect the medical decision-making process for determining the eligibility of competitive athletes who have cardiovascular abnormalities.

INTRODUCTION

Participation in physical activity and sport yields positive effects on an individual's physical, mental, and social health, but participation in any physical activity has inherent risks of injury. Preparticipation physical examinations (PPEs) often can identify conditions that may predispose an individual to injury. Even with a PPE, however, certain conditions may go undetected. As such, the chance exists for severe—and even catastrophic—injury because of preexisting conditions. Blood disorders (e.g., anemia and hemophilia) and cardiovascular disorders (e.g., syncope, hypertension, and hypotension) are conditions that warrant medical attention. If left untreated, these conditions can have serious physical effects on the body and can become even more problematic if they occur during exercise.

This chapter will provide a basic overview of the anatomy of the cardiovascular system, with a focus on the heart. (Discussion on the bronchial trees and lungs is included with Chapter 26.) Next, the causes, identification, and management of various cardiovascular diseases and disorders in the physically active population will be discussed. Recommendations are provided to reduce the risk of these conditions by means of a thorough cardiovascular history as part of preparticipation screening. Finally, issues concerning counseling individuals at risk for sudden death are discussed.

ANATOMY OF THE CIRCULATORY SYSTEM

The circulatory system includes the cardiovascular system and the lymphatic system. The heart and lungs have an intimate relationship both physically and functionally. The heart is positioned obliquely to the left of the midline of the body and is divided into four chambers: the right and left atria superiorly, and the right and left ventricles inferiorly (**Fig. 24.1**). The heartbeat consists of a simultaneous contraction of the two atria, followed immediately by a simultaneous contraction of the two ventricles. The contraction phase is known as systole; the phase in which the chambers relax and fill with blood is known as diastole. Two pairs of valves within the heart ensure that blood flow is unidirectional. The atrioventricular valves seal off the atria during contraction of the ventricles to prevent the backflow of blood. The aortic and pulmonary semilunar valves prevent the flow of blood from the aorta and pulmonary artery back into the ventricles.

The right side of the heart pumps blood to the lungs, where carbon dioxide and oxygen are exchanged. The left side of the heart receives the freshly oxygenated blood from the lungs and pumps it out to the systemic circulation. The vessels interconnecting the heart and lungs are known as the

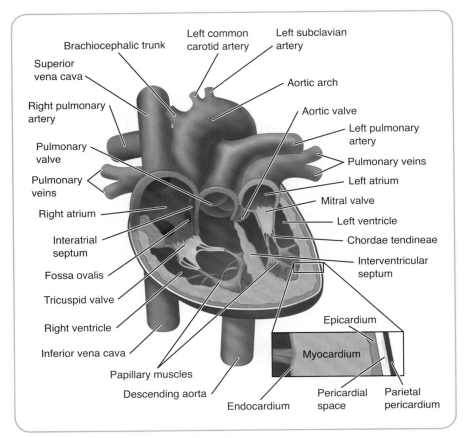

Figure 24.1. Heart.

pulmonary circuit; the vessels that supply the body are known as the systemic circuit (**Fig. 24.2**). The systemic circulation is composed of numerous and different circuits in parallel, which allows wide variations in regional blood flow without changing the total systemic flow. The heart and blood vessels (e.g., arteries, arterioles, veins, venules, and capillaries) transport oxygen, nutrients, and hormones to cells; remove waste products and carbon dioxide from cells; defend the body against infections; and prevent blood loss through clotting.

Functioning as part of the immune system, the lymphatic system is composed of lymph capillaries (i.e., lacteals), nodes, vessels, and ducts (**Fig. 24.3**). This one-way system transports fluids, nutrients (e.g., fats and proteins), and tissue waste back into the bloodstream via connections with major veins, and it flows only toward the heart.

BLOOD AND LYMPH DISORDERS

> **?** A 30-year-old female recreational golfer is diagnosed with iron-deficiency anemia attributed to an inadequate diet. What implications will this have on her ability to continue participating in golf on a weekly basis, and what is the management for this condition?

Blood flow delivers nutrients to and delivers wastes from cells and is involved in gas exchange, absorbing nutrients, and forming urine. Lymphatic vessels return fluids that have leaked from the vascular system back to the blood, protect the body by removing foreign material from the lymph stream, and provide a site for immune surveillance. Blood and lymph disorders presented in this chapter include anemia, hemophilia, Reye syndrome, and lymphangitis.

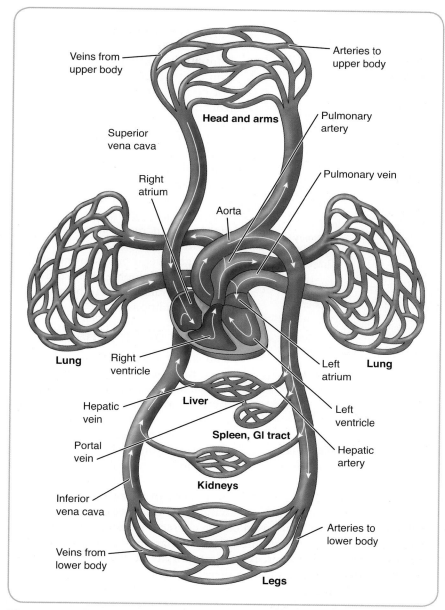

Veins from upper body

Arteries to upper body

Head and arms

Pulmonary artery

Superior vena cava

Pulmonary vein

Right atrium

Aorta

Lung

Lung

Right ventricle

Left atrium

Hepatic vein

Liver

Left ventricle

Portal vein

Spleen, GI tract

Hepatic artery

Inferior vena cava

Kidneys

Veins from lower body

Arteries to lower body

Legs

Figure 24.2. Pulmonary and systemic circulation in an adult.

Anemia

Iron, which is present in all human cells, serves several functions, including carrying oxygen from the lungs to the tissues in the form of hemoglobin, facilitating oxygen use and storage in the muscles as myoglobin, serving as a transport medium for electrons within the cells in the form of cytochromes, and playing an integral part of enzyme reactions in various tissues. Insufficient amounts of iron can interfere with these vital functions and lead to serious illness or even death. A reduction in either the red blood cell (RBC) volume (i.e., hematocrit) or the hemoglobin concentration is called **anemia**. Although anemia has five separate classifications, each one is caused by impaired RBC formation, excessive loss, or destruction of RBCs.

The recommended dietary allowance (RDA) for iron in men is 8 mg per day and in women 18 mg per day except for pregnant women, in which case the RDA is 27 mg per day. The average diet contains 5 to 7 mg of iron per 1,000 kcal. Therefore, it is necessary to consume 3,000 kcal per day

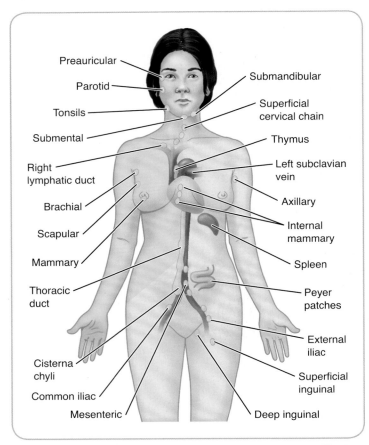

Figure 24.3. Lymphatic system with major lymph nodes. The *pale green area* denotes the body area drained by the right lymphatic duct; the rest of the body is drained by the thoracic duct.

to meet the RDA. A major concern is that many physically active females consume less than 2,000 kcal per day. In addition, individuals consuming a modified vegetarian diet that is low in iron content and low in iron bioavailability may not be receiving sufficient iron. Good sources of iron include lean animal meat (e.g., liver, beef roasts, tenderloin, lamb, and chicken or turkey legs), tuna, oysters, shrimp, enriched raisin bran or corn flakes, bagels, bran muffins, dried apricots, baked potatoes with the skin, peas, kidney beans, chickpeas, tofu, and molasses.

Anemia reduces maximum aerobic capacity, decreases physical work capability at submaximal levels, increases lactic acidosis, increases fatigue, and decreases exercise time to exhaustion.[1] Although several predisposing factors can increase the risk of developing anemia (**Box 24.1**), physically active individuals tend to be more prone to specific anemic conditions.

Stages of Anemia

Iron status is assessed through several laboratory tests. Because each test assesses a different aspect of iron metabolism, the results of one test may not always agree with those of other tests. The hemoglobin concentration and hematocrit commonly are tested, because they measure the amount of functional iron in the body. The concentration of hemoglobin in circulating RBCs is the more direct and sensitive measure. The hematocrit indicates the proportion of whole blood that is occupied by the RBCs, and it decreases only after the hemoglobin concentration falls. Hematological tests based on the characteristics of RBCs (i.e., hemoglobin, hematocrit, and total iron-binding capacity) are more popular and less expensive than biochemical tests. The biochemical tests (e.g., free erythrocyte protoporphyrin concentration, serum ferritin concentration, and transferrin saturation), however, detect earlier changes in iron status.

BOX 24.1 Predisposing Factors for Development of Anemia

- Personal or family history of anemia, bleeding disorders, or chronic disease
- Intermittent jaundice early in life
- Excessive menstrual flow; increased duration, frequency, or volume
- Chronic blood loss through gastrointestinal bleeding
- Certain drugs and toxins (e.g., chronic use of aspirin or nonsteroidal anti-inflammatory drugs)

- Childbirth
- Disadvantaged socioeconomic background
- Poor diet or dietary restriction (e.g., vegetarian diet, weight loss diets, or fad diets)
- Cancer
- Volunteer blood donor
- Diminished hepatic, renal, or thyroid function

Adapted from Harris SS. Helping active women avoid anemia. *Phys Sportsmed.* 1995;23(5):35–48; with permission.

Iron deficiency develops gradually, progressing through several stages before anemia is evident. These stages include the following:

- **Stage I.** Iron depletion is characterized by less than 12 mg per mL of an iron–protein complex known as ferritin, which is an indicator of reduced iron stores in the bone marrow. Other components of iron status—hemoglobin, hematocrit, free erythrocyte protoporphyrin, serum iron, iron-binding capacity, and transferrin saturation—remain normal.

- **Stage II.** Iron-deficiency erythropoiesis follows several months of iron depletion and is characterized by decreased levels of circulating iron, but hemoglobin and hematocrit remain normal.

- **Stage III.** Iron-deficiency anemia follows several weeks of iron-deficient erythropoiesis. Hemoglobin production diminishes, and the individual develops clinically recognized iron-deficiency anemia, which is referred to as frank anemia.

Iron-Deficiency Anemia

■ Etiology

Iron deficiency is the most common nutritional deficiency worldwide. Among men 18 years and older and postmenopausal women in the United States, however, iron-deficiency anemia is uncommon. During infancy and childhood, inadequate diet may be an underlying factor. In adults, blood loss through heavy menstrual bleeding or through slow, chronic bleeding associated with gastrointestinal ulcers, intestinal polyps, hemorrhoids, or cancer (e.g., uterine, colon) can lead to the condition. Other conditions that may increase the risk of anemia include alcoholism, use of certain medications (e.g., chemotherapy drugs, HIV medications, and seizure medications), autoimmune diseases, and insecticide exposure. The condition also is seen in endurance athletes and individuals who maintain a low percentage of body fat.

■ Signs and Symptoms

Early symptoms include exercise fatigue, tachycardia, blood mixed with feces, pallor, and epithelial abnormalities, such as a sore tongue. Symptoms that can develop at a later time include cardiac murmurs, congestive heart failure, loss of hair, and pearly sclera. Additional signs and symptoms of iron-deficiency anemia include the following:

- Muscle burning

- Nausea

- Shortness of breath

- Appetite for substances that have little or no nutritional value (e.g., starch, ice, or clay)

- Palpitations

- Spoon-shaped nails (koilonychia)

- Dry scaling and fissures of the lips (angular cheilosis)

- Inflammation of the tongue (glossitis)

■ Management

Treatment includes dietary iron supplementation (e.g., ferrous sulfate or ferrous gluconate) and ascorbic acid (i.e., vitamin C) to enhance iron absorption. Because caffeine hampers iron absorption, avoid colas, coffee, tea, chocolates, and other caffeine products. If active bleeding is attributed to polyps, ulcers, malignancies, or hemorrhoids, surgery may be necessary.

Exercise-Induced Hemolytic Anemia

■ Etiology

Exercise-induced hemolytic anemia, sometimes referred to as **runner's anemia**, occurs during exercise when RBCs are destroyed and hemoglobin is liberated into the medium in which the cells are suspended. This process of intravascular hemolysis can occur in both high- and low-impact sports and physical activities. In high-impact activities, such as running, it is posited that the trauma of repetitive, hard foot strikes destroys the RBCs. This condition, which sometimes is referred to as **foot strike hemolysis**, is more commonly observed in marathoners and middle-age distance runners, particularly those who are overweight, run on hard surfaces, wear poorly cushioned shoes, and run with a stomping gait. Intravascular hemolysis, however, also has been reported in competitive swimmers and rowers. As such, damage to the cells could be attributed to other possibilities, including muscle contraction, acidosis, or increased body temperature.

■ Management

Runner's anemia rarely is severe enough to cause appreciable loss of iron. In general, the condition may be of more concern to highly competitive, world-class athletes, for whom a fractional physiological difference can result in a competitive disadvantage. Prevention and treatment focuses on encouraging runners to be lean, to run on soft surfaces, to avoid running with a stomping gait, and to wear well-cushioned shoes and insoles.

Sickle Cell Anemia

■ Etiology

The sickle cell gene is common in people whose origin is areas where malaria is widespread, such as in Africa, the Mediterranean, the Middle East, India, the Caribbean, and South and Central America, hence the required screening of all newborns in the United States.[2] **Sickle cell anemia** is more common in African Americans and results from abnormalities in hemoglobin structure producing a characteristic sickle- or crescent-shaped RBC that is fragile and unable to transport oxygen. The condition is attributed to inheriting an autosomal recessive gene or to possessing two sickle genes as opposed to having the sickle cell trait, in which only one sickle gene is inherited. Because of their rigidity and irregular shape, sickle cells clump together and block small blood vessels, leading to vascular occlusions, or infarcts, in the central nervous system and organs, such as the heart, lungs, kidneys, and spleen (**Fig. 24.4**). Although an individual with sickle cell trait may be asymptomatic for one's entire life, exercising excessively in high heat or humidity or at high altitude may lead to dehydration, increased body temperature, hypoxia, and acidosis, which are predisposing factors for increased protein concentration in the circulating blood cells. This high concentration of protein increases blood viscosity and impairs blood flow, which can lead to a stroke, congestive heart failure, acute renal failure, pulmonary embolism, or sudden death.

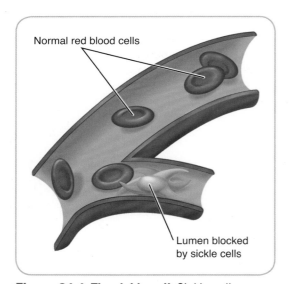

Normal red blood cells

Lumen blocked by sickle cells

Figure 24.4. The sickle cell. Sickle cells are abnormal RBCs that are fragile and unable to transport oxygen. Because of their rigidity and irregular shape, they often clump together and block small blood vessels, leading to vascular occlusions in the vital organs.

■ Signs and Symptoms

Individuals with sickle cell anemia may be asymptomatic. When manifested, signs and symptoms may include recurrent bouts of swollen, painful, and inflamed hands and feet, irregular heartbeat, severe fatigue, headache, pallor, muscle cramping, and severe pain because of oxygen deprivation. The sclera of the eye also may appear to be jaundiced. Confusion may exist in differentiating between sickling and heat cramping. Heat cramping is often preceded by muscle twinges; sickling has none. People with heat cramps hobble to a stop, whereas sickling individuals collapse to the ground with weak muscles. Those with heat cramps yell in pain and contracted, rock hard muscles are noticeable, whereas sickling individuals lie still, do not yell in pain, and the muscles look normal.[2]

■ Management

Currently, no treatment is known to reverse the condition. Because dehydration can complicate the condition, individuals should hydrate maximally before, during, and after exercise or physical exertion. Liquids with caffeine should be avoided because of their diuretic effect. Individuals should build up slowly during their physical training, allowing for longer periods of rest and recovery between repetitions. Because ambient heat stress, dehydration, asthma, illness, and altitude predispose an athlete with sickle cell trait to an onset of crisis due to physical exertion, efforts should be made to emphasize hydration, control asthma, prohibit exertion if the athlete is ill, adjust the work/rest cycles during environmental heat stress, and provide supplemental oxygen for competitions in individuals new to altitude.[3]

Hemophilia

■ Etiology

Hemophilia is a bleeding disorder characterized by a deficiency of selected proteins in the body's blood-clotting system. Three categories of blood proteins play a role in blood clotting:

1. Procoagulant proteins help to form clots.

2. Anticoagulant proteins prevent the formation of clots.

3. Fibrinolytic proteins help to dissolve clots that have formed.

The clotting process involves blood particles, called platelets, and procoagulant plasma proteins, called clotting factors. The process begins with the platelet phase, during which the platelets stick to a blood vessel at the site of an injury. An intricate cascade of enzyme reactions occurs, producing a web-like protein network that encircles the platelets and holds them in place. This is followed by the coagulation phase in which clot formation begins. In this cascade, each clotting factor is transformed from an inactive to an active form.

Hemophilia occurs in three types, which are differentiated by the deficient clotting factor. Hemophilias A, B, and C are inherited diseases. Because of the pattern of inheritance, hemophilias A and B occur almost always in males; hemophilia C can occur in both males and females. All three types, however, can cause prolonged bleeding. Complications may occur from the disease or from treatment of the disease (**Box 24.2**).[4]

■ Signs and Symptoms

Signs and symptoms may include large or deep bruises, joint pain and swelling caused by internal bleeding, intramuscular bleeding, blood in the urine or stool, and prolonged bleeding from cuts or injuries, surgical procedures, or tooth extraction. During infancy, hemophilia appears to be asymptomatic because of limited mobility. As the child begins to fall and bump into things, superficial bruises occur. Soft-tissue bleeding becomes more frequent as the child becomes more active. In most

---

BOX 24.2 Complications of Hemophilia

- **Deep internal bleeding.** Hemophilia may cause deep muscle bleeding. Swelling of a limb may press on nerves and lead to numbness or pain, which may result in reluctance to use the limb.

- **Damage to joints.** Internal bleeding may put pressure on and damage joints. Pain may be severe, resulting in reluctance to use a limb or joint. If bleeding occurs frequently and goes untreated, the irritation to a joint may lead to destruction of that joint or to the development of arthritis.

- **Infection.** People with hemophilia are more likely to receive blood transfusions and, as such, are at a greater risk of receiving contaminated blood products. Although risk of infection through blood products has decreased substantially since the introduction of genetically engineered clotting products, called recombinant factors, that are free of infection, it is still possible for people who rely on blood products to contract other diseases, such as infection with the HIV and hepatitis.

- **Adverse reaction to clotting factor treatment.** Some people with hemophilia develop proteins in their blood that inactivate the clotting factors used to treat bleeding.

cases, the bumps and bruises do not require medical treatment. Signs and symptoms that would indicate an emergency situation include the following:

- Suspected bleeding into the head, neck, or digestive tract

- Sudden pain, swelling, and warmth of extremity muscles and large joints, such as the knees, elbows, hips, and shoulders

- Persistent bleeding from an injury, especially if the individual has a severe form of hemophilia

■ Management

Treatment of hemophilia varies with its severity. Referral to a physician is necessary to ensure proper medication, and if the bleeding is serious enough, potential repeated infusions of blood plasma may be necessary.

Reye Syndrome

■ Etiology

Reye syndrome is a rare but serious, acute disease that almost exclusively affects individuals between 2 and 16 years of age.[5] The condition tends to occur in previously healthy children and almost always follows an upper respiratory viral infection. In particular, the condition is associated with type B influenza and varicella (chickenpox), but it may develop after a common cold. The precise cause of the condition is unknown, but using aspirin to treat the viral illness or infection may trigger the condition in children by disrupting the body's urea cycle. The result is an accumulation of ammonia and acidity in the blood, while the level of sugar drops (hypoglycemia). At the same time, the liver may swell and develop fat deposits. Severe brain edema may lead to critically high intracranial pressure or convulsions and, eventually, to a coma and brain death.

■ Signs and Symptoms

Reye syndrome progresses quickly and can result in permanent liver damage, irreversible neurological damage, coma, and even death. The signs and symptoms typically begin approximately 1 week after a viral infection (e.g., influenza, chickenpox, or a cold). Following appearance of recovery from an illness, a child may become much more seriously ill. The condition typically progresses through five stages[5]:

- **Stage I.** Lethargy, vomiting, and hepatic dysfunction, followed by a few days of recovery

- **Stage II.** Hyperventilation, delirium, and hyperactive reflexes

- **Stage III.** Coma and rigidity of organ cortices

- **Stage IV.** Deepening coma, large and fixed pupils, and loss of cerebral functions

- **Stage V.** Seizures, loss of deep tendon reflexes, flaccidity, and respiratory arrest

■ Management

Suspected cases of Reye syndrome should be immediately referred to a physician for advanced care. Children often require hospitalization and intensive treatment to restore blood sugar levels, control cerebral edema, and correct acid-base imbalances.

Lymphangitis

■ Etiology

Lymph nodes or glands filter the lymph fluid. **Lymphangitis** is an inflammation of the lymphatic channels that occurs as a result of infection at a site distal to the channel. Pathogenic organisms invade the lymphatic vessels, either directly, through an abrasion, or wound, or as a complication of an infection, and then spread along these channels toward regional lymph nodes.

■ Signs and Symptoms

Once the organisms enter the channels, local inflammation and subsequent infection ensue, manifesting as red streaks that are visible along the course of the vessels. The inflammation or infection then extends proximally, toward regional lymph nodes. Individuals often complain of headache, loss of appetite, fever, chills, malaise, and muscle aches. The condition can progress rapidly, particularly when caused by group A streptococci, to bacteremia and disseminated infection and sepsis.

■ Management

Immediate referral to a physician is required, and hospitalization usually is necessary. If possible, the affected area should be elevated and immobilized to reduce swelling, pain, and spread of infection. Hot, moist compresses may help to reduce inflammation and pain. Prescribed antimicrobial and antibiotic agents should be administered, and analgesics or anti-inflammatory medications can be used to reduce pain, inflammation, and swelling. An abscess may require surgical drainage.

 Anemia can reduce maximum aerobic capacity, decrease physical work capability at submaximal levels, increase lactic acidosis, increase fatigue, and decrease exercise time to exhaustion. Because the golfer's anemia was attributed to her eating habits, management of the condition should include a diet rich in iron content as well as dietary iron supplementation and ascorbic acid to enhance iron absorption.

SYNCOPE

 Following 60 minutes of an intense, running workout on a treadmill, a healthy, 25-year-old man steps off the treadmill, suddenly collapses, and loses consciousness. What might explain this sudden unconsciousness, and how should this condition be managed?

Syncope is a sudden, transient loss of consciousness (T-LOC), described as "fainting," that often occurs in healthy individuals and is not associated with seizures, coma, shock, or other states of altered consciousness. **Presyncope** is a sense of impending LOC, light-headedness, or weakness. It appears more frequently than syncope and provides a better source of injury/illness history, because the patient usually has better recollection of the event.[6] Questions concerning syncope should be part of the medical history during the PPE. If a history of syncope is noted, the individual should be referred to a physician for further evaluation. Syncope and presyncope have three primary classifications (**Box 24.3**).[6]

Of the various conditions that can lead to neurally mediated reflex faints, the best known is the common or vasovagal faint. Other neurally mediated reflex faints include carotid sinus syndrome and situational faints such as those triggered by blood draws, emotional upset, pain, micturition, defecation, coughing, and swallowing.[7] The common orthostatic (postural) hypotensive faints are associated with movement from lying or sitting to a standing position. Cardiac arrhythmias may cause faints if the heart rate is excessively rapid or too slow, such as during the onset of a paroxysmal supraventricular tachycardia (SVT). Structural cardiopulmonary diseases are relatively infrequent causes of faints. A common cause in this category is fainting due to an acute myocardial infarction or ischemic event. Although quite rare, cerebrovascular disease may lead to fainting during a vertebrobasilar transient ischemic attack (TIA).[7]

Etiology

Decreased blood flow to the brain can occur because (1) the heart fails to pump the blood, (2) the blood vessels don't have enough tone to maintain blood pressure to deliver the blood to the brain, (3) there is not enough blood or fluid within the blood vessels, or (4) a combination of these reasons. The end result is a sudden drop in blood pressure that reduces blood circulation to the brain and leads to LOC. This condition is more common in children and young adults, although it can occur at any age.

 See **Causes of Syncope and Near Syncope**, available on the companion Web site at thePoint.

BOX 24.3 Classification of Syncope

Reflex (Neurally Mediated) Syncope

Vasovagal

- Mediated by emotional distress: fear, pain, instrumentation, blood phobia
- Mediated by orthostatic stress

Situational

- Cough, sneeze
- Gastrointestinal stimulation (swallow, defecation, visceral pain)
- Micturition (post-micturition)
- Postexercise
- Postprandial
- Others (e.g., laugh, brass instrument playing, weight lifting)

Carotid sinus syncope

Atypical forms (without apparent triggers and/or atypical presentation)

Syncope Due to Orthostatic Hypotension

Primary autonomic failure

- Pure autonomic failure, multiple system atrophy, Parkinson disease with autonomic failure, Lewy body dementia

Secondary autonomic failure

- Diabetes, amyloidosis, uremia, spinal cord injuries

Drug-induced orthostatic hypotension:

- Alcohol, vasodilators, diuretics, phenothiazines, antidepressants

Volume depletion

- Hemorrhage, diarrhea, vomiting, etc.

Cardiac Syncope (Cardiovascular)

Arrhythmia as primary cause

Bradycardia

- Sinus node dysfunction (including bradycardia/tachycardia syndrome)
- Atrioventricular conduction system disease
- Implanted device malfunction

Tachycardia

- Supraventricular
- Ventricular (idiopathic, secondary to structural heart disease or to channelopathies)

Drug-induced bradycardia and tachyarrhythmia

Structural disease

Cardiac

- Cardiac valvular disease, acute myocardial infarction/ischemia, hypertrophic cardiomyopathy, cardiac masses (atrial myxoma, tumors, etc.), pericardial disease/tamponade, congenital anomalies of coronary arteries, prosthetic valves dysfunction

Others

- Pulmonary embolus, acute aortic dissection, pulmonary hypertension

Signs and Symptoms

Typical neurally mediated syncope occurs while standing and often is preceded by prodromal symptoms, including restlessness, pallor, weakness, sighing, yawning, diaphoresis, and nausea. These symptoms may be followed by light-headedness, blurred vision, collapse, and LOC. Occasionally, mild clonic seizures occur, but unless other signs indicate, a detailed seizure evaluation is not indicated. Other signs and symptoms may include dizziness, profuse sweating, paresthesia of the hands or feet, and unilateral or bilateral chest pain. Some forms of syncope suggest a serious disorder, including those occurring with exercise, those associated with palpitations or irregularities of the heart, and those associated with a family history of recurrent syncope or sudden death.

Management

Neurally mediated syncope usually responds well to avoidance of stimuli that trigger the event. If syncope does occur, initial management includes assessment of the patient's vital signs. The patient should be placed in a safe, lying-down position. Recovery usually occurs within minutes. If the patient does not regain consciousness within a few minutes or demonstrates signs of breathing or cardiac impairment, the emergency action plan (EAP), including summoning emergency medical services (EMS), should be activated.

A thorough medical evaluation should be conducted in the following cases:

- Syncope recurs.
- Syncope occurs with exercise.
- Syncope is associated with palpitations or irregularities of the heart.
- Family history of syncope

In cases of severe syncope, β-blockers, cardiac pacing, and antidepressants may be recommended; however, the success rate is poor.

The exerciser may have experienced syncope as a result of dehydration or heat illness. The patient's vital signs should be measured and monitored. If he does not regain consciousness within a few minutes, the EAP, including summoning EMS, should be activated.

SHOCK

Following a slide into home plate that resulted in a collision with the catcher, a baseball player sustains a compound fracture to the tibia. The athletic trainer activated the EAP, including summoning EMS. The athletic trainer also immobilized the leg. What possible complications might occur as a result of this traumatic injury? What other treatment should the athletic trainer provide while waiting for EMS to arrive?

Shock occurs with injuries involving severe pain, bleeding, the spinal cord, fractures, or intra-abdominal or intrathoracic regions, but shock also may occur, to some degree, with minor injuries. The severity of shock depends on one's age, physical condition, pain tolerance, fatigue, dehydration, presence of any disease, extreme cold or heat exposure, or handling of an injured area. Types of shock include anaphylactic, cardiogenic, hypovolemic, metabolic, neurogenic, respiratory, psychogenic, and septic (**Box 24.4**).

Etiology

Shock occurs if the heart is unable to exert adequate pressure to circulate enough oxygenated blood to the vital organs. This condition may result from a damaged heart that fails to pump properly, low blood volume from blood loss or dehydration, or dilation of blood vessels that leads to blood pooling in larger vessels away from vital areas (**Fig. 24.5**). The result is a lack of oxygen and nutrition at the cellular level. The heart pumps faster, but because of reduced volume, the pulse rate is weakened and the blood pressure drops (i.e., **hypotension**). A rapid, weak pulse is the most prominent sign of shock. As an individual's condition deteriorates, breathing becomes rapid and shallow, and sweating is profuse. Vital body fluids pass through weakened capillaries, thereby causing further circulatory distress. If not corrected, circulatory collapse can lead to unconsciousness and even death.

BOX 24.4 Types and Causes of Shock

- **Hypovolemic.** From excessive blood or fluid loss leading to inadequate circulation and oxygen supply to all body organs. Possible causes include hemorrhage, dehydration, multiple trauma, and severe burns.

- **Respiratory.** From insufficient oxygen in the blood as a result of inadequate breathing. Possible causes are spinal injury to the respiratory nerves, airway obstruction, or chest trauma, such as from a pneumothorax, hemothorax, or punctured lung.

- **Neurogenic.** Occurs when peripheral blood vessels dilate and an insufficient blood volume cannot supply oxygen to the vital organs. This may occur in a spinal or head injury when nerves that control the vascular system are impaired, thereby altering the integrity of blood vessels.

- **Psychogenic.** Refers to a temporary dilation of blood vessels, resulting in the draining of blood from the head with pooling of blood in the abdomen. A common example is an individual fainting from the sight of blood.

- **Cardiogenic.** Occurs when the heart muscle is no longer able to sustain enough pressure to pump blood through the system. Possible causes are injury to the heart or previous heart attack.

- **Metabolic.** Results from a severe loss of body fluids because of an untreated illness that alters the biochemical equilibrium. Possible causes are insulin shock, diabetic coma, vomiting, or diarrhea.

- **Septic.** Derives from severe, usually bacterial, infection whereby toxins attack the walls of small blood vessels, causing them to dilate, thereby decreasing blood pressure.

- **Anaphylactic.** Refers to a severe allergic reaction of the body to a foreign protein that is ingested, inhaled, or injected (e.g., foods, drugs, or insect stings).

Signs and Symptoms

Signs and symptoms of shock can develop over time (**Box 24.5**). Initially, the individual may have a feeling of uneasiness or restlessness, increased respirations, and increased weakened heart rate. The skin turns pale and clammy, which usually is accompanied by profuse sweating. The lips, nail beds, and membranes of the mouth appear to be cyanotic. Thirst, weakness, nausea, and vomiting may then become apparent. During later stages, a rapid, weak pulse and labored, weakened respirations may lead to decreased blood pressure and possible unconsciousness.

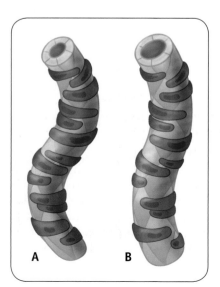

Figure 24.5. Shock. The diameter of an arteriole blood vessel is controlled by circular layers of smooth muscles that either constrict or relax to regulate peripheral blood flow (**A**). Blood vessels dilate during shock. This action increases the size of the vascular bed and decreases the resistance to blood flow, resulting in blood pooling in larger vessels, depriving the brain and vital organs of needed oxygen. As a result, heart rate increases, giving the characteristic rapid, weak pulse that often is the first sign of shock (**B**).

BOX 24.5 Signs and Symptoms of Shock

- Restlessness, anxiety, fear, or disorientation
- Nausea and/or vomiting
- Cold, clammy, moist skin
- Shallow, irregular breathing; breathing also may be labored, rapid, or gasping
- Profuse sweating
- Extreme thirst
- Dizziness
- Eyes are dull, sunken, and with the pupils dilated
- Rapid and weak pulse
- Skin that is chalklike but that later may appear to be cyanotic

---

Management

The EAP, including summoning EMS, should be activated. While waiting for EMS to arrive, the clinician should maintain the airway, control any bleeding, splint any fractures, and maintain normal body temperature. If a head or neck injury is not suspected, the feet and legs should be elevated 8 to 12 in. Vital signs should be taken and recorded every 5 minutes. **Application Strategy 24.1** summarizes the immediate care of shock.

 The compound fracture sustained by the baseball player can lead to shock. Shock is considered to be a medical emergency. As such, the EAP, including summoning EMS, should be activated. While waiting for EMS to arrive, the clinician should maintain the airway, maintain normal body temperature, and position the athlete lying down with the leg raised after—and only if—it has been properly immobilized. The management of shock is explained in **Application Strategy 24.1**.

APPLICATION STRATEGY 24.1

Management of Shock

- Activate EAP, including summoning EMS. Secure and maintain an open airway. Control any major bleeding. Monitor vital signs.
- If a head or neck injury or a leg fracture is not suspected, elevate the feet and legs 8–12 in. With breathing difficulties, the patient might be more comfortable with the head and shoulders raised in a semireclining position. If a head injury is suspected, elevate the head and shoulders to reduce pressure on the brain. The feet also may be slightly elevated. In a suspected neck injury, keep the patient lying flat.
- A patient who vomits or is unconscious should be placed on one's side to avoid blocking the airway with any fluids. This allows the fluids to drain from the mouth.
- Splint any fractures. This reduces shock by slowing bleeding and helps to ease pain. If the patient has a leg fracture, keep the leg level while splinting the fracture. Raise the leg only after it has been properly immobilized.
- Maintain normal body temperature. This action may require removing any wet clothing, if possible, and covering the patient with a blanket. Keep the patient quiet and still. Avoid rough or excessive handling of the patient.
- Do not give the patient anything by mouth.
- Monitor vital signs every 2–5 minutes until EMS arrives.

BLOOD PRESSURE DISORDERS

 A senior athlete reports feeling dizzy when getting up from a lying position and when suddenly changing body positions while playing tennis. What might this person be experiencing, and what is the management for this condition?

Blood pressure is the force per unit area exerted on the walls of an artery, generally considered to be the aorta. It is the result of two factors—namely, cardiac output and total peripheral resistance. Cardiac output is determined by heart rate, myocardial contractility (i.e., force of contraction), blood volume, and venous return. Peripheral resistance is determined by arteriolar constriction. As one of the most important vital signs, blood pressure reflects the effectiveness of the circulatory system.

Although blood pressure varies among individuals, normal blood pressure is considered to be 120 mm Hg systolic blood pressure and 80 mm Hg diastolic blood pressure. **Systolic blood pressure** (SBP) is measured when the left ventricle contracts and expels blood into the aorta. **Diastolic blood pressure** (DBP) is the residual pressure in the aorta between heartbeats. It is not unusual for a relatively physically fit person to have a blood pressure of 90/70 mm Hg. Blood pressure may be affected by gender, weight, race, lifestyle, and diet, and it can vary throughout the day, depending on the time of day and the individual's fitness level. Blood pressure is measured in the brachial artery with a sphygmomanometer and stethoscope (refer to **Application Strategy 2.1**).

Any change in either cardiac output or peripheral resistance results in an increase or decrease in blood pressure. **Hypertension** is defined as a sustained, elevated blood pressure greater than 140 mm Hg SBP or greater than 90 mm Hg DBP. A fall of 20 mm Hg or more from a person's normal baseline SBP characterizes hypotension.

Hypertension

Hypertension affects approximately 50 million individuals in the United States and approximately 1 billion individuals worldwide.[8] The higher the blood pressure, the greater the chance of myocardial infarction, heart failure, stroke, and kidney disease. For individuals 40 to 70 years of age, each increment of 20 mm Hg in SBP or of 10 mm Hg in DBP doubles the risk of cardiovascular disease across the entire blood pressure range of 115/75 to 185/115 mm Hg.[8,9]

Several factors increase the risk of developing hypertension (**Table 24.1**). Onset generally is between the ages of 20 and 50 years, with the frequency being greatest in African Americans. Hypertension can be caused by a variety of substances, including the following:

- Certain prescribed medications
- Oral contraceptives
- Anabolic steroids
- Amphetamines
- Chronic alcohol use
- Nasal decongestants containing sympathomimetic amines
- Some nonsteroidal anti-inflammatory drugs
- Sleep apnea
- Chronic kidney disease
- Renovascular disease
- Coarctation of the aorta
- Thyroid or parathyroid disease

Hypertension is classified into prehypertension, stage 1 hypertension, and stage 2 hypertension (**Table 24.2**). This categorization applies to adults 18 years of age and older who are not taking antihypertensive medication and are not acutely ill. When SBP and DBP fall into different categories, the

TABLE 24.1 Risk Factors for Developing Hypertension

RISK FACTOR	REASON
Age	Arteries lose their elasticity, and blood pressure increases with age. High incidence of hypertension after age 60 years
Diabetes	High incidence in those with diabetes is attributed to insulin resistance promoted by abdominal obesity.
Heredity	Higher incidence with a family history of hypertension and heart disease in women (<65 years) and men (<55 years)
High blood	High blood lipids contribute to atherosclerosis and hypertension. A high-fat diet also contributes to lipids hypertension.
Obesity	Excess body fat, especially abdominal fat, is closely associated with hypertension.
Race	Prevalence differs among racial and ethnic groups, but incidence in African Americans is among the highest in the world.
Sex	Higher incidence in men and postmenopausal women
Smoking	Smoking increases the workload of the heart and, as such, increases blood pressure.

higher category is used to classify the individual's blood pressure status. For more detailed standards in children and adolescents, refer to Chapter 2.

Categories of Hypertension

Classifications of hypertension are based on the mean of two or more properly measured, seated blood pressure readings on each of two or more occasions. In contrast to past standards, new standards classify a designated prehypertension category to identify patients who are at increased risk for progression to hypertension. Individuals in the 130/80 to 139/89 mm Hg range are at twice the risk of developing hypertension compared with those who have lower values.[8]

Hypertension is divided into two categories. Primary, or essential, hypertension is a chronic, progressive disorder with no identifiable cause that often attacks the heart, brain, kidneys, and eyes and that is associated with increased morbidity and mortality. The condition can be treated successfully with medication, diet modification, and exercise. Secondary hypertension has an identified cause, which often is associated with chronic renal disease, renovascular disease, **coarctation**, and other conditions. If the cause is identified, secondary hypertension can be controlled.

Clearance for Sport and Physical Activity Participation

An individual who has mild or moderate hypertension should not participate in competitive sports and physical activity until cleared by a physician. These individuals often are given physician clearance to participate in activity if their blood pressure is well controlled and no target organ damage

TABLE 24.2 Classification of Blood Pressure in Adults

CLASSIFICATION	SYSTOLIC (mm Hg)[a]		DIASTOLIC (mm Hg)[a]	LIFESTYLE MODIFICATION
Normal	<120	and	<80	Encourage
Prehypertension	120–139	or	80–89	Yes
Stage 1 hypertension	140–159	or	90–99	Yes
Stage 2 hypertension	≥160	or	≥100	Yes

[a]Treatment determined by highest category.

From James PA, Oparil S, Carter BL, et al. 2014 evidence-based guideline for the management of high blood pressure in adults report from the panel members appointed to the Eighth Joint National Committee (JNC 8). *JAMA*. 2014;311(5):507–520. http://jama.jamanetwork.com/article.aspx?articleid=1791497. Accessed July 1, 2015.

or heart disease is present. These individuals should have their blood pressure rechecked by the athletic trainer on a weekly basis and by the physician every 2 to 4 months. For individuals with stage 2 hypertension, physical activity is restricted, especially in sports or activities with a high static component (e.g., wrestling, gymnastics, weight lifting, rock climbing, and rowing) until the hypertension is well controlled.

Management of Hypertension

Treatment of hypertension focuses on reducing SBP and DBP as well as on preventing long-term complications. Target blood pressure readings of less than 140/90 mm Hg are associated with a decrease in cardiovascular complications. The target for a patient with hypertension along with diabetes or renal disease is less than 130/80 mm Hg.[8] Nonpharmaceutical treatment includes lifestyle modifications and aerobic exercise. Pharmaceutical treatment may involve antihypertensive medications.

■ Lifestyle Modifications

Because hypertension has a significant impact on risk for cardiovascular disease, individuals with hypertension should be encouraged to establish lifestyle modifications in collaboration with an exercise program. These steps may include measures such as the following[8,10]:

- Lose weight if overweight or obese (body mass index 18.5 to 24.9 kg per m^2).

- Engage in regular aerobic physical activity, such as brisk walking.

- Limit alcohol intake. For most males, alcohol intake should be no more than two drinks per day (<1 oz per day of ethanol; e.g., 24 oz of beer, 10 oz of wine, or 3 oz of 80-proof whiskey); females and lighter weight males should not have more than one drink per day.

- Avoid consuming sugar-containing beverages and energy-dense snacks.

- Reduce sodium intake to less than 2,300 mg per day.

- Consume a diet rich in fruits, vegetables, and low-fat dairy products, with a reduced content of saturated and total fats.

- Maintain adequate dietary potassium, calcium, and magnesium intake.

- Do not smoke cigarettes.

   Diet modifications should include a diet low in saturated fats, with total dietary fat not exceeding 30% of total caloric intake, and increased potassium, calcium, and magnesium intake. In severe cases of hypertension, more significant sodium and alcohol restrictions, weight loss, and reduction of other cardiovascular risk factors must be incorporated into the program.

■ Exercise Program

Aerobic exercise has a positive effect on the blood pressure of individuals with hypertension by lowering resting SBP an average of 4 to 9 mm Hg and DBP an average of 6 mm Hg. Specific mechanisms for this response are still unknown, but significant contributing factors may include the following[8]:

- Reduced activity of the sympathetic nervous system, which decreases peripheral resistance and blood flow

- Altered renal function, which facilitates the elimination of sodium by the kidneys, subsequently reducing fluid volume and blood pressure

- Decreased body fat

- Decreased smoking and alcohol consumption that often accompany exercise conditioning

- Increased relaxation during exercise

   According to the U.S. Department of Health and Human Services, adults who wish to attain substantial health benefits should perform aerobic exercise a minimum of 150 minutes (2 hours and 30 minutes) per week at a moderate intensity, such as brisk walking, or 75 minutes (1 hour and

15 minutes) a week of vigorous-intensity aerobic physical activity, or an equivalent combination of moderate- and vigorous-intensity aerobic activity. Aerobic activity should be performed in episodes of at least 10 minutes, and preferably, be spread throughout the week. Children and adolescents should do 60 minutes (1 hour) or more of physical activity daily including primarily moderate- or vigorous-intensity at least 3 days a week. The sessions should include primarily moderate or vigorous aerobic physical activity, muscle strengthening, and bone strengthening.[11] Individuals with hypertension should avoid isometric exercises and heavy resistance training.

■ Pharmaceutical Medications

When lifestyle modifications, diet, and physical activity fail to control hypertension, diuretics and antihypertensive agents often are prescribed. Most patients require two or more antihypertensive medications to achieve a desirable blood pressure. Thiazide-type diuretics, which are used in the initial therapy for most patients, enhance the antihypertensive efficacy of multidrug regimens, can be useful in achieving blood pressure control, and are more affordable than other antihypertensive agents. Diuretics lower blood pressure by increasing fluid loss; however, some diuretics can lead to a potassium deficiency. As such, individuals should be aware of the signs of potassium imbalance, including weakness (particularly of the legs), unexplained numbness or tingling sensations, cramps, irregular heartbeats, and excessive thirst and urination.[8]

Hypotension

When arterial blood pressure is lower than normal, inadequate blood is circulated to the heart, brain, and other vital organs. The result often is a collapse of bodily functions. Hypotension, or low blood pressure, is defined as a decrease of 20 mm Hg or more in an individual's normal SBP. It can be caused by a variety of factors, including shock, acute hemorrhage, dehydration, orthostatic hypotension, **postural hypotension**, or overtreatment of hypertension (**Box 24.6**).

Orthostatic hypotension is not unusual. Estimated to occur in approximately half of all elderly people, it can lead to fainting and falls. In the absence of symptoms, however, treatment is not required. Symptoms that indicate a medical referral include dimming or loss of vision, light-headedness, dizziness, excessive perspiration, diminished hearing, pallor, nausea, and weakness. It should be noted that certain medications (e.g., vasodilators and antidepressants) may cause orthostatic hypotension. This complication can be addressed by having a physician change the medication or dosage.

BOX 24.6 Nonneurogenic Causes of Hypotension

- Shock as a response to stress or trauma
- Heat (e.g., hot environments, hot showers and baths, or fever)
- Hemorrhage
- Drug toxicity (e.g., alcohol, anesthesia, diuretics, analgesics, or vasodilators)
- Diabetes mellitus
- Overtreatment of hypertension (e.g., diuretics, antihypertensives, or vasodilators)
- Allergic drug reaction
- Dehydration
- Orthostatic or postural hypotension
- Low-salt diets
- Straining on heavy lifting, urination, or defecation
- Diarrhea
- Vasovagal syncope (fainting)

Physically active people do not usually need to be concerned about hypotension. In general, the lower the blood pressure, the better—as long as the person feels well. Older individuals, however, should always check with their physician before performing heavy resistance exercises. Non-pharmaceutical steps that can be taken to reduce the effects of orthostatic hypotension include the following:

■ Avoid prolonged standing, vigorous exercise, alcohol, hot environments, hot showers or baths.

■ Execute slow, careful changes in position, especially when arising in the morning.

■ Eat multiple, small meals.

■ Schedule physical activities in the afternoon.

■ Increase salt and fluid intake.

> The senior athlete most likely has experienced orthostatic hypotension. Management for this condition can include avoiding prolonged standing, vigorous exercise, alcohol, and hot environments; slowly and carefully changing body positions; eating multiple, small meals; scheduling physical activities in the afternoon; and increasing salt and fluid intake.

SUDDEN CARDIAC DEATH

> **?** A Little League Baseball pitcher receives a line drive to his chest. He immediately collapses. What condition should be suspected, and how should this condition be managed?

Sudden cardiac death (SCD) has been termed the "silent killer." It is defined as an unexpected death resulting from sudden cardiac arrest within 6 hours of an otherwise normal, healthy clinical state.[12]

Epidemiology

The prevalence of SCD during physical activity is rare, yet it is the leading cause of death in young athletes. It is estimated that sudden death in athletes occurs approximately once every 3 days in the United States.[13–15] Males have an increased death rate from SCD than that of females, with the highest rates being seen in basketball and football players.[16] Explanation for the low occurrence in female athletes is inconclusive; however, some researchers postulate that the decreased incidence can be attributed to the following[17,18]:

■ Fewer females participate in sports.

■ Fewer females participate in highly intense sports that require full-body protective equipment (e.g., football or ice hockey).

■ Gender differences exist regarding cardiac adaptation to training demands.

■ Females have smaller hearts.

SCD often is precipitated by physical activity and may be caused by an array of cardiovascular conditions. The age of the individual appears to dictate the underlying physiological pathology for the occurrence of SCD. The most common causes of SCD in athletes younger than 35 years of age in the United States are hypertrophic cardiomyopathy, commotio cordis, and anomalous coronary arteries.[16,18] Noncardiac causes, a small percentage of sudden death in athletes, may be due to death from heat stroke, asthma, cerebral artery rupture, and exertional rhabdomyolysis secondary to sickle cell trait.[16,18] Atherosclerotic coronary artery disease, such as myocardial ischemia and myocardial infarction, is the leading cause for individuals older than 35 years.

Cardiac Causes of Sudden Cardiac Death

Cardiac anomalies are the most direct cause of SCD in individuals younger than 35 years, with hypertrophic cardiomyopathy being the most common. Other reported cardiac-related causes include cardiac mass, mitral valve prolapse, myocarditis, acquired valvular heart disease, coronary artery anomalies, ruptured aortic aneurysm (often from intrinsic aortic weakness with Marfan syndrome), Wolff-Parkinson-White syndrome, and arrhythmogenic right ventricular dysplasia. Other rare cardiac conditions that can contribute to sudden death involve abnormalities of the cardiac conduction system (i.e., long QT syndrome), which can result in lethal cardiac rhythm problems.

Hypertrophic Cardiomyopathy

Hypertrophic cardiomyopathy (HCM), characterized by an abnormal thickening of the left ventricle wall, is the most common inherited cardiac disorder, occurring in 1:500 of the general population.[19] The condition typically goes undetected during routine physical examination. By definition, HCM is a hypertrophied, nondilated left ventricle in the absence of another cardiac or systemic disease capable of producing the degree of hypertrophy that is present. A normal left ventricle is approximately 1 cm thick. In HCM, the wall thickness typically ranges from 2 to 4 cm—and can be greater than 15 cm.[20] This abnormal thickness can lead to electrical problems and abnormal rhythms, including ventricular fibrillation and lethal rhythm.

Physical examinations should include a thorough cardiac history and cardiac examination (see "Cardiovascular Preparticipation Screening" section). Unfortunately, HCM often goes undetected during routine physical examinations. HCM should be suspected in a young athlete who presents with exertional dyspnea, chest pain, unexplained syncope, or prior recognition of a heart murmur. A family history of HCM, SCD, heart disease in a close relative younger than 50 years of age, or unexplained syncope should also raise red flags during the assessment of the patient. During the physical examination, the most important finding is a systolic murmur increased/elicited by provocative maneuvers such as Valsalva, standing, or exertion.[19] As a result, periods of arrhythmia or blood flow obstruction may produce syncope during physical exertion. Any individual exhibiting these signs or symptoms should be seen immediately by a physician or a cardiologist.

Mitral Valve Prolapse

Mitral valve prolapse (MVP) is not a frequent cause of sudden death but can affect a small portion of the population, spanning all ages.[21] MVP is a condition in which redundant tissue is found on one or both leaflets of the mitral valve. During a ventricular contraction, a portion of the redundant tissue on the mitral valve pushes back beyond the normal limit and, as a result, produces an abnormal sound. This sound is followed by a systolic murmur as blood is regurgitated back through the mitral valve into the left atrium. Because of the characteristic sound, this condition often is referred to as a "click-murmur syndrome." Individuals with MVP usually experience some degree of chest pain, dyspnea, palpitations, and fatigue with exertion.[21] Athletes with MVP can engage in all competitive sports unless any of the following features is present, in which case the individual should participate in only low-intensity competitive sports[22]:

■ Prior syncope judged to be arrhythmogenic in origin

■ Sustained or repetitive and nonsustained SVT or frequent and/or complex ventricular tachyarrhythmias on ambulatory monitoring

■ Severe mitral regurgitation

■ Left ventricular (LV) systolic dysfunction

■ Prior embolic event

■ Family history of MVP-related sudden death

Myocarditis

Myocarditis is an inflammatory condition of the muscular walls of the heart that can result from a bacterial or viral infection. The condition is characterized by the infiltration of inflammatory cells into the myocardium, leading to an abnormally enlarged left ventricle. SCD occurs when the inflammatory changes in the myocardium lead to degeneration or death of adjacent muscle cells, resulting in electrical instability and life-threatening arrhythmias. Although some individuals may be asymptomatic, others exhibit symptoms commonly associated with viral infections, including fever, body aches, fatigue, cough, or vomiting; this similarity often impedes establishing the diagnosis. Exercise intolerance, shortness of breath, and more serious cardiac symptoms, including **palpitations** or syncope, may occur without warning.

Any sport participant with probable or definitive evidence of myocarditis should be withdrawn from all competitive sports and undergo a thorough medical examination, which may lead to 6 months of total rest following the onset of clinical manifestations. Return to training and competition may occur after the following[22]:

- LV function, wall motion, and cardiac dimensions return to normal.

- Clinically relevant arrhythmias are absent on ambulatory monitoring and graded exercise testing.

- Serum markers of inflammation and heart failure have normalized.

- The 12-lead electrocardiogram (ECG) has normalized.

Acquired Valvular Heart Disease

Acquired valvular heart disease stems from a defect or insufficiency in a heart valve that can lead to improper blood flow through the heart. The condition is manifested as either **valvular stenosis**, which is a narrowing of the orifice around the cardiac valves, or **regurgitation**, which involves a backward flow of blood. The condition is named according to the affected valve (e.g., mitral valve, aortic valve, and tricuspid valve). If more than one valve is affected, the condition is called **multivalvular disease**, which occurs in the context of rheumatic heart disease. The characteristic murmurs associated with this condition are detected during a physical examination.

Individuals with mild-to-moderate mitral and tricuspid valve stenosis or regurgitation typically can participate in sports and physical activity. Each case, however, must be evaluated on an individual basis.

Initially, experts posited that aortic stenosis was a common cause of sudden death; however, new research has not supported their theory. Aortic stenosis, like other valve conditions, often can be detected early through physical examination. Individuals with mild aortic stenosis may participate in physical activity and competitive sports. Individuals with mild or moderate asymptomatic aortic stenosis and a history of **supraventricular tachycardia** (i.e., rapid heartbeats proximal to the ventricles in the atrium or atrioventricular node) or ventricular arrhythmias at rest should participate only in low-intensity physical activity and sports. Individuals with severe aortic stenosis or aortic regurgitation and significant dilation of the proximal ascending aorta associated with Marfan syndrome should not engage in any competitive sport.[22]

Coronary Artery Disease

The most common cause of sudden death in individuals older than 35 years is coronary artery disease (CAD), also referred to as **atherosclerosis**. An excessive buildup of cholesterol within the coronary arteries narrows the diameter of the arteries and impedes the flow of blood, which in turn reduces the amount of oxygen supplied to the heart. Subsequent to the diminished oxygen, **angina** is a common symptom. If excessive cholesterol buildup blocks a coronary artery, the person is at risk for a **myocardial infarction**. If the blockage is in a major coronary artery, death often occurs.

Unlike young individuals, who rarely know if they have a cardiac anomaly that may put them at risk for sudden death, physically active individuals older than 35 years usually have experienced prodromal cardiovascular symptoms or have a known medical history of CAD. Therefore, individuals older than 35 years can choose to ignore the symptoms and continue participating at the same level, placing them at risk for sudden death; change their lifestyle according to CAD recommendations and continue to participate in limited activity; or stop physical activity.

The American College of Sports Medicine (ACSM) has developed a list of risk factors for CAD and recommends an exercise ECG before beginning a moderate or vigorous exercise program for anyone who has had a history of angina, palpitations, syncope, or dyspnea during physical activity

TABLE 24.3 American College of Sports Medicine Coronary Artery Disease Risk Factors

POSITIVE RISK FACTORS	DEFINING CRITERIA
Family history	Myocardial infarction, coronary revascularization, or sudden death before 55 years of age in father or other male first-degree relative (i.e., brother or son) or before 65 years of age in mother or other first-degree female relative (i.e., sister or daughter)
Cigarette smoking	Current cigarette smoker or someone who quit within the previous 6 months
Hypertension	Systolic blood pressure ≥140 mm Hg or diastolic blood pressure ≥90 mm Hg confirmed by measurements on at least two separate occasions, or using antihypertensive medication
Hypercholesterolemia	Total serum cholesterol >200 mg/dL (5.2 mmol/L) or high-density lipoprotein cholesterol <35 mg/dL (0.9 mmol/L), or on lipid-lowering medication; if low-density lipoprotein cholesterol is available, use >130 mg/dL (3.4 mmol/L) rather than total cholesterol >200 mg/dL.
Impaired fasting glucose	Fasting blood glucose of ≥110 mg/dL (6.1 mmol/L) confirmed by measurements on at least two separate occasions
Obesity	Body mass index ≥30 kg/m^2, or waist girth >100 cm
Sedentary lifestyle	Persons making up the least active 25% of the population, as defined by the combination of a sedentary job involving sitting for a large part of the day and no regular exercise or active recreational pursuits
NEGATIVE RISK FACTOR	**DEFINING CRITERIA**
High serum high-density	>60 mg/dL (1.6 mmol/L) lipoprotein cholesterol

From American College of Sports Medicine. *ACSM's Guidelines for Exercise Testing and Prescription.* 7th ed. Baltimore, MD: Lippincott Williams & Wilkins; 2010; with permission.

(**Table 24.3**).[23] For individuals with CAD, regular and recreational physical activity and moderate-intensity exercise training are recommended.[22]

Marfan Syndrome

Marfan syndrome does not necessarily lead to SCD. When SCD does occur, it usually is caused by the condition's hallmark characteristic—namely, a weakened aorta. Marfan syndrome is a genetic disorder of the connective tissue that can affect the skeleton, lungs, eyes, heart, and blood vessels. A single mutant gene is linked to the condition. Although usually inherited, 25% of all cases have no family history.[24]

Individuals with Marfan syndrome are tall in stature, with overly long extremities; the arm span exceeds the person's height. Joints usually are hypermobile, and the person may have a pigeon (sunken) chest, stretch marks, scoliosis, and increased incidence of hernias. A positive thumb test and wrist test are classic signs of Marfan syndrome. The thumb test involves adduction of the thumb across the palm of the hand and flexion of the fingers around the thumb; the test is positive if the thumb extends past the fifth finger. The wrist test involves the person encircling a wrist with the thumb and fifth finger of the opposite hand; the test is positive if the thumb and fifth finger overlap. In addition to orthopedic anomalies, it is not unusual to find an excessively high palate, eye defects (i.e., myopia or nearsightedness), MVP, and defects in the connective tissue layers of the aorta. As a result of the defect in the aorta tissues, death from Marfan syndrome usually is associated with an aortic dissection or rupture.

Screening for Marfan syndrome includes a musculoskeletal and eye examination as well as an echocardiogram to determine abnormalities of the aorta. Marfan syndrome has no cure, but with careful medical management, most people can live a normal life. An individual with Marfan syndrome should avoid contact activities because of the risk of injury to the eyes and aorta. Individuals can participate in low and moderate static/low dynamic competitive sports, such as brisk walking, leisure bicycling, golf, slow jogging, and slow-paced tennis if they do not have aortic root dilation, moderate-to-severe mitral regurgitation, or a family history of dissection causing sudden death in a Marfan relative.[22]

See **Screening for Marfan Syndrome**, available on the companion Web site at thePoint.

Rare Cardiac Conditions

Other rare cardiac conditions, such as a long QT syndrome and right ventricular dysplasia, may contribute to SCD. Both conditions produce serious arrhythmias. Long QT syndrome, which usually affects children and young adults, is a hereditary disorder of the heart's electrical system. The individual is susceptible to arrhythmia, which produces inefficient contraction of the heart. The result is the reduction of normal blood volume in the body and the brain. Inability of the heart to regain its normal rhythm can lead to ventricular fibrillation, which is a fatal arrhythmia.

Right ventricular dysplasia, a disorder of the right ventricle, is characterized by the formation of adipose or fibrous tissue extending from the epicardium to the endocardium. This abnormal growth of tissue increases the risk of ventricular fibrillation. Any unstable ventricular heart rhythm, such as ventricular tachycardia or ventricular fibrillation, can lead to death. In fact, most cardiac conditions that produce SCD are the result of an abnormal ventricular rhythm.[21,22]

Wolff-Parkinson-White syndrome is an abnormality of cardiac rhythm that manifests as an SVT. The condition is associated with an accessory electrical pathway in the heart proximal to the ventricles that can spontaneously produce episodes of rapid twitching of the atrium muscle fibers within a range of 200 to 300 heartbeats per minute. The condition often is seen in asymptomatic, healthy individuals during electrocardiographic examination. Although rarely associated with sudden death, the condition may complicate other heart conditions, such as myocarditis or ischemic heart disease.

Congenital coronary artery anomalies are another cause of sudden death in young athletes. The most common anomaly is an abnormal origin of the left coronary artery. The anomaly necessitates an acute takeoff angle, forcing the artery to pass between the aorta and the pulmonary artery, both of which can decrease blood flow to the heart. Other anomalies may involve an abnormal origin of the right coronary artery, presence of a right coronary artery without a left coronary artery, and abnormal coronary artery spasm. Congenital coronary artery anomalies may not be detected during exercise because symptoms, such as syncope, near syncope, and chest pain, are intermittent and unpredictable.

Noncardiac Causes of Sudden Death

SCD usually is directly related to cardiac conditions. Noncardiac conditions, however, also can lead to SCD; these include commotio cordis, substance abuse, head injuries, heat illness, exertional hyperthermia, exercise-induced anaphylaxis, exertional rhabdomyolysis, and sickle cell trait. Often, noncardiac conditions are more easily identifiable through physical examination and field evaluation. As such, if a condition can be identified, it usually can be treated.

Commotio Cordis

Cardiac arrest from a low-impact, blunt blow to the chest in the absence of a structural cardiovascular disease is rare in sports. According to the U.S. Commotio Cordis Registry, since 1995, 188 athletes have died from blunt force injury to the heart (commotio cordis). The mean age was 14.7 years, and 96% were males.[25] The leading mechanism of injury was from a projectile striking the chest, including baseballs, softballs, hockey pucks, and lacrosse balls. Other less frequent projectiles were a soccer ball and a cricket ball.[26] Also, many deaths occur around the home or on the playground in informal activities related or unrelated to recreational sports (often involving close relatives) in which the chest impact is delivered in an innocent fashion (e.g., light blows during playful "shadow boxing").[22] Postmortem analyses of individuals dying from commotio cordis often reveal no structural damage to the heart or overlying protective structures (e.g., sternum or ribs), but soft-tissue contusions of the left chest wall are commonly visualized.[27] This suggests that sudden death in these cases resulted from blunt force–induced conduction abnormalities.

Upon impact, collapse may be instantaneous or preceded by brief periods of consciousness and physical activity. Resuscitation efforts were previously rarely successful; however, resuscitation has been proven to be more successful (35%).[28,29] Because commotio cordis usually is a fatal event, focus has been aimed at prevention. Possible prevention strategies include the use of protective padded equipment that covers the area of the chest over the heart, switching to age-appropriate safety balls or pucks made of softer materials, and encouraging all coaches and officials to become trained in cardiopulmonary resuscitation (CPR), automated external defibrillator (AED) use, and first aid.

Substance Abuse

Many nutritional supplements and drugs are marketed to improve exercise duration or physical strength, to shorten recovery time from exertion, to reduce fat, or to enhance athletic performance in other ways. Certain types of drug abuse can lead to cardiac changes that predispose an individual to SCD. Amphetamines are central nervous system stimulants that increase heart rate, respiration rate, and blood pressure. Cocaine, which is an anesthetic, constricts coronary arteries and has been known to lead to myocardial infarction in those with and in those without CAD. In addition, myocarditis has been found in autopsy reports of cocaine-related SCD cases. It must be noted that a massive dose of cocaine is not required to produce cardiac or respiratory consequences. Several reported cases of SCD have involved anabolic steroid users, although a direct relationship between steroid use and sudden death has not yet been established.

Produced in the kidneys, **erythropoietin** is a hormone that stimulates bone marrow to increase production of RBCs. Erythropoietin (EPO/EPOGEN) became synthetically available in the late 1980s when its use as an ergogenic aid for endurance athletes was first documented. The use of EPO is equal to blood doping and, like blood doping, can increase blood volume and viscosity of the blood, leading to decreased circulation, thrombosis, and myocardial infarction. These adverse cardiovascular effects have led to SCD; EPO may be one of the most deadly ergogenic aids available.[30]

Head Injuries

Catastrophic brain injuries that can lead to SCD include skull fracture, epidural hematoma, acute and subacute subdural hematoma, second-impact syndrome, or various other brain hemorrhage conditions. Individuals should be observed closely after sustaining any type of head injury, regardless of the level of consciousness. Signs of rapidly increasing intracranial pressure include a dilated or irregular pupil or pupils, reduced pulse, nausea or vomiting, dyspnea, **photophobia**, mood swings, muscle weakness, and decreased level of consciousness. **Decortication**, a condition that presents as extension of the legs with flexion of the elbows, wrists, and fingers, or **decerebration**, a condition that presents as extension of all four extremities, often is present in severe injuries (see Chapter 7). An individual who is unable to remember events leading up to (i.e., **retrograde amnesia**) or following the injury (i.e., **anterograde amnesia**) should not be permitted to continue activity and should be referred immediately to a physician. Additional information concerning head injuries can be found in Chapter 20.

Heat Illness

Heat illness is one of the most preventable causes of SCD, yet individuals die from exertional hyperthermia each year. In football, heat stroke is second only to head injuries as the most frequent cause of death. The condition also is seen in distance runners and wrestlers who are dehydrated through weight loss. Heat stroke almost always is preceded by prolonged, strenuous physical exercise in individuals who are poorly acclimatized or in situations during which evaporation of sweat is inhibited.

The individual often complains of a feeling of "burning up." Deep breaths, irritability, hysterical behavior, and an unsteady gait may be present. As the condition deteriorates, the skin is hot and dry and appears to be red or flushed, and the pulse becomes rapid and strong (as high as 150 to 170 heartbeats per minute). Brain tissue damage by excessive body heat leads to vasomotor collapse, shallow breathing, decreased blood pressure, and a rapid and weak pulse. Muscle twitching or seizures may occur just before the individual lapses into a coma. This condition is a medical emergency and, as such, warrants activation of the EAP, including summoning EMS. Further information concerning heat illness is presented in Chapter 29.

Sickle Cell Trait

Sickle cell trait is an inherited disorder in which RBCs tend to form into a sickle-shaped structure (**Fig. 24.4**). This sickling formation of RBCs prevents efficient transportation of oxygen to the tissues and can lead to vascular occlusion, coagulation, and even death. Eight percent of all African Americans have sickle cell trait, and individuals in the 23- to 30-year-old age range have a 1.3 in 1,000 chance of dying from sudden death during exertional activities, particularly during extreme conditions of heat, humidity, and increased altitude.[31] Unexpected death is almost always associated with severe exertional **rhabdomyolysis**, a fatal disease stemming from renal failure caused when cellular contents of damaged skeletal muscle (myoglobin) enter the circulation. Sickle cell anemia is easily screened through laboratory testing. As such, recommendations can be made to ensure that individuals with sickle cell anemia can safely participate in sport and physical activity.

 Following the collapse of the Little League Baseball, an immediate assessment of airway, breathing, and circulation (ABCs) is essential. If the athlete is not breathing or does not have a pulse, the EAP, including summoning EMS, should be activated and CPR administered. The player may have experienced cardiac arrest from the blow to the chest. The condition, known as commotio cordis, results in conduction abnormalities. Because it usually is fatal, focus has been on prevention rather than treatment.

CARDIOVASCULAR PREPARTICIPATION SCREENING

 In preparation for PPEs of high school and college athletes, several areas must be addressed, including obtaining a cardiovascular history. What questions should be asked as part of the medical history to assist in screening for those at risk of sudden death?

Identification of the risks associated with SCD requires a two-tiered approach. First, a standard screening examination should be done 6 to 8 weeks before engaging in physical activity or sport and be performed by a health care provider with the medical skills, requisite training, and clinical experience to obtain a detailed cardiovascular history, to perform an extensive physical examination, and to recognize potential heart disease or cardiac anomalies. In an attempt to improve the screening and identification of individuals at potential risk of SCD, the American Heart Association (AHA) recommends 12 items (8 for personal and family history and 4 for physical examination) be investigated (**Box 24.7**). At the discretion of the primary care physician, a positive response or finding in any 1 or more of the 12 items may be judged sufficient cause to refer the individual for cardiovascular evaluation. Parental verification is recommended for high school and middle school age children.

Although these guidelines present a somewhat standard approach for reducing the incidence of SCD, no universal standard for screening high school athletes exists. Most preparticipation standards are set by state legislation, state athletic associations, or individual school districts, and most often consist of a medical history review and basic physical examination.[32] Identification of a possible cardiovascular abnormality during the cardiac history or standard physical examination is the first tier of recognition. Many of these conditions were listed in **Box 2.3**. The second tier involves referral to a cardiologist for more extensive screening, including an echocardiogram.

 See **Diagnostic Testing for Various Causes of Sudden Cardiac Death**, available on the companion Web site at thePoint.

The decision regarding whether to permit an individual to participate after identifying a cardiovascular abnormality must be resolved on an individual basis under the Americans with Disabilities Act of 1990, the Rehabilitation Act of 1973, and similar state statutes prohibiting unjustified discrimination against the physically impaired. These laws permit an individual with the physical capabilities and skills to participate in a sport despite the fact that a cardiovascular abnormality is present. Exclusion from participation must be based on reasonable medical judgments, given the state of scientific research on the specific condition. These laws require careful balancing of the individual's right to participate, the physician's evaluation of the medical risks of participation, and an organization's interest in conducting a safe athletic program.

Many health care professionals, including members of the National Athletic Trainers' Association, believe that emergency preparedness and management of sudden cardiac arrest are a priority for every sport venue, including high school and college athletic programs.[33] As part of a well-defined EAP, every facility should establish catastrophic incident guidelines that address the immediate action plan, chain of command responsibilities, standards for documentation of the event,

BOX 24.7 The 12-Element American Heart Association Recommendations for Preparticipation Cardiovascular Screening of Competitive Athletes

Medical History[a]

Personal history

1. Exertional chest pain/discomfort

2. Unexplained syncope/near syncope[b]

3. Excessive exertional and unexplained dyspnea/fatigue associated with exercise

4. Prior recognition of a heart murmur

5. Elevated systemic blood pressure

Family history

6. Premature death (sudden and unexpected, or otherwise) before age 50 years due to heart disease in at least one relative

7. Disability from heart disease in a close relative younger than 50 years of age

8. Specific knowledge of certain cardiac conditions in family members: hypertrophic or dilated cardiomyopathy, long QT syndrome or other ion channelopathies, Marfan syndrome, or clinically important arrhythmias

Physical examination

9. Heart murmur[c]

10. Femoral pulses to exclude aortic coarctation

11. Physical stigmata of Marfan syndrome

12. Brachial artery blood pressure (sitting position)[d]

[a]Parental verification is recommended for high school and middle school athletes.

[b]Judged not to be neurocardiogenic (vasovagal); of particular concern when related to exertion.

[c]Auscultation should be performed in both supine and standing positions (or with Valsalva maneuver), specifically to identify murmurs of dynamic left ventricular outflow tract obstruction.

[d]Preferably taken in both arms.

From American Heart Association. Preparticipation cardiovascular screening of young competitive athletes: policy guidance (June 2012). https://www.heart.org/idc/groups/ahaecc-public/@wcm/@adv/documents/downloadable/ucm_443945.pdf.

and long-term support for individuals who may be affected by SCD. This action plan should include CPR and AED training for all targeted first responders, and it recommends that access to early defibrillation is essential within 3 to 5 minutes from the time of the collapse to the first shock. The review of equipment readiness and the EAP by on-site personnel for each athletic event is desirable, as is the annual review of the EAP.[33] It is critical to have an EAP in place to help any facility or sport program work through an emotional and highly visible situation.

 The medical history for cardiovascular conditions should include questions regarding previous chest pain during physical exertion; exercise-induced syncope or near syncope; excessive, unexplained shortness of breath, fatigue, and dizziness with exercise; history of heart murmur; history of hypertension; family history of death from cardiovascular disease in a relative younger than 50 years; and family history of HCM, dilated cardiomyopathy, long QT syndrome, or Marfan syndrome.

SUMMARY

1. Anemia is a reduction in either the RBC volume (hematocrit) or hemoglobin concentration. Anemia reduces maximum aerobic capacity, decreases physical work capability at submaximal levels, increases lactic acidosis, increases fatigue, and decreases exercise time to exhaustion.

2. Hemophilia occurs in three types—namely, A, B, and C. These types are distinguished by the clotting factor that is deficient. All three types can cause prolonged bleeding.

3. Reye syndrome is a rare but serious, acute illness that disrupts the body's urea cycle, resulting in the accumulation of ammonia in the blood, hypoglycemia, severe brain edema, and critically high intracranial pressure. The disease almost exclusively affects individuals from 2 to 16 years of age. It is linked to the use of aspirin to treat a viral infection.

4. Syncope is a transient LOC, described as "fainting," that often occurs in healthy individuals.

5. Shock occurs when the heart is unable to exert adequate pressure to circulate enough oxygenated blood to vital organs.

6. A rapid and weak pulse is the most prominent sign of shock, but other signs include rapid and shallow breathing, profuse sweating, and cold, clammy skin.

7. Reflex (neurally mediated) syncope is the most common type of syncope that produces fainting and results from a sudden drop in blood pressure, which reduces blood circulation to the brain, leading to an LOC.

8. Blood pressure is the force per unit area exerted on the walls of an artery, generally considered to be the aorta. It is the result of two factors—namely, cardiac output and total peripheral resistance.

9. Blood pressure varies among individuals, but normal is considered to be 120 mm Hg SBP over 80 mm Hg DBP. Hypertension is defined as a sustained, elevated blood pressure of greater than 140 mm Hg SBP or greater than 90 mm Hg DBP. Hypotension is characterized by a fall of 20 mm Hg or more from a person's normal baseline SBP.

10. An individual in stage 1 or 2 hypertension should not participate in sport and physical activity until cleared by a physician. Individuals with stage 1 hypertension usually can participate if the blood pressure is well controlled and no target organ damage or heart disease is present. The blood pressure should be rechecked every week by a qualified specialist (e.g., athletic trainer) and every 2 to 4 months by the physician.

11. For individuals in stage 2 hypertension, restrictions are placed on physical activity, especially in sports or activities with a high static component.

12. Diet modifications for hypertension include limiting sodium and saturated fats, with the total dietary fat not to exceed 30% of the total caloric intake, and increasing potassium, calcium, and magnesium intake.

13. Aerobic exercise has been shown to reduce blood pressure among individuals in the prehypertension stage and in stage 1 hypertension.

14. Orthostatic hypotension is not unusual; however, a physician should be consulted if dizziness or light-headedness becomes more frequent with a sudden change in body position.

15. Physically active people do not usually need to be concerned with hypotension. In general, a lower blood pressure is desirable as long as the person feels well.

16. SCD is rare. When it does occur, however, the on-site personnel should immediately activate the EAP and begin CPR.

17. HCM is the most common cardiac-related cause of sudden death.

18. Other cardiac-related causes of SCD include MVP, myocarditis, acquired valvular heart disease, CAD, Marfan syndrome, long QT syndrome, Wolff-Parkinson-White syndrome, and arrhythmogenic right ventricular dysplasia.

19. Noncardiac causes of SCD include commotio cordis, heat illness, head injuries, substance abuse, exertional hyperthermia, exercise-induced anaphylaxis, exertional rhabdomyolysis, and sickle cell anemia.

20. The risk of SCD in physically active individuals can be reduced by using a two-tiered system. First, a PPE should include an extensive cardiac medical history and physical examination. If a cardiac abnormality is identified, the individual should then be referred to a specialist for further evaluation.

21. Determination of continued participation in sports should rest with the individual and the team physician after consultation with expert cardiologists, family, and team officials.

APPLICATION QUESTIONS

1. You are employed as an athletic trainer at a high school. During a preseason meeting with athletes and their parents, one of the parents expresses concern about recent news stories reporting an increased incidence of SCD in young athletes. The parent asks you to describe the screening process for SCD as it pertains to the student athletes at your school and discuss the effectiveness of the screening process. How would you respond to the parent's questions?

2. You are providing athletic training services for a high school lacrosse tournament. A 17-year-old goalie takes a line drive shot to his chest. He immediately collapses. What condition might be suspected? What is the immediate management for this potential condition?

3. A senior athlete reports feeling dizzy when getting up from a lying-down position and when suddenly changing body positions while playing tennis. What open-ended questions might you use to gather a thorough medical history? What might this person be experiencing? How would you manage this situation?

4. A collegiate wrestler has been diagnosed with sickle cell anemia. What implications will this have on his sport performance? What can be done to lessen the impact of this disease on the individual?

5. You are the athletic trainer for a National Collegiate Athletic Association (NCAA) Division I football program. During the preparticipation examination, one of the players was found to have a blood pressure of 150/90 mm Hg. Should you be concerned with this measurement? Why or why not? What implications might this blood pressure have on athletic participation? What is your immediate course of action?

REFERENCES

1. Fields KB. Anemia in athletes. In: Mellion MB, Walsh WM, Madden C, et al, eds. *Team Physician's Handbook*. Philadelphia, PA: Hanley & Belfus; 2002:249–253.

2. Eichner ER. Sickle cell trait. *J Sport Rehabil*. 2007;16(3):197–203.

3. National Athletic Trainers' Association. Consensus statement: sickle cell trait and the athlete. http://www.nata.org/sites/default/files/SickleCellTraitAndTheAthlete.pdf. Accessed July 1, 2015.

4. Bolton-Maggs PH, Pasi KJ. Haemophilias A and B. *Lancet*. 2003;361(9371):1801–1809.

5. Tamparo CD, Lewis MA. *Diseases of the Human Body*. Philadelphia, PA: FA Davis; 2011.

6. Moya A, Sutton R, Ammirati F, et al. Guidelines for the diagnosis and management of syncope (version 2009). *Eur Heart J*. 2009;30(21):2631–2671. Accessed July 1, 2015.

7. Jhanjee R, van Dijk JG, Sakaguchi S, et al. Syncope in adults: terminology, classification, and diagnostic strategy. *Pacing Clin Electrophysiol*. 2006;29(10):1160–1169.

8. James PA, Oparil S, Carter BL, et al. 2014 evidence-based guideline for the management of high blood pressure in adults report from the panel members appointed to the Eighth Joint National Committee (JNC 8). *JAMA*. 2014;311(5):507–520. Accessed July 1, 2015.

9. U.S. Department of Health and Human Services, National Institutes of Health. Description of high blood pressure. http://www.nhlbi.nih.gov/health/health-topics/topics/hbp. Accessed July 15, 2015.

10. U.S. Department of Agriculture, U.S. Department of Health and Human Services. *Dietary Guidelines for Americans, 2010.* 7th ed. Washington, DC: U.S. Government Printing Office; 2010. http://health.gov/dietaryguidelines/dga2010/DietaryGuidelines2010.pdf. Accessed July 15, 2015.

11. U.S. Department of Health and Human Services, National Institutes of Health. 2008 physical activity guidelines for Americans. www.health.gov/paguidelines. Accessed July 15, 2015.

12. Van Camp SP, Bloor CM, Mueller FO, et al. Nontraumatic sports death in high school and college athletes. *Med Sci Sports Exerc.* 1995;27(5):641–647.

13. Casa DJ, Guskiewicz KM, Anderson SA, et al. National Athletic Trainers' Association position statement: preventing sudden death in sports. *J Athl Train.* 2012;47(1):96–118. http://www.nata.org/sites/default/files/Preventing-Sudden-Death-Position-Statement_2.pdf. Accessed July 15, 2015.

14. Casa DJ, Anderson SA, Baker L, et al. The Inter-Association Task Force for preventing sudden death in collegiate conditioning sessions: best practices recommendations. *J Athl Train.* 2012;47(4):477–480. Accessed July 15, 2015.

15. Casa DJ, Almquist J, Anderson SA, et al. The Inter-Association Task Force for preventing sudden death in secondary school athletics programs: best practices recommendations. *J Athl Train.* 2013;48(4):546–553. Accessed July 15, 2015.

16. Maron BJ, Haas TS, Murphy CJ, et al. Incidence and causes of sudden death in U.S. college athletes. *J Am Coll Cardiol.* 2014;63(16):1636–1643. http://content.onlinejacc.org/article.aspx?articleID=1838312. Accessed July 15, 2015.

17. Maron BJ. Sudden death in young athletes. *N Engl J Med.* 2003;349(11):1064–1075.

18. Maron BJ, Doerer JJ, Haas TS, et al. Sudden deaths in young competitive athletes: analysis of 1866 deaths in the United States, 1980–2006. *Circulation.* 2009;119(8):1085–1092. http://circ.ahajournals.org/content/119/8/1085.long. Accessed July 15, 2015.

19. Wever-Pinzon OE, Myerson M, Sherrid MV. Sudden cardiac death in young competitive athletes due to genetic cardiac abnormalities. *Anadolu Kardiyol Derg.* 2009;9(suppl 2):17–23.

20. Pelliccia A, Maron BJ, Culasso F, et al. Athlete's heart in women. Echocardiographic characterization of highly trained elite female athletes. *JAMA.* 1996;276(3):211–215.

21. Hayek E, Gring CN, Griffin BP. Mitral valve prolapse. *Lancet.* 2005;365(9458):507–518.

22. Maron BJ, Zipes DP. 36th Bethesda Conference: eligibility recommendations for competitive athletes with cardiovascular abnormalities. *J Am Coll Cardiology.* 2005;45(8):1311–1375.

23. American College of Sports Medicine. *ACSM's Guidelines for Exercise Testing and Prescription.* Baltimore, MD: Lippincott Williams & Wilkins; 2010.

24. Ho NC, Tran JR, Bektas A. Marfan's syndrome. *Lancet.* 2005;366(9501):1978–1981.

25. National Athletic Trainers' Association. NATA official statement on commotio cordis. http://www.nata.org/sites/default/files/CommotioCordis.pdf. Accessed July 1, 2015.

26. Maron BJ, Gohman TE, Kyle SB, et al. Clinical profile and spectrum of commotio cordis. *JAMA.* 2002;287(9):1142–1146.

27. Maron BJ, Poliac LC, Kaplan JA, et al. Blunt impact to the chest leading to sudden death from cardiac arrest during sports activities. *N Engl J Med.* 1995;333(6):337–342.

28. Link MS. Commotio cordis: ventricular fibrillation triggered by chest impact–induced abnormalities in repolarization. *Circ Arrhythm Electrophysiol.* 2012;5(2):425–432. Accessed July 15, 2015.

29. Maron BJ, Doerer JJ, Haas TS, et al. Commotio cordis and the epidemiology of sudden death in competitive lacrosse. *Pediatrics.* 2009;124(3):966–971.

30. Eichner ER. Blood doping: infusions, erythropoietin and artificial blood. *Sports Med.* 2007;37(4–5):389–391.

31. Harris KM, Haas TS, Eichner ER, et al. Sickle cell trait associated with sudden death in competitive athletes. *Am J Cardiol.* 2012;110(8):1185–1188.

32. O'Connor DP, Knoblauch MA. Electrocardiogram testing during athletic preparticipation physical examinations. *J Athl Train.* 2010;45(3):265–272.

33. Inter-Association Task Force Recommendations on Emergency Preparedness and Management of Sudden Cardiac Arrest in High School and College Athletic Programs: A Consensus Statement. https://www.nata.org/sites/default/files/sudden-cardiac-arrest-consensus-statement.pdf

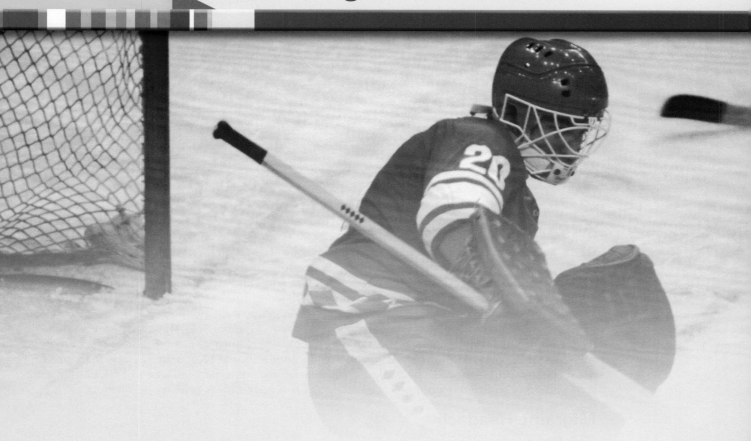

STUDENT OUTCOMES

1. Describe the pathophysiology of migraine headaches.

2. List the signs and symptoms of various types of migraine headaches.

3. Describe the prevention and management of migraine headaches.

4. Differentiate between a seizure disorder and epilepsy.

5. Identify the causes of epilepsy.

6. List the types of generalized and partial seizures.

7. Describe the characteristics and management of common seizures.

8. Describe the seizure situations that constitute a medical emergency.

9. Explain the exercise guidelines for individuals with controlled seizures.

INTRODUCTION

The body's nervous system includes the brain, spinal cord, and nerves. It regulates and coordinates body activities, and it brings about responses by which the body adjusts to changes in its internal and external environment. Initially, this chapter explores migraine headaches—namely, their types, signs, symptoms, and management. Next, the various types of seizure disorders are presented followed by signs, symptoms, management, and physical activity guidelines for those who suffer from a seizure disorder. Finally, information is presented regarding infections of the central nervous system and reflex sympathetic dystrophy.

HEADACHES

 A female collegiate basketball player complains of a pounding headache with nausea. Two weeks earlier, she reported a similar headache that was accompanied by light sensitivity. Should this individual be referred to a physician for further assessment and care?

It is estimated that a majority of men and women have experienced one or more severe headaches. Migraine headaches in particular afflict women more than men.[1] In addition, headaches are the most common pain reported in adolescent children.[2] Headaches may be chronic or acute, and they often signal nothing more than fatigue, stress, or tension. In some cases, however, headaches can indicate a serious disease (**Box 25.1**).

Headaches are caused by irritation of one or more of the pain-sensitive structures or tissues in the head and neck including the cranial arteries and veins, the cranial and spinal nerves, the cranial and cervical muscles, and the meninges. The condition may stem from organic disorders (e.g., toxins, systemic diseases, or diseases in specific systems of the body), psychoneurological problems (e.g., nervous tension, fatigue, worry, excitement, or psychoneuroses), or environmental insults (e.g., head trauma, bright lights, noise, rapid altitude change, sunstroke, motion sickness, or irritants such as smoke, dust, or pollen).[3] According to the International Headache Society, there are four main classifications of headaches: migraine headache, tension-type headache (TTH), cluster headache and other trigeminal autonomic cephalalgias (TACs), and other primary headaches.[4]

Migraine Headache

Etiology

A migraine headache is defined by the International Headache Society as an idiopathic, episodic headache disorder with attacks lasting from 4 to 72 hours and is classified into two major subtypes, migraine without aura and migraine with aura with four additional subgroups that include symptoms from one of the two major subtypes (**Box 25.2**).[4] Women with a history of migraines show a relationship between their headaches and menstrual cycle. Menstrual migraines are thought to be triggered by a change in estrogen levels that accompanies the menstrual cycle.[5] This fluctuation in hormone level is considered one of many **triggers** or conditions that hasten, worsen, or lengthen the

---

BOX 25.1 Red Flags That Require Further Examination

- Serious headaches after 50 years of age
- Headache associated with focal neurological deficits
- Sudden onset of a headache
- Papilledema (i.e., edema of the optic disc)
- Change in pattern in a headache (e.g., increased severity and frequency)
- Headache associated with trauma

- Headache associated with antalgic gait, amnesia, or altered consciousness
- New-onset headache in immunocompromised patients
- Headache associated with systemic illness, fever, or neck stiffness
- Early morning nausea and vomiting without headache

BOX 25.2 Classifications of Migraine Headaches

- **Migraine without aura.** Recurrent headache disorder manifesting in attacks lasting 4–72 hours. Typical characteristics of the headache are unilateral location, pulsating quality, moderate or severe intensity, aggravation by routine physical activity, and association with nausea and/or photophobia and phonophobia.

- **Migraine with aura.** Recurrent disorder manifesting in attacks of reversible focal neurological symptoms that usually develop gradually more than 5 minutes and last 60 minutes. Attacks include unilateral visual, sensory, or other central nervous system symptoms such as reversible changes in speech, motor, or visual changes. Headache with the features of migraine without aura usually follows the aura symptoms. Less commonly, headache lacks migrainous features or is completely absent.

- **Chronic migraine.** Headache occurring on 15 or more days per month for more than 3 months with symptoms occurring at least 8 days per month. This migraine is classified because of the inability to differentiate individual headache episodes and difficulty in keeping individuals medication-free in order to assess the headache history.

- **Complications with migraine.** A debilitating migraine lasting more than 72 hours that may include migrainous aura and/or non–aura-debilitating symptoms. Such migraines include persistent aura without infarction, migrainous infarction, and migraine aura-triggered seizures.

- **Probable migraine.** Previously termed migrainous disorder, probable migraines are classified as migraine-like headaches that are secondary to another disorder. This attack is usually missing one of the features required for the two major subgroups of migraine.

- **Episodic syndromes that may be associated with migraine.** Episodes can occur from excessive, frequent crying in a baby from birth to 4 months who shows signs of colic, or childhood period syndromes such as motion sickness and periodic sleep disorders (sleep walking, sleep talking, night terrors, bruxism), recurrent gastrointestinal disturbance, cyclic vomiting syndrome, abdominal migraine, benign paroxysmal vertigo, and benign paroxysmal torticollis.

Headache Classification Committee of the International Headache Society. The international classification of headache disorders, 3rd edition (beta version). *Cephalalgia.* 2013;33(9):629–808. http://www.ihs-classification.org/_downloads/mixed/International-Headache-Classification-III-ICHD-III-2013-Beta.pdf.

duration of a migraine. Other common triggers include aspartame, caffeine (i.e., use or withdrawal), monosodium glutamate, nicotine, nitrates, alcohol, cheese, chocolate, missed meals, perfume, red grapes, too much or too little sleep, stress, bright lights, strong odors, or a change in altitude.[4,6]

Signs and Symptoms

Migraine with aura, commonly referred to as a classic migraine, is characterized by a forewarning, also known as an aura that usually precedes the onset of a migraine roughly 5 to 60 minutes before the headache. Some of the most common auras include seeing flashes, losing part of the visual field, smelling a specific odor, tasting a specific taste, or feeling dizzy. Migraine headaches typically are unilateral (but also can be bilateral), pulsating, of moderate to severe intensity, exacerbated by activity, and associated with nausea, vomiting, photophobia, phonophobia, and the desire to lie down in a dark, quiet room. Migraine headaches can last from 4 hours to 3 days.[4]

Tension-Type Headache

Etiology

This is the most common type of primary headache; its lifetime prevalence in the general population ranges in different studies from 30% to 78%. Previously, little was known about this type of headache, however, several studies have recently been completed strongly suggesting a neurobiological cause.[4]

Signs and Symptoms

This type of headache is characterized by bilateral, mild to moderate pain that is of a "pressing" or "tightening" quality in the bitemporal or occipital region. Pain lasts from 30 minutes to 7 days and may be associated with mild nausea, phonophobia, and photophobia. Chronic TTHs are present at least 15 days per month for at least 6 months.[4]

Cluster Headache

Etiology

Cluster headaches present as severe unilateral pain, either orbitally, supraorbitally, or temporally, that lasts from 15 to 180 minutes. They occur from every other day to eight times per day and often wake the patient from sleep.[4] Although less common than migraines, cluster headaches onset is between 20 and 40 years of age and tend to occur more often in males.

Signs and Symptoms

The pain is often described as unilateral "stabbing," "boring," or "burning." Pain is clustered, or grouped, and can last from 2 weeks to 3 months, followed by headache-free periods that last from months to years.[4] The episodes are associated with at least two of the following, all of which are ipsilateral: conjunctival injection, lacrimation, nasal congestion, rhinorrhea, forehead and facial sweating, pupillary contraction (miosis), lid drooping (ptosis), and eyelid edema. Most patients are restless or agitated during an attack. Alcohol may trigger the headache.

Other Primary Headaches

Etiology

This category of headaches is used when a new headache occurs for the first time in close temporal relation to another disorder that is a known cause of headache, and this new headache is coded according to the causative disorder as a secondary headache. This group can include the following[4]:

- Headaches precipitated by coughing or straining in the absence of any intracranial disorder (coughing headache)

- Headache precipitated by any form of exercise. Subforms such as "weight lifters' headache" are recognized (exertional headache).

- Headache precipitated by sexual activity, usually starting as a dull bilateral ache as sexual excitement increases and suddenly becoming intense at orgasm, in the absence of any intracranial disorder

- Attacks of dull headache that always awaken the patient from sleep

- High-intensity headache of abrupt onset mimicking that of ruptured cerebral aneurysm

- Persistent strictly unilateral headache responsive to indomethacin

- Headache that is daily and unremitting from very soon after onset (within 3 days at most). The pain is typically bilateral, pressing or tightening in quality, and of mild to moderate intensity. There may be photophobia, phonophobia, or mild nausea.

Signs and Symptoms

Because of the very nature of the diverse causes of headaches in this category, signs and symptoms are also varied.

Management of Headaches

Treatment begins with a history and description of the headache while ruling out metabolic and structural etiologies. Most headaches are treated with drug therapy; however, the longer the symptoms go untreated, the less likely that medication will relieve the pain. Over-the-counter pain relievers, such as ibuprofen, naproxen, and caffeine, or nonsteroidal anti-inflammatory drugs (NSAIDs) may be sufficient. Prescription medications used for intense headaches include drugs intended to prevent the migraine from occurring and abortive drugs to stop the headache after it begins.

Preventive treatment may be warranted if headaches interfere with daily activities or occur more than four times per month. A number of drugs and alternative therapeutic techniques can be used, including β-blockers, calcium channel blockers, antidepressants, selective serotonin-reuptake inhibitors, monoamine oxidase inhibitors, NSAIDs, and corticosteroids.[1,4] Stress reduction and biofeedback techniques also have been successful for some patients.[4] If medications and stress reduction techniques are not helpful, a computed tomographic scan or magnetic resonance imaging may be necessary to determine if a structural disorder of the central nervous system is causing the pain.

> The female basketball player most likely has a migraine headache. Her history is consistent with a migraine headache, including throbbing or pounding headache pain associated with light sensitivity, loss of appetite, and/or nausea four or more times per month. If the headache does not respond to an over-the-counter anti-inflammatory or analgesic medication, referral to a physician is warranted.

SEIZURE DISORDERS AND EPILEPSY

? What issues should be addressed in determining the sport participation level of an individual with a seizure disorder?

A seizure is an abnormal electrical discharge in the brain. A **seizure disorder** entails recurrent episodes of sudden, excessive charges of electrical activity in the brain, whether from known or idiopathic causes. **Epilepsy** is a general term used to describe only recurrent (at least two) idiopathic episodes of sudden, excessive discharges of electrical activity in the brain. The discharge may trigger altered sensation, perception, behavior, mood, level of consciousness, or convulsive movements. Seizures and epilepsy often are used interchangeably; however, it is important to understand their definitions.

Causes of Epilepsy

Epilepsy appears to be directly related to age of onset and generally is categorized as provoked or unprovoked (**Box 25.3**). Seizures that begin before 5 years of age usually are associated with mental or neurological impairment. Seizures that begin between 5 and 15 years of age are not usually associated

---

BOX 25.3 Causes of Epilepsy

1. Unprovoked or idiopathic (no cause of the seizure is identified)
2. Provoked
   - Posttraumatic (e.g., skull fracture, intracranial hematoma)
   - Metabolic (e.g., hyponatremia, hypocalcemia, hypoglycemia, hypomagnesemia, dehydration)
   - Drug and drug withdrawal (e.g., alcohol, cocaine)
   - Infections (e.g., meningitis, encephalitis, brain abscess)
   - Anoxia and hypoxia
   - Cerebrovascular (e.g., stroke, intracerebral or subarachnoid hemorrhage, sinus thrombosis)
   - Hyperthermia
   - Sleep deprivation
   - Febrile seizures
   - Neoplasms (e.g., primary intracranial, carcinomatous meningitis, metastatic, lymphoma, leukemia)
   - Perinatal or hereditary (e.g., congenital anomalies, genetic and hereditary disorders, perinatal trauma)

with a known metabolic or structural cause and are called idiopathic or unprovoked seizures. These seizures respond very well to treatment, and individuals usually can participate in physical activity with little to no restrictions. Trauma and tumors are responsible for most seizures in young adults; strokes are the most frequent cause in those 40 years and older.[7]

Types of Seizures

Seizures can be divided into three basic types:

1. Partial or focal

2. Generalized

3. Special epileptic syndromes

Box 25.4 summarizes the classifications of seizures.

Partial or Focal Seizures

■ Etiology

Partial or focal seizures have a localized onset, are focused in one particular area of the brain, and are restricted to specific areas of the body. Partial seizures may be subdivided into simple, in which consciousness is retained, and complex, in which consciousness is impaired.

■ Signs and Symptoms

A simple partial seizure is relatively common. It is classified according to the main clinical manifestations. The sensory manifestation includes bodily sensations and discomforts, such as tingling, numbness, "pins and needles," or loss of feeling. A motor manifestation is characterized by involuntary movements of the face, limbs, or head and may involve an inability to speak. The seizures, which can last for minutes or hours, may be followed by localized weakness or paralysis of the body part in which the seizure occurs; this condition is termed **Todd paralysis**. The patient may experience powerful emotions, such as fear, anxiety, depression, or embarrassment, for no apparent reason. In some cases, a feeling of the mind and body separating may be reported. The person also may experience visual, olfactory, and auditory hallucinations. Psychic symptoms may include disturbing memory flashbacks or frequent, disconcerting feelings of déjà vu, in which something or someone unfamiliar seems to be familiar, or jamais vu, in which something or someone familiar seems to be unfamiliar. Time distortions, out-of-body experiences, sudden nausea, or stomach pain may occur. Consciousness is not impaired; however, a partial or focal seizure may precede a generalized seizure and serve as an aura that consciousness is about to be altered.[8]

Complex partial seizures affect a larger area of the brain and, therefore, impair consciousness. They also are referred to as temporal lobe epilepsy or psychomotor seizures and are characterized

---

BOX 25.4 Classification of Seizures

1. **Partial or focal seizures**
   - Simple (i.e., consciousness not impaired)
   - Complex (i.e., impairment of consciousness)
   - Partial with secondary generalization

2. **Generalized seizures**
   - Tonic–clonic (i.e., grand mal)
   - Intermittent seizure
   - Continuous seizure (i.e., status epilepticus)
   - Absence (i.e., petit mal)
   - Myoclonic epilepsy
   - Posttraumatic

3. **Special epileptic syndromes**
   - Febrile seizures
   - Hysterical seizures
   - Reflex epilepsy

by attacks of purposeful movements or experiences followed by impairment of consciousness. In other words, although appearing to be conscious, the patient is in an altered state of consciousness, an almost trancelike state. These purposeful activities and experiences may include the following[7]:

- Emotions (e.g., depression, fear, paranoia, or crying out)

- Simple automatism (e.g., chewing, swallowing, lip smacking, or saying the same words over and over)

- Complex automatism (e.g., walking into a room, undressing, or arranging objects)

- Hallucinations (e.g., auditory, visual, gustatory, or olfactory)

If engaged in activity, an individual's movements usually are disorganized, confused, and unfocused, but observers may find it hard to believe that the individual does not know of his or her actions. The average seizure lasts from 1 to 5 minutes. The individual is unresponsive to verbal stimuli and may exhibit disorientation or confusion. Afterward, the individual is unable to recall the actions that took place. These types of seizures usually start between 10 and 30 years of age.

Generalized Seizures

Generalized seizures can affect the entire brain. These seizures may be further subdivided into convulsive and nonconvulsive types.

The tonic–clonic, or grand mal, seizure is the most common and severe seizure of the convulsive type. It may occur in an intermittent or a continuous form. Tonic refers to prolonged contractions of skeletal muscles, whereas clonic refers to rhythmic contractions and relaxation of muscles in rapid succession.

An intermittent seizure may be tonic, clonic, or both, and it often is associated with loss of consciousness. Many individuals experience a sensory phenomenon (aura), such as a particular taste or smell, before the seizure. The average seizure lasts from 50 to 90 seconds but may extend up to 5 minutes. Because the unconscious, seizing individual is overtaken by the excessive electrical discharge during the seizure, control of bladder and bowel functions may be lost, resulting in urination or defecation. This action typically is embarrassing and unpleasant but not unexpected. When the seizure ends, the brain may shift into a sleep pattern. As such, the individual may be unarousable for a brief period of time (i.e., seconds to a few minutes). The muscles relax during this period, and the person awakens. Following the seizure, the person often is disoriented, confused, and lethargic and may not remember what happened.

> A continuous tonic–clonic seizure (status epilepticus) is a medical emergency. Continuous convulsions can last 30 minutes or longer, or recurrent generalized convulsions can occur without the person regaining full consciousness between attacks. If the convulsions exceed 60 minutes, irreversible neuronal damage may occur. Any seizure that lasts longer than 5 minutes should be seen as indicating a serious problem. Accordingly, the emergency action plan, including summoning of emergency medical services (EMS), should be activated.

Myoclonic seizures are characterized by sporadic or continuous clonus of muscle groups. They are associated with progressive mental deterioration. These types of seizures are seldom seen in the physically active population.

Posttraumatic seizures are provoked by head trauma and are classified as impact, immediate, early, and late. Impact seizures occur at the time of trauma and are considered to result from electrochemical changes induced by the trauma. Immediate seizures occur within the first 24 hours of trauma. Early seizures occur within the first week after head trauma and often are associated with prolonged posttraumatic amnesia lasting more than 24 hours. A late seizure occurs after the first week of head trauma but primarily within 1 year, and it may be associated with a history of childhood epilepsy.

The typical absence, or petit mal, attack is characterized by a slight loss of consciousness, or blank staring into space, for 3 to 15 seconds without loss of body tone or falling. Slight twitching of the facial muscles, lip smacking, or fluttering of the eyelids may occur. Onset of the condition usually is between 4 and 8 years of age; it tends to resolve by age 30 years.

Special Epileptic Syndromes

A third category of seizures includes febrile seizures during infancy and childhood. Febrile seizures have their onset during the course of a fever usually greater than 38.9°C (102°F) and are most likely to happen while the temperature is rising rapidly. Other seizures in this category include hysterical seizures and reflex epilepsy. These conditions represent a small subgroup of seizures that occur only in response to specific stimuli, such as flickering lights, specific sounds, sudden movements, eating, or reading of words or numbers.

Immediate Management of Seizures

It is important that the clinician note the time at the onset and the end of a seizure. Seconds may seem like minutes; unless accurately timed, the actual length of the seizure may be exaggerated. Management of any seizure is directed toward protecting the individual from injury. Nearby objects should be removed or padded so that the individual does not strike them during uncontrollable muscle contractions. The individual should not be restrained, but the head should be protected at all times. Although the individual may bite the tongue during the seizure, nothing (e.g., fingers or any object) should be placed into the mouth. In an effort to avoid embarrassment to the individual, any observers or spectators should be removed from the area, if possible, to allow privacy. When the seizure ends, it is not unusual for the individual to fall into a sleep pattern. The clinician should ensure an adequate airway and wait until the individual awakens.

Medications and Epilepsy

Antiepileptic and anticonvulsive medications are the agents of choice for those with seizure disorders and epilepsy. These medications should be taken at least 1 to 2 hours before physical activity. The long-term goal is to control or eliminate seizure activity with the lowest doses of the fewest medications. Because anticonvulsive agents have long half-lives, they clear the body slowly and take time to build up to the therapeutic range. As such, regular, long-term administration (i.e., months to years to a lifetime) of medication is needed to keep the body level of the medication in the therapeutic range. Failure to take medication over several days can result in falling out of the effective therapeutic range. Serum levels should be checked frequently for two reasons:

It is essential to document the length of time of the seizure and the amount of time the patient sleeps. If a single, continuous seizure or a series of intermittent seizures exceeds 5 minutes, the emergency action plan, including summoning EMS, should be activated. If the patient has a known seizure disorder, the athletic trainer should attempt to discern the reason for the seizure. If possible, the patient should be questioned about the use of prescribed medication; this information should be provided to EMS on their arrival. **Application Strategy 25.1** summarizes the management of a seizure.

1. To ensure that the medication is within the therapeutic range

2. If the patient is physically active, to ensure that increased fitness levels have not altered the drug metabolism

If serum levels are too low, the risk of seizures is increased. If levels are too high, the toxic effects of the medication may depress brain activity, and as such, vital functions may not be supported. Side effects of some of the medications may cause sedation, dizziness, nausea, vision changes, concentration difficulties, and fatigue.[8] These agents should be avoided in competitive athletes, although many anticonvulsive agents are approved by the National Collegiate Athletic Association (NCAA) and the United States Olympic Committee (USOC).

Physical Activity Guidelines

In nearly all instances, seizure disorders can be controlled with proper medication. Traditionally, good seizure control has been identified as being seizure-free for 6 months or a year. Patients should be carefully evaluated by a neurologist before participation in physical activity and sports, particularly those sports with a danger of falling, contact sports, and water sports, is allowed. Several issues must be addressed in determining participation levels:

■ What type of physical or sport activity is being performed?

■ Is there a risk of death or severe injury if the patient has a seizure during activity?

■ Is there a preexisting brain injury or any neurological dysfunction?

■ Is there a risk of potential brain injury from participation in the activity (e.g., concussion or intracranial hematoma)?

APPLICATION STRATEGY 25.1

Management of Seizures

During the Seizure

1. Note the time that the seizure began.
2. Help the patient to a supine position; protect the head and remove glasses and loosen clothing.
3. Do not stop or restrain the person or place your fingers or any object in the mouth.

After the Seizure

1. Ensure an adequate airway.
2. Turn the patient to one side to allow saliva to drain from mouth.
3. Protect the person from curious bystanders.
4. Do not leave until the patient is fully awake.
5. If this is

A first-time seizure
   The patient should be seen by a physician.

A continuous seizure or if another seizure occurs in rapid succession
   Activate the emergency action plan, including summoning EMS.

6. Send documentation, including a written description of the following:
   - Type of seizure; localized or generalized
   - How it started
   - Length of time from onset until return of consciousness
   - Number of seizures

- Will exercise adversely affect seizure control?

- What are the potential effects of anticonvulsive medications on performance (e.g., impaired judgment or delayed reaction time)?

Head injury during activity participation can certainly precipitate seizures. Individuals with epilepsy, however, are no more prone to seizures after a head injury than are individuals without epilepsy. In addition, epilepsy does not increase the risk of injury while participating in sports, although certain activities (e.g., football, scuba diving, mountain climbing, and automobile racing) should be discouraged if they put the individual or others at risk should a seizure occur. Any individual with a history of seizures should be prohibited from boxing, regardless of seizure control. Individuals who experience frequent seizures should choose physical activities accordingly. It is highly recommended that children with seizure disorders be allowed to participate in physical activity and sports provided that good seizure control and proper supervision are available at all times.

 In determining the sport participation level of an individual with a seizure disorder, the following areas should be addressed: the type of sport being played (i.e., contact or collision versus noncontact), the risk of death or severe injury if the individual has a seizure during activity, the presence of a preexisting brain injury or any neurological dysfunction, the risk of potential brain injury from participation in the sport (e.g., concussion, intracranial hematoma), any adverse effect of exercise on seizure control, and the potential effects of anticonvulsive medications on sport performance (e.g., impaired judgment or delayed reaction time).

OTHER CENTRAL NERVOUS SYSTEM DISORDERS

> **?** A 35-year-old male recreational soccer player sustained an ankle injury. He reported to a sports medicine clinic for evaluation and treatment. Assessment indicated a mild inversion ankle sprain, and standard acute management was initiated. During the 2 weeks postinjury, the pain intensified (related as a 10+ on a scale of 1 to 10); he was unable to walk, to put any pressure on the left leg, to ascend or descend stairs, or to put any type of material (e.g., sheets, blankets, or clothes) on the ankle. He reports getting only 2 to 4 hours of sleep each night. He has been taking naproxen for the pain, but the naproxen appears to be causing nausea, vomiting, and dizziness. After completing a thorough reassessment of the ankle, the presence of an injury that supports the level of pain and dysfunction cannot be confirmed. How should this condition be managed?

Three rare but serious central nervous system disorders can impact the physically active participant. Meningitis, an infection and inflammation of the membranes (i.e., meninges) and fluid (i.e., cerebrospinal fluid) surrounding the brain and spinal cord, most often is caused by bacteria or viruses. Encephalitis is an inflammation of the brain caused by a viral infection; the disease often is spread by insects, particularly mosquitoes that feed on infected birds and animals. Complex regional pain syndrome (CRPS), sometimes referred to as reflex sympathetic dystrophy, is an uncommon disturbance of the sympathetic nervous system (i.e., the part of the nervous system that controls blood flow and sweat glands). If not recognized early and treated immediately, each condition can have devastating effects on an individual.

Meningitis

Etiology

Most cases of meningitis are caused by bacteria or a virus, but meningitis also can result from a fungal infection; parasites; a blow to the head; some types of cancer; inflammatory diseases, such as lupus; a sensitivity reaction to certain medications, especially ibuprofen (e.g., Advil or Motrin); and an infusion of gamma globulins used to treat other conditions.

Viral meningitis, also called aseptic meningitis, usually is mild and often clears on its own in 1 to 2 weeks. Common intestinal viruses cause approximately half the cases in the United States. Viruses associated with mumps, herpes infection, or other diseases as well as polluted water also can cause viral meningitis.

Acute bacterial meningitis, caused primarily by the bacterium *Streptococcus pneumoniae* (pneumococcus), is considered to be a medical emergency. Most cases occur when bacteria from an infection in another part of the body (e.g., osteomyelitis, pneumonia, or endocarditis) travels through the bloodstream to the brain and spinal cord. Bacteria also can spread directly to the brain or spine from a severe head injury (e.g., skull fracture); from an infection in the paranasal sinus, middle ear, nose, or teeth; neurosurgical procedures (e.g., cerebrospinal fluid diversion shunts); or penetrating wounds.[9] The condition is contagious through exposure to the bacteria when someone with meningitis coughs or sneezes. The bacteria also can be spread through kissing or sharing eating utensils, a toothbrush, or a cigarette.

 See **Causes of Acute Bacterial Meningitis**, available on the companion Web site at thePoint.

Cryptococcal meningitis is a fungal form of the disease that affects approximately 10% of people with AIDS. Although cryptococcal meningitis can be treated effectively with antifungal medications, it tends to recur in nearly half of those affected. In these cases, a physician may recommend long-term antifungal therapy with drugs such as fluconazole (e.g., Diflucan).

Signs and Symptoms

Early symptoms of bacterial and viral meningitis are similar to those of the flu but tend to have a sudden onset (**Box 25.5**). Symptoms may include a sudden high fever, severe headache, cervical rigidity, vomiting, sensory disturbances, and mental confusion.[10] During assessment, a positive Kernig or Brudzinski sign may be present (see Chapter 21). In older patients, nuchal rigidity is a classic sign.

BOX 25.5 Signs and Symptoms of Acute Bacterial Meningitis

- High fever that prevents one from eating or drinking
- Irritability
- Delirium
- Severe headache
- Progressive lethargy
- Chills
- Drowsiness
- Photophobia

- Nuchal rigidity associated with positive Kernig and Brudzinski signs
- Nausea and vomiting
- An accompanying skin rash, especially near the axilla or on the hands or feet
- Confusion
- Convulsion or seizure
- Rapid progression of small hemorrhages under the skin

As the disease progresses, the brain swells and may begin to bleed. Initial drowsiness may progress to stupor or coma. Meningitis is fatal in approximately 10% of cases. Unfortunately, those who survive may have serious long-term neurological complications (e.g., deafness, blindness, loss of speech, learning disabilities, and behavior problems) or nonneurological complications (e.g., kidney and adrenal gland failure).[9]

Chronic (ongoing) forms of meningitis occur when slow-growing organisms, such as the microorganisms that cause tuberculosis, invade the membranes and fluid surrounding the brain. Although acute meningitis strikes suddenly, chronic meningitis develops over weeks or months. Nevertheless, the symptoms of chronic meningitis (i.e., headaches, fever, vomiting, and mental cloudiness) are similar to those of acute meningitis.

Management

Acute bacterial meningitis requires prompt treatment with intravenous antibiotics to ensure recovery and reduce the risk of complications. The choice of antibiotics depends on the degree of penetration of the agent through the blood–brain barrier and the bactericidal effect of the agent. Often, analyzing a sample of cerebrospinal fluid can help to identify the causative agent. In general, antibiotic treatment should be administered as soon as possible following the cerebrospinal fluid collection and treatment against *S. pneumoniae* should extend for 10 to 14 days, followed by a course of oral antibiotics.[10,11] Also, corticosteroids can be administered to help prevent hearing loss, which is the most common complication of the disease.

Meningitis is a medical emergency. The recovery rate depends on the length of time that elapses before the patient receives treatment. If meningitis is suspected, the emergency action plan should be activated.

Mild cases of viral meningitis usually are treated with bed rest, plenty of fluids, and analgesics to reduce fever and relieve body aches. If meningitis is caused by the herpes virus, treatment may include a herpes group antiviral medication. Not all viruses that cause meningitis, however, have antiviral agents available for use.

Encephalitis

Etiology

Encephalitis is an inflammation of the brain, especially the cerebral hemisphere, cerebellum, or brainstem, caused by a viral infection. It may occur in epidemic outbreaks. The disease often is spread by insects, particularly mosquitoes that feed on infected birds and animals. Encephalitis takes two forms:

- **Primary.** Caused by a direct viral invasion of the brain and spinal cord, the condition can be sporadic or epidemic. The most common sporadic form, herpes simplex encephalitis, may start as a minor illness with headache and fever, followed by more serious symptoms. Epidemic varieties commonly are caused by mosquito-borne viruses. The major types of mosquito-borne encephalitis that infect people in the United States are Eastern equine encephalitis, Western equine encephalitis, St. Louis encephalitis, La Crosse encephalitis, and more recently, West Nile encephalitis.

■ **Secondary (postinfectious).** This form follows or occurs with a viral infection in another part of the body, such as chickenpox, measles (rubeola), mumps, rubella, or polio. The cause of encephalitis in some secondary cases may be a hypersensitivity reaction manifested as an overreaction of the immune system to a foreign substance.

Primary encephalitis is the most serious kind of encephalitis, but the secondary form is more common. A few thousand cases of encephalitis are reported annually in the United States. In addition, many cases likely go unreported, because people experience only mild or nonspecific symptoms. Even though mosquito-borne encephalitis is rare, encephalitis is the most common mosquito-borne disease in the United States.

Signs and Symptoms

Signs and symptoms vary with the age of the patient but, in most cases, generally appear within 5 to 15 days of being bitten by an infected mosquito. In infants, there may be a sudden onset of fever, convulsions, and bulging in the soft spots (i.e., fontanelles) of the skull. Children may experience headache, fever, and drowsiness, followed by nausea, vomiting, photophobia, muscular pain, and nuchal rigidity. Adults often experience a sudden onset of fever, nausea, and vomiting accompanied by severe headache, muscle aching that may progress to tremors, and photophobia. Mental confusion and disorientation are hallmark symptoms in adults.

Management

In treating herpes simplex encephalitis, an antiviral agent, such as acyclovir, may be prescribed initially. In some cases, an anticonvulsant medication is prescribed. Anti-inflammatory drugs or medications that reduce pressure within the skull may be used as well. Because viruses that cause encephalitis do not respond to antibiotics, supportive treatment may consist of rest and a healthy diet, including plenty of liquids to help the immune system fight the virus. In some cases, physical and speech therapy may be a part of the treatment plan.

Complex Regional Pain Syndrome

Etiology

CRPS is the new term for pain disorders formerly called **reflex sympathetic dystrophy**. CRPS requires the presence of regional pain and sensory changes following a noxious event. The pain is associated with findings such as abnormal skin color, temperature changes, abnormal sweating, hypersensitivity in the affected area, abnormal edema, and significant impairment of motor function (e.g., muscle weakness in the affected limb). The combination of these findings exceeds their expected magnitude in response to known physical damage.[12] CRPS is more likely to affect women (~75%) than men, and although the condition can occur at any age, it is most common in people between 50 and 70 years of age.[13]

CRPS occurs in two types, with similar signs and symptoms but different causes. Type I, previously known as reflex sympathetic dystrophy, occurs following an illness or injury that has not directly damaged the nerves in the affected limb. This injury could be as simple as a splinter, ankle sprain, intravenous catheter insertion, or back strain or as complex as a myocardial infarction, surgery, or infection. Type II, once referred to as causalgia, follows a distinct nerve injury.[13] The diagnosis of CRPS is excluded by the existence of painful conditions with known pathology that could account for the degree of pain and dysfunction at the injured site.

The nature of CRPS is puzzling, and the cause is not clearly understood. It is thought that the initiating event, often minor trauma, sensitizes C-nociceptive fibers. These small-diameter axons with slow conduction velocities are polymodal, responding to mechanical, thermal, and chemical stimuli. The activation of the sympathetic nervous system permits the body to respond appropriately to injury by activating the inflammatory response. Normally, this activity decreases within minutes to hours after the injury. In CRPS, however, the sympathetic impulses do not shut off. This triggers a constant inflammatory response, causing vessels to spasm and leading to continual release of neurotransmitters, increased pain, and tissue destruction.

Signs and Symptoms

Signs and symptoms of both types of CRPS develop in three stages (**Box 25.6**). Some people never progress past stage 1, and only a small percentage of those affected advance to stage 3. Signs and symptoms initially appear only near the site of the injury. Pain, usually located in the distal part of an extremity, is described as burning or aching and is aggravated by movement or lowering the affected limb. Tapping on the skin (i.e., Tinel sign) may increase pain, or sudden jolts of sharp pain may occur, especially at trigger points.[13]

Initially, the affected limb usually is warmer, shows a red and sometimes mottled discoloration, and has pronounced distal edema. Skin temperature can shift from hyperthermic to hypothermic during the later course of the disease. Substantial muscle weakness in the affected limb that is disproportionate to the injury also can be reported. Nails become brittle and grooved, and regional hair growth increases. The skin appears to be thin and glossy; eventually, hyperkeratosis and palmar or plantar fibrosis may be present.[13]

BOX 25.6 Signs and Symptoms of Complex Regional Pain Syndrome

Stage 1: Generally lasts from 1 to 3 months and is characterized by the following:

- Severe burning or aching pain, tenderness, and swelling limited to the site of injury
- Changes in skin temperature, color, and texture. The skin may be sweaty or cold. Skin color can range from white and mottled to red or blue. The skin may become tender, thin, or shiny in the affected area.
- Increased hair and nail growth
- Muscle cramps or spasms
- Edema and joint stiffness restrict mobility.

Stage 2: Generally lasts from 3 to 6 months and is marked by the following:

- Pain intensifies and spreads; pain is disproportionate to the injury.
- Edema increases.
- More pronounced changes in skin color and texture
- Hair becomes coarse, then scant; nails become brittle, cracked, and grooved.
- Muscle and joint stiffness increases; atrophy occurs.

Stage 3: Permanent damage occurs. Signs and symptoms may include the following:

- Debilitating pain that may now affect an entire limb
- Muscle atrophy and advanced joint damage, causing reduced mobility in the affected body part
- Flexion tendon contractures
- Irreversible skin damage
- Osteoporosis

The illness can spread from its source to elsewhere in the body in the following patterns:

■ **Continuity type.** Symptoms may migrate from the initial site of the pain, for example, from the hand to the shoulder, trunk, and face, affecting a quadrant of the body.

■ **Mirror-image type.** Symptoms may spread from one limb to the opposite limb.

■ **Independent type.** Symptoms may leap to a distant part of the body.

Management

Dramatic improvement and even remission of CRPS are possible if treatment begins within a few months of the initial symptoms. The main goal of the treatment plan is pain relief, functional recovery, and psychological improvement. Over-the-counter NSAIDs, such as aspirin, ibuprofen (e.g., Advil or Motrin), and naproxen sodium (e.g., Aleve), may ease pain and inflammation. Prescription pain relievers may be recommended in some cases. Because hypersensitivity to heat is one of the most consistent symptoms in patients with acute CRPS, cryotherapy may provide substantial relief of pain, swelling, and sweating. If the affected area is cool, applying heat may offer relief. Gentle, guided exercising of the affected limbs may improve range of motion and strength.

If the preceding treatments are not effective, the supervising physician may recommend use of the corticosteroid prednisone to reduce inflammation or may inject an anesthetic to block pain fibers in the affected nerves. Vasodilators, which traditionally are used to treat high blood pressure, may help to relieve pain in affected areas by easing blood vessel constriction. Transcutaneous electrical nerve stimulation (TENS) may be used to ease chronic pain, or biofeedback techniques may help the patient to relax the body and relieve pain symptoms. In rare cases, surgically cutting the nerves in the affected area may be recommended. This procedure is controversial, however, because it also may destroy other sensations.[13]

The 35-year-old male recreational soccer player sustained an ankle inversion sprain that did not correspond to the level of the reported symptoms. The individual may be experiencing CRPS. As such, the individual should be referred to a physician for further evaluation.

SUMMARY

1. Migraine headaches are characterized by moderate to severe throbbing or pounding pain often accompanied by light sensitivity, nausea or vomiting, loss of appetite, and abdominal pain.

2. Treatment for migraine headaches is based on the type, frequency, and cause of the migraine. Most often, migraines are treated with various drug therapies.

3. A seizure disorder entails recurrent episodes of sudden, excessive charges of electrical activity in the brain, whether from known or unknown (idiopathic) causes. Epilepsy is a general term used to describe only recurrent idiopathic episodes (at least two) of sudden, excessive discharges of electrical activity in the brain. The discharge may trigger altered sensation, perception, behavior, mood, or level of consciousness or may lead to convulsive movements.

4. Seizures are classified as partial, generalized, or special epileptic syndromes.

5. The most serious seizure is the tonic–clonic seizure, which may occur in an intermittent or a continuous form. An intermittent seizure, which usually lasts only from 50 to 90 seconds but may extend to 5 minutes, often is preceded by a particular taste or smell (aura).

6. The typical absence (petit mal) attack is characterized by a slight loss of consciousness or blank staring into space for 3 to 15 seconds without loss of body tone or falling.

7. The simple partial seizure is characterized by involuntary movements of the face, limbs, or head, and the individual may experience tingling or numbness. The localized motor seizures may be followed by localized weakness or paralysis of the body part in which the seizure occurs.

8. Complex partial (psychomotor) seizures are characterized by purposeful movements or experiences followed by impairment in consciousness.

9. Management of any seizure is directed toward protecting the individual from injury. The area surrounding the individual should be clear of objects; immovable objects should be padded. The individual should not be restrained, but the head should be protected at all times. Nothing should be placed in the mouth of an individual having a seizure. When the seizure ends, an adequate airway should be ensured. If the time of the seizure exceeds 5 minutes, activation of the emergency action plan is warranted.

10. In the majority of cases, individuals with a seizure disorder can be allowed to participate in certain physical activities and sports provided that good seizure control and proper supervision are available at all times.

11. Certain activities (e.g., football, scuba diving, mountain climbing, and automobile racing) may put the individual or others at risk if a seizure occurs. Participation in these activities should be discouraged.

12. Meningitis, an infection and inflammation of the membranes (meninges) and fluid (cerebrospinal fluid) surrounding the brain and spinal cord, most often is caused by bacteria or viruses.

13. Encephalitis is an inflammation of the brain caused by a viral infection. The disease often is spread by insects, particularly mosquitoes that feed on infected birds and animals.

14. CRPS, sometimes referred to as reflex sympathetic dystrophy, is an uncommon disturbance of the sympathetic nervous system. The condition often is associated with intense pain, abnormal skin color, temperature changes, hypersensitivity to touch, edema, and motor dysfunction not proportionate to the injury.

APPLICATION QUESTIONS

1. A high school baseball player reports to the preseason physical examination with a history of partial seizures. Should this individual be permitted to participate in baseball? Explain your response. If the individual wanted to play on the school ice hockey team, would your response be the same or different? Why?

2. Your high school soccer team participated in a weekend tournament sponsored by a school district in a neighboring state. The Tuesday following the tournament, the parent of a member of your soccer team calls to report that her daughter will not be in school today, having just been seen by a doctor who diagnosed the young girl with meningitis. How would you respond to the parent about this news? What is your obligation, as an athletic trainer, to notify other individuals about this condition? Why? Will any follow-up management be required on your part?

3. You are an athletic trainer employed at a university. A member of the women's gymnastics team complains of a pounding headache with nausea. How would you immediately manage this condition? Should this individual be immediately referred to a physician for further assessment and care, or can she wait to be seen tomorrow? Explain your response.

4. During field hockey practice, one of the athletes has a partial seizure. The athlete has no previous history of seizures. How would you manage this condition to safeguard the athlete?

REFERENCES

1. Smitherman TA, Burch R, Sheikh H, et al. The prevalence, impact, and treatment of migraine and severe headaches in the United States: a review of statistics from national surveillance studies. *Headache*. 2013;53:427–436.

2. Rapoff MA, Connelly M, Bickel JL, et al. Headstrong intervention for pediatric migraine headache: a randomized clinical trial. *J Headache Pain*. 2014;15:12.

3. Tamparo CD, Lewis MA. *Diseases of the Human Body*. Philadelphia, PA: FA Davis; 2000.

4. Headache Classification Committee of the International Headache Society. The international classification of headache disorders, 3rd edition (beta version). *Cephalalgia*. 2013;33(9):629–808. http://www.ihs-classification.org/_downloads /mixed/International-Headache-Classification-III -ICHD-III-2013-Beta.pdf. Accessed July 15, 2015.

5. Newman LC. Understanding the causes and prevention of menstrual migraine: the role of estrogen. *Headache*. 2007;47(suppl 2):S86–S94.

6. Andress-Rothrock D, King W, Rothrock J. An analysis of migraine triggers in a clinic-based population. *Headache*. 2010;50(8): 1366–1370.

7. Jordan BD, Sundell R. Epilepsy and the athlete. In: Mellion MB, Walsh WM, Madden C, Putukian M, Shelton GL, eds. *The Team Physician's Handbook*. Philadelphia, PA: Hanley & Belfus; 2002:294–298.

8. Parka ED. Seizure disorders ID athletes. *Athl Ther Today*. 2006;11(4):36–38.

9. Donovan C, Blewitt J. Signs, symptoms and management of bacterial meningitis. *Paediatr Nurs*. 2010;22(9):30–35.

10. Nudelman Y, Tunkel AR. Bacterial meningitis: epidemiology, pathogenesis and management update. *Drugs*. 2009;69(18):2577–2596.

11. Jawień M, Garlicki AM. Bacterial meningitis—principles of antimicrobial treatment. *Przegl Epidemiol*. 2013;67:421–427.

12. Rand SE. Complex regional pain syndrome in the adolescent athlete. *Curr Sports Med Rep*. 2009;8(6):285–287.

13. de Rooij AM, de Mos M, van Hilten JJ, et al. Increased risk of complex regional pain syndrome in siblings of patients? *J Pain*. 2009;10(12):1250–1255.

26

Respiratory Tract Conditions

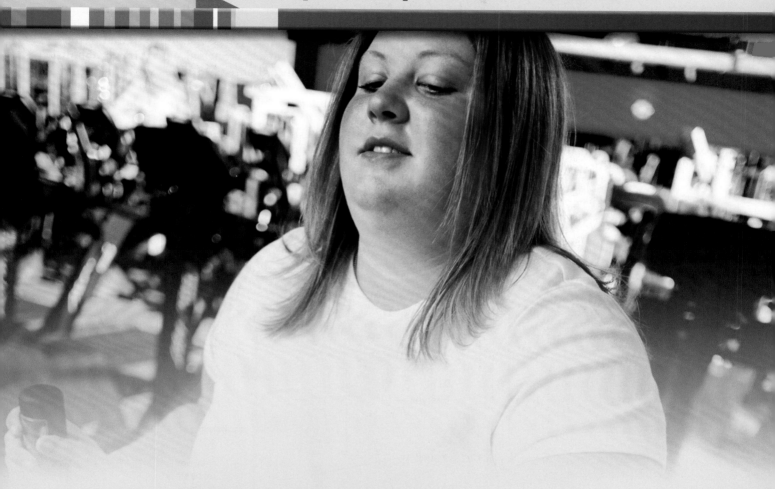

STUDENT OUTCOMES

1. Explain the physiological factors associated with common respiratory tract conditions.

2. Identify the signs and symptoms of common upper respiratory tract conditions, including the common cold, sinusitis, pharyngitis, laryngitis, tonsillitis, and allergic rhinitis.

3. Describe the strategies that can be used to prevent the common cold.

4. Identify the signs and symptoms of general respiratory conditions, including bronchitis, bronchial asthma, exercise-induced bronchospasm, influenza, and pneumonia.

5. Describe the management of common respiratory tract conditions.

6. Explain the use of metered-dose inhalers and peak flow meter in the management of asthma.

INTRODUCTION

Healthy lungs consist of an elastic network of air passageways and spaces that are bound together by connective tissue. Although the lungs occupy the majority of the thoracic cavity, each lung weighs only approximately 0.6 kg (1.25 lb). The left lung is smaller than the right lung, because it contains a concavity known as the cardiac notch, in which the heart is nestled. The lungs extend distally to the level of, or slightly below, the 12th rib in 80% of people and to the L1 spinal level in approximately 18% of individuals. The primary bronchial tubes branch obliquely downward from the trachea and then branch into approximately 23 levels until the terminal bronchioles are reached (**Fig. 26.1**). These tiny air sacs, called alveoli, serve as diffusion chambers where oxygen from the lungs enters adjacent capillaries and carbon dioxide from the blood is returned to the lungs.

Conditions of the respiratory tract are common. Resistance to these conditions can be suppressed by a variety of factors, including fatigue, chronic inflammation from a localized infection, environment (e.g., allergens, dust, and smog), and psychological stress. In this chapter, common upper respiratory tract infections and general respiratory conditions are discussed.

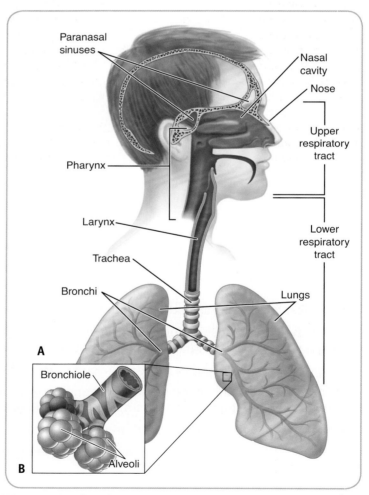

Figure 26.1. Respiratory system. A, The trachea, bronchi, and lungs. **B,** The terminal ends of the bronchial tree are alveolar sacs, where oxygen and carbon dioxide are exchanged.

UPPER RESPIRATORY TRACT INFECTIONS

 A swimmer appears to have a common cold. What additional signs and symptoms would suggest that the swimmer has sinusitis?

Viral conditions are often referred to as upper respiratory infections (URIs). These conditions, although minor, can clearly impact one's performance, especially if a fever is present. In general, individuals should not participate in physical activity if they have a fever (≥100.5°F/38.0°C), severe malaise, **myalgia**, weakness, shortness of breath, and/or severe cough or if they are dehydrated.[1,2] Fever decreases strength, aerobic power, endurance, coordination, and concentration, and it can lead to injury or heat illness. Dehydration magnifies the effects of fever and also can lead to heat illness. In this section, the common cold, sinusitis, pharyngitis, laryngitis, tonsillitis, and allergic rhinitis (i.e., hay fever) are discussed.

Common Cold

Etiology

The average adult has from one to six colds each year, with human rhinoviruses accounting from 40% to 50% of these infections. The coronavirus, respiratory syncytial virus, parainfluenza virus, and adenovirus also cause colds. These RNA viruses cause URI when they spread in oral or nasal secretions. The viruses stay in the cooler upper airways because they prefer temperatures below 98.6°F/37.0°C.[2,3] The majority of colds occur during the fall and spring months. The condition may be triggered by aspirin sensitivity, use of oral contraceptives, topical decongestant abuse, cocaine abuse, presence of nasal polyps or a deviated septum, or allergic conditions. A cold can be quite contagious and can be transmitted either by person-to-person contact or by airborne droplets; however, several strategies can be implemented to reduce the risk of getting a cold (**Box 26.1**).

Upper respiratory symptoms usually begin 1 to 2 days after exposure and generally last for 7 to 10 days. Viral shedding and contagion, however, can continue for another 2 or 3 weeks. Although many individuals feel that performance in sport and physical activity is hindered by a

---

BOX 26.1 Strategies to Reduce the Risk of Getting a Cold

- Avoid contact with individuals who have URIs, particularly children, who tend to have more frequent URIs.

- In the presence of individuals who have URIs, avoid touching objects or sharing objects that they have touched.

- Wash the hands frequently during cold season and avoid touching the eyes and nose with the fingers. This will prevent many viruses from reaching the mucous membranes.

- Drink plenty of clear, nonalcoholic fluids.

- Although vitamin C supplements will not decrease the incidence of colds, they will decrease the duration and severity of symptoms.

- Reduce environmental factors (e.g., dust, smog, allergens) that may be a predisposing factor for rhinitis.

- Reduce stress.

- If using a topical decongestant, follow the instructions carefully. Do not prolong its use because rebound rhinitis may occur. Use decongestants during the day and, because of their sedative effect, antihistamines at night.

- If cold symptoms are mild, exercise is safe. If, however, symptoms include headache, fever, muscle aches, hacking productive cough, or loss of appetite, then exercise should cease. Rest is best.

cold, the majority of clinicians suggest resuming regular training a few days after the symptoms' cessation.[2,4]

Signs and Symptoms

Symptoms include a rapid onset of **rhinorrhea**, nasal itching, sneezing, nonproductive cough, and associated itching and puffiness of the eyes. **Malaise**, a mild sore throat, chills, and in some cases, low-grade fever also may be present. Although most cold symptoms are benign and confined to the upper respiratory tract, colds can lead to middle ear infections and bacterial sinusitis when airflow is obstructed by swollen nasal membranes.

Management

Although no cure for the viral common cold is known, over-the-counter (OTC) medications can alleviate or lessen the symptoms. These may include antihistamines, antitussives, expectorants, decongestants, and antipyretics. Treatment is mainly supportive and symptomatic. OTC medications are not recommended for use in children.[5,6] Zinc has been shown in clinical studies involving children to perform well in reducing the number of colds.[6] Caution should be observed when any medications are used by competitive athletes because an agent may be on the list of banned substances, particularly at high competitive levels.

Sinusitis

Etiology

Sinusitis is an inflammation of the paranasal sinus caused by a bacterial or viral infection, allergy, or environmental factors (**Fig. 26.2**). Sinusitis can be acute, lasting for less than 30 days; subacute, lasting for 3 weeks to 2 months; or chronic, lasting for longer than 2 months. The condition often is triggered by an obstruction of the passageway between the sinuses (i.e., ostium) because of local mucosal swelling and insult or by mechanical obstruction. Local mucosal swelling may be secondary to an upper respiratory tract infection, allergy, or direct trauma. Mechanical obstruction may be caused by a deviated septum; concha bullosa, which is the vesicle of serum or blood located on the concha inside the nose; or nasal masses from polyps or tumors.

Signs and Symptoms

A sinus infection should be suspected when cold symptoms last for longer than 7 to 10 days or if cold symptoms start to improve but then become worse once again. Nasal congestion, facial pain or pressure over the involved sinus, pain in the upper teeth, or pain and pressure behind the eyes (i.e., retro-orbital) are present. Other symptoms may include purulent nasal discharge, palpable pain over the involved sinus, night- and daytime coughing, and in severe cases, perinasal and eyelid swelling, fever, and chills. Drainage with bacterial infections most likely is dark in color, whereas drainage from other causes usually is clear. Chronic sinusitis is characterized by chronic nasal congestion, rhinorrhea or postnasal discharge accompanied by perinasal pressure, and headache not associated with migraine or muscle tension. The individual often pinches the bridge of the nose to demonstrate the area of discomfort or reports discomfort that is aggravated by eyeglasses.

Management

Treatment involves controlling the infection, reducing mucosal edema, and allowing nasal discharge. Oral antibiotics, such as amoxicillin, penicillin, or

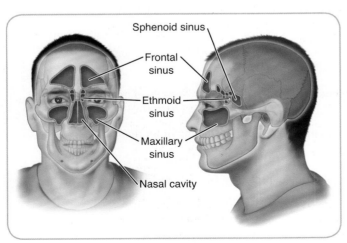

Figure 26.2. Facial sinuses. The frontal and ethmoid sinuses are more commonly involved in sinusitis.

erythromycin, may be prescribed; however, some patients may not see significant benefits with antibiotics.[7] Topical agents, such as phenylephrine hydrochloride (e.g., Neo-Synephrine) or oxymetazoline hydrochloride (e.g., Afrin), can be used during the first 3 to 4 days of treatment to facilitate drainage. Longer use of decongestants, however, can lead to a rebound effect, whereby production of mucus and edema is increased. In severe cases, surgical intervention may be necessary to drain the sinuses.

Pharyngitis (Sore Throat)

Etiology

Pharyngitis may be caused by a viral, bacterial, or fungal infection of the pharynx, leading to a sore throat. The condition may result from a common cold, influenza, streptococcal infection, diphtheria, herpes simplex virus types 1 and 2, Epstein-Barr virus, gonococcal bacteria, chlamydia, or candidiasis. If caused by the bacteria *Streptococcus pyogenes* (i.e., strep throat) and inadequately treated, peritonsillar abscess, scarlet fever, rheumatic fever, or rheumatic heart disease may result. Peak seasons for pharyngitis include the late winter and early spring.[7,8]

Signs and Symptoms

The throat typically appears to be dark red and the tonsils red and swollen, and a pus discharge may be present. Throat pain is aggravated by swallowing and may radiate along the distribution of the glossopharyngeal nerve (i.e., cranial nerve IX) to the ears. Other symptoms include rhinorrhea, swollen lymph glands, hoarseness, headache, cough, conjunctivitis, low-grade fever, and malaise. Individuals with bacterial pharyngitis generally do not have rhinorrhea, cough, or conjunctivitis.[7,8]

Management

Treatment for streptococcal pharyngitis includes antibiotics, such as penicillin or erythromycin. Other antibiotics that may be used are amoxicillin, cephalosporins, macrolides, or clindamycin.[7] The Infectious Diseases Society of America (IDSA) adopted strict guidelines for the treatment of acute pharyngitis, which include laboratory confirmation of *Streptococcus* infection with either a rapid antigen detection test (RADT) or throat culture before antibiotics are prescribed.[9] In cases that do not involve streptococcal pharyngitis, treatment involves bed rest, drinking fluids, warm saline gargles, throat lozenges, and mild analgesics (e.g., aspirin or ibuprofen).[7]

Laryngitis

Etiology

In **laryngitis**, tissues inferior to the epiglottis are swollen and inflamed, leading to swelling around the vocal cords so that they cannot vibrate normally, resulting in a characteristic hoarseness of the voice. Laryngitis is common and often occurs during a URI (e.g., cold). The condition also can be caused by direct trauma to the throat, gastroesophageal reflux disease (GERD), allergies, or cigarette smoke or from general irritation of straining the vocal cords, as may occur in singers, politicians, cheerleaders, or other individuals who shout excessively while playing or working.

Signs and Symptoms

Laryngitis is characterized by a weak, hoarse, gravelly voice; sore throat; fever; cough (usually dry and nonproductive); a tickling in the back of the throat; and difficulty swallowing. Children's croup, or acute epiglottis, can, however, present like laryngitis. Similar to a cough, laryngitis may persist after the acute infection is over. This can be recognized by noting that the fever and ill feeling subside but the hoarseness continues for another several days to a week or longer.

Management

Laryngitis is self-limiting under most conditions. The patient should attempt to rest the voice. Drinking warm liquids; sucking on a cough drop, throat lozenge, or hard candy; or gargling with a warm salt solution (half a teaspoon of salt in 1 cup of water) may relieve some of the symptoms. One should avoid smoking or places where cigarettes are smoked. Use of a humidifier, preferably a cool mist ultrasonic humidifier, may ease symptoms. This type of humidifier is more expensive than the usual vaporizer, but it is also safer and more effective. Standing for extended periods in a hot, steamy shower also may be helpful. Aspirin, ibuprofen, or acetaminophen may be used to reduce the fever, muscle discomfort, and pain. Aspirin, however, should not be used in someone younger than 19 years, because it can trigger an attack of Reye syndrome.

The patient should be seen by a physician if any of the following conditions are present, because these symptoms may indicate a more serious underlying problem:

- Difficulty breathing or swallowing
- Fever of greater than 101.0°F/38.3°C
- In a young child, a deep cough like the bark of a seal
- Presence of brown, green, or yellow sputum
- Hoarseness that lasts for 1 month without any identifiable cause

Tonsillitis

Etiology

The tonsils are lymph glands or nodes located at the back of the throat that help to protect the pharynx by filtering disease-producing bacteria before they enter the breathing passage. During the filtering process, the tonsils themselves may become inflamed and acutely or chronically infected. This condition, called **tonsillitis**, is most often caused by a bacterial streptococcal infection but may result from viral infections, such as the flu, common cold, mononucleosis, or herpes simplex. All forms of tonsillitis are contagious and generally spread from person to person in coughs, sneezes, and nasal fluids.

Signs and Symptoms

Tonsillitis is characterized by inflamed and enlarged tonsils, fever, painful swallowing, sore throat, and a slight change in voice. Tissues surrounding the tonsils frequently form pus during acute attacks of tonsillitis, particularly streptococcal tonsillitis, causing the tonsils to show white specks or become coated with whitish exudate. Other symptoms include swollen lymph nodes, headache, and bad breath. Nausea, vomiting, and abdominal pain may occur in younger children. Pharyngitis often occurs along with tonsillitis.

Management

Acute cases of bacterial tonsillitis can be treated with antibiotics, such as penicillin, but viral tonsillitis cannot. Chronic recurrent tonsillitis may be treated by surgical removal of the tonsils, a procedure known as a tonsillectomy.

Allergic Rhinitis (Hay Fever)

Etiology

Allergic rhinitis (AR) is an inflammation of the nasal mucous membranes that affects 10% to 20% of children and adults in the United States and often coexists with asthma.[7,10] The risk of rhinitis increases throughout childhood and adolescence and then peaks during the late 20s and early 30s. Rhinitis may be classified into nonallergic and allergic; AR is further divided into seasonal (hay fever) and perennial (all-year-round). Hay fever usually involves a specific period of symptoms during successive years caused by airborne pollens or fungal spores associated with that season. In contrast, perennial AR occurs year-round if the patient is continually exposed to allergens such as food (e.g., shellfish or bread mold), dust, and animal emanations (e.g., hair or feathers).

Signs and Symptoms

Postnasal drainage leads to a chronic sore throat and bronchial infection. In addition, the pharyngeal openings of the eustachian tubes can become blocked by swollen mucosa, enlarged lymphoid tissue, or exudate. Without normal airflow, increasing negative pressure in the middle ear results in fluid accumulation, leading to partial hearing loss and recurrent middle ear infections.

Taking a complete history is the key to differentiate AR from other respiratory conditions. Questions should focus on the relationship of symptoms to seasons or exposures that trigger symptoms. For example, if symptoms increase while the individual is outdoors, pollen may be the triggering agent; if symptoms increase while the individual is indoors, mold could be the culprit. In addition, certain geographic areas may have more environmental allergens than others. Individuals should try to limit their exposure to allergens when participating in different environments. Allergy tests (i.e., skin or intradermal testing) may not be necessary if a history uncovers allergens to specific environmental factors.

Management

Management involves limiting exposure to the allergen or irritant, suppressive medication to alleviate symptom severity, and specific hypersensitization to reduce responsiveness to unavoidable allergens. For example, if dust is an allergen, then having bare floors, having pillows and mattresses encased in plastic covers, minimizing cloth curtains, and avoiding cluttered tabletops can reduce the amount of dust in a home. Oral and topical antihistamines are effective in reducing histamine-related symptoms such as itching, rhinorrhea, and sneezing; however, drowsiness, lethargy, mucous membrane dryness, and occasional nausea and light-headedness may be unwanted side effects.[7,11] Intranasal steroids used to relieve nasal obstruction are the treatment of choice for persistent moderate to severe AR and may also improve nonallergic rhinitis.[7,11] Caution should be observed when any of the preceding medications are used by competitive athletes, however, because an agent may be on the list of banned substances, particularly at high competitive levels.

  In addition to the signs and symptoms associated with the common cold, sinusitis would be suggested if the swimmer exhibits nasal congestion, facial pain over the sinus region, pain behind the eyes, and coughing.

GENERAL RESPIRATORY CONDITIONS

  A softball player has exercise-induced bronchospasm. What conditions might contribute to the severity of this respiratory problem?

General respiratory conditions may result from infection or irritation from inhaled particles and substances. Bronchitis, bronchial asthma, exercise-induced bronchospasm (EIB; formerly called exercise-induced asthma), influenza, and pneumonia are discussed.

Bronchitis

Etiology

Bronchitis is the inflammation of the mucosal lining of the tracheobronchial tree. The condition results from infection or inhaled particles and substances and may be acute or chronic (chronic obstructive pulmonary disease). The most common causes stem from viruses (e.g., parainfluenza, respiratory syncytial, adenoviruses, rhinoviruses, influenza viruses, or enteroviruses) and bacteria (e.g., *Mycoplasma pneumoniae*, *Chlamydia pneumoniae*, or *Bordetella pertussis*).[1]

Signs and Symptoms

Acute bronchitis, which is commonly seen in physically active individuals, involves bronchial swelling, mucus secretion, and increased resistance to expiration. Coughing, wheezing, and large amounts of purulent mucus are present. Once the stimulus is removed, however, the swelling decreases and the airways return to normal.

Chronic bronchitis is characterized by a productive daily cough for at least 3 consecutive months in 2 successive years. Irritation may result from cigarette smoke, air pollution, or infections. This condition can progress to increased airway obstruction, heart failure, and cellular

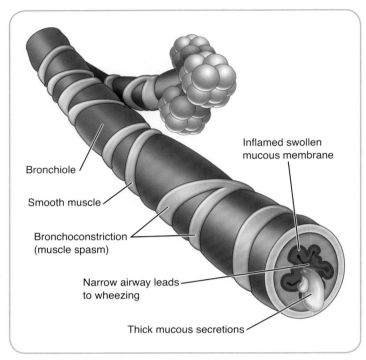

Figure 26.3. Bronchospasm. An asthma attack is caused by bronchospasm that constricts the bronchiolar tubes. This spasm, combined with increased bronchial secretions and mucosal swelling, results in a characteristic, loud wheezing sound that is heard during expiration.

changes in respiratory epithelial cells that may become malignant. Signs and symptoms include marked cyanosis, edema, large production of sputum, and abnormally high levels of carbon dioxide as well as low levels of oxygen in the blood. This condition is often seen simultaneously with emphysema.

Management

No specific therapy is available for most types of viral bronchitis. Most cases, however, subside after a few days or a week. Limited prescribed medication is available if the cause stems from influenza viruses. Bacteria-related bronchitis is treated more effectively with macrolides. Fever associated with the conditions may be managed with acetaminophen or ibuprofen. Aspirin, however, should not be used for individuals younger than 19 years, because it increases the incidence of Reye syndrome.[1]

Bronchial Asthma

Etiology

Asthma is caused by a constriction of bronchial smooth muscles (bronchospasm), increased bronchial secretions, and mucosal swelling, all leading to an inadequate airflow during respiration (especially expiration) (**Fig. 26.3**). The condition is classified as intermittent, seasonal, or chronic. Intermittent asthma usually is of relatively short duration, occurring less than 5 days per month with extended, symptom-free periods. Symptoms of seasonal asthma occur for prolonged periods as a result of exposure to seasonal inhalant allergens. Chronic asthma occurs daily or near daily, with an absence of extended, symptom-free periods.

Signs and Symptoms

Patients with asthma experience episodic, paroxysmal attacks of shortness of breath and wheezing, which result from air squeezing past the narrowed airways. Because the airways cannot fill or empty adequately, the diaphragm tends to flatten, and the accessory muscles must work harder to enlarge the chest during inspiration. This increased workload leads to a rapid onset of fatigue when the patient can no longer hyperventilate enough to meet the increased oxygen need. Acute attacks may occur spontaneously, but they are often provoked by a viral infection.

A large amount of thick, yellow, or green sputum is produced by the bronchial mucosa. As dyspnea continues, anxiety, loud wheezing, sweating, rapid heart rate, and labored breathing develop. In severe cases, respiratory failure may be indicated by cyanosis, decreased wheezing, and decreased levels of consciousness.

Management

Current guidelines for asthma management concur that inhaled corticosteroids (ICS) are the mainstays of anti-inflammatory therapy in asthma. However, asthma is often inadequately controlled, even with high doses of ICS, warranting additional therapies. Accordingly, long-lasting β_2-agonists (LABAs) delivered by a compressor-driven nebulizer or inhaler are used in combination with ICS. However, short-term treatment includes using short-acting β_2-agonists to give quick relief to symptoms.[7,12] The value of bronchodilators in children and young adults, however, continues to be debated. Once the attack has subsided, the lungs usually return to normal.

Exercise-Induced Bronchospasm

Etiology

EIB has been observed in 35% to 78% of patients with asthma, most commonly in the form of a reaction 3 to 12 minutes after exercise is completed.[11] Factors contributing to the severity of EIB include ambient air conditions (e.g., cold air, low humidity, and pollutants); duration, type, and intensity of exercise; exposure to allergens in sensitized individuals; overall control of asthma; poor physical conditioning; respiratory infections; time since the last episode of EIB; and any underlying bronchial hyperreactivity. Individuals suffering from allergies, sinus disease, or hyperventilation may be at increased risk for EIB, and symptoms can be exacerbated for those with bronchitis, emphysema, and other diseases affecting the bronchial tubes.

Despite the prevalence of EIB, the mechanism of bronchospasm remains unclear. One theory emphasizes the significance of a rise in osmolarity in the respiratory tract, resulting in the release of mediators during exercise, whereas the other main theory stresses the activity of the vascular system resulting in air passage narrowing.[7,13] Regardless of the mechanism, the amount of ventilation and the temperature of the inspired air both during and after exercise are important factors in determining the severity of EIB. The greater the ventilations (i.e., volume of air inspired) in cold, dry air, the greater the risk of EIB, and the more strenuous the exercise, the greater the ventilations.

Recently, EIB has been diagnosed according to forced expiratory volume at 1 second (FEV_1) using a peak flow meter. Normally, individuals can have up to a 10% decrease in FEV_1 postexercise. When FEV_1 drops by 15%, however, the individual is considered to have mild EIB. A drop of 20% to 40% indicates moderate to severe EIB, and a drop of more than 40% indicates severe EIB. Several questions can be asked during the history to help screen for EIB (**Box 26.2**).

See **Application Strategy: Use of a Peak Flow Meter**, available on the companion Web site at thePoint.

Signs and Symptoms

EIB occurs in three distinct phases. In the first phase, symptoms peak 5 to 10 minutes after exercise begins, lasting for 30 to 60 minutes. Common signs and symptoms include chest pain, chest tightness, or a burning sensation with or without wheezing; a regular, dry cough; shortness of breath shortly after or during exercise; and stomach cramps after exercise. Approximately 50% of individuals with EIB experience the second phase, a "refractory" period. This phase starts 30 minutes to 4 hours after exercise begins and is associated with limited to no bronchospasm. During this period, it may be possible to exercise longer and more strenuously without difficulty. The final phase involves symptoms similar to those experienced during the first phase, but these symptoms are less severe. Symptoms recur 12 to 16 hours after exercise is completed and usually remit within 24 hours.[14]

Management

Pharmacological therapy includes inhaled β-agonists, steroids, cromolyn, nedocromil, ipratropium or tiotropium, and oral leukotriene antagonists. Competitive athletes, however, should consult with appropriate governing

See **Application Strategy: Use of a Metered-Dose Inhaler**, available on the companion Web site at thePoint.

BOX 26.2 History Questions to Screen for Exercise-Induced Bronchospasm

- Have you ever been told that you have asthma or EIB?

- Do you ever have chest pain or tightness during or following exercise?

- Do you ever wheeze during or after moderate exercise?

- Do you ever have shortness of breath during or after exercise?

- Do you ever have itching of the nose or throat or sneezing episodes during or after exercise?

- Have you ever experienced stomach cramps after exercise?

- Have you ever missed work or school because of chest pain, chest tightness, coughing, wheezing, or prolonged shortness of breath?

APPLICATION STRATEGY 26.1

Management Algorithm for Exercise-Induced Bronchospasm

General Recommendations

- Consult a physician before beginning an exercise program.
- Take medication for asthma as prescribed to achieve overall control of asthmatic symptoms, including those caused by exercise and airborne allergens.
- Use a peak flow meter as directed by a physician.
- Avoid exposure to air pollutants and allergens whenever possible.
- Avoid exercise during the early morning hours, when the concentration of ragweed is highest.

Exercise Routine

- Use a bronchodilator before exercise.
- Perform a 5- to 10-minute warm-up period of moderate stretching and work out slowly for another 10–15 minutes, keeping the pulse rate below 60% of maximum heart rate.
- Increase the time and intensity of the workout as tolerated, especially if the activity is new.
- Breathing
  - Breathe slowly through the nose to warm and humidify the air. Exercise in a warm, humid environment, such as a heated swimming pool.
  - In cold, dry environments, breathe through a mask or a scarf. Alternatively, consider different locations and types of exercise during winter months, such as swimming, running, or cycling indoors.
- Perform a gradual 10- to 30-minute cooldown period after a vigorous workout.
  - This avoids rapid thermal changes in the airways.
  - This can be achieved by slowing to a less intense pace while jogging, cycling, swimming, and stretching.

sport bodies to ensure the medication is legal for competition. Nonpharmacological therapy includes high intensity warm-up exercise to help reduce EIB, but it is not as effective as albuterol or other medications. There are also some data indicating that a low-salt diet or fish oil supplementation to the diet will reduce EIB and the inflammation associated with the condition.[15]

Application Strategy 26.1 presents a management algorithm for individuals with EIB.

Influenza

Etiology

Influenza, or "the flu," is a specific viral bronchitis caused by *Haemophilus influenza* type A, B, or C. It often occurs in epidemic proportions, particularly among school-aged children. Immunization for the type A and B viruses is available for individuals who are at high risk, including pregnant women; individuals with chronic illness, such as diabetes mellitus and disorders of the pulmonary or cardiovascular system; children; and those with immunocompromised systems. Individuals with a fever should not be immunized until the fever has passed.

Signs and Symptoms

A fever of 39.0° to 39.5°C (102° to 103°F), chills, malaise, headache, general muscle aches, hacking cough, and inflamed mucous membranes may be present. Rapid onset of symptoms can occur within 24 to 48 hours after exposure to the virus. Sore throat, watery eyes, photophobia, and a nonproductive cough may linger for up to 5 days. In some cases, the cough may progress to bronchitis.

Management

Initial treatment consists of rest, plenty of fluids, salt water gargles, cough medication, and analgesics to control fever, aches, and pains. If the temperature does not return to near normal within

24 hours, the patient should be seen immediately by a physician to rule out other infectious conditions.

Pneumonia

Etiology

Pneumonia is an inflammation and infection of the lungs that may be caused by bacteria, viruses, mycoplasmas, or other infectious agents, such as fungi, including *Pneumocystis* sp., and by various chemicals. Individuals at an increased risk of pneumonia include those age 65 years or older; very young children, whose immune systems are not fully developed; those with an immunodeficiency disease (e.g., AIDS) or a chronic illness (e.g., cardiovascular disease, emphysema, or diabetes); individuals who have had their spleen removed; and individuals whose immune system has been impaired by chemotherapy or long-term use of immunosuppressant drugs. Smoking and abusing alcohol or drugs can also place one at higher risk. Smoking damages the airways, and alcohol interferes with the action of the white blood cells that fight infection. Use of intravenous drugs can lead to injection site infections that can travel through the bloodstream to the lungs. In addition, exposure to air pollutants or toxic fumes from certain agricultural, construction, and industrial chemicals may contribute to some types of pneumonia.

Pneumonia bacteria are present in some healthy throats. When body defenses are weakened in some way, such as by illness, old age, malnutrition, general debility, or impaired immunity, the bacteria can multiply and cause serious damage. Usually, when a person's resistance is lowered, bacteria work their way into the lungs and inflame the alveoli. The alveoli then fill with pus and other liquids, preventing oxygen from transferring into the bloodstream. The tissue from either part of a lobe of the lung, an entire lobe, or most of the lung's five lobes becomes completely filled with liquid. The infection quickly spreads through the bloodstream, and the whole body is invaded. In some cases, this may lead to death. *Streptococcus pneumoniae* is the most common cause of bacterial pneumonia, and it is one form of pneumonia for which a vaccine is available. Pneumonia can affect one or both lungs. Infection of both lungs is popularly referred to as double pneumonia.

Signs and Symptoms

The signs and symptoms of pneumonia vary greatly, depending on the type of organism causing the infection and any underlying conditions that may be present. Bacterial pneumonia often follows a URI, such as a cold or flu. Signs and symptoms are likely to present suddenly and include shaking, chills, high fever, sweating, chest pain (pleurisy), and a cough that produces thick phlegm that is rust, green, or yellow in color. Symptoms may be fewer or milder in older adults or in those with a chronic illness.[1,7]

Viral pneumonia, which is caused by some of the same viruses that cause influenza, strikes primarily during the fall and winter and tends to be more serious in people with cardiovascular or lung disease. It usually starts with a dry and nonproductive cough, headache, fever, muscle pain, and fatigue. As the condition progresses, the patient may become breathless, develop a cough that produces phlegm, and run the risk of developing a secondary bacterial pneumonia as well.

Mycoplasmas are tiny organisms that cause symptoms similar to those of both bacterial and viral pneumonia, although these symptoms appear more gradually and often are milder. Mycoplasmas often cause the type of pneumonia seen in individuals with walking pneumonia. The patient is not sick enough to stay in bed and, therefore, may not seek medical care. This type of pneumonia spreads easily in situations where people congregate and is common in child care centers and among school children and young adults.

Certain types of fungus also can cause pneumonia, especially *Histoplasma capsulatum*, which is common in the Mississippi and Ohio River valleys. Some people experience no symptoms after inhaling this fungus. Others develop symptoms of acute pneumonia, and still others may develop a chronic pneumonia that persists for months.

Pneumonia caused by a parasite, *Pneumocystis carinii*, commonly affects Americans with AIDS. The signs and symptoms of *P. carinii* pneumonia include an ongoing cough, fever, and trouble breathing.

Management

Treatment for pneumonia varies, depending on the type of pneumonia and on the severity of symptoms. Bacterial pneumonia is usually treated with antibiotics; however, antibiotics are not effective against viral forms of pneumonia. Although viral pneumonia may be treated with antiviral medications, the recommended treatment is the same as that for the flu (i.e., rest and plenty of fluids). Mycoplasmal pneumonias are treated with antibiotics. Regardless, it may take 4 to 6 weeks to recover completely if the pneumonia is serious. In some cases, fatigue may continue long after the infection itself has cleared. In addition to these treatments, the physician may recommend OTC medications to reduce fever, treat aches and pains, and soothe the cough associated with pneumonia. The aim is not to suppress the cough completely, however, because coughing helps to clear the lungs.

 Conditions that could contribute to the severity of EIB include ambient air conditions, exposure to allergens, poor physical conditioning, respiratory infections, and amount of time since the last episode of EIB.

SUMMARY

1. Viral conditions are often referred to as URIs.

2. The common cold is an acute viral infection that may be triggered by aspirin sensitivity, use of oral contraceptives, abuse of topical decongestants, abuse of cocaine, presence of nasal polyps or a deviated septum, and allergic conditions.

3. Sinusitis is an inflammation of the paranasal sinus caused by a bacterial or viral infection, an allergy, or environmental factors.

4. If pharyngitis is caused by the bacteria *S. pyogenes* and is inadequately treated, peritonsillar abscess, scarlet fever, rheumatic fever, or rheumatic heart disease may result.

5. In laryngitis, the tissues below the level of the epiglottis are swollen and inflamed, preventing the vocal cords from vibrating normally, which results in hoarseness of the voice.

6. Tonsillitis is an infectious condition characterized by inflamed and enlarged tonsils, fever, painful swallowing, sore throat, and a slight change in voice.

7. Hay fever may be seasonal (i.e., caused by airborne pollens and fungal spores associated with that season) or perennial (i.e., occurs year-round if the patient is continually exposed to allergens).

8. Bronchitis may be acute or chronic, and it is characterized by bronchial swelling, mucus secretion, and increased resistance to expiration.

9. Asthma is caused by a constriction of bronchial smooth muscles (bronchospasm), increased bronchial secretions, and mucosal swelling, each leading to inadequate airflow during respiration (especially during expiration). Wheezing, a common sign of asthma, results from air squeezing past the narrowed airways. The condition is classified as intermittent, seasonal, or chronic, and it is managed with bronchodilators, aerosol corticosteroids, and cromolyn sodium.

10. EIB affects up to 90% of those with asthma and up to 35% of those without known asthma. Key signs are a dry, regular cough within 8 to 10 minutes of the start of moderate exercise as well as stomach cramps after exercise.

11. Rapid onset of fever, chills, malaise, headache, general muscle aches, hacking cough, and inflamed mucous membranes indicates the onset of influenza, or "the flu." Initial treatment consists of rest, plenty of clear fluids, salt water gargles, cough medication, and analgesics to control fever, aches, and pains.

12. Viral pneumonia, which strikes primarily during the fall and winter, tends to start with a dry and nonproductive cough, headache, fever, muscle pain, and fatigue. As the condition progresses, the patient becomes short of breath, develops a cough that produces phlegm, and runs the risk of developing a secondary bacterial pneumonia.

APPLICATION QUESTIONS

1. Athletes often get colds and influenza during their competitive season. What strategies in the athletic training facility can be used to decrease the risk of getting a cold or decreasing the severity of a cold?

2. A 15-year-old previously diagnosed with asthma would like to improve his cardiovascular endurance without triggering exercise-induced bronchospasm. What activities might be recommended, and what guidelines should be followed in developing an exercise program for this individual?

3. A volleyball player has suddenly developed a headache, queasy stomach, general body aches, and has a slight body chill. What open-ended questions might you ask to confirm your suspicion that the individual may be developing the flu?

4. You are providing athletic training coverage for a recreational soccer tournament. Prior to the start of the first game, a 17-year-old male has an asthma attack. The individual does not have his inhaler. However, one of his teammates has an inhaler. Would you suggest that the individual use his teammate's inhaler? Explain your response.

REFERENCES

1. Martin TJ. Infections in athletes. In: Mellion MB, Walsh WM, Madden C, et al, eds. *The Team Physician's Handbook*. 3rd ed. Philadelphia: Hanley & Belfus; 2002:225–243.
2. Ahmadinejad Z, Alijani N, Mansori S, et al. Common sports-related infections: a review of clinical pictures, management and time to return to sports. *Asian J Sports Med*. 2014;5(1):1–9.
3. Saremi J. Upper respiratory viral infections in the athlete. *American Fitness*. 2007;25(6):60–64.
4. Mišigoj-Duraković M, Duraković Z, Baršić B. To exercise or not to exercise in acute upper respiratory tract infections? *Kinesiology*. 2005;37(1): 5–12.
5. Shefrin AE, Goldman RD. Use of over-the-counter cough and cold medications in children. *Can Fam Physician*. 2009;55(11):1081–1083.
6. Allan GM, Arroll B. Prevention and treatment of the common cold: making sense of the evidence. *CMAJ*. 2014;186(3):190–199.
7. Kamat D, Adam HM, Cain KK, et al, eds. *American Academy of Pediatrics: Quick Reference Guide to Pediatric Care*. Elk Grove Village, IL: American Academy of Pediatrics; 2010.
8. Vincent MT, Celestin N, Hussain AN. Pharyngitis. *Am Fam Physician*. 2004;69(6):1465–1470.
9. Undeland DK, Kowalski TJ, Berth WL, et al. Appropriately prescribing antibiotics for patients with pharyngitis: a physician-based approach vs a nurse-only triage and treatment algorithm. *Mayo Clin Proc*. 2010;85(11):1011–1015.
10. Brożek JL, Bousquet J, Baena-Cagnani CE, et al. Allergic rhinitis and its impact on asthma (ARIA) guidelines: 2010 revision. *J Allergy Clin Immunol*. 2010;126(3):466–476.
11. Kemp AS. Allergic rhinitis. *Paediatr Respir Rev*. 2009;10(2):63–68.
12. Virchow JC, Mehta A, Ljungblad L, et al. Add-on montelukast in inadequately controlled asthma patients in a 6-month open-label study: the MONtelukast In Chronic Asthma (MONICA) study. *Respir Med*. 2010;104(5):644–651.
13. Wolanczyk-Medrala A, Dor A, Szczepaniak W, et al. Exercise-induced bronchospasm among athletes in Lower Silesia Province. *J Sports Sci*. 2008;26(13):1467–1471.
14. Hermansen CL, Kirchner JT. Identifying exercise-induced bronchospasm. Treatment hinges on distinguishing it from chronic asthma. *Postgrad Med*. 2004;115(6):15–25.
15. Storms WW. Exercise-induced bronchospasm. *Curr Sports Med Rep*. 2009;8(2):45–46.

Gastrointestinal Conditions

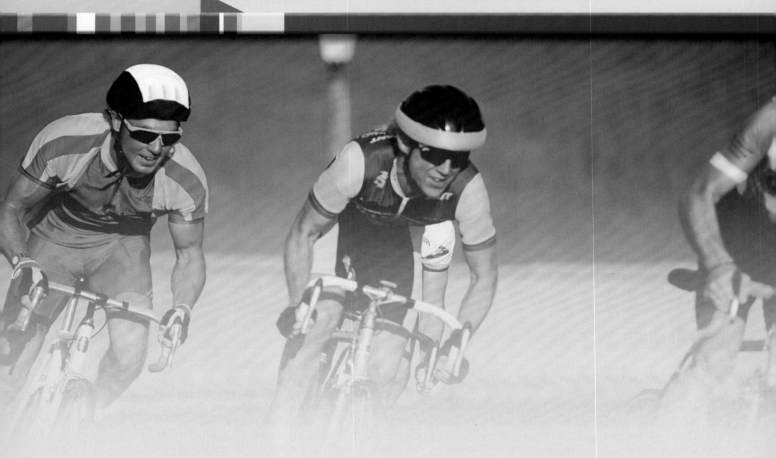

STUDENT OUTCOMES

1. Explain the physiological factors associated with common gastrointestinal (GI) conditions.

2. Identify the common signs and symptoms associated with upper GI conditions, including dysphagia, gastroesophageal reflux, dyspepsia (indigestion), gastric (peptic) ulcers, gastritis, and gastroenteritis.

3. Identify the common signs and symptoms associated with lower GI conditions, including irritable bowel syndrome, Crohn disease, ulcerative colitis, diarrhea, constipation, and hemorrhoids.

4. Describe the general management of upper and lower GI conditions.

5. Explain the factors that may not be related to an injury or condition specific to the upper or lower GI tract but that can adversely affect the entire GI tract.

INTRODUCTION

The gastrointestinal (GI) tract extends from the mouth to the anus. It functions to absorb nutritional substances from ingested food and to expel waste (**Fig. 27.1**). In an active population, exercise alone can induce both upper and lower GI symptoms and problems. During the first few minutes of exercise, up to 15% of the central blood volume is shunted away from the visceral organs to the working muscles. As core temperature rises, 20% of central blood volume is shunted to the skin for cooling. This can result in the reduction of normal intestinal blood flow by as much as 80% for the purpose of maintaining an adequate central blood volume.[1] Exercise-induced shunting, as it often is called, can lead to decreased esophageal motility, erosive hemorrhagic gastritis, delayed gastric emptying, diarrhea, or intestinal bleeding. Dehydration, high ambient temperature, and lack of acclimatization

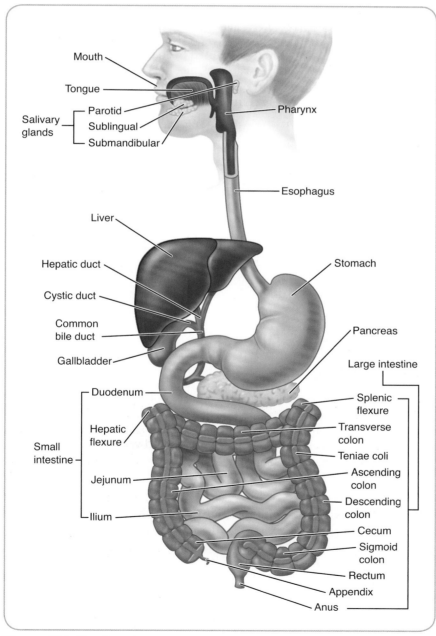

Figure 27.1. The digestive system.

to exercise in the heat can exacerbate this hypoperfusion of the GI tract. Nervous tension also can lead to indigestion, diarrhea, or constipation and can adversely affect sport and physical activity. Many disorders may appear to be minor, but they can be the first sign of more serious underlying conditions.

In this chapter, disorders affecting the upper and lower GI region are discussed. Factors not specific to the upper or lower GI tract but affecting the entire GI tract also are presented.

UPPER GASTROINTESTINAL DISORDERS

 Before the start of a rehabilitation session at a sports medicine clinic, a middle-aged man indicates that he has a mild fever, upset stomach, and abdominal cramps. He also states that during the previous night, he had diarrhea and experienced nausea but did not vomit. What condition might be present, and how should this situation be managed?

Upper GI disorders (i.e., stomach and above) are caused by local irritation resulting from a variety of factors, including stress and the ingestion of caffeine, alcohol, and tomato and citric acid products. This irritation can lead to nausea, emesis (i.e., vomiting), bloating, abdominal cramps, and heartburn. General management includes agents containing antacids and diet modification.

Dysphagia
Etiology
Dysphagia is associated with labored swallowing actions. Predisposing factors include a narrowing of the esophagus as well as paralysis or muscle spasms of the esophageal or pharyngeal muscles.

Signs and Symptoms
The patient will have difficulty swallowing or be unable to swallow.

Management
Any patient who exhibits dysphagia should discontinue activity and be referred immediately to a physician for further evaluation.

Gastroesophageal Reflux Disease
Etiology
When gastric juice, an extremely acidic substance, regurgitates into the esophagus, it is called **gastroesophageal reflux disease** (GERD). The condition often occurs when an individual eats or drinks to excess, but it also is caused by conditions that force abdominal contents superiorly, such as obesity, pregnancy, and running. In the condition referred to as runner's reflux, the stomach contents splash upward with each step. Increasing the intensity of exercise can result in a decrease in the frequency, amplitude, and duration of esophageal contractions.

Signs and Symptoms
Gastroesophageal reflux is associated with mild heartburn, which is a burning, radiating, substernal pain. When gastroesophageal reflux is caused by a chronic exposure to gastric juices, reflux leads to physical complications, such as severe heartburn and upper chest pain. Symptoms are so similar to those of a heart attack that many first-time sufferers are rushed to the nearest medical facility.

Management
Initial management involves use of antacids 4 hours before exercise as well as changes in diet, timing of meals before exercise, and type of activity.

Dyspepsia (Indigestion)

Etiology

Dyspepsia, or indigestion, is associated with upper GI pain that has no identified etiology but has been attributed to excessive acid accumulation in the stomach and overconsumption of alcohol.

Signs and Symptoms

Irregularly occurring symptoms can range from a sense of fullness after eating to feeling as though something is lodged in the esophagus to heartburn, nausea, vomiting, and loss of appetite. Pain and discomfort at the xiphoid region during digestion are the most common symptoms.

Management

Use of antacids 4 hours before exercise and activity modification may help with the discomfort. If symptoms persist, immediate referral to a physician is warranted to rule out more serious abdominal conditions or diseases.

Gastric (Peptic) Ulcer

Etiology

Gastric ulcers occur at the lower end of the esophagus, in the stomach, or in the duodenum. Excessive production of gastric acid usually is a precursor, along with consumption of excessive alcohol, spicy or salty foods, pepper or caffeinated drinks, or salicylates and use of tobacco products, particularly cigarettes and cigars.[2] The resulting open lesion is further exposed to the effects of gastric acids and pepsins released within the stomach. In essence, the stomach begins digesting itself.

Signs and Symptoms

The most common symptom is a gnawing epigastric pain that typically occurs within 1 to 3 hours of eating and after the consumption of orange juice, coffee, aspirin, or alcohol. The pain often is relieved by eating again. Dyspepsia, nausea, vomiting, heartburn, and diarrhea also may be present. The danger with a peptic ulcer is perforation of the stomach wall, followed by peritonitis and, potentially, massive hemorrhage.

Management

Treatment is aimed at reducing acid secretions, healing the mucosal lining, and relieving symptoms. When taken on an empty stomach or 1 hour after a meal, antacids reduce acidity within 30 minutes and continue to reduce it for up to 3 hours. Bland diets may have some limited benefit. In addition, patients should be advised to avoid alcohol, caffeine, and smoking. If over-the-counter (OTC) antacids fail to reduce the pain and discomfort, the patient should be referred to a physician. Hemorrhaging and perforations, which may be present, can result in an emergency situation; these patients should be under a physician's supervision.

Gastritis

Etiology

Gastritis, the most common stomach ailment, occurs when the stomach lining becomes inflamed, leading to erosion of the gastric mucosa. It may be induced by anxiety, exercise-related hypoperfusion, use of nonsteroidal anti-inflammatory drugs, or excessive consumption of caffeine or alcohol.

Signs and Symptoms

After consumption of an offending substance, acute gastritis may present with GI bleeding, belching, epigastric pain, and vomiting, including **hematemesis**. Chronic gastritis may exhibit similar symptoms, mild discomfort, or no symptoms. When present, symptoms range from a loss of appetite to a "full" feeling in the stomach or vague epigastric pain.

Management

Symptoms are relieved by eliminating the irritant or cause. Anticholinergics and antacids may relieve distress, but with severe bleeding, blood replacement may be necessary. Antacids may be contraindicated if gastric bleeding is present. If gastric bleeding does occur, exercise is contraindicated, and the patient should be referred to a physician.

Gastroenteritis

Etiology

The incidence of gastroenteritis, an acute inflammation of the mucous membrane of the stomach or small intestine, is second only to that of upper respiratory tract infections in adolescents and young adults.[1] The condition also may be called intestinal flu, traveler's diarrhea, or food poisoning. The condition may be caused by a viral or bacterial infection, allergic reaction, medication, parasites, contaminated food (food poisoning), or emotional stress.

Signs and Symptoms

In mild cases, increased secretion of hydrochloric acid in the stomach may lead to indigestion, nausea, flatulence (gas), and a sour stomach. In moderate to severe cases, abdominal cramping, diarrhea, fever, and vomiting can lead to fluid and electrolyte imbalance.

Management

The condition often is self-limiting and usually clears in 2 to 3 days. Treatment includes eliminating irritating foods from the diet, avoiding factors that bring on anxiety and stress, and avoiding dehydration by drinking clear fluids or electrolyte-containing fluids. Antimotility drugs (e.g., Imodium, Lomotil, and Diasorb) reduce movement in the small intestine and may be effective for abdominal cramps and diarrhea, but these drugs also may prolong some infections. The patient's return to activity is limited by hydration status, the nature of the infection, the complexity of the symptoms (e.g., frequent diarrhea), and reconditioning. Children and senior athletes should be carefully monitored for fluid and electrolyte imbalance during exercise.

 The male patient had a mild fever, upset stomach, abdominal cramps, diarrhea, and nausea. He may have gastroenteritis. He should be encouraged to rest and increase his intake of clear or electrolyte-containing fluids. He also should be advised to see a physician if the condition does not improve in 2 to 3 days.

LOWER GASTROINTESTINAL DISORDERS

 What treatment should be suggested to a triathlete who is experiencing chronic diarrhea while running?

Lower GI disorders occur distal to the stomach. Common conditions associated with lower GI problems include irritable bowel syndrome, Crohn disease, ulcerative colitis, diarrhea, constipation, and hemorrhoids. Many lower GI disorders are managed by increasing dietary fiber and avoiding irritating foods.

Irritable Bowel Syndrome

Etiology

Irritable bowel syndrome (IBS) is marked by abdominal pain and altered bowel function (i.e., constipation, diarrhea, or alternating constipation and diarrhea) for which no organic cause can be determined. It affects up to 20% of the North American population, with women twice as likely as men to be affected.[3] This chronic condition, which sometimes is referred to incorrectly as "spastic colon," usually begins during early adulthood, lasting intermittently for years. It commonly presents with symptoms between ages 20 and 50 years.[4] Although originally thought to be psychological in origin, physiological etiology may include errors in GI tract motility, alterations in autonomic regulation, increased visceral sensitivity, abnormal brain-gut interaction, and flora changes.[4]

Signs and Symptoms

The most prominent symptom with IBS is abdominal pain or discomfort that lasts for at least 12 weeks (which need not be consecutive) of the preceding 12 months and includes at least two of the three following features: Relief is achieved with defecation, onset is associated with a change in frequency of stool, and/or onset is associated with a change in the form and appearance of the stool.[3] The stool may be covered with mucus. Heartburn, abdominal distension, back pain, weakness, and faintness also may occur. Acute attacks may subside within 1 day, but recurrent exacerbation is likely.

Management

This patient should be referred to a physician to rule out more serious conditions. A complete blood count and stool examination should be administered to identify occult blood, ova, parasites, and pathogenic bacteria that may be linked to related conditions. No single successful treatment is available for IBS. Dietary modification may involve eliminating irritating foods (i.e., dairy products, gas-forming foods, caffeine, and artificial sweeteners) or, if constipation is a symptom, adding fiber. Adequate rest and exercise is encouraged, along with reduction of stress. A sedative or antispasmodic medication may be used.[4,5]

Crohn Disease

Etiology

Crohn disease (i.e., regional enteritis) is a serious, chronic inflammation, usually of the ileum, although it may affect any portion of the intestinal tract. Its cause is unknown. The condition is distinguished from IBS by its inflammatory pattern. The inflammation extends through all layers of the intestinal wall, resulting in a characteristic thickening or toughening of the wall and a narrowing of the intestinal lumen. The inflammation tends to be patchy or segmented. The disease may be mild, moderate, severe, or in remission.

Signs and Symptoms

The patient often experiences colicky or chronic abdominal pain in the right lower quadrant, diarrhea 10 to 20 times per day, loss of appetite, and weight loss. A variety of sores, fissures, or fistulas may appear in the anal region. The disease can lead to complications outside the digestive tract, such as joint pain, eye problems, skin rash, or liver disease, suggesting a possible immune system response.

Management

This patient should be referred to a physician. A barium enema, sigmoidoscopy, and colonoscopy may be necessary to rule out other conditions. Only a biopsy, however, can provide a definitive diagnosis. Treatment is symptomatic and supportive. It involves medications to prevent flare-ups or maintain remission of the disease. Mild symptoms may respond to an antidiarrheal medication, such as loperamide (e.g., Imodium), which slows or stops the painful spasm. For mild to moderate symptoms, aminosalicylates (e.g., sulfasalazine or mesalamine) also may be used to manage the condition or to prevent relapses. Corticosteroids, which can be administered orally, rectally, or by injection, are given when symptoms are more severe.[2] Fistulas are treated with antibiotics. If the immune system is impacted, immunomodulator medications may be prescribed.

Ulcerative Colitis

Etiology

Colitis is another chronic, inflammatory ulceration of the colon, often beginning in the rectum or sigmoid colon and extending upward into the entire colon. Unlike Crohn disease, in which the inflammatory pattern extends into all layers of the intestinal wall and is patchy or segmented, the inflammation in ulcerative colitis tends to involve only the mucosal lining of the colon. The affected part of the colon is uniformly involved and exhibits erythema and numerous hemorrhagic ulcerations, with no patches of healthy mucosal tissue being evident.[2]

Signs and Symptoms

Recurrent bloody diarrhea is a classic symptom and can lead to anemia. The stool often contains pus and mucus. Abdominal pain and severe urgency to move the bowels also are characteristic. Other symptoms include fever, weight loss, and signs of dehydration. Periodic exacerbation of the disease followed by remission of symptoms is common.

Management

Management of colitis focuses on suppressing the inflammatory response to relieve symptoms and permit healing. Mild symptoms may respond to an antidiarrheal medication, such as loperamide (e.g., Imodium A-D), and to changes in the diet. Usually, corticosteroids (e.g., hydrocortisone or prednisone) are given for a few weeks to control the active disease. When symptoms are under control, aminosalicylates (e.g., sulfasalazine or mesalamine) may be used to keep the disease in remission. Moderate to severe symptoms usually require corticosteroids to control inflammation. Anti-inflammatories and corticosteroid treatment also can be effective.[2] If the immune system is impacted, immunomodulator medications may be prescribed.

Diarrhea

Etiology

Anxiety and precompetition jitters commonly result in "nervous diarrhea." A common and troublesome disorder, **diarrhea** is characterized by abnormally loose, watery stools. This is caused by food residue running through the large intestine before the organ has had sufficient time to absorb the remaining water. Diarrhea in adults may result from malabsorption syndrome, gastritis, lactose intolerance, IBS, Crohn disease, ulcerative colitis, GI tumors, diverticular disease, viral and bacterial infections of the intestine, parasitic infections, psychogenic disorders, food allergies, and a variety of medications.[2] Prolonged diarrhea can lead to dehydration and depletion of electrolytes, particularly sodium, bicarbonate, and potassium. Common among runners, runner's diarrhea, or runner's trots, is caused by increased intestinal motility that can lead to several patterns of bowel dysfunction (**Box 27.1**). If this is a known problem, the patient should perform light exercise before activity to help empty the bowels and drink extra water to maintain hydration.

Signs and Symptoms

Abnormally loose and watery stools may be accompanied by flatulence, abdominal distension, fever, headache, vomiting, malaise, and **myalgia**.

Management

Diarrhea may respond to certain antidiarrheal medications, which reduce intestinal movement, increase fluid absorption, modify intestinal bacteria, or reduce inflammation associated with diarrhea. Pepto-Bismol, loperamide (e.g., Imodium), or diphenoxylate with atropine (e.g., Lomotil) may help; however, these products should not be used on a regular basis. An attempt should be made to defecate at a regular daily time, taking advantage of the morning gastrocolic reflex, a propulsive reflex in the colon that stimulates defecation. Peristalsis and defecation can be stimulated by drinking coffee or tea, having a light meal before competition, and jogging to stimulate the gastrocolic reflex. Exercise—specifically, more than what the body is accustomed to—increases intestinal activity; therefore, individuals may want to do the following:

■ Immediately decrease the level of training and competition by 20% to 40% in both mileage and intensity until the episode passes and then build back up slowly.

■ Eliminate foods that trigger bowel irritation, including dairy products if lactose intolerance is involved, excessive juices, fresh fruits, raisins and other dried fruits, beans, and lentils.

BOX 27.1 Patterns of Bowel Dysfunction Found in Runners

1. **Nervous diarrhea before competition**
   - More common in women
   - Occurs in runners with
     - Irregular bowel function when not running
     - History of lactose intolerance

2. **The need to stop and have a bowel movement while training**
   - More common in men during the first few miles of a run
   - Occurs in runners
     - With irregular bowel function
     - Who eat before running
     - Who take a morning run before breakfast

3. **Cramps and diarrhea without blood in the stool after hard run**
   - Common in runners; associated with severe lower abdominal cramps, nausea, and vomiting

4. **Cramps and diarrhea with blood in the stool after hard run**
   - Associated with diarrhea, severe lower abdominal cramps, and rectal bleeding

---

- Limit the amount of sugar-free gum and hard candies that contain sorbitol, which can cause diarrhea.

- Improve hydration before and during exercise to increase plasma volume and decrease intestinal mucosal ischemia.

Individuals on a low-fiber diet may benefit from adding fiber to absorb excess fluids. In contrast, individuals on a high-fiber diet may benefit by reducing fiber to decrease stimulation of intestinal motility. Food triggers can be identified by keeping a food/diarrhea chart. This can be done by taking away any suspected food for a few days, followed by eating a large portion of the food and observing any changes in bowel movements. Food usually moves through the intestines in 2 to 4 days. A simple way to identify the body's "transit time" is to eat foods that can be seen in the feces, such as corn, sesame seeds, or beets. An increase in clear liquids for 24 to 48 hours should be followed by readjustment to a regular diet.[1]

Constipation

Etiology

Constipation occurs when stools are difficult to pass. Some people are overly concerned with the frequency of their bowel movements, because they have been taught that a healthy person has a bowel movement every day. This is not true. Most people pass stools anywhere from 3 times a day to 3 times a week. If the stools are soft and pass easily, a patient is not constipated.

Signs and Symptoms

Constipation is present if a patient has two or fewer bowel movements each week. Infrequent or incomplete bowel movements are not a disease but, rather, are a description of symptoms that may indicate a more serious underlying condition. Potential causes include lack of fiber in the diet, improper bowel habits, lack of exercise, emotional distress, diabetes mellitus, pregnancy, laxative abuse, and drug effects from narcotics or nonsteroidal anti-inflammatory pain relievers and antidepressant medicines.

Management

Management depends on the origin of the condition. Individuals who have a low-fiber diet should gradually increase their intake of high-fiber foods. Fiber absorbs water and makes feces softer and easier to eliminate. Bran cereals are rich in fiber, even superior to salads, vegetables, and fruits. Increasing daily exercise, particularly aerobic exercise, and ensuring adequate fluid intake can help to alleviate symptoms. Laxatives or suppositories are useful but should be used sparingly and only for short-term treatment because they stimulate and promote bowel emptying. They work by holding water and swelling in the intestines, whereas stool softeners work by mixing fat and water into fecal matter. Some common OTC stool softeners include Dulcolax, Senokot, Metamucil, and Citrucel.

In addition to medications, drinking warm, clear fluids (e.g., juice, soda, or broth), particularly in the morning, can stimulate bowel activity. The body naturally wants to defecate approximately half an hour after consuming a warm beverage in the morning. Time should be allotted to relax and honor this urge. It is advisable to drink plenty of fluids throughout the day but no more than half a cup of prune juice. Signs suggesting that sufficient fluid is being consumed include urination every 2 to 4 hours and urine that is light in color, like lemonade, and not dark, like apple cider. Surgical intervention may be necessary in cases of chronic constipation.

Hemorrhoids (Piles)

Etiology

Hemorrhoids are dilations of the venous plexus surrounding the rectal and anal area. They are most common during pregnancy and in those who are older than 30 years. The dilated sacs become exposed if they protrude internally into the rectal and anal canals (i.e., polyps) or externally around the anal opening. Several factors increase the incidence of hemorrhoids, including constipation, diarrhea, straining during physical exertion, pelvic congestion, enlargement of the prostate, uterine fibroids, rectal tumors, varicose veins, and pregnancy.

Signs and Symptoms

Pain, itching, and passing small amounts of bright red blood on defecation, separate from the feces, are the most common signs and symptoms. Athletes who participate in contact or collision sports (e.g., boxing, football, and ice hockey) normally may experience small amounts of blood on defecation. In many endurance runners, blood in fecal material is caused by GI bleeding and is quite common and normal. This bleeding can lead to iron-deficiency anemia. If moderate amounts of blood are mixed with feces, however, a full evaluation by a physician should be conducted.

Management

The condition normally heals within 2 to 3 weeks. Medicated rectal anesthetic preparations can be used to relieve pain, itching, and irritation. Forms of medication include suppository, cream, ointment, and aerosol foam. Preparation-H, Proctofoam, Tucks Pads, and Tronolane are OTC rectal preparations. Pain or swelling also can be relieved by following the suggestions listed in **Box 27.2**.

BOX 27.2 Reducing the Inflammation of Hemorrhoids

- Take warm sitz baths for 15 minutes several times a day, especially after bowel movements.
- Use stool softeners to prevent constipation and products to ease friction (i.e., petroleum jelly applied around the anus).
- Increase fiber in the diet by adding unprocessed bran to breakfast cereals and eating other high-roughage food.
- Drink plenty of water and other clear fluids.
- Do not ignore the urge for bowel movements because a delay allows pressure to build up in the rectum and increases the chance of constipation and development of hemorrhoids.
- Exercise to promote good abdominal muscle tone.
- Avoid pushing too hard or long during bowel movements.

If these suggestions are not successful, physician referral is indicated. Prescribed nitroglycerin ointment applied over the inflamed area has been found to relieve hemorrhoid pain in approximately 5 minutes. In severe cases, however, surgery may be necessary.

Treatment for the triathlete experiencing chronic diarrhea while running should include taking antidiarrheal medications (e.g., Pepto-Bismol, Imodium, or Lomotil), eliminating foods that trigger bowel irritation, improving hydration before and after exercise, eating a low-fiber diet 24 to 36 hours before exercise, and decreasing the intake of coffee or tea before exercise. If the condition continues, refer the patient to a physician for further evaluation.

OTHER GASTROINTESTINAL PROBLEMS

Two hours after eating at a fast-food restaurant, while on the bus trip home from a game, several baseball players report varying levels of abdominal gas and pain, nausea, vomiting, low-grade fever, and diarrhea. What condition should be suspected, and what is the management for this condition?

Certain factors, although they may not be related to an injury or condition specific to the upper or lower GI tract, may affect the entire GI tract. Anxiety and stress, vomiting, and food poisoning are such conditions.

Anxiety and Stress Reaction

Etiology

Performance anxiety and pregame stress are common in competing athletes. Upper GI tract function can be affected through decreased acid secretion in the stomach, slowed intestinal motility, or decreased blood flow. Continued anxiety can lead to hypersecretion of stomach acids, increased motility, or decreased transit time.

Signs and Symptoms

Common symptoms include dry mouth, dyspepsia, gastroesophageal reflux, heartburn, abdominal cramping, or diarrhea.

Management

Treatment involves reassurance and education about the body's processes; relaxation techniques, such as deep breathing, passive and active relaxation, soothing music, and therapeutic massage; and behavior modification using cognitive restructuring, concentration skills, confidence training, coping rehearsal, imagery, and positive self-talk. Many of these intervention strategies are discussed in Chapter 7.

Vomiting

Etiology

Nausea is an unpleasant, wavelike feeling in the back of the throat and/or stomach that may or may not result in vomiting. Vomiting is the forceful elimination of the contents of the stomach through the mouth. Retching is the movement of the stomach and esophagus without vomiting and is also called "dry heaves."

Signs and Symptoms

Vomiting involves the oral ejection of stomach contents from reverse peristaltic contractions of voluntary and involuntary muscles. It often is preceded by a watering mouth and nausea. It often results from the intake of irritating foods and other intestinal irritants, stress, excessive consumption of alcohol or other drugs, or food poisoning.

Management

Vomiting is best managed by comforting the patient and maintaining a clear airway. The mouth should be rinsed and monitored for repeated vomiting, followed by administration of antinausea medication and clear fluids to prevent dehydration. If food poisoning is expected or blood is found in the vomit, immediate referral to a physician is necessary. Vomiting also can be an early sign of pregnancy, particularly if it occurs in the morning hours.

Food Poisoning

Etiology

The most common cause of food poisoning is contaminated food. Food poisoning, however, also can stem from insecticides or infectious organisms (e.g., bacteria from the salmonella group, certain staphylococci, streptococci, or dysentery bacilli) from food that is undercooked or decomposed.

Severe cases of food poisoning require activation of the emergency action plan, including summoning emergency medical services. Fluids must be replaced intravenously, and pumping of the stomach contents may be necessary. If possible, samples of the vomitus should be provided to the physician; the sample can aid in identifying the food that is responsible for the poisoning.

Signs and Symptoms

Food poisoning includes varying levels of abdominal gas and pain, nausea, vomiting, low-grade fever, and diarrhea. These signs and symptoms can begin from 1 to 6 hours after ingestion of contaminated foods and may last for 1 to 3 days. Dehydration from the vomiting and diarrhea can lead to weakness, fatigue, and increased risk of heat illness.

Management

Mild symptoms are treated conservatively with rapid replacement of fluids and electrolytes and administration of an antidiarrheal agent. If tolerated, light fluids, such as broth or bouillon with a small amount of salt, may be eaten. Poached eggs or bland cereals may also be given as tolerated. Severe cases of food poisoning require activation of the emergency action plan.

 The symptoms reported by the baseball players suggest food poisoning. The athletes should continue to be monitored to determine the severity of the condition. Mild symptoms are treated conservatively, with rapid replacement of fluids and electrolytes and administration of an antidiarrheal agent. Severe cases require intravenous fluid replacement, and pumping of the stomach contents may be necessary. As such, activation of the emergency action plan, including summoning emergency medical services, is warranted.

SUMMARY

1. Exercise-induced shunting can lead to decreased esophageal motility, erosive hemorrhagic gastritis, delayed gastric emptying, diarrhea, or intestinal bleeding. Dehydration, high ambient temperatures, and lack of acclimatization can exacerbate hypoperfusion of the GI tract.

2. Many upper GI tract disorders are caused by irritation attributed to stress or to the ingestion of caffeine, alcohol, or tomato and citric acid products, leading to nausea, vomiting, bloating, abdominal cramps, and heartburn.

3. Gastroesophageal reflux is associated with regurgitation of gastric juices into the esophagus. Dyspepsia, or indigestion, is associated with upper GI pain that has no identified etiology. Both are treated with antacids taken 4 hours before physical activity.

4. Peptic ulcers generally occur at the lower end of the esophagus, in the stomach, or in the duodenum. Antacids may reduce or neutralize stomach acids and prevent them from moving into the esophagus, reducing heartburn and discomfort.

5. Gastroenteritis is second in incidence only to upper respiratory tract infections in adolescents and adults. It is caused by viral or bacterial infection, allergic reaction, medication, contaminated food, or emotional stress. The condition is self-limiting and usually clears in 2 to 3 days. Treatment includes eliminating irritating foods from the diet, avoiding factors that bring on anxiety and stress, and avoiding dehydration.

6. Diarrhea, which is common among runners, is caused by increased intestinal motility. Antidiarrheal medications reduce intestinal movement, increase fluid absorption, modify intestinal bacteria, or reduce inflammation associated with diarrhea. If this is a known problem, the patient should try to defecate before exercise and should not eat before running.

7. Hemorrhoids are dilations of the venous plexus surrounding the rectal and anal area. Pain, itching, and passing small amounts of bright red blood on defecation, separate from the feces, are the most common signs and symptoms. Medicated rectal anesthetic preparations can be used to relieve pain, itching, and irritation. The condition normally heals within 2 to 3 weeks.

8. Anxiety and stress can lead to decreased acid secretion in the stomach, slower intestinal motility, or decreased blood flow. Continued anxiety can lead to hypersecretion of stomach acids, increased motility, or decreased transit time. Treatment involves reassurance and education about the body's processes, relaxation techniques, and behavior modification.

9. Vomiting may be caused by irritating foods and other intestinal irritants, stress, excessive alcohol or drug consumption, or food poisoning. Although it often can be treated conservatively with antinausea medication and clear fluids to prevent dehydration, vomiting may be an early sign of pregnancy, particularly if it occurs in the morning hours. Persistent vomiting signals a more serious condition, in which case immediate referral to a physician is warranted.

APPLICATION QUESTIONS

1. A 17-year-old swimmer reports to practice with a mild fever, upset stomach, and abdominal cramps. He also reports experiencing diarrhea and nausea for the past 3 days. What condition(s) might be suspected? How would you manage this condition?

2. A distance runner has reported the consistent need to stop and have a bowel movement while training. Is this normal for runners? What suggestions would you make to the runner?

3. Three hours after eating a pregame meal, several members of a softball team develop stomach cramping, nausea, and diarrhea. Given these signs and symptoms, how will you manage the situation? What detrimental effects, if any, will this situation have on the players' performance? What is your obligation, as an athletic trainer, to notify health authorities about this incident?

4. What is the potential effect of high levels of performance anxiety and pregame stress on the upper GI tract? How would you manage a situation in which an athlete develops upper GI tract problems as a result of anxiety and stress?

REFERENCES

1. Balakrishnan N, Torres JL, Mellion MB. Gastrointestinal problems. In: Mellion MB, Walsh WM, Madden C, et al, eds. *Team Physician's Handbook*. Philadelphia, PA: Hanley & Belfus; 2002:244–248.
2. Tamparo CD, Lewis MA. *Diseases of the Human Body*. Philadelphia, PA: FA Davis; 2011.
3. Brandt LJ, Bjorkman D, Fennerty MB, et al. Systematic review on the management of irritable bowel syndrome in North America. *Am J Gastroenterol*. 2002;97(11 suppl):S7–S26.
4. Blesse LC. Irritable bowel syndrome: relieving the symptoms, and the frustration. *JAAPA*. 2010;23(11):46–51.
5. Ehrenpreis ED. Irritable bowel syndrome. 10% to 20% of older adults have symptoms consistent with diagnosis. *Geriatrics*. 2005;60(1):25–28.

Endocrine Conditions

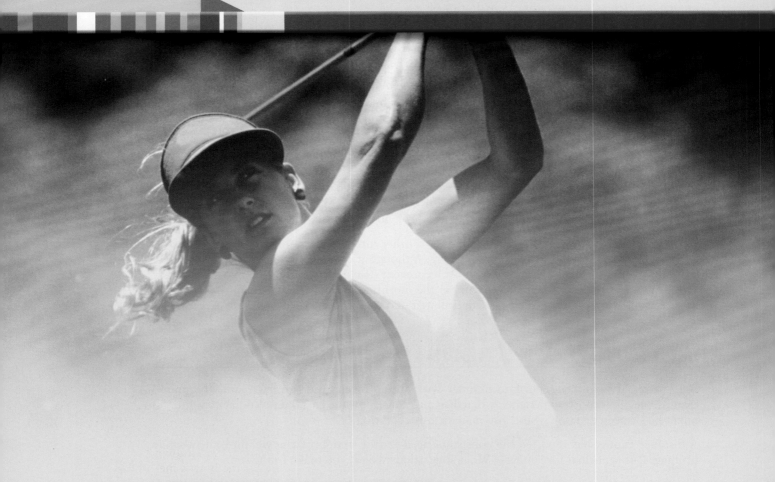

STUDENT OUTCOMES

1. Describe the signs and symptoms of hyperthyroidism and hypothyroidism and explain the management of thyroid disorders.

2. Describe the signs and symptoms of acute and chronic pancreatitis and explain the management of both conditions.

3. Explain the insulin regulation of blood glucose levels.

4. Explain the physiological basis of diabetes.

5. Describe the four types of diabetes mellitus.

6. Describe the circulatory and neural complications that can result from diabetes mellitus.

7. Describe the signs and symptoms of insulin shock and diabetic coma and explain the management of insulin shock and diabetic coma.

8. Explain the nutritional recommendations for physically active individuals with type 1 and type 2 diabetes.

9. Identify physical activities that are indicated and contraindicated for a physically active individual with diabetes.

INTRODUCTION

The endocrine system is one of the most critical systems for maintaining a healthy body. The system is a series of ductless organs that secrete hormones into the blood to be transported throughout the body (**Fig. 28.1**). Endocrine glands include the pituitary, thyroid, parathyroid, adrenal, pineal, and thymus glands. In addition, several organs contain discrete areas of endocrine tissue and produce hormones. Such organs include the pancreas, gonads (i.e., ovaries and testes), and hypothalamus. When hormones are not produced in the proper level, serious conditions may occur. In this chapter, thyroid disorders, such as hyperthyroidism and hypothyroidism, are discussed, as are pancreatitis and diabetes mellitus.

THYROID DISORDERS

The thyroid is a butterfly-shaped gland located at the base of the neck, just below the Adam's apple. The thyroid gland produces two main hormones: thyroxine and triiodothyronine. These hormones maintain the rate at which the body uses fats and carbohydrates, regulate the body temperature, influence the heart rate, and help to regulate the production of protein. The thyroid gland also produces calcitonin, a hormone that regulates the amount of calcium in the blood. The rate at which these hormones are released is controlled by the pituitary gland and the hypothalamus, an area at the base of the brain that acts as a thermostat for the body.

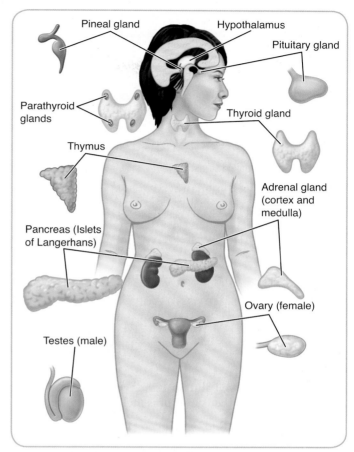

Figure 28.1. Location of the major endocrine glands.

As long as the thyroid produces the necessary amount of hormones, metabolism functions normally. Occasionally, the thyroid gland produces too much thyroxine causing a condition known as hyperthyroidism (i.e., overactive thyroid disease). This condition can accelerate the body's metabolism by as much as 60% to 100%, causing sudden weight loss, rapid or irregular heartbeat, nervousness, or irritability. In contrast, if too little thyroxine is produced, hypothyroidism occurs.

Hyperthyroidism

Etiology

Hyperthyroidism is caused by the overproduction of thyroxine. This condition frequently produces a cluster of symptoms called thyrotoxicosis. Hyperthyroidism can result from a number of conditions and diseases, most commonly **Graves disease**. In turn, Graves disease may result from genetic and immunological factors and is marked by an enlarged thyroid gland (i.e., goiter), characteristic changes in the structure of the eyes (i.e., ophthalmopathy), and rarely, characteristic skin lesions (i.e., dermopathy).[1] Graves disease usually occurs in people younger than 40 years of age and affects women seven to eight times more than men, and is the most common cause of pediatric hyperthyroidism.[2,3]

Signs and Symptoms

The classic manifestations of hyperthyroidism are goiter, symptoms of thyrotoxicosis, ophthalmopathy, and dermopathy (**Table 28.1**). The symptoms of thyrotoxicosis include nervousness, increased heart rate, loss of sleep, fatigue during ordinary activities, excessive perspiration, and heat intolerance. As a result, sport and physical activity may be contraindicated. Ophthalmopathy results in the eyeball protruding beyond its normal protective orbit when the tissues and muscles behind the eyes

TABLE 28.1 Signs and Symptoms of Thyroid Disorders

HYPERTHYROIDISM	HYPOTHYROIDISM
Sudden weight loss, even when appetite and food intake remain normal or increase	Unexplained weight gain
Rapid or irregular heartbeat (arrhythmia) or pounding of the heart	Elevated blood cholesterol levels
Nervousness, irritability, tremor	Depression
Sweating	Pale, dry skin; puffy face
Changes in menstrual patterns	Heavier than normal menstrual periods
Increased sensitivity to heat	Increased sensitivity to cold
Changes in bowel patterns, especially more frequent bowel movements	Constipation
An enlarged thyroid (goiter), which may appear as a swelling at the base of the neck	Goiter
Fatigue, muscle weakness	Headache
Difficulty sleeping	Sleep apnea Brittle nails; coarse hair Hypertension Paresthesia

swell and push the eyeball forward; this can cause the front surface of the eyeball to become very dry. Other symptoms include the following:

■ Red or swollen eyes

■ Widening of the space between the eyelids

■ Excessive tearing or discomfort in one or both eyes

■ Light sensitivity, blurry or double vision, and inflammation or reduced eye movement

■ Inflammation of the muscles surrounding the eye leading to persistent blinking

Dermopathy is marked by the appearance of thickened patches of skin, usually on the feet or legs, having an "orange skin" texture and uneven pigmentation.[4]

Management

Several treatments are available for hyperthyroidism. The choice of a specific approach depends on the individual's age, sex, physical condition, and severity of the disorder. One approach involves the use of antithyroid medication (i.e., drugs that block hormone production within the thyroid gland). Symptoms usually improve in 6 to 8 weeks, but it may be necessary to continue the use of antithyroid medications for a year or more.[1]

Another approach is to alter the structure of the thyroid gland, either through surgery or with **radioactive iodine**. Radioactive iodine, which is the most common treatment method in the United States, is taken orally. It is absorbed by the thyroid gland, causing the gland to shrink and the symptoms to subside. The process usually occurs within 2 to 3 months. Because this treatment causes thyroid activity to slow considerably, however, the individual eventually may need to take a medication every day to replace thyroxine.[1,2]

Hypothyroidism

Etiology

Hypothyroidism may be caused by an insufficient quantity of thyroid tissue or by the loss of functional thyroid tissue. An insufficient quantity of thyroid tissue may result from thyroid surgery, in which a portion of the gland is removed; radioactive iodine therapy for another thyroid disease, such as hyperthyroidism or Graves disease; or a congenital thyroid abnormality. The progressive loss of functional thyroid tissue generally is idiopathic, but it is thought to have strong ties to an autoimmune disorder, such as Hashimoto thyroiditis, which is the leading cause of hypothyroidism.[5] The principal symptom of Hashimoto thyroiditis is goiter. Other causes may include iodine deficiency, radiation therapy for cancers of the head and neck, a pituitary disorder whereby the pituitary gland fails to produce enough thyroid-stimulating hormone, or pregnancy. Some women develop hypothyroidism during or after pregnancy, often because they produce antibodies to their own thyroid gland. Left untreated, hypothyroidism increases the risk of miscarriage, premature delivery, and preeclampsia. It also can seriously affect the developing fetus.[4]

Hypothyroidism occurs mainly in women older than 40 years, and the risk of developing the disorder increases with age.[6,7] Others at risk for the condition include those with a close relative, such as a parent or grandparent, who has an autoimmune thyroid disorder; those with previous head and neck or thyroid irradiation or surgery; those with other autoimmune endocrine conditions, such as type 1 diabetes mellitus, adrenal insufficiency, and ovarian failure; and those with some other nonendocrine autoimmune disorders (e.g., celiac disease, vitiligo, pernicious anemia, and multiple sclerosis), primary pulmonary hypertension, and Down and Turner syndromes.[6]

Signs and Symptoms

The signs and symptoms of hypothyroidism vary widely, depending on the severity of the hormone deficiency and on the age of the patient (**Table 28.1**). In children, retarded growth, delayed emergence of secondary sexual characteristics, impaired intelligence, and one or more of the adult symptoms of hypothyroidism may be present. In adults, the initial onset of symptoms such as fatigue, constipation, intolerance to cold, muscle cramps, menorrhagia (prolonged or profuse menses), and sluggishness are barely noticeable and may be attributed simply to the individual getting older. Additional symptoms, however, develop as the metabolism continues to slow; these additional symptoms include mental clouding, diminished appetite, and weight gain. The skin may become dry, and the hair and nails may become brittle. During the advanced stages of the disease, the affected individual may have an expressionless face, sparse hair, and an enlarged thyroid (goiter).[5] Hypothyroidism also may be associated with increased risk of heart disease, primarily because high levels of low-density lipoprotein (LDL) cholesterol (considered to be the "bad" cholesterol) can occur in people with an underactive thyroid. Hypothyroidism also can lead to an enlarged heart, bouts of depression, dementia, and decreased sexual desire (libido).

Management

The treatment of choice for hypothyroidism involves hormone replacement therapy with the synthetic thyroxine. The medication restores adequate hormone levels, reduces fatigue, gradually lowers cholesterol levels elevated by the disease, and may reverse any weight gain.[5] Overtreatment of the synthetic thyroxine may cause subclinical hyperthyroidism, which increases the risk of osteoporosis and atrial fibrillation. Undertreatment causes subclinical hypothyroidism, which may increase cardiovascular risk.[7,8]

PANCREATITIS

The pancreas is a long, flat gland that lies horizontally behind the stomach. The head of the pancreas rests against the upper part of the small intestine (duodenum), and its tail reaches toward the spleen. The pancreas has two main functions:

1. Produce digestive juices and enzymes to help break down fats, carbohydrates, and proteins (pancreatic exocrine function). Once produced, these juices and enzymes are then transported through a small duct that opens into the duodenum.

2. Secrete the hormones insulin and glucagon into the bloodstream, along with somatostatin, another hormone that helps to regulate their function. The primary role of insulin and glucagon is to regulate the metabolism of carbohydrates and to control the level of blood sugar.

When inflammation develops in the pancreas, these functions are disrupted. The inflammation can be acute or chronic. Symptoms in most cases are mild to moderate but can be severe causing permanent tissue damage.[9]

Acute Pancreatitis

Etiology

Gallstones are the leading cause of acute pancreatitis.[9] These stones migrate out of the gallbladder through the common bile duct, which merges with the pancreatic duct near the entrance to the duodenum. At this junction, gallstones can lodge in or near the pancreatic duct and block the flow of pancreatic juices into the duodenum thus causing inflammation. Digestive enzymes then become active in the pancreas instead of in the digestive tract, causing acute pancreatitis.

Alcohol abuse typically is cited as the second major cause of acute pancreatitis. Other causes of the disorder include drug reactions, viral infections, systemic immunological disorders, pancreatic cancer, or complications from a duodenal ulcer. In some cases, the cause is unknown.

Signs and Symptoms

The main symptom of acute pancreatitis is the sudden onset of persistent, mild to severe abdominal pain centered over the epigastric region that may radiate to the back and, occasionally, the chest. It can persist for hours or days without relief. Drinking alcohol or eating worsens the pain. Many people with acute pancreatitis sit up and bend forward or curl up in a fetal position, because these positions seem to relieve the pain. Severe attacks also may cause abdominal distention or bruises from internal bleeding, nausea or vomiting, fever, and tachycardia. Vital signs show a rapid pulse, low blood pressure, and elevated temperature.

Management

Acute pancreatitis requires immediate medical care to avoid possibly fatal complications. Treatment largely is symptomatic. The aim is to maintain circulation and fluid volume, decrease pain and pancreatic secretions, antibiotics and control any complications. Analgesic drugs, intravenous administration of fluids, and fasting may be necessary. Acute pancreatitis usually is self-limiting, and pancreatic function eventually is restored.

Chronic Pancreatitis

Etiology

Unlike acute pancreatitis, which may improve spontaneously and without long-term complications, chronic pancreatitis is characterized by permanent damage in terms of structure, function, or both because of progressive inflammation. Alcohol abuse is thought to be the leading cause. Less common causes include autoimmune disease, systemic immunological disorders, obstruction of the pancreatic duct by tumor, and genetic abnormalities. The disease usually presents itself in adults between 30 and 40 years of age, but some patients present before the age of 30 years.[9]

As the inflammation persists, it slowly destroys the pancreas, and the organ becomes less able to secrete the enzymes and hormones that are needed for proper digestion. This leads to poor absorption (malabsorption) of nutrients, particularly fat, causing weight loss and passage of fat-containing stools that are loose, malodorous, and oily in appearance. Eventually, the cells that produce insulin are impaired, causing diabetes. Chronic pancreatitis, especially the hereditary form, also is linked to increased risk for pancreatic cancer.[9]

Signs and Symptoms

Chronic pancreatitis differs from acute pancreatitis in that the inflammation is a slow, progressive destruction of the tissues, often over many years. This disease usually is less obvious, and during its early stages, the signs and symptoms can be difficult to recognize. Some people with chronic pancreatitis have no pain. Others have intermittent periods of mild to moderate abdominal pain linked to recurrent bouts of acute pancreatitis, often worsening after drinking alcohol or eating a meal. Other symptoms may include nausea, vomiting, fever, bloating, gas, weight loss, malabsorption, and hyperglycemia.

Management

Treatment of chronic pancreatitis is aimed at managing pain and correcting any nutritional disorders that result from malabsorption. A low-fat diet is recommended. Pain may be relieved through medication or various surgical procedures. Pancreatic enzyme replacement therapy may help to correct malabsorption problems and provide additional pain relief. If the condition is caused by alcoholism, the mortality rate is high.[1,9]

DIABETES MELLITUS

> **?** During a rehabilitation session, a patient becomes very dizzy, complains of a headache, and reports being very hungry. The patient is sweating profusely, the skin appears to be pale and clammy, and movement is somewhat clumsy. In addition, the person appears to be swallowing an excessive number of times. What condition should be suspected, and how should the condition be managed?

Diabetes mellitus (DM) is a chronic metabolic disorder characterized by a near or absolute lack of the hormone insulin, insulin resistance, or both. The disease affects approximately 30 million children and adults in the United States—9.3% of the population—and ranks fifth among the leading causes of death in the United States. The most life-threatening consequences of diabetes are heart disease and stroke, which strike people with diabetes more than twice as often as they do those without the disorder.[10] Several factors increase the risk and severity of diabetes, including heredity, increasing age, minority ethnicity, obesity, female gender, stress, infection, a sedentary lifestyle, and a diet high in carbohydrates and fat.

Physiological Basis of Diabetes

Carbohydrates in human nutrition supply the body's cells with glucose to deliver energy to the body's systems. Eating causes the blood glucose (BG) to rise, stimulating the pancreas to release insulin. Under normal conditions, BG ranges between 80 and 120 mg per dL. The main effect of insulin is lowered blood sugar levels, but it also stimulates amino acid uptake, fat metabolism, and protein synthesis in muscle tissue. Insulin lowers blood sugar by enhancing membrane transport of glucose and other simple sugars from the blood into body cells, especially the skeletal and cardiac muscles (**Fig. 28.2**). It does not accelerate the entry of glucose into liver, kidney, and brain tissue, all of which have easy access to BG regardless of insulin levels. After glucose enters the target cells, insulin

- Promotes the oxidation of glucose for adenosine triphosphate production.

- Joins glucose together to form glycogen.

- Converts glucose to fat for storage, particularly in adipose tissue.

As a general rule, energy needs are met first, and then liver and muscle cells can assemble the excess single glucose cells into long, branching chains of glycogen for storage. The liver cells also are able to convert excess glucose to fat for export to other cells. High BG levels return to normal as excess glucose is stored as glycogen, which can be converted back to glucose, and as fat, which cannot be converted back to glucose.

When BG falls, as occurs between meals, other special cells of the pancreas respond by secreting glucagon into the blood. Glucagon raises BG by stimulating the liver to dismantle its glycogen stores and release glucose into the blood for use by the body's cells. Epinephrine, another hormone, also can stimulate the liver cells to return glucose to the blood from liver glycogen. This "fight-or-flight" response often is triggered when a person experiences stress.

When insulin activity is absent or deficient, as in those with diabetes, the level of blood sugar remains high after a meal, because glucose is unable to move into most tissue cells, causing BG levels to increase to abnormally high levels. Increased osmotic blood pressure drives fluid from the cells into the

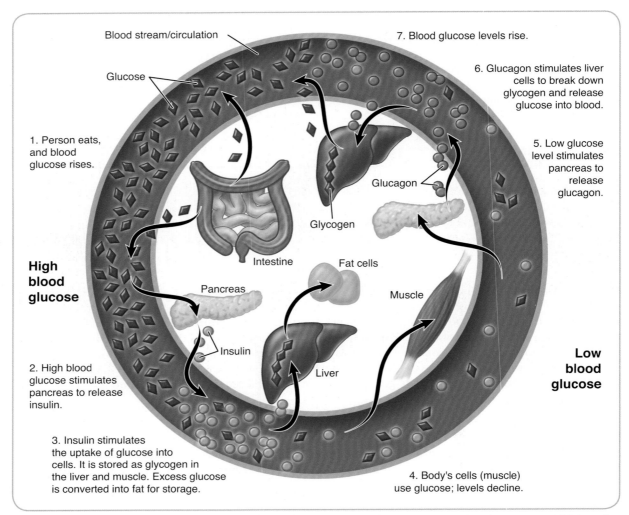

Figure 28.2. Maintaining a balance of blood glucose. Insulin must be available to stimulate uptake of BG into the body's cells. As the cells use glucose, blood levels decline, and the liver responds by releasing glucagon into the bloodstream. Glucagon stimulates liver cells to break down stored glycogen and releases glucose into the blood and, in doing so, raises BG to normal levels.

vascular system, leading to cell dehydration. The excess glucose is passed into the kidneys, resulting in **polyuria**, a huge urine output of water and electrolytes that leads to decreased blood volume and further dehydration. Serious electrolyte losses also occur as the body rids itself of excess ketones. Because ketones are negatively charged ions, they carry positive ions out with them; as a result, sodium and potassium ions are lost. An electrolyte imbalance leads to abdominal pains and possible vomiting, and the stress reaction spirals. Dehydration stimulates the hypothalamic thirst centers, causing **polydipsia**, or excessive thirst. In response, the body shifts from carbohydrate metabolism to fat metabolism for energy. The final cardinal sign, **polyphagia**, refers to excessive hunger and food consumption—a sign that the person is "starving." As such, although plenty of glucose is available, it cannot be used. In severe cases, blood levels of fatty acids and their metabolites rise dramatically, producing an excess of ketoacids that, in turn, results in acidosis. Acetone, a by-product of fat metabolism, is volatile and blown off during expiration, which gives the breath a sweet or fruity odor. If the condition is not rectified with insulin injection, further dehydration and ketoacidosis result as the ketones begin to spill into the urine (i.e., ketonuria). If untreated, ketoacidosis disrupts virtually all physiological processes, including heart activity and oxygen transport. Severe depression of the nervous system leads to confusion, drowsiness, coma, and finally, death.

Types of Diabetes

The National Diabetes Data Group and the World Health Organization recognize four types of DM:

1. Type 1

2. Type 2

3. Gestational DM

4. Other specific types of diabetes

Each group is characterized by high BG levels, or hyperglycemia. For individuals with symptoms of DM, such as excessive thirst and urination or unexplained weight loss, only an elevated fasting plasma glucose of greater than 126 mg per dL, or a random venous plasma glucose of greater than 200 mg per dL, is required to confirm the diagnosis. High blood pressure, LDL cholesterol, and glucose levels are linked to serious complications in the diabetic. Recently, the American College of Physicians, National Institutes of Health, and American Diabetes Association established new guidelines for monitoring those with diabetes. In addition to traditional glucose testing that measures blood sugar levels, a new gold standard is the A1C test, which measures levels of a substance in the blood called hemoglobin A1C. The A1C test reports control of glucose levels for the past 2 to 3 months. The U.S. Food and Drug Administration has approved several A1C monitors for home use, and the ideal parameters for diabetics are as follows[10,11]:

- A1C <7%

- Blood pressure <135/80 mm Hg

- LDL cholesterol <100 mg per dL

Because athletic trainers most likely encounter physically active individuals with type 1 or type 2 DM, these conditions receive more focus and are compared in **Table 28.2**.

Type 1 Diabetes Mellitus

In type 1 DM, the pancreas cannot synthesize insulin. As such, the individual must obtain insulin to assist the cells in taking up the needed fuels from the blood. This insulin must be injected. It cannot be taken orally, because insulin is a protein and the gastrointestinal enzymes would digest it.

TABLE 28.2 Comparison of Type 1 and Type 2 Diabetes Mellitus

	TYPE 1	TYPE 2
Former names	Juvenile-onset diabetes Insulin-dependent diabetes mellitus	Adult-onset diabetes Non–insulin-dependent diabetes mellitus
Age of onset	Usually before 30 years	Usually after 30 years
Type of onset	Abrupt (i.e., days to weeks)	Usually gradual (i.e., weeks to months)
Nutritional status	Almost always lean	Usually obese
Insulin production	Negligible to absent	Present but may be in excess and ineffective because of obesity
Insulin	Needed for all patients	Necessary in only 20%–30% of patients
Diet	Mandatory, along with insulin for control of blood glucose	Diet alone frequently is sufficient to control blood glucose.
High incidence	White population	Women with a history of gestational diabetes, blacks, Native Americans, Hispanics
Family history	Minor	Common link

Type 1 DM (formerly called insulin-dependent diabetes or juvenile diabetes) is considered to be an autoimmune disorder and is one of the most frequent chronic childhood diseases. The onset usually is acute, developing over a period of a few days to weeks. Individuals who develop type 1 DM are usually younger than 25 years, with an equal incidence in both sexes and an increased prevalence in the white population.[11] A family history of type 1 DM or other endocrine disease is found in a small number of cases. The disease typically has an onset before 30 years of age in people who typically are not obese; however, it can begin at any age. Obese individuals generally have a more difficult time balancing glucose levels. In addition, the effects of exercise on the metabolic state are more pronounced in these individuals, and the management of exercise-related problems is more difficult.

Type 2 Diabetes Mellitus

Type 2 DM is the most common form of diabetes and is associated with a family history of diabetes, older age, obesity, and lack of exercise. It is more common in women with a history of gestational diabetes and in African Americans, Latinos, Native Americans, Asian Americans/Pacific Islanders.[10] Although the exact cause of type 2 DM is unknown, high BG and insulin resistance are major contributing factors. The body cannot use insulin correctly and the resistance is related to an insulin secretory defect, which prohibits or limits the transfer of insulin across the cellular membrane. As in type 1 DM, BG rises to an inappropriate level (i.e., hyperglycemia). The high BG stimulates the pancreas to make insulin, exhausting the insulin secretory cellular defect and reducing the cell's ability to continue making insulin. Therefore, type 2 DM appears to be a self-aggravating condition.

Onset is typically after 40 years of age, but type 2 DM also is seen in obese children. Obesity, a major factor in adults, affects nearly 90% of adults with type 2 DM. Compared to normal-weight individuals, obese people require much more insulin to maintain a normal BG level. More insulin is produced, but as body fat increases, insulin receptors are reduced in number and ability to function. Consequently, insulin resistance increases, and adipose and muscle tissues become less able to take up glucose. At some point, the body cannot supply enough insulin to keep up, and type 2 DM develops.

Gestational Diabetes Mellitus

Gestational DM is an operational classification (rather than a pathophysiological condition) that identifies women who develop DM during gestation. The condition is associated with older age, obesity, and a family history of diabetes. Women who are diagnosed with DM before pregnancy are not included in this group. Women who develop type 1 DM during pregnancy and women with undiagnosed, asymptomatic, type 2 DM that is discovered during pregnancy are classified as having gestational DM. Most women classified with gestational DM have normal glucose homeostasis during the first half of the pregnancy, but the mother's BG rises because of hormones secreted during the latter half of the pregnancy. As a result, the mother cannot produce enough insulin to handle the higher BG, leading to hyperglycemia. The hyperglycemia usually resolves after delivery, but it places the woman at risk for developing type 2 DM later in life.

Other Specific Types of Diabetes

Types of DM from various known causes are grouped together to form the classification called "other specific types." This group includes those with genetic defects of β-cell function or with defects of insulin action and persons with pancreatic disease, hormonal disease, and drug or chemical exposure.[10]

Complications of Diabetes Mellitus

In both type 1 and type 2 DM, glucose fails to enter into the cells and accumulates in the blood, which can lead to both acute and chronic complications. **Figure 28.3** illustrates some of the metabolic consequences of untreated diabetes. Over the long term, these metabolic changes can lead to serious chronic complications. Chronically elevated BG levels can damage the blood vessels and nerves, leading to circulatory and neural damage. Failure to adequately balance nutrition, exercise, insulin injections, and BG levels also can cause a physically active individual to experience insulin shock or diabetic coma.

Circulatory Complications

Coronary heart disease, the most common form of cardiovascular disease, usually involves atherosclerosis and hypertension. Atherosclerosis is the accumulation of lipids and other materials in the arteries. The condition begins with the accumulation of soft, fatty deposits along the inner arterial wall, especially at branch points. These deposits eventually enlarge and become hardened with minerals, forming plaque, which in turn hardens and narrows the arteries. Blood platelets cause clots to form whenever an injury occurs. Under normal conditions, these clots form and dissolve in blood all the time, but with atherosclerosis, clots form faster than they are dissolved. In those with diabetes, atherosclerosis tends to develop early, progress rapidly, and be more severe. More than 84% of people with diabetes die as a result of cardiovascular diseases, especially heart attacks.[10] Complications in the capillaries also may lead to impaired kidney function and retinal degeneration with accompanying loss of vision. Approximately 75% of people with diabetes have impaired kidney function, loss of vision, or both.[10] Consequently, diabetes is the leading cause of kidney failure and blindness.

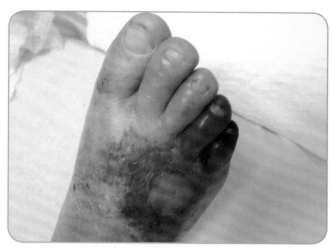

Figure 28-3. Metabolic consequences of untreated diabetes. The metabolic consequences of type 1 diabetes mellitus are more rapid and severe than those of type 2 diabetes mellitus. In type 1, no insulin is available to allow glucose to enter the cells, resulting in a cascade of metabolic changes. In type 2, some glucose enters the cells. Because the cells are not "starved" for glucose, the body does not shift into the metabolism of fasting (i.e., losing weight and producing ketones).

Nerve Complications

Diabetes causes nerves to deteriorate. The initial symptom often is a painful, prickling sensation in the arms and legs. Later, loss of sensation may occur in the hands and feet. Injuries to these areas may go unnoticed, and infections can progress rapidly. Undetected injuries and infection may lead to aseptic necrosis of tissue (i.e., **gangrene**), necessitating amputation of the involved limbs (most often the feet or legs). For this reason, it is critical that those with diabetes take very good care of their feet and visit a podiatrist regularly. As a preventive measure, silica gel shoe inserts should be used and cotton polyester socks worn to prevent blisters and keep the feet dry. All open wounds should be treated promptly, cleaned daily, and carefully checked for infection.

Nerve damage also can retard gastric emptying. When the stomach empties slowly after a meal, the person may experience a premature feeling of fullness. This can lead to bloating, nausea, vomiting, weight loss, and poor control of BG resulting from irregular nutrient absorption.

Hypoglycemia

Hypoglycemia, which is common in those with type 1 insulin-treated diabetes, can range from very mild, lower levels of glucose (60 to 70 mg per dL) with minimal or no symptoms to severe hypoglycemia with very low levels of glucose (< 40 mg per dL) and neurological impairment. Although hypoglycemia can occur with any individual, it is critical in a person with type 1 DM, because the ability to recover from it is limited. In a person with diabetes, hypoglycemia associated with insulin therapy may be related to errors in dosage, delayed or skipped meals, exercise, intensity of BG control, variation in absorption of insulin from subcutaneous injection sites, variability of insulin binding, and impairment of counterregulation. When left untreated, this condition can lead to insulin shock.

Insulin Shock

■ Etiology

Exercise lowers blood sugar; as such, any exercise must be counterbalanced with increased food intake or decreased amounts of insulin. Hypoglycemia results if BG falls below normal levels. Although any individual can experience hypoglycemia, it is particularly critical for the physically active person with diabetes to address the situation immediately.

■ Signs and Symptoms

Contrary to the slow onset of a diabetic coma, hypoglycemia has a rapid onset. Signs and symptoms include dizziness; headache; intense hunger; aggressive behavior; pale, cold, and clammy skin; profuse perspiration; salivation; drooling; and tingling in the face, tongue, and lips. Other observable signs may include a staggering gait, clumsy movements, confusion, and a general decrease in performance.

■ Management

Because glucose levels in the blood are low compared to high levels of insulin, treatment focuses on getting 10 to 15 g of a fast-acting carbohydrate into the system quickly. This can be found in 4 oz (one-half cup) of juice or regular soda, 1 tablespoon of honey or corn syrup, 2 tablespoons of raisins, 4 packets or 4 teaspoons of sugar, and four or five saltine crackers.[10] Chocolates, which contain a high level of fat, should not be used for treating a hypoglycemic reaction, because the fat interferes with the absorption of sugar. If the person is unconscious or unable to swallow, the patient should be rolled on his or her side, and close attention should be given to the airway so that saliva drains out of the mouth, not into the throat. Sugar or honey should be placed under the tongue, because it is absorbed through the mucous membrane. Recovery usually is rapid.

After initial recovery, the patient should wait 15 minutes and check the blood sugar level. If the level is still less than 70 mg per dL or no meter is available and the patient still has symptoms, another 10 to 15 g of carbohydrates should be administered. Blood testing and treatment should be repeated until the BG level has normalized. Even when the BG level has returned to normal, however, physical performance and judgment may still be impaired, or the patient may relapse if the quick sugar influx is rapidly depleted. After the symptoms resolve, the patient should be instructed to have a good meal as soon as possible to increase carbohydrates in the body.

Many individuals with diabetes who experience repeated bouts of hypoglycemia have glucagon injection kits that contain a syringe prefilled with a diluting solution and a vial of glucagon powder. Once the solution and powder are mixed, they are injected into the upper arm, thigh, or buttock. Although the individual may instruct friends and family members on how to mix, draw up, and inject the glucagon, athletic trainers may not automatically be included in the process. It is critical, however, that athletic trainers know whether and under what circumstances a glucagon injection should be administered as well as when to activate the emergency plan. The athletic trainer should be properly trained by the individual's physician or designee, and permission to administer the solution should be documented.

Diabetic Coma

■ Etiology

Without insulin, the body is unable to metabolize glucose, leading to hyperglycemia. As the body shifts from carbohydrate metabolism to fat metabolism, an excess of ketoacids in the blood can lower the blood pH to 7.0 (i.e., normal pH is 7.35 to 7.45), leading to a condition called diabetic ketoacidosis. This is manifested by ketones in the breath, **ketonemia**, and **ketonuria**.

As the name implies, diabetic coma is a serious condition and is considered to be a medical emergency. The emergency plan, including summoning emergency medical services (EMS), should be activated.

■ Signs and Symptoms

Symptoms appear gradually and often occur over several days. The patient becomes increasingly restless and confused and complains of a dry mouth and intense thirst. Abdominal cramping and vomiting are common. As the patient slips into a coma, signs include dry, red, warm skin; eyes that appear deep and sunken; deep, exaggerated respirations; a rapid, weak pulse; and a sweet, fruity acetone breath similar to nail polish remover.

■ Management

It is not usually possible to diagnose with certainty whether a patient is in a diabetic coma or insulin shock. As such, a conscious patient should be given glucose or orange juice. If recovery is not rapid, a medical emergency exists, and the emergency plan should be activated. The additional glucose will not worsen the condition provided that the patient is transported immediately. If the person is unconscious or semiconscious, nothing should be given orally. Instead, an open airway should be maintained, the person treated for shock, and the emergency plan activated. **Application Strategy 28.1** summarizes the management of insulin shock and diabetic coma.

Nutrition and Exercise Recommendations

Control of diabetes depends on a balance of glucose levels, insulin production, nutrition, and exercise. Before initiating an exercise program, a physician should be consulted about diet and normal BG levels documented, because strenuous exercise is contraindicated for some individuals with diabetes. With the advent of BG self-monitoring, exercise is encouraged if certain precautions are followed. BG levels should be taken 30 minutes before and 1 hour after exercise to determine the effects of exercise on BG; this allows better regulation of food intake and insulin dosage.

Nutritional Recommendations for Type 1 Diabetes

Normally, the body secretes a constant, baseline amount of insulin at all times, and it secretes more insulin as the BG level rises following meals. Individuals with type 1 DM must learn to

---

APPLICATION STRATEGY 28.1

Management Algorithm for Diabetic Emergencies

Look for a medic alert tag.

Is the person conscious?

Yes	**No**
Administer 10–15 g of fast-acting carbohydrate:	Activate the emergency plan, including summoning EMS.
■ 4 oz of regular cola	
■ 6 oz of ginger ale	Roll the patient on to the side so that saliva will drain out of the mouth.
■ 4 oz of apple or orange juice	
■ 4 packets of table sugar	
■ 2 tablespoons of raisins	

Does the patient show signs of improvement after the initial carbohydrates?   Maintain an open airway.

Yes	**No**	
Wait 15 minutes, and check the blood sugar level.	*Activate the emergency plan, including summoning EMS.*	Place sugar or fast-acting carbohydrates under the tongue.
		Do not give liquids.

If the blood glucose level is still below 70 mg per dL or if symptoms persist,

■ Give another 10–15 g carbohydrates.
■ Repeat blood testing and treatment until blood glucose is normalized.

After the symptoms resolve,

The patient should eat a good meal as soon as possible.

adjust their insulin doses and administration schedule to accommodate meals, physical activity, and health status. Recommendations for maintaining optimal nutritional status focus on controlling BG levels, achieving a desirable blood lipid profile, controlling blood pressure, and preventing and managing complications from diabetes. The diet should provide a consistent daily intake of carbohydrates at each meal and each snack to minimize fluctuations in the BG level. A meal should be ingested 1 to 3 hours before physical activity, and the individual should have approximately 10 to 15 g of additional carbohydrates 30 minutes before moderate activity or approximately 20 to 30 g of carbohydrates before vigorous activity. During intense exercise, 15 to 30 g of carbohydrates should be ingested every 30 minutes. A snack of carbohydrates should follow the exercise period; carbohydrates are readily available from fruits, fruit juices, yogurt, crackers, and other starches.

When exercise lasts for several hours, insulin requirements decrease; as such, total insulin dosage should be decreased 20% to 50%. Injection administration should be timed so that peak activity does not take place when high insulin levels are present (i.e., 2 to 4 hours after injection). If this is not possible, the individual should eat a high-carbohydrate snack, such as juice and crackers or milk and cookies, approximately 30 minutes before the resumption of activity.[10] In addition, food should always be available for supplemental feeding (e.g., in the locker room, on the bus, and in the athletic training kit).

Nutritional Recommendations for Type 2 Diabetes

As with type 1 DM, an individual with type 2 DM must maintain a near-normal BG level by delivering the same amount of carbohydrates each day, spaced evenly throughout the day. Eating too much carbohydrate at one time can raise BG too high, stressing the already compromised insulin-producing cells. Eating too little carbohydrate can lead to hypoglycemia. In addition, those who have elevated blood lipids may need to watch not only their carbohydrates but also their fat intake. When an individual lowers fat intake, the percentage of calories from carbohydrates increases. A high-carbohydrate diet raises triglycerides and lowers high-density lipoprotein. For those individuals accustomed to a high-fat diet, complying with a low-fat diet may be difficult. When combined with regular exercise, even moderate weight loss (i.e., 10 to 20 lb) can improve BG control and blood lipid profiles, help to reverse insulin resistance, and reduce blood pressure.[10]

Exercise Recommendations

Exercise is a critical component in managing diabetes. Aerobic exercise can decrease the requirements of insulin and increase the body's sensitivity to it. Exercise also can help an individual to attain and maintain ideal body weight; decrease the risk for hypertensive diseases, including cardiovascular and peripheral vascular disease; and slow the progression of **diabetic nephropathy**. It is recommended that people with prediabetes or diabetes or the general adult public should aim for a minimum of 30 minutes most days. Children and teens should aim for at least 60 minutes most days. The goal is to increase the heart rate and cause the individual to break a light sweat.[10] It is recommended that physically active individuals with diabetes follow the guidelines listed in **Box 28.1**.

Despite the benefits of exercise, individuals with type 2 DM who have lost protective neural sensation should not participate in treadmill walking, prolonged walking, jogging, or step exercises. Recommended exercises include low-resistance walking, swimming, bicycling, rowing, chair exercises, arm exercises, and other non–weight-bearing exercises. Activities that require resistance strength training are permissible as long as no indications of retinopathy or nephropathy are present. Scuba diving, rock climbing, and parachuting are strongly discouraged.

 Hypoglycemia, or low blood sugar, should be suspected. It is necessary to get sugar into the system quickly. This can be accomplished by giving the patient table sugar, honey, sugared candy, orange juice, or a regular soda. Recovery should be rapid. The patient should be instructed to have a good meal as soon as possible. Finally, the patient should be closely monitored for any relapse.

BOX 28.1 Guidelines for Safe Exercise by Physically Active Individuals with Diabetes

- Have a routine medical examination and be cleared for activity.
- Develop a balanced program of diet and exercise under a physician's supervision.
- Wear identification (e.g., bracelet or necklace) indicating that the individual has diabetes.
- Eat at regular times throughout the day.
- Avoid exercising at the peak of insulin action and in the evening, when hypoglycemia is more apt to occur.
- Adjust carbohydrate intake and insulin dosage before physical activity.
- Check blood glucose levels before, during (if possible), and after physical activity.
- Prevent dehydration by consuming adequate fluids before, during, and after physical activity.
- Have access to fast-acting carbohydrates during exercise to prevent hypoglycemia.
- Avoid alcoholic beverages or drink them in moderation.
- Avoid cigarette smoking.

SUMMARY

1. Hyperthyroidism is caused by overproduction of thyroxine, leading to a cluster of symptoms called thyrotoxicosis. The symptoms of thyrotoxicosis include nervousness, increased heart rate, loss of sleep, fatigue during ordinary activities, excessive perspiration, and heat intolerance.

2. Hypothyroidism may be caused by an insufficient quantity of thyroid tissue or by the loss of functional thyroid tissue. In adults, the initial onset of symptoms such as fatigue, constipation, intolerance to cold, muscle cramps and menorrhagia, and sluggishness are barely noticeable. As the metabolism continues to slow, however, symptoms include mental clouding, diminished appetite, and weight gain.

3. Gallstones are the leading cause of acute pancreatitis. Alcohol abuse also is a leading cause of the disease.

4. The main symptom of acute pancreatitis is the sudden onset of persistent, mild to severe abdominal pain centered over the epigastric region that may radiate to the back and, occasionally, the chest.

5. Alcohol abuse is thought to be the leading cause of chronic pancreatitis.

6. Insulin is needed after carbohydrate ingestion to transfer glucose from the blood into the skeletal and cardiac muscles. It also promotes glucose storage in the muscles and liver in the form of glycogen. If little or no insulin is secreted by the pancreas, glucose bypasses the body cells and rises to abnormally high levels in the blood. The excess glucose is excreted in the urine, drawing with it large amounts of water and electrolytes and leading to weakness, fatigue, malaise, and increased thirst.

7. When glucose cannot enter the cells, the cells shift from carbohydrate metabolism to fat metabolism for energy, resulting in dehydration and ketoacidosis, which can depress cerebral function. Acetone, formed as a by-product of fat metabolism, is volatile and blown off during expiration, giving the breath a sweet or fruity odor.

8. There are four types of DM:

- Type 1 (insulin-dependent) DM has an onset before age 30 years in people who are not obese.

- Type 2 (non–insulin-dependent) DM is the most common form. It is highly associated with a family history of diabetes, older age, obesity, and lack of exercise.

- Gestational DM occurs when a pregnant woman cannot produce enough insulin to handle the higher BG level because of hormones secreted during the latter half of pregnancy. The condition usually resolves after delivery, but it places the woman at risk for developing type 2 DM later in life.

- Other specific types of diabetes include individuals with genetic defects of β-cell function or with defects of insulin action and persons with pancreatic disease, hormonal disease, and drug or chemical exposure.

9. Chronic diabetes can lead to atherosclerosis and coronary heart disease, kidney failure, blindness, and impaired neural function, whereby the individual may become unaware of injuries or infections of the hands and feet.

10. Severe hypoglycemia can lead to insulin shock. The signs and symptoms include a rapid onset with dizziness; headache; intense hunger; aggressive behavior; pale, cold, and clammy skin; profuse perspiration; salivation; drooling; and tingling in the face, tongue, and lips.

11. An individual progresses into a diabetic coma (i.e., hyperglycemia) over a long period of time. Common symptoms include dry mouth, intense thirst, abdominal pain, confusion, and fever. Severe signs include deep respirations; rapid, weak pulse; dry, red, warm skin; and a sweet, fruity acetone breath.

12. Because it may be difficult to determine which condition is present, a fast-acting carbohydrate should be given to the individual. If the individual is in insulin shock, recovery usually is rapid. If recovery does not occur, the emergency plan should be activated.

13. An individual with diabetes should have a consistent daily intake of carbohydrates at each meal and snack to minimize BG fluctuations. A preactivity meal should be eaten 1 to 3 hours before activity, and 10 to 15 g of carbohydrates should be ingested 30 minutes before moderate activity or 20 to 30 g before vigorous activity. In addition, 15 to 30 g of carbohydrates should be ingested every 30 minutes during activity.

14. Aerobic, low-resistance exercise is recommended for the individual with diabetes. The program should be established under the guidance of a supervising physician.

APPLICATION QUESTIONS

1. As an athletic trainer at an National Collegiate Athletic Association (NCAA) Division I University that fields 26 athletic teams, you can expect that several student athletes will have type 1 diabetes. In an effort to ensure effective care of these individuals, a management plan should be initiated as part of the preparticipation examination (PPE). Within the medical history component of a PPE, what questions might you include as part of a supplemental questionnaire to identify individuals with type 1 diabetes?

2. Travel demands associated with away contests may be more demanding for the collegiate athlete than the high school athlete due to a higher frequency of longer distances of travel, overnight, or weekend trips. As the athletic trainer for a NCAA Division II women's basketball team, you are aware that one of the team members has type 1 diabetes. Specific to events that involve traveling both prior to and during travel, what strategies might you employ to ensure effective care for that student athlete?

3. Twenty minutes after the start of soccer practice, a 16-year-old male with type 1 diabetes suddenly feels lethargic and faint. It is not readily apparent whether the individual is experiencing a diabetic coma or insulin shock. How would you manage this condition?

REFERENCES

1. Ginsberg J. Diagnosis and management of Graves' disease. *CMAJ.* 2003;168(5):575–585.

2. Chao M, Jiawei X, Guoming W, et al. Radioiodine treatment for pediatric hyperthyroid Grave's disease. *Eur J Pediatr.* 2009;168(10):1165–1169.

3. National Endocrine and Metabolic Diseases Information Service. *Graves' Disease.* NIH Publication No. 12-6217. Bethesda, MD: National Institute of Diabetes and Digestive and Kidney Diseases, National Institutes of Health; 2012. http://www.niddk.nih.gov/health-information/health-topics/endocrine/graves-disease/Documents/Graves_508.pdf. Accessed June 29, 2015.

4. Tamparo CD, Lewis MA. *Diseases of the Human Body.* Philadelphia, PA: FA Davis; 2011.

5. National Endocrine and Metabolic Diseases Information Service. *Hypothyroidism.* NIH Publication No. 13-6180. Bethesda, MD: National Institute of Diabetes and Digestive and Kidney Diseases, National Institutes of Health; 2013. http://www.niddk.nih.gov/health-information/health-topics/endocrine/hypothyroidism/Documents/Hypothyroidism_508.pdf. Accessed June 29, 2015.

6. Roberts CG, Ladenson PW. Hypothyroidism. *Lancet.* 2004;363(9411):793–803.

7. Fatourechi V. Subclinical hypothyroidism: an update for primary care physicians. *Mayo Clin Proc.* 2009;84(l):65–71.

8. Pearce EN, Bergman DA. Toward optimal health: the experts discuss thyroid dysfunction. *J Womens Health (Larchmt).* 2004;13(2):141–146.

9. National Digestive Diseases Information Clearinghouse. *Pancreatitis.* NIH Publication No. 08–1596. Bethesda, MD: National Institute of Diabetes and Digestive and Kidney Diseases, National Institutes of Health; 2008. http://www.niddk.nih.gov/health-information/health-topics/liver-disease/pancreatitis/Documents/Pancreatitis_508.pdf. Accessed June 29, 2015.

10. American Diabetes Association. Diabetes basics. http://www.diabetes.org. Accessed June 29, 2015.

11. Diabetes: new ways to deal with an old problem. *Ebony.* 2003;58(5):64–68.

Environmental Conditions

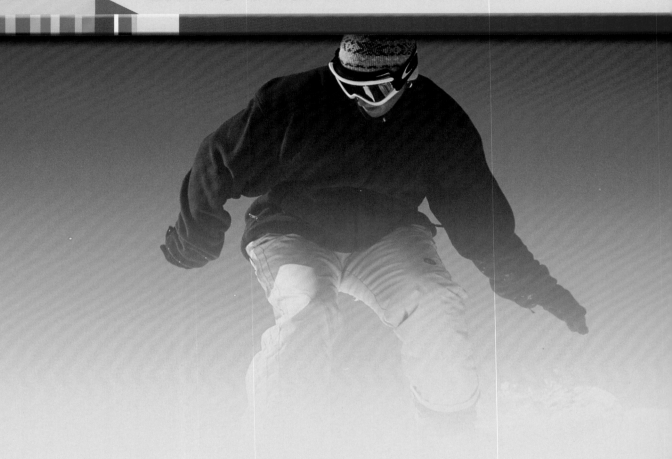

STUDENT OUTCOMES

1. Describe the activation of heat-regulating mechanisms in the body, including the methods used to generate heat via internal and external sources.

2. Demonstrate measurement of the heat stress index using a sling psychrometer.

3. Explain the methods used to prevent heat illness.

4. Identify the signs and symptoms of heat-related conditions.

5. Describe the appropriate management of heat-related conditions.

6. Describe the body's production of internal heat during cold ambient temperatures.

7. Differentiate between frostbite and systemic cooling and describe the appropriate management of each condition.

8. Explain the impact of high altitude and poor air quality on exercise and sport performance.

9. Explain the dangers of lightning and list the lightning safety guidelines for sport and exercise participation.

INTRODUCTION

Environmental conditions affect even the best conditioned individuals. Athletic practices and contests can be held on hot, humid days or on cold, windy days, which predisposes individuals to hyperthermia and hypothermia, respectively. In addition, exercising during thunderstorms that produce lightning can be extremely dangerous. These environmental conditions as well as altitude and air quality are discussed in this chapter.

HEAT-RELATED CONDITIONS

 Field hockey practice is scheduled for this afternoon. The U.S. Weather Bureau is forecasting 90°F (air temperature), with a relative humidity of 80% during the practice time. Based on this information, what measures should be taken to reduce the risk of heat-related illness?

The process by which the body maintains body temperature is called **thermoregulation**. It is controlled primarily by the **hypothalamus**, which is a region of the diencephalon forming the floor of the third ventricle of the brain. **Hyperthermia**, or elevated body temperature, occurs when internal heat production exceeds external heat loss (**Fig. 29.1**). The hypothalamus is a gland that maintains **homeostasis**, or a state of equilibrium within the body, by initiating cooling or heat-retention mechanisms to achieve a relatively constant body core temperature between 36.1° and 37.8°C (97° and 100°F). The body core encompasses the skull, thoracic, and abdominal area. Heat-regulating mechanisms, such as perspiring or shivering, are activated by two means:

1. Stimulation of peripheral thermal receptors in the skin

2. Changes in blood temperature as it flows through the hypothalamus

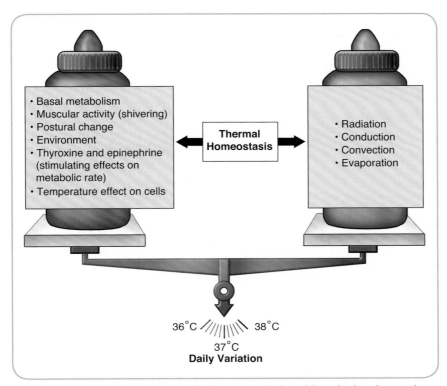

Figure 29.1. Thermal homeostasis. Homeostasis is achieved when internal heat production and heat loss are properly balanced to maintain a relatively constant body core temperature.

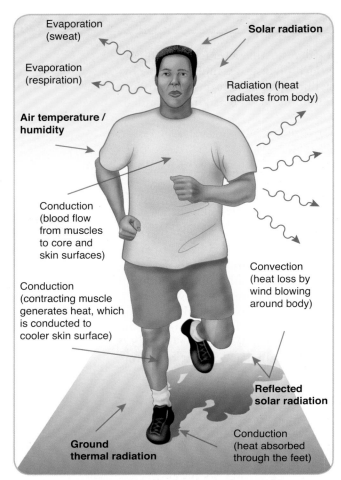

Figure 29.2. Heat gain and loss. Heat produced within working muscles is transferred to the body's core and skin. During exercise, body heat is dissipated into the surrounding environment by radiation, conduction, convection, and evaporation. *Straight lines* represent heat gain, and *wavy lines* indicate heat loss.

Internal Heat Regulation

During exercise, the body gains heat either from external sources (i.e., environmental temperatures) or from internal processes (**Fig. 29.2**). Much of the internal heat is generated during muscular activity through energy metabolism. The act of shivering can increase the total metabolic rate by threefold to fivefold. During sustained, vigorous exercise, the metabolic rate can increase by 20- to 25-fold above the resting level. Theoretically, such a rate can increase core temperature by approximately 1°C (1.8°F) every 5 to 7 minutes.

During exercise, the circulatory system must deliver oxygen to the working muscles and heated blood from deep tissues (i.e., core) to the periphery (i.e., shell) for dissipation. The increased blood flow to the muscles and skin is made possible by increasing cardiac output and redistributing regional blood flow (i.e., blood flow to the visceral organs is reduced). As exercise begins, heart rate and cardiac output increase while superficial venous and arterial blood vessels dilate to divert warm blood to the skin surface. Heat is dissipated when the warm blood flushes into skin capillaries. This is evident when the face becomes flushed and reddened on a hot day or after exercise. When the individual is in a resting state and the air temperature is less than 30.6°C (87°F), approximately two-thirds of the body's normal heat loss results from conduction, convection, and radiation. As air temperature approaches skin temperature and exceeds 30.6°C (87°F), evaporation becomes the predominant means of heat dissipation.

Radiation

Radiation is the loss of heat from a warmer object to a cooler object in the form of infrared waves (i.e., thermal energy) without physical contact. Usually, body temperature is warmer than the environment, and radiant heat is dissipated through the air to surrounding solid, cooler objects. When the temperatures of surrounding objects, such as hot artificial turf, exceed skin temperature, radiant heat is absorbed. Participating in a shaded area is one means of reducing the effects of radiant heat during activity.

Conduction

Conduction is the direct transfer of heat through a liquid, solid, or gas from a warm to a cooler object. For example, a football player can absorb heat through the feet simply by standing on hot artificial turf. The rate of conductive heat loss depends on the temperature gradient (i.e., difference) between the skin and surrounding surfaces and on the thermal qualities of both surfaces. For example, heat loss in water can be considerable.

Convection

Convection depends on conduction from the skin to the water or the air next to it. The effectiveness of heat loss by convection is dependent on the speed at which the air (or water) next to the body is exchanged. If air movement is slow, air molecules next to the skin are warmed and act as insulation. In contrast, if warmer air molecules are continually replaced by cooler air molecules, as occurs on a breezy day or in a room with a fan, heat loss increases as the air currents carry heat away.

Convection cools the body as air currents pass by while the individual is running or cycling. For example, air currents at 4 miles per hour are approximately twice as effective for cooling as air currents moving at 1 mile per hour. This is the basis of the wind-chill index (**Fig. 29.4**), which shows the equivalent still-air temperature for a particular ambient temperature at different wind velocities. In water, the body loses heat more rapidly by convection while swimming than lying motionless in the water.

Evaporation

Evaporation is the most effective heat loss mechanism for cooling the body. During rest, sweat glands assist thermoregulation by secreting unnoticeable amounts of sweat (i.e., ~500 mL per day). Sweat is a weak saline solution, largely composed of water (99%), which evaporates when molecules in the water absorb heat from the environment and become energetic enough to escape as a gas. As core temperature rises during exercise or illness, peripheral blood vessels dilate and sweat glands are stimulated to produce noticeable amounts of sweat. On a hot, dry day, sweating is responsible for more than 80% of heat loss. Sweating, however, does not cool the body; the evaporation of the sweat is what cools the body. The total sweat that is vaporized from the skin depends on three factors:

1. The skin surface exposed to the environment

2. The temperature and relative humidity of the ambient air

3. The convective air currents around the body

Relative humidity is the most important factor in determining the effectiveness of evaporative heat loss. Relative humidity is the ratio of water in the ambient air to the total quantity of moisture that can be carried in air at a particular ambient temperature. It is expressed as a percentage. For example, 65% relative humidity means that ambient air contains 65% of the air's moisture-carrying capability at the specific temperature. When humidity is high, the ambient vapor pressure approaches that of the moist skin, and evaporation is greatly reduced. Therefore, this avenue for heat loss is closed, even though large quantities of sweat bead on the skin and, eventually, roll off. In this form, sweating represents a useless water loss that can lead to a dangerous state of dehydration and overheating.

In addition to heat loss through sweating, a basal level of body heat loss exists because of the continuous evaporation of water from the lungs, from the mucosa of the mouth, and through the skin. This averages approximately 350 mL of water as it seeps through the skin every day, as well as another 300 mL of water vaporized from mucous membranes in the respiratory passages and mouth. The latter is illustrated when you "see your breath" in very cold weather.

In total, it is not uncommon for an individual to lose 1.5 to 2.5 L per hour of water during exercise. This translates into a loss of 3 to 6 lb of body weight per hour. During a 2- to 3-hour workout, an individual can become dehydrated by losing 1% to 2% of body weight, which could compromise physiological function and negatively influence performance. Dehydration of >3% of body weight further compromises physiological function and increases the risk of developing an exertional heat illness (i.e., heat cramps, heat exhaustion, or heat stroke).[1,2] Although an individual may continually drink water throughout an exercise bout, less than 50% of the fluid lost is replenished. This "voluntary dehydration" was recognized long ago and continues to be characterized by researchers. Accordingly, a physically active individual should drink as much fluid as possible before exercise and before thirst is perceived during exercise. It is critical to drink beyond the perception of satisfying one's thirst to **hyperhydrate** the body to prevent voluntary dehydration.

Measuring the Heat-Stress Index

The heat-stress index is a measure of ambient air temperature, humidity, and solar radiant energy. The most commonly used heat-stress index, the Wet-Bulb-Globe Temperature (WBGT) Index, consists of the measurement of ambient temperature (T_a), wet-bulb temperature (T_w), and black globe temperature (T_g) as follows:

1. For outdoor use,

$$\text{WBGT} = (0.1 \times T_a) + (0.7 \times T_w) + (0.2 \times T_g)$$

2. For indoor use,

$$WBGT = (0.3 \times T_a) + (0.7 \times T_w)$$

Currently, the WBGT is the most widely used index of determining heat stress for indoor and outdoor use. It is used in military and industrial settings to determine safe limits for physical activity. The index is limited, however, in that it fails to take into account the impact of wearing clothing. Clothing that is impermeable or semipermeable can impede or prevent sweat evaporation, and as such, a higher heat stress level is generated.

 See **Application Strategy: Using a Sling Psychrometer to Determine Relative Humidity**, available on the companion Web site at thePoint, for further information on use of a sling psychrometer.

T_w is the temperature recorded by a thermometer with the mercury bulb surrounded by a wet wick. T_g is the temperature recorded by a thermometer with a mercury bulb encased in a sphere that is painted black. The black globe absorbs radiant energy from the environment to obtain a measure that is not available using dry- and wet-bulb thermometers.

A sling psychrometer measures heat stress by exposing dry- and wet-bulb thermometers to rapid airflow. One thermometer is ordinary (i.e., a dry-bulb thermometer); the other thermometer has a cloth wick over its bulb (i.e., a wet-bulb thermometer). After whirling the instrument in the air for several minutes, the temperatures of both thermometers are read. If the surrounding air is holding as much moisture as possible (i.e., relative humidity of 100%), no difference exists between the two temperatures. In contrast, greater differences in the recorded temperatures indicate a high rate of evaporation and low humidity.

In 2002, the National Athletic Trainers' Association (NATA) published a position statement on exertional heat illnesses.[3] This statement served as a basis for an additional document in 2003 released by the Inter-Association Task Force on Exertional Heat Illness,[4] a group that convened at the request of the NATA to develop universal guidelines for reducing the risk of heat illness. The document from the Inter-Association Task Force received the support of the American Academy of Pediatrics, the American College of Emergency Physicians, the American Orthopaedic Society for Sports Medicine, and the American College of Sports Medicine, among other prestigious organizations. Because of the inception of these documents, these organizations including the Korey Stringer Institute are continuously providing updated evidence to promote the prevention of sudden death in sport through health and safety initiatives. The NATA provides the public with position and consensus statements providing various recommendations for ensuring a safe exercise environment for sport participants. For example, in certain geographic locations, such as the Southeastern United States, the WBGT is routinely high, extreme, or hazardous throughout a large portion of the year; as such, appropriate steps should be taken to reduce increased risk of heat illness. **Table 29.1** lists recommendations for activities when temperature, humidity, and radiation are measured using the WBGT index.

Factors That Modify Heat Tolerance

Several factors can affect an individual's tolerance to heat. Acclimatization and proper hydration are among the most critical in preventing heat illness.

TABLE 29.1 Wet-Bulb-Globe Temperature Risk Chart

WET-BULB-GLOBE TEMPERATURE	FLAG COLOR	LEVEL OF RISK	COMMENTS
<65°F (<18°C)	Green	Low	Risk is low but still exists on the basis of risk factors.
65°–73°F (18°–23°C)	Yellow	Moderate	Risk increases as the event progresses through the day.
73°–82°F (23°–28°C)	Red	High	Everyone should be aware of injury potential; individuals at risk should not participate in physical activity.
>82°F (28°C)	Black	Extreme or hazardous	Consider rescheduling or delaying the event until safer conditions prevail; if the event must take place, a high alert condition exists.

> **BOX 29.1 Physiological Changes Seen After 10 Days of Heat Exposure**
>
> ■ Heart rate and body temperature decrease.
>
> ■ Sweat becomes more diluted (i.e., less salt is lost).
>
> ■ Peripheral blood flow and plasma volume increase.
>
> ■ Sweat is distributed more evenly over the skin surface.
>
> ■ The increased perspiration rate is sustained over a longer period of time.
>
> ■ Sweating capacity nearly doubles.

Acclimatization

Exercising moderately during repeated heat exposures can result in physiological adaptation to a hot environment, which can improve performance and heat tolerance (**Box 29.1**). In general, the major acclimatization occurs during the first week of heat exposure and is complete after 14 days. Only 2 to 4 hours of daily heat exposure is required. The first several exercise sessions should be light and last approximately 15 to 20 minutes. Thereafter, exercise sessions can progressively increase in duration and intensity. Well-acclimatized individuals should train for 1 to 2 hours under the same heat conditions that will be present during their competitive event.[3] Proper hydration is essential for the acclimatization process to be effective. In 2009, the NATA released the preseason heat-acclimatization guidelines for secondary school athletics. This guideline provides several recommendations for a 14-day heat-acclimatization period.[5]

Heat acclimatization is lost rapidly, however. As a general rule, 1 day of heat acclimatization is lost over 2 to 3 days without heat exposure, with the major benefits being lost within 2 to 3 weeks after returning to a more temperate environment.

Fluid Rehydration

The primary objective of fluid replacement is to maintain plasma volume so that circulation and sweating occur at optimal levels. Dehydration progressively decreases plasma volume, peripheral blood flow, sweating, and stroke volume (i.e., the quantity of blood ejected with each heartbeat), and it leads to a compensatory increase in heart rate. The general deterioration in circulatory and thermoregulatory efficiency increases the risk of heat illness, impairs physiological functions, and decreases physical performance.

Thirst is not an adequate indicator of water needs during exercise. Physically active individuals may not become thirsty until systemic water loss equals 2% of body weight.[6] Rather, thirst develops in response to increases in osmolality and blood sodium concentrations and decreases in plasma volume caused by dehydration.

It is essential that physically active individuals begin an exercise session when they are well hydrated and have ready access to adequate water replacement throughout the exercise session to prevent dehydration. Cold beverages of 10° to 15°C (50° to 59°F) are recommended because cooler drinks, especially water, empty from the stomach and small intestine significantly faster than warm fluids.[1] Fluid replacement guidelines include the following[1]:

■ Preexercise hydration: 500 to 600 mL (17 to 20 fl oz) of water or a sports drink 2 to 3 hours before exercise and 200 to 300 mL (7 to 10 fl oz) of water or a sports drink 10 to 20 minutes before exercise

■ Exercise hydration: 200 to 300 mL (7 to 10 fl oz) of water or a sports drink every 10 to 20 minutes

■ Postexercise hydration: Within 2 hours of exercise, rehydrate with water to restore hydration status, CHOs to replenish glycogen stores, and electrolytes to speed rehydration. Ingestion equal to 150% of weight loss can result in optimal rehydration 6 hours after exercise.

See **Recommended Fluid Intake for a Strenuous 90-Minute Exercise Bout**, found on the companion Web site at thePoint.

BOX 29.2 Strategies to Reduce the Risk of Dehydration

Healthy population

- Have unlimited fluid available during exercise.

- When exercising for 1 hour or more, drink at least 7–10 oz of fluid every 10–20 minutes. Drink beyond thirst.

- Drink cool fluids containing less than 8% CHOs.

- Use individual water bottles to accurately measure fluid consumption.

- Freeze fluid in plastic bottles before exercise; the bottles will thaw and stay cool during exercise sessions.

- Record preexercise and postexercise weight to determine if excessive and unsafe weight loss has occurred.

- Replenish lost fluid with at least 24 oz of fluid for every pound of body weight lost.

- Avoid caffeine, alcohol, and carbonated beverages.

Children (in addition to previous)

- Allow 10–14 days of acclimatization.

- Reduce intensity of prolonged exercise.

Several steps can be taken to ensure adequate hydration before, during, and after exercise (**Box 29.2**).

To prevent dehydration, fluids must be ingested and absorbed by the body. Running through sprinklers or pouring water over the head may feel cool and satisfying, but it does not prevent dehydration. A standard rule is to drink until thirst is quenched—and then drink a few more ounces.

An easy method to determine if enough fluids are being consumed is to monitor the color and volume of the urine. An average adult's urine amounts to 1.2 quarts in a 24-hour period. Urination of a full bladder usually occurs four times each day. Within 60 minutes of exercise, passing light-colored urine of normal to above-normal volume is a good indicator of adequate hydration. If the urine is dark yellow in color, of a small volume, and of strong odor, the individual needs to continue drinking. Ingesting vitamin supplements often can result in a dark-yellow urine; as such, urine color, volume, and odor must all be considered when determining hydration status.[4,6]

Carbohydrate Replacement

Consuming carbohydrates (CHOs) during the preexercise hydration session along with a healthy daily diet can increase glycogen stores and benefit optimal performance. If exercise is intense, additional CHOs should be consumed 30 minutes before exercise and after exercise. During exercise, 1 L of a 6% CHO drink per hour of exercise is recommended.[1] CHO concentrations greater than 8% may compromise the rate of fluid emptying from the stomach and absorbed from the intestine. Fruit juices, CHO gels, sodas, and some sport drinks have CHO concentrations greater than 8% and are not recommended during an exercise session as the sole beverage.[1] While maintaining hydration, the participant should avoid diuretics, such as excessive amounts of protein, caffeinated drinks (e.g., soda, tea, and coffee), chocolate, and alcoholic beverages.

Clothing

Light-colored, lightweight, and porous clothing is preferred to dark, heavy weight, and nonporous material. Clothing made of 100% cotton is not recommended, especially in hot climates, because moisture in sweat-soaked cotton does not evaporate easily. Evaporative heat loss occurs only when clothing is thoroughly wet and perspiration can evaporate. Changing into a dry shirt simply prolongs the time between sweating and cooling. Heavy sweat suits or rubberized plastic suits produce high relative humidity close to the skin and retard evaporation, severely increasing the risk of heat illness. Even when wearing only football helmets and loose-fitting, porous jerseys and shorts, 50% of the body surface of football players can be sealed and evaporative cooling is limited. The increased metabolic rate that is needed to carry the weight of the equipment and the increased temperature on artificial surfaces also can increase the risk of heat illness. As such, football players should initially practice in t-shirts, shorts, and low-cut socks. On hot, humid days, uniforms should not be worn, and if possible, shoulder pads and helmets should be removed often to allow radiation and evaporative cooling. Because much of the body's heat escapes through the head, helmets used in noncontact sports (e.g., cycling) should allow adequate airflow and evaporation.

Age

Children have a lower sweating capacity and a higher core temperature during exposure to heat as compared to adolescents and adults. This occurs even though children have a higher number of heat-activated sweat glands per unit of skin. Sweat composition in children also differs. Children excrete higher concentrations of sodium and chlorine and lower concentrations of lactate and potassium. Therefore, children do not benefit from electrolyte beverages and should use only cool water for fluid replacement.[7] In addition, children require a longer time to acclimatize to heat as compared to adolescents and young adults.

In general, middle-aged and older men and women are less tolerant to exercising in heat. When compared to younger men and women, older men and women develop higher heart rates, higher skin and core temperatures, and lower sweat rates during exercise in heat. Aging can lead to a limited peripheral vascular response that can impair local vasodilation. The onset of sweating also appears to be delayed with advancing age, and the sweating response appears to be blunted. This may result from either a limitation in sweat gland output or a dehydration-limited sweat output if fluid replacement is insufficient. In addition, older individuals do not recover from dehydration as effectively as younger individuals do, which may be related to a blunted thirst drive. This may make older individuals more prone to dehydration that could adversely affect the thermoregulatory capacity.

Sex

The general consensus is that women can tolerate the physiological and thermal stress of exercise at least as well as men of comparable fitness and level of acclimatization. Both sexes can acclimatize to a similar degree; however, sweating does differ. Although women possess more heat-activated sweat glands per unit of skin area as compared to men, women sweat less than men do. Compared with men, women begin to sweat at higher skin and core temperatures, produce less sweat for a comparable heat-exercise load, and yet show an equivalent heat tolerance. Women probably rely more on circulatory mechanisms for heat dissipation, whereas men rely on evaporative cooling. The production of less sweat to maintain thermal balance can provide women with significant protection from dehydration during exercise at a high ambient temperature.

Diuretics, Supplements, and Medications

Individuals taking diuretics or laxatives should be carefully observed for dehydration. These agents increase fluid loss, reduce plasma volume, and may adversely affect thermoregulation and cardiovascular function. Substances used to induce vomiting and diarrhea also lead to dehydration and may cause excessive electrolyte loss with accompanying muscle weakness. Some nutritional supplements, such as creatine phosphate, require additional fluids to decrease the risk of heat cramps and other associated heat illnesses. Medications, such as β-adrenergics, anticholinergics, antihistamines, β-blockers, calcium channel blockers, and tricyclic antidepressants, can impair the body's normal mechanisms of dissipating heat, which may result in a dangerously high core temperature.[8] Before taking supplements or medications, an individual should be fully informed regarding the proper use and possible side effects of the substances.

Practice Schedules

On hot, humid days, workouts, practices, and competitions should be scheduled during early morning or evening hours to avoid the worst heat of the day (i.e., 11:00 a.m. to 3:00 p.m.). It also may be necessary to allow frequent water breaks (i.e., 10 minutes every half an hour), shorten practices, and lessen the exercise intensity. Whenever possible, participants should be moved out of direct sunlight (e.g., shade trees and tents), and restrictive equipment (e.g., pads and helmets) should be removed frequently.

Weight Charts

Measuring pre- and postexercise weight can decrease the risk of heat illness. Measurement of the athlete's sweat rate (sweating rate = preexercise body weight − postexercise body weight + fluid intake − urine volume / exercise time in hours) should be a representative range of environmental conditions, practices, and competitive events. Begin by weighing a large number of athletes prior to an intense 1-hour practice session and then reweigh them at the end of the 1-hour practice. Do not allow any rehydration or urination during the 1-hour postpractice session when the sweat rate is being calculated. When water loss reaches 3% of body mass, a definite impairment is noted in physical work capacity, physiological function, and thermoregulation. A rule of thumb is that for every pound of water lost, 24 oz (i.e., 3 cups) of fluid should be ingested, meaning that 150% of the fluid loss during exercise is replenished.

Identifying Individuals at Risk

Healthy individuals at risk for heat illness include those who are poorly acclimated or conditioned, those who are inexperienced with heat illness, those with large muscle mass, children, wheelchair athletes, Special Olympians, and elderly people. Others who are at risk are listed in **Box 29.3**.

Heat Illnesses

If the signs and symptoms of heat stress (e.g., thirst, fatigue, lethargy, flushed skin, headache, and visual disturbances) are not treated, cardiovascular compensation begins to fail, and a series of progressive complications, termed heat illness, can result. The various forms of heat illness, in order of severity, include exercise-associated muscle (heat) cramps, exercise (heat) exhaustion, and exertional heat stroke. Although symptoms often overlap between the conditions, failure to take immediate action can result in severe dehydration and possible death.

Exercise-Associated Muscle (Heat) Cramps

■ Etiology

Heat cramps are painful, involuntary muscle spasms caused by excessive water and electrolyte loss during and after intense exercise in the heat. Paradoxically, the condition most frequently occurs in well-conditioned, acclimatized, physically active individuals who have overexerted themselves in hot weather and rehydrated only with water. Predisposing factors include lack of acclimatization, use of diuretics or laxatives, neuromuscular fatigue, and sodium depletion in the normal diet. The condition can be prevented by ingesting copious amounts of water and increasing the daily intake of salt through a normal diet several days before the period of heat stress.[9]

■ Signs and Symptoms

Exercise-associated muscle cramps commonly occur in the calf and abdominal muscles, but they also may involve the muscles of the upper extremity. Signs and symptoms mimic dehydration and include thirst, sweating, transient muscle cramps, and fatigue. Body temperature is not usually elevated, and the skin remains moist and cool. Pulse and respiration may be normal or slightly elevated. Dizziness may be present.

■ Management

The patient should stop activity, replace lost fluids with sodium-containing fluids, and begin mild, passive stretching of the involved muscle(s) and ice massage over the affected area. The patient should ingest enough cool CHO fluids to drink beyond the point of satisfying thirst. A recumbent position may allow more rapid redistribution of blood flow to cramping leg muscles.[3] The patient should be watched carefully, because this condition may precipitate heat exhaustion or heat stroke.

BOX 29.3 Individuals at Risk for Heat Illness

Healthy individuals

- Age extremes (children, elderly persons)
- Excessive muscle mass, large, or obese
- Poorly acclimatized or conditioned
- Previous history of heat illness
- Salt or water depletion
- Sleep deprived

Those with acute illnesses

- Illnesses that involve fever
- Gastrointestinal illnesses

Those with chronic illnesses

- Alcoholism and substance abuse (e.g., amphetamines, cocaine, hallucinogens, laxatives, diuretics, narcotics)
- Cardiac disease
- Certain nutritional supplements (e.g., creatine phosphate)
- Cystic fibrosis
- Eating disorders
- Medications (e.g., anticholinergics, antidepressants, antihistamines, diuretics, neuroleptics, β-blockers)
- Skin problems with impaired sweating (e.g., miliaria rubra or miliaria profunda)
- Uncontrolled diabetes mellitus or hypertension
- Using oil- or gel-based sunscreens that block evaporative cooling

Wheelchair athletes who

- Have a spinal cord injury (alters thermoregulation)
- Limit water intake to avoid going to the bathroom

Exercise (Heat) Exhaustion

■ Etiology

Exercise (heat) exhaustion usually occurs in individuals who are not acclimatized during the first few intense exercise sessions on a hot day. Those who wear protective equipment or heavy uniforms also are at greater risk, because evaporation through the material may be retarded. It is a "functional" illness and is not associated with organ damage. Heat exhaustion is caused by ineffective circulatory adjustments compounded by a depletion of extracellular fluid, especially plasma volume, as a result of excessive sweating. Blood pools in the dilated peripheral vessels, which dramatically reduces the central blood volume necessary to maintain cardiac output.

■ Signs and Symptoms

Thirst, headache, dizziness, light-headedness, mild anxiety, fatigue, profuse sweating, weak and rapid pulse, and low blood pressure in the upright position are common signs and symptoms (**Fig. 29.3A**). The patient may appear to be ashen and gray, with cool, clammy skin. An uncoordinated gait often is

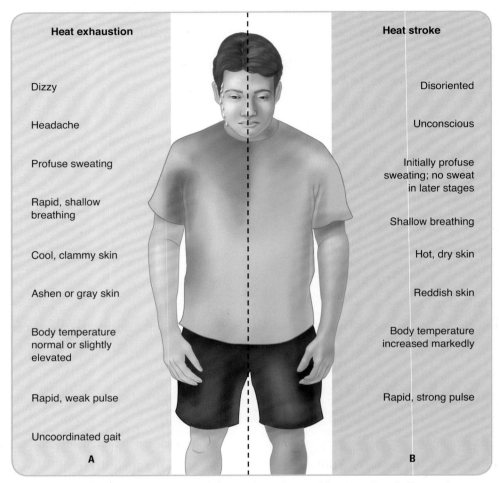

Heat exhaustion	Heat stroke
Dizzy	Disoriented
Headache	Unconscious
Profuse sweating	Initially profuse sweating; no sweat in later stages
Rapid, shallow breathing	Shallow breathing
Cool, clammy skin	Hot, dry skin
Ashen or gray skin	Reddish skin
Body temperature normal or slightly elevated	Body temperature increased markedly
Rapid, weak pulse	Rapid, strong pulse
Uncoordinated gait	
A	**B**

Figure 29.3. Signs and symptoms of heat exhaustion and heat stroke. A, Heat exhaustion. **B,** Heat stroke.

present. Urine output may be small. Sweating may be reduced if the person is dehydrated, but body temperature generally does not exceed 40°C (104°F).[9] The patient may have an urge to defecate or may experience diarrhea. Significant neurological impairment is absent.

■ Management

The patient should be moved immediately to a cool place. All equipment and unnecessary clothing should be removed. Rapid cooling of the body should be initiated. Two effective cooling methods are evaporative cooling and ice immersion. Evaporative cooling involves spraying copious amounts of tap water over the patient's skin with air fanning. The average cooling rate through this technique is 0.14°C per minute.[10] Ice immersion involves placing the patient into a pool or tub of cold water (~1° to 15°C [35° to 59°F]). Circulation of the water may enhance cooling. If immersion in ice water is not available, other cooling methods should be used. These may include wrapping in cool, wet, iced towels; using fans; and applying crushed ice packs to the neck, axilla, and groin. Fans and cool-mist machines, however, have limited use during humid conditions. It is essential to administer copious amounts of cool fluids with a diluted electrolyte solution as quickly as possible. Elevating the legs to reduce postural hypotension also can be effective. If recovery is not rapid and uneventful, the patient should be transported to the closest medical facility; intravenous fluids may need to be administered. Some patients, particularly endurance athletes exercising in the heat, may require as much as 4 L of fluid replacement.[11] Physical activity should not be resumed until the patient has returned to the pre-dehydrated state and been cleared by a physician.

Exertional Heat Stroke

■ Etiology

Exertional heat stroke is the least common, but most serious, heat-related illness. In football, heat stroke is second only to head injuries as the most frequent cause of death. The condition also is seen in dehydrated distance runners and wrestlers. Unlike classic heat stroke, which involves prolonged heat exposure in infants, elders, or unhealthy sedentary adults in whom body heat-regulation mechanisms are inefficient, exertional heat stroke occurs during physical activity.[3]

During exercise, metabolic heat continues to rise. Decreased blood plasma volume causes the heart to beat faster and work harder to pump blood through the circulatory system. The thermoregulatory system is overloaded, and the body's cooling mechanisms fail to dissipate the rising core temperature. The hypothalamus shuts down all heat-control mechanisms, including the sweat glands, in an effort to conserve water loss. A vicious circle is created in which, as temperature increases, the metabolic rate increases, which in turn increases heat production. The skin becomes hot and dry. As the temperature continues to rise, permanent brain damage may occur. Core temperature can rise to 40.6°C (105°F), and it has been known to reach 41.7° to 42.2°C (107° to 108°F). If untreated, death is imminent. Mortality is directly related to the magnitude and duration of the hyperthermia.

■ Signs and Symptoms

By definition, the condition occurs when body temperature is elevated to a level that causes characteristic clinical and pathological damage to body tissues and affects multiple organs. Initial symptoms include a feeling of burning up, confusion, disorientation, irrational behavior, agitation, profuse sweating, and an unsteady gait. As the condition deteriorates, sweating ceases. The skin is hot and dry and appears to be reddened or flushed (**Fig. 29.3B**). The patient hyperventilates or breathes deeply and has dilated pupils, giving the appearance of a glassy stare. As core temperature rises, the pulse becomes rapid and strong (as high as 150 to 170 beats per minute). The patient may become hysterical or delirious. Tissue damage by excessive body heat leads to vasomotor collapse, shallow breathing, decreased blood pressure, and a rapid pulse. Muscle twitching, vomiting, or seizures may occur just before the patient lapses into a coma.[9]

■ Management

Mortality and organ damage appear to be directly proportional to the length of time between elevation of core body temperature and initiation of cooling therapy.

The emergency medical plan, including summoning emergency medical services (EMS), should be activated.

The patient should be moved immediately to a cool place. All equipment and unnecessary clothing should be removed, and rapid cooling of the body should be initiated. Core temperature should be measured every 5 to 10 minutes and, to avoid hypothermia, should not fall below 38°C (100.4°F).[3] Victims of exertional heat stroke usually require airway management, intravenous fluids, and in severe cases, circulatory support. Physical activity should not be resumed until the patient has returned to the predehydrated state and been cleared by a physician.

Other Heat Conditions

Four other common conditions may result from exercising in the heat. These include heat syncope, exertional hyponatremia, miliaria rubra, and miliaria profunda. Although not usually life threatening, they can be bothersome to a competitive individual. **Table 29.2** lists the signs, symptoms, and immediate care for all heat-related conditions.

Heat Syncope

■ Etiology

Heat syncope, or orthostatic dizziness, can occur when a person is exposed to high environmental temperatures, or it can be seen at the end of a race in individuals who are not acclimatized who may or may not be under heat stress. The condition is usually attributed to vasodilation, postural pooling of blood, diminished venous return, dehydration, reduction in cardiac output, and cerebral

TABLE 29.2 Management of Heat-Related Conditions

CONDITION	SIGNS/SYMPTOMS	TREATMENT
Heat cramps	Involuntary muscle spasms or cramps, normal pulse and respirations, profuse sweating and dizziness	Rest in cool place; massage the cramp with ice and passive stretching; drink cool water with diluted electrolyte solution.
Heat syncope	Weakness, fatigue, hypotension, blurred vision, fainting, elevated skin and core temperature	Place supine in cool place; elevate legs; give oral saline if conscious; record blood pressure and body temperature.
Miliaria rubra and miliaria profunda	Pruritic, inflamed skin eruptions	Cool and dry the affected skin; control infection; avoid reexposure until lesions have healed.
Heat exhaustion	Thirst; headache; weakness; confusion; profuse sweating; skin is wet, cool, and clammy and may appear ashen; breathing is rapid and shallow; pulse is weak.	Rest in cool place; remove equipment and clothing; execute rapid cooling of body; sponge or towel with cool water, or use a fan; intravenous fluids; discontinue activity until thoroughly recovered and cleared by a physician.
Heat stroke	Sweating ceases; irritability progresses to confusion and hysteria; unsteady gait; pulse is rapid and strong; skin is hot, dry, red, or flushed; blood pressure falls; convulsions; seizures; coma	Activate the emergency medical plan, including summoning EMS; rapidly cool body with immersion in ice water, or place crushed ice packs on the neck, axilla, and groin.

ischemia.[3,9] The condition is often seen during the first 5 days of acclimatization or in individuals with heart disease or those taking diuretics. Predisposing factors include dehydration, lack of acclimatization, ending the exercise bout without a cooldown, or moving quickly from the cold (e.g., a cold bath) into a hot sauna or whirlpool.

■ Signs and Symptoms

Signs and symptoms include dizziness, low blood pressure (hypotension), blurred or tunnel vision, pale or sweaty skin, weakness or fatigue, reduced pulse rate, and elevated skin temperature. Core temperature may not be elevated.[3]

■ Management

Treatment involves placing the patient in a supine position in a shaded or cool area, elevating the legs above the level of the head, monitoring vital signs, and replacing any water deficit.

Exertional Hyponatremia

■ Etiology

Exercising for long periods may cause low blood sodium (i.e., **hyponatremia**), which is a potentially fatal condition. Low blood sodium occurs when an individual drinks excessive amounts of water, thus diluting the sodium content of blood. Inadequate sodium intake also may play a role; however, low blood sodium is most likely to occur during prolonged exercise in dehydrated individuals who lose large amounts of sodium through sweating.

The emergency medical plan, including summoning EMS, should be activated. Blood sodium levels need to be monitored. Use of certain diuretics or intravenous solutions may be necessary.

■ Signs and Symptoms

Hyponatremia is characterized by headache, confusion, nausea, cramping, bloated stomach, altered consciousness, significant mental compromise, swelling in the extremities (e.g., fingers and ankles), and seizures. In severe cases, the individual may experience respiratory changes as a result of cerebral and/or pulmonary edema.[4]

■ **Management**

The patient should not resume activity until cleared by a physician and instructed in an individual-specific hydration protocol to ensure that the proper level and type of beverages and meals are consumed before, during, and after exercise.[4]

Miliaria Rubra and Miliaria Profunda

■ **Etiology**

Miliaria rubra and miliaria profunda are seen in humid climates or with skin that is totally covered by clothing, resulting in a highly humid environment. The sweat glands are occluded with organic debris and can no longer produce sweat for evaporation, which may predispose the individual to heat conditions. If the resulting heat rash is localized, it is called miliaria rubra; if the condition becomes generalized and prolonged, it is called miliaria profunda.

■ **Signs and Symptoms**

Miliaria rubra (i.e., heat rash or prickly heat) is an inflamed, itchy (i.e., **pruritic**) skin eruption that arises when active sweat glands are blocked. The lesions are truncal, noninflamed, and **papular**. Individuals with profunda are less heat tolerant than the general population due to the prolonged suppression of heat loss; therefore, they are at a higher risk for heat illnesses.

■ **Management**

Treatment involves cooling and drying the skin and relieving the itching. Cool baths and topical antipruritics, such as pramoxine and calamine lotion, can provide relief. The rash usually subsides if a person avoids sweating for 1 or 2 days.

 Because the U.S. Weather Bureau is forecasting 90°F (air temperature) with a relative humidity of 80% during the scheduled time for field hockey practice, the following measures should be taken to reduce the risk of heat-related illness: Practice should be shortened and the intensity of some activities reduced; water should be available at any time throughout practice; and scheduled water breaks should take place every 20 minutes.

COLD-RELATED CONDITIONS

 The weather for a scheduled soccer game is forecasted to be in the low 40s, with winds gusting up to 25 miles per hour. What measures can be taken to prevent cold-related conditions?

Hypothermia, or reduced body temperature, occurs when the body is unable to maintain a constant core temperature. In cold weather, three primary heat-promoting mechanisms attempt to maintain or increase core temperature. The initial response is cutaneous vasoconstriction to prevent blood from shunting to the skin. Because the skin is insulated with a layer of subcutaneous fat, heat loss is reduced. The second response is to increase metabolic heat production by shivering, which is an involuntary contraction of skeletal muscle, or to increase physical activity. During vigorous exercise, skeletal muscles can produce 30- to 40-fold the amount of heat produced at rest. During gradual, seasonal changes, an increased amount of the hormone thyroxine is released by the thyroid gland, which serves as the third avenue to increase metabolic rate.

Because of their larger ratio of surface area to body mass and smaller amount of subcutaneous fat, children are more prone to heat loss during cold exposure than adults are. Cold exposure also increases the risk for exercise-induced bronchospasm, which is being seen increasingly in children. Women are less able to produce heat through exercise or shivering because of their lower percentage of lean body mass, although the additional subcutaneous fat does provide more tissue insulation. Men tend to maintain lower heart rate, higher stroke volume, and higher mean arterial blood

---

BOX 29.4 Predisposing Factors for Cold-Related Injuries

- Inadequate insulation from cold and/or wind
- Restrictive clothing or arterial disease that prevents peripheral circulation, especially in the feet
- Diet lacking adequate CHOs or fat
- Presence of chronic metabolic disorders
- Spinal cord injury (cannot vasoconstrict peripheral arterioles in the skin and has a blunted shivering response to cold)
- Preexisting fatigue or general weakness
- Use of alcohol, tobacco products (especially smoking tobacco), and other medications, such as barbiturates, phenothiazines, reserpine, and narcotics
- Age (very young or old)
- Decreased circulation

---

pressure than women do, but no distinct differences are seen in cold tolerance when genders are matched for aerobic fitness at the same relative workload. Elderly people, however, have a decreased capacity for metabolic heat production and vasoconstriction. Alcohol dulls mental awareness of cold and inhibits shivering, perhaps by causing hypoglycemia.[12]

Preventing Cold-Related Injuries

During cold weather, body heat is lost through respiration, radiation, conduction, convection, and evaporation. Although the body attempts to generate heat through heat-producing mechanisms, this may be inadequate to maintain a constant core temperature. **Box 29.4** lists predisposing factors that contribute to cold-related injuries.

Several steps that can be taken to prevent heat loss are summarized in **Box 29.5**. The "layered principle" of clothing allows several (i.e., three or more) thin layers of insulation rather than one or two thick ones. Fabrics should be light yet porous enough to allow free exchange of perspiration, and they should not restrict movement. Fabrics may include wool, wool/synthetic blends, polypropylene, treated polyesters (e.g., Capilene), and hollow polyesters (e.g., ThermoStat).[13] Cotton has poor insulating ability that is markedly decreased when saturated with perspiration. Pile garments that contain down (e.g., Dacron, Hollofil, Thinsulate, or Quallofil) are more useful when worn during warm-up, time-outs, or cooldown periods following exercise. Jackets with a hood and drawstring as well as pants made of wind-resistant material (e.g., Gore-Tex, nylon, or 60/40 cloth) can protect against the wind.

A ski cap, face mask, and neck warmer can protect the face and ears from frostbite. Ski goggles can protect the eyes; goggles must be well ventilated to prevent fogging and be treated with antifog preparations. Polypropylene gloves or, in extreme temperatures, woolen mittens can be worn with windproof outer mittens of Gore-Tex or nylon. Athletic shoes should be large enough to accommodate an outer pair of heavy wool socks. It is important to avoid getting wet, because heat loss can be increased by evaporation. The insulating ability of clothing can be decreased by as much as 90% when saturated either with external moisture or condensation from perspiration. If weather conditions are bad enough, it is better to cancel the practice or event for the day.

Cold Conditions

People tend to adapt less readily to cold than to heat. Even inhabitants of cold regions show only limited evidence of adaptation, such as a higher metabolic rate. Like heat illness, cold-related injuries range from minor problems, such as Raynaud syndrome, cold-induced bronchospasm, or frostbite, to the more severe, general systemic cooling, or hypothermia, which can be life threatening. Cold emergencies occur in two ways. In one, the core temperature remains relatively constant, but the

BOX 29.5 Reducing the Risk of Cold-Related Injuries

- Check weather conditions and consider possible deterioration.

- Identify individuals who may be susceptible to cold and observe closely.

- Dress in several light layers.

- Wear windproof, dry, well-insulated clothing that allows water evaporation; wool, polypropylene, or polyesters (e.g., Capilene, ThermoStat) are recommended.

- Carry windproof pants and jacket if conditions warrant; keep the back to the wind.

- Wear well-insulated, windproof mittens, gloves, hats, and scarves.

- Wear well-insulated footwear that keeps the feet dry.

- Avoid dehydration. Do not drink alcoholic beverages or eat snow because these worsen hypothermia.

- Carry nutritious snacks that contain predominantly CHOs.

- Eat small amounts of food frequently.

- Do not stand in one position for extended periods of time. Wiggle the toes and keep moving to bring warm blood to various areas of the body.

- Stay dry by wearing appropriate rain gear or protective clothing. If wet, change into dry clothing as soon as possible.

- Breathe through the nose, rather than the mouth, to minimize heat and fluid loss.

- Watch the face, ears, and fingers for signs of frostbite.

shell temperature decreases. This results in localized injuries from frostbite. In the other, both core temperature and shell temperature decrease, leading to general body cooling. All body processes slow down, and systemic hypothermia results. If left unabated, death is imminent.

Raynaud Syndrome

■ Etiology

Raynaud syndrome is seen in young individuals, especially females. It can be caused by an underlying disease or anatomical abnormality, and it can be a long-term complication of frostbite. Usually, however, its source is unknown.

■ Signs and Symptoms

The condition is characterized by bilateral episodes of spasms of the digital blood vessels in response to emotion or cold exposure. Initially, during the ischemic phase, the affected digits (usually the fingers) become cold, pale, and numb. This is followed by hyperemia with redness, throbbing pain, and swelling.

■ Management

Treatment involves warming the affected extremity. A physician should evaluate the patient to rule out an underlying condition. Cigarette smoking should be avoided, because it compromises circulation.

Cold-Induced Bronchospasm

■ Etiology

Cold-induced bronchospasm is also a condition seen frequently in young people. It is brought on by exposure to cold, dry air during cold-weather sports.

■ Signs and Symptoms

Linked to exercise-induced bronchospasm, the patient experiences difficulty breathing, as manifested by shortness of breath, coughing, chest tightness, and wheezing.

■ Management

Attacks can be prevented by the use of bronchodilators or cromolyn sodium. Salmeterol, a more recent, long-acting bronchodilator, administered 30 to 60 minutes before exercise appears to protect many individuals for up to 12 hours. Chapter 26 provides information on exercise-induced bronchospasm.

Frostbite Injuries

■ Etiology

Frostbite is caused by the freezing of soft tissue. Individuals who have cold urticaria (cold allergy) or Raynaud syndrome are at higher risk for frostbite. Frostbite is classified on a continuum of three degrees (**Table 29.3**). First-degree, or superficial, frostbite involves the skin and underlying tissues, but the deeper tissues are soft and pliable. If damage extends into the subcutaneous tissues, it is classified as second-degree frostbite. Third-degree, or deep, frostbite involves the tissues deep to the subcutaneous layers and may result in complete destruction of the injured tissue, including damage to bones, joints, and tendons.[14] Damage depends on the depth of cold penetration that results from the duration of exposure, temperature, and wind velocity. Areas commonly affected are the fingertips, toes (especially when wearing constricting footwear), earlobes, and tip of the nose.

■ Signs and Symptoms

In superficial frostbite, the area may feel firm to the touch, but the tissue beneath is soft and resilient. The skin initially appears red and swollen, and the patient complains of diffuse numbness, transient tingling, or burning. If the frostbite extends into the subcutaneous or deep layers, the skin feels hard, because it actually is frozen tissue. The area then turns white, with a yellow or blue tint that looks waxy.

■ Management

A person with superficial frostbite should be removed from the cold and taken indoors immediately and then treated with careful, slow warming of the area. Clothing and jewelry should be removed and the injured area immersed in water heated to between 37° and 40°C (98° and 104°F) for 15 to 30 minutes.[15] A whirlpool is ideal, but if one is unavailable, a basin large enough to prevent the skin from touching the sides of the container should be used. Hot water should be avoided, because it may cause burns. If frostbite is superficial, rewarmed skin may have clear blisters, whereas with deep frostbite, the rewarmed skin has hemorrhagic blisters.[14] The involved area should be dried and a sterile dressing applied. If fingers or toes are involved, sterile dressings should be placed between the digits before covering. The entire area can be covered with towels or a blanket to keep it warm, and the patient should be transported to the nearest medical center, with the affected limb slightly elevated.

 Deep frostbite is best rewarmed under controlled conditions in a hospital. The emergency medical plan, including summoning EMS, should be activated. During transport, the patient should be kept warm, but active rewarming of the frozen part should not occur.

If the frostbite is severe, hemorrhagic blisters may form over the area, and gangrene may develop within 2 to 3 weeks. Throbbing, aching pain as well as burning sensations may last for weeks. The skin may remain permanently red, tender, and sensitive to reexposure to cold.

TABLE 29.3 Signs and Symptoms of Frostbite

First degree	Skin is soft to the touch and appears initially red, then white, and usually is painless. The condition typically is noticed by others first.
Second degree	Skin is firm to the touch, but tissue beneath is soft and initially appears red and swollen. Diffuse numbness may be preceded by an itchy or prickly sensation. White or waxy skin color may appear later.
Third degree	Skin is hard to the touch, totally numb, and appears blotchy white to yellow-gray or blue-gray.

Systemic Body Cooling (Hypothermia)

Hypothermia is more of a danger to individuals who are exposed to cold for long periods of time, such as long distance runners and Nordic ski racers, especially those who are slowing down late in a race because of fatigue or injury. Any injured or ill individual who has been exposed to cold weather or cold water should be suspected of having hypothermia until proved otherwise.

■ Etiology

Most of the body heat is lost through radiation involving the exposed surfaces on the hands, face, head, and neck. When the temperature is 4.4°C (40°F), more than half the body's generated heat can be lost from an uncovered head. If the temperature is −15°C (5°F), up to 75% of the body's heat is lost through the head. Air movement coupled with cold produces a wind-chill factor that causes heat loss from the body much faster than occurs in still air. The faster the wind, the higher the wind-chill factor (**Fig. 29.4**).

When core temperature falls below 35°C (95°F), essential biochemical processes begin to slow. Heart and respiration rates slow, cardiac output and blood pressure fall, and as the skin and muscles cool, shivering increases violently. Numbness sets in, and even the simplest task becomes difficult to perform. If core temperature continues to drop below 32°C (90°F), shivering ceases, and muscles become cold and stiff. Cold diuresis (i.e., polyuria) occurs as blood is shunted away from the shell to the core in an effort to maintain vascular volume. This leads to excessive excretion of urine by the kidneys. If intervention is not initiated, death is imminent.

 See **Signs and Symptoms of Hypothermia**, available on the companion Web site at thePoint, for highlights of the stages of systemic hypothermia.

■ Signs and Symptoms

Patients with hypothermia are divided into those with mild hypothermia (rectal temperature between 37° and 35°C [98.6° and 95°F]) and those with moderate-to-severe hypothermia (rectal temperature between 34° and 32°C [93.2° and 90°F]). Rectal temperatures obtained through either a digital or mercury thermometer that can read below 34° (93.2°F) are preferred over using

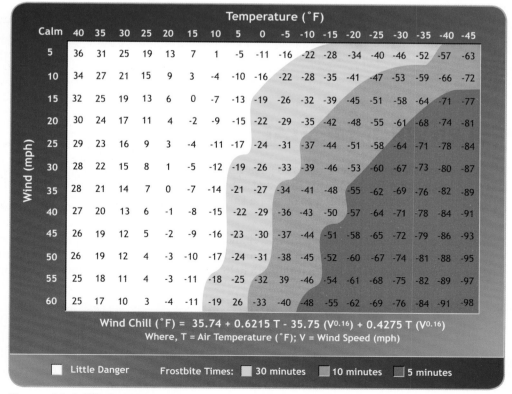

Figure 29.4. Wind-chill index.

a tympanic, axillary, or oral temperature due to environmental concerns, such as exposure to air temperatures.[15]

In mild hypothermia, the patient is vigorously shivering. The patient may appear to be clumsy, apathetic, or confused and have slurred speech, stumble, and drop things. Blood pressure is within normal limits. A patient with moderate-to-severe hypothermia does not feel any sensation or pain, is not shivering, and presents with depressed respiration and pulse. The patient's movements will become jerky, and the patient becomes unaware of the surroundings. Blood pressure will be decreased and difficult to measure. Cardiac arrhythmias, dilated pupils, and muscle rigidity may lead to bradycardia, severely depressed respirations, and hypotension; pulmonary edema progresses to a comatose state and eventually cardiac arrest.[15]

■ Management

In cases of mild hypothermia, the patient should be moved carefully into a warm shelter. Any wet or damp clothing should be removed. Rewarming can be accomplished by insulating the patient with dry clothes (remember to cover the head) and allowing the patient to shiver inside a blanket or sleeping bag or by using external rewarming devices, such as hot-water bottles or heating pads. Apply external heat only to the trunk and other areas of heat transfer, such as the axilla, chest

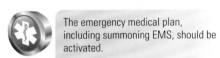
The emergency medical plan, including summoning EMS, should be activated.

wall, and groin. Warm drinks (preferably nonalcoholic and noncaffeinated) and foods containing 6% to 8% CHOs to sustain metabolic heat production may be useful after the patient is partly rewarmed and able to swallow. The patient should continue to be rewarmed en route to the nearest medical facility.

If hypothermia is moderate to severe, on-site rewarming should not be attempted. Once rewarming begins, serious electrolyte, metabolic, and cardiovascular changes occur that cannot be treated in the field. As such, while waiting for EMS to arrive, treatment involves preventing any further cooling and monitoring and treating for shock as necessary. As in mild hypothermia, remove any wet or damp clothing; insulate the patient with warm, dry clothing or blankets; and apply heat to the trunk, axilla, chest wall, and groin. Continue to monitor vital signs and be prepared for airway management.[15]

The effects of cold can be minimized by dressing in several layers of insulating clothing under the uniforms. Jackets with a hood and drawstring as well as pants made of wind-resistant material can protect against the wind. Wool socks and gloves also may keep the player warm.

OTHER ENVIRONMENTAL CONDITIONS

> **?** The threat exists for thunderstorms to pass through the area during a scheduled afternoon lacrosse game. Based on this information, what actions should be taken before the game, and how should a decision to suspend the game be determined?

The ever-changing environment presents a unique challenge for individuals participating in sport and physical activity. Individuals must cope with heat, humidity, cold, rain, lightning, altitude, and air pollution. A basic understanding of these situations can help to facilitate the performance of participants.

Altitude Disorders

The percentage of oxygen in the atmosphere at an altitude of 10,000 ft is exactly the same as that at sea level. The density of air, however, decreases progressively with ascension above sea level. The decreased partial pressure of ambient oxygen, or density of oxygen molecules, makes it more difficult to deliver oxygen to working muscles of the body. This leads to a reduction in work capacity that is directly proportional to altitude. This factor has little, if any, effect on short bursts of energy, but it can have significant impact on sustained aerobic activities. In some cases, individuals are unaware of the impact that altitude exposure can have on their performance and, in compensating for the decrease in maximum oxygen uptake, experience hyperventilation or tachycardia. As a result, stroke volume is reduced, and fewer red blood cells are available to transport needed oxygen.

High-altitude illness is a collective term for the syndromes that affect individuals who are not acclimatized shortly after their ascent to high altitude. The term encompasses the primary cerebral syndromes of acute mountain sickness (AMS) and high-altitude cerebral edema (HACE) as well as the pulmonary syndrome high-altitude pulmonary edema (HAPE). Both HACE and HAPE occur much less frequently than AMS, but these two syndromes are potentially fatal. Risk factors for developing high-altitude illness include the rate of ascent, the altitude reached, and the individual's susceptibility.[16]

Acute Mountain Sickness

■ Etiology

Altitude sickness is a disorder related to **hypoxia** at high altitudes. Predisposing factors include cold temperatures, strenuous exercise, use of cigarettes or alcohol, respiratory infections or a blunted ventilatory response, the water-retaining phase of the menstrual cycle, and a family history of AMS. The mildest form of altitude sickness, AMS arises after rapid ascent (i.e., <24 hours) to altitudes above 8,200 ft (2,500 m). A time lag of 8 or more hours occurs between arrival at the altitude and onset of symptoms.[17]

■ Signs and Symptoms

Signs and symptoms are directly proportional to the rapidity of the ascent and both the duration and degree of physical exertion, and they are inversely proportional to acclimatization and physical conditioning. Symptoms usually start 4 to 8 hours after arrival at high altitude. Headache is the cardinal symptom but may not be sufficiently distinctive to differentiate it from other causes of headache. Other symptoms include dizziness, fatigue, nausea, vomiting, suppressed appetite, insomnia, dyspnea, decreased urine output, and tachycardia during physical exertion. Appetite suppression can be severe during the onset of a high-altitude stay, and this suppression can result in an average reduction of energy intake by approximately 40%, with an accompanying loss of body mass. The nonspecific symptoms of AMS can result in diagnostic confusion with those of other disorders, such as exhaustion, dehydration, hypothermia, alcohol hangover, and migraine headache.[16]

■ Management

Acclimatization and physical conditioning can enhance altitude tolerance, reduce the severity of AMS, and decrease the physical performance decrements that occur during the early stages of altitude sickness. In addition, diets that are high in CHOs (i.e., >70% of total kilocalories) and low in salt can lessen the impact of AMS. If AMS occurs, treatment involves a reduction in altitude, physical rest, eating frequent small meals, avoiding alcohol, and taking acetaminophen for the headache. Recovery normally is seen within a few days, with no residual effects.

High-Altitude Cerebral Edema

■ Etiology

HACE, often thought of as the end stage of AMS, rarely occurs below 10,000 ft. It usually happens in people who ascend rapidly to significant altitudes.

■ Signs and Symptoms

Several days after the onset of mild AMS, increased brain cell volume leads to a severe headache, nausea and vomiting, ataxia, impaired judgment, inability to make decisions, irrational behavior, and in some cases, altered consciousness. Without treatment, coma usually develops within 1 to 2 days, and death occurs rapidly because of brain herniation.[17]

■ Management

An immediate descent is mandatory. High-flow supplemental oxygen or a portable hyperbaric bag should be used while descending or if descent is delayed.

High-Altitude Pulmonary Edema

■ Etiology

For unknown reasons, some individuals experience a severe aspect of AMS at altitudes greater than 9,000 ft. The condition is referred to as HAPE. Individuals at greatest risk include those who ascend rapidly, perform strenuous exercise on arrival, are obese, are male, and have a previous history of pulmonary edema.[17] HAPE may develop during the first exposure but often develops after descent and reascent or occurs during the second night after ascent. The lungs accumulate fluid within the alveolar walls that may progress to pulmonary edema.

■ Signs and Symptoms

Initial signs and symptoms include shortness of breath (**dyspnea**), decreased performance, cough, and reduced exercise tolerance greater than expected for the altitude.[16,17] A dry cough with substernal chest pains becomes productive, with blood-stained sputum, later in the illness. During rest, headache, decreased concentration, fatigue, **tachycardia**, and abnormal breath sounds (i.e., **rales**) in the middle right lobe also may be present. Later, **cyanosis**; extreme weakness; mild fever (rarely exceeding 38.3°C [101°F]); productive cough with bloody, frothy sputum; irrational behavior; and coma may occur.

■ Management

A rapid return to a lower altitude is imperative. The patient should be given oxygen as soon as possible. Exertion should be kept to a minimum. If oxygen is unavailable and descent impossible, treatment in a portable hyperbaric chamber may be lifesaving, although the recumbent position that is necessary for operation of the chamber may not be tolerated by the patient. The condition resolves rapidly.

Preventing Altitude Illness

Acclimatization is the single most important factor in preventing the onset of altitude sickness. In general, the length of the acclimatization period depends on the altitude. Individuals who are native to areas of high altitude have a larger chest capacity, more alveoli, more capillaries that transport blood to tissues, and a higher red blood cell level. As a result, these individuals have an advantage in endurance activities at higher altitudes. Training for aerobic activities (i.e., events lasting longer than 3 or 4 minutes) at altitudes above 6,800 ft (2,000 m) requires acclimatization for 10 to 20 days for maximal performance. Highly anaerobic activities at intermediate altitudes do not require arrival in advance of the event. The benefits of acclimatization probably are lost within 2 to 3 weeks after returning to sea level.

Air Pollution and Exercise

Chemicals that make up air pollution typically are classified as either primary pollutants (i.e., those emitted directly into the environment) or secondary pollutants (i.e., those that develop from the interactions of the primary pollutants). Most primary pollutants essentially come from the combustion of petroleum-based fuels, including carbon monoxide, sulfur oxides, nitrogen oxides, hydrocarbons, and particulates. Secondary pollutants include ozone, peroxyacetyl nitrate, sulfuric acid, aldehydes, and sulfates. Smog usually contains both primary and secondary pollutants. Certain individuals are more susceptible to the adverse effects of air pollution. Even what would be subthreshold concentrations of air pollutants for healthy adults can compromise respiratory and cardiovascular function in children and elderly people. Others who are more affected by air pollution include individuals with respiratory disorders (e.g., asthma or chronic obstructive pulmonary disease) and heart disease.

Carbon Monoxide

The most frequent air pollutant is carbon monoxide. It is a colorless, odorless gas that reduces the ability of hemoglobin to transport oxygen and restricts the release of oxygen at the cellular level. In an individual who smokes cigarettes, carbon monoxide reduces both aerobic power and the ability to sustain strenuous, submaximal exercise. It not only interferes with maximal performance during exercise but also can impair attentiveness; decision making; and psychomotor, behavioral, or attention-related tasks, and it may result in higher core temperatures during prolonged exercise. The major group at risk from carbon monoxide exposure includes individuals with cardiovascular disorders (e.g., angina pectoris, ischemic cardiovascular disease, and intermittent **claudication**), pulmonary diseases (e.g., chronic bronchitis and emphysema), or anemia.

Sulfur Oxides

Sulfur oxides are produced from burning coal or petroleum products. They include sulfur dioxide, sulfuric acid, and sulfate, with 98% of the sulfur released into the atmosphere being in the form of sulfur dioxide. By itself, sulfur dioxide has little effect on lung function in normal individuals, but it can be a potent bronchoconstrictor in those with asthma. Exposure to just a trace amount of the gas during brief periods of strenuous exercise (i.e., 10 minutes) can produce a marked decrease in airway conductance in people with asthma. Individuals with asthma can prevent problems in breathing by using disodium cromoglycate before exposure or by breathing through the nose.

Nitrogen Oxides

Nitrogen oxide is a combination of nitrogen and oxygen that develops from high-temperature combustion. It is seen in several forms—namely, nitrous oxide, nitric oxide, nitrogen dioxide (NO_2), dinitrogen dioxide, dinitrogen pentoxide, and nitrate ions. Oxide levels in the air are particularly high during peak traffic periods, at airports, and in the smoke associated with cigarette smoking and firefighting. High NO_2 levels (i.e., 200 to 4,000 ppm) can cause severe pulmonary edema and even death. In lower concentrations (i.e., 2 to 5 ppm), NO_2 increases airway resistance and reduces pulmonary diffusion capacity.

Ozone

Ozone (i.e., triatomic oxygen) is a complex union of oxygen, nitrogen oxides, hydrocarbons, and sunlight and is therefore designated a photochemical oxidant. Ozone is classified as either ground level or atmospheric. Atmospheric ozone is produced naturally and protects the earth from the sun's ultraviolet waves. The ozone that interferes with functional capacity is ground level, which stays close to the earth's surface and originates in automobile and factory emissions. Ground-level ozone is an irritant that can exacerbate existing respiratory conditions, such as emphysema and asthma. The effects of ground-level ozone normally are short term, but they can diminish work production and may produce shortness of breath and early fatigue. When maximal exertion is required, ozone may lead to coughing, chest tightness, shortness of breath, pain during deep breaths, nausea, eye irritation, fatigue, and lowered resistance to lung infections.

Ozone levels are indexed as low, moderate, or high (**Table 29.4**). The ozone index can be found on the weather page of most newspapers or on the Web (e.g., https://weather.com/). Individuals who reside in regions of high ozone levels may become desensitized to the irritating effects after repeated exposures and, as such, do not develop symptoms or changes in functional abilities.

Primary Particulates

Primary particulates, which include dust, soot, and smoke, can impair pulmonary function when inhaled into the lungs. The fine dust from charcoal and cigarette smoke increases airway resistance

TABLE 29.4 Ozone Level	
LEVEL	**ACTIVITY PRECAUTIONS**
Low	No precautions are necessary.
Moderate	Individuals with respiratory conditions should minimize outdoor exposure and decrease prolonged exercise or work.
High	Individuals with respiratory conditions should stay indoors. Individual without respiratory conditions should minimize outdoor exposure.

and reduces forced expiratory volume. The ability of fine dust to infiltrate the lungs depends on the particle size, amount of air inspired and expired in a single breath (i.e., **tidal volume**), frequency of breathing, and whether the particle was inhaled nasally or orally. During strenuous exercise, the breathing rate significantly increases, and breathing tends to be oral. Therefore, exercise likely increases the impact of these pollutants on breathing effectiveness.

Exercising in Thunderstorms

Another environmental threat is inclement weather conditions, such as rain, lightning, and thunderstorms. Most organized outdoor sport practices and competitions are held between 3:00 p.m. and 9:00 p.m., which are peak periods for the development of thunderstorms and lightning. If the lightning (flash) to thunder (bang) occurs within 30 seconds, all outdoor activities should end, and all participants should seek shelter, preferably in a sturdy building.

Lightning Injuries

■ **Etiology**

Lightning poses a triple threat of injury—namely, burns from the high temperature of the lightning strike, injury caused by the elicited mechanical forces activated by the intense levels of electricity (electromechanical forces), and the resulting concussive forces that can propel objects through the air, causing blunt trauma (e.g., fracture and concussion). Lightning injuries usually are the result of five different mechanisms[18]:

1. Direct strike

2. Contact injury

3. Side flash (splash)

4. Ground current (step voltage)

5. Blunt trauma

If a patient is not breathing and is in cardiac arrest, the emergency medical plan, including summoning EMS, should be activated. Rescue breathing and cardiopulmonary resuscitation should be initiated. Unless ruled out, a cervical spine injury should always be suspected, and treatment should proceed accordingly. Any person struck by lightning should be immediately transported to the nearest medical facility.

■ **Signs and Symptoms**

The most common burn from lightning is a Lichtenberg figure, which resembles a feathering pattern on the skin. A Lichtenberg figure is not actually a burn; rather, it is a pattern on the skin from the electron avalanche that strikes the body hit by lightning, which causes an inflammatory dermal response. The pattern is transient and fades after 24 hours.

Direct strikes are the most deadly, particularly when the person is in contact with metal (e.g., golf club, shoe cleats, belt buckle, bra clips, watch band, or metal bleachers), with the burn normally appearing where the person's body is in contact with that metal object. Additional symptoms are cardiac asystole (cardiac standstill) and respiratory arrest. Fortunately, the heart is likely to restart spontaneously if the victim is not experiencing respiratory arrest. The most critical factor in determining morbidity and mortality associated with a lightning strike is the duration of apnea rather than cardiac asystole. It is not uncommon for a person to become unconscious or confused or to develop amnesia following a lightning strike. Other medical conditions that have been reported include blunt trauma, including fractures and internal organ damage; brain lesions because of hypoxia caused by cardiac asystole; ruptured tympanic membranes; ocular problems, including hyphema as well as fixed and dilated pupils; seizures; subdural and epidural hematomas; anterior compartment syndromes; and transitory lower extremity paralysis.[19]

■ **Management**

Lightning strikes claim the lives of approximately 100 people each year. Prior to moving into action, survey the scene and determine if it is safe to respond to the situation. Activate the EMS plan. Move the victim to a safer location, if available. The priority is to assess and treat for apnea and asystole. If the person is conscious and has normal cardiorespiratory function, a secondary assessment should be conducted to assess and treat any burns, fractures, or other trauma that may have been sustained.

Lightning Safety Policy

As mentioned, most organized outdoor sport practices and competitions are conducted between the hours of 3:00 p.m. and 9:00 p.m. Most lightning casualties occur between May and September, with July having the greatest number of casualties. There are 45% of deaths and 80% of casualties occurred in these months between 10:00 a.m. and 7:00 p.m.[19,20] Thunderstorms can become threatening within 30 minutes of the first sign of thunder. All athletic and recreational facilities should have a formalized emergency action plan specific to lightning safety prior to the start of the thunderstorm season. This plan should include the following[19]:

See **Lightning Safety Policy for All Outdoor Activities, Including Swimming**, available on the companion Web site at thePoint.

- Specific chain of command to identify an individual with the authority to remove participants from athletic venues or activities

- Weather watcher to actively look for signs of developing local thunderstorms, such as high winds, darkening clouds, and any lightning or thunder

- Specific plan to monitor local weather forecasts from either local weather radio stations or the National Weather Service

- Clearly defined and listed safe structures or locations to evacuate to in the event of lightning. Ideally, this structure should have plumbing, electric wiring, and telephone service. If unavailable, an alternative is the use of a fully enclosed vehicle with a metal roof and the windows completely closed.

- Specific criteria for suspension and resumption of activities. (By the time the flash-to-bang count approaches 30 seconds or less, all individuals should be inside or should immediately seek a safe structure or location. To determine distance of the storm, begin counting at the first sight of the flash. Stop counting when the associated bang [thunder] is heard. Divide by 5 to determine the distance in miles. For example, a flash-to-bang count of 30 seconds equates to a distance of 6 miles.) Wait at least 30 minutes after the last sound of thunder or lightning flash before resuming the activity.

- Recommended lightning safety strategies. If caught outside, assume the lightning-safe position (i.e., crouched on the ground, weight on the balls of the feet, feet together, head lowered, and ears covered). Do not lie flat on the ground.

All coaches, athletic trainers, athletic directors, athletic supervisors, managers, and physically active individuals should understand the development of thunderstorms and lightning strikes. This lightning safety policy can decrease the risk of injury and death as well as protect the organization or institution from litigation if the policy is referred to and heeded.

Before the start of the lacrosse game, the athletic trainer should review the school's lightning safety emergency plan, determine who will serve as the designated weather watcher, and meet with the game officials and visiting team's athletic trainer (or coach) to explain the lightning safety plan. The game should be suspended if the "flash-to-bang" is within 30 seconds or if a thunderstorm appears imminent.

SUMMARY

1. The body generates heat by cutaneous vasoconstriction, increasing the metabolic heat production by shivering or physical activity, and the increase of the hormone thyroxine during gradual, seasonal changes. The body loses heat through respiration, radiation, conduction, convection, and evaporation.

2. During exercise, the body gains heat from external sources (e.g., environmental temperatures) or internal processes (e.g., muscle activity).

3. During rest, approximately two-thirds of the body's normal heat loss results from conduction, convection, and radiation. As air temperature approaches skin temperature and exceeds 30.6°C (87°F), evaporation becomes the primary means of heat dissipation.

4. Sweating places a high demand on the body's fluid reserves and can create a relative state of dehydration. If sweating is excessive and fluids are not continually replaced, plasma volume falls, and core temperature may rise to lethal levels.

5. Acclimatization and proper hydration are among the most critical factors in preventing heat illness. Minerals lost through sweating generally can be replaced through the diet. During prolonged exercise, drinking a small amount of electrolytes added to a rehydration beverage replaces fluids more effectively than drinking plain water.

6. To prevent dehydration, fluids must be ingested and absorbed by the body. Cold liquids, especially water, empty from the stomach and small intestines faster than warm fluids do.

7. Exercise-associated muscle (heat) cramps are caused by excessive loss of water and electrolytes during and after intense exercise in the heat. Treatment involves passive stretching of the involved muscles and ice massage over the affected area. The patient also should drink fluids containing an electrolyte solution to beyond the point of satisfying thirst.

8. Exercise (heat) exhaustion is a functional illness and is not associated with organ damage. Treatment involves moving the patient to a cool place and rapidly cooling the body. The patient also should drink fluids containing an electrolyte solution to beyond the point of satisfying thirst. Intravenous fluids may need to be administered if the dehydrated state is moderate to severe.

9. Exertional heat stroke signifies a significantly elevated core temperature and dehydration. The emergency medical plan, including summoning EMS, should be activated, because the patient may require airway management, intravenous fluids, and in severe cases, circulatory support. While waiting for EMS to arrive, the patient should be moved to a cool place, and efforts should be made to rapidly cool the body. Immersion in ice water is the most effective method to cool the body; however, to avoid hypothermia, the core temperature should not fall below 38°C (100.4°F). If conscious, the patient should drink copious amounts of fluid.

10. In the prevention of cold-related injuries, the principle of layering clothing has proven to be effective through providing several thin layers of insulation. In addition, a ski cap, face mask, and neck warmer can protect the face and ears from frostbite.

11. Frostbite occurs when the core temperature remains relatively constant but the shell temperature decreases. Superficial frostbite is treated by moving the patient indoors, removing any wet or damp clothing, and rapidly rewarming the involved body part in water heated to between 39° and 42°C (102.2° and 107.6°F) for 30 to 45 minutes. Deep frostbite is best rewarmed under controlled conditions in a hospital. The emergency medical plan should be activated.

12. Hypothermia occurs when both core and shell temperatures decrease, leading to general body cooling. If hypothermia is mild, the patient can be rewarmed; if hypothermia is moderate to severe, on-site rewarming should not be attempted. The emergency medical plan, including summoning EMS, should be activated.

13. Altitude sickness may involve AMS, HAPE, or HACE. The latter two conditions can lead quickly to death; therefore, oxygen therapy and immediate descent are mandatory.

14. Carbon monoxide, the most frequent air pollutant, interferes with the ability of hemoglobin to transport oxygen to the cells. Other air pollutants that can affect sport performance include sulfur oxides, nitrogen oxides, ozone, and primary particulates.

15. Lightning poses a double threat of injury—namely, burns from the high temperature of the lightning strike and concussive injuries caused by the elicited electromechanical forces.

16. Most thunderstorms occur between 10:00 a.m. and 7:00 p.m. during the months of May through September. Schools and sport organizations should have a detailed lightning safety policy to prevent injury or death from storms.

APPLICATION QUESTIONS

1. A new soccer coach has joined the athletic staff at your high school. What guidelines should be provided to the coach to prevent heat illness during preseason practice sessions?

2. The WGBT in the wrestling room is 85°F. A wrestler leaves the mat during the match complaining of dizziness. Assessment indicates rapid and weak pulse; ashen, cool, and clammy skin; and dizziness. What condition should be suspected? How might his condition be managed?

3. Although it is not raining, the rumble of thunder can be heard in the distance during a softball game. Should the umpires be advised to suspend the game, or is it better to wait and see if any lightning is associated with the storm? What criteria would indicate that the game should be suspended?

4. You have been asked to speak to a group of hikers in an outdoor pursuits class who are going backpacking in the Smokey Mountains in January. What suggestions might you provide to help the hikers prevent hypothermia during their trip?

5. A cross-country skier complains of pain and numbness in the fingers and toes. Observation reveals red and swollen toes and fingers, but palpation finds the areas to be cold and firm to the touch. What condition should be suspected? What is the management for this condition?

REFERENCES

1. Casa DJ, Armstrong LE, Hillman SK, et al. National Athletic Trainers' Association position statement: fluid replacement for athletes. *J Athl Train*. 2000;35(2):212–224.
2. Sawka MN, Burke LM, Eichner ER, et al. American College of Sports Medicine position stand. Exercise and fluid replacement. *Med Sci Sports Exerc*. 2007;39(2):377–390.
3. Binkley HM, Beckett J, Casa DJ, et al. National Athletic Trainers' Association position statement: exertional heat illnesses. *J Athl Train*. 2002;37 (3):329–343.
4. Casa DJ, Almquist J, Anderson S. Inter-Association Task Force on Exertional Heat Illnesses consensus statement. *NATA News*. 2003;6:24–29.
5. Casa DJ, Csillan D. Preseason heat-acclimatization guidelines for secondary school athletics. *J Athl Train*. 2009;44(3):332–333.
6. Mellion MB, Shelton GL. Safe exercise in the head and heat injuries. In: Mellion MB, Walsh WM, Madden D, et al., eds. *The Team Physician's Handbook*. Philadelphia, PA: Hanley & Belfus; 2002:133–143.
7. Meyer F, Bar-Or O, MacDougall D, et al. Drink composition and electrolyte balance of children exercising in the heat. *Med Sci Sports Exerc*. 1995;27(6):882–887.
8. Wexler RK. Evaluation and treatment of heat-related illnesses. *Am Fam Physician*. 2002;65 (11):2307–2314.
9. Raukar N, Lemieux R, Finn G, et al. Heat illness—a practical primer. *R I Med J (2013)*. 2015;98 (7):28–31.
10. Hadad E, Rav-Acha M, Heled Y, et al. Heat stroke: a review of cooling methods. *Sports Med*. 2004;34(8):501–511.
11. Coris EE, Ramirez AM, Van Durme DJ. Heat illness in athletes: the dangerous combination of heat, humidity and exercise. *Sports Med*. 2004;34(1):9–16.
12. Moran DS. Potential applications of heat and cold stress indices to sporting events. *Sports Med*. 2001;31(13):909–917.
13. Bowman WD. Safe exercise in the cold and cold injuries. In: Mellion MB, Walsh WM, Madden C, et al., eds. *The Team Physician's Handbook*. Philadelphia, PA: Hanley & Belfus; 2002:144–151.
14. Biem J, Koehncke N, Classen D, et al. Out of the cold: management of hypothermia and frostbite. *CMAJ*. 2003;168(3):305–311.
15. Cappaert TA, Stone JA, Castellani JW, et al. National Athletic Trainers' Association position statement: environmental cold injuries. *J Athl Train*. 2008;43(6):640–658.

16. Basnyat B, Murdoch DR. High-altitude illness. *Lancet*. 2003;361(9373):1967–1974.

17. Bärtsch P, Saltin B. General introduction to altitude adaptation and mountain sickness. *Scand J Med Sci Sports*. 2008;18(suppl 1):1–10.

18. Whitcomb D, Martinez JA, Daberkow D. Lightning injuries. *South Med J*. 2002;95(11): 1331–1334.

19. Walsh KM, Cooper MA, Holle R, et al. National Athletic Trainers' Association position statement: lightning safety for athletics and recreation. *J Athl Train*. 2013;48(2):258–270.

20. Casa DJ, Guskiewicz KM, Anderson SA, et al. National Athletic Trainers' Association position statement: preventing sudden death in sports. *J Athl Train*. 2012;47(1):96–118.

30

Athletes with Physical Disabilities

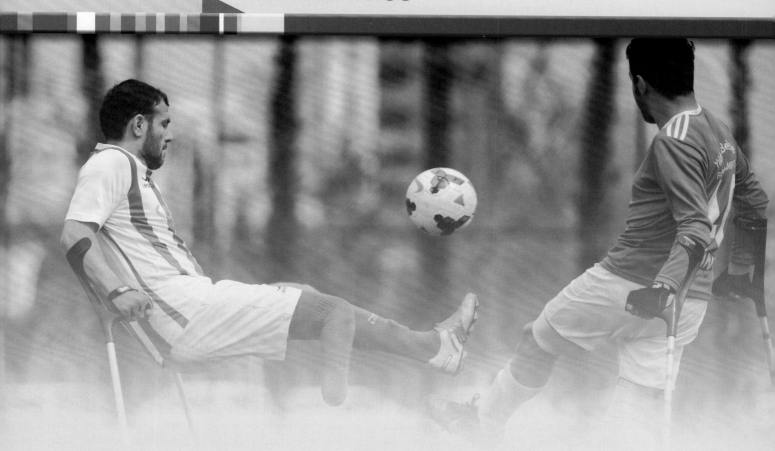

STUDENT OUTCOMES

1. Identify the disability groupings of athletes participating in Paralympic sports.

2. Define spinal cord injury (SCI) in terms of complete or incomplete.

3. Utilize the American Spinal Injury Association (ASIA) Impairment Scale level to describe spinal cord injury by level of neurological impairment.

4. Explain tetraplegia, thoracic paraplegia, and lumbar paraplegia and implications for participation in activities of daily living and sports.

5. Describe why persons with SCI are at higher risk for developing urinary tract infections, neurogenic bowel, pressure sores, blood clots, and respiratory complications and provide strategies for preventing, identifying, and treating the condition.

6. Define autonomic dysreflexia.

7. Describe specificity in terms of cause, type, and complications.

8. Explain effects of spinal cord injury on exercise.

9. Educate others regarding the pathophysiology and impairments experienced by an individual with cerebral palsy (CP).

10. Provide examples of how using the tools for classifying cerebral palsy assist the athletic trainer in caring for athletes with CP.

11. Explain the effects of CP on exercise and the evaluation and treatment of sport-related injury.

12. Educate others regarding the causes of amputation and pathophysiology and impairments experienced by individuals with amputation.

13. Explain the effects of amputation on exercise and the evaluation and treatment of sport-related injury.

INTRODUCTION

Sports participation by athletes with disabilities originated as a key component of rehabilitation programs designed for those who had been severely injured and impaired in World War II. By 1960, the first Paralympic Games took place, with 400 athletes from 23 countries participating.[1] It is estimated that in the 2016 Paralympic Games, more than 4,350 athletes will compete at this elite international competition.[2] Athletes participating in Paralympic sports are grouped based on disability: physical impairment, visual impairment, and intellectual impairment.[3] Physical impairment includes impaired muscle power, impaired passive range of motion, loss of limb or limb deficit, leg length difference, short stature, hypertonia, ataxia, and athetosis.[3] Today, about 15% of the world's population experiences some sort of disability.[4] In the United States, there are 26 organizations for persons with disabilities who desire to participate in competitive and recreational sports (**Table 30.1**).[5] For athletes participating at the highest level, the Paralympic Games, injury rates are similar to those found for able-bodied (AB) participants competing in similar elite level events.[6] Overuse injuries are more prevalent than acute injuries, although acute injuries are frequently seen in ball-handling sports.[6] Wheelchair athletes have the highest risk of sustaining upper extremity injuries, whereas athletes with spinal cord injury are at risk for sustaining lower leg fractures due to poor bone density.[6] Due to altered biomechanics and issues related to prosthetics, amputee athletes appear to have the highest incident of injury and pain. Athletes with cerebral palsy experience the highest number of musculoskeletal soft-tissue injury.[6] This chapter will cover the most common physical disability groups represented in the Paralympic Games: spinal cord injury, cerebral palsy, and amputation. Information regarding classification, typing, complications, and exercise and treatment concerns for athletes with physical disabilities within each of these categories is presented.

SPINAL CORD INJURY

? Mary is about to conduct an assessment of an athlete with a spinal cord injury. During the history portion of the examination, what information will be most useful in helping her to obtain a comprehensive picture of his injury? After obtaining the history, what potential complications might this patient experience based on his level of spinal cord injury? Could these complications impact the physical examination?

Spinal cord injury (SCI) can be defined as a lesion to the neural elements within the spinal canal (i.e., the cervical, thoracic, lumbar, and sacral segments of the spinal cord, including the conus medullaris and caudal equina). These injuries can occur due to trauma or congenital in nature, as in spina bifida. For the purpose of this chapter, traumatic and congenital SCI will be treated in the same manner. Estimates of the number of individuals with SCI currently living in the United States have been

TABLE 30.1 Disability Sports

ORGANIZATION	CONTACT INFORMATION
Adaptive snow sports a. Alpine skiing b. Sit skiing c. Adaptive snowboarding d. Cross country skiing e. Sledge hockey	a. http://www.disabledsportsusa.org/adaptive-skiing-alpine/ b. http://www.spinalcord.org/access-sit-ski-solutions/ c. http://www.disabledsportsusa.org/snowboarding/ d. http://www.disabledsportsusa.org/cross-country-skiing/ e. http://www.usahockey.com/sledhockey
Blind sports a. Alpine skiing b. Archery c. Athletics d. Chess e. Football f. Goalball g. Judo h. Nine-pin bowling i. Cycling j. Shooting k. Showdown l. Swimming	http://www.disabledsportsusa.org/adaptive-skiing-alpine/
Wheelchair sports a. Basketball b. Curling c. Racing d. Rugby e. Tennis f. Dance g. Fencing h. Power hockey i. Netball j. Soccer	http://www.wheelchairsportsfederation.org/
Adaptive water sports a. Sailing b. Scuba diving c. Skiing d. Fishing	http://wnyadaptivewatersports.org/wp/

reported as high as 400,000 with approximately 12,000 new injuries each year.[7] The most common cause of traumatic SCIs is motor vehicle accidents, representing approximately 42% of the injuries in the United States. The majority of persons living with SCI are male (82%).[7] Common sports for athletes with SCI include track and field, basketball, and rugby. Athletes with SCI utilize wheelchairs specifically designed for their chosen sport, with the exception being swimming.

Types of Spinal Cord Injury

SCI can be classified into two categories: complete and incomplete. Individuals who have sustained a complete SCI have no sensory or motor function below the level where the injury occurred (**Fig. 30.1**). Individuals who have sustained an incomplete SCI have partial sensory and motor function below the level where the injury occurred. SCI is also described by the *Neurological Level of Injury*, or the lowest or most caudal, fully intact and functioning spinal nerve segment, for both sensory and motor function, after SCI.

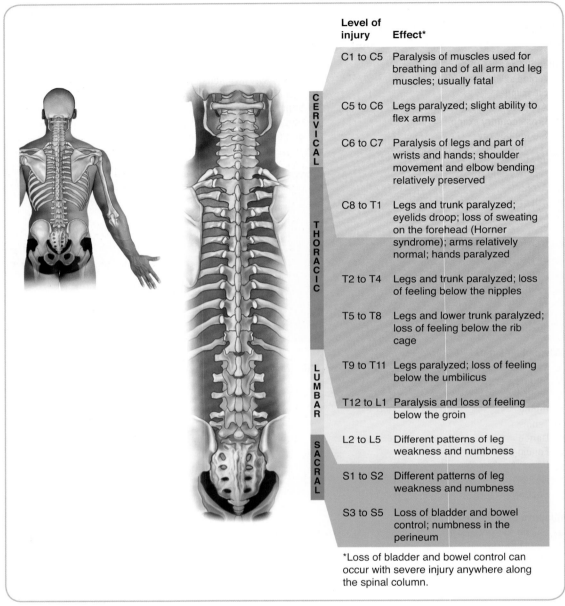

Level of injury	Effect*
C1 to C5	Paralysis of muscles used for breathing and of all arm and leg muscles; usually fatal
C5 to C6	Legs paralyzed; slight ability to flex arms
C6 to C7	Paralysis of legs and part of wrists and hands; shoulder movement and elbow bending relatively preserved
C8 to T1	Legs and trunk paralyzed; eyelids droop; loss of sweating on the forehead (Horner syndrome); arms relatively normal; hands paralyzed
T2 to T4	Legs and trunk paralyzed; loss of feeling below the nipples
T5 to T8	Legs and lower trunk paralyzed; loss of feeling below the rib cage
T9 to T11	Legs paralyzed; loss of feeling below the umbilicus
T12 to L1	Paralysis and loss of feeling below the groin
L2 to L5	Different patterns of leg weakness and numbness
S1 to S2	Different patterns of leg weakness and numbness
S3 to S5	Loss of bladder and bowel control; numbness in the perineum

*Loss of bladder and bowel control can occur with severe injury anywhere along the spinal column.

Figure 30.1. Neurological levels of impairments.

Neurological Level of Injury

The American Spinal Injury Association (ASIA) Impairment Scale describes the neurological levels of injury based on the resulting functional impairments due to SCI.[8] The classifications include the following:

A = Complete: no motor or sensory function in the lowest sacral segment (S4 to S5)

B = Sensory incomplete: some sensory function below neurological level and in S4 to S5

C = Motor incomplete: There is voluntary anal sphincter contraction, with some motor function to three levels below the motor level of the injury, but most of the key muscles are weak.

D = Motor incomplete: the same as C, with the exception that most of the key muscles are fairly strong

E = Normal: Although hyperreflexia may be present, normal sensory and motor recovery are exhibited.

Complete Spinal Cord Injury (Tetraplegia)

Tetraplegia results in impairment of both motor and sensory function of the arms, trunk, legs, and pelvic organs and is caused by complete SCI within the cervical region. Previously, tetraplegia was known as quadriplegia, but both refer to the same condition.[7] Complete SCI at the C1 to C3 level results in the most significant amount of impairment. A person who has sustained a complete SCI between C1 and C3 will need a ventilator in order to breath and will have no motor or sensory function of any of the four extremities. Complete SCI below C3 may require initial use of a ventilator, but eventually, the patient will regain control over lung function, as the lungs are innervated from the C4 nerve root. Patients sustaining complete SCI at the C1 to C4 level are able to control power wheelchairs by manipulating the control stick with the chin or mouth.[8]

Complete SCI at the C5 level results in the ability to flex elbows and the possibility of using hand controls to steer a power wheelchair. It is possible that a person with C5-level SCI may be able to utilize a manually powered wheelchair but will still need assistance with transferring from the wheelchair to another chair or bed.[9]

Persons with complete SCI at the C6 level are able to flex the elbows, flex and extend the wrists, are able to use assistive devices to grasp objects, and provide assistance during transfers. It is also possible for individuals with C6 SCI to drive adaptive vehicles designed with acceleration and breaking controls on the steering wheel.[9]

Persons with complete SCI at the C7/C8 level have the greatest ability to engage in independent living because wrist extension (C7) and finger flexion (C8) is still possible. Assistive devices enable the patient to engage in activities of daily living, including personal care, driving, and even typing.[9]

Incomplete Spinal Cord Injury

Individuals with incomplete SCI will have some degree of sensory and motor function below the point of injury. However, the extent of damage is not known until 6 to 8 weeks after the initial injury. Depending on how the cord has been damaged, an individual may have some sensory function and limited to no motor function, or may have limited to no sensory function but retain motor function. There are five categories of incomplete SCI, and each is named for the portion of the spinal cord that has been damaged (**Box 30.1**).

Thoracic Paraplegia

The majority of individuals with SCI who participate in recreational and competitive sports are thoracic paraplegics, meaning they have full motor and sensory function of the upper extremities

---

BOX 30.1 Classification of Incomplete Spinal Cord Injuries

- **Anterior cord syndrome:** results in an impaired ability to correctly detect temperature, touch, and pain sensations below the point of injury. Eventually, some movement may later be recovered.

- **Central cord syndrome:** results in loss of motor function in the arms but some leg movement is retained. Some recovery is possible.

- **Posterior cord syndrome:** The patient will retain good muscle power, pain, and temperature sensation but have poor coordination.

- **Brown-Sequard syndrome:** results in opposing bilateral function because the damage is to the lateral aspect of the spinal cord. The patient will have unilateral impaired loss of movement but preserved sensation on one side of the body and preserved movement and loss of sensation on the other side of the body.

- **Cauda equina lesion:** results in loss of full or partial sensation below L1 and L2. It is possible that function may eventually be restored.

Adapted from BrainAndSpinalCord.org. Spinal cord injury. http://www.brainandspinalcord.org/spinal-cord-injury.html. Accessed November 24, 2015.

and some of the torso. Individuals with SCI damage between T1 and T6 may obtain a high degree of independency with regard to self-care and wheelchair control. Individuals with damage between T6 and T12 are able to balance and engage quite successfully in recreational and competitive sports and may even walk with the assistance of canes, crutches, or walkers.

Lumbar Paraplegia

Individuals with lumbar paraplegia will have full motor and sensory function of the torso and upper extremities but have varying degrees of motor and sensory deficits in the lower extremities. People who have lumbar and/or sacral spinal cord injuries can obtain full independence, ambulate using walking assistive devices, and even drive. However, spinal cord damage at any level may result in loss of bladder, bowel, and sexual function.

Complications Associated with Spinal Cord Injury

Patients with tetraplegia need varying levels of assistance with feeding, personal hygiene, dressing, toiletry needs, transportation/mobilization, and transfers. Patients with paraplegia may be functionally independent and encounter fewer medical complications associated with their SCI. Depending on the level within the spinal cord where the impairment occurs, attention should be focused on preventing secondary complications from occurring. From a prevention, recognition, possible treatment, and referral perspective, the athletic trainer, as part of the health care team, needs to be aware of several complications associated with SCI.

Urinary Tract Infection and Neurogenic Bowel

Depending on the level of injury, people with tetraplegia have differing levels of bowel and bladder control. **Urinary tract infections** (UTIs) are common among individuals with SCI and may be life threatening if not recognized early and treated.[9] A UTI describes any infection that begins in the urinary system. Although many cases are simply painful and annoying, the condition can become a serious health problem if the infection spreads to the kidneys. Although any structure in the genitourinary system can be infected, most infections occur in the lower tract. **Cystitis** (inflammation of the bladder) and **urethritis** (inflammation of the urethra) are the most common basis for UTIs. Most cases are caused by *Escherichia coli*, which ascend the urinary tract from the opening in the urethra. The bacteria also may be introduced during urinary tract catheterization. Elite athletes competing with complete SCI catheterize an average of four times a day and often reuse the same catheter multiple times, increasing the risk of developing UTIs.[10] Some individuals may present with very few symptoms, yet have significant **bacteriuria**. An individual with cystitis may complain of pain during urination (**dysuria**), urinary frequency and urgency, and pain superior to the pubic region. However, in the athlete with SCI, the patient has no or limited sensory function, so may be unable to feel the pain or the need to void. Therefore, care should be taken to inspect the urine for cloudiness, blood, or a foul-smelling odor. Other symptoms, such as high fever, shaking, chills, nausea, and vomiting, may indicate a simultaneous upper UTI of the kidney (**acute pyelonephritis**).

Following complete SCI, **neurogenic bowel** occurs due to impaired sphincter muscle control and disruption of normal ambulation impacting normal bowel motility. As a result, constipation or fecal incontinence may occur, posing serious health concerns for the individual with SCI.[10] Clinically, neurogenic bowel presents one of two ways, depending on the level of spinal cord impairment. The ability to voluntarily control the external anal sphincter muscle is impaired, resulting in the rectum being constantly constricted, and an inability to voluntarily expel fecal matter. This is due to injury to the spinal cord above the conus medullaris (lower end of the spinal cord between T12 and L1) and is referred to as **upper motor neuron (UMN) bowel syndrome**. In order for the stools to be evacuated, the rectum must be externally stimulated. Injury to the spinal cord below the conus medullaris and cauda equina causes a loss in control over anal muscles that control the opening to the rectum and is referred to as **lower motor neuron (LMN) bowel syndrome**. LMN bowel syndrome is characterized by both constipation and fecal incontinence.[11]

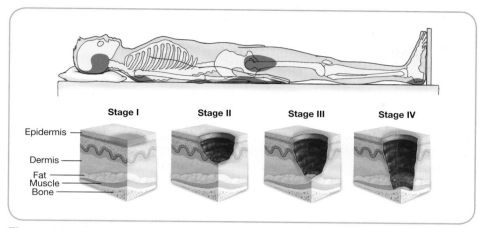

Figure 30.2. Classification of pressure sores by stage.

Pressure Sores

Pressure sores are also referred to as bedsores or decubitus ulcers. As the name implies, the lesions are caused by constant pressure applied over a period time, most often in areas of boney prominences. Pressure sores are frequently found over the ischial tuberosity, greater trochanter, medial epicondyle of the femurs, and the posterior aspect of the calcaneus and elbows. The skin is able to withstand pressure for short periods of time before the tissue begins to break down. Because of the sensory deficits experienced by individuals with SCI, the brain does not receive the pressure or pain impulses, nor can the individual redistribute the weight in order to relieve the pressure on the affected area. The rate of blood flow is decreased as well, and as a result, the healing process is impaired.[12] The skin begins to break down after about 15 minutes of constant pressure, with the first sign being redness. Tissue break down occurs in four stages (**Fig. 30.2**). **Application Strategy 30.1** describes the signs of pressure sores as well as the management of each stage. If left untreated, bedsores can be life threatening, as the infection may spread to the vital organs. Other causes of bedsores include prolonged exposure to wet skin from sweat, stool or urine, and bruises, burns, or scrapes that go untreated.[12]

Blood Clots

Individuals with SCI are at risk for developing a blood clot, or **deep vein thrombosis** (DVT), due to the lack of muscle contraction and decreased blood flow, especially during the acute phase of an injury and when bedridden.[13,14] Preventive measures include the use of compression stockings and blood thinners. Blood clots form most often in the veins of the thigh and lower leg. If the clot becomes dislodged, it may travel through the body to the lungs, resulting in a pulmonary embolism. DVTs may present with or without symptoms. In the SCI population, DVTs may be even more difficult to recognize because the patient may not experience the pain and tenderness that can be present with this condition. The affected area may become swollen and red in the absence of any known trauma.[15] If a DVT is suspected, refer the patient to the nearest medical facility immediately.

Respiratory Considerations

As mentioned in the discussion on DVTs, individuals with SCI are at risk for developing a **pulmonary embolism** (PE) secondary to a DVT. Again, the risk is highest during the acute phase of the initial injury but should always be a concern in any SCI patient. A patient experiencing a PE may present with difficulty breathing, arrhythmia, tachycardia, chest pain or discomfort, excessive coughing or coughing up blood, light-headedness, low blood pressure, and fainting.[15] For patients with SCI, signs are dependent on the level at which the spine has been damaged. A more common respiratory complication is **pneumonia**. Preventative measures include working with a respiratory therapist on breathing exercises. Please refer to Chapter 26 for a full discussion on the causes, sign and symptoms, complications, and management options of pneumonia.

APPLICATION STRATEGY 30.1

Stages of Pressure Sore Progression and Management Strategies

Stage 1

Signs

- Redness or discoloration appearing within 15 minutes that does not resolve or fade within 30 minutes

Management

- If area is wet, clean with mild soap and water, patting the skin dry (not wiping) with a soft cloth. Ensure that clothing and padding are also dry.
- Continue to monitor the area. If redness/discoloration does not resolve within 2 days, refer the patient for further medical evaluation.

Prevention

- Keep the area clean and dry.
- Check for sources of friction, such as worn out padding and replace as needed. Inspect any protective equipment, seat cushions, and straps and replace as needed.
- Immediately attend to bruises, scraps, and burns.

Stage 2

Signs

- The epidermis appears broken, and a wound begins to appear. Drainage may or may not be present.

Management

- The wound should be cleaned with saline and patted dry using a soft, sterile cloth. If little to no drainage is present, use a bio-occlusive, self-adherent hydrocolloid dressing to prevent infection. This may be left in place for up to 5 days, but the patient should be inspected frequently for signs of infection.

Prevention

- Consult frequently with a medical director during this period and immediately refer the patient if the condition deteriorates. Keep the area dry and reduce the amount of pressure placed on the area if possible.

Stage 3

Signs

- The depth of the wound extends into the dermis and underlying tissues.

Management

- Contact a medical director for instructions on special cleaning and debriding techniques. The wound may need to be packed and antibiotics administered.

Prevention

- May be necessary to utilize a mechanical pneumatic mattress or chair seats that constantly change the pressure of the surface in contact with the affected area. Continue to monitor, keeping the area dry and clean.

Stage 4

Signs

- Tissue damage extends into the muscle and the bone may be visible. Dead and damaged tissue is clearly seen and may be accompanied by a foul smell.

Treatment

- Consult your medical director immediately as surgery is needed.

Autonomic Dysreflexia

Autonomic dysreflexia is a life-threatening condition seen in both the acute and chronic phases of injury for individuals having sustained SCI above the T6 level. Pain or irritation due to abnormal conditions below the damaged spinal segment attempt to send a signal to the brain that is interrupted and/or interpreted incorrectly. The most common trigger is irritation of the bladder or colon.[16] In response, the blood pressure rises and heart rate may increase or decrease. The patient may have no symptoms or may complain of a headache and mild discomfort. However, if the blood pressure continues to rise and causes increasing intracranial pressure, the condition may become a life-threatening emergency. Potential outcomes include intracranial hemorrhage, retinal detachment, seizures, and death.[16] Two important factors that influence the severity and occurrence are the level of injury and the completeness of a SCI. There is a greater cardiovascular response at higher levels of injury. About 27% of tetraplegics with incomplete SCI will present with autonomic dysreflexia as compared to 91% of tetraplegics with complete lesions. One way to prevent an occurrence of autonomic dysreflexia is eliminating the cause of the irritation. Because a common cause of the condition is from bowel or bladder irritation, it is imperative that anticholinergic drugs and clean intermittent catheterization techniques are utilized.[10]

Spastic Muscles

In the months following the initial SCI, the patient may experience muscle **hypertonus**, **hyperreflexia**, **clonus**, and muscle spasm.[17] In fact, 80% of people who have suffered SCI develop muscle spasticity. Acute prolonged spasmodic episodes may be triggered by superficial cutaneous stimulation, exposure to heat or cold, and bladder distention. Episodes may be so violent and forceful that the patient may be thrown out of his or her wheelchair or fracture bones. Spasticity eventually results in permanent muscle contraction and shortening. Management is rendered in the form of physical, pharmaceutical, surgical, and electrical interventions.

Diminished, Absent, or Altered Pain Response

A diminished or absent pain response[18] may contribute to the development of pressure sores and the failure to notice the presence of wounds, injuries, infections, and other conditions for which pain is the first indication. However, persons with SCI also may develop chronic pain as well as experience pain arising from different areas within the body that is manifested differently than before the injury occurred. **Table 30.2** describes the different types of pain individuals with SCI most often experience.

TABLE 30.2 Pain Experienced by Individual with Spinal Cord Injury		
TYPE	**DESCRIPTION/CAUSE**	**TREATMENT**
Neurogenic pain	Burning, tingling, or stabbing pain arising from areas of the body that no longer have sensory innervation. This results as a failure of the brain to receive all the needed information to properly interpret the origin and cause of the pain.	Neurogenic pain is difficult to treat as the origin is unknown. Onset of neurogenic pain years after the initial injury is cause for alarm, because it may indicate the onset of a new pathology.
Musculoskeletal pain	Aching, dull throbbing pain that increases with activity and is relieved by rest. Pain can usually be traced to repetitive motions such as using the upper extremity to propel a wheelchair, throwing motions in sports, and so forth.	Musculoskeletal pain is treated through activity modification, ergonomic corrections to equipment, as well as therapeutic pain management interventions.
Visceral or referred pain	Cramping, aching, stabbing pain located in the stomach or abdomen and low to mid back may indicate complications with the digestive system. The pain may not be experienced over the organ that is involved but referred to another part of the viscera.	Onset of referred pain warrants patient referral for further medical assessment.
Chronic pain	Pain that is constant, lasting for months and even years in areas that have normal sensation, as well as noninnervated areas is considered chronic pain.	Chronic pain has a psychological component, often contributing to depression. Work in consultation with a medical director and mental health provider to treat the patient's chronic pain.

Patients may describe a burning, tingling, or stabbing pain arising from areas of their body that no longer have sensory innervation. This type of pain is called **neurogenic pain** and is a result of a failure of the brain to receive all the needed information to properly interpret the origin and cause of the pain. This type of pain is difficult to treat because the origin is unknown. Onset of neurogenic pain years after the initial injury is cause for alarm, because it may indicate the onset of a new pathology.

Effects on Exercise

There are several physiological changes which may occur following SCI that can affect exercise training and testing. Many changes occur due to associated damage to the sympathetic nervous system. The heart may be affected due to sympathetic outflow from the medulla to the SA node being partially interrupted between T1 and T4 nerve roots and completely interrupted above T1. With these individuals, increases in heart rate will occur due to the vagus nerve and the Frank-Starling mechanism being intact.[19] Heart rate, blood pressure, and blood vessel constriction may also be affected due to the separation of the adrenal medullae from normal innervation. SCI above T5 completely separates the adrenal medullae from normal innervation and SCI between T5 and T9 results in partial innervation. Leg vasomotor control can also be compromised; normally, vasoconstriction facilitates shunting of blood to active muscles during exercise and venoconstriction aids venous return from the legs to the heart when upright. SCI above L1 results in complete separation of the leg vasculature from the central nervous system (CNS), and SCI between L1 and L2 can lead to partial separation. The accumulated effects of this is often referred to as **sympathetic decentralization** which can result in venous pooling, orthostatic and exercise hypotension, edema, and thermoregulation issues.[19] Due to these issues, most adaptations during exercise with SCI individuals are more peripheral in nature (e.g., increased size, strength, endurance, aerobic power, anaerobic power, blood flow, enzymes, and glycogen) as opposed to central adaptations (e.g., increased stroke volume, cardiac output, blood volume, oxygen delivery, and high-density lipoprotein cholesterol). Medications, such as muscle relaxants, anticonvulsants, and antibiotics, may also have an effect on one's response to exercise.[19]

Injury Diagnosis, Treatment, and Rehabilitation Considerations

Sensory dysfunctions can make the SCI individual more susceptible to easy burning of the skin in areas of sensory impairments. When stimuli are applied to sensory-compromised areas, decubitus ulcers, pain, and dysesthesia may also occur. Motor dysfunction can lead to muscle atrophy and deterioration, flaccid or spastic paralysis, cardiovascular deconditioning, and osteoporosis in areas where motor control has been compromised. Taking these into account, it is very difficult to diagnose and treat injuries that occur in a sensory-compromised area. *The use of heat and cold modalities must be monitored very closely.* The use of the upper extremity for ambulation by individuals with SCI must be a concern when designing exercise treatment and rest protocols. **Table 30.3** contains the most common injuries seen in individuals with SCI.[19]

There are several considerations that must be made during the rehabilitation process due to the sympathetic nervous system, sensory, and motor deficits. Many individuals with SCI will have pronounced orthostatic and postexercise hypotension.[19] All exercise sessions must take place in a safe environment taking into account compromised balance due to motor dysfunction. Autonomic dysreflexia may also be a concern for individuals with quadriplegia. Many individuals may have a compromised

TABLE 30.3 Common Injuries Sustained by Athletes with Spinal Cord Injury

OVERUSE INJURIES	OVEREXERTION INJURIES	SOFT TISSUE INJURIES	LOW BACK PAIN
Shoulder impingement	Muscle strains	Blisters	Soft tissue: muscle or ligament
Tendinitis and bursitis	Sprains	Abrasions	Mechanical or biomechanical: joint
Carpal tunnel syndrome	Contusions	Lacerations	Neurological: nerve root impingement

thermoregulatory system that can result in impaired perspiration mechanisms; therefore, exercise environment temperature will be a concern. Surgical issues such as fusions, internal fixation devices, and shunts must be addressed when designing a rehabilitation program.[19]

During the history portion of the examination process, Mary should ask if the patient had a complete or incomplete SCI and if the patient knows his ASIA neurological level of impairment. If the patient responds that he has an incomplete SCI, Mary can then determine the classification of the incomplete SCI. Individuals with SCI are at a higher risk than AB individuals for developing UTIs and neurogenic bowel. During the history, Mary should ask specific questions about the patient's bladder and bowel function as well as perform abdominal percussion and auscultation. Urinalysis and temperature assessment will provide useful information regarding these conditions. Lung auscultations and percussions will assist in assessing for the presence of respiratory complications. A vital sign and cranial nerve assessment should be performed to rule out possible autonomic dysreflexia. Mary should also inquire about potential hot spots that may develop into pressure sores and inspect the skin in areas that are more susceptible to developing these sores. Finally, a musculoskeletal assessment that includes range of motion and manual muscle testing along with myotome, dermatome, and deep tendon reflexes would be beneficial for assessing spasticity associated with SCI. Depending on the patient's level of neurological impairment, the area needing treatment may have sensory and motor deficits. In patents with sensory deficit, care should be taken to avoid using modalities that may burn the skin because the patient will be unable to detect the painful stimuli. If working on core stabilization or dynamic strength in a rehabilitation program, the patient needs to be supported and secured to prevent falling. Another concern is orthostatic hypertension, so it is imperative to slowly progress the patient through positional changes in posture.

CEREBRAL PALSY

Tyrese is providing athletic training services at a cerebral palsy (CP) race walking event. A coach has asked him to look at one of her athletes. Tyrese confirms that this is not an emergent situation with the athlete and asks the coach what type of CP the athlete has. How will the knowledge of the type of CP that the athlete has impact the history taking and physical examination of the athlete?

Athletes with CP will compete as ambulatory athletes or utilize wheelchairs specifically designed for their sports. Common sports for athletes with CP include 7-a-side football (soccer), race running, athletics, snow skiing, and table cricket.[20] In race running, participants use three-wheeled tricycles designed to support the upper body, yet allow appropriate space for using the legs to run (**Fig. 30.3**). The different stresses on the body during training and competition must be considered when working with athletes with CP.

Pathophysiology, Common Causes, and Risk Factors

CP is defined as a nonprogressive lesion or malformation of the brain that interferes with normal brain development before, during, or immediately after birth.[20] The condition damages areas of the brain that control muscle tone and spinal reflexes and results in limited ability to move and maintain posture and balance. CP is not one disease with a single cause, but a group of disorders that are related. About 85% of CP cases occur before birth and it occurs in as many as 5 out of 1,000 live births.

CP has several suspected causes: infections during pregnancy, such as German measles or rubella, which can cause damage to the developing nervous system; Rh incompatibility in which the mother's body produces immune cells (antibodies) that destroy the fetus's blood cells leading to

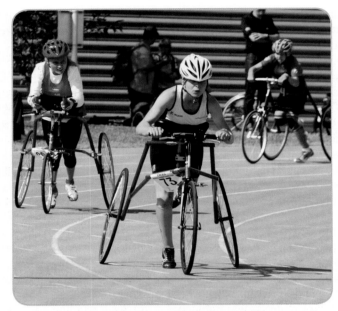

Figure 30.3. **Race walking with assistance from a modified wheel chair.** (Used with permission, Hannah Dines/Matthew Hamilton [photographer].)

jaundice, which can damage brain cells and lead to severe oxygen shortage in the brain; or trauma to the head during labor and delivery. Medical mistakes are also commonly blamed for cases of CP. Impairments may include cognitive, visual, hearing, speech, and swallowing difficulties. Factors that increase the risk for CP include breech presentation, complicated labor and delivery, low Apgar score (heart rate, breathing, muscle tone, reflexes, and skin color), low birth weight, multiple births, nervous system malformations, such as microcephaly, and maternal bleeding, or severe proteinuria late in pregnancy.

Types of Cerebral Palsy

CP may be described by the body part that has been impacted by the condition, how a person's movements are affected, and by the severity of impairments (**Fig 30.4**).[21] **Quadriplegia CP** is used to describe bilateral involvement of both the upper and lower extremity, as well as the muscles of the trunk, face, and mouth.[20] **Diplegia CP** describes involvement of both legs, with some involvement of the arms. When the arm and leg on the same side are affected, the term used to describe the condition is **hemiplegia**. Spastic, dyskinetic, and ataxic are terms used to describe CP by how movement is impaired.

Spastic CP occurs when there is damage to the motor cortex of the brain and accounts for 70% to 80% of all CP.[22] Spasticity is an abnormal increase in muscle tone or stiffness, limiting range of motion and normal muscle length and function. A person with spastic CP may present with increased muscle tone (*hypertonicity*), rapid, serial muscle contractions (*clonus*), involuntary crossing of the legs (*scissoring*), or fixed joints due to sustained muscle *contracture*.

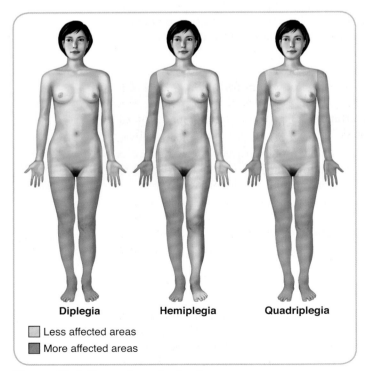

Diplegia   Hemiplegia   Quadriplegia

☐ Less affected areas
■ More affected areas

Figure 30.4. **Types of cerebral palsy.**

Additional impairment may include muscle spasm and exaggerated deep tendon reflexes.[23] Spasticity may result in permanent flexion contractures of the elbows, wrists, and fingers in the upper extremity and of the hip and knees in the lower extremity. As the gastrocnemius–soleus complex shortens, an equinovarus foot posture may occur. Overtime, specificity will result in atrophy of the soft tissue, joint contractures, and skeletal deformity and pain.[22]

Dyskinetic CP occurs in about 6% of persons with CP and is caused by damage to the basal ganglia of the brain.[24] A person with dyskinetic CP presents with involuntary motion that occurs when the person is attempting voluntary movement. Slow twisting movements or repetitive movements are referred to as **dystonia** or dyskinesia. **Athetosis** is alternating episodes of hypotonus and extreme motion. Athetosis is sometimes described as slow, writhing, restless movements. Individuals with **chorea**, a third form of dyskinesia, present with brief, abrupt, irregular, and unpredictable movements that may at times appear wild and violent.[24]

Ataxic CP results when the centers within the cerebellum that control posture have been damaged.[25] A person with ataxic CP will appear clumsy, uncoordinated, shaky, and unsteady. Hand tremors, imprecise movement, and difficulty grasping small objects are commonly seen in the upper extremity, whereas a wide-base gait, staggering, and frequent falling is seen in the lower extremity. Ataxic CP will also affect speech, swallowing, and eye movement.

Knowing the type of CP an individual has should provide the athletic trainer with a better understanding of the potential complications and concerns the person may encounter during athletic and recreational activities. Understanding these classification systems, in particular, knowing the impact on gross motor function, fine motor function, and communication function, will allow for appropriate modifications to sports and protective equipment based on the needs of the individual.[21]

The Gross Motor Function Classification System–Expanded & Revised

This classification system uses the ability to self-initiate mobility with regard to standing, walking, and wheeled conveyance to assess gross motor function and ability. Testing is conducted in the individual's own environment (home, school, work, community) making this a true functional assessment.[26] The Gross Motor Function Classification System–Expanded & Revised (GMFCS–E&R) has five distinct classifications that can serve to clarify the appropriate assistive technologies the individual needs. Although this tool is designed to assess persons in age bands 6 to 12 years old and 12 to 18 years old, the GMFCS–E&R classification rarely changes older than 5 years. Therefore, it is likely that once the initial needed assistive devices are identified, a person with CP will most likely need the same assistance/adaptations throughout the lifespan.[21] The GMFCS–E&R classifications are presented in **Table 30.4**.

The Manual Ability Classification System

The Manual Ability Classification System (MACS) is a classification system for children with CP ages 4 to 18 years and examines fine motor skills when engaging in activities of daily living.[27] The system includes five categories describing how the child attempts to self-initiate manipulation of everyday objects and their most frequently used fine motor skills. See **Table 30.5** for MACS classification descriptors.

The Communication Function Classification System

This classification system is used to classify everyday communication needs based on five areas of effective communication.[28] Consistent with the MACS and GMFCS, the Communication Function Classification System (CFCS) also incorporates activity and participation levels as described in the World Health Organization's (WHO) International Classification of Functioning, Disability, and Health (ICF). CFCS classification levels can be viewed in **Table 30.6**.

Effects on Exercise

There has been very little research involving CP and exercise due to the fact that individuals with CP historically didn't participate in exercise.[29] With spasticity and inefficient mobility present, higher than expected exercise response values are seen. Individuals with CP will have higher heart rate, blood pressure, expired air, and blood lactate levels than AB individuals at equal work rates. Reduced mechanical efficiency will also be seen due to the extra energy required to overcome muscle

TABLE 30.4 Gross Motor Function Classification System—Extended & Revised

FOR CHILDREN/YOUTH BETWEEN THEIR 6TH AND 18TH BIRTHDAY

LEVEL	DESCRIPTORS
1	Can walk indoors and outdoors and climb stairs without using hands for support Can perform usual activities such as running and jumping Has decreased speed, balance, and coordination
2	Has the ability to walk indoors and outdoors and climb stairs with a railing Has difficulty with uneven surfaces, inclines, or in crowds Has only minimal ability to run or jump
3	Walks with assistive mobility devices indoors and outdoors on level surfaces May be able to climb stairs using a railing May propel a manual wheelchair (may require assistance for long distances or uneven surfaces)
4	Walking ability is severely limited even with assistive devices. Uses wheelchairs most of the time and may propel their own power wheelchair May participate in standing transfers
5	Has physical impairments that restrict voluntary control of movement and the ability to maintain head and neck position against gravity Is impaired in all areas of motor function Cannot sit or stand independently, even with adaptive equipment Cannot independently walk although may be able to use powered mobility

Adapted from Figoni S. Spinal cord disabilities: paraplegia and tetraplegia. In: Durstine JL, Moore GE, eds. *ACSM's Exercise Management for Persons with Chronic Diseases and Disabilities*. Champaign, IL: Human Kinetics; 2009; Cerebral Palsy International Sports and Recreation Association. Sports. http://cpisra.org/dir/sports/. Accessed December 10, 2015.

tonus in spastic CP. Maximal physiological responses to exercise have been shown to be 10% to 20% lower than AB individuals with physical work capacity as much as 50% lower.[29] This low work capacity and maximal responses may be related to low fitness levels and poor exercise habits. However, they may also be presented due to difficulty performing movements, muscle imbalances, and poor functional strength. Considering the nature of disability, there is no reason not to expect benefits from exercise. The limited research has observed some benefits, such as increased heart and lung efficiency and increased strength, flexibility, mobility, and coordination. Exercise can also be expected to help maintain bone mineral density, assist in weight control, and reduce the risk of chronic diseases as seen in AB individuals.

TABLE 30.5 Manual Abilities Classification System

LEVEL	DESCRIPTOR
1	Objects are handled easily and successfully.
2	Handles most objects but with some reduced quality and/or speed
3	Handles objects with difficulty—the child will need help to prepare and/or modify activities.
4	Handles a limited selection of easily managed objects and always requires some help from others
5	The child is not able to handle objects or to complete even simple actions with their hands.

Adapted from Figoni S. Spinal cord disabilities: paraplegia and tetraplegia. In: Durstine JL, Moore GE, eds. *ACSM's Exercise Management for Persons with Chronic Diseases and Disabilities*. Champaign, IL: Human Kinetics; 2009; Cerebral Palsy Alliance. Types of cerebral palsy. https://www.cerebralpalsy.org.au/what-is-cerebral-palsy/types-of-cerebral-palsy/. Accessed December 10, 2015.

LEVEL	DESCRIPTOR
TABLE 30.6 Communication Function Classification System	
1	A person independently and effectively alternates between being a sender and receiver of information with most people in most environments
2	A person independently alternates between being a sender and receiver with most people in most environments but the conversation may be slower
3	A person usually communicates effectively with familiar communication partners, but not unfamiliar partners, in most environments
4	The person is not always consistent at communicating with familiar communication partners.
5	A person is seldom able to communicate effectively even with familiar people.

Adapted from Figoni S. Spinal cord disabilities: paraplegia and tetraplegia. In: Durstine JL, Moore GE, eds. *ACSM's Exercise Management for Persons with Chronic Diseases and Disabilities*. Champaign, IL: Human Kinetics; 2009; Cerebral Palsy Alliance. Spastic cerebral palsy. https://www.cerebralpalsy .org.au/what-is-cerebral-palsy/types-of-cerebral-palsy/spastic-cerebral-palsy/. Accessed December 12, 2015.

Injury Diagnosis, Treatment, and Rehabilitation Considerations

Injury diagnosis can be very difficult with individuals with CP due to the irregularities of muscle tone and movement. Range of motion and manual muscle testing can be of little use when diagnosing an injured individual with CP. Palpation can often be difficult due to excessive neuromuscular excitability seen in many individuals. Therefore, the athletic trainer must often rely almost exclusively on the history, mechanism of injury, and visual observation when diagnosing the injury.[29] The aforementioned irregularities will also have an effect on the treatment of individuals. The application of modalities may trigger episodes of spasticity and neuromuscular excitability. Additionally, these irregularities may inhibit the athlete's ability to keep body parts in certain positions for extended periods of time.

Athletes with CP may compete in wheelchair activities or ambulatory events depending on the severity of their movement dysfunction. Athletes utilizing wheelchairs will experience many of the injuries common to athletes with SCI, whereas ambulatory athletes will commonly incur many of the injuries seen with AB athletes.[29]

The irregularities of muscle tone and movement must be considered when designing an injury treatment protocol for athletes with CP. Modes of exercise will be very dependent on ability. Leg cycle, wheelchair, and arm crank ergometers may be used for aerobic conditioning, as well as traditional ambulatory methods. Muscular strength and endurance can be increased using traditional methods, such as free weight and weight machines, and have also been found to have some positive effect on specificity.[29] Many athletes with CP may have compromised balance which must be considered at all times. Rehabilitation should focus on flexibility to prevent joint contractures. Traditional therapies such as massage, stretching, hydrotherapy, cryotherapy, thermotherapy, and neuromuscular inhabitation may be useful.[30] Keep in mind that many athletes with CP may be taking antiseizure, as well as muscle relaxant medications, which may slow the physiological responses to exercise.[29]

 By knowing if the athlete has quadriplegia, hemiplegia, or diplegia CP, Tyrese will have an expectation of where he should see impairment. Likewise, knowing if the individual has spastic, dyskinetic, or ataxic CP provides Tyrese with baseline information on the athlete's gross motor function, fine motor function, and communication function. Individuals with CP often have irregularities in muscle tone and movement, as well as hyper- or hyponeurological responses. Because range of motion, manual muscle testing, and palpation will be of little use when diagnosing an injured individual with CP, the athletic trainer must rely almost exclusively on the history, mechanism of injury, and visual observation when diagnosing the injury.

AMPUTATION

 What biomechanical factors can increase the risk of injury for an amputee?

Within the United States, there are approximately 2 million people who have experienced amputation of a limb. Common causes of amputations include vascular disease, trauma, and cancer.[31] Athletes with amputation may compete using a wheelchair or with or without prosthetics. Common sports for athletes with amputation included track and field, swimming, basketball, volleyball, and cycling. When working with individuals with amputations, having a shared language is important for increased communication. Commonly used terms are presented in **Table 30.7**.

Pathophysiology, Common Causes, and Risk Factors

Amputations may be a surgical amputation and removal of any part of the body, or a congenital amputation where an individual is born without a limb or limbs. The more common causes for surgical amputation are diabetes (50%), injuries, infections, tumors, and insufficient blood supply.[32] Congenital amputation occurs in approximately 1 in 2,000 newborns, and the cause is rarely known. Modern technology has significantly helped individuals who have incurred an amputation through improved rehabilitation of badly damaged limbs and the increased technology of prosthetic devices.

Effects on Exercise

Physiological adaptations to exercise training are similar to AB individuals. The effect on exercise training and testing in individuals with amputation is very individualized depending on where the amputation has occurred, therefore individualization is the key.[33] Testing and training should be focused

TABLE 30.7 Common Terminology in Amputee Sports	
TERM	**DEFINITION**
Acquired amputation	Surgical removal of a limb (i.e., traumatic, elective, disease)
AE	Above the elbow amputation; transhumeral
AK	Above the knee amputation; transfemoral
Amputee/limb loss athlete	At least one major joint or part of an extremity missing
BE	Below the elbow amputation; transradial
BK	Below the knee amputation; transtibial
Blade runners	Term for amputee sprinters
Congenital amputation	Born missing a limb, "limb deficient"
Day leg	Prosthetic designed for everyday activity, occasionally worn for some of the field events
DBK	Double below knee amputation (bilateral)
Intact limb	Nonamputated limb
Phantom limb	Sensation that the missing limb is still attached
Phantom pain	Pain sensation arising from missing limb
Residual limb	Portion of limb remaining after amputation (i.e., stump or residuum)

Adapted from Hetzler T, Smith AE, Rempe D. Amputee athletes, part I: foundational knowledge. *Int J Athl Ther Train*. 2014;19(2):33–38.

on mobilization of all available muscle mass. Depending on the area of amputation, testing and training can be conducted using an arm crank or wheelchair ergometer, bicycle, or treadmill. Depending on the area and level of the amputation, scar tissue in the knee, hip, shoulder, or elbow may be a limiting factor to exercise with the affected area.

Injury Diagnosis, Treatment, and Rehabilitation Considerations

The biomechanics of individuals with amputations will be altered placing the individual at greater risk for sustaining chronic, overuse, and stress-related injury. There are three primary reasons why biomechanical function is a major factor for amputees and injury. First, the intact limb (if one exists) and core must compensate for loss of power, control, endurance, and force no longer generated by the lost limb.[34] The individual must develop and refine new/altered patterns of movement as he or she learn how to compete at increasing levels of competition. Second, depending on the prosthetic worn, changes to the individual's center of gravity may occur, as well as alteration in the running gait.[35] Stress will be generated and transmitted differently, to which the body must adapt. If increased stress and adaptation do not occur together or are not addressed through appropriate preventative and treatment measures, the individual is at greater risk for developing stress response or overuse injury such as low back pain, chronic hamstring strains, and lateral hip pain for athletes with lower limb amputation.[34,35] Athletes with upper extremity amputations have a higher incidence of shoulder, cervical, and thoracic conditions.[34] Finally, the skin should be inspected frequently for deterioration associated with constant pressure applied by the prosthetic and/or securing straps. Pressure sores, addressed earlier in this chapter, as well as blisters, rashes, and wounds frequently occur in areas where a constant load is applied. Individuals will attempt to alter biomechanics in order to relieve the pressure being applied to the involved area.

Injury rehabilitation considerations are similar to AB individuals with the exception of the increased incidence of scar tissue at the distal end of the limb. Muscle imbalances, flexibility, and proper gait mechanics must be addressed. Core stabilization exercises, increasing proprioception, and improving balance also decrease risk of injury.[33–35] Phantom limb pain may be present in some athletes with amputations. This is due to a reorganization of the cerebral cortex in which the area of the cortex serving the amputated limb enlarges and the neurons cause pain. Although phantom pain is commonly experienced by individuals with amputations, the pain should not be dismissed but instead, requires the clinician to rule out other causes. Multiple treatment options are available to treat phantom pain, ranging from basic physical therapy to pharmaceutical interventions, although none have been found to be more successful than another.

With an amputation, the intact limb and core must compensate for loss of power, control, endurance, and force no longer generated by the lost limb, thereby making it necessary to develop and refine new/altered patterns of movement as they learn how to compete at increasing levels of competition. Depending on the prosthetic worn, changes to the individual's center of gravity may also occur, as well as alterations in the running gait leading to stress being generated and transmitted differently throughout the body. If increased stress and adaptation do not occur together or are not addressed through appropriate preventative and treatment measures, the individual is at greater risk for developing stress response or overuse injuries. Finally, constant pressure applied by the prosthetic and/or securing straps may lead to pressure sores, blisters, rashes, and wounds. Individuals may then attempt to alter biomechanics in order to relieve the pressure being applied to the involved area, thus increasing the risk for further injury.

SUMMARY

1. Athletes participating in Paralympic sports are grouped based on disability: physical impairment, visual impairment, and intellectual impairment. Physical impairment includes impaired muscle power, impaired passive range of motion, loss of limb or limb deficit, leg length difference, short stature, hypertonia, ataxia, and athetosis.

2. Individuals who have sustained a complete SCI have no sensory or motor function below the level where the injury occurred. Individuals who have sustained an incomplete SCI have partial sensory and motor function below the level where the injury occurred.

3. The ASIA Impairment Scale describes the neurological level of injury based on the resulting functional impairments due to the SCI.

   A = Complete: no motor or sensory function in the lowest sacral segment (S4 to S5)

   B = Sensory incomplete: some sensory function below neurological level and in S4 to S5

   C = Motor incomplete: There is voluntary anal sphincter contraction, with some motor function to three levels below the motor level of the injury, but most of the key muscles are weak.

   D = Motor incomplete: the same as C, with the exception that most of the key muscles are fairly strong

   E = Normal: Although hyperreflexia may be present, normal sensory and motor recovery are exhibited.

4. Tetraplegia results in impairment of both motor and sensory function of the arms, trunk, legs, and pelvic organs and is caused by complete SCI within the cervical region. Persons with tetraplegia need assistance with most personal care needs and activities of daily living.

5. The majority of individual with SCI who participate in recreational and competitive sports are thoracic paraplegics, meaning they have full motor and sensory function of the upper extremities and some of the torso.

6. Individuals with lumbar paraplegia will have full motor and sensory function of the torso and upper extremities but have varying degrees of motor and sensory deficits in the lower extremities.

7. Because of limited mobility and impaired innervation to the muscles controlling bladder and bowel function, persons with SCI are at greater risk for developing UTIs and neurogenic bowel.

8. Lack of mobility and impaired innervation in SCI individuals contribute to the increased risk for developing pressure sores, blood clots, DVT, and potential PEs.

9. Autonomic dysreflexia is a life-threatening condition seen in both the acute and chronic phases of injury for individuals having sustained SCI above the T6 level. Inability to receive and/or accurately analyze pain originating from below the injury causes an exaggerated increase in blood pressure and heart rate, thus increasing intracranial pressure that may lead to death.

10. Spasticity is an abnormal increase in muscle tone or stiffness, limiting range of motion and normal muscle length and function. A person with spastic CP may present with increased muscle tone (hypertonicity); rapid, serial muscle contractions (clonus); involuntary crossing of the legs (scissoring); fixed joints due to sustained muscle contracture; and exaggerated deep tendon reflexes. Overtime, specificity will result in atrophy of the soft tissue, joint contractures and skeletal deformity, and pain.

11. Physiological changes in the SCI patient due to associated damage to the sympathetic nervous system, referred to as sympathetic decentralization, can result in venous pooling, orthostatic and exercise hypotension, edema, and thermoregulation issues.

12. CP is defined as a nonprogressive lesion or malformation of the brain that interferes with normal brain development before, during, or immediately after birth. The condition damages areas of the brain that control muscle tone and spinal reflexes and results in limited ability to move and maintain posture and balance.

13. The ability to make appropriate modifications to sports and protective equipment based on the needs of the individual requires the athletic trainer to understand CP classification systems relating to gross motor function, fine motor function, and communication function. The three primary classifications systems are GMFCS–E&R, the MACS, and the CFCS.

14. Due to spasticity and inefficient mobility present, higher than expected exercise response values are seen in individuals with CP, such as a higher heart rate, blood pressure, expired air, and blood lactate levels than AB individuals at equal work rates.

15. Athletic trainers must rely almost exclusively on history, mechanism, and visual observation when diagnosing an injury in CP patients.

16. Common causes of amputations include vascular disease, trauma, cancer, and congenital factors. Amputations are classified by body part and proximity to the nearest joint.

17. The biomechanics of individuals with amputations will be altered and, therefore, place the individual at greater risk for sustaining chronic, overuse, and stress-related injury, such as low back pain, chronic hamstring strains, and lateral hip pain for athletes with lower limb amputation. Upper extremity amputees experience shoulder, thoracic, and cervical pathology.

18. The skin at the site of the amputation should be inspected frequently for deterioration associated with constant pressure applied by the prosthetic and/or securing straps. Pressure sores, blisters, rashes, and wounds frequently occur in areas where a constant load is applied.

REFERENCES

1. International Paralympic Committee. Paralympics: history of a movement. http://www.paralympic.org/the-ipc/history-of-the-movement. Accessed September 24, 2015.

2. International Paralympic Committee. Annual report: 2013. http://www.paralympic.org/sites/default/files/document/140722154927621_Annual+Report+2013_FINAL_V2.pdf. Accessed September 24, 2015.

3. Wikipedia. Paralympic sports. https://en.wikipedia.org/wiki/Paralympic_sports. Accessed December 12, 2015.

4. The World Bank. Disability overview. http://www.worldbank.org/en/topic/disability/overview. Accessed September 24, 2015.

5. American Academy of Physical Medicine and Rehabilitation. Directory of athletes with disabilities organizations. http://www.aapmr.org/about-physiatry/about-physical-medicine-rehabilitation/patient-resources/directory-of-organizations-for-athletes-with-disabilites---listing. Accessed September 24, 2015.

6. Fagher K, Lexell J. Sports-related injuries in athletes with disabilities. *Scand J Med Sci Sports.* 2014;24(5):e320–e331.

7. BrainandSpinalCord.org. Spinal cord injury. http://www.brainandspinalcord.org/spinal-cord-injury.html. Accessed November 24, 2015.

8. BrainandSpinalCord.org. Levels of spinal cord injury. http://www.brainandspinalcord.org/content/levels_of_spinal_cord_injury. Accessed November 24, 2015.

9. McKinley W, Pai AB, Kulkarni U, et al. Functional outcomes per level of spinal cord injury. http://emedicine.medscape.com/article/322604-overview. Updated July 27, 2015. Accessed November 24, 2015.

10. Krassioukov A, Cragg JJ, West C, et al. The good, the bad and the ugly of catheterization practices among elite athletes with spinal cord injury: a global perspective. *Spinal Cord.* 2015;53(1):78–82.

11. Krassioukov A, Eng JJ, Claxton G, et al. Neurogenic bowel management after spinal cord injury: a systematic review of the evidence. *Spinal Cord.* 2010;48(10):718–733.

12. Spinal Injury Network. Pressure sores. http://www.spinal-injury.net/pressure-sores-sci.htm. Accessed December 6, 2015.

13. BrainandSpinalcord. Spinal cord injury treatment. http://www.brainandspinalcord.org/spinal-cord-injury-treatment.html. Accessed December 6, 2015.

14. Christopher and Dana Reeves Foundation. Deep vein thrombosis. http://www.christopherreeve.org/site/c.mtKZKgMWKwG/b.8776955/k.6933/Deep_Vein_Thrombosis.htm. Accessed December 6, 2015.

15. Centers for Disease Control and Prevention. Venous thromboembolism (blood clots): facts. http://www.cdc.gov/ncbddd/dvt/facts.html. Accessed December 6, 2015.

16. Krassioukov A, Warburton DE, Teasell R, et al. A systematic review of the management of autonomic dysreflexia after spinal cord injury. *Arch Phys Med Rehabil.* 2009;90(4):682–695.

17. Elbasiouny SM, Moroz D, Bakr MM, et al. Management of spasticity after spinal cord injury: current techniques and future directions. *Neurorehabil Neural Repair.* 2010;24(1):23–33.

18. Richards SJ, Dyson-Hudson T, Bryce TN, et al. Pain after spinal cord injury. http://www.msktc.org/lib/docs/Factsheets/SCI_Pain_after_SCI.pdf. Accessed December 6, 2015.

19. Figoni S. Spinal cord disabilities: paraplegia and tetraplegia. In: Durstine JL, Moore GE, eds. *ACSM's Exercise Management for Persons with Chronic Diseases and Disabilities.* Champaign, IL: Human Kinetics; 2009:298–305.

20. Cerebral Palsy International Sports and Recreation Association. Sports. http://cpisra.org/dir /sports/. Accessed December 10, 2015.

21. Cerebral Palsy Alliance. Types of cerebral palsy. https://www.cerebralpalsy.org.au/what-is -cerebral-palsy/types-of-cerebral-palsy/. Accessed December 10, 2015.

22. Cerebral Palsy Alliance. Spastic cerebral palsy. https://www.cerebralpalsy.org.au/what-is -cerebral-palsy/types-of-cerebral-palsy/spastic -cerebral-palsy/. Accessed December 12, 2015.

23. National Institute of Neurological Disorders and Stroke. NINDS spasticity information page. http://www.ninds.nih.gov/disorders/spasticity /spasticity.htm. Accessed December 12, 2015.

24. Cerebral Palsy Alliance. Dyskinetic cerebral palsy. https://www.cerebralpalsy.org.au/what-is -cerebral-palsy/types-of-cerebral-palsy/dyskinetic -cerebral-palsy/. Accessed December 12, 2015.

25. Cerebral Palsy Alliance. Ataxic cerebral palsy. https://www.cerebralpalsy.org.au/what-is-cerebral -palsy/types-of-cerebral-palsy/ataxic-cerebral -palsy-ataxia/. Accessed December 12, 2015.

26. CanChild. Gross Motor Function Classification System–Expanded & Revised (GMFCS–E&R). https://canchild.ca/en/resources/42-gross-motor -function-classification-system-expanded-revised -gmfcs-e-r. Accessed December 12, 2015.

27. Eliasson AC, Krumlinde-Sundholm L, Rösblad B, et al. The Manual Ability Classification System (MACS) for children with cerebral palsy: scale development and evidence of validity and reliability. *Dev Med Child Neurol.* 2006;48: 549–554.

28. Hidecker MJ, Paneth N, Rosenbaum PL, et al. Developing and validating the Communication Function Classification System for individuals with cerebral palsy. *Dev Med Child Neurol.* 2011;53(8):704–710.

29. Laskin J. Cerebral palsy. In: Durstine JL, Moore GE, Painter PL, et al, eds. *ACSM's Exercise Management for Persons with Chronic Diseases and Disabilities.* 3rd ed. Champaign, IL: Human Kinetics; 2009:343–349.

30. Thibaut A, Chatelle C, Ziegler E, et al. Spasticity after stroke: physiology, assessment and treatment. *Brain Inj.* 2013;27(10):1093–1105. http:// www.coma.ulg.ac.be/papers/vs/Spastic_BI.pdf. Accessed December 12, 2015.

31. Ziegler-Graham K, MacKenzie EJ, Ephraim PL, et al. Estimating the prevalence of limb loss in the United States: 2005 to 2050. *Arch Phys Med Rehabil.* 2008;89(3):422–429.

32. Ziegler-Graham K, MacKenzie EJ, Ephraim PL, et al. Estimating the prevalence of limb loss in the United States: 2005 to 2050. *Arch Phys Med Rehabil.* 2008;89(3):422–429.

33. Pitetti KH, Pedrotti MH. Lower limb amputation. In: Durstine JL, Moore GE, eds. *ACSM's Exercise Management for Persons with Chronic Diseases and Disabilities.* Champaign, IL: Human Kinetics; 2009:280–284.

34. Pepper M, Willick S. Maximizing physical activity in athletes with amputations. *Curr Sports Med Rep.* 2009;8(6):339–344.

35. Hetzler T, Smith AE, Rempe D. Amputee athletes, part 2: biomechanics and common running injuries. *Int J Athl Ther Train.* 2014;19(2): 39–42.

Common Infectious Diseases

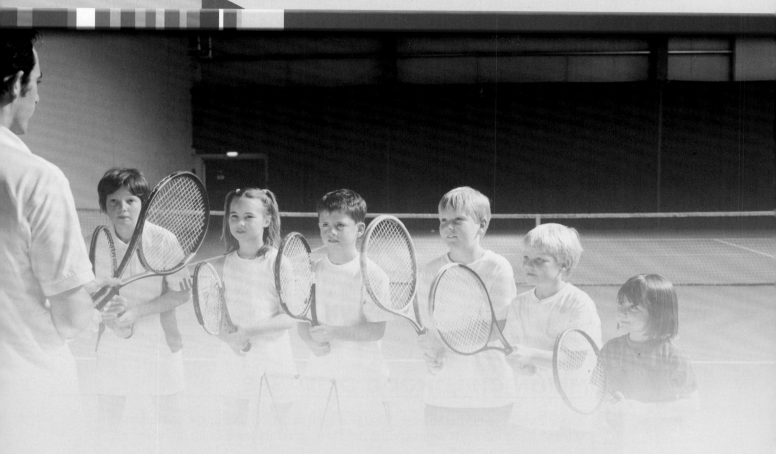

STUDENT OUTCOMES

1. Identify the common childhood diseases that can be prevented through early vaccinations.

2. Describe the characteristic lesions and associated symptoms of specific childhood diseases.

3. Explain the mode of transmission, incubation period, common signs and symptoms, and treatment of infectious mononucleosis.

4. Describe the signs and symptoms of viral meningitis.

5. Differentiate the signs and symptoms of the common sexually transmitted diseases and describe the treatment for these conditions.

6. Identify the five different classifications of hepatitis and differentiate the modes of transmission for each.

7. Describe the early signs and symptoms of hepatitis and explain the progression of severity of symptoms.

8. Identify the common signs and symptoms of AIDS.

9. Explain the safety precautions that can be taken to minimize the transmission of highly infectious diseases.

INTRODUCTION

Although it is not the intention of this chapter to discuss all infectious diseases to which sport and physical activity participants may be exposed, several common diseases may confront the athletic trainer. For some childhood diseases, vaccines exist that can prevent infection. In older populations, however, individuals may not have received the necessary booster shots to prevent the onset of various illnesses. Chickenpox, mumps, measles (i.e., rubeola), rubella (i.e., German measles), and influenza are among the more commonly transmitted infections.

Sexually transmitted diseases (STDs) continue to be a major concern for health care providers, particularly clinicians working with teenagers and college students, because many individuals in these populations are sexually active. Chlamydia, candidiasis, and trichomoniasis are common STDs that can affect sport and physical activity performance. If diagnosed and treated early, these conditions tend to be annoying rather than troublesome. Several serious STDs, however, such as hepatitis and AIDS, deserve special attention.

This chapter addresses the signs and symptoms, identification, and treatment of common childhood diseases, STDs, and other common infectious conditions. Although definitive diagnosis and treatment are completed by a physician, it is critical that the athletic trainer recognize a potential condition and immediately refer the patient to the primary care physician or team physician.

COMMON CHILDHOOD DISEASES

 In reviewing the medical history of high school students planning to participate in the upcoming fall sport season, what information would identify an increased risk for contracting influenza?

Most bacterial and viral infectious diseases of childhood are prevented through a series of early vaccinations given between birth and 18 months of age. A vaccine is a suspension of infectious agents, or some part of them, that is given to establish resistance to an infectious disease. Vaccines are divided into four general classes:

1. Those containing living infectious organisms, which are either disabled or otherwise nonvirulent strains.

2. Those containing infectious agents killed by physical or chemical means.

3. Those containing solutions of toxins from microorganisms that may be used directly but that usually are treated to neutralize their toxic potential.

4. Those containing substances extracted from a portion of an infectious agent. Effective antiviral vaccines often are made by extracting only a small portion of the virus' protein coat.

Whatever its makeup, the vaccine stimulates the body to develop specific defensive mechanisms that result in near-permanent protections from the disease. Booster shots are given on entry into school (age 4 to 6 years) and again in adolescence (age 11 to 12 and/or 14 to 16 years). Maintaining immunity against diphtheria and tetanus requires that booster vaccinations be given every 10 years. Because of its bloodborne transmission and significance to athletic trainers, however, hepatitis is discussed in more detail later in the chapter.

Bacterial Childhood Diseases

In the United States, infants are immunized against diphtheria, tetanus, and pertussis (DTP) and against *Haemophilus influenzae* type b (Hib). Even so, a few cases of diphtheria and tetanus are reported each year in nonimmunized or partially immunized adults. Prior to effective vaccination, Hib was one of the leading causes of invasive bacterial disease in children younger than 5 years and was the leading cause of meningitis in this age group.[1]

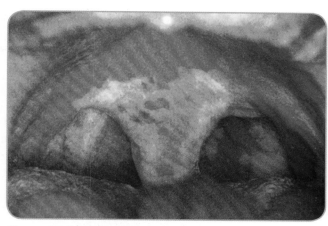

Figure 31.1. Diphtheria.

Diphtheria

■ Etiology

Diphtheria, which is caused by the organism *Corynebacterium diphtheriae*, is an acute, life-threatening, infectious disease that invades the upper respiratory region. The bacterium has an incubation period of 2 to 5 days. As it multiplies along mucous membrane surfaces, the organism irritates the tissue, producing a very distinctive, leathery, blue-white pseudomembrane (i.e., false membrane) that is composed of bacteria, necrotized tissue, inflammatory cells, and fibrin.[1–3] This membrane may grow to the extent that it impairs respiratory function.

■ Signs and Symptoms

The characteristic symptom is a thick, patchy, gray or blue-white membrane that forms over the mucous membranes of the pharynx, larynx, tonsils, soft palate, and nose (**Fig. 31.1**). Other symptoms include a mild fever (100° to 101°F), sore throat, rasping cough, hoarseness, and enlarged, tender cervical lymph nodes. There may be a strong, foul odor to the breath. If untreated, the pseudomembrane, along with swelling, may occlude the air passages, leading to death by suffocation, or the infection may spread throughout the body, leading to death from its adverse effects on the heart (i.e., myocarditis), nerves (i.e., neuritis), and kidneys. Transmission is by direct contact, droplet spread, and indirect contact with articles soiled by discharges from infected persons.

■ Management

Immediate referral to a physician is warranted. Treatment involves administration of a diphtheria antitoxin and antibiotics to destroy the organism. The patient must be isolated, and bed rest is required. A soft or liquid diet is recommended.

Tetanus (Lockjaw)

■ Etiology

The tetanus bacillus, *Clostridium tetani*, grows in the absence of oxygen in soil, dust, feces, and saliva. Tetanus spores invade the body, usually through a puncture wound or through lacerations, burns, trivial or unnoticed wounds, or injected contaminated street drugs. The spores produce a powerful toxin that attacks the central nervous system, which acts directly on voluntary muscles to produce contraction. The disease may affect anyone at any time, but children are at greater risk because of their tendency to develop skin wounds as a result of play activities.

■ Signs and Symptoms

The onset of symptoms may be gradual or abrupt. Abdominal rigidity usually is followed by painful muscle contractions, primarily of the masseter and neck muscles, although the trunk muscles also may be involved. Later, in the most common manifestation of tetanus, the jaws become rigidly fixed (i.e., lockjaw). In addition, the voice is altered, and the facial muscles contract, contorting the patient's face into a grimace. Finally, muscles in the back and extremities may become rigid, or the patient may experience extremely severe convulsive spasms of the muscles.

The final phase of the disease may be accompanied by tachycardia, profuse sweating, high fever, and intense pain.[1,2,4]

■ Management

Because of the serious nature of tetanus, all wounds should be cleansed thoroughly following standard protocol (see Chapter 6). In puncture wounds, bite wounds, and more significant lacerations or burns, a booster shot is recommended as soon as possible (within 72 hours) if the time from the previous booster is greater than 5 years. The toxin is neutralized if the tetanus antitoxin is administered before the toxin becomes attached to nerve tissue. Muscle relaxants also may be prescribed.

Pertussis (Whooping Cough)

■ Etiology

Pertussis is caused by the bacillus *Bordetella pertussis* and has an incubation period of 7 to 10 days. It is an extremely contagious respiratory infection common in children; yet, it remains the most common of all the diseases that can be preventable by routine childhood immunization.[1,5,6]

■ Signs and Symptoms

Whooping cough occurs in three stages—namely, catarrhal, paroxysmal, and convalescent. The catarrhal state begins with an insidious onset of an irritating cough, particularly at night, which may be accompanied by anorexia, sneezing, listlessness, conjunctivitis, and low-grade fever. The cough becomes progressively more irritating, violent, and eventually, paroxysmal within 1 to 2 weeks. The repeated episodes of violent coughing are interspersed with inhalations that feature a crowing or high-pitched whoop. In older children and adults, the whoop may be absent, but persistent coughing spells are present. These attacks frequently end with the expulsion of clear mucus followed by vomiting caused by choking on mucus. The coughing can be violent enough to cause nosebleed, detached retina, and hernia. During this stage, the child also is highly susceptible to secondary infections, such as otitis media, pneumonia, or encephalopathy. This stage lasts from 3 to 4 weeks. The final stage, the convalescent stage, may last from 1 to 2 months, with even a mild upper respiratory infection triggering symptoms.[1,5,6]

■ Management

Immediate referral to a physician is warranted. Antibiotics are effective only during the early stages (i.e., before the persistent coughing spells); if administration is delayed past this stage, antibiotics have little effect.

Haemophilus Influenzae *Type B*

■ Etiology

In children younger than 5 years, Hib is one of the leading causes of invasive bacterial disease and the leading cause of meningitis in this age group. The disease also can cause pneumonia, cellulitis, septic arthritis, otitis, sinusitis, and bronchitis. The bacteria are transmitted through respiratory droplets or other person-to-person contact. The following groups are at high risk:

- Those older than 65 years

- Those with chronic disorders of the pulmonary or cardiovascular system, including those with asthma

- Those with chronic metabolic diseases (e.g., diabetes), renal dysfunction, or immunosuppression

- Children and teenagers receiving long-term aspirin therapy (i.e., risk of Reye syndrome)

■ Signs and Symptoms

Symptoms usually come on rapidly, and they can include headache, muscle soreness, fatigue, loss of appetite, nasal congestion, sore throat, cough, and chest pains (**Fig. 31.2**). The virus also can lead to pneumonia and encephalitis, an infection of the meninges of the brain. If the organism leads to meningitis, the symptoms generally include fever, chills, malaise, headache, and vomiting. As the meninges become more irritated, other signs and symptoms occur, such as a stiff neck, exaggerated deep tendon reflexes, and back spasm in which the back arches backward so that the body rests on the head and heels.

■ Management

When the condition is identified, immediate referral to a physician is warranted. Typically, antibiotics are administered intravenously for at least 2 weeks, followed by oral antibiotics. Prophylactic treatment of close contacts with rifampin also is indicated.

Viral Childhood Diseases

In 1955, Jonas Salk introduced the first killed virus vaccine for poliomyelitis, one of the most feared diseases of the time because of its potential for permanent crippling, disability, and death. Shortly thereafter, Albert B. Sabin introduced the first live virus vaccine for poliomyelitis, and because of its widespread success, this vaccine became the preferred protection against poliomyelitis. By 1969, vaccines also were available for measles, mumps, and rubella. Vaccines for chickenpox and influenza soon followed. **Table 31.1** summarizes the incubation period, signs and symptoms, and duration of the more common viral childhood diseases.

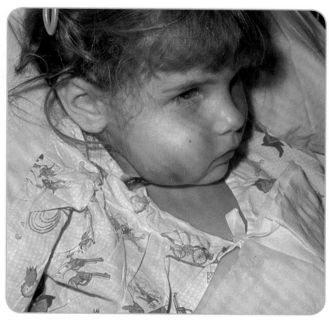

Figure 31.2. *Haemophilus influenzae* **type b.**

TABLE 31.1 Common Viral Infections

DISEASE	TRANSMISSION	INCUBATION PERIOD	CLINICAL SYMPTOMS	DURATION
Chickenpox (varicella)	Direct contact with respiratory secretions and fluid from lesions	10–21 days (typically 14–16 days)	Fever, headache, profuse rash on trunk, and oral mucosa that leads to blisters that turn cloudy and become encrusted with scabs	1–2 weeks
Influenza	Airborne droplets; indirect contact with contaminated objects	1–4 days	Chills, fever, headache, muscle aches and pains, nonproductive cough, sore throat, hoarseness, rhinitis	2–7 days
German measles (rubella)	Nasopharyngeal droplets; direct contact with throat and nasal secretions of infected person	12–23 days (typically 14 days)	Light rash on face that spreads to trunk and extremities, low-grade fever, and enlarged lymph nodes; can cause congenital heart defects in an infant if acquired by the mother during the first trimester of pregnancy	1–5 days
Measles (rubeola)	Airborne droplets; direct contact with nasal and throat secretions of infected person	10–12 days	Fever, photophobia, malaise, rhinitis, Koplik spots, swollen throat, progressive brownish-pink rash on face and body	4–7 days
Mumps	Airborne droplets; direct contact with saliva of infected person	12–21 days	Enlarged salivary glands, fever, headache, malaise, and males may have swollen and tender testes	10 days

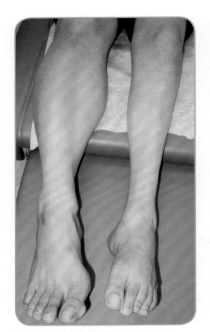

Figure 31.3. Polio.

See **Vaccines and Toxoids Recommended for Adults in the United States**, which identifies the vaccines and booster shots recommended for adults, by age groups, in the United States, at the companion Web site at thePoint.

Poliomyelitis (Polio)

■ Etiology

Polio is an inflammation of the gray matter of the spinal cord. It often results in spinal and muscle paralysis. The virus is spread by direct contact via fecal–oral and oral–oral routes.

■ Signs and Symptoms

The site of paralysis depends on the location of nerve cell destruction in the spinal cord or brainstem. Muscle paralysis may involve only one leg, leading to visible muscle wasting (**Fig. 31.3**). Sensation, however, may be intact, or the patient may have progressive paralysis that affects the vital organs and leads to death. In general, the infection has several possible outcomes[1,7]:

- Asymptomatic illness occurs in a majority of poliovirus infections.

- Minor flulike symptoms with fever, headache, malaise, sore throat, stomach pain, and nausea/vomiting occurs in a low percentage of the population.

- Nonparalytic polio with back pain and muscle spasms in addition to symptoms of minor illness occurs in 1% to 2% of the population.

- Paralytic polio with spinal and/or cranial paralysis occurs 3 to 4 days after minor illness has subsided in up to 2% of infected patients.

■ Management

Although the disease has been eradicated in the Western hemisphere by widespread immunization, polio remains a potentially serious disease in developing countries. Other than analgesics to relieve pain, no treatment exists for polio.

Chickenpox (Varicella)

■ Etiology

Most individuals have chickenpox by age 10 years. It is a mild, but very contagious, disease in children. In adults, however, the disease can have severe effects. Chickenpox is caused by the varicella zoster virus. The incubation period may be 10 days to 3 weeks following exposure, but it generally runs from 14 to 16 days. The disease is spread by direct contact with respiratory secretions and fluid from lesions of the infected person. It may be communicable from 1 to 2 days before the rash onset ending when all lesions are crusted.[1,8]

■ Signs and Symptoms

Chickenpox has a sudden onset of slight fever, mild headache, malaise, and loss of appetite for approximately 24 to 36 hours before the skin rash appears. The rash begins as flat, red spots (macules) that develop on the trunk and scalp and that, in a day or two, develop into raised papules and then clear vesicles containing a clear fluid surrounded by a red base (**Fig. 31.4**). Within 24 to 48 hours, the blisters turn cloudy and encrusted with a granular scab. They erupt in crops so that all three stages are present at the same time, beginning first on the back and chest and then spreading to the face, neck, and limbs.

■ Management

Immediate referral to a physician is warranted. Treatment is limited to relief of the symptoms, because no cure exists for chickenpox. Isolation is important during the infectious period, usually until all the scabs disappear. Bicarbonate of soda baths, calamine lotion, or antihistamine lotions may help to relieve the pruritus. Scratching the lesions should be avoided. In severe cases,

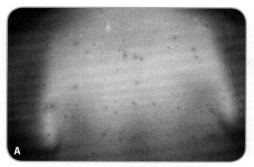
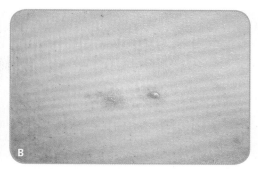

Figure 31.4. Varicella (A and B).

an antiviral agent, acyclovir, may be used. Because of its association with an increased incidence of Reye syndrome, aspirin should not be used to treat fever in cases of chickenpox among children and adolescents.[1]

Mumps

■ Etiology

Mumps is most prevalent in the adolescent age group. In contrast to chickenpox, mumps is characterized by swelling of the salivary glands near the neck. The incubation period generally is 12 to 25 days, and the disease is communicable from 6 days before symptoms appear to as long as 9 days after symptoms appear. Mumps is spread by airborne droplets and by direct contact with the saliva of an infected person.[1]

■ Signs and Symptoms

The classic symptoms of mumps are unilateral or bilateral swollen parotid glands (**Fig. 31.5**). Initially, there may be loss of appetite, headache, discomfort, and mild fever. These signs are followed by earache, salivary gland swelling, and a fever.[1] The glands may become so swollen that it hurts to drink sour liquids or chew food. Complications, which tend to occur more frequently in males, may include epididymitis, meningitis, and rarely, a number of other serious illnesses, such as pancreatitis and various central nervous system manifestations.

■ Management

Immediate referral to a physician is warranted. Because of the viral nature of the disease, antibiotics are ineffective. Analgesics, fluids, and rest are the main forms of treatment.

Measles (Rubeola)

■ Etiology

Measles is known to spread rapidly among unimmunized individuals and those who have not received booster shots against the childhood disease. It is spread by airborne droplets, direct contact with the nasal or throat secretions of infected patients, and articles that have been freshly contaminated. The incubation period generally ranges from 10 to 12 days.[1]

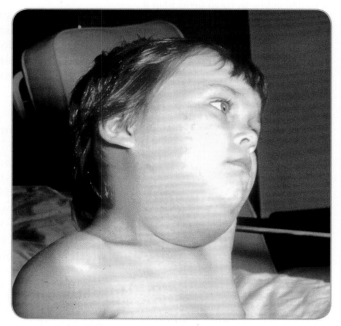

Figure 31.5. Mumps.

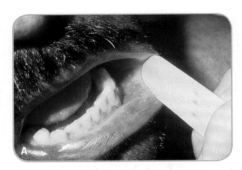

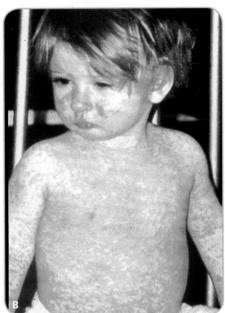

Figure 31.6. Rubeola (measles).
A, Koplik spots. **B,** Rash gives skin a
blotchy appearance.

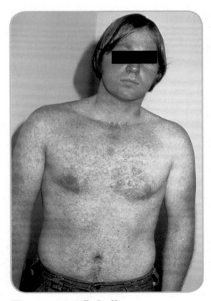

Figure 31.7. Rubella.

■ Signs and Symptoms

The onset of symptoms usually is gradual. Early symptoms include fever, photophobia, malaise, conjunctivitis, rhinitis, and cough. The disease is characterized by small white spots (i.e., Koplik spots) inside the cheeks that appear 4 to 5 days after the initial symptoms and 1 to 2 days before the onset of rash. Koplik spots are found on the oral mucosa opposite the molars (**Fig. 31.6A**). They look like tiny, bluish-gray specks surrounded by a red halo. Throat swelling is present. The temperature may rise to 39.4° to 40.6°C (103° to 105°F). The rash first appears as irregular, brownish-pink spots around the hairline, ears, and neck. Within 24 to 48 hours, it spreads to the body, arms, and legs, giving the skin a blotchy appearance (**Fig. 31.6B**). In certain areas, the lesions may be clustered so densely that the skin surface appears generally swollen and red. Within 3 to 5 days, the fever decreases, and the spots flatten, turn a brownish color, and begin to fade. Encephalitis is the most serious complication.

■ Management

Immediate referral to a physician is warranted. Treatment is symptomatic. Bed rest, usually in a darkened room to alleviate the discomfort of photophobia, is indicated. Fluids and acetaminophen are recommended for fever. Aspirin is not recommended for children because of the chance of developing Reye syndrome. The patient should be kept isolated until the rash disappears.

Rubella (German Measles)

■ Etiology

Normally, rubella is a mild disease in both children and adults, with one attack giving lifelong vaccination, but the disease can be extremely dangerous for an unborn child when a woman is infected during the first trimester of pregnancy. Birth defects may include heart disorders, eye clouding (i.e., cataracts), deafness, and mental retardation. The disease is transmitted by droplets or direct contact with the throat and nasal secretions of infected patients. The incubation period ranges from 12 to 23 days with typical incubation of 14 days. The disease is communicable for approximately 1 week before and at least 4 days after the onset of the rash.

■ Signs and Symptoms

Rubella is marked by fever, symptoms of a mild upper respiratory tract infection, malaise, headache, swollen lymph nodes, joint pain, and a fine, red rash on the face that spreads to the body (**Fig. 31.7**). The rash is composed of pale-red, slightly elevated, discrete papules, or the rash may be highly diffuse and bright red. The rash begins on the face, spreads rapidly to other portions of the body, and usually fades so rapidly that the face may clear before the extremities are affected. The symptoms usually last only 2 to 3 days except the joint pain, which may last longer or return.

■ Management

Referral to a physician is warranted. Treatment is symptomatic. Bed rest is indicated. Topical antipruritic or warm water baths may be recommended to relieve itching.

In reviewing the medical history of high school students planning to participate in the upcoming fall sport season, the following conditions would indicate an increased risk for contracting influenza: chronic disorders of the pulmonary or cardiovascular system (e.g., asthma); chronic metabolic diseases (e.g., diabetes), renal dysfunction, or immunosuppression; and long-term aspirin therapy (i.e., risk of Reye syndrome).

INFECTIOUS MONONUCLEOSIS

 What is the inherent danger associated with participation in contact or collision sports for a patient diagnosed with infectious mononucleosis?

Etiology

The Epstein-Barr virus, which is in the herpes family, causes infectious mononucleosis, an acute viral disease manifested by a general feeling of malaise and fatigue. Commonly called the kissing disease, mononucleosis is transmitted in saliva by the oral–pharyngeal route. It also may be spread by sharing the drinking container of an infected patient. Infectious rates are highest among individuals between 15 and 25 years of age; after age 40 years, the condition is rare. The incubation period for infectious mononucleosis is 4 to 6 weeks.[9] "Chronic fatigue syndrome" and the Epstein-Barr virus have similar signs and symptoms, but the association of the two continues to be debated.

Signs and Symptoms

Initial symptoms include headache, malaise, and fatigue. After 3 to 5 days, fever, swollen lymph glands, and a sore throat develop. Patients often describe the sore throat as "the worst sore throat I've ever had." In 10% to 15% of patients, jaundice and a rubella-like rash also may be present. Complications may arise if enlarged tonsils or adenoids obstruct the airway or if neurological or cardiac changes occur.

Management

A patient suspected of having mononucleosis should be immediately referred to a physician. Anti-inflammatory medication may be used to control headaches, fever, and general muscle aches and pains. Lozenges, saltwater gargles, and viscous lidocaine (Xylocaine) can ease throat pain. The overwhelming majority of patients recover uneventfully. Corticosteroid therapy (prednisone) is used only for patients with severe cases or specific indications, such as imminent airway obstruction or severe mono-hepatitis, or in the presence of neurological, hematological, or cardiac complications.

Patients with mononucleosis should not participate in any contact or collision activities during which trauma could rupture the enlarged and vulnerable spleen.[9] In some individuals, an ultrasonography may be indicated to better assess the size of the spleen. Enlarged spleens have been known to rupture up to 3 weeks after initial symptoms appear. If the spleen is not markedly enlarged or painful, and if liver function is normal, as determined by appropriate laboratory tests, limited physical training may be resumed 3 weeks after onset of the illness, with strenuous exercise and return to contact activities occurring in another 1 to 2 weeks. A flak jacket can be worn to protect the spleen from injury.

 The inherent danger associated with participation in contact or collision sports for a patient diagnosed with mononucleosis is the risk of splenic rupture. Enlarged spleens have been known to rupture up to 3 weeks after appearance of the initial symptoms of mononucleosis.

VIRAL MENINGITIS

 What practices should be followed to reduce the risk of athletic team members contracting viral meningitis?

Viral infections of the nervous system are rare in athletes. Athletes and physically active individuals are at a greater risk for viral meningitis, however, when poor hygienic measures are used with drink-dispensing machines, water bottles, and water coolers.

Signs and Symptoms

Signs and symptoms of viral meningitis include fever, headache, nausea, vomiting, myalgia, neck pain, **nuchal rigidity,** decreased coordination, malaise, photophobia, and altered mental status. Because the meninges are inflamed, stretching them through neck flexion produces pain.

Management

The most important step in treating this condition is immediate referral to a physician for an accurate diagnosis. Drug therapy is used to control symptoms. The condition usually resolves on its own. The patient should not return to activity until 2 to 3 weeks after symptoms have eased. Activity should be resumed in a gradual progression. If symptoms recur, the virus is still present, and activity should cease until the patient has been reevaluated by a physician.

 In an effort to reduce the risk of athletic team members contracting viral meningitis, practices should be employed that ensure that proper hygienic measures are used with drink-dispensing machines, water bottles, and water coolers.

SEXUALLY TRANSMITTED DISEASES

 Why is the diagnosis of STDs more complicated with female patients?

Infections of the genital tract are called STDs. It is suggested that almost half of the nearly 20 million cases of STDs occurring annually in Americans are acquired in persons aged 15 to 24 years.[10] Chlamydia is the most common bacterial STD in the United States.[10] Unlike herpes and the human papillomavirus, chlamydia is highly preventable, because transmission can be interrupted through the use of condoms. In addition, chlamydia is easily treated with antibiotic therapy.

 See **Common Sexually Transmitted Diseases**, found on the companion Web site at thePoint, for a summary of the modes of transmission, incubation periods, signs and symptoms, and general treatments of the more common STDs.

In females, chlamydia often is asymptomatic and undiagnosed, leading to potentially dangerous health and fertility problems. Some experts suggest that chlamydia screening should become a routine part of annual gynecological examinations.

Gonorrhea, the second most common STD in the United States, is characterized in males by a pungent, thick, milky yellow or greenish discharge and a burning sensation during urination. In women, the condition often is asymptomatic until it progresses to pelvic inflammatory disease. Genital ulcers commonly result from herpes, syphilis, and chancroids (**Fig. 31.8**).

 In women, many STDs are asymptomatic, and they remain as such until a more serious disease develops. An undiagnosed STD can lead to potentially dangerous health and fertility problems.

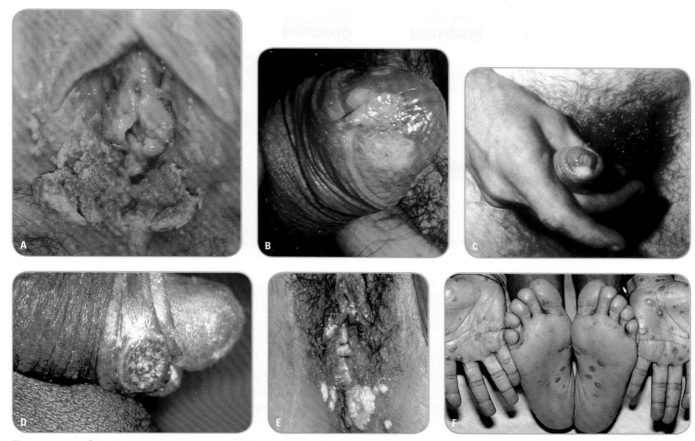

Figure 31.8. Symptoms of sexually transmitted diseases (A–F).

HEPATITIS

? What is the mode of transmission for hepatitis B?

Hepatitis is divided into six types, each of which is caused by a different virus. **Table 31.2** compares the five major hepatitis viruses. Hepatitis G virus has been discovered, but little is known about the virus, which is a bloodborne RNA virus. The American Medical Association, American Academy of Family Physicians, and American Academy of Pediatrics advocate that all children should receive a complete series of hepatitis B virus (HBV) vaccinations during the first 18 months of life. Vaccination as a prophylactic measure is required of an employer at no cost to an employee if that employee may be exposed to bloodborne pathogens.

All older children and adolescents at high risk for HBV infection, in addition to those listed in **Box 31.1**, should receive a complete series of the vaccination. Although not specifically mentioned, coaches, referees, officials, recreational sport supervisors, and personal trainers also should be vaccinated, because they often are first on the scene of an acute injury involving hemorrhage.

Etiology

Hepatitis B, the most common form of viral hepatitis, has an incubation period of 60 to 150 days and is transmitted by blood or blood products (i.e., posttransfusion hepatitis), semen, vaginal secretions, and saliva. Manual, oral, or penile stimulation of the anus is strongly associated with the spread of this virus. It is possible that an individual who is infected with HBV will exhibit no signs

TABLE 31.2 Major Viruses Known to Cause Hepatitis in Humans

	HEPATITIS A	HEPATITIS B	HEPATITIS C	HEPATITIS D	HEPATITIS E
Transmitted	Fecal–oral; contaminated food and water (epidemics)	Bloodborne; sexual contact; contaminated needles	Bloodborne; sexual contact	Bloodborne	Fecal–oral
Incubation period	15–50 days	60–150 days	15–150 days	30–60 days	20–60 days
Special features	Immunoglobulin prophylaxis is effective	Preexposure and postexposure prophylaxis available	Asymptomatic in many; main cause of posttransfusion hepatitis; often becomes chronic	Coinfection with active hepatitis B virus or infection superimposed on chronic hepatitis B	High mortality in pregnant women. Large epidemics caused by contaminated water supplies

Adapted from Bartlett JB. *Pocket Book of Infectious Disease Therapy*. Baltimore, MD: Lippincott Williams & Wilkins, 1997; with permission.

or symptoms, and the virus may go undetected. The HBV antigen is still present, however, and can be transmitted unknowingly to others through exposure to blood and other body fluids or through sexual contact. HBV can survive for at least 1 week in dried blood or on contaminated surfaces.[1]

Signs and Symptoms

Hepatitis primarily attacks the liver, severely impairing its function. Early symptoms include mild, flulike symptoms, such as malaise, fatigue, and loss of appetite. Progressive signs include severe fatigue, anorexia, nausea, vomiting, diarrhea, general muscle and joint pain, high fever, vomiting, severe abdominal pain, and dark urine. The most notable signs include a yellowing of the whites of the eyes and a yellowish or jaundiced skin appearance in light-complexioned individuals (**Fig. 31.9**). Hepatitis may increase the risk of developing cancer of the liver. In rare cases, hepatitis is fatal.

Management

Immediate referral to a physician is warranted if the individual has been exposed, or is suspected of having been exposed, to the virus. Currently, no specific drug therapy exists that will cure viral hepatitis. Postexposure vaccination also is available when individuals have come into direct contact with the body fluids of an infected person. Bed rest and adequate fluid intake can prevent dehydration, but the disease must run its course.

BOX 31.1 Individuals at Risk for Infection with Hepatitis B Virus and HIV

- All health care workers, including athletic trainers, athletic training students, nurses, and physicians
- Gay men
- Persons with multiple sex partners
- Caregivers of the developmentally disabled
- Inmates in correctional facilities
- Patients undergoing dialysis
- Anyone who has resided in Haiti or Central Africa (HIV)
- Injection drug users
- Household contacts of adoptees who are surface antigen positive

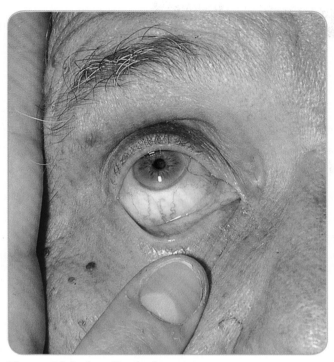

Figure 31.9. Jaundice in the eyes.

 Hepatitis B is transmitted by blood or blood products, semen, vaginal secretions, and saliva. Manual, oral, or penile stimulation of the anus is strongly associated with the spread of this virus.

AIDS

 Should an individual who has tested positive for infection with HIV be permitted to participate in an organized sports program?

Etiology

Acquired immunodeficiency syndrome results from infection with HIV, which falls within a special category called **retroviruses**. An individual can be HIV-positive and, as such, infectious for years before any signs of AIDS appear. HIV attacks and destroys cells in the body's immune system, particularly the lymphocyte known as the helper T cell. In a healthy individual, these cells stimulate the immune system to fight disease. In an infected individual, a gradual deterioration of the immune system leaves the body vulnerable to a variety of infections and cancers, such as herpes, oral candidiasis, pneumonia, encephalitis, and retinitis.

Currently, HIV has been found to be transmitted only in blood, semen, and vaginal secretions. In sports, the risk of AIDS is rare. In boxing, football, or wrestling, where participants may have a bloody nose or open cuts, close contact with the competitor may pose a health risk. To date, however, no documented case of HIV transmission through participation in sport has been published. Small amounts of bloodstain on a uniform do not require removal of the participant from the game or a uniform change; however, uniforms that become saturated with blood should be changed before returning to participation.

BOX 31.2 **Common Signs and Symptoms Associated with AIDS**

- Persistent fever or night sweats
- A persistent, dry cough unrelated to smoking
- Unexplained weight loss and loss of appetite
- Persistent, unexplained diarrhea or bloody stools
- Extreme fatigue not explained by physiological activity or mental depression
- Easy bruising or atypical bleeding from any body opening
- Blotches or bumps on or under the skin
- White spots or unusual blemishes in the mouth
- Persistent, severe headaches

Signs and Symptoms

Signs and symptoms of AIDS vary, depending on the degree to which the immune system is impaired. Common symptoms include those listed in **Box 31.2**. Some researchers suggest that AIDS is more severe in women, with HIV infection progressing much faster.

Management

Immediate referral to a physician is warranted if the individual has been exposed, or is suspected of having been exposed, to the virus. To date, no effective cure or vaccine exists for AIDS. Various drug therapies have been developed for controlling the symptoms and decreasing the progression of the disease, but the success of drug therapy appears to be related to the stage of the virus and the time at which the drug therapy is initiated. Healthy HIV-positive athletes and those with AIDS may continue physical activity. The Americans with Disabilities Act of 1991 states that individuals infected with HIV cannot be discriminated against and may be excluded from participation only on sound medical grounds. In some cases, fatigue may not allow participation in intensive exercise or competition. The best defenses against the virus remain education about safe-sex practices and use of condoms as well as practicing universal precautions when dealing with blood and blood products (see **Application Strategy 10.1**).

 The Americans with Disabilities Act of 1991 states that athletes infected with HIV cannot be discriminated against and may be excluded from participation only on sound medical grounds.

SUMMARY

1. Childhood diseases can be prevented by early immunization (between birth and 18 months of age). Booster shots are given on entry into school and at adolescence.

2. Childhood bacterial diseases that can be prevented through vaccinations include diphtheria, tetanus, pertussis (whooping cough), and Hib. Childhood viral diseases that can be prevented through vaccinations include poliomyelitis (polio), chickenpox (varicella), mumps, measles (rubeola), rubella (German measles), and hepatitis.

3. Adults between 18 and 24 years of age should receive booster shots for measles, mumps, rubella, varicella, and tetanus. Diphtheria and tetanus shots should be repeated every 10 years.

4. Mononucleosis is transmitted in saliva. Infection rates are highest among individuals aged 15 to 25 years. Signs and symptoms include headache, fatigue, loss of appetite, enlarged lymph nodes, swollen glands, and an enlarged spleen.

5. Individuals are at a greater risk of viral meningitis when poor hygienic measures are used around water bottles and watering stations.

6. Chlamydia is the most common bacterial STD in the United States, followed by gonorrhea and genital ulcers from herpes, syphilis, and chancroids. In males, common signs and symptoms of an STD include a mild itching and burning during urination and a discharge from the penis. In females, a vaginal discharge may be present, but many STDs are asymptomatic until the more serious pelvic inflammatory disease occurs.

7. Hepatitis B is the most common form of viral hepatitis, but it can be prevented with proper vaccination. The condition primarily attacks the liver, severely impairing function. Signs and symptoms include severe fatigue, malaise, and loss of appetite progressing to anorexia, nausea, vomiting, high fever, and a jaundiced appearance.

8. AIDS results from infection with HIV, which has been found to be transmitted in blood, semen, and vaginal secretions.

9. Most common viral diseases, including hepatitis and AIDS, can be prevented in the settings of athletics and physical activity by following universal precautions when dealing with blood and blood products.

10. If an individual is suspected of contracting an infectious disease, a physician referral is always recommended so that drug therapy can be prescribed along with other treatment. If the infection can be spread from person to person, individuals who are infected should be isolated from others until the physician determines that cross-infection is no longer possible.

APPLICATION QUESTIONS

1. As the community high school athletic trainer, you have received inquiries from several parents about vaccination requirements for participation in middle and high school athletics. What are the vaccination requirements for athletic participation in a public school setting?

2. A male cross-country runner is complaining of a swollen throat, difficulty in swallowing, and a mild fever. There are also notable irregular, brownish-pink spots around the hairline and extending down the neck onto the shoulders and arms. As part of the history component of an assessment, what questions would you ask the athlete regarding this condition?

3. During a preseason meeting with parents of the high school student athletes, several parents express concerns about students with HIV being allowed to participate on the school's athletic teams. They expect that, at a minimum, they should be informed of the name of any HIV-positive student so that they can decide whether or not their child will remain on the team. How would you respond to the parents' concerns and expectations?

4. An 18-year-old collegiate swimmer has been diagnosed with infectious mononucleosis. What is the treatment protocol for this athlete and how will return to full activity be determined?

REFERENCES

1. Hamborsky J, Kroger A, Wolfe C, eds. *Epidemiology and Prevention of Vaccine—Preventable Diseases*. 13th edition. Washington, DC: Centers for Disease Control and Prevention; 2015. http://www.cdc.gov/vaccines/pubs/pinkbook/index.html. Accessed June 30, 2015.
2. Tamporo CD, Lewis MA. *Diseases of the Human Body*. Philadelphia, PA: FA Davis; 2011.
3. Centers for Disease Control and Prevention, National Center for Immunization and Respiratory Diseases, Division of Bacterial Diseases. Diphtheria. http://www.cdc.gov/diphtheria/index.html. Updated May 13, 2013. Accessed June 30, 2015.
4. Centers for Disease Control and Prevention, National Center for Immunization and Respiratory Diseases, Division of Bacterial Diseases. Tetanus. http://www.cdc.gov/tetanus/index.html. Updated January 9, 2013. Accessed June 30, 2015.
5. Tiwari T, Murphy TV, Moran J. Recommended antimicrobial agents for the treatment and postexposure prophylaxis of pertussis: 2005 CDC guidelines. *MMWR Recomm Rep*. 2005; 54(RR-14):1–16.
6. Centers for Disease Control and Prevention, National Center for Immunization and Respiratory Diseases, Division of Bacterial Diseases. Pertussis (whooping cough). http://www.cdc.gov/pertussis/. Updated December 1, 2014. Accessed June 30, 2015.
7. Centers for Disease Control and Prevention, National Center for Immunization and Respiratory Diseases, Division of Bacterial Diseases. Polio vaccination. http://www.cdc.gov/vaccines/vpd-vac/polio/default.htm. Updated October 30, 2014. Accessed June 30, 2015.
8. Centers for Disease Control and Prevention, National Center for Immunization and Respiratory Diseases, Division of Bacterial Diseases. Chickenpox (varicella). http://www.cdc.gov/chickenpox/. Updated November 18, 2014. Accessed June 30, 2015.
9. Centers for Disease Control and Prevention, National Center for Immunization and Respiratory Diseases, Division of Bacterial Diseases. Epstein-Barr virus and infectious mononucleosis. http://www.cdc.gov/epstein-barr/about-mono.html. Updated January 7, 2014. Accessed June 30, 2015.
10. U.S. Department of Health and Human Services. Sexually transmitted diseases. http://www.hhs.gov/ash/oah/adolescent-health-topics/reproductive-health/stds.html. Accessed June 30, 2015.

32

Dermatology

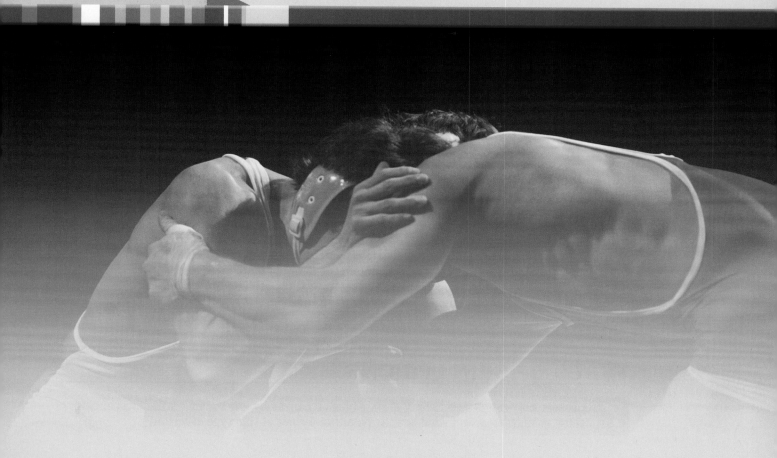

STUDENT OUTCOMES

1. Describe the common skin lesions.

2. List the signs and symptoms of an abscess, acne, onychia, paronychia, folliculitis, furuncles, carbuncles, cellulitis, and impetigo contagiosa.

3. List the signs and symptoms of tinea unguium, tinea pedis, tinea cruris, tinea corporis, tinea capitis, tinea versicolor, and candidiasis.

4. List the signs and symptoms of herpes gladiatorum, herpes zoster, verrucae, and molluscum contagiosum.

5. Describe the general management of bacterial, fungal, and viral skin infections.

6. Describe the common skin irritations caused by mechanical reactions, such as intertrigo, athlete's nodules, acne mechanica, and striae distensae, and explain the management of each condition.

7. List the signs and symptoms of sunburn, pernio, miliaria, eczema, psoriasis, and hyperhidrosis, and explain the management of each condition.

8. List the signs and symptoms of bites or stings from a mosquito, bee, wasp, ant, spider, flea, tick, and lice.

9. Explain the management of an insect bite or sting.

10. Differentiate between allergic contact dermatitis and irritant contact dermatitis, and explain the management of both conditions.

11. Describe the three types of urticaria and explain the management of each.

INTRODUCTION

Dermatology is the study of the skin. Any individual can occasionally contract skin conditions, but several are more commonly seen in the physically active population. Skin infections may be caused by bacteria, fungi, or viruses. Related inflammatory skin conditions may result from mechanical, environmental, allergic, or chemical skin reactions. Early identification of the ensuing lesions and specific treatment minimize the healing time and prevent both the spread and the recurrence of the condition.

This chapter first provides an overview of the various types of skin lesions and then discusses the more common skin infections and conditions that are seen in the physically active population. When appropriate, individual management plans are provided. Many of these conditions can be seen in the color plates included with this chapter. It is important to note that many systemic diseases are manifested in skin lesions or rashes. Therefore, it is critical for the athletic trainer to identify potentially serious lesions and refer the patient immediately to a physician, particularly if any uncertainty exists regarding the nature of the skin lesion.

TYPES OF SKIN LESIONS

 A soccer player has a transient, elevated lesion caused by local edema. What type of skin lesion is suggested, and what are the potential causes of this type of lesion?

The skin is the largest organ of the body. It serves four major functions:

1. The skin protects the body from bacteria, fungi, various viruses, and other germs in the outside environment.

2. The skin helps to regulate body temperature.

3. The skin prevents the loss of fluids and nutrients through the cutaneous surface.

4. The skin aids in the transmission of information from the outside environment to the brain.

The outer layer of skin, called the epidermis, contains the germinal layer, in which the production of new skin cells occurs and **sebum** is produced. The underlying dermis contains the sweat glands, hair follicles, sebaceous glands, blood vessels, and a complex array of nerve endings (see **Fig. 10.6**). The deepest layer, called the subcutaneous tissue, is composed primarily of fat (for insulation and energy storage).

The skin can be damaged by direct trauma, allergic reactions, chemical irritants, heat, cold, bacteria, fungi, and viruses. Whenever the skin is damaged, a lesion appears. These lesions are identified by their size and by their depth (**Table 32.1**).

 The soccer player has a transient, elevated lesion caused by local edema. This indicates a possible wheal. The wheal could be a common allergic reaction to an insect bite, sunlight, or pressure.

TABLE 32.1 Basic Types of Skin Lesions

PRIMARY LESIONS (MAY ARISE FROM PREVIOUSLY NORMAL SKIN)

Circumscribed, flat, nonpalpable changes in skin color

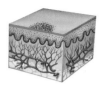

Macule—small, flat spot up to 1 cm (freckle, mole, rubella)

Patch—flat spot; 1 cm or larger

Palpable, elevated, solid masses

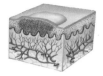

Papule—solid, elevated lesion less than 10 mm (wart, psoriasis)

Plaque—elevated superficial lesion 1 cm or larger, often formed by coalescence of papules

Nodule—marble-like lesion; larger than 0.05 cm; often deeper and firmer than a papule (lipoma, cysts, tumors)

Wheal—transient, irregular superficial area of localized skin edema (mosquito bite, hive, sunlight, or pressure)

Circumscribed, superficial elevations of the skin formed by free fluid in a cavity within the skin layers

Vesicle—up to 1 cm; filled with serous fluid (contact dermatitis, herpes simplex, herpes zoster)

Bulla—1 cm or larger; filled with serous fluid (second-degree burn)

Pustule—elevated lesion containing pus (acne, furuncle [boil], carbuncle)

SECOND LESIONS (RESULT FROM CHANGES IN PRIMARY LESIONS)

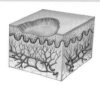

Erosion—Loss of the superficial epidermis; surface is moist but does not bleed (moist area after the rupture of a vesicle, as in chickenpox).

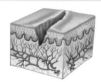

Ulcer—deeper loss of epidermis and dermis; may bleed and scar (stasis ulcer of venous insufficiency, syphilitic chancre)

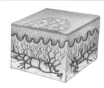

Fissure—a linear crack in the skin (athlete's foot)

Crust—dried residue of serum, pus, or blood (impetigo, scab)

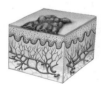

Scales—a thin flake of exfoliated epidermis (dandruff, psoriasis, tinea versicolor)

SKIN INFECTIONS

 A wrestler received treatment for an open sore on the right thigh. Three days later, observation reveals a honey-colored crust with surrounding erythema. Impetigo is suspected. What signs and symptoms would confirm this suspicion?

Skin infections may stem from bacteria, fungi, or viruses. Bacterial or fungal infections can cause pustules on or within the skin or its associated structures, such as the sweat glands and the hair follicles. Although most infections tend to be painful, superficial irritations also can be extremely itchy. The three main bacteria are staphylococci, streptococci, and bacilli. Staphylococci commonly appear in clumps on the skin, in upper respiratory tract infections, and in lesions which contain pus. Streptococci are associated with serious systemic diseases, such as scarlet fever. Many bacilli are not pathological, but some can lead to major systemic diseases, such as tetanus. Fungi, such as yeast and molds, often attack the skin, hair, and nails. Fungi fall into three basic categories: dermatophytes, candidiasis (moniliasis), and tinea versicolor. Viruses invade the living cells and may multiply until they kill the cell, burst out to reinfect other cells, or lie dormant within the cell without ever causing an infection.

Skin infections can preclude an individual from participating in physical activity. Participation should not be permitted if open wounds or infectious skin conditions cannot be adequately protected, thus preventing exposure to others. The National Collegiate Athletic Association (NCAA) has identified several skin infections that would lead to medical disqualification from practice or competition if not adequately protected. As per the NCAA definition, the skin condition or open wound must be noninfectious, appropriately covered, and treated. These include bacterial infections (i.e., impetigo, erysipelas, carbuncles, staphylococcal disease, folliculitis, and hidradenitis suppurativa), viral skin infections (i.e., herpes simplex, herpes zoster [chickenpox], and molluscum contagiosum), fungal skin infections (i.e., tinea corporis), and parasitic skin infections (i.e., pediculosis and scabies).[1]

Bacterial Skin Conditions

Bacterial lesions typically are caused by a staphylococcal or streptococcal infection. Hot tubs or whirlpools that are not adequately chlorinated may harbor *Pseudomonas* sp.; most infections are self-limiting and need no treatment other than regulating pool chlorination. The more common bacterial infections in the physically active population are abscesses, acne vulgaris, onychia and paronychia, folliculitis, furuncles (boils) and carbuncles, hidradenitis suppurativa, erysipelas, cellulitis, and impetigo contagiosa.

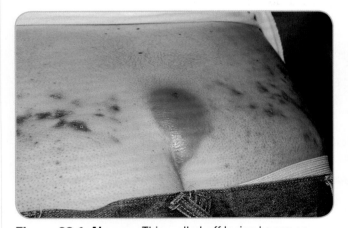

Figure 32.1. Abscess. This walled-off lesion began as folliculitis that became a furuncle and then an abscess. Note the older scar from previous furuncles and cystic acne lesions.

Abscess

■ Etiology

An **abscess** is a circumscribed collection of pus appearing in an acute or chronic, localized infection. The abscess may be a cavity formed by liquefaction necrosis within solid tissue and may affect any tissue of the body, such as bone, tooth root, appendix, brain, gums, lungs, abdominal wall, gastrointestinal tract, ears, tonsils, sinuses, breasts, kidneys, and prostate gland.

■ Signs and Symptoms

An abscess usually is associated with tissue destruction, so the lesion appears as an encapsulated pocket of pus (**Fig. 32.1**). Pain, redness, swelling, and a fever typically are present.

Acne

■ Etiology

Nearly all adolescents experience acne at one time or another. Although the etiology is unknown, acne is believed to be caused by excessive sebum production secondary to a hormonal imbalance, abnormal follicular keratinization that results in follicular blockage, proliferation of *Propionibacterium acnes*, and inflammation. At 8 or 9 years of age, the adrenal glands begin producing increasing amounts of an androgen that causes the sebaceous glands to enlarge and produce more sebum. Sebum secretion peaks during adolescence and declines after the teenage years. Two types of lesions occur in acne: noninflammatory lesions, such as open or closed comedones, and inflammatory (popular, nodular, or cystic) lesions.[2]

■ Signs and Symptoms

The obstructed follicle may become apparent as a blackhead (i.e., open follicle) or whitehead (i.e., closed follicle). The blackhead is not dirt, so scrubbing or washing will not remove it. Whiteheads represent follicles that have become dilated with cellular debris but possess only a microscopic opening to the skin surface. When the oil and other material in the whitehead break through the pore wall and cause irritation under the skin, a pimple results. Pimples can be erythematous papules, pustules, or nodules and commonly are seen on the face, neck, and back. Papules and pustules are small (diameter, 5 mm), whereas nodules are larger. The superficial pustules eventually dry, whereas the deeper nodules may become chronic and form disfiguring scars.

Onychia and Paronychia

■ Etiology

Onychia is inflammation of the matrix of the nail plate, whereas **paronychia** involves only the lateral border or nail fold (**Fig. 32.2**). The conditions may develop from staphylococcal, streptococcal, or fungal organisms; with fungal organisms, the infection is called onychomycosis. The conditions also may occur secondary to diabetes or vaginal candidal infection or, occasionally, from endocrine problems, such as hypoparathyroidism, hypothyroidism, and adrenocortical deficiency.[3]

■ Signs and Symptoms

If onychia is present, the nail fold becomes red, swollen, and painful and can produce purulent drainage. Paronychia often follows a hangnail and is seen in individuals whose hands frequently are immersed in water or mud (e.g., football linemen, chefs, and nurses). Occasionally, the feet may be affected if they are immersed frequently. Inflammation and swelling is centralized on the lateral border of the nail plate or nail fold. Small amounts of pus may be extruded from the nail fold, particularly with secondary infection.

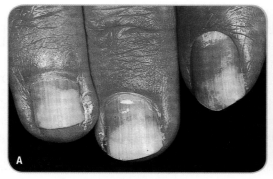 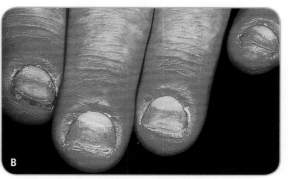

Figure 32.2. Nail conditions. A, Onycholysis is a painless separation of the distal nail plate from the nail bed. **B,** Paronychia is an inflammation of the proximal and lateral nail folds and may be acute or chronic.

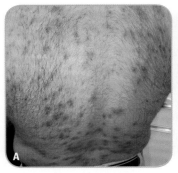
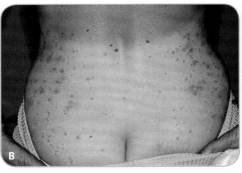
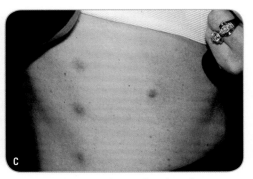

Figure 32.3. Folliculitis. A, Folliculitis commonly is called an "ingrown" hair, whereby the hair grows inward and curls up to form an infected nodule. **B,** Pustular rashes can occur where occlusive bathing suits are worn. **C,** Hot tub folliculitis can result from high water temperatures in the presence of *Staphylococcus*.

Folliculitis

■ Etiology

Folliculitis is an infection of the upper portion of the hair follicle and surrounding areas caused by staphylococci. Commonly referred to as an "ingrown" hair, the hair grows inward and curls up to form an infected nodule (**Fig. 32.3**). It tends to occur in areas with short, coarse hair (e.g., facial hair, nape of the neck, chest, back, buttocks, thighs, or skin under protective padding) and can develop from friction with pads or during shaving. Pustular rashes on the trunk have been reported where occlusive bathing suits are worn. Chemical irritants, inadequate chlorination, and superhydration of the skin caused by high water temperatures (i.e., hot tubs) also are causative factors.[4,5]

■ Signs and Symptoms

The inflammation begins with a pustule forming at the mouth of the hair follicle; a crust forms and, eventually, sloughs off, along with the hair. This relatively painless pustule heals without scarring. If associated with staphylococci, swelling and erythema with or without a pustule may be present on the skin surface. These lesions are painful and may scar. "Hot tub" folliculitis, caused by *Pseudomonas aeruginosa*, may present with multiple pustular lesions on the trunk and extremities within 6 hours to 2 days after exposure.[6] Mild fever and malaise also may occur.

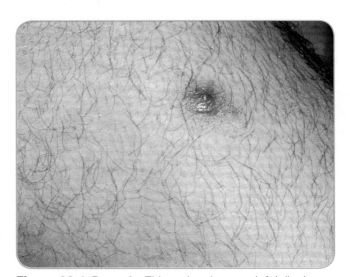

Figure 32.4. Furuncle. This patient has a painful, "pointing" furuncular nodule on the thigh.

Furuncles and Carbuncles

■ Etiology

Furuncles (boils) and carbuncles are complications of folliculitis that stem from friction or repeated blunt trauma. The infection progresses deeper and extends out from the follicle and the lesions usually contain pus. Common sites include the buttocks, belt line, anterior thigh, back of the neck, face, and axilla.

■ Signs and Symptoms

Commonly called an abscess or boil, a furuncle is a large, well-defined, deep erythematous nodule that progresses into a pustule of walled-off, purulent material, turning hard and tender when staphylococci invade the subcutaneous tissue (**Fig. 32.4**). The furuncle develops into a fluctuant mass and, eventually, opens to the skin surface, allowing the purulent contents to drain, either spontaneously or following incision of the furuncle. A carbuncle is several furuncles that have merged into a deep, communicating purulent mass.

Hidradenitis Suppurativa

■ Etiology

Hidradenitis suppurativa is a potentially serious, chronic inflammatory, **suppurative** disorder affecting the follicles and apocrine sweat glands (**Fig. 32.5**). The condition is not present before puberty, because the sweat glands are not active. At a later age, however, it can appear. *Staphylococcus aureus* usually is involved in the condition, but in chronic cases, *Proteus* sp. may be involved. Seen more commonly in women than in men, it develops primarily in the sweat glands located in the armpits, in the groin, around the breasts, and in the anal region. The condition also is seen at a higher rate in extremely overweight individuals and cigarette smokers.[7]

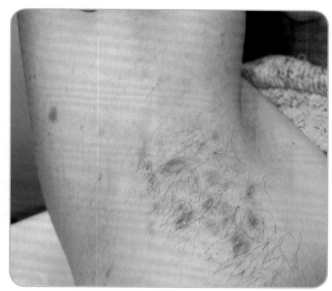

Figure 32.5. Hidradenitis suppurativa. This chronic inflammatory, pus-producing disorder affects the follicles and apocrine sweat glands.

■ Signs and Symptoms

Stage 1 hidradenitis suppurativa presents with solitary or multiple isolated, firm, red nodules without scarring or sinus tract. In stage 2, pustules and abscesses may discharge pus spontaneously and heal slowly, resulting in scar tissue. Stage 3 is characterized by extensive, multiregion involvement, with multiple interconnected sinus tracts and scarring. The appearance of nodules recurs periodically throughout the year. Heat, perspiration, and being overweight can aggravate the condition.

Pain is a common symptom in chronic conditions. Over time, extensive scarring can lead to restrictive, tight skin and vaginal, urethral, and anal strictures. If the sweat glands in the armpits or groin are involved, this can limit motion of the arms or legs. Secondary bacterial infection with staphylococci, streptococci, pseudomonas, and *Escherichia* sp. is common and produces a foul-smelling odor.[7] Infection and inflammation can spread beyond the sweat glands into the deep layers of the skin and muscle tissue, leading to cellulitis. Patients with hidradenitis suppurativa often feel socially isolated, suffering severe psychological impact because of this physically painful and disabling disease.

Cellulitis

■ Etiology

Cellulitis is a painful infection of the deep dermis caused by group A β-hemolytic streptococci (GABHS) or *S. aureus*. Some people are at risk for infection by other types of bacteria. They include people with weak immune systems and those who handle fish, meat, poultry, or soil without using gloves.

■ Signs and Symptoms

Lesions appear as an ill-defined area of tender erythema on the trunk or extremities, usually around a break in the skin, such as surgical wounds, trauma, tinea infections, or ulcerations (**Fig. 32.6**). Intense pain may be present, as may malaise, fever, and lymphangitis. Sport participation is contraindicated, because trauma to the site can cause bacteremia.

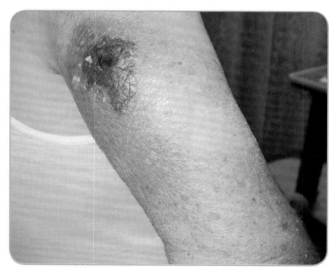

Figure 32.6. Cellulitis. This painful infection of the deep dermis and subcutaneous tissue usually occurs around a break in the skin.

Erysipelas

■ Etiology

Erysipelas is an acute, superficial, bacterial infection of the dermis and hypodermis that characteristically extends into the cutaneous lymphatics. It is considered to be a specific clinical type of cellulitis caused more frequently by streptococcal bacteria.[8] The leg is the clinical site most frequently encountered; other common sites are the face, arm, and upper thigh.

Bacterial inoculation into an area of skin trauma is the initial event in developing erysipelas. A common portal of entry is athlete's foot. Other portals include superficial wounds, stasis ulcerations, inflammatory dermatoses, dermatophyte infections, insect bites, and surgical incisions. Other predisposing factors include diabetes, alcohol abuse, infection with HIV, nephrotic syndrome, other immunocompromising conditions, and vagrant lifestyle.

Cases of erysipelas have been reported in all age groups, but it appears that infants, young children, and elderly patients are the most commonly affected groups. The peak incidence has been reported to occur between 60 and 80 years of age, especially in patients who are considered to be high risk and immunocompromised or in those with lymphatic drainage problems (e.g., after mastectomy, pelvic surgery, and bypass grafting).[8]

■ Signs and Symptoms

Erysipelas usually has a sudden onset with patients unable to recall an inciting event but can report a history of recent trauma or pharyngitis. Prodromal symptoms, such as malaise, chills, and high fever, often begin before onset of the skin lesions and usually are present within 48 hours of cutaneous involvement. Initially, a small erythematous patch progresses to a fiery-red, indurated, tense, and shiny plaque. Pruritus, burning, and tenderness are typical complaints. A well-demarcated plaque may extend by 2 to 10 cm each day. The infection rapidly invades and spreads through the lymphatic vessels, producing overlying skin "streaking" and regional lymph node swelling and tenderness. Systemic symptoms may include drowsiness or disorientation, tachypnea, tachycardia, hypotension, and oliguria.

Impetigo Contagiosa

■ Etiology

Impetigo is a highly contagious, bacterial skin inflammation most often seen in those participating in wrestling, football, rugby, swimming, and gymnastics (**Fig. 32.7**). Caused by *S. aureus* either alone or in combination with GABHS, the condition may be transmitted by direct contact; through sharing unclean towels, clothing, and equipment; or after a minor skin injury, such as an insect bite, abrasion, or dermatitis.[5,9]

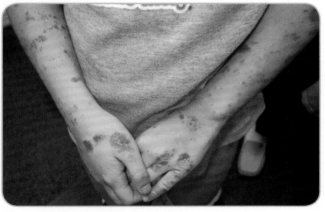

Figure 32.7. Impetigo. This highly contagious skin condition often is seen in wrestlers, swimmers, and gymnasts.

■ Signs and Symptoms

Impetigo has two different presentations—namely, bullous and nonbullous.[5,6] The bullous type, linked to *S. aureus*, begins as multiple, fluid-filled vesicles that either combine or individually enlarge to form blister-like lesions that eventually collapse centrally. The center has the characteristic of a honey-crusted lesion that, when removed, reveals reddened plaques draining serous fluid. Nonbullous impetigo caused by GABHS begins as small vesicles or pustules with erythematous bases and honey-colored crusts, which also drain fluid. The lesions may itch or burn but generally are painless. Eventually, the crust disappears, leaving a red mark that heals without scarring. Common sites are the face, buttocks, extremities, or perineum.

Ecthyma, a more serious form of impetigo, occurs when the infection penetrates deep into the skin's second layer (i.e., the dermis). Signs and symptoms include painful, fluid- or pus-filled sores that turn into deep ulcers, usually on the legs and feet. A hard, thick, gray-yellow crust covers the sores. Lymph glands may be swollen in the affected area. Scars may remain after the ulcers heal. Several conditions can be complicated by impetigo, including the following:

■ Abrasions

■ Atopic dermatitis

   ■ Individuals with a history of asthma, hay fever, or eczema

   ■ Frequent crusts on the face, popliteal region, or antecubital fossae

   ■ Contact dermatitis (especially from shoe materials and rubberized pads)

   ■ Irritant dermatitis (hands chapped from frequent immersion in or handling of irritating substances)

Methicillin-Resistant Staphylococcus aureus

■ Etiology

Methicillin-resistant *Staphylococcus aureus* (MRSA) is caused by a strain of staph bacteria that has become resistant to antibiotics commonly used to treat ordinary staph infections. Individuals who develop MRSA infections in hospitals or other health care settings, such as nursing homes and dialysis centers, are said to have a health care–associated MRSA (HA-MRSA). Another type of MRSA occurring in the wider community among healthy people is called community-associated MRSA (CA-MRSA).[5] Under normal conditions, *S. aureus* colonizes on the skin and inside the nose of an estimated 20% to 40% of healthy people.[10] Individuals who have no symptoms are called carriers. When a breakdown of the skin occurs, this bacterium invades the body, producing a skin infection (e.g., abscess or cellulitis) or a systemic infection (e.g., pneumonia and blood infection).[11] The infection is spread by skin-to-skin contact. At-risk populations include groups such as high school wrestlers, child care workers, and people who live in crowded conditions.

■ Signs and Symptoms

The most common presentation is small red bumps that resemble pimples, boils, or spider bites. These can quickly turn into deep, painful abscesses that require surgical draining. Sometimes, the bacteria remain confined to the skin, but although rare, they can also burrow deep into the body, causing potentially life-threatening infections in bones, joints, surgical wounds, the bloodstream, heart valves, and lungs.

General Management of Bacterial Infections

Most infectious bacterial skin conditions (e.g., folliculitis, acne, cellulitis, furuncles, and carbuncles) should be cleansed with soap, water, and **astringents** and are treated initially with over-the-counter (OTC) topical antibacterial agents that are applied several times per day. A physician referral may be necessary for incision, drainage, and in some instances, debridement. Patients with any suspicious lesions should be immediately referred to a physician to culture and test the lesion for any antimicrobial sensitivity. If the condition is more severe, systemic antibiotics may need to be prescribed.

Patients should be withheld from physical activity and competition if satellite lesions, cellulitis, purulent conjunctivitis, weeping lesions, or large or multiple, honey-crusted lesions are present. Patients who have cellulitis, furuncles, or carbuncles are not significantly contagious to others but should not participate in sports, because continued trauma to the involved areas can lead to systemic complications, such as bacteremia and progressive soft-tissue infections. Prior to being cleared for return to play, patients should have no new skin lesions for 48 hours, have completed a 72-hour course of directed antibiotic therapy, and have no further drainage or exudate from any lesion.[5] **Application Strategy 32.1** summarizes the general treatment of bacterial infections.

Fungal Skin Conditions

Fungal skin infections are quite common among physically active individuals. Fungus grows and thrives in dark, warm, moist environments, such as the areas between the toes or between the skin of the groin and scrotum. During activity, perspiration often accumulates in these areas. Augmented with the wearing of constrictive clothing, such as an athletic supporter, tight shorts, or spandex, the perspiration often enhances and encourages fungal growth.

Fungal infections are identified by small patches of erythema, scaling, and severe itching. Dermatophytes, also known as ringworm (tinea) fungi, and yeasts cause most fungal infections, including tinea unguium (nails), tinea pedis (feet), tinea cruris (groin), tinea corporis (body), tinea capitis (scalp), candidiasis, and tinea versicolor (**Fig. 32.8**). All but tinea versicolor are contagious and spread from person to person by sharing towels or socks and by walking with no shoes in the locker rooms and shower stalls. Fungal infections can be prevented by taking several precautionary measures (**Box 32.1**).

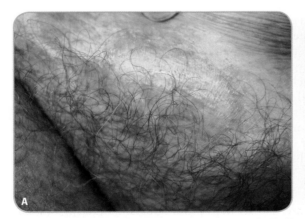 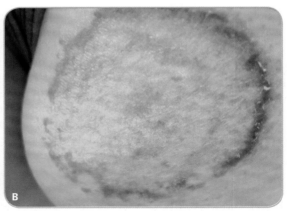

Figure 32.8. Fungal infections. A, Tinea cruris. **B,** Tinea corporis.

> **BOX 32.1 Prevention of Fungal Infections**
>
> - Shower after every practice and competition.
>
> - After each shower, thoroughly dry the feet, groin, and areas between the toes as well as under the arms and breasts.
>
> - Apply absorbent antifungal powder to the shoes, socks, and feet, between the toes, under the arms and breast, and in the groin area.
>
> - Change socks and underwear daily; allow wet shoes to dry thoroughly before wearing them.
>
> - Wear street shoes that allow some ventilation to the feet.
>
> - Clean and disinfect the floors in the shower room, dressing room, and athletic training room daily.
>
> - Never go barefoot in a shower or locker room.

Tinea Unguium

Etiology

Tinea unguium (nail), or onychomycosis, as it is more properly known, is a fungal infection of the nail beds and nails. It is common among physically active individuals, particularly those who swim in pools, use communal showers, or have chronic tinea pedis and wear occlusive footwear.[10] The fungus invades the hyponychium at the most distal attachment of the nail plate or a lateral nail fold. It migrates to the undersurface of the nail plate, leading to a nail bed infection that causes discoloration of the nail plate. The most common form, distal subungual onychomycosis, usually is associated with athlete's foot (tinea pedis).

The fingernails are more commonly affected by the fungus *Candida albicans*, which leads to *Candida* onychomycosis. Although the fungus can cause primary nail infection in people with chronic mucocutaneous candidiasis or other immunological disorders, it usually occurs as a secondary infection in otherwise healthy nails.

Signs and Symptoms

Infections usually start distally, with yellow streaks in the nail plate that gradually extend to include the entire nail. The nails become thickened, with a marked subungual hyperkeratosis that can be painful and can separate the nail plate from the bed. Over time, the nail plate becomes brittle and crumbles. Clinically, *Candida* onychomycosis may be similar in appearance to distal subungual onychomycosis, except that the entire thickness of the nail plate is affected and appears yellow, green, or opaque. The patient usually will complain of pain with activity and have some aesthetic concerns.[12]

Tinea Pedis

Etiology

Tinea pedis (i.e., athlete's foot) is the most frequent fungal infection in the physically active population. It can spread in the locker room during casual handling of contaminated socks, or it can be picked up by another player on the floor or shower stall. Infection is based on individual susceptibility, however, and may not affect certain people. Although 1% to 3% of the population are carriers of tinea pedis, prepubertal children rarely are affected.

Signs and Symptoms

Tinea pedis is divided into three types. The most common type is found in the intertriginous web spaces as a scaly, peeling eruption with or without erythema, maceration, or fissuring. When the toe webs are **macerated** and infected, *Candida* yeast usually is present in addition to the original dermatophyte. It is common for the eruptions to extend to the plantar or dorsal surface of the toe. The second type includes an eruption of vesicles and bullae on the midfoot. Dry, vesicular lesions may exude a yellowish serum. Scratching the area leads to scaling, peeling, and cracking fissures in the skin, particularly if the condition extends between the toes and can spread the problem to other parts of the body. The third type produces a hyperkeratotic scale with minimal erythema on the plantar surface. All three types are recognized by extreme **pruritus**, redness, and scaling on the sole of the feet and between the toes.

Tinea Cruris

■ Etiology

Tinea cruris (i.e., jock itch) involves the genitalia but often originates in the feet; therefore, the feet should always be examined when this condition is present.[13] Although typically seen in obese adult men and male athletes, women are reporting an increase in the incidence of the condition because of the increased use of panty hose, spandex, and other tight, restricting clothing. It rarely is seen in children. *Trichophyton rubrum* is the most common source of tinea cruris.

■ Signs and Symptoms

Perspiration can accumulate between the genitals and skin of the thigh. The crural or perineal folds between the scrotum and inner thighs usually are the first areas to exhibit small patches of erythema and scaling. Other signs and symptoms include diffuse, thick, dark lesions; weeping vesicles or pustules on the margins of inflammation; and severe itching. The infection can spread to the thighs, perineal area, buttocks, and abdomen. When scrotal redness or scaling occurs, it typically is the result either of an allergic reaction to skin medications used before seeing a physician or of chronic skin inflammation caused by scratching or long-term irritation. It is important to note that a patient with tinea cruris can infect bedding, towels, and clothing; these should be changed daily and thoroughly washed in hot water.

Tinea Corporis

■ Etiology

Tinea corporis (i.e., tinea of the body) is caused by dermatophytes, usually of the genus *Trichophyton*. It affects both humans and animals.

■ Signs and Symptoms

The condition is characterized by one or more circular, pruritic patches that are slightly erythematous, dry, scaly, and usually, hypopigmented.[5,14] The lesions may be slightly elevated at the border, where they are more inflamed and scaly compared with the central part of the lesion. A well-defined, central ring generally is found on the upper extremities, axillae, and trunk. Certain individuals can carry the spores without the rash; the degree of rash depends on the host's cellular-based immune response, which can vary widely. Tinea corporis is common in prepubertal children, because they often contract the condition from infected pets. Wrestlers are at a high risk for outbreaks because of improper or inadequate cleansing of the mats and uniforms, skin-to-skin contact, occlusive equipment, and macerated skin.[5,15] Among wrestlers, the condition is referred to as tinea gladiatorum.

Tinea Capitis

■ Etiology

Tinea capitis, or ringworm of the scalp, is very common in children. Primary sources of the infection are contaminated hair brushes, combs, and animals.

■ Signs and Symptoms

The condition begins as a small papule on the scalp and then spreads peripherally. The lesions appear as small, gray scales resulting in scattered bald patches.[5]

Tinea Versicolor

■ Etiology

Tinea versicolor, also known as pityriasis versicolor, is one of the most common pigmentary disorders worldwide. It stems from a yeast, known as *Malassezia furfur*, that is a normal part of the skin flora.

Excessive heat, humidity, and oily skin promote the growth of this organism in the stratum corneum. It is seen more often on the trunk, primarily the back, and on the upper extremities rather than on the lower extremities. It is commonly seen during adolescence and young adulthood when sebaceous activity is high.

■ Signs and Symptoms

Referred to as "sun spots," tinea versicolor is best noticed after exposure to the sun. Although the rest of the skin tans, the area with tinea versicolor does not. The patient usually will have many irregularly shaped, slightly scaling macules and patches, generally covering large areas of the body and separated by normal skin. The macules are yellowish-brown, pale yellow, or dark-brown, and occasionally reddish or pinkish, appearing to be either hypopigmented or hyperpigmented.[16] In dark-skinned individuals, the infection appears as well-defined, white patches. The area may be asymptomatic or mildly pruritic. Scratching detaches sheets of epidermis, leaving patches of raw base. The patches develop and resolve without treatment. Unlike other fungal infections, it is not contagious.

Candidiasis

■ Etiology

Candidiasis, which is caused by the yeast fungus *C. albicans*, can produce infections on the skin or mucous membranes or in the vagina. Skin infections tend to be found in skinfolds, such as the axillae, groin, and below the breasts, when friction occurs within a hot, moist, humid environment. The condition is more common in women who wear a swimsuit or a competition uniform for long periods of time.

■ Signs and Symptoms

The lesion appears as a deep, beefy-red color and is bordered with small, red, satellite pustules. In skinfolds, a white, macerated border may surround the red area. Later, deep and painful fissures may develop where the skin creases. If left untreated, the infection can lead to a life-threatening systemic disease.

General Management of Fungal Skin Infections

Treatment of fungal skin infections involves antifungal medication and changing the warm, moist environment. The two main classes of antifungals are allylamines and azoles. Use of either an allylamine or azole antifungal treatment depends on patient compliance and cost; allylamines are more costly but allow shorter treatment periods. Dry infections of athlete's foot, jock itch, and tinea capitis respond well to OTC topical azoles, such as clotrimazole (e.g., Lotrimin and Mycelex), one of the oldest antifungal treatments. Others include miconazole (e.g., Mictrin and Monistat) or tolnaftate (e.g., Tinactin). These typically are applied twice daily for at least 1 month. Moderate cases are best treated with allylamines, such as terbinafine, butenafine, or naftifine, twice daily for 2 to 4 weeks.[5,12,13] For individuals who continue the type of activity that can lead to the infection, topical treatment should continue for 2 weeks after signs of the infection are gone. During treatment, the area should be kept clean and dry. Loose, absorbent clothing (e.g., cotton socks and underwear) should be worn, and shower and locker rooms should be kept clean.[1,5]

Patients with widespread fungal infections (e.g., tinea corporis or tinea capitis) should be treated with griseofulvin, but this agent is not always effective. Resistant cases may respond better to systemic ketoconazole, fluconazole, and itraconazole; however, long-term use of these drugs, especially ketoconazole, may cause liver toxicity. Patients with tinea corporis should not return to play until completing a minimum of 72-hour topical fungicide treatment. The lesions must be covered with a gas-permeable dressing followed by underwrap and stretch tape. Patients with tinea capitis should complete a minimum of 2-week systemic antifungal therapy.[5] The general management of fungal skin conditions can be seen in **Application Strategy 32.2.**

Viral Skin Conditions

Skin lesions caused by viruses, such as herpes simplex, herpes gladiatorum, herpes zoster (i.e., shingles), verrucae (i.e., warts), and molluscum contagiosum, can be difficult to treat, because

APPLICATION STRATEGY 32.2

Management of Fungal Skin Conditions

- Wash the involved region four to five times daily and after physical exertion.
- Rinse all soap residue from the region and completely dry the area. With dry tinea infections, apply antifungal powder liberally before an exercise period.
- Apply topical antifungal agents, such as Halotex, Lotrimin, Mycelex, and Tinactin, twice daily for 1 month.
- If the condition does not clear up, see a physician to rule out candidiasis, dermatitis, psoriasis, or other skin disorders.
- In resistant infections, prescribed allylamines, such as terbinafine, butenafine, or naftifine, may be used twice daily for 2–4 weeks.
- Follow proper personal hygiene as listed in **Box 32.1**.

they often require long-term therapy and activity restrictions. Routine hygienic measures, such as showering immediately after activity and keeping individuals with open lesions on exposed skin from participating in contact sports, may reduce or eliminate transmission of these pathogens.

Herpes Simplex

■ Etiology

Herpes simplex virus (HSV) encompasses more than 80 different viruses and is extremely contagious. The two most common types are HSV-1 and HSV-2. HSV-1 (i.e., cold sores) normally infects the area of the lips, nose, and chin and orally recurs, on average, one to three times per year (**Fig. 32.9**). It has been known to be transmitted by direct skin-to-skin contact during participation in sports such as wrestling, in which it is called herpes gladiatorum.[17] It also causes approximately one-third of new cases of genital herpes and is transmitted most often through oral sex. HSV-2 causes two-thirds of all new genital herpes cases and 95% of recurrences of genital herpes.[18] HSV-1 recurs genitally approximately once every other year, whereas on average, HSV-2 recurs genitally approximately five times per year.

■ Signs and Symptoms

The incubation period for primary infection (2 to 12 days) usually begins with a burning and stinging pain, tenderness, or itching at the infected site, followed by clusters of vesicles on an erythematous base. The lesions are capable of latency as they migrate to the dorsal ganglions in the spinal cord. There may be no other symptoms, or there may be fever, localized lymphadenopathy, malaise, myalgia, dysuria, pharyngitis, or rarely, keratoconjunctivitis. Preexisting abrasions or other underlying skin conditions will increase the likelihood of transmission.[5,18]

It is critical to identify the condition at an early stage and immediately refer the patient to a physician for care. During the latent state, the patient has no blisters, sores, or other symptoms. During the shedding stage, the virus begins to multiply in the nerves and can enter into body fluids, such as saliva, semen, or vaginal fluids. No symptoms are present at this stage, but the virus can be easily spread during this time.

A tendency exists to recur regularly—even monthly—at the site of the primary lesion. Several factors can trigger recurrences, particularly of the HSV-1 strain. These include sunlight exposure (especially on the lips), stress, fatigue, food allergies, other infections (e.g., cold or influenza), impaired immune system, hormonal changes caused by a woman's menstrual cycle, or pregnancy.[18]

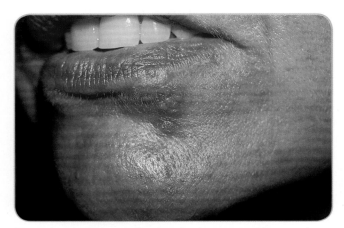

Figure 32.9. Herpes simplex. Lesions are evident on the vermillion border of the lip and beyond.

Herpes Zoster

■ Etiology

Herpes zoster, or shingles, as it is more commonly known, is rare. Local trauma that occurs during contact sports occasionally can precipitate reactivation of the varicella virus, which, after a case of chickenpox, can retreat into the nerve roots, where it lies dormant. Participation should be prohibited, both for pain relief and to lessen transmission to others who have never had chickenpox.

■ Signs and Symptoms

Herpes zoster is characterized by unilateral, blister-like lesions that erupt along dermatomes, usually T3–L3 in the trunk or, less commonly, in the area of the 5th cranial nerve.[19] Migrating along the dermatomes, the

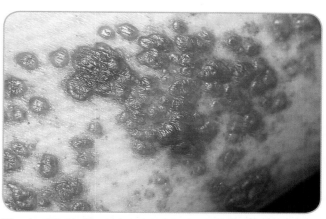

Figure 32.10. Herpes zoster. These grouped vesicles of various sizes are on an erythematous base.

condition initially causes pain, burning, tingling, or itching, followed by eruptions of fluid-filled vesicles in strips on one side of the body 1 to 3 days later (**Fig. 32.10**). Other signs and symptoms include headache, malaise, swollen lymph nodes near the site of the eruption, and a low-grade fever. A few days after the vesicles form, they burst and crust over. Fluids from the lesions contain live viruses, so the patient remains infectious until the lesions crust over. The rash and blisters also can occur around the eye, on the face or scalp, inside the mouth, or down an arm or leg. Although the rash and blisters may resemble chickenpox, shingles typically is limited to a small area on one side of the body.

Verrucae Virus

■ Etiology

More than 60 types of the human papillomavirus can lead to a rapid growth of cells on the outer layer of skin, resulting in a wart, of which verrucae plana (i.e., flat wart) and verrucae plantaris (i.e., plantar wart) are only two of the more common ones. Incubation is several weeks to 5 years after exposure.

■ Signs and Symptoms

The common wart is prevalent on the hands and appears as a small, round, elevated lesion with a rough, dry surface (**Fig. 32.11**). They do not retain the normal fingerprint lines on the hands and feet that corns and calluses do.[20] Pressure on the wart increases the pain. Because of its location, the common wart often is subjected to secondary bacterial infection. A plantar wart, which grows into the thick stratum corneum of the foot, has tiny, dark red or black dots, representing thrombosed

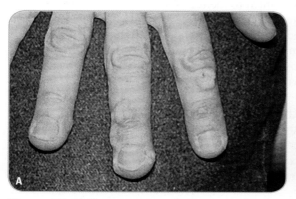
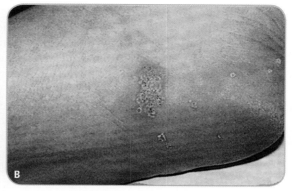

Figure 32.11. Verrucae virus. A, Verruca vulgaris produces dry, rough warts on the hands. **B,** Verruca plantaris leads to plantar warts.

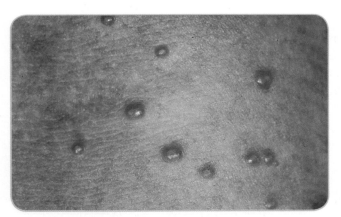

Figure 32.12. Molluscum contagiosum. This highly contagious poxvirus produces characteristic dome-shaped, shiny, waxy papules with a central white core.

capillaries that have been penetrated by the root of the wart. Verrucae plantaris likely is transmitted from swimming pool decks or shower rooms.

Molluscum Contagiosum

■ Etiology

A poxvirus, molluscum contagiosum, is commonly reported by swimmers, wrestlers, gymnasts, and younger children who have immature immune systems. The virus is spread by personal contact and by contaminated swimming pools and gymnastic equipment.

■ Signs and Symptoms

Lesions, which are multiple, pearly papules 1 to 10 mm in diameter, appear flesh-colored to yellow and have a tiny, round spot on the surface (**Fig. 32.12**).[5] They commonly are found on the trunk, axilla, face, thighs, and genital areas. The condition is primarily a cosmetic problem; however, blunt trauma can rupture a papule, causing a disabling local inflammatory reaction that can mimic cellulitis. It is moderately contagious and is spread by skin-to-skin contact and autoinoculation. The lesions usually resolve in 6 to 12 months.

General Management of Viral Skin Infections

Some viral conditions will dry up and heal without treatment. The virus, however, cannot be eradicated from the body. For herpes simplex and herpes zoster, treatment with oral antiviral medications should begin promptly. Patients with herpes simplex should not be cleared for return to play until they are free of systemic symptoms (e.g., fever, malaise), have no new lesions for at least 72 hours, have no moist lesions, and have completed a minimum of 120 hours of systemic antiviral therapy.[5] Although painful, a case of shingles usually heals entirely within a month with or without treatment. Because infection with HIV can precipitate herpes zoster in a young person, an HIV test is appropriate.

Recurrences of verrucae virus are frequent, and no single method of treatment is effective for all lesions. Options include mechanical, chemical, or immunological methods. Within 6 months, most young people develop an immunological reaction to the virus, and the wart may disappear with or without treatment. For others, any treatment will be ineffective. During the competitive season, a doughnut pad can be worn to alleviate some of the pressure to the area. After the season, under the direction of a physician or podiatrist, treatment may involve injections into the wart to kill the virus, cryosurgery (liquid nitrogen), electrocautery, excision, or laser treatment. Immunological methods used to induce an immune response to suppress warts include injected agents (e.g., *Candida* or mumps antigen), topical agents, or oral agents.[5,20]

Treatment for molluscum contagiosum involves immediate referral to a physician who may employ a destructive mechanical modality (e.g., curettage, electrotherapy, or cryotherapy with liquid nitrogen), chemical treatments (e.g., physician-applied trichloroacetic acid), or immunological methods (e.g., topically applied immune enhancer that stimulates cytokines).[20] Full activity can be resumed 2 to 4 days after resolution of the curetted or removed lesions. Any localized lesions may be covered with a gas-permeable dressing followed by underwrap and stretch tape.[5]

 The open sore that presented on the right thigh of the wrestler 3 days earlier has a honey-colored crust with surrounding erythema. The signs and symptoms that would indicate impetigo include itching or burning, but the area is not usually painful. The sore ruptures quickly, oozing either fluid or pus that forms a honey-colored crust, and eventually, the crust disappears, leaving a red mark that heals without scarring. Common sites for impetigo are the face, most often around the nose and mouth, body folds, and areas subject to friction and occlusion (e.g., thighs and axillae).

OTHER SKIN REACTIONS

> **?** During a summer field hockey camp for high school girls, one of the players comes off the field and reports being stung by a bee. This is the first time the individual has ever been stung. What signs and symptoms would suggest an allergic reaction to the venom?

Unlike skin infections caused by bacteria, fungi, and viruses, other skin problems caused by mechanical, environmental, allergic, or chemical reactions are not infectious and generally are mild in nature. Once identified, they can be treated easily with topical medications.

Chafing of the Skin

Etiology

Chafing of the skin, or **intertrigo**, is a superficial dermatitis more often caused by the friction of fabric rubbing against moist, warm skin rather than by skin rubbing against skin. The condition may occur between the creases of the neck, in the axillary and buttocks area, or beneath large breasts but is seen primarily in the groin region of individuals with muscular thighs or in obese individuals.

Signs and Symptoms

The condition is characterized by erythema, maceration, burning, and itching (**Fig. 32.13**). In severe cases, the skin becomes eroded and weeping. The condition can be prevented by wearing loose, soft, cotton underwear to keep the skin dry, clean, and free of friction or by wearing shorts with longer legs made of low-friction fabric.

Management

Treatment involves initial application of a cold compress. The area should be cleansed daily with mild soap and water, followed by application of a soothing ointment. Talcum powders should be avoided, because they can be abrasive and do not effectively absorb moisture.

Athlete's Nodules

Etiology

Also referred to as surfer's nodules, athlete's nodules are asymptomatic, dermal nodules found at various sites of the body that encounter repeated minor trauma, such as the feet of surfers and runners, knees of canoeists, and knuckles of boxers.

Signs and Symptoms

They generally occur at sites of recurrent trauma or friction and present as a solitary dermal nodule that is asymptomatic, symmetrical, and flesh-colored; they range in size from 0.5 to 4.0 cm. Location is dependent on the particular sport that the patient participates in. For example, boxers have them located on their knuckles from hitting the speed bag and they are referred to as "knuckle pads," surfers have them on the dorsal aspect of the feet and they are referred to as "surfer's nodules," and they are found on football players' ankles.

Management

Protective pads at the trauma sites can help to decrease pain. Otherwise, high-potency topical or intralesional corticosteroids can be applied. If this does not provide relief, the nodules can be incised.

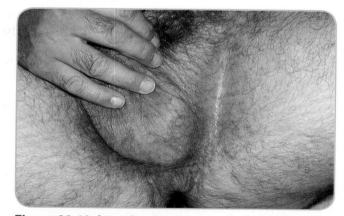

Figure 32.13. Intertrigo. Intertrigo, or chafing of the skin, is a superficial dermatitis more often caused by the friction of fabric rubbing against moist, warm skin rather than by skin rubbing on skin. This condition often is confused with tinea cruris and cutaneous candidiasis.

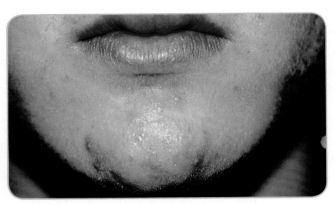

Figure 32.14. Acne mechanica. This young male developed acne-like lesions that appeared under his football chin strap. The bacterial culture was positive for *S. aureus*.

Acne Mechanica

Etiology

Characterized by a local exacerbation of acne vulgaris caused by heat, occlusion, pressure, and friction, acne mechanica presents with erythematous crops of papules and pustules in areas of mechanical trauma.

Signs and Symptoms

Sometimes referred to as football acne, the acne develops wherever skin is exposed to prolonged causative factors, such as under chin straps, forehead bands, shirt collars, football shoulder pads, backpack straps, automobile seats, bras, wide belts, and orthopaedic casts and braces. Like regular acne, the signs are whiteheads, blackheads, and pimples in the affected area (**Fig. 32.14**). If left unattended, the acne may develop into a cyst—a thick lump beneath the surface of the skin formed by the buildup of secretions deep within hair follicles.

Management

Treatment and prevention include thoroughly cleansing the area after activity with a mildly abrasive cleanser and back brush. Application of a topical astringent or 10% benzoyl peroxide agent, a topical antibiotic, and in severe cases, a systemic antibiotic may be prescribed. The condition usually improves or resolves after the season. Prevention involves wearing a clean, absorbent t-shirt under the football pads and treating any underlying acne vulgaris. If an exercise leotard is worn during exercise, it should be removed immediately after the workout.

Striae Distensae

Etiology

Stretch marks, or **striae distensae**, often are seen in individuals who participate in high-intensity weight training. Although the origin is unclear, it is most often seen after rapid growth of a body part, which is believed to result in fragmented elastic skin fibers.

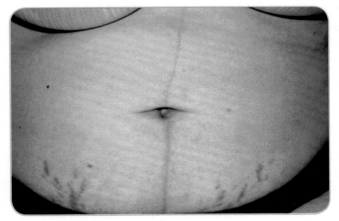

Figure 32.15. Striae. Striae occurs after rapid growth of a body part, such as during high-intensity weight training or during pregnancy. The initial purplish color will fade over time, but the striae are permanent.

Signs and Symptoms

The condition is characterized by linear pink or flesh-colored patches most often seen on the chest, shoulders, and upper outer arms (**Fig. 32.15**).

Management

No treatment exists for striae distensae.

Sunburn

Etiology

Sunburn is an inflammatory response of the skin to excessive exposure to the ultraviolet radiation in the sun's rays. Repeated overexposure can lead to an increased risk of premature aging, cutaneous melanoma, and cancer.[21] Sunscreens applied to the skin prior to sun exposure can prevent many of the damaging effects of ultraviolet radiation. The effectiveness of the sunscreen is based

BOX 32.2 Prevention of Sunburn

- Use a sunscreen with an appropriate sun protection factor (SPF) for your skin type (preferably one with an SPF of 15 or higher).
- Apply sunscreen 20–30 minutes before exposure to the sun.
- Apply sunscreen evenly over all exposed skin to avoid isolated areas of sunburn.
- Reapply sunscreen every 2–4 hours, especially if sweating profusely.
- Select sunscreen that has a high rate of efficacy when subjected to moisture.
- Be careful when applying the sunscreen around the eyes.
- Sunscreen sprays work well for the top of the head; lip protectors also should be used.
- Avoid midday exposure to the sun (10:00 a.m.–4:00 p.m.).
- While in the sun, wear loose, woven, light, cotton clothing.
- Hats with brims are much better than caps or visors.
- Sunburn can occur on cloudy days, so sunscreen should be worn at all times.
- Be aware of the reflective photo-energy potential when around water or snow.
- Several medications (e.g., antibiotics, antiseptics, anesthetics, and certain nonsteroidal anti-inflammatory drugs) increase sensitivity to the sun. Read the instructions for use of any medications before sun exposure. If there are questions, consult a pharmacist or physician.
- Drink plenty of nonalcoholic beverages to prevent dehydration.

on the SPF. For example, an SPF of 15 indicates that an individual can be exposed to ultraviolet light 15-fold longer than without a sunscreen before the skin will begin to burn. Higher numbers provide better protection: SPF 15 is good, SPF 30 is better, and SPF 50 provides a complete sun block. A minimum SPF of 15 is recommended. The degree of sunburn depends on the length of exposure to the sun, the sun's relative level of intensity, and personal skin type. Although sunburns are easily treated, it is best to prevent them from occurring (**Box 32.2**).

Signs and Symptoms

Sunburns are classified as first, second, or third degree. The full extent of the injury may not be assessed until 24 to 48 hours after exposure. First-degree sunburns have mild erythema throughout the area of exposure and may have associated pain and discomfort (**Fig. 32.16**). Second-degree sunburns have vesicles or blisters in addition to the erythema. Peeling of the skin usually begins after 2 to 3 days, and the skin is dry and itchy. Third-degree sunburns will exhibit skin ulcerations. Systemic symptoms of burns, regardless of their degree, include fever, chills, nausea, and exhaustion. Acute sunburn (i.e., actinic dermatitis) can be painful and disfiguring and, depending on the severity, can prevent participation in sport and physical activities.[1,21]

Management

If sunburn occurs, apply a cold compress, topical hydrocortisone 1% cream or spray, and aloe vera to decrease pain and discomfort. If systemic aspirin or nonsteroidal anti-inflammatory drugs (NSAIDs) are used, they must be taken immediately after exposure to the sun to be effective. Serious second- and third-degree sunburns require immediate referral to a physician to ensure proper treatment and prevention of infection. Oral corticosteroids may be prescribed to relieve the pain.

Pernio (Chilblains)

Etiology

Excessive exposure to cold can lead to **pernio**, a condition whereby the skin tissue does not freeze but, rather, reacts with erythema, itching, and burning. This happens especially on the dorsa of the

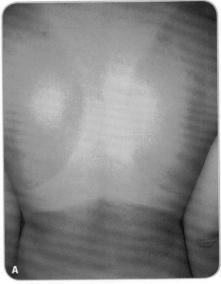
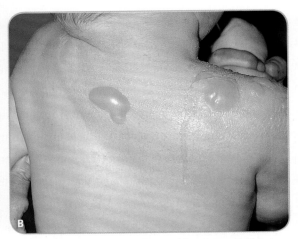

Figure 32.16. **Sunburn. A,** First-degree sunburn. **B,** Second-degree sunburn with substantial blisters.

fingers and toes and on the heels, nose, and ears. More commonly seen in young women, the condition often occurs with the first exposure to lower temperatures in highly humid conditions.

Signs and Symptoms

The affected area appears reddish, and it itches and burns (**Fig. 32.17**). Lesions may be single or multiple and, in severe cases, may appear blistered or ulcerated.

Management

Treatment involves gradual warming of the body part. Topical steroids may help to reduce inflammation, but the potency must be low enough to prevent further vasoconstriction. Heavy woolen socks may need to be worn at all times, including when indoors and while sleeping.

Miliaria Rubra

Etiology

Miliaria, or "prickly heat," is caused when active sweat glands become blocked by organic debris, leading to an inflamed and pruritic skin eruption. It was discussed in detail in Chapter 29.

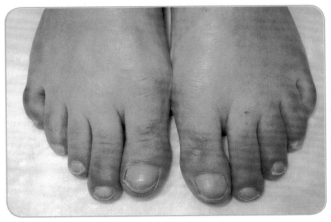

Figure 32.17. **Chilblains.** Excessive exposure to cold can lead to pernio, in which the tissue does not freeze, but, rather, appears reddish, itches, and burns.

Management

Treatment involves cooling and drying the skin, controlling the itching, and watching for infection. Individuals should avoid occlusive topical ointments and close-fitting, poorly absorbent fabrics on the skin.

Dry (Xerotic) Skin

Etiology

Dry skin is common during the winter months. Individuals who must shower frequently are particularly prone to this condition. Xerotic skin can be caused by a number of factors, but decreased skin lipids appear to be the major cause (**Box 32.3**). In the winter, dry and cold winds increase evaporation from convection, and low temperatures decrease skin flexibility and, in doing so, exacerbate the condition.

> ## BOX 32.3 Causes of Dry (Xerotic) Skin
>
> - Genetic predisposition to dry skin
> - Repetitive trauma from scratching already dry skin
> - Decreased skin lipids because of the following:
>   - Age
>   - Chronic illness
>   - Malnutrition
>
> - Environmental factors, such as the following:
>   - Decreased humidity
>   - Winter weather (dry, cold winds)
>   - Indoor heating and air conditioning
>   - Dry environments (airplanes)
> - Use of industrial or domestic cleansers or solvents
> - Frequent bathing

Signs and Symptoms

The skin appears dry, with variable erythema and scaling. Usually appearing first on the shins, it is also common on the forearms and dorsum of the hands. For individuals who exercise outdoors in the winter, the face can also be affected. Localized or generalized pruritus is the most common symptom. When severe, the dry skin loses its suppleness and cracks, fissures, and erythema appear.

Management

Treatment is focused on preventing skin dehydration. Tepid, rather than hot, water should be used for bathing, and time spent in the shower should be limited. Moisturizing soaps may be used; however, xerotic areas should be avoided. If possible, use of soap should be limited to the genitalia, underarms, hands, feet, and face. Bubble baths and brisk scrubbing should be avoided. Emollient lotions containing high concentrations of lipids increase and maintain hydration by occluding the skin surface and help to insulate against the cold. These should be applied frequently and liberally, especially after each hand washing and immediately after bathing to minimize water loss from evaporation. Swimmers should moisturize the whole body after bathing. In severe cases, antipruritics may be used to decrease pruritus and scratching, thus enabling the outer skin layer to heal. α-Hydroxy acids and topical corticosteroids can be used to decrease the inflammation associated with fissures and severely dry skin.

Eczema

Etiology

Eczema is a generic term for acute or chronic inflammatory conditions of the skin. The condition can have an onset during the first few years of life, and a history of asthma or hay fever may be reported.[22] Eczema can take a physical as well as an emotional toll.

Signs and Symptoms

The condition is characterized by poorly marginated erythema with scaling and exudate (**Fig. 32.18**). Persistent itching and burning can lead to evidence of excoriation. The condition is aggravated by an increase in body heat and perspiration, both of which occur during physical activity. Patients may report that the itching and scratching disrupt their sleep.

Management

Topical corticosteroids in an emollient cream or ointment base can serve as a substitute for soap, bath oils,

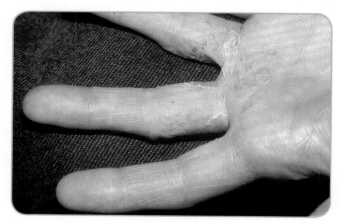

Figure 32.18. Eczema. This inflammatory condition of the skin is characterized by poorly marginated erythema with scaling and exudate. In this patient, the vesicles are beginning to dry, and the lesions are becoming scaly.

and moisturizers. These are active ingredients intended to support the dermal layer and reduce itching. Consistent use of the steroid should be applied to the affected area after bathing. Use of very potent steroid applications should not exceed 3 weeks; use of moderate to mild steroid application should not exceed 3 months at a time without reexamination of the affected region.[22] Antihistamines may provide relief from the itching but, during acute flares, systemic corticosteroids most often are used.

Psoriasis

Etiology

Psoriasis is a chronic, distressing skin disorder that can affect the skin, tendons, ligaments, and joints and is characterized by a rapid buildup of rough, dry, dead skin cells, forming thick scales. Normally, it takes approximately a month for new skin cells to move from the lowest layer of skin, where they first form, to the outermost layer, where they die and scale off in flakes. In psoriasis, the life cycle of skin cells speeds up, resulting in a multitude of dead cells on the outermost layer of skin. The scales tend to flare periodically and may go into remission, but they usually remain active for years. The most common form of psoriasis, plaque psoriasis, occurs in more than 80% of affected individuals.[23]

Factors that may trigger psoriasis include a systemic infection (e.g., strep throat), an immune system response to disease, injury to the skin, certain medications (e.g., lithium, β-blockers, antimalarial drugs, NSAIDs, and oral steroid withdrawal), alcohol, and environmental factors, such as overexposure to sun or prolonged contact with chemicals (e.g., disinfectants and paint thinners).[23,24]

Signs and Symptoms

Plaque psoriasis is characterized by sharply demarcated, dry, red patches of skin covered with silvery scales that typically affect the elbows, knees, scalp, and intergluteal cleft (**Fig. 32.19**). Scales from scalp patches of psoriasis may resemble dandruff. In some cases, there may be pitting, ridging, and discoloration of fingernails and toenails. Individuals lose many of the protective functions of skin, including its ability to protect against infection, regulate body temperature, and prevent loss of fluids and nutrients through the cutaneous surface.[25]

Management

Psoriasis is difficult to control because of the wide variation in type, severity, and response to treatment. It is a chronic disease without a cure. Three broad categories of treatment options exist, including topical modalities, phototherapy, and systemic therapy. Topical therapies are effective for mild to moderate cases, whereas phototherapy and systemic medications are more appropriate for more severe cases. Topical treatments include topical steroids, tar, anthralin, vitamin D derivatives, retinoids (e.g., tazarotene), immunosuppressants (e.g., tacrolimus and pimecrolimus), and salicylic acid. Newer topical treatments (e.g., Elidel cream and Protopic) have been especially effective in treating children with the disorder.[24] Phototherapy with broadband ultraviolet B light, narrowband ultraviolet B light, and psoralen with ultraviolet A light as well as oral acitretin, methotrexate, and cyclosporin also are highly effective.[23] Alefacept (e.g., Amevive) is a treatment option for more severe cases of psoriasis or for those cases that do not respond to other treatments.

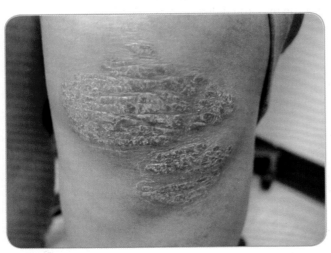

Figure 32.19. Psoriasis. This chronic skin condition is characterized by a rapid buildup of rough, dry, dead skin cells forming thick scales.

Hyperhidrosis

Etiology

Hyperhidrosis is a condition involving excessive perspiration, particularly on the palms and axillary region. The condition can interfere with sports that require holding various objects (e.g., balls, discus, bars, oars, and sticks) or that require gripping (e.g., tennis and racquetball).

The plantar sweat glands often are stimulated when the extremities are used and during times of emotional excitement, which also stimulates the axillary apocrine glands.

A number of factors can affect how much an individual sweats and even how the sweat smells. Some people sweat more than others for no apparent reason; however, other factors can cause intense sweating. These may include heredity, certain foods (i.e., spicy foods, hot beverages, and beverages containing caffeine or alcohol), and certain drugs (i.e., some antipsychotic medications, morphine, excess doses of the thyroid hormone thyroxine, and overdoses of analgesics [e.g., aspirin and acetaminophen]). Women going through menopause may experience hot flashes (i.e., a rise in skin temperature accompanied by sweating and a feeling of intense heat) because of a drop in estrogen levels. Some menopausal women also may be awakened at night by soaking sweats followed by chills.

Signs and Symptoms

Patients describe excessive perspiration triggered by emotion that began in childhood or adolescence. It is most likely to occur on the face, underarms, palms, and soles of the feet. Palmar hyperhidrosis usually is accompanied by plantar hyperhidrosis, which is easier to conceal, but may cause **bromhidrosis**, infection, and skin maceration. Excessive palm perspiration can make it difficult to grasp common objects and, if one avoids handshakes or chooses not to touch other individuals, can lead to professional embarrassment.

Management

For some individuals, OTC antiperspirants used on the underarms, hands, and feet may limit the production of perspiration. Antiperspirants block the sweat ducts with aluminum salts, thereby reducing the amount of perspiration that reaches the skin. Deodorants, which can eliminate odor but not perspiration, turn the skin acidic, which makes it less attractive to bacteria. Antiperspirants can cause irritation or contact dermatitis. For more severe cases, an individual may apply, as prescribed, 20% aluminum chloride hexahydrate with anhydrous ethyl alcohol. The solution must be applied to dry skin, typically before sleep, and washed off 6 to 8 hours later.[26] Physically active individuals may wish to wear gloves to help absorb the sweat, or they may choose not to participate in activities that require a prolonged hand grip. If OTC products are not strong enough, other recommended treatments may include iontophoresis, botulinum toxin (e.g., Botox) injections to block the nerves that trigger the sweat glands, or surgery to remove troublesome sweat glands.

Bites and Stings

Bites and stings come from a variety of insects, including mosquitoes, flies, spiders, ants, bees, fleas, and ticks. Although many are just annoying pests that can be discouraged with standard insect repellent, their bites and stings can be painful or even life threatening if the individual develops an allergic reaction to the venom (i.e., anaphylaxis).

Anaphylaxis

■ Etiology
Anaphylaxis is an immediate, shock-like, and frequently fatal hypersensitivity reaction that occurs within minutes of administration of an allergen unless appropriate first-aid measures are taken immediately. The condition is characterized by contraction of smooth muscle and dilation of capillaries because of the release of pharmacologically active substances (e.g., histamine, bradykinin, and serotonin).

■ Signs and Symptoms
Signs and symptoms include respiratory distress, cyanosis, rapid and weak pulse, weakness, low blood pressure, localized urticaria or edema, paresthesia, dilated pupils, choking, wheezing, sudden collapse, involuntary loss of bowel and bladder control, headache, dizziness, seizures, and unconsciousness.

■ Management
A patient with a history of such reactions may wear a medical identification tag and have a self-administered epinephrine device (Epipen). An Epipen auto-injector is an epinephrine-delivery system

Use of an Epipen Auto-Injector

1. Check the expiration date to make sure the pen is usable.
2. Check the fluid for cloudiness or discoloration (discard if cloudy or discolored).
3. Remove the gray safety cap.
4. Hold the Epipen firmly with the black tip against the skin of the thigh.
5. Push the pen into the thigh and apply moderate pressure for 10 seconds to inject the fluid.
6. Discard the used pen using universal precautions.
7. Call emergency medical assistance to provide further care for the injured party.

with a spring-activated needle. It is used to treat severe allergic reactions to insect bites or stings, foods, drugs, and other allergens. It also may be used as treatment for basic life support of individuals suffering from a severe asthma attack.

Epipen comes in two strengths—namely, Epipen Jr. for children up to 33 lb and Epipen Adult. It is best used when injected directly into the skin, preferably the thigh, but it can be injected through clothing if necessary. Once in the system, epinephrine constricts blood vessels to improve blood circulation and blood pressure and relaxes smooth muscles to improve breathing. Epinephrine also stimulates the heartbeat and reverses swelling and hives. The effects of epinephrine take place within seconds and can last for 10 to 20 minutes. Epipen should not be stored in extreme heat or direct sunlight, be refrigerated, or be used if the liquid is cloudy or discolored or the expiration date has passed. **Application Strategy 32.3** describes the proper use of a self-administered epinephrine device.

Mosquitoes, Gnats, and Flies

■ Etiology
Mosquitoes, gnats, and a variety of flies feed on human blood and are considered to be biting insects.

■ Signs and Symptoms
Most bites appear as erythematous, macular or papular, pruritic, painful lesions. The lesion may not be apparent immediately but may appear as a delayed hypersensitive response to the saliva of the biting organism.

■ Management
Immediate application of a cold compress can relieve pain, or an OTC topical corticosteroid or systemic antihistamine may be used. Systemic corticosteroids are used in severe cases. Once a lesion has appeared, it should be monitored closely for secondary infection.

Bees, Wasps, and Ants

■ Etiology
It is estimated that more than 20% of the U.S. population is allergic to the hymenopteran venom from bees, wasps, and ants, which in turn carries a higher risk of allergic and anaphylactic reactions. Individuals involved in outdoor activities are at special risk for insect stings. Yellow jackets and honeybees, for example, are fond of sweets and can be drawn to rehydration stations stocked with sugar-containing sport drinks. Fire ants, especially in the southern United States, can be found on practice and game fields where individuals may sit on the ground.

■ Signs and Symptoms
The sting results in a painful wheal or hive caused by the venom. The site rapidly becomes pruritic, and itching can last for several hours. Occasionally, an exaggerated local reaction can occur in which the swelling and itching extend beyond the sting site to the involved extremity and may be associated with dyspnea, tachycardia, hypotension, and anaphylaxis.

APPLICATION STRATEGY 32.4

Management of a Bee Sting

Prevention Note

For sensitive athletes who participate outdoors, suggest that they do the following:
1. Refrain from wearing bright, colorful, or floral clothing.
2. Refrain from using scented soaps, lotions, or aftershaves.

After Sustaining a Bee Sting

1. Immediately refrain from strenuous exercise.
2. Remove the stinger with a fingernail. Do not squeeze it, because this will inject more venom.
3. Apply ice to the site.
4. Systemic antihistamines may help with local reactions.
5. Observe closely for signs of anaphylactic shock:

   - Faintness, deteriorating consciousness, or other signs of shock
   - Generalized urticaria or edema
   - Paresthesia
   - Choking or signs of laryngeal edema
   - Pupillary dilation
   - Wheezing, coughing, or difficulty breathing

If Anaphylaxis Occurs

1. Place the patient supine with the feet elevated.
2. Apply a constricting band a few inches proximal to the sting site that

   - Occludes superficial venous and lymphatic return.
   - Does not obstruct arterial flow.

3. Continue ice application to further reduce venom absorption.
4. Check for a medical identification tag.
5. If the person has an Epipen or other allergy kit, inject the epinephrine into the thigh as instructed.
6. If respiratory or cardiac arrest occurs, begin cardiopulmonary resuscitation.

◼ Management

This situation may result in a medical emergency. When a sting occurs, the guidelines in **Application Strategy 32.4** should be followed.

Spiders

◼ Etiology

The venom from several spiders also can lead to painful lesions (**Fig. 32.20**).

◼ Signs and Symptoms

Black widow spiders are found throughout the United States; however, only the female—a dark-black, globular-shaped spider with the characteristic ventral, reddish marking (typically an "hourglass") on her abdomen—is large enough to bite through human skin. Because the webs typically are built in relatively undisturbed, protected areas, most sport-related bites occur in storage areas for equipment. The bite often is felt as a "pinprick" and may be slightly red. Significant symptoms usually start 1 hour after the bite, with the most common symptom being spasmodic muscle pain. The spasms may progress to regional muscle groups of the trunk, with pain and spasm lasting from 12 to 48 hours. Other reactions may include an increased respiratory rate, tachycardia, hypertension, fever, headache, nausea, vomiting, restlessness, and anxiety.

Activate the emergency plan, including summoning emergency medical services (EMS).

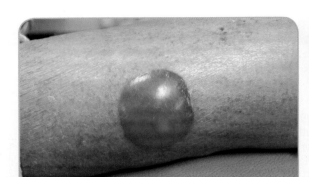
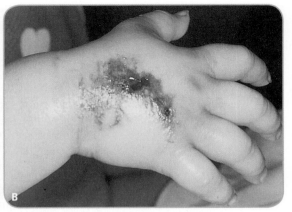

Figure 32.20. Spider bites. A, This spider bite resulted in a large, fluid-filled bullous. **B,** Necrotizing skin damage resulted from a brown recluse spider bite.

The brown recluse spider is found predominantly in the Southern and Midwestern United States. Bites cause the most severe form of arthropod-induced tissue necrosis, yet these bites are relatively painless at first and may go undetected. In the ensuing hours, the site becomes pruritic, red, and mildly swollen. Local pain, resulting from vasospasm and ischemia, begins within 2 to 8 hours. After 12 to 18 hours, a small, central vesicle develops, surrounded by an irregular border of erythema, ecchymosis, and edema. If the blister ruptures, the erythema darkens and may spread distally. After 5 to 7 days of progressive aseptic necrosis, the bite area becomes depressed and covered with a black crust that eventually sloughs off, leaving an open ulcer that tends to heal over a period of several weeks. Healing is slow, requiring 2 to 4 months.[27]

The bark scorpion, which is native to Arizona and adjacent regions, is a nocturnal spider that tends to hide in dark areas during the day. The small tooth at the base of its stinger distinguishes the bark scorpion from other less toxic species. Individuals involved with outdoor activities are most at risk. Individuals who are stung by a scorpion feel immediate, intense pain that significantly worsens with light pressure over the site. The pain may radiate throughout the extremity. Systemic reactions include restlessness, hypersalivation, dysphagia, visual changes, roving eye movements, respiratory distress (with stridor or wheezing), hypertension, fever, loss of bowel or bladder control, muscle spasms, and paralysis.

■ Management

The majority of spider bites and stings occurring in healthy, young adults can be managed on-site. Management includes cleaning the site with soap and water, application of ice, elevation of the affected limb to approximately heart level, and administration of aspirin or Tylenol as needed for minor discomfort. Application of ice or cold packs to bite sites has been shown to significantly reduce inflammation and slow the evolution of the lesion.[27] Prophylactic antibiotics usually are given to prevent secondary infection. Antihistamines are administered mainly to relieve pruritus and swelling. Children who have been stung or any patient who is experiencing severe symptoms, such as respiratory distress, should be transported immediately to the nearest medical facility for evaluation and management.

Fleas and Ticks

■ Etiology

Bites from fleas cause only minor discomfort. Ticks are parasites that attach their heads onto people or animals and then absorb blood. Deer ticks, in particular, are frequent carriers of **Lyme disease**, whereas other wood ticks carry a specific type of bacteria that leads to an infectious disease called Rocky Mountain spotted fever. Ticks are easily picked up on clothing when the individual is in tall grass, shrubs, or a wooded area.

◼ Signs and Symptoms

Most fleas bite in patterns of three and tend to attack the ankle and foot. Scratching the area could complicate the condition by developing a secondary infection.

Common symptoms from a tick bite include generalized malaise, myalgia (especially in the back and legs), fever, frontal headaches, nausea, and vomiting. Other symptoms may include nonproductive cough, sore throat, pleuritic chest pain, and abdominal pain.[28] An allergic reaction to tick saliva will occur at the bite site. The resulting rash usually occurs within hours to a few days after the bite, usually does not expand, and disappears within a few days.

Deer ticks are considerably smaller than an American dog tick, but the deer tick needs to stay attached to the host for 24 to 36 hours to transmit the disease-causing bacteria. The disease occurs in two stages: localized and disseminated.[28] The localized stage is characterized by a bull's-eye rash (a round ring with central clearing that may expand to a diameter of up to 50 cm) (**Fig. 32.21**). Common sites for the rash are the thigh, groin, trunk, and armpit. Other possible symptoms include low-grade fever, fatigue, headache, arthralgia, cough, and regional lymphadenopathy. Flulike symptoms including malaise, myalgia, arthralgia, headache, and fever may occur. Lymphadenopathy is also likely to occur during the localized stage. The disseminated stage is seen a few weeks after the initial infection when symptoms progress to multiple secondary cutaneous annular lesions, fever, cough, pharyngitis, adenopathy, and changes in the central nervous system symptoms. For dark-complexioned individuals, the rash looks like a bruise. During this stage, rheumatological (pain in tendons, bursae, muscle, and bones), cardiac (conduction abnormalities, myocarditis, and pericarditis), neurological (Bell palsy, meningitis, encephalitis, and cognitive difficulties), and additional manifestations (conjunctivitis, splenomegaly, and keratitis) may occur.[28]

In Rocky Mountain spotted fever, a bacterium is unlikely to be transmitted to a person by a tick that is attached for less than 20 hours. Symptoms develop 2 to 14 days after the bite and include chills, fever, severe headache, muscle pain, mental confusion, and a rash initially appearing on the wrists and ankles as spots that are 1 to 5 mm in diameter and then spreading to most parts of the body. About one-third of infected people do not get a rash. Other symptoms may include photophobia, diarrhea, excessive thirst, hallucinations, loss of appetite, nausea, and vomiting.[28]

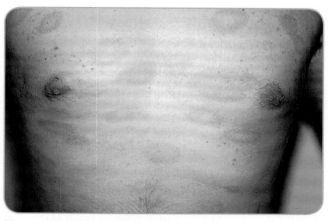

Figure 32.21. Lyme disease. The characteristic bull's-eye rash appears 3 days to 1 month after infection and presents itself as multiple annular lesions of erythema with central clearing.

◼ Management

For flea bites, treatment is limited to applying an antipruritic lotion over the area. For tick bites, the tick should be removed by applying a substance that blocks the tick's access to the air (e.g., petroleum jelly, mineral oil, or fingernail polish). The substance should make the tick withdraw its head. No attempt should be made to pull the tick from the body because doing so may leave the head embedded under the skin. If signs and symptoms of Rocky Mountain spotted fever or Lyme disease appear, the patient should be referred immediately to a physician for treatment. Routine antibiotic prophylaxis is not indicated; however, if symptoms develop, antibiotic treatment for 14 to 21 days is curative in most cases.[28]

Scabies

◼ Etiology

Scabies is a skin disease caused by a tiny, eight-legged burrowing mite, *Sarcoptes scabiei*, that produces severe, intensely itching lesions in the area of its burrows. The condition can lead to a "miniepidemic" in sports that involve physical contact, such as wrestling, rugby, or football. The mite can be spread on towels, uniforms, or equipment. Once on the skin surface, the mite burrows into the epidermis, but symptoms may not arise until 3 to 4 weeks after exposure.[12] Because of the contagious nature, physicians often recommend treatment for entire families, sexual partners, athletic teams, groups, or school classes to eradicate the mite.

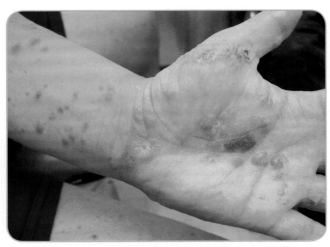

Figure 32.22. Scabies. Scabies is caused by a burrowing mite, which produces severe, intensely itching lesions in the area of its burrows.

■ Signs and Symptoms

The affected area appears as small, dark burrows and tiny vesicles in a linear distribution between the fingers and in toe web spaces, in axillary skinfolds, around the waist, or on the elbows, wrist, ankles, lateral foot, breasts, buttocks, periumbilical skin, and genitalia (**Fig. 32.22**). Intense itching, which often is severe, is usually worse at night. In first-time infections, pruritus may not develop for several weeks, whereas recurring infections may lead to symptoms within 24 hours.[15]

■ Management

Immediate referral to a physician is essential. Treatment involves eliminating the scabies infestation with medications. Topical creams and lotions, such as permethrin (e.g., Acticin) and lindane (e.g., Kwell), can be applied over the body and left on for 8 to 12 hours before being washed off. Lindane is not recommended for infants, small children, women who are pregnant or nursing, or people who have seizures or other neurological disorders. The locker room and game equipment should be disinfected. Bedding and clothing must be washed daily in hot water. Although these medications kill the mites, the itching may not subside for several weeks.

Lice (Pediculosis)

■ Etiology

Pediculus corporis (i.e., body lice), pediculus capitis (i.e., head lice), and pediculus pubis (i.e., genital lice) affect 6 to 12 million people each year and are spread by close physical contact, which makes outbreaks among those who participate in physical activities and sports problematic.[12]

■ Signs and Symptoms

Once infected, it can take up to 10 days for the nit (louse egg) to hatch. Based on the location of the infestation, patients may describe nighttime itching and, through subsequent scratching, pustules and excoriation. Head lice cause itching when they bite the skin of the scalp and neck. Egg sacks, or nits, can adhere firmly to the hair shafts and be seen behind the ears, on the back of the neck, and on the head. Body lice (length, 2 to 4 mm) are clearly visible, live in the folds of clothing, and tend to bite in areas of close contact with clothing. Pubic lice (e.g., crab lice [length, 1 to 2 mm]) typically are seen in the genitals, anal region, and lower abdomen but also can be found on the chest or axillary hair (**Fig. 32.23**).

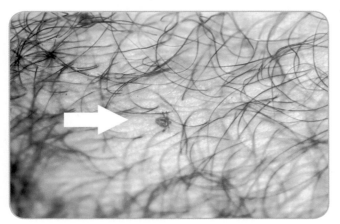

Figure 32.23. Lice. A pubic louse is a small, brown, living crab louse that can be seen here at the base of the pubic hairs (*arrow*).

■ Management

Treatment of head and pubic lice involves a 7-day regimen of permethrin lotion (either 1% or 5%), lindane 1% shampoo, petrolatum for eyelashes, and/or shampoo containing pyrethrin and piperonyl butoxide. Nit combs are available to help remove nits from hair, and all clothing, bed linens, and sporting equipment should be washed in boiling water and dried in a hot dryer or discarded.

Contact Dermatitis
Etiology

Contact dermatitis is classified as either allergic or irritant dermatitis (**Fig. 32.24**). **Allergic contact dermatitis,**

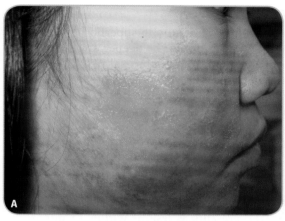 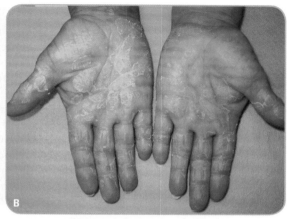

Figure 32.24. Contact dermatitis. A, Allergic contact dermatitis results when a substance comes in direct contact with the skin, leading to a simple inflammatory reaction. **B,** Irritant contact dermatitis results when the substance causes direct skin damage, pain, or ulceration, such as with tight shoes or prolonged used of latex gloves.

which accounts for almost one-third of all contact dermatitis, results when a substance comes in direct contact with the skin, leading to a simple inflammatory reaction. Common agents that contribute to the condition include adhesive tape, rubber articles (e.g., straps, pads, swim goggles, swim fins, swim caps, and shoes), tape adherent and remover, soap, detergent, and deodorant. In contrast, **irritant contact dermatitis** results when the substance causes direct skin damage, pain, or ulceration. Contact dermatitis affects only the area in direct contact with the causative agent, leading to a sharp line of demarcation between normal skin and affected skin. For example, reacting to a watch band or swimming goggles leads to characteristic patterns of erythema and irritation.

Signs and Symptoms

Allergic dermatitis remains localized to the affected area and is identified by dry vesicles that are accompanied by pain, erythema, and pruritic conditions. Heat, whether internal or external (e.g., hot bath), intensifies symptoms and accelerates the skin's reaction. Irritant dermatitis also presents with erythema, pruritus, pain, and swelling. It often occurs secondary to physical and mechanical agents, such as burns from dry ice, abrasions from artificial turf, friction burns caused by poorly fitted equipment, **striae**, or increased sweating between skinfolds (e.g., groin or under breast tissue), as well as during skin loss secondary to an application of a causative agent (e.g., adhesive tape). Diagnosis of either type of contact dermatitis relies on the history and distribution of the rash.

Management

During acute reactions, a cold compress should be applied to the affected area. Systemic antihistamines are used to reduce itching and inflammation along with topical agents (e.g., corticosteroids) for acute cases. Topical antihistamines and benzocaine products never should be used for these conditions. In more severe cases with vesiculation and blistering, oral prednisone therapy may be prescribed.[29] The causative agent should be identified and contact with the agent eliminated. Disqualification from activity is dependent on the degree of skin involvement, severity of symptoms, and type of sport (i.e., contact versus noncontact).

Urticaria

Etiology

Urticaria (i.e., hives) usually is systemic in origin. It is caused by a hypersensitivity to foods or drugs, infection, physical agents (e.g., heat, cold, light, and friction), or psychic stimuli (**Fig. 32.25**).

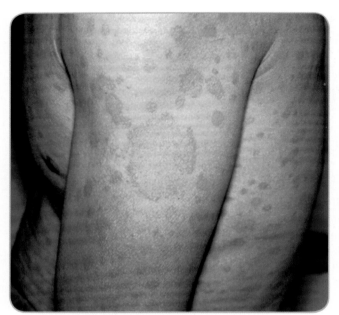

Figure 32.25. Urticaria. Hives may result from hypersensitivity to foods or drugs, infection, physical agents, or psychic stimuli.

Signs and Symptoms

The condition may present with superficial swellings of the dermis, called **wheals**, or deeper swellings of the dermis, subcutaneous, or submucosal tissues, known as **angioedema**. Wheals are smooth, slightly elevated areas on the body that appear red with a pale center and are accompanied by severe itching. They may mature into pink, superficial plaques that usually resolve within 24 hours without sequela. Angioedema tends to be pale and painful and to last longer than wheals, and it also may affect the mouth and, rarely, the bowel.[30] Urticaria commonly is seen in allergies to mechanical or chemical irritants.

Cholinergic urticaria, also known as generalized heat urticaria, presents as lesions within 15 minutes of sweat-inducing stimuli, such as physical exertion, a hot bath, fever, alcohol, or sudden emotional stress. Clinical presentation reveals small papules that appear first in the upper thorax and neck, then spread inferiorly to involve the entire body. Systemic symptoms, although rare, include generalized sweating, abdominal cramps, dizziness, wheezing, and bradycardia. The inner aspects of the arms, legs, and lateral flanks are common sites. Some medical experts believe that **exercise-induced urticaria** may be a variation of cholinergic urticaria, but the lesions are much larger. Systemic signs are limited to wheezing and hypotension. **Cold urticaria** is very common in those who are physically active, is nonallergic, and is characterized by localized or generalized wheals that develop in minutes in response to cold exposure. The condition often becomes apparent when a cold pack is placed on an individual who is hypersensitive to cold.

Management

Based on the cause, aggravating factors should be identified and eliminated. Currently, no cure is available for heat urticaria, but antihistamines, such as hydroxyzine and cyproheptadine, generally are used to relieve symptoms. Although individuals are symptomatic, they may wish to avoid physical activity and sports participation. Simple cooling lotions, such as menthol in aqueous cream, often are used. Unlike heat urticaria, exercise-induced urticaria can be successfully treated with prescribed antihistamines, anticholinergics, or β-agonists. Epinephrine generally is the treatment of choice when systemic signs are present. Avoid NSAIDs and aspirin in favor of acetaminophen, because analgesics can aggravate the symptoms.[30] In cold urticaria, the condition responds well to small doses of oral corticosteroids.

 If the field hockey player is having an allergic reaction to the venom, she could experience anaphylactic shock. The signs and symptoms of anaphylaxis include respiratory distress, cyanosis, weakness, rapid and weak pulse, low blood pressure, localized urticaria or edema, paresthesia, dilated pupils, choking, wheezing, sudden collapse, involuntary loss of bowel and bladder control, headache, dizziness, seizures, and unconsciousness. This condition is life threatening and represents a medical emergency.

SUMMARY

1. Whenever skin is damaged, a lesion appears. Skin lesions are identified by their size and depth. Recognizing the type of lesion can help to identify the cause of the skin damage.

2. Skin infections may stem from fungi, bacteria, or viruses.

3. Bacterial lesions typically are caused by a staphylococcal or streptococcal infection. Impetigo is highly contagious and is characterized by small vesicles that form pustules and, eventually, honey-colored, weeping crustaceans. Bacterial skin conditions are treated with OTC antibacterial topical agents.

4. Fungi thrive in dark, warm, moist environments and often attack the fingernails, toenails, foot, groin, body, and scalp. Common signs and symptoms include pruritus, redness, and scaling. Antifungal medication is used to treat the condition.

5. Viral skin conditions can range from the common wart to the highly contagious herpes gladiatorum and molluscum contagiosum, which can infect an entire team. Any lesions on the trunk, axilla, face, and thigh should be referred immediately to a physician.

6. Sunburns are classified as first, second, or third degree. Prevention involves using a sunscreen with an SPF of 15 or higher and avoiding exposure to the sun during the midday.

7. Miliaria, or prickly heat, occurs when active sweat glands become blocked by organic debris. Treatment involves cooling and drying the skin, controlling the itching, and watching for secondary infection.

8. Bites and stings from insects can be painful and itchy. Immediate application of cold can relieve pain, or a topical corticosteroid or systemic antihistamine may be used. In severe cases, systemic corticosteroids are used. The patient should be watched carefully for signs of anaphylactic shock.

9. Allergic contact dermatitis results when a substance comes in direct contact with the skin and causes a simple inflammatory reaction. Irritant contact dermatitis results when the substance causes direct skin damage, pain, or ulceration. Treatment involves removal of the substance, application of a cold compress, possible use of topical corticosteroids, and systemic antihistamines to reduce itching and inflammation.

10. Urticaria, or hives, is caused by hypersensitivity to foods or drugs, infection, physical agents, or psychic stimuli. The resulting wheal is accompanied by severe itching and is treated with antihistamines, anticholinergics, or β-agonists.

APPLICATION QUESTIONS

1. There has been an outbreak of impetigo among members of the high school wrestling team. How would you manage this situation? What strategies could be implemented to prevent the condition from recurring?

2. An 18-year-old football player has several small, raised, pus-filled skin lesions on the underside of his jaw. Based on the location and appearance, what type of skin lesion may be present? What can be done to treat this condition?

3. A lacrosse player is complaining of an irritating itch on the bottom of the feet and between the toes. The skin appears red and scaly. What condition should be suspected? Is this condition preventable? What can be done to treat this condition and prevent the spread of the infection?

4. A gymnast notices small itching bumps covering her lower leg and foot after removing tape applied to her sprained ankle. The area is extremely red and itchy. What condition might you suspect? What can be done immediately for this condition? What strategies can be used to prevent the condition from recurring?

REFERENCES

1. National Collegiate Athletic Association. Skin infections. In: Parsons JT, ed. *2014–15 NCAA Sports Medicine Handbook*. Indianapolis, IN: National Collegiate Athletic Association; 2014:65–71. http://www.ncaapublications.com/product downloads/MD15.pdf. Accessed July 15, 2015.

2. Frith M, Harmon CB. Acne scarring: current treatment options. *Dermatol Nurs*. 2006;18(2):139–142.

3. Watkins J. Independent nurse: clinical—management guide—chronic paronychia. *Gen Pract*. 2006; 17:101.

4. Stulberg DL, Penrod MA, Blatny RA. Common bacterial skin infections. *Am Fam Physician*. 2002;66(1):119–124.

5. Zinder SM, Basler RS, Foley J, et al. National Athletic Trainers' Association position statement: skin diseases. *J Athl Train*. 2010;45(4):411–428.

6. Levy JA. Common bacterial dermatoses: protecting competitive athletes. *Phys Sportsmed*. 2004;32(6):33–39.

7. Trent JT, Kerdel FA. Tumor necrosis factor alpha inhibitors for the treatment of dermatologic diseases. *Dermatol Nurs*. 2005;17(2):97–107.

8. Bonnetblanc JM, Bédane C. Erysipelas: recognition and management. *Am J Clin Dermatol*. 2003; 4(3):157–163.

9. Studdiford J, Stonehouse A. Bullous eruption on the posterior thigh. *J Fam Pract*. 2005;54(12): 1041–1044.

10. Kirkland EB, Adams BB. Methicillin-resistant *Staphylococcus aureus* and athletes. *J Am Acad Dermatol*. 2008;59(3):494–502.

11. Saben BR. MRSA in athletes: what athletic trainers and therapists need to know. *Athl Ther Today*. 2009;14(6):33–36.

12. Winokur RC, Dexter WW. Fungal infections and parasitic infestations in sports: expedient identification and treatment. *Phys Sportsmed*. 2004;32(10):23–33.

13. Nadalo D, Montoya C, Hunter-Smith D. What is the best way to treat tinea cruris? *J Fam Pract*. 2006;55(3):256–258.

14. Tosanger M, Crutchfield CE III. Tinea corporis. *Dermatol Nurs*. 2004;16(5):453.

15. Adams BB. Dermatologic disorders of the athlete. *Sports Med*. 2002;32(5):309–321.

16. Schwartz RA. Superficial fungal infections. *Lancet*. 2004;364(9440):1173–1182.

17. Landry GL, Chang CJ. Herpes and tinea in wrestling: managing outbreaks, knowing when to disqualify. *Phys Sportsmed*. 2004;32(10): 34–41.

18. Centers for Disease Control and Prevention. Genital herpes—CDC fact sheet (detailed). http://www.cdc.gov/std/herpes/stdfact-herpes -detailed.htm. Accessed June 30, 2015.

19. Snow M. Shutting down shingles. *Nursing*. 2006;36(4):18–19.

20. Cyr PR. Viral skin infections: preventing outbreaks in sports settings. *Phys Sportsmed*. 2004; 32(7):33–38.

21. Centers for Disease Control and Prevention. Skin cancer. http://www.cdc.gov/cancer/skin/. Accessed June 30, 2015.

22. Peter J. Managing mild to moderate eczema. *Practice Nurse*. 2006;31(6):24–28.

23. Centers for Disease Control and Prevention. Psoriasis. http://www.cdc.gov/psoriasis/. Accessed June 30, 2015.

24. Luba KM, Stulberg DL. Chronic plaque psoriasis. *Am Fam Physician*. 2006;73(4):636–644.

25. Petrou I. Managing psoriasis in pediatric cases. *Dermatology Times*. 2006;27(4):38.

26. Eisenach JH, Atkinson JL, Fealey RD. Hyperhidrosis: evolving therapies for a well-established phenomenon. *Mayo Clin Proc*. 2005;80(5): 657–666.

27. Leach J, Bassichis B, Itani K. Brown recluse spider bites to the head: three cases and a review. *Ear Nose Throat J*. 2004;83(7):465–470.

28. Centers for Disease Control and Prevention. *Tickborne Diseases of the United States: A Reference Manual for Health Care Providers*. 3rd ed. Fort Collins, CO: U.S. Department of Health and Human Services, Centers for Disease Control and Prevention; 2015.

29. Freiman A, Barankin B, Elpern DJ. Sports dermatology part 2: swimming and other aquatic sports. *CMAJ*. 2004;171(11):1339–1341.

30. Guldbakke KK, Khachemoune A. Classification and treatment of urticaria: a brief review. *Dermatol Nurs*. 2005;17(5):361–364.

Glossary

A

A-angle   The angle between a vertical line dividing the patella in half and a second line drawn from the tibial tubercle to the apex of the inferior pole of the patella. An angle of 35° or greater has been linked to increased patellofemoral pain.

Abscess   A circumscribed collection of pus appearing in an acute or chronic, localized infection.

Abscessed tooth   A painful infection at the root of a tooth or between the gum and a tooth.

Absorption   Occurs when an electrical wave passes through a medium and its kinetic energy is either partially or totally assimilated by the tissue.

Absorption rate   How quickly a drug gets into the tissues to produce a therapeutic effect.

Accessory movements   Movements within a joint that cannot be performed voluntarily by the patient.

Acclimatization   Physiological adaptations of an individual to a different environment, especially climate or altitude.

Acne mechanica   A local exacerbation of acne vulgaris caused by heat, occlusion, pressure, and friction.

Acromegaly   A disorder marked by progressive enlargement of peripheral parts of the body, especially the head, face, hands, and feet.

Active inhibition   A technique whereby a patient consciously relaxes a muscle before stretching.

Active movement   Joint motion performed voluntarily by the patient through muscular contraction.

Acute injury   An injury with rapid onset because of a traumatic episode but with short duration.

Adhesions   Tissues that bind the healing tissue to adjacent structures, such as other ligaments or bone.

ADLs   Activities of daily living.

Administration of medication   Providing one dose of a medication to a patient.

Affective   Pertaining to feelings or a mental state.

Afferent nerves   Nerves carrying sensory input from receptors in the skin, muscles, tendons, and ligaments to the central nervous system.

Agonist muscles   Muscles that perform the desired movement; primary movers.

Albuminuria   Protein in the urine.

Allergic contact dermatitis   Results when a substance comes in direct contact with the skin and leads to a simple inflammatory reaction.

Alveoli   Air sacs at the terminal ends of the bronchial tree where oxygen and carbon dioxide are exchanged between the lungs and surrounding capillaries.

Amenorrhea   The absence or abnormal cessation of menstruation.

Amplitude   A measure of the force, or intensity, that drives an electrical current; the maximum amplitude is the top or highest point of each phase.

Analgesia   A conscious state in which normal pain is not perceived, such as a numbing or sedative effect.

Analgesic   An agent that produces analgesia.

Anaphylaxis   An immediate, shock-like, frequently fatal, hypersensitivity reaction that occurs within minutes of the administration of an allergen unless appropriate first aid measures are taken immediately.

Anastomosis   A network of communicating blood vessels that supply a joint.

Anatomical position   Used as a universal reference to determine anatomic direction; it is a position whereby the body is erect, facing forward, with the arms at the side of the body, and the palms facing forward.

Anatomical snuff box   The site directly over the scaphoid bone in the wrist; pain here indicates a possible fracture.

Anchor strip   The first strips of tape applied directly to the skin, for which subsequent strips are attached. Anchor strips "secure or anchor" the individual strips together to increase the strength of the overall technique.

Androgen   A class of hormones that promotes the development of male genitals and secondary sex characteristics and that influences sexual motivation.

Anemia   An abnormal reduction in red blood cell volume or hemoglobin concentration.

Anesthesia   A partial or total loss of sensation.

Anesthetic   An agent that produces anesthesia.

Angle of inclination   The angle of depression formed by the meeting of a line drawn through the shaft of the femur with a line passing through the long axis of the femoral neck; normally about 125° in the frontal plane.

Angle of torsion In the transverse plane, the relationship between the femoral head and the femoral shaft, which normally is rotated 15°.

Anisocoria A condition in which the two pupils are not of equal size.

Anisotropic Having different strengths in response to loads from different directions.

Annulus fibrosus The ring of fibrocartilage and fibrous tissue forming the circumference of the intervertebral disk.

Antacid An agent that neutralizes stomach acid.

Antagonist muscles Muscles that oppose or reverse a particular movement.

Antalgic gait A noticeable limp.

Anterograde amnesia The loss of memory of events following a head injury.

Anteversion The forward displacement or the turning forward of a body segment without bending.

Antibiotic A soluble substance derived from a mold or bacterium that inhibits the growth of other microorganisms.

Antihistamine A medication used to counteract the effects of histamine; one that relieves the symptoms of an allergic reaction.

Antipyretic A medication used to relieve or reduce a fever.

Antiseptic A substance that inhibits the growth of infectious agents.

Apnea The temporary cessation of breathing.

Apneustic breathing Characterized by prolonged inspirations unrelieved by attempts to exhale, which indicates trauma to the pons.

Aponeurosis A flat, expanded, tendon-like sheath that attaches a muscle to another structure.

Apophysis An outgrowth or projection on the side of a bone, usually where a tendon attaches.

Apophysitis The inflammation of an apophysis.

Appendicitis The inflammation of the appendix.

Arrhythmia A disturbance in the heartbeat rhythm.

Arthralgia Severe joint pain.

Arthrogram A diagnostic tool whereby a radiopaque material is injected into a joint to facilitate obtaining a radiograph.

Arthrokinematics An accessory motion, or an involuntary joint motion, that occurs simultaneously with physiological motion but that cannot be measured precisely.

Arthroscopy A diagnostic tool whereby the inside of a joint is viewed through a small camera lens (arthroscope) to facilitate the surgical repair of the joint and/or joint structures.

Aseptic necrosis The death or decay of tissue because of a poor blood supply in the area.

Asthma A disease of the lungs characterized by constriction of the bronchial muscles, increased bronchial secretions, and mucosal swelling, all leading to airway narrowing and inadequate airflow during respiration.

Astringent An agent that causes contraction of the tissues, an arrest of secretion, or control of bleeding.

Ataxia An inability to coordinate the muscles in the execution of voluntary movement.

Ataxic (Biot's) breathing Characterized by unpredictable irregularity, whereby breaths may be shallow or deep and stop for short periods, indicating respiratory depression and brain damage, typically at the medullary level.

Atherosclerosis A condition whereby irregularly distributed lipid deposits are found in the large- and medium-sized arteries.

Atrophy A wasting away or deterioration of tissue because of disease, disuse, or malnutrition.

Aura A peculiar sensation that precedes an epileptic attack.

Auricular hematoma An ear injury caused when repeated blunt trauma pulls the cartilage away from the perichondrium; "cauliflower ear."

Auscultation Listening for sounds, often with a stethoscope, to denote the condition of the lungs, heart, pleura, abdomen, and other organs.

Autogenous Originating within the body.

Autoinoculation The spreading of an infection from one body part to another by touching the lesion and then scratching or rubbing somewhere else.

Autonomic dysreflexia A rare but dangerous condition in wheelchair athletes; commonly triggered by an obstructed bowel or bladder, which disturbs the regulation of blood pressure and heart rate.

Axial force Loading directed along the long axis of a body.

Axonotmesis Damage to the axons of a nerve followed by the complete degeneration of the peripheral segment without severance of the supporting structure of the nerve.

B

Bacteremia The presence of viable bacteria in the circulating blood.

Ballistic stretch Increasing flexibility by using repetitive bouncing motions at the end of the available range of motion.

Bankart lesion An avulsion or damage to the anterior lip of the glenoid as the humerus slides forward in an anterior dislocation.

Battery Unpermitted or intentional contact with another individual without his or her consent.

Battle sign A delayed discoloration behind the ear because of a basilar skull fracture.

Bending Loading that produces tension on one side of an object and compression on the other side.

Bennett fracture A fracture dislocation to the proximal end of the 1st metacarpal at the carpometacarpal joint.

Bimalleolar fracture   Fractures of both the medial and the lateral malleolus.

Bioavailability   The amount of the drug's concentration when it reaches the target site within a certain time frame.

Bipartite   Having two parts.

Blood oxygen levels   Measurement of the amount of oxygen in the blood using a pulse oximeter.

Blood–brain barrier   The barrier that protects the brain against toxic substances.

Blowout fracture   Fracture of the floor of the eye orbit, without fracture to the rim; produced by a blow on the globe, with the force being transmitted via the globe to the orbital floor.

Boutonnière deformity   A rupture of the central slip of the extensor tendon at the middle phalanx, resulting in no active extensor mechanism at the proximal interphalangeal joint.

Bowler's thumb   A compression of the digital nerve on the medial aspect of the thumb, leading to paresthesia in the thumb.

Boxer's fracture   A fracture of the 5th metacarpal, resulting in a flexion deformity because of the rotation of the head of the metacarpal over the neck.

Brachial plexus   A complex web of spinal nerves (C5–T1) that innervates the upper extremity.

Bradykinin   Normally present in blood; a potent vasodilator. It increases blood vessel wall permeability and stimulates nerve endings to cause pain.

Bradypnea   An abnormal slowness of respiration.

Break test   Used to test resistance; an overload pressure is applied in a stationary or static position.

Bronchitis   Inflammation of the mucosal lining of the tracheobronchial tree characterized by bronchial swelling, mucus secretions, and dysfunction of the cilia.

Bronchospasm   A contraction of the smooth muscles of the bronchial tubes causing a narrowing of the airway.

Buccal   Pertaining to, adjacent to, or in the direction of the cheek.

Bucket-handle tear   A longitudinal meniscal tear of the central segment that can displace into the joint, leading to locking of the knee.

Burner   Burning or stinging sensation characteristic of a brachial plexus injury.

Bursa   A fibrous sac membrane containing synovial fluid typically found between tendons and bones; acts to decrease friction during motion.

Bursitis   Inflammation of the bursae.

C

Calcific tendinopathy   The accumulation of mineral deposits in a tendon.

Callus   The localized thickening of skin (epidermis) because of physical trauma. Fibrous tissue containing immature bone tissue that forms at fracture sites during repair and regeneration.

Cancellous tissue   Bone tissue of relatively low density.

Cardiac asystole   Cardiac standstill.

Cardiac tamponade   An acute compression of the heart because of effusion of fluid or blood into the pericardium from a rupture of the heart or penetrating trauma.

Carpal tunnel syndrome   Compression of the median nerve as it passes through the carpal tunnel, leading to pain and tingling in the hand.

Carrying angle   The angle between the humerus and ulna when the arm is in anatomical position.

Cathode   Negatively charged electrode in a direct current system.

Cauda equina   The lower spinal nerves that course through the lumbar spinal canal; resembles a horse's tail.

Cauliflower ear   A hematoma that forms between the perichondrium and cartilage of the auricle (ear) because of repeated blunt trauma.

Causalgia   A persistent, severe, and burning sensation of the skin, usually following direct or indirect (vascular) partial injury of a sensory nerve and accompanied by cutaneous changes (temperature and sweating).

Cavitation   Gas bubble formation because of nonthermal effects of ultrasound.

Celiac plexus   The nerve plexus that innervates the abdominal region.

Checkrein   A technique to limit range of motion by using one or more strips of tape placed one on top of each other to increase tensile strength or a series of strips placed in an X pattern to increase shear, tensile, and flexure forces.

Chemosensitive   Sensitivity to chemical stimulation.

Cheyne-Stokes breathing   Periods of deep breathing alternating with periods of apnea.

Chondral fracture   A fracture involving the articular cartilage at a joint.

Chondromalacia patellae   A degenerative condition in the articular cartilage of the patella caused by abnormal compression or shearing forces.

Chronic injury   An injury with long onset and long duration.

Chyme   A semifluid mass of partly digested food passed from the stomach into the duodenum.

Circumduction   The movement of a body part in a circular direction.

Cirrhosis   A progressive inflammation of the liver, usually caused by alcoholism.

Claw toes   Toe deformity characterized by hyperextension of the metatarsophalangeal joint and hyperflexion of the interphalangeal joints.

Clonic   A movement marked by repetitive muscle contractions and relaxation in rapid succession.

Close-packed position   The joint position in which contact between the articulation structures is maximal.

Closed-cell foam The foam material whereby air cannot pass from one cell to another, allowing the material to rebound and return to its original shape quickly but offering less cushioning at low levels of impact.

Coach's finger A fixed flexion deformity of the finger caused by dislocation at the proximal interphalangeal joint.

Coarctation A constriction, stricture, or stenosis.

Coccygodynia Prolonged or chronic pain in the coccygeal region because of irritation of the coccygeal nerve plexus.

Cognitive The quality of knowing or perceiving.

Cognitive model A model that seeks to explain how an athlete approaches the rehabilitation process and encompasses personal factors such as performance anxiety, self-esteem/motivation, extroversion/introversion, psychological investment in the sport, coping resources, history of past stressors, and previous intervention strategies.

Cold diuresis The excretion of urine in cold weather because of blood being shunted away from the skin to the core to maintain vascular volume.

Cold urticaria A condition characterized by redness, itching, and large, blister-like wheals on skin that is exposed to cold.

Collateral ligaments The major ligaments that cross the medial and lateral aspects of a hinge joint to provide stability from valgus and varus forces.

Colles fracture A fracture involving a dorsally angulated and displaced and a radially angulated and displaced fracture within 1.5 in of the wrist.

Commission A committing of an act that is not legally your duty to perform.

Comparative negligence The relative degree of negligence on the part of the plaintiff and the defendant, with damages awarded on a basis proportionate to each person's carelessness.

Compartment syndrome A condition in which increased intramuscular pressure brought on by activity impedes blood flow and function of tissues within that compartment.

Compression A pressure or squeezing force directed through a body in such a way as to increase density.

Concentric A shortening of the muscle fibers that decreases the angle of the associated joint.

Concussion The violent shaking or jarring action of the brain, resulting in immediate or transient impairment of neurological function.

Conduction The direct transfer of energy between two objects in physical contact with each other.

Conductors Mediums that facilitate the movement of ions such as water, blood, and electrolyte solutions (e.g., sweat).

Congenital Existing at birth.

Conjunctivitis A bacterial infection that leads to itching, burning, watering, and an inflamed eye; pinkeye.

Constipation Infrequent or incomplete bowel movements.

Contracture A permanent muscular contraction because of tonic spasm, fibrosis, loss of muscular equilibrium, or paralysis.

Contraindication A condition that will be adversely affected if a particular action is taken.

Contralateral Pertaining to the opposite side.

Contranutation The anterior rotation of the ilium on the sacrum, indicating anterior torsion of the joint, or the posterior rotation of the sacrum on the ilium on one side; the limb on that side probably is medially rotated.

Contrecoup injuries Injuries away from the actual injury site because of rotational components during acceleration.

Contusion A compression injury involving the accumulation of blood and lymph within a muscle; a bruise.

Convection The transfer of energy between two objects via a medium, such as air or water, as it moves across the body, creating temperature variations.

Conversion Involves the changing of another energy form (e.g., sound, electricity, a chemical agent) into heat.

Coordination The body's ability to execute smooth, fluid, accurate, and controlled movements.

Cortical tissue Compact bone tissue of relatively high density.

Cosine law As the angle deviates from 90°, the energy varies with the cosine of the angle: effective energy = energy × cosine of the angle of incidence.

Counterirritant A substance causing irritation of superficial sensory nerves to reduce pain transmission from another underlying irritation.

Coup injuries Injuries at the site where direct impact occurs.

Coxa valga An alteration of the angle made by the axis of the femoral neck to the axis of the femoral shafts so that the angle exceeds 135°; the femoral neck is in more of a straight line relationship to the shaft of the femur.

Coxa vara An alteration of the angle made by the axis of the femoral neck to the axis of the femoral shaft so that the angle is less than 135°; the neck becomes more horizontal.

Cramp A painful involuntary muscle contraction that is either clonic or tonic.

Crepitus A crackling sound or sensation characteristic of a fracture when the bone's ends are moved.

Cruciate ligaments Major ligaments that crisscross the knee in the anteroposterior direction, providing stability in that plane.

Cryokinetics The use of cold treatments before an exercise session.

Cryotherapy Cold application.

Cubital fossa Relating to the anterior elbow.

Cubital recurvatum Extension beyond 0° at the elbow.

Cubital tunnel syndrome Entrapment of the ulnar nerve in the cubital tunnel at the elbow.

Cubital valgus At the elbow, a valgus angle greater than 20°.

Cubital varus At the elbow, a valgus angle less than 10°.

Current The actual movement of ions.

Curvatures A bending, as in the spine (kyphosis, scoliosis, or lordosis).

Cyanosis A dark blue or purple skin color because of deficient oxygen in the blood.

Cyclist's nipples A nipple irritation because of the combined effects of perspiration and wind chill, producing cold, painful nipples.

Cyclist's palsy Seen when a biker leans on the handlebar for an extended period of time, resulting in paresthesia in the ulnar nerve distribution.

Cystitis Inflammation of the bladder.

D

Dead arm syndrome A common sensation felt with a recurrent anterior shoulder subluxation and multidirectional instability.

Decerebrate rigidity The extension of all four extremities.

Decompression The surgical release of pressure from fluid or blood accumulation.

Decorticate rigidity The extension of the legs with flexion of the elbows, wrists, and fingers.

de Quervain tenosynovitis An inflammatory stenosing tenosynovitis of the abductor pollicis longus and extensor pollicis brevis tendons.

Dermatome A region of skin supplied by cutaneous branches of a single spinal nerve.

Dermis The corium of the skin that contains blood and lymphatic vessels, nerves and nerve endings, glands, and, except for glabrous skin, hair follicles.

Detached retina A condition in which the neurosensory retina is separated from the retinal epithelium by swelling.

Detraining The loss of the benefits gained in physical training, which can occur after only 1 to 2 weeks of nonactivity, with significant decreases measured in both metabolic and working capacity.

Diabetes mellitus A metabolic disorder characterized by near or absolute lack of the hormone insulin, insulin resistance, or both.

Diabetic ketoacidosis A condition whereby an excess of ketoacids in the blood can lower the blood pH to 7.0; manifested by ketones in the breath, blood, and urine.

Diagnosis The definitive determination of the nature of the injury or illness made by a physician.

Diarrhea Loose or watery stools.

Diastolic blood pressure Arterial blood pressure reached either during or as a result of diastole; the lowest level of any given ventricular cycle.

Diathermy A local elevation of temperature in the tissues produced by the therapeutic application of high-frequency electrical current, ultrasound, or microwave radiation.

Diffuse injuries An injury over a large body area, usually because of low velocity–high mass forces.

Disease-oriented evidence Physiological information (e.g., blood pressure, range of motion) or symptoms (e.g., headache, nausea).

Diplopia Double vision.

Disinfectant A chemical agent applied to nonliving objects; most commonly used to disinfect surgical instruments and cleanse medical equipment and facilities.

Disposition The immediate and long-term management of an injury or illness.

Diuretic A chemical that promotes the excretion of urine.

Drug A therapeutic agent used in the prevention, diagnosis, cure, treatment, or rehabilitation of a disease, condition, or injury.

Drug dispensing Providing more than one individual dose to a person.

Drug interaction The ability of one drug to alter the effects of another drug; it may either intensify (synergistic action) or reduce (inhibit) the effects of the other drug.

Drug metabolism The enzymatic alteration of a drug's structure whereby the original drug is broken down into metabolites (an altered product of metabolism).

Dural sinuses Formed by tubular separations in the inner and outer layers of the dura mater; these sinuses function as small veins for the brain.

Duty of care The standard of care measured by what is learned, or should have been learned, in the professional preparation of an individual charged with providing health care.

Dysesthesia A disagreeable sensation or a sensation short of anesthesia produced by ordinary stimuli.

Dysmenorrhea Difficult or painful menstruation; menstrual cramps.

Dyspepsia Gastric indigestion.

Dysphagia Difficulty in swallowing.

Dysplasia Abnormal tissue development.

Dyspnea Labored or difficult breathing.

Dysrhythmia A serious irregularity of the heart rate.

Dysuria Pain during urination.

E

Eccentric Movement in which the muscle resists its own lengthening so that the joint angle increases during the contraction.

Ecchymosis Superficial tissue discoloration.

Echocardiogram An ultrasonic record obtained by echocardiography in the investigation of the heart and great vessels.

Ecthyma A more serious form of impetigo, which occurs when the infection penetrates deep into the skin's second layer (dermis).

Ectopic bone The proliferation of bone ossification in an abnormal place.

Edema Swelling from a collection of exuded lymph fluid in interstitial tissues.

Effective radiating area In ultrasound, the portion of the transducer's surface area that actually produces the ultrasound wave.

Efferent nerves Nerves carrying motor impulses from the central nervous system to the muscles.

Effleurage Superficial, longitudinal massage strokes used to relax the patient.

Effusion The escape of fluid from blood vessels into the surrounding tissues or joint cavity.

Elastic limit A material's yield point.

Elasticity The ability of a muscle to return to normal length after either lengthening or shortening has taken place.

Electrocardiogram A graphic record of the heart's action currents obtained with an electrocardiograph.

Electromagnetic radiation The energy emitted by an object.

Electromagnetic spectrum A graphic presentation of electromagnetic radiation based on its wavelength or frequency.

Embolism The obstruction or occlusion of a vessel by bacteria or other foreign body.

Emergency action plan A blue print for how to respond to emergency situations at an activity site.

Emergency medical services A well-developed process that activates the emergency health care services of the athletic training facility and community to provide immediate health care to an injured patient.

Emesis Vomiting.

Emmetropia 20/20 vision, indicating that the light rays are focused precisely on the retina.

Encephalitis Inflammation of the brain, especially of the cerebral hemisphere, cerebellum, or brain stem, caused by a viral infection.

End feel The sensation felt in the joint as it reaches the end of the available range of motion.

Endometriosis The ectopic occurrence of endometrial tissue, frequently forming cysts containing altered blood.

Enteric coated preparations Drugs covered by acid-resistant materials (e.g., fatty acids, waxes, shellac) that protect the drug from the acid and pepsin in the stomach.

Epicondylitis Inflammation and microrupturing of the soft tissues on the epicondyles of the distal humerus.

Epidermis The outer epithelial portion of the skin.

Epilepsy A disorder of the brain characterized by recurrent episodes of sudden, excessive discharges of electrical activity in the brain.

Epiphyseal fracture An injury to the growth plate of a long bone in children and adolescents; may lead to arrested bone growth.

Epistaxis Profuse bleeding from the nose; nosebleed.

Erb point Located 2 to 3 cm above the clavicle at the level of the transverse process of the C6 vertebra; compression over the site may injure the brachial plexus.

Erythema Inflammatory redness of the skin.

Erythropoietin A hormone produced in the kidneys that stimulates bone marrow to increase production of red blood cells.

Estrogens Hormones that produce female secondary sex characteristics and that affect the menstrual cycle.

Evidence-based health care Health care practice that aims to provide patients with the best quality care by integrating the best evidence with clinical expertise and the individual patient's values and circumstances.

Excitability A muscle's ability to respond to a stimulus; irritability.

Excoriation A scratch mark; a linear break in the skin surface, usually covered with blood or serous crusts.

Exculpatory waiver Based on the athlete's assumption of risk, a release that is signed by the athlete or by the parent of an athlete younger than the age of 18 years that releases the physician from liability of negligence.

Exercise-induced urticaria Hives brought on by exercise; a variation of cholinergic urticaria but with lesions that are much larger.

Exertional sickling When a red blood cell (RBC) changes shape from round to sickle or half-moon shape.

Expressed warranty A written guarantee that states the product is safe for consumer use.

Extensibility The ability of a muscle to be stretched or to increase in length.

Extensor mechanism A complex interaction of muscles, ligaments, and tendons that stabilize and provide motion at the patellofemoral joint.

Extrasynovial Structures found outside the synovial cavity and synovial fluid.

Extrinsic An origination outside the part where it is found or on which it acts; denoting, especially, a muscle.

Extruded disk A condition in which the nuclear material bulges into the spinal canal and runs the risk of impinging adjacent nerve roots.

Extruded tooth A tooth driven in an outwardly direction.

Exudate Material composed of fluid, pus, or cells that has escaped from blood vessels into the surrounding tissues following an injury or inflammation.

F

Facet joint A joint formed when the superior and inferior articular processes mate with the articular process of the adjacent vertebrae.

Failure A loss of continuity; a rupture of soft tissue or fracture of bone.

Fasciitis The inflammation of the fascia surrounding portions of a muscle.

Fibroblast A cell that is present in connective tissue and capable of forming collagen fibers.

Fibrositis The inflammation of fibrous tissue.

First-pass effect The drug metabolism that takes place first in the liver via hepatic enzymes.

Fistulas An abnormal passage from a hollow organ to the surface or from one organ to another.

Flat back A decreased anterior lumbar curve.

Flatulence The presence of an excessive amount of gas in the stomach and the intestines.

Flexibility The total range of motion at a joint; dependent on normal joint mechanics, mobility of soft tissues, and muscle extensibility.

Focal injuries An injury in a small, concentrated area, usually because of high velocity–low mass forces.

Focus The ability to perceive and address various internal (thoughts, emotions, and physical responses) and external (sights and sounds) cues, and, when needed, to shift one's attention to other cues in a natural, effortless manner.

Follicular phase Days 1 to 14 of the ovarian cycle, in which the follicle (spheroidal cell cluster in the ovary contain an ovum or egg) grows.

Foot strike hemolysis A condition in which red blood cells are thought to be destroyed by repetitive, hard foot strikes.

Foreseeability of harm A condition whereby danger is or should have been apparent, resulting in an unreasonably unsafe condition.

Fracture A disruption in the continuity of a bone.

Freiberg disease Avascular necrosis that occurs to the 2nd metatarsal head in some adolescents.

Friction The deepest form of massage, consisting of deep, circular motions performed by the thumb, knuckles, or ends of the fingers at right angles to the involved tissue.

Frontal plane A longitudinal (vertical) line that divides the body or any of its parts into anterior and posterior portions.

G

Gamekeeper's thumb A sprain of the metacarpophalangeal (MP) joint of the thumb when it is in near extension and the thumb is forcefully abducted away from the hand, tearing the ulnar collateral ligament at the MP joint.

Ganglion cyst A benign tumor mass commonly seen on the dorsal aspect of the wrist.

Gangrene Necrosis because of the obstruction, loss, or diminution of blood supply; may be localized to a small area or involve an entire extremity or organ.

Gastritis Inflammation, especially mucosal, of the stomach.

Gastrocolic reflex A propulsive reflex in the colon that stimulates defecation.

Gastroenteritis Inflammation of the mucous membrane of the stomach and/or small intestine.

Genu recurvatum A condition of hyperextension of the knee.

Genu valgum A deformity marked by the abduction of the leg in relation to the thigh; knock-knee.

Genu varum A deformity marked by the adduction of the leg in relation to the thigh; bowleg.

Gestation Pregnancy.

Gingivitis Inflammation of the gums.

Glenoid labrum A soft-tissue lip around the periphery of the glenoid fossa that widens and deepens the socket to add stability to the joint.

Glucagon A polypeptide hormone secreted by pancreatic alpha cells. It activates hepatic phosphorylase, thereby increasing glycogenolysis; decreases gastric motility and gastric and pancreatic secretions; and increases urinary excretion of nitrogen and potassium.

Goniometer A protractor used to measure joint position and available joint motion (range of motion).

Graves disease A toxic goiter characterized by diffuse hyperplasia of the thyroid gland; a form of hyperthyroidism.

Gross negligence Committing, or not committing, an act with total disregard for the health and safety of others.

Grotthus-Draper law An inverse relationship that exists between the amount of penetration and absorption. The more energy absorbed by superficial tissues, the less energy is available to be transmitted to the underlying tissues.

Gynecomastia The excessive development of the male mammary glands.

H

Half-life The period during which an agent decreases to half its original strength. The longer the half-life of an agent, the slower it leaves the body.

Halitosis Bad breath.

Hallux The first toe or great toe.

Hammer toes A flexion deformity of the distal interphalangeal joint of the toes.

Heat cramps Painful, involuntary muscle spasms caused by excessive water and electrolyte loss.

Heel bruise A contusion to the subcutaneous fat pad located over the inferior aspect of the calcaneus.

Hemarthrosis A collection of blood within a joint or cavity.

Hematemesis The vomiting of blood.

Hematocele A rapid accumulation of blood and fluid in the scrotum around the testicle and cord.

Hematoma A localized mass of blood and lymph confined within a space or tissue.

Hematuria Blood or red blood cells in the urine.

Hemoglobinuria Hemoglobin in the urine; in sufficient quantities, hemoglobin results in the urine being colored from light red-yellow to fairly dark red.

Hemophilia   A bleeding disorder characterized by a deficiency of selected proteins in the body's blood clotting system.

Hemorrhoids   Dilations of the venous plexus surrounding the rectal and anal area that can become exposed if they protrude internally or externally.

Hemothorax   A condition involving a loss of blood into the pleural cavity but outside the lung.

Heparin   An anticoagulant that is a component of various tissues and mast cells.

Hepatitis   Inflammation of the liver.

Hernia   The protrusion of abdominal viscera through a weakened portion of the abdominal wall.

High-density material   Materials that absorb more energy from higher impact intensity levels through deformation, thus transferring less stress to a body part.

Hill-Sachs lesion   A small defect usually located on the posterior aspect of the articular cartilage of the humeral head and caused by the impact of the humeral head on the glenoid fossa as the humerus dislocates.

Hip pointer   Contusions caused by direct compression to an unprotected iliac crest that crushes soft tissue and, sometimes, the bone itself.

Histamine   A powerful stimulant of gastric secretion, a constrictor of bronchial smooth muscle, and a vasodilator (capillaries and arterioles) that causes a fall in blood pressure.

Homeostasis   The state of a balanced equilibrium in the body's various tissues and systems.

Hydrocele   Swelling in the tunica vaginalis of the testes.

Hyperemia   Increased blood flow into a region or body part once treatment has ended.

Hyperesthesia   Excessive tactile sensation.

Hyperglycemia   Abnormally high levels of glucose in the circulating blood that can lead to diabetic coma.

Hyperhidrosis   Excessive or profuse sweating.

Hyperhydrate   Overhydration; excess water consumption of the body.

Hypermetropia   Farsightedness; occurs when the light rays are focused at a point behind the retina.

Hypermobile patella   Movement of the patella equal to three or more quadrants of the patella, indicating laxity of the restraints, which can predispose an athlete to a laterally subluxating or dislocating patella.

Hypermobility   Increased motion at a joint; joint laxity.

Hyperreflexia   A condition in which the reflexes are exaggerated.

Hypertension   Sustained elevated blood pressure above the norms of 140 mm Hg systolic or 90 mm Hg diastolic.

Hyperthermia   Elevated body temperature.

Hypertrophic cardiomyopathy   Excessive hypertrophy of the heart, often of obscure or unknown origin.

Hypertrophy   A general increase in the bulk or size of an individual tissue not resulting from tumor formation.

Hyphema   A hemorrhage into the anterior chamber of the eye.

Hypoesthesia   Decreased tactile sensation.

Hypoglycemia   Abnormally low levels of glucose in the circulating blood that can lead to insulin shock.

Hypomobile patella   Movement of the patella equal to one quadrant or less.

Hypomobility   Decreased motion at a joint.

Hyponatremia   Abnormally low concentrations of sodium ions in the circulating blood.

Hypotension   Characterized by a fall of 20 mm Hg or more from a person's normal baseline systolic blood pressure.

Hypothalamus   A region of the diencephalon forming the floor of the third ventricle of the brain; responsible for thermoregulation and other autonomic nervous mechanisms underlying moods and motivational states.

Hypothenar   The fleshy mass of muscle and tissue on the medial side of the palm.

Hypothermia   Decreased body temperature.

Hypovolemic shock   Shock caused by a reduction in blood volume, as from hemorrhage or dehydration.

Hypoxia   Having a reduced concentration of oxygen in air, blood, or tissue, short of anoxia.

I

Idiopathic   Of unknown origin or cause.

Impetigo   A highly contagious bacterial infection characterized by small vesicles that form pustules and, eventually, honey-colored, weeping crustaceans.

Impingement syndrome   Chronic condition caused by repetitive overhead activity that damages the supraspinatus tendon, the glenoid labrum, the long head of the biceps brachii, and the subacromial bursa.

Implied warranty   An unwritten guarantee that the product is reasonably safe when used for its intended purpose.

Indication   A condition that could benefit from a specific action.

Infarcts   The clumping together of cells that block small blood vessels, leading to vascular occlusion, ischemia, and necrosis in organs.

Infectious mononucleosis   An acute illness associated with the Epstein-Barr herpetovirus and characterized by fever, sore throat, enlargement of the lymph nodes and spleen, and leukopenia, which changes to lymphocytosis.

Infiltrative anesthesia   A process that produces numbness by interfering with nerve function in a localized, subcutaneous, soft-tissue area. It is commonly used for the treatment of soft-tissue injuries or as an anesthetic before minor surgical procedures.

Inflammation   Pain, swelling, redness, heat, and loss of function that accompany musculoskeletal injuries.

Influenza An acute, infectious respiratory tract condition characterized by malaise, headache, dry cough, and general muscle aches.

Informed consent Consent given by a person of legal age who understands the nature and extent of any treatment and the available alternative treatments before agreeing to receive treatment.

Innominate Without a name; used to describe anatomic structures.

Inspection Refers to factors seen at the actual site of injury such as redness, bruising, swelling, cuts, or scars.

Instability A joint's inability to function under the stresses encountered during functional activities.

Interpulse interval The period within a discrete pulse when the current is not flowing. The duration of the intrapulse interval cannot exceed the duration of the interpulse interval.

Interrater reliability The consistent reliability of measurements made between several researchers or instruments.

Intersection syndrome A tendinitis or friction tendinitis in the 1st and 2nd dorsal compartments of the wrist.

Intertrigo Dermatitis occurring between folds of the skin because of sweat retention, moisture, warmth, and concomitant overgrowth of resident microorganisms.

Intracapsular Structures found within the articular capsule; intra-articular.

Intrarater reliability Values that determine how consistent measurements by a single researcher or instrument are.

Intrinsic In anatomy, denoting those muscles of the limbs for which the origin and insertion are both in the same limb.

Intruded tooth A tooth driven deep into the socket in an inward direction.

Inverse square law The intensity of radiant energy striking the tissues (E) is directly proportional to the square of the distance (D) between the source of the energy (E_S) and the tissues ($E = E_S/D^2$).

Ion An atom or group of atoms carrying a charge of electricity by virtue of having gained or lost one or more electrons.

Iontophoresis A technique whereby direct current is used to drive charged molecules from certain medications into damaged tissue.

Ipsilateral Situated on, pertaining to, or affecting the same side (as opposed to contralateral).

Irritant contact dermatitis Results when a substance causes direct skin damage, pain, or ulceration.

Ischemia Local anemia because of decreased blood supply.

Ischemic necrosis Death of a tissue because of decreased blood supply.

J

Jaundice A yellowish discoloration of the skin, sclera, and deeper tissues, often resulting from liver damage.

Jersey finger A rupture of the flexor digitorum profundus tendon from the distal phalanx because of the rapid extension of the finger while actively flexed.

Jones fracture A transverse stress fracture of the proximal shaft of the 5th metatarsal.

Joule's law The greater the resistance or impedance, the more heat that will be developed. Tissues with a high fluid content, such as skeletal muscle and areas surrounding joints, absorb more of the energy and, therefore, are heated to a greater extent, whereas fat is not heated as much.

K

Kehr sign Referred pain down the left shoulder; indicative of a ruptured spleen.

Keloids A nodular, firm, movable, and often linear mass of hyperplastic scar tissue.

Ketoacidosis A condition caused by excess accumulation of acid or a loss of base in the body; characteristic of diabetes mellitus.

Ketonemia A recognizable concentration of ketone bodies in the blood plasma.

Ketonuria Enhanced urinary excretion of ketone bodies.

Kienböck disease Avascular necrosis of the lunate, often seen in young athletes and thought to be caused by repetitive trauma or an unrecognized lunate fracture.

Kinematic chain A series of interrelated joints that constitute a complex motor unit so that motion at one joint produces motion at the other joints in a predictable manner.

Kinematics The study of the spatial and temporal aspects of movement.

Kinesthesia The sensation of position, movement, tension, and so on of parts of the body as perceived through nerve end organs in the muscles, tendons, and joints.

Kinetics The study of the forces causing and resulting from motion.

Kyphosis An excessive curve in the thoracic region of the spine.

L

Laryngospasm The spasmodic closure of the glottic aperture, leading to shortness of breath, coughing, cyanosis, and even a loss of consciousness.

Laxity The amount of "give" within a joint's supportive tissue.

Legg-Calvé-Perthes disease An avascular necrosis of the proximal femoral epiphysis, seen especially in young males aged 3 to 8 years.

Leukoplakia A disease of the mouth characterized by white patches and oral lesions on the cheeks, gums, and/or tongue that can lead to oral cancer.

Level of evidence Pyramid that demonstrates which pieces of evidence are stronger or weaker than others.

Licensure An act that gives permission for an individual to practice a profession by a governmental body.

Lipid solubility Fat soluble; denoting the ability of fat-soluble vitamins to be absorbed better than water-soluble vitamins and to accumulate in the body because of their increased ability to cross cell membranes.

Lisfranc injury Involves the disruption of the tarsometatarsal joint, with or without an associated fracture caused by a severe twisting injury. The 1st metatarsal typically is dislocated from the first cuneiform, whereas the other four metatarsals are displaced laterally, usually in combination with a fracture at the base of the 2nd metatarsal.

Little League elbow A tension stress injury of the medial epicondyle; seen in adolescents.

Little League shoulder A fracture of the proximal humeral growth plate caused by repetitive rotational stresses during the act of pitching; seen in adolescents.

Loose-packed position The resting position where the joint is under the least amount of strain.

Lordosis An excessive convex curve in the lumbar region of the spine.

Low-density material Materials that absorb energy from low impact intensity levels.

Lumbar plexus The interconnected roots of the first four lumbar spinal nerves.

Lyme disease An inflammatory disorder that typically occurs during the summer months and is characterized by a specific lesion and accompanied by fever, malaise, fatigue, headache, and stiff neck.

Lymph nodes Small lymphatic organs that filter lymph and contain macrophages and lymphocytes.

Lymphangitis Inflammation of the lymphatic vessels.

M

Macerated To soften skin with moisture by steeping or soaking.

Macrotrauma When a single force produces an acute injury.

Maisonneuve fracture An external rotation injury of the ankle with an associated fracture of the proximal third of the fibula.

Malaise A lethargic feeling of general discomfort; an out-of-sorts feeling.

Malfeasance Committing an act that is not your responsibility to perform.

Mallet finger The rupture of the extensor tendon from the distal phalanx because of forceful flexion of the phalanx.

Mallet toe A toe in a neutral position at the metatarsophalangeal and proximal interphalangeal joints but flexed at the distal interphalangeal joint.

Malocclusion An inability to bring the teeth together in a normal bite.

Malpractice Committing a negligent act while providing care.

Marfan syndrome An inherited connective tissue disorder affecting many organs but commonly resulting in dilation and weakening of the thoracic aorta.

Mast cells The connective tissue cells that carry heparin, which prolongs clotting, and histamine.

Maximal efficacy The drug dose at which a response occurs and continues to increase in magnitude before reaching a plateau or threshold.

McBurney point A site one-third of the distance between the anterior superior iliac spines and the umbilicus that, with deep palpation, produces rebound tenderness and indicates appendicitis.

Mechanosensitive Sensitive to mechanical stimulation.

Menarche The onset of menses.

Meninges Three protective membranes that surround the brain and spinal cord.

Meningitis Inflammation of the meninges of the brain and spinal column.

Menisci The fibrocartilaginous disks found within a joint that serve to reduce joint stress.

Menorrhagia Prolonged or profuse menses.

Metabolites Any altered product of metabolism, especially of catabolism.

Metatarsalgia A condition involving general discomfort around the metatarsals heads.

Microalbuminuria Minute particles of albumin in the urine, signifying the first stage of kidney disease.

Microtrauma An injury to a small number of cells because of the accumulative effects of repetitive forces.

Miliaria An eruption of minute vesicles and papules that occurs when active sweat glands become blocked by organic debris; prickly heat.

Minimum effective concentration The minimum concentration of a drug that must be present for that drug to be effective.

Misfeasance While committing an act that is your responsibility to perform, following the wrong procedure or performing the right procedure in an improper manner.

Mitral valve prolapse A condition in which redundant tissue is found on one or both leaflets of the mitral valve. During a ventricular contraction, a portion of the redundant tissue on the mitral valve pushes back beyond the normal limit and, as a result, produces an abnormal sound, followed by a systolic murmur as blood is regurgitated back through the mitral valve into the left atrium; often called a click-murmur syndrome.

Modality   A therapeutic agent that promotes optimal healing while reducing pain and disability.

MRI   A diagnostic technique using magnetism to produce high-quality, cross-sectional images of organs or structures within the body without X-rays or other radiation.

Multivalvular disease   An acquired valvular heart disease stemming from a defect or insufficiency in more than one heart valve; manifested as either valvular stenosis or regurgitation.

Muscle cramps   A painful, involuntary contraction that may be clonic (alternating contraction and relaxation) or tonic (continued contraction over a period of time).

Muscle spasms   An involuntary contraction of short duration caused by reflex action biochemically derived or initiated by a mechanical blow to a nerve or muscle.

Myalgia   Pain in a muscle.

Myelogram   A radiograph of the spinal cord taken after the injection of an opaque substance that shows contrast on the developed photograph.

Myocardial infarction   A heart attack.

Myocarditis   An inflammatory condition of the muscular walls of the heart that can result from a bacterial or viral infection.

Myopia   Nearsightedness.

Myositis   The inflammation of connective tissue within a muscle.

Myositis ossificans   The accumulation of mineral deposits within muscle tissue.

Myotome   A group of muscles primarily innervated by a single nerve root.

N

Near syncope   A sense of impending loss of consciousness or weakness.

Necrosis   Death of a tissue resulting from the deprivation of blood supply.

Negligence   A breach of one's duty of care that causes harm to another individual.

Neoplasm   A mass of tissue that grows more rapidly than normal and that may be benign or malignant.

Nephropathy   Any disease of the kidney.

Neuralgia   Pain of a severe throbbing or stabbing character in the course or distribution of a nerve.

Neurapraxia   An injury to a nerve that results in temporary neurological deficits followed by a complete recovery of function.

Neuroma   A nerve tumor.

Neurotmesis   The complete severance of a nerve.

Nightstick fracture   A fracture to the ulna because of a direct blow; commonly seen in football players.

Nociceptor   A receptor that is sensitive to potentially damaging stimuli that results in pain.

Nonfeasance   Failing to perform one's legal duty of care.

Nonunion fracture   The failure of normal healing of a fractured bone.

Nuchal rigidity   Stiffness in the nape or back of the neck.

Nucleus pulposus   The soft fibrocartilage in the central portion of the intervertebral disk.

Nutation   The backward rotation of the ilium on the sacrum. When occurring on only one side, the anterior superior iliac spine is higher and the posterior superior iliac spine is lower on that side, resulting in an apparent or functional short leg on the same side.

Nystagmus   Abnormal jerking or involuntary eye movement.

O

Observation   A visual analysis of overall appearance, symmetry, general motor function, posture, and gait.

Ohm law   Current (I) in a conductor increases as the driving force (V) becomes larger or as resistance (R) is decreased ($I = V/R$).

Oligomenorrhea   Infrequent menstrual cycles or menstruation involving scant blood flow.

Omission   The failure to perform a legal duty of care.

Onychia   Inflammation of the nail matrix.

Open-cell foam   Foam with cells that are connected to allow air passage from cell to cell, allowing the foam to deform quickly under stress, which limits its shock-absorbing qualities.

Organomegaly   The abnormal enlargement of an organ.

Orthostatic hypotension   Low blood pressure caused by a sudden change in body position, such as moving from a lying to a standing position.

Osgood-Schlatter disease   Inflammation or partial avulsion of the tibial apophysis because of traction forces.

Osteitis pubis   A stress fracture to the pubic symphysis caused by repeated overload of the adductor muscles or repetitive stress activities.

Osteochondral fracture   A fracture involving the articular cartilage and underlying bone.

Osteochondritis dissecans   A localized area of avascular necrosis resulting in complete or incomplete separation of the joint cartilage and the subchondral bone.

Osteochondrosis   Any condition characterized by degeneration or aseptic necrosis of the articular cartilage because of limited blood supply.

Osteolysis   The softening, absorption, and destruction of bony tissue.

Osteomyelitis   The inflammation or an infection of the bone and bone marrow.

Osteopenia   A condition of reduced bone mineral density that predisposes the individual to fractures.

Osteoporosis   A pathological condition of reduced bone mass and strength.

Otitis externa A bacterial infection involving the lining of the auditory canal; swimmer's ear.

Otitis media A localized infection in the middle ear secondary to upper respiratory infections.

Ovarian cycle A cycle associated with the maturation of an egg.

Overload principle Physiological improvements occur only when a patient physically demands more of the muscles than is normally required.

Ovulation The release of the egg occurring at midcycle, when the ballooning ovarian wall ruptures and expels the egg.

P

Painful arc Pain located within a limited number of degrees in the range of motion.

Palpitations A perceptible, forcible pulsation of the heart, usually with an increase in frequency or force, with or without irregularity in rhythm.

Papules A small, red, elevated, and painful bump on the skin.

Paresis A partial paralysis of a muscle, leading to a weakened contraction.

Paresthesia Abnormal sensations such as tingling, burning, itching, or prickling.

Paronychia A fungal/bacterial infection in the folds of skin surrounding a fingernail or toenail.

Parrot-beak tear A horizontal meniscal tear, typically in the middle segment of the lateral meniscus.

Passive movement The movement of an injured limb or body part through the range of motion with no assistance from the injured patient.

Patella plica A fold in the synovial lining that may cause medial knee pain without associated trauma.

Patellofemoral joint The gliding joint between the patella and patellar groove of the femur.

Patellofemoral stress syndrome A condition whereby the lateral retinaculum is tight or the vastus medialis oblique is weak, leading to lateral excursion and pressure on the lateral facet of the patella, causing a painful condition.

Pathology The cause of an injury, its development, and the functional changes that result.

Pericardial tamponade The compression of venous return to the heart because of increased volume of fluid in the pericardium; usually results from direct trauma to the chest.

Perilunate dislocation The dorsal dislocation of the lunate relative to the other carpals.

Perimenopausal The period of time between ages 46 and 55 years when the menstrual cycle may shorten and become irregular in both frequency and bleeding; precedes menopause.

Periodontitis Inflammation of the deeper gum tissues that normally hold the teeth in place.

Periorbital ecchymosis Swelling and hemorrhage into the surrounding eyelids; black eye.

Periostitis Inflammation of the periosteum (the outer membrane covering the bone).

Peristalsis The periodic waves of smooth muscle contraction that propel food through the digestive system.

Peritonitis An irritation of the peritoneum that lines the abdominal cavity.

Pernio Chilblain; a condition in which the tissue does not freeze but rather reacts with erythema, itching, and burning.

Pes cavus A high arch.

Pes planus Flat feet.

Pétrissage A massage technique that consists of pressing and rolling the muscles under the fingers and hands.

Phagocytosis The process by which white blood cells surround and digest foreign particles such as bacteria, necrotic tissue, and foreign particles.

Pharmacokinetics The study of how a drug moves through the body to produce the desired effects.

Pharyngitis A viral, bacterial, or fungal infection of the pharynx, leading to a sore throat.

Phlebothrombosis Thrombosis, or clotting, in a vein without overt inflammatory signs and symptoms.

Phonophobia A morbid fear of one's own voice or of any sound.

Phonophoresis The introduction of anti-inflammatory drugs through the skin with the use of ultrasound.

Photophobia An abnormal sensitivity to light.

Plantar fascia A specialized band of fascia that covers the plantar surface of the foot and helps to support the longitudinal arch.

Plyometric training A type of explosive exercise that maximizes the myotactic on-stretch reflex.

Pneumothorax A condition whereby air is trapped in the pleural space, causing a portion of a lung to collapse.

Polydipsia Frequent drinking because of extreme thirst.

Polyphagia Excessive hunger and food consumption; gluttony.

Polyuria The excessive excretion of urine, leading to a huge urinary output of water and electrolytes and, in turn, to decreased blood volume and further dehydration.

Postconcussion syndrome A delayed condition characterized by persistent headaches, blurred vision, irritability, and an inability to concentrate.

Premenstrual syndrome A series of physical and psychological symptoms, such as headaches, breast tenderness, back pain, bloating, irritability, depression, fatigue, and certain food cravings, that occurs during the luteal phase (days 15 to 28) of the menstrual cycle.

Prodromal symptoms An early symptom of a disease.

Progesterone The hormone responsible for thickening the uterine lining in preparation for the fertilized ovum.

Progressive resistance exercise A method to improve strength by increasing resistance using the overload principles as the patient's strength increases.

Prolapsed disk A condition in which the eccentric nucleus produces a definite deformity as it works its way through the fibers of the annulus fibrosus.

Proliferation phase In the menstrual cycle, days 6 to 14, when the endometrium rebuilds itself.

Pronation An inward rotation of the forearm; the palms face posteriorly. At the foot, the combined motions of calcaneal eversion, foot abduction, and dorsiflexion.

Pronator syndrome A condition in which the median nerve is entrapped by the pronator teres, leading to pain on activities involving pronation.

Prophylactic To prevent or protect.

Proprioception A sensory response that aids a person in sensing movement and location of their body.

Proprioceptive neuromuscular facilitation Exercises that stimulate proprioceptors in muscles, tendons, and joints to improve flexibility and strength.

Prostaglandins Active substances found in many tissues, with effects such as vasodilation, vasoconstriction, and the stimulation of intestinal or bronchial smooth muscle.

Proteinuria Abnormal concentrations of protein in the urine.

Pruritus Intense itching.

Pseudo-boutonnière deformity A flexion deformity of the proximal interphalangeal joint, which resembles a boutonnière deformity, but the central slip of the extensor tendon is not involved.

Pulmonary contusion A contusion to the lungs because of compressive force.

Pulmonary embolism A blood clot that travels through the circulatory system to lodge in the lungs.

Pupillary light reflex The rapid constriction of pupils when exposed to intense light.

Purulent Containing, consisting of, or forming pus.

Pyarthrosis Suppurative pus within a joint cavity.

Q

Q-angle The angle between the line of quadriceps force and the patellar tendon.

R

Raccoon eyes A delayed discoloration around the eyes from a fracture of the anterior cranial fossa.

Radial tunnel syndrome A condition caused by direct trauma or entrapment at the elbow as the radial nerve passes anterior to the cubital fossa, pierces the supinator muscle, and runs posterior again into the forearm.

Radiation The transfer of energy in the form of infrared waves (radiant energy) without physical contact.

Rales Abnormal breath sounds.

Rate of dissolution A condition by which the more rapidly a drug dissolves, the faster the onset of its effects will be; for example, drugs that dissolve quickly (liquid medications) have a more rapid onset of effects compared with drugs that dissolve more slowly (enteric coated preparations).

Raynaud syndrome A condition characterized by intermittent, bilateral attacks of ischemia of the fingers or toes and marked by severe pallor, numbness, and pain.

Receptor The functional macromolecule, or target site, to which a drug binds to produce its effects.

Reciprocal inhibition A technique using an active contraction of the agonist to cause a reflex relaxation in the antagonist, allowing it to stretch; a phenomenon resulting from reciprocal innervation.

Referred pain A type of visceral pain that travels along the same nerve pathways as somatic pain and that is perceived by the brain as somatic in origin.

Reflection Occurs when an energy wave strikes an object and is bent back away from the material, as in an echo.

Reflex An action involving the stimulation of a motor neuron by a sensory neuron in the spinal cord without the involvement of the brain.

Reflex sympathetic dystrophy A complex regional pain syndrome in which pain is associated with findings such as abnormal skin color, temperature changes, abnormal sweating, hypersensitivity in the affected area, abnormal edema, and often significant impairment of motor function.

Refraction The deflection of an energy wave because of a change in the speed of absorption as the wave passes between mediums of different densities.

Registration Used in some states, it requires that individuals who wish to practice a profession within the state must register with a governmental agency.

Regurgitation A backward flow, as of blood through an incompetent heart valve; the return of contents in small amounts from the stomach.

Reliability How reproducible the results are when the measurement should be the same when done by multiple people.

Resilience The ability to bounce or spring back into shape or position after being stretched, bent, or impacted.

Resistors Media that inhibit the movement of ions such as skin, fat, and lotion.

Resting position A slightly flexed position of a joint that allows maximal volume to accommodate any intraarticular swelling.

Retinopathy A noninflammatory, degenerative disease of the retina.

Retrograde amnesia Forgetting events that occurred before an injury.

Retroversion A turning backward; a decreased angle between the femoral condyles and femoral head, usually less than 15°.

Retroviruses Any virus of the family *Retroviridae* known to reverse the usual order of reproduction within the cells they infect.

Reverse piezoelectric effect In ultrasound, the conversion of an electrical current into mechanical energy as it passes through a piezoelectric crystal (e.g., quartz, barium titanate, lead zirconate, titanate) housed in the transducer head.

Reye syndrome A severe disorder of young children following an acute illness, usually influenza or varicella infection, and characterized by recurrent vomiting beginning within a week after the onset of the condition, from which the child either recovers rapidly or lapses into a coma with intracranial hypertension; death may occur because of edema of the brain and resulting cerebral herniation.

Rhabdomyolysis An acute, fulminating, and potentially fatal disease of skeletal muscles that entails the destruction of skeletal muscles, as evidenced by the release of myoglobin into the blood and urine.

Rhinitis An inflammation of the nasal membranes with excessive mucus production resulting in nasal congestion and postnasal drip.

Rhinorrhea Clear nasal discharge.

Rotator cuff The supraspinatus, infraspinatus, teres minor, and subscapularis (SITS) muscles, which hold the head of the humerus in the glenoid fossa and produce humeral rotation.

Runner's anemia Exercise-induced hemolytic anemia, which occurs when the red blood cells are destroyed and the hemoglobin is liberated into the medium in which the cells are suspended.

Runner's nipples Nipple irritation resulting from friction as the shirt rubs over the nipples.

S

Sacral plexus Interconnected roots of the L4–S4 spinal nerves that innervate the lower extremities.

Saddle joint A biaxial-like condyloid joint with both concave and convex areas but with freer movement; the carpometacarpal joints of the thumbs.

Sagittal plane A longitudinal (vertical) line that divides the body or any of its parts into right and left portions.

Salicylates Any salt of salicylic acid; used in aspirin.

Scapulohumeral rhythm The coordinated rotational movement of the scapula that accompanies abduction and adduction of the humerus.

Scheuermann disease Osteochondrosis of the spine because of abnormal epiphyseal plate behavior that allows for herniation of the disk into the vertebral body, giving a characteristic wedge-shaped appearance.

Sciatica The compression of a spinal nerve because of a herniated disk, annular tear, myogenic or muscle-related disease, spinal stenosis, facet joint arthropathy, or compression from the piriformis muscle.

Scoliosis A lateral rotational spinal curvature.

Scope of care The roles and responsibilities of an individual in a profession; delineates what should be learned in the professional preparation of that individual.

Screwing-home mechanism The rotation of the tibia on the femur at the end of extension to produce a "locking" of the knee in a close-packed position.

Sebum Secretions of the sebaceous glands; an oily substance that binds epidermal cells.

Seizure An abnormal electrical discharge in the brain.

Seizure disorder Recurrent episodes of sudden, excessive charges of electrical activity in the brain, whether from known or unknown (idiopathic) causes.

Sensitivity The ability of the diagnostic test to detect an injury.

Sequestrated disk The nuclear material from an intervertebral disk that is separated from the disk itself and potentially migrates.

Serous otitis The fluid buildup behind the eardrum associated with otitis media and upper respiratory infections.

Sever disease A traction-type injury, or osteochondrosis, of the calcaneal apophysis seen in young adolescents.

Shear force A force directed parallel to a surface.

Shin bruise A contusion to the tibia; sometimes referred to as tibial periostitis.

Shock A collapse of the cardiovascular system when insufficient blood cannot provide circulation for the entire body.

Sickle cell anemia Abnormalities in hemoglobin structure, resulting in characteristic sickle- or crescent-shaped red blood cells that are fragile and unable to transport oxygen.

Sign An objective, measurable physical finding that you can hear, feel, see, or smell during the assessment.

Sinding-Larsen-Johansson disease The inflammation or a partial avulsion of the apex of the patella because of traction forces.

Sinusitis The inflammation of the paranasal sinuses.

SLAP lesion An injury to the superior labrum that typically begins posteriorly and extends anteriorly, disrupting the attachment of the long head of the biceps tendon to the superior glenoid tubercle.

Smith fracture The volar displacement of the distal fragment of the radius; sometimes called a reversed Colles fracture.

Snapping hip syndrome A snapping sensation either heard or felt during motion of the hip.

Snowball crepitation The sound similar to that heard when crunching snow into a snowball; indicative of tenosynovitis.

Solar plexus punch A blow to the abdomen with the muscles relaxed, resulting in an immediate inability to catch one's breath.

Somatic pain Pain arising from the skin, ligaments, muscles, bones, and joints.

Spasm Transitory muscle contractions.

Spear tackler's spine A condition caused by a history of using a spear-tackling technique, whereby the athlete uses the top or crown of the helmet as the initial point of contact, placing the cervical spine at risk for serious injury because of excessive axial loading.

Specificity The ability of a diagnostic test to detect health.

Spica A pattern of applying tape or elastic wrap that consists of a continuous figure eight pattern around two adjoining body parts (e.g., torso and thigh/hip, torso and upper arm/shoulder, or the thumb and wrist).

Spina bifida occulta A spinal defect characterized by the absence of vertebral arches in which there is no protrusion of the cord or its membrane.

Spinal stenosis A loss of cerebrospinal fluid around the spinal cord because of deformation of the spinal cord or a narrowing of the neural canal.

Spondylolisthesis The anterior slippage of a vertebrae resulting from complete bilateral fracture of the pars interarticularis.

Spondylolysis A stress fracture of the pars interarticularis.

Sports medicine The area of health and special services that applies medical and scientific knowledge to prevent, recognize, manage, and rehabilitate injuries related to sports, exercise, or recreational activity.

Sprain An injury to ligamentous tissue.

Standard of care What another minimally competent professional who is educated and practicing in the same profession would have done in the same or similar circumstance to protect an individual from harm.

Static stretch A stretching movement that is slow and deliberate and lasts for at least 15 seconds.

Status epilepticus A condition in which one major attack of epilepsy succeeds another with little or no intermission.

Stenosing The narrowing of an opening or stricture of a canal; stenosis.

Step deformity A change in direction resembling a stairstep in a line, a surface, or the construction of a solid body.

Steroids A large family of chemical substances including endocrine secretions and hormones.

Sticking point Insufficient strength to move a body segment through a particular angle.

Stitch in the side A sharp pain or spasm in the chest wall, usually on the lower right side, during exertion.

Strain The amount of deformation with respect to the original dimensions of the structure; injury to the musculotendinous unit.

Stress The distribution of force within a body; quantified as force divided by the area over which the force acts.

Stress fracture A fracture resulting from repeated loading with relatively low magnitude forces.

Striae distensae Bands of thin, wrinkled skin, initially red but becoming purple and white, that commonly occur on the abdomen, buttocks, and thighs during and following pregnancy and that result from atrophy of the dermis and overextension of the skin.

Strict liability A manufacturer's absolute liability for any and all defective or hazardous equipment that unduly threatens an individual's personal safety.

Stirrup strip Used specifically when taping ankles whereby one strip of tape that, when applied correctly, resembles the stirrup of a saddle.

Subconjunctival hemorrhage Minor capillary ruptures in the eye globe.

Subcutaneous emphysema The presence of air or gas in subcutaneous tissue; characterized by a crackling sensation on palpation.

Subungual hematoma A hematoma beneath a fingernail or toenail.

Sudden death A nontraumatic, unexpected death that occurs instantaneously or within a few minutes of an abrupt change in a patient's previous clinical state.

Supination The outward rotation of the forearm, with the palms facing forward. At the foot, the combined motions of calcaneal inversion, foot adduction, and plantar flexion.

Supraventricular tachycardia The rapid beating of the heart, proximal to the ventricles, in the atrium or the atrioventricular node.

Sustained-release preparations A capsule or tablet filled with tiny spheres that contain a drug. The sphere is coated and designed to dissolve at variable rates, ranging from 8 to 24 hours.

Sustentaculum tali The anteromedial surface of the calcaneus that largely supports the talus.

Swayback A decrease of the anterior lumbar curve and increase in the posterior thoracic curve from neutral.

Symptom Subjective information provided by a patient regarding his or her perception of the problem.

Syncope Fainting or light-headedness.

Syndrome An accumulation of common signs and symptoms characteristic of a particular injury or disease.

Systolic blood pressure Pressure exerted by blood on the blood vessel walls during ventricular contractions.

T

Tachycardia The rapid beating of the heart; usually applied to rates more than 100 beats per minute.

Tachypnea Rapid breathing.

Tackler's exostosis Irritative exostosis on the anterior or lateral humerus.

Tapotement A massage technique that uses sharp, alternating, and brisk hand movements, such as hacking, slapping, beating, cupping, and clapping, to increase blood flow and to stimulate peripheral nerve endings.

Tendinitis Inflammation of a tendon.

Tendinosis A tendinous condition associated with degeneration rather than with inflammation.

Tenosynovitis Inflammation of a tendon sheath.

Tensile force A pulling or stretching force directed axially through a body or body part.

Tension pneumothorax A condition in which air continuously leaks into the pleural space, causing the mediastinum to displace to the opposite side, compressing the uninjured lung and the thoracic aorta.

Testosterone The primary androgen produced by the testes. Testosterone stimulates the growth and maturation of the internal and external genitalia at puberty and is responsible for sexual motivation.

Thenar The fleshy mass of muscle and tissue on the lateral palm; the ball of the thumb.

Therapeutic medications Prescription or over-the-counter medications used to treat an injury or illness.

Therapeutic range The range between the minimum effective concentration and toxic concentration.

Thermoregulation The process by which the body maintains body temperature; primarily controlled by the hypothalamus.

Thermotherapy Heat application.

Thoracic outlet syndrome A condition whereby nerves and/or vessels become compressed in the root of the neck or axilla, leading to numbness in the arm.

Thrombophlebitis The acute inflammation of a vein.

Tibiofemoral joint The dual condyloid joints between the tibial and femoral condyles that function primarily as a modified hinge joint.

Tidal volume The amount of air inspired and expired in a single breath.

Tinea Ringworm; fungal infection of the hair, skin, or nails characterized by small vesicles, itching, and scaling; types include tinea pedis (athlete's foot), tinea cruris (jock itch), and tinea capitis (ringworm of the scalp).

Tinnitus A ringing or other noises in the ear because of trauma or disease.

Todd paralysis A paralysis of temporary duration (normally not more than a few days) that occurs in the limb or limbs involved in epilepsy after the seizure.

Tomogram A cross-sectional image of an organ or body part at various depths of field produced by an X-ray technique.

Tonic Steady, rigid muscle contractions with no relaxation.

Torque A rotary force; the product of a force and its moment arm, or moment.

Torsion force The twisting around an object's longitudinal axis in response to an applied torque.

Tort A wrong done to an individual whereby the injured party seeks a remedy for damages suffered.

Torticollis A congenital or acquired spasm of the sternocleidomastoid muscle; "wry neck."

Toxic concentration A concentration of drug levels in the blood plasma that is too high and, therefore, increases the risk of toxic effects.

Toxic synovitis Occurring largely in children, a transient, inflammatory condition characterized by a painful hip joint accompanied by an antalgic gait and limp.

Translation The anterior gliding of the tibial plateau on the femur.

Transverse plane A horizontal line that divides the body into superior and inferior portions.

Traumatic asphyxia A condition involving extravasation of blood into the skin and conjunctiva because of a sudden increase in venous pressure.

Triage Assessing all injured patients to determine priority of care.

Trigger An event or system in which a relatively small input hastens, worsens, or lengthens the duration of a condition, the magnitude of which is unrelated to the magnitude of the input.

Trigger finger A condition whereby the finger flexors contract but are unable to reextend because of a nodule within the tendon sheath or due to the sheath being too constricted to allow for free motion.

Tunics Three layers of protected tissues that surround the eye.

U

Unconsciousness An impairment of brain function wherein the patient lacks conscious awareness and is unable to respond to superficial sensory stimuli.

Urethritis Inflammation of the urethra.

Urticaria Hives; an eruption of itching wheals, usually of systemic origin, which may result from a state of hypersensitivity to foods or drugs, infection, physical agents, or psychic stimuli.

V

Vaginitis Inflammation of the vagina.

Valgus An opening on the medial side of a joint caused by the distal segment moving laterally.

Validity The assurance that measurements represent what we think they represent.

Valsalva maneuver Holding one's breath against a closed glottis, resulting in sharp increases in blood pressure.

Valvular stenosis A narrowing of the orifice around the cardiac valves.

Varicocele An abnormal dilation of the veins of the spermatic cord, leading to an engorgement of blood into the spermatic cord veins when standing.

Varus An opening on the lateral side of a joint caused by the distal segment moving medially.

Vasoconstriction A narrowing of the blood vessels; the opposite of vasodilation.

Vasodilation The enlarging of the blood vessels; the opposite of vasoconstriction.

Vehicles   Substances combined with medications that use enteral routes to facilitate entry into the body; may include tablets, capsules, liquids, powders, suppositories, enteric-coated preparations, and sustained-release preparations.

Vertigo   A balance disturbance characterized by a whirling sensation of one's self or external objects.

Vibration   A massage technique using finite, gentle, and rhythmic movement of the fingers to vibrate the underlying tissues for relaxation or stimulation.

Visceral pain   Pain resulting from disease or injury to an organ in the thoracic or the abdominal cavity.

Viscoelastic   Responding to loading over time with changing rates of deformation.

Volkmann contracture   Ischemic necrosis of the forearm muscles and tissues caused by damage to the blood flow.

Voltage   The force that causes ions to move.

W

Watt   A unit of electrical power. For an electrical current: watts = voltage × amperage.

Wedge fracture   A crushing compression fracture that leaves a vertebra narrowed anteriorly.

Wheal   A smooth, slightly elevated area on the body that appears red or white and is accompanied by severe itching; commonly seen in allergies to mechanical or chemical irritants.

Wolff law   A law that states that bone and soft tissue will respond to the physical demands placed on them, causing the formation of collagen to remodel or realign along the lines of stress, thus promoting healthy joint biomechanics.

Wrist drop   A weakness and/or paralysis of the wrist and finger extensors because of radial nerve damage.

Y

Yield point (elastic limit)   The maximum load that a material can sustain without permanent deformation.

Z

Zone of primary injury   The region of injured tissue before vasodilation.

Zone of secondary injury   The region of damaged tissue following vasodilation.

Index

Page numbers followed by *f* denote figures, those followed by *t* denote tables, those followed by *b* indicate boxed material, and those followed by *as* indicate Application Strategies.